Osteoarthritis

DIAGNOSIS AND MEDICAL/SURGICAL MANAGEMENT

FOURTH EDITION

Osteoarthritis

DIAGNOSIS AND MEDICAL/SURGICAL MANAGEMENT

FOURTH EDITION

▬ ROLAND W. MOSKOWITZ, MD, MS(MED)

Professor of Medicine
Case Western Reserve University School of Medicine
Co-Director, Arthritis Translational Research Program
University Hospitals Case Medical Center
Cleveland, Ohio

▬ ROY D. ALTMAN, MD

Professor of Medicine, Rheumatology and Immunology
The David Geffen School of Medicine
University of California at Los Angeles
Los Angeles, California

▬ MARC C. HOCHBERG, MD, MPH

Professor of Medicine
Head, Division of Rheumatology & Clinical Immunology
University of Maryland School of Medicine
Baltimore, Maryland

▬ JOSEPH A. BUCKWALTER, MD, MS

Arthur Steindler Chair and Head of Orthopaedics and Rehabilitation
University of Iowa Healthcare
Iowa City, Iowa

▬ VICTOR M. GOLDBERG, MD

Professor of Orthopaedic Surgery
Department of Orthopaedics
Case Western Reserve University School of Medicine
Cleveland, Ohio

⬛ Wolters Kluwer | Lippincott Williams & Wilkins
Health
Philadelphia · Baltimore · New York · London
Buenos Aires · Hong Kong · Sydney · Tokyo

Acquisitions Editor: Susan Rhyner
Managing Editor: Nancy Winter
Development Editor: Franny Murphy
Project Manager: Fran Gunning
Marketing Manager: Kimberly Schonberger
Manufacturing Coordinator: Kathleen Brown
Creative Director: Doug Smock
Production Services: International Typesetting & Composition
Printer: RR Donnelley

© 2007 by LIPPINCOTT WILLIAMS & WILKINS, a Wolters Kluwer business

530 Walnut Street
Philadelphia, PA 19106 USA
LWW.com

1st, 2nd, 3rd Editions, W. B. Saunders Company, 1984, 1992, 2001

Printed in the USA

Library of Congress Cataloging-in-Publication Data

Osteoarthritis : diagnosis and medical/surgical management / [edited by]
    Roland W. Moskowitz ... [et al.].—4th ed.
      p. ; cm.
    Includes bibliographical references and index.
    ISBN-13: 978-0-7817-6707-1
    ISBN-10: 0-7817-6707-5
    1. Osteoarthritis.   I. Moskowitz, Roland W.
    [DNLM: 1. Osteoarthritis.   WE 346 O848 2007]
  RC931.O67O88 2007
  616.7'22—dc22
                           2006030158

To purchase additional copies of this book, call our customer service department at (800) 638-3030 or fax orders to (301) 223-2320. International customers should call (301) 223-2300.

Visit Lippincott Williams & Wilkins on the Internet: at LWW.com. Lippincott Williams & Wilkins customer service representatives are available from 8:30 am to 6 pm, EST.

10 9 8 7 6 5 4 3 2 1

Dedication

Previous editions of this text have been dedicated to Drs. Leon Sokoloff, Jonas H. Kellgren, and John S. Lawrence whose pioneering contributions to our understanding of osteoarthritis (OA) are still routinely referred to many decades later. Dr. Sokoloff's conceptual contributions related to the pathology and pathophysiology of OA, and to the study of animal models remain as relevant today as when first reported. Similarly, the epidemiologic studies performed by Drs. Kellgren and Lawrence, and their classification of OA radiologic stages, are a living standard on which OA clinical studies continue to be based.

It has been said that advances in knowledge are based on the ability of others to stand on the shoulders of those who came before them, seeing further beyond the horizon to new, otherwise unattainable vistas. Accordingly, we recognize and additionally dedicate this textbook to more recent leaders in the field of osteoarthritis research, Drs. David S. Howell, Henry J. Mankin, and Robert B. Salter. Drs. Howell and Mankin are former editors of this textbook. Dr. Howell is internationally recognized for his contributions to the pathophysiology of articular hyaline cartilage and the growth plate, as well as, to the role of calcification in bone and joint pathology. He represents the classic triple-threat academician excelling as a clinician, educator, and basic investigator. His original paintings of seaside landscapes further identify his renaissance character. Dr. Howell mentored Dr. Altman in the clinical and basic sciences in osteoarthritis. Dr. Mankin, similarly internationally recognized, has led the way in our understanding of cartilage biochemistry and disease pathophysiology; as a mentor to others in the field, he is without peer. The Mankin classification for OA pathology remains a standard of OA histopathologic classification. We are honored by and indebted to him for the foreword to this fourth edition; his impact on the editors of this text, and on the field in general, has, and continues to be, immense. Dr. Salter's contributions to disease modeling, experimental surgical approaches, and biomechanics as related to joint therapeutics are legendary; who has not prescribed his "Continuous Passive Motion" postoperatively to patients undergoing orthopedic surgery. Dr. Salter has played a special role in the initiation of Dr. Moskowitz's interest in the field of osteoarthritis; his presentation of studies related to a compression-immobilization and other models of OA some four decades ago ignited Dr. Moskowitz's interest in the field, an interest which has continued to this day. It is with a sense of privilege that we add these names to the dedication of our book—mentors who have influenced the lives not only of the authors of this text, but OA investigators throughout the world.

A special appreciation goes to our wives, Peta, Linda, Susan, Kitty, and Harriet for their continuing support. One of these days they are going to believe us when we say "this is the last edition we'll work on!" We know that, should future editions hopefully follow, they will continue to be as much on our side as ever—we love you for that.

Foreword

It is a great pleasure to have an opportunity to review and introduce this fourth edition of a really great book on an incredibly important subject . . . osteoarthritis! The book is edited by world authorities in the field of rheumatology but I note with pleasure that several contributing authors are orthopedists, suggesting as we all know that the two specialties are joined together on the altar of the inflamed or damaged joint.

These are modern times in the world and life is in many ways better than it was in the "olden days." In the year 1903 the average age of survival was 47 and the patients' lives were dominated by tuberculosis, polio, trauma, and an array of cardiac and neurologic disorders that contributed to miserable lives and short survival. By 2003, the mean survival was 30 years longer and the average age until death was 77. Patients have a much better life and in many ways a happier and more productive one. Having said that however, they now have other disorders . . . such as HIV, Alzheimer's, osteoporosis, and multiple sites of osteoarthritis. This last mentioned disorder now dominates the lives of many old people, limits their activities, demands that they take sometimes dangerous medications, use canes, crutches, walkers, or wheelchairs, and in fact have operative procedures that often make them better . . . but not always.

The causes of osteoarthritis are not really well understood. There is no doubt that trauma to a joint is a problem, and certainly the knee joint is most often damaged by what sometimes seem to be minor injuries. Athletes have problems with partial tears of muscles, torn menisci, cruciate ligament injuries, subchondral fractures and, at times, repeated effusions. Older persons who develop osteoporosis may have tiny stress fractures, or may develop abnormal structure based on alteration in joint alignment. Patients with an array of metabolic bone and soft tissue diseases may be prone to cartilage injury or bone problems. These include osteomalacia, hyperparathyroidism, osteonecrosis, and fibrous dysplasia amongst others. We still, however, need to know more about the possible genetic causes or alterations in cartilage structure that may lead to the disease. There is no doubt that chondrocytes and the cartilage matrix change with advancing age, and some of this is related to collagen types, glycosaminoglycan distribution, water content, apoptotic activity, and changes in the aggrecan structure. Perhaps of equal concern is the effect of the synovium and agents such as interleukin-1 on cartilage structure or the possibility of alterations in the subchondral bone structure, which allow damage to the cartilage tidemark.

What a great accomplishment it would be if people could have a reduced frequency and severity of this disease; and if we could find ways of preventing it or reducing its effect and eliminating some of the major impairments that now cause people to be far less functional.

The group of authors presenting chapters in this volume are extraordinary in their commitment to the subject of osteoarthritis, some for many years, and in their ability to write with substance, clarity, and hope. They review the etiology, the pathology, the epidemiology, the biochemistry, and the genetics of the disease and define how these various factors alter and affect the presentation and the patient's fate. Imaging is crucial, particularly using new technology such as that associated with special gadolinium MRIs. The section on treatment is particularly rewarding since it describes in great detail the pharmacologic agents, nonpharmacologic approaches, and intra-articular injection therapies. The final phase is to review the various anatomical sites and the methods of surgical and other treatments currently in use or soon to be introduced.

Of particular importance are the suggestions that the biologic and, more importantly, the genetic approaches to the disease may in the future provide new methods of early diagnosis, genetic predisposition, and ultimately treatment methods that can slow, stabilize, or even eliminate the disease. Biochemical interference with the actions of the MMPs and the interleukins, stabilization of the cell structure, diminution of apoptotic activity, increases in chondrocyte cell division and collagen, and proteoglycan synthesis are really the wave of the future and, according to the chapter authors, are possible and probable with further research. Identification of very early disease by special imaging effects or biologic studies may allow us to introduce earlier treatment protocols which will allow the cartilage to heal and restore the joint to better function.

Of great importance is the rational approach expressed by the authors of the chapters on operative procedures. These are often very effective . . . for a while. It seems logical to assess the competence of these systems by careful evidence-based result analysis and to establish some guidelines for choosing the correct procedure to be performed and best patients to have such surgery.

This is a great book—a treasure for the physician and basic scientist and indeed an important contribution to the successful diagnosis and treatment of patients with osteoarthritis. It describes the disease in detail, provides insight into the cause of the problems; but most of all it defines the way we treat it now and, much more importantly, the way we will treat it in the future. There is hope here for new methods, which will make osteoarthritis less of a problem and ultimately will diminish the suffering and disability of mankind.

Henry J. Mankin MD
Former Chief of Orthopaedic Surgery
Massachusetts General Hospital
Edith M. Ashley Professor of Orthopaedics Emeritus
Harvard Medical School

Preface

This fourth edition of *Osteoarthritis* comes some 22 years after its first appearance in 1984. At that time, interest in osteoarthritis (OA) was only beginning its ascendancy in both the scientific and lay universe. This interval between the third and fourth editions, 6 years, is significantly less than that between each of the first three editions (8 and 9 years respectively). This shortened interval clearly defines the rapid pace of our understanding of OA as a disease and cartilage as a target, not only with respect to basic and clinical aspects, but also to its impact on society. OA is an entity of high priority emphasis by the National Institute of Arthritis, Musculoskeletal and Skin Diseases (NIAMS); the Arthritis Foundation (AF); the Centers for Disease Control and Prevention (CDC); the Osteoarthritis Research Society International (OARSI); and participants in the World Health Organization (WHO) Bone and Joint Decade interplays.

Publication of subspecialty books has become less attractive to publishing companies, given the easy accessibility today of updates on any and all diseases on the web throughout the world.

We are pleased that our publisher Lippincott Williams & Wilkins (LWW), an internationally recognized publishing house of the highest integrity, was enthusiastically supportive of our moving ahead with the fourth edition. LWW has a strong history in the field of rheumatic diseases, publishing *Arthritis and Allied Conditions: A Textbook of Rheumatology* which addresses the entire broad rheumatologic field. Support of this publication on OA broadens their outreach in the musculoskeletal disease field, especially for a disease in which it is anticipated that 40 million or more people in the United States will be afflicted, by the year 2020.

The text is designed to be of use to multiple medical disciplines including, rheumatologists, basic investigators in the field of OA and cartilage, orthopedists, physiatrists, and primary care physicians whose practices include significant numbers of patients with OA.

The textbook provides a comprehensive overview; it is not meant to be encyclopedic but, rather, to provide a comprehensive overview of the disease and its ramifications, of benefit to a diverse population of readers. As will be noted for those who have copies of the previous text, there are a number of new authors with a significantly increased international representation. This broader authorship reflects increased communication amongst physicians and investigators throughout the world, who share a common interest in the diffusion of OA knowledge.

The editorship of the text has also undergone changes. Dr. David Howell, a founding editor of the text, has elected to discontinue participation following his retirement; he is one of three individuals to whom this edition is dedicated. His advice, creativity, and sagacity will be missed. Dr. Roy Altman has assumed the role of senior co-editor with Dr. Moskowitz, with plans to assume increasing responsibility in future editions. Dr. Marc Hochberg, Professor of Medicine at the University of Maryland and Chief of the Rheumatic Disease Unit at that institution, is an internationally recognized expert in clinical and investigative rheumatology; we welcome the strengths his participation brings to this text.

The text is divided into major subsections: Basic Considerations; General Aspects of Diagnosis; General Aspects of Management; and Surgical Considerations. New chapters include a discussion of ultrasound and alternative imaging for OA; a chapter on the ever-increasing interest in complementary and alternative medicine; and a discussion of new frontiers in surgical orthopedics related to Osteoarthritis. Recognition of the multiplicity of factors related to the etiopathogenesis of OA seen in the multiauthorship of this chapter by individuals with expertise in cartilage biochemistry, inflammatory pathways, and joint biomechanics. The chapter on biochemistry and molecular and cellular biology of articular cartilage has been expanded, recognizing the major gains we have seen in our understanding of these processes. In addition to detailed discussion of radiologic presentations in OA, MRI, a modality taking its place of increased importance in OA investigations, has been expanded and includes not only traditional MRI technology, but interesting new approaches such as dGEMRIC (delayed gadolinium-enhanced MRI). The chapter on noninvasive markers similarly has been expanded to note our increased knowledge in this area. Recognizing that we still need additional answers before such biomarkers can be used in disease diagnosis, measurement of disease progression, and responses to therapy, the advent of new biomarkers and a better understanding now available auger well that biomarker relevance to OA will have increasing value. The chapter on pharmacologic treatment of OA has been materially revised, recognizing not only the gains we have made in pharmacologic approaches for symptomatic relief, but also addressing controversies in overall safety of both selective and nonselective NSAIDs. The sections on orthopedics have been revised so as to present an approach concentrating not only on surgical techniques but, rather, on a general understanding of surgical indications, outcomes, and expectations so as to be of value to clinicians no matter what their subspecialty discipline.

Despite all the advances that have been made, and these have been significant, much needs yet to be learned if we are to achieve our goals to provide optimal symptomatic relief with the highest efficacy and least toxicity; to relieve pain, improve function, and prevent disability; and, hopefully, to one day be able to effectively retard, reverse, and prevent the osteoarthritic process itself. Efforts at disease modification are hampered not only by lack of positive comparators for use in trials of new agents but, also, uncertainty as to the best outcomes to define disease-modification responses. Exciting initiatives such as the osteoarthritis initiative (OAI) funded by the NIAMS, a multi-year study to better understand the osteoarthritic process including risk factors for incident OA and for disease progression, and the relationships of biochemical and imaging markers in assessment of the disease process, will significantly advance our clinical understanding of OA. Plans by the AF and CDC to increase awareness of arthritis amongst the general population, and to advise self-help programs whereby risk factors can be modified and disease onset/ progression minimized will significantly impact awareness of the disease and, subsequently, disease prevention. Organizations such as OARSI, comprised of the leading international investigators and clinicians with an interest in this disease entity, will help to further foster advances in this field. The authors of this text (and, we suspect, everyone interested in this disease) hope that by the time of the fifth edition, many of these questions will have been answered and therapeutic targets achieved!

Roland W. Moskowitz, MD
Roy D. Altman, MD
Marc C. Hochberg, MD
Joseph A. Buckwalter, MD
Victor M. Goldberg, MD

Contributors

STEVEN B. ABRAMSON, MD Professor of Medicine and Pathology, Department of Medicine, Division of Rheumatology, New York University School of Medicine; Director, Division of Rheumatology, NYU Hospital for Joint Diseases, New York, New York, *Etiopathogenesis of Osteoarthritis*

ROY D. ALTMAN, MD Professor of Medicine, Rheumatology and Immunology, The David Geffen School of Medicine, University of California at Los Angeles, Los Angeles, California, *Intra-articular Therapy, Laboratory Findings in Osteoarthritis*

JOHN-ERIK BELL, MD Center for Shoulder, Elbow and Sports Medicine, New York Presbyterian Hospital, Columbia University Medical Center, New York, New York, *Upper Extremity Considerations: Shoulder*

RICHARD BERGER, MD Assistant Professor, Department of Orthopaedic Surgery, Rush Medical College and Rush Presbyterian–St. Luke's Medical Center, Chicago, Illinois, *Lower Extremity Considerations: Knee*

DANIEL J. BERRY, MD Professor of Orthopaedic Surgery, Mayo Medical School and Rochester Methodist Hospital and St. Mary's Hospital, Rochester, Minnesota, *Lower Extremity Considerations: Hip*

LOUIS U. BIGLIANI, MD Frank E. Stinchfield Professor and Chairman, Department of Orthopaedic Surgery, Columbia University Medical Center, Center for Shoulder, Elbow and Sports Medicine, New York Presbyterian Hospital, Columbia University Medical Center, New York, New York, *Upper Extremity Considerations: Shoulder*

RODERICK J. BRUNO, MD Clinical Instructor, Tufts University, Department of Orthopaedics, New England Medical Center, Boston, Massachusetts, *Upper Extremity Considerations: Hand, Wrist, and Elbow*

JOSEPH A. BUCKWALTER, MD, MS Professor, Head and Steindler Chair, Department of Orthopaedics & Rehabilitation, University of Iowa Healthcare & Clinics, Iowa City, Iowa, *Secondary Osteoarthritis*

VIJAY CHANDNANI, MD Chief, Musculoskeletal Radiology, Grant Hospital, Columbus, Ohio, *Radiologic Diagnosis*

KAY CHAPMAN, PHD University Lecturer in Musculoskeletal Sciences, Nuffield Department of Orthopaedic Surgery, University of Oxford, Oxford, United Kingdom, *Molecular Genetics of Osteoarthritis*

LAN CHEN, MD, PHD Clinical Assistant Professor, Department of Medicine, University of Pennsylvania; Attending Physician, Rheumatology/Department of Medicine, University of Pennsylvania Medical Center, Philadelphia, Pennsylvania, *Secondary Osteoarthritis*

BRIAN J. COLE, MD, MBA Assistant Professor, Department of Orthopaedic Surgery, Rush Medical College and Rush Presbyterian–St. Luke's Medical Center, Chicago, Illinois, *Lower Extremity Considerations: Knee*

PHILIP G. CONAGHAN, MBBS, PHD, FRACP, FRCP Professor of Musculoskeletal Medicine, Academic Unit of Musculoskeletal Disease, University of Leeds, Leeds, UK, *Ultrasound and Alternatives Imaging Outcomes*

JULIE C. DICARLO, PHD Scientist, Synarc, Inc., San Francisco, California, *Magnetic Resonance Imaging*

SARA L. EDWARDS, MD Center for Shoulder, Elbow and Sports Medicine, New York Presbyterian Hospital, Columbia University Medical Center, New York, New York, *Upper Extremity Considerations: Shoulder*

PAUL EMERY, MA, MD, FRCP, ARC Professor of Rheumatology, Academic Unit of Musculoskeletal Disease, University of Leeds, Leeds, UK, *Ultrasound and Alternatives Imaging Outcomes*

SANFORD E. EMERY, MD Professor and Chairman, Department of Orthopaedics, West Virginia University, School of Medicine; Morgantown, West Virginia, *Osteoarthritis of the Spine*

PATRICK GARNERO, DSC, PHD Vice President, Molecular Markers, Synarc; Director of Research, INSERM Unit 403, Lyon, France, *Noninvasive Biochemical Markers in Osteoarthritis*

GARRY E. GOLD, MD Associate Professor, of Radiology, Stanford University School of Medicine, Stanford, California, *Radiologic Diagnosis*

STEVEN H. GOLDBERG, MD Robert E. Caroll Hand and Microvascular Fellow, Department of Orthopaedic Surgery, Columbia University Medical Center, New York-Presbyterian Hospital, New York, New York, *Upper Extremity Considerations: Hand, Wrist, and Elbow*

VICTOR M. GOLDBERG, MD   Professor of Orthopaedic Surgery, Department of Orthopaedics, Case Western Reserve University School of Medicine, Cleveland, Ohio, *General Considerations, Indications, and Outcomes, Lower Extremity Considerations: Knee*

ANDREAS H. GOMOLL, MD   Instructor, Harvard Medical School; Department of Orthopedic Surgery, Brigham & Women's Hospital, Boston, Massachusetts, *New Frontiers in Surgery of Osteoarthritis*

FARSHID GUILAK, PHD   Laszlo Normandy Professor of Orthopaedic Surgery; Director, Orthopaedic Research, Duke University Medical Center, Duke University, Durham, North Carolina, *Etiopathogenesis of Osteoarthritis*

DICK HEINEGARD, MD   Professor, Department of Cell and Molecular Biology; Section for Connective Tissue Biology, Lund Sweden, *Cell Biology, Biochemistry, and Molecular Biology of Articular Cartilage in Osteoarthritis*

THOMAS M. HERING, PHD   Associate Professor, Departments of Orthopaedics, Medicine, and Anatomy, Case Western Reserve University, Cleveland, Ohio, *Cell Biology, Biochemistry, and Molecular Biology of Articular Cartilage in Osteoarthritis*

MARC C. HOCHBERG, MD, MPH   Professor of Medicine, Head, Division of Rheumatology & Clinical Immunology, University of Maryland School of Medicine, Baltimore, Maryland, *Design of and Outcome Measures for Use in Clinical Trials in Patients with Osteoarthritis, Baseline Program*

MICHELE M. HOOPER, MD   Assistant professor, Department of Medicine, Case Western Reserve University School of Medicine, University Hospitals of Cleveland, Cleveland, Ohio, *Osteoarthritis: Clinical Presentations*

AUBREY J. HOUGH, JR., MD   Distinguished Professor, Department of Pathology, Associate Dean for Translational Research and Special Programs, College of Medicine, University of Arkansas for Medical Sciences; Little Rock, Arkansas, *Pathology of Osteoarthritis*

MICHAEL N. KANG, MD   Fellow, Department of Orthopaedic Surgery, Stanford University Medical Center, Stanford Hospital & Clinics, Stanford, California, *Lower Extremity Considerations: Hip*

DIPALI KAPOOR, MD   Fellow, Division of Rheumatology, Northwestern University Medical School, Chicago, Illinois, *Epidemiology of Osteoarthritis*

HELEN I KEEN, MBBS, FRACP   Research Fellow, Academic Unit of Musculoskeletal Disease, University of Leeds, Leeds, UK, *Ultrasound and Alternatives Imaging Outcomes*

SHARON L. KOLASINSKI, MD   Associate Professor of Clinical Medicine, Division of Rheumatology, University of Pennsylvania; Chief of Clinical Service, Department of Medicine, Division of Rheumatology, Hospital of the University of Pennsylvania, Philadelphia, Pennsylvania, *Complementary and Alternative Medicine*

MANISH KOTHARI, PHD   Vice President, Business Development & New Services, Scientific Client Services, Synarc, Inc., San Francisco, California, *Magnetic Resonance Imaging*

WILLIAM N. LEVINE, MD   Associate Professor, Columbia University; Director, Sports Medicine, and Associate Director, The Shoulder Service, Columbia-Presbyterian Medical Center, New York, New York, *Upper Extremity Considerations: Shoulder*

CHRISTOPHER B. LITTLE, BVMS, PHD, DIP, ACVS   Director and Associate Professor, Raymond Purves Bone and Joint Research Laboratories, Department of Surgery (Orthopaedics), University of Sydney at Royal North Shore Hospital, Sydney, Australia, *Experimental Models of Osteoarthritis*

JOHN LOUGHLIN, PHD   University Lecturer in Musculoskeletal Sciences, Nuffield Department of Orthopaedic Surgery, University of Oxford, Oxford, United Kingdom, *Molecular Genetics of Osteoarthritis*

WILLIAM J. MALONEY III, MD   Professor and Chair, Department of Orthopaedic Surgery, Stanford University Medical Center, Stanford Hospital & Clinics, Stanford, California, *Lower Extremity Considerations: Hip*

JASON M. MCKEAN, MD   Trauma Training Center Research Fellow, Department of Orthopaedic Surgery, Columbia University Medical Center, New York-Presbyterian Hospital, New York, New York, *Upper Extremity Considerations: Hand, Wrist, and Elbow*

JAMES MICHELSON, MD   Professor, Orthopaedic Surgery, Director of Clinical Informatics, The George Washington University School of Medicine and Health Sciences, George Washington University Hospital, Washington, DC, *Lower Extremity Considerations: Foot and Ankle*

TOM MINAS, MD, MS   Associate Professor, Harvard Medical School; Director, Cartilage Repair Center, Department of Orthopedic Surgery, Brigham & Women's Hospital, Boston, Massachusetts, *New Frontiers in Surgery of Osteoarthritis*

ROLAND W. MOSKOWITZ, MD   Professor of Medicine, Case Western Reserve University School of Medicine, Co-Director, Arthritis Translational Research Program, University Hospitals Case Medical Center, Cleveland, Ohio, *Osteoarthritis: Clinical Presentations*

DAVID H. NEUSTADT, MD, FACP, MACR   Clinical Professor of Medicine, University of Louisville School of Medicine, Louisville, Kentucky, *Intra-articular Therapy*

CHARLES PETERFY, MD, PHD   Chief Medical Officer, Scientific Client Services, Synarc, Inc., San Francisco, California, *Magnetic Resonance Imaging*

A. ROBIN POOLE, PHD, DSC   Professor Emeritus, Department of Surgery, McGill University; Director, Joint Diseases Laboratory, Shriners Hospitals for Children, Montreal, Quebec, Canada, *Etiopathogenesis of Osteoarthritis*

DONALD RESNICK, MD   Professor of Radiology, University of California, San Diego, Medical School and VA Medical Center, San Diego, California, *Radiologic Diagnosis*

VYTAUTAS M. RINGUS, MD   Resident, Department of Orthopaedics, West Virginia University, School of Medicine; Department of Orthopaedics, University Hospitals of Cleveland, Case Western Reserve University, Cleveland, Ohio, *Osteoarthritis of the Spine*

AARON ROSENBERG, MD   Professor, Department of Orthopaedic Surgery, Rush Medical College and Rush Presbyterian–St. Luke's Medical Center, Chicago, Illinois, *Lower Extremity Considerations: Knee*

MELVIN P. ROSENWASSER, MD   Robert E. Carroll Professor of Hand Surgery, Columbia University College of Physicians and Surgeons; Attending Orthopedic Surgeon and Chief of Hand and Trauma Service, New York Presbyterian Hospital, New York, New York, *Upper Extremity Considerations: Hand, Wrist, and Elbow*

LINDA J. SANDELL, PHD   Professor and Director of Research, Department of Orthopaedic Surgery, Department of Cell Biology and Physiology, Washington University School of Medicine; Attending, Barnes-Jewish Hospital, St. Louis, Missouri, *Cell Biology, Biochemistry, and Molecular Biology of Articular Cartilage in Osteoarthritis*

H. RALPH SCHUMACHER, JR., MD   Professor, Department of Medicine (Rheumatology), University of Pennsylvania School of Medicine; Chief of Rheumatology, VA Medical Center, Philadelphia, Pennsylvania, *Secondary Osteoarthritis*

LEENA SHARMA, MD   Professor of Medicine, Department of Medicine, Division of Rheumatology, Feinberg School of Medicine at North Western University, Chicago, Illionois, *Epidemiology of Osteoarthritis*

LEE S. SIMON, MD   Associate Professor of Medicine, Harvard Medical School; Associate Chief of Medicine, Director of Graduate Medical Education, Director of Rheumatology Clinical Research, Beth Israel Deaconess Medical Center, Boston, Massachusetts, *The Pharmacologic Treatment of Osteoarthritis*

MARGARET M. SMITH, PHD   Senior Research Fellow, Raymond Purves Bone and Joint Research Laboratories, Department of Surgery (Orthopaedics), University of Sydney at Royal North Shore Hospital, Sydney, Australia, *Experimental Models of Osteoarthritis*

TODD STITIK, MD   Professor, Physical Medicine and Rehabilitation, UMDNJ—New Jersey Medical School, Newark, New Jersey, *Baseline Program*

VIBEKE STRAND, MD   Adjunct Clinical Professor, Immunology and Rheumatology, Stanford University School of Medicine, Stanford, California, *The Pharmacologic Treatment of Osteoarthritis, Design of and Outcome Measures for Use in Clinical Trials in Patients with Osteoarthritis*

ROBERT J. STRAUCH, MD   Associate Professor, Department of Orthopedic Surgery, Columbia University College of Physicians and Surgeons; Attending Surgeon, New York Presbyterian Hospital, New York, New York, *Upper Extremity Considerations: Hand, Wrist, and Elbow*

Acknowledgments

The support of our managing editor, Nancy Winter, of Lippincott Williams & Wilkins, is deeply appreciated. The publication of a multiauthored textbook requires a great deal of administrative support; Nancy was always there, unquestioning, and anxious to be as helpful as possible no matter what the issue. Similarly, we note our appreciation for the roles of Kimberly Schonberger, Fran Gunning and Susan Rhyner for project, marketing concepts and production. Ms. Michele Sawicki, Program Assistant in the Arthritis Translational Research Program at University Hospitals Case Medical Center, provided invaluable assistance in coordinating author-editing interplays, and together with Ms. Charu Dutt, Composition editor for LWW, were instrumental in achieving our targeted publication goals. The Osteoarthritis Research Society International (OARSI), the preeminent international organization dedicated to increasing our understanding of basic and clinical aspects of osteoarthritis and fostering guidelines for disease classification and therapy, provided academic and administrative support, and encouragement as to the importance of this fourth edition in furthering knowledge in this field. An educational grant from Pfizer Inc. was instrumental in support of production and publication costs, and in augmenting the availability of the text to clinicians, researchers, and libraries.

Contents

Basic Considerations

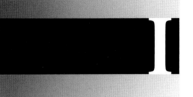

Epidemiology of Osteoarthritis

Leena Sharma   *Dipali Kapoor*

INTRODUCTION

Osteoarthritis (OA) is the most common form of arthritis and a leading cause of chronic disability, in large part due to knee and/or hip involvement. The societal burden of OA relates to its pervasive presence. For example, in the Rotterdam study, only 135 of 1040 persons 55 to 65 years of age were free of radiographic OA (definite osteophyte presence or more severe) in the hands, knees, hips, or spine.[1] Not all OA is symptomatic; still, the World Health Organization estimates that OA is a cause of disability in at least 10% of the population over age 60 years[2] and OA affects the lives of more than 20 million Americans.[3] Knee OA alone was as often associated with disability as were heart and chronic lung disease.[4] Current treatments for OA may improve symptoms but do not delay progression. Progression of OA to advanced and disabling stages is the leading indication for joint replacement.

The increase in the prevalence of symptomatic OA with age, coupled with the inadequacy of symptom-relieving or disease-modifying treatment, contributes to its impact. The number of persons in the U.S. with arthritis is anticipated to rise from 15% of the population (40 million) in 1995 to 18% of the population (59 million) by 2020.[3] A better understanding of the factors that contribute to disease and disability in OA is a high priority, especially given the lack of disease-modifying treatment options.

Epidemiologic studies, in addition to incidence and prevalence data, have supplied much of what is known about the natural history of OA and predisposing or protective factors. In addition, epidemiologic investigation has provided information to aid the performance and interpretation of clinical trials; such background information is critical in a disease like OA, which is heterogeneous in its expression and variably progressive.

The following chapter will provide an overview of the areas in which epidemiologic investigation of OA has occurred or has spurred methodologic development: defining OA for study, identifying typical patterns of disease (intra-articular localization, inter-articular joint clustering), developing approaches to assess OA progression, identifying risk factors for OA development and progression, identifying factors that mediate the effect of other factors, and understanding pathogenesis in terms of both anatomic and functional outcomes. This chapter focuses on knee, hip, and hand OA: knee and/or hip OA bear most of the responsibility for the burden of OA; hand OA may also be a source of symptoms, and may be a marker of a systemic predisposition toward OA.

DEFINING OSTEOARTHRITIS

Consensus Definition

Over the twentieth century, the definition of OA has evolved from "hypertrophic arthritis" to the most recent current consensus definition:[5] "OA diseases are a result of both mechanical and biologic events that destabilize the normal coupling of degradation and synthesis of articular cartilage chondrocytes and extracellular matrix, and subchondral bone. Although they may be initiated by multiple factors, including genetic, developmental, metabolic, and traumatic, OA diseases involve all of the tissues of the diarthrodial joint. Ultimately, OA diseases are manifested by morphologic, biochemical, molecular, and biomechanical changes of both cells and matrix which lead to a softening, fibrillation, ulceration, loss of articular cartilage, sclerosis and eburnation of subchondral bone, osteophytes, and subchondral cysts. When clinically evident, OA diseases are characterized by joint pain, tenderness, limitation of movement, crepitus, occasional effusion, and variable degrees of inflammation without systemic effects."

Classification of Osteoarthritis

OA is usually classified as primary (idiopathic) or secondary to metabolic conditions, anatomic abnormalities, trauma, or inflammatory arthritis (Table 1–1).

Diagnostic Criteria

Diagnostic criteria have been developed for knee,[6] hip,[7] and hand[8] OA. Recursive partitioning yielded criteria sets with the best combination of sensitivity and specificity (Table 1–2). In the studies in which these criteria were developed, comparison groups were patients with causes of joint pain other than OA. The American College of Rheumatology (ACR) criteria are intended to distinguish OA from other causes of symptoms and are best suited to recruit participants from clinical settings in which a high prevalence of other arthritides or soft tissue conditions and a higher (than the general population) likelihood of having symptomatic OA is expected. Of note, in community-based studies, the ability to distinguish OA from the absence of joint disease is paramount,[9–11] and definitions of OA for epidemiologic study

TABLE 1–1
CLASSIFICATION OF OSTEOARTHRITIS

PRIMARY (IDIOPATHIC)
Peripheral joints
Spine
    Apophyseal joints
    Intervertebral joints
Subsets
    Generalized osteoarthritis
    Erosive inflammatory osteoarthritis
    Diffuse idiopathic skeletal hyperostosis
    Chondromalacia patellae
Hereditary

SECONDARY
Trauma
    Acute
    Chronic (occupational, sports)
Underlying joint disorders
    Local (fracture, infection)
    Diffuse (rheumatoid arthritis)
Systemic metabolic or endocrine disorders
    Ochronosis (alkaptonuria)
    Wilson disease
    Hemochromatosis
    Kashin-Bek disease
    Acromegaly
    Hyperparathyroidism
Crystal deposition disease
    Calcium pyrophosphate dihydrate (pseudogout)
    Basic calcium phosphate (hydroxyapatite–octacalcium
        phosphate–tricalcium phosphate)
    Monosodium urate monohydrate (gout)
Neuropathic disorders (Charcot joints)
    Tabes dorsalis
    Diabetes mellitus
    Intra-articular corticosteroid overuse
Miscellaneous
    Bone dysplasia (multiple epiphyseal dysplasia, achondroplasia)
    Frostbite

have been developed with this in mind. These definitions are discussed in the following paragraphs.

Patterns of Disease

Specific inter- and intra-articular patterns of OA may represent subsets that have distinctive risk factor profiles and disease course, and, in theory, respond differently to treatment.

Knee Osteoarthritis

Unilateral and bilateral knee OA may represent not different subsets as much as different stages within the same subset. Bilateral knee OA is more common than unilateral disease, affecting 5% versus 2%, respectively, of persons 45 to 74 years of age in NHANES I.[12] Having OA in one knee increases the likelihood of having OA in the contralateral knee.[13,14] Among Chingford study participants with unilateral knee OA, 34% developed contralateral OA within 2 years.[15] In a clinic-based study of 63 patients with knee OA, 12 of 13 with unilateral OA at baseline developed contralateral OA over 11 years.[16]

Based on x-ray data, it is believed that tibiofemoral OA is more common than patellofemoral OA. In the Framingham cohort, patellofemoral OA was found in 5%, tibiofemoral OA in 23%, and mixed tibiofemoral and patellofemoral OA in 20%.[17] In a community study in the United Kingdom, men with symptomatic OA most often had isolated medial disease (21%, vs. patellofemoral in 11%, mixed in 7%).[18] In women, however, patellofemoral OA was most common (24% vs. medial in 12%, mixed in 6%).

Studies which have examined whether OA is more likely on the right or left side revealed no difference in one study[19] and, in a recent study, a slightly greater prevalence of tibiofemoral OA on the right side.[20]

Hip Osteoarthritis

In persons with hip OA, bilateral involvement was reported in 35%[21] and 42%.[22] Involvement of one hip increased the likelihood of contralateral hip OA in the Chingford study.[14] Hip OA appears to be equally common on the right and left sides.[19,20]

Superior or lateral involvement is more common than medial involvement. In 6000 patients who had bowel x-rays, 4.7% had hip OA; of these, involvement was lateral in 50% and medial in 24%.[23] In a hospital-based study, Ledingham et al. found superior pole migration in 82%, medial/axial migration in 8%, and an indeterminate pattern in 10%.[22] Superomedial and medial/axial patterns were more common in women, and superolateral patterns were more common in men.[22]

Hand Osteoarthritis

There is strong evidence for clustering of hand joint involvement in OA. Having OA in either distal interphalangeal (DIP) or proximal interphalangeal (PIP) joints at baseline increased the risk of incident OA in all other hand joints.[24] Having thumb base OA at baseline increased the risk of developing metacarpophalangeal (MCP) OA and, to

TABLE 1–2
OSTEOARTHRITIS CLASSIFICATION CRITERIA

Joint	Clinical and Laboratory	Clinical, Laboratory, and Radiographic
Knee	Knee pain AND Crepitus, and morning stiffness ≤30 minutes, and age ≥38 years OR Crepitus, and morning stiffness >30 minutes, and bony enlargement OR No crepitus, and bony enlargement	Knee pain AND Osteophytes OR OA synovial fluid (clear, viscous, WBC <2000/mm^3), and morning stiffness ≤30 minutes, and crepitus
Sensitivity	89%	94%
Specificity	88%	88%
Hand	1. Hand pain, aching, or stiffness AND 2. Hard tissue enlargement of 2 or more of 10 selected hand joints* AND 3. Metacarpophalangeal swelling in fewer than 2 joints AND 4a. Hard tissue enlargement involving 2 or more distal interphalangeal joints (second and third distal interphalangeal joints may be counted in both 2 and 4a) OR 4b. Deformity of 2 or more of 10 selected hand joints*	
Sensitivity	93%	
Specificity	97%	
Hip	1. Hip pain AND 2a. Hip internal rotation <14° AND 2b. ESR ≤15 mm/h (hip flexion ≤115° if no ESR available) OR 3a. Range of motion ≥15° internal rotation AND 3b. Morning stiffness of the hip ≤60 minutes AND 3c. Age >50 years	Hip pain AND At least two of the following: ESR less than 20 mm/hr Radiographic femoral or acetabular osteophytes Radiographic joint space narrowing (superior, axial, or medial)
Sensitivity	87%	89%
Specificity	75%	91%

*Second and third distal interphalangeal, second and third proximal interphalangeal, and first carpometacarpal joints. ESR, erythrocyte sedimentation rate.

a lesser extent, DIP and PIP OA.[24] After adjusting for age, the risk of hand OA was increased by having contralateral hand OA,[25] prevalent OA in one or more joints in the same row,[24,25] or prevalent OA in the same ray.[24,25] DIP OA was more common on the right than on the left side;[20] a previous study revealed no differences between dominant and non-dominant hands.[26]

A study of 53-year-old men and women from a large general population sample revealed evidence of a polyarticular hand OA subset that involved the DIP, PIP, and thumb base joints.[27] Clustering was most apparent by row (rather than by ray) and by symmetric involvement of the same joint in both hands. There was clear evidence of clustering in the men as well, and the patterns were indistinguishable between men and women.[27]

Clustering of Osteoarthritis Involvement of the Knee, Hip, and Hand

Multiple involvement of five joint groups—DIP, PIP, carpometacarpal (CMC), knee, and hip—occurred more frequently than could be expected by chance in the Chingford population.[14] However, the association between contralateral joints was stronger than the associations between different joint groups. Knee and hip OA are each associated with the presence of hand OA.[28–30] When examined within the same population, the link between knee and hand OA appeared stronger.[14,31] In BLSA participants, an association was found between knee OA and DIP OA, PIP OA, and OA in two or more hand joint groups, adjusting for age and BMI (ORs 1.71 to 2.16).[28] Of patients who had undergone meniscectomy, those with hand OA had more frequent and more severe knee OA in both operated and unoperated knees than did those without hand OA, adjusting for sex and age.[32,33] The presence of hand OA was associated with a threefold increase in the risk of hip OA.[29,30]

Defining Osteoarthritis for Epidemiologic Study

Much effort has been devoted toward developing a definition of OA for epidemiologic study that encapsulates symptoms, disability, and joint pathology. At the heart of the difficulty is the issue that, while there is some correlation between radiographic disease severity and both symptoms and disability, the relationships are not as strong as one would expect.

As noted above, in epidemiologic studies, a key distinction is between OA and the absence of arthritis. For this reason, and the frequency of mild or intermittent symptoms, epidemiologic studies have tended to rely upon radiographic definitions of OA. *Symptomatic*, radiographic OA has been defined by a radiographic criterion coupled with a positive response to a question, e.g., pain, in that joint, on most days of a month within the preceding year. The use of a definition combining symptom and x-ray criteria reflects a desire to capture persons with clinically significant OA. A potential limitation of this approach is that a subset of persons with OA may have physically limiting disease but self-reported symptoms that fall below the applied "symptomatic" cut-off.

The most widely used system to grade radiographic severity continues to be the Kellgren and Lawrence grading system,[34] by which 1 of 5 grades is assigned with the aid of atlas reproductions, according to the following definitions: 0 for normal, 1 for possible osteophytic lipping, 2 for definite osteophytes and possible joint space narrowing, 3 for moderate or multiple osteophytes, definite joint space narrowing, some sclerosis, and possible bony attrition, and 4 for large osteophytes, marked joint space narrowing, severe sclerosis, and definite bony attrition. The K/L system is osteophyte driven; it is unclear how to handle knees with joint space narrowing without osteophytes. Also, the K/L system is limited by incorrect assumptions, including the following: that change in any one feature is linear and constant, and that the relationship between features is constant.[35] Most investigators assess individual radiographic features in addition to a global score.

Although x-ray continues to be used heavily, MRI is common in epidemiologic studies, and provides rich opportunities to assess articular cartilage, subarticular bone, menisci, ligaments, and, aided by contrast, synovium. An MRI-based definition of OA has not as yet been established.

Knee Osteoarthritis

The presence of definite osteophytes is the recommended definition for radiographic knee OA.[36,37] Further validating an osteophyte-based definition, tibiofemoral osteophytes predicted cartilage defects on MRI, whether or not radiographic joint space narrowing (as defined by <3 mm) was present, in individuals 49 to 58 years of age.[38,39] In the

patellofemoral joint however, osteophytes predicted MRI cartilage defects only in narrowed patellofemoral joints, suggesting that osteophytes alone may not be sufficient to identify cases of patellofemoral OA.[39]

Hip Osteoarthritis

A definition including joint space width appears to be valid and practical for epidemiologic study of hip OA.[9,40] In men, an overall grade, minimal joint space width, and thickness of subchondral sclerosis were most predictive of hip pain.[40] Minimal joint space was best associated with other radiographic features, and measures of joint space were more reproducible than other indices.[40] However, there are caveats with a joint space width definition: the cut-off for what is a normal joint space width at the hip may differ between ethnic groups and change with age; it is unclear how to handle osteophytes without joint space narrowing; a less stringent cut-off increases sensitivity but sacrifices specificity.[9] Specificity may be enhanced by requiring at least one other radiographic feature or by using a global system.[9] Of note, minimum joint space width 2 mm or less was more closely associated (than global radiographic scoring approaches) with hip pain.[41] The effect of using alternative definitions of disease on estimates of prevalence has been demonstrated.[42]

Hand Osteoarthritis

Defining hand OA is important to advance the investigation of hand OA itself and to document its presence as a marker of a systemic predisposition towards OA. Most epidemiologic studies have relied on the presence of definite osteophytes, or K/L 2. Alternative global radiographic scoring systems were developed.[43,44] While Heberden's node presence and DIP osteophytes had similar sensitivity, the specificity and positive predictive value of radiographic osteophytes was higher for detecting knee, CMC, and PIP OA, and OA in more than two groups of joints.[45]

At present there is no agreement on the best definition of generalized OA; Cooper et al. demonstrated that thresholds could be defined for the number of involved joint groups that distinguished a polyarticular subset of OA; these thresholds varied with age and other factors.[14]

INCIDENCE

Knee Osteoarthritis

In the Framingham study (participant mean age 70.8 years), 2% of women per year developed radiographic knee OA, and 1% per year developed symptomatic, radiographic knee OA, versus 1.4% and 0.7% of men, respectively.[13] In a Dutch population-based study (participant age 46 to 66 years), about 2% of women and 0.8% of men developed radiographic knee OA per year.[46] In the Goteborg study (participant age 75 years), the incidence of knee OA was 0.9% per year.[47]

Two incidence studies were restricted to patients seeking medical care with symptomatic joint disease. Oliveria et al. evaluated incident symptomatic, radiographic knee OA rates in a large HMO in central Massachusetts, mostly involving white, blue-collar workers, and found higher rates in women (female to male ratio for hand, hip, and knee OA 2:1), and an increase in incidence with age until 80 years.[48] The age- and sex-standardized incidence rate for knee OA was 240 per 100,000 person-years (95% confidence interval (CI) 218.00-262.00). The incidence of clinical knee OA was over 1% per year in women of age 70 to 89 years. Wilson et al. found equal rates of incident symptomatic OA in men and women of Olmstead County Minnesota (mostly northern European).[49] The age- and sex-adjusted rate for knee OA was 163.8 per 100,000 person-years (95% CI 127.1-200.6). The difference in results between these two studies may relate in part to broader exclusions for secondary OA in the latter study.

Hip Osteoarthritis

Over 8 years, 3.5% to 11.9% (depending on the radiographic definition used) of women of age 65 years and older in the study of osteoporotic fractures (SOF) developed hip OA.[50] The age- and sex-standardized incidence rate for symptomatic, radiographic hip OA was reported to be 88 per 100,000 person-years (95% CI 75-101) by Oliveria et al.[48] and 47.3 per 100,000 person-years (95% CI 27.8 -66.8) by Wilson et al.[49]

Hand Osteoarthritis

In the Tecumseh Community Health Study, 1.8% of participants (of age 27 to 51 years) developed hand OA per year.[51] In the Goteborg study (participant age 75 years), 2.7% of participants developed DIP or PIP OA per year.[47] In the Framingham study (mean age 55 years), Chaisson et al. found that 3.6% of women and 3.2% of men developed radiographic OA in at least one hand joint per year.[24] Women had more incident disease than men in all hand joints except the MCP group for which rates were comparable between men and women. The most frequently affected joints were, in decreasing order, DIP-2 (57% in women, 36% in men), thumb IP, CMC-1, and DIP-5.[24] The higher overall rate in the older Framingham cohort versus the younger Tecumseh cohort (51) most likely reflects an increase in the incidence of hand OA with age, but also may relate to differences in how OA was defined.

In a cohort of men of age 60 years and above in the Baltimore Longitudinal Study of Aging (BLSA), the incidence was highest at the DIP joints and increased with age in all hand joints.[52] Oliveria et al. reported an age- and sex-standardized incidence rate for symptomatic, radiographic hand OA of 100 per 100,000 person-years (95% CI 86-115).[48]

PREVALENCE

Studies of the prevalence of knee OA are summarized in Table 1–3.[19,53–55] The prevalence of radiographic knee OA rises in women from 1% to 4% in those 24 to 45 years of age to 53% to 55% in those of age 80 years and older. In men, the prevalence rises from 1% to 6% in those 45 years and younger to 22% to 33% in those 80 years and

TABLE 1–3
PREVALENCE OF KNEE OSTEOARTHRITIS

Study	Age Range of Participants	Age Subset	Radiographic Knee OA in Women	Symptomatic Radiographic Knee OA in Women	Radiographic Knee OA in Men	Symptomatic Radiographic Knee OA in Men
Lawrence,[53] 1966	>35	35–44	4.0	2.8	5.6	2.5
		45–54	13.1	5.4	8.2	4.1
		55–64	40.0	21.8	28.2	9.7
		65+	49.1	28.6	26.4	14.3
Felson,[54] 1987	63–94	<70	25.1	7.6	30.4	6.2
		70–79	36.2	13.0	30.7	7.8
		≥80	52.6	15.8	32.6	5.4
Anderson,[55] 1988	35–74	35–44	1.2		1.2	
		45–54	3.6		2.2	
		55–64	7.5		5.1	
		65–74	20.3		9.0	
van Saase,[19] 1989	>45	45–49	12.7		7.7	
		50–54	16.1		11.2	
		55–59	14.0		11.8	
		60–64	24.2		23.0	
		65–69	33.3		13.1	
		70–74	40.2		24.7	
		75–79	40.2		22.0	
		≥80	54.6		22.2	

TABLE 1–4
PREVALENCE OF HIP OSTEOARTHRITIS

Study	Age Range of Participants	Age Subset	Radiographic Hip OA in Women	Symptomatic Radiographic Hip OA in Women	Radiographic Hip OA in Men	Symptomatic Radiographic Hip OA in Men
Lawrence,[53] 1966	>55		6.2	3.4	16.5	5.5
Maurer,[60] (1979)	55–74		2.8	0.7	3.5	0.7
Danielsson,[21] 1984	40–89	40–44	0.4		*	
		45–49	0.4		0.4	
		50–54	0.4		0.8	
		55–59	1.2		1.2	
		60–64	1.6		1.6	
		65–69	0.8		2.8	
		70–74	5.2		2.4	
		75–79	4.7		6.4	
		80–84	5.0		11.5	
		85–89	10.0		5.6	
van Saase,[19] 1989	>45	45–49	2.6		2.8	
		50–54	2.0		2.2	
		55–59	2.6		5.9	
		60–64	3.8		10.1	
		65–69	10.9		11.2	
		70–74	14.8		4.7	
		75–79	14.5		10.2	
		80+	26.0		11.1	

*no cases found

TABLE 1–5
PREVALENCE OF RADIOGRAPHIC HAND OSTEOARTHRITIS

Study	Age Range of Participants	Age Subset	DIP OA in Women	PIP OA in Women	MCP OA in Women	CMC-1 OA in Women	DIP OA in Men	PIP OA in Men	MCP OA in Men	CMC-1 OA in Men
Lawrence,[53] 1966	>15	15–24	*	*	*		*	*	*	
		25–34	*	*	0.6		1.8	*	1.8	
		35–44	7.7	*	2.2		5.5	2.4	*	
		45–54	22.9	5.9	6.5		22.5	5.5	12.0	
		55–64	54.8	28.7	25.2		47.1	10.6	17.3	
		65+	80.4	49.1	43.8		65.6	32.3	43.0	
van Saase,[19] 1989	>20	20–24	1.0	*	0.7	0.3	0.3	0.3	0.7	*
		25–29	0.5	*	1.0	*	0.3	0.3	1.8	*
		30–34	0.3	0.3	2.9	*	2.2	0.3	3.7	0.9
		35–39	4.2	1.0	4.2	1.5	2.3	1.0	4.4	1.0
		40–44	8.9	1.4	8.2	5.8	8.6	1.0	9.6	3.5
		45–49	22.0	3.6	15.5	10.9	14.1	3.0	9.7	4.4
		50–54	41.6	9.7	22.5	16.4	24.0	5.4	16.7	11.5
		55–59	55.5	20.5	29.2	24.5	40.5	12.3	29.1	15.5
		60–64	68.9	29.6	45.6	34.5	48.9	11.8	40.5	20.8
		65–69	76.0	31.1	54.6	42.1	51.7	18.1	40.5	18.1
		70–74	74.7	35.2	56.6	46.7	58.8	20.0	50.6	23.5
		75–79	73.5	44.4	63.2	53.0	64.4	32.2	45.8	42.4
		80+	72.7	48.1	55.8	57.1	48.1	18.5	37.0	25.9

*no cases found

older. Other studies report a prevalence of 12% (Chingford, women 45 to 64 years),[56] 3.6% (Michigan Bone Health Study, women 24 to 45 years),[57] and 29% (Rotterdam, >55 years).[58] In the Beijing Osteoarthritis study, prevalence of radiographic OA in Chinese men rose from 10% at 60 to 64 years to 45.7% at ages over 80 years, similar to findings in Framingham men.[59] Rates in Beijing women in these age groups were 39.6% and 59.1% respectively, about 40% higher than what was found in Framingham women, applying the same case definitions and radiographic methods.

Studies of the prevalence of hip OA are summarized in Table 1–4.[19,21,53,60] An increase in hip OA with age is seen in both genders, especially in women. Other studies report a prevalence of 3% in women and 3.2% in men (NHANES I, 55 to 74 years),[61] and 15.9% in women and 14.1% in men (Rotterdam, >55 years).[58] Hoaglund et al. found only five cases of hip OA (graded K/L 3-4) in 500 Hong Kong southern Chinese hospital patients.[62] A subsequent study similarly found a lower prevalence of hip OA in Hong Kong Chinese men.[63] Prevalence of hip OA in men and women was substantially lower in Beijing men and women than in U.S. cohorts assessed using the same methods.[64] For radiographic hip OA, prevalence ratios were 0.07 (Chinese women to white women in the SOF), 0.22 (Chinese women to women in the NHANES I), and 0.19 (Chinese men to white men in the NHANES I).

Though reported differences may relate to study methodology, the prevalence of hip OA may be lower in Jamaicans,[65] Asian Indians,[66] and Nigerians[67] than in European populations.

Two studies of the prevalence of hand OA are summarized in Table 1–5.[53,69] The prevalence of radiographic and also of symptomatic, radiographic hand OA at all sites rises with age, and is greater in women. Plato and Norris provide age-specific prevalence rates for individual hand joints for men in the BLSA, and summarize several previous U.S. studies.[68] Other studies report a prevalence of 14% in the DIP and 16% in CMC-1 (Chingford, women 45 to 64 years);[56] 3% in DIP joints, 1.0% in PIP, 0.7% in MCP, 0 in CMC-1, 0.5% in IP-1 (Michigan Bone Health Study, women 24 to 45 years);[57] 35% in DIP joints in women, and 24% in men (Hong Kong southern Chinese, >54 years);[62] and 30%, for symptomatic hand OA in women, and 29% in men (National Household Education Surveys [NHES] 25 to 74 years).[69]

RISK FACTORS FOR INCIDENT OSTEOARTHRITIS

Individual studies have traditionally sought to identify risk factors for incident disease or OA progression but not both, in large part due to the cost and logistics of powering both outcomes. The current era is witness to the development and initiation of large-scale studies that will have power to look at incidence, progression, and disability within the same study: the Rotterdam study MOST (Multicenter Osteoarthritis Study), and the OAI (Osteoarthritis Initiative).

A candidate's risk factor's effect on each outcome—incidence and progression—should be specifically and separately examined. It is widely believed that the risk factor profiles for each of these key outcomes may overlap but are not identical. Also, the magnitude of the effect of a given risk factor may differ according to the stage of OA disease present in a given joint, i.e., prior to definite OA (the stratum for study of incident OA), or after OA is definitely present (the stratum for progression). As is the case in these studies, it is ideal that the examination of effect on incident and progressive OA occurs within the same study. Otherwise, if the effect on incidence differed from that on progression when these outcomes were examined in separate studies, it would remain possible that the difference was linked to methodologic differences between studies.[70] An additional key design element of MOST and the OAI reflects evolution in views of the basic OA condition that is of highest priority to study in terms of potential intervention and/or prevention strategy development: the cohorts of each of these studies includes individuals with symptomatic radiographic knee OA or those at higher (than the general population) risk to develop it.[70]

To identify risk factors for incident OA, longitudinal studies, which allow determination of the relationship of a risk factor at baseline to new disease development over time, are of course optimal, but are more expensive to perform. Cross-sectional studies of the relationship between exposure to a given factor and risk of having disease have been more common. OA development is often attributed to a joint-specific local mechanical environment within a systemic milieu, leading to categorization of risk factors as either systemic or local. However, certain risk factors like age, a systemic factor that may act in part by altering the mechanical environment, illustrate that categorization may oversimplify what are complex risk factor effects. Unless otherwise specified, the following studies have focused on a radiographic definition of OA (i.e., K/L ≥2).

Body Weight

In Framingham participants of median age 37 years, weight predicted the presence of knee OA 36 years later.[71] The age-adjusted relative risk for knee OA in the heaviest quintile of baseline weight versus the lightest three quintiles was 2.07 (95% CI 1.67-2.55) for women and 1.51 for men. Results were unaffected by adjustment for serum uric acid level and physical activity. Weight change in Framingham women affected the risk for developing knee OA.[72] A decrease in BMI of 2 units over the previous 10 years decreased the odds of knee OA (OR 0.46, 95% CI 0.24-0.86). Analyses were adjusted for age, baseline BMI, knee injury, smoking, job physical labor, habitual physical activity, and educational level.

A subsequent Framingham study (mean subject age 70.5 years) in subjects free of disease at baseline confirmed that higher BMI increased the risk of OA (OR 1.6/5 unit increase, 95% CI 1.2-2.2) and weight change was directly related to risk of OA (OR 1.4/10 lb change in weight).[73] These findings were present in women; per the authors, the absence of relationship in men may reflect a gender difference or the small number of incident cases in men.

In a longitudinal study of the Chingford population (women, mean age 54 years), belonging to the top BMI tertile was associated with an increased risk of knee OA (OR

2.38, 95% CI 1.29-4.39), adjusting for hysterectomy, estrogen replacement therapy, physical activity, knee pain, and social class.[74] In Chingford participants with unilateral knee OA, 46% in the top BMI tertile developed OA in the uninvolved knee over 2 years versus 10% in the lowest tertile.[15]

Obesity was more strongly associated with bilateral (OR 6.6, 95% CI 4.71-9.18) than unilateral OA (OR 3.4 in right knees), adjusting for injury, age, and gender in 45 to 74 year old NHANES I participants.[12] There is little evidence of a metabolic link between body weight and knee OA. With one exception,[75] population-based studies have not revealed an independent relationship of a metabolic correlate of obesity (e.g., serum lipids, glucose or glucose tolerance test, body fat distribution, and blood pressure) with knee OA.[76-79]

In both the Framingham and Chingford populations, while BMI was linked to all patterns of knee OA (tibiofemoral, patellofemoral, and mixed), odds ratios were highest for mixed involvement.[17,80]

The possibility remains, albeit small, that knee symptoms preceding OA lead to lower levels of activity which contribute to obesity, and that other factors cause OA. However, analysis of NHANES I data[55] revealed no evidence that the association between BMI and knee OA is stronger for those with knee symptoms. In Framingham women, the association between weight and knee OA was stronger in those *without* symptoms; in men, the association appeared to be stronger in those with symptomatic disease.[71]

In contrast to the knee, a more modest association between body weight and hip OA has been described. In NHANES I, neither obesity nor fat distribution was associated with hip OA.[61] However, being overweight was more closely associated with bilateral (OR 2.0, 95% CI 0.97-4.15) than unilateral hip OA (OR 0.54, 95% CI 0.26-1.16), adjusting for gender, age, race, and education. In the Zoetermeer study, obesity was linked to OA in the right but not the left hip in men, and was not associated with hip OA in women[81] In another study involving farmers, the risk of hip OA was highest in the tallest and heaviest members of the sample though the association with weight, height, or BMI did not achieve significance.[82] In an early report from the Rotterdam study it was stated that being overweight increased the risk of incident knee OA but not incident hip OA.[83]

Support for a link between obesity and hand OA comes from one longitudinal study[51] and some cross-sectional studies[76,79,81] but not others.[57,84,85] In the Tecumseh study, mean age- and smoking-adjusted baseline weight was higher among those who developed hand OA than among those who remained free of disease.[51] Blood pressure, cholesterol, uric acid, and glucose were not linked to the development of hand OA. A cross-sectional relationship was detected in men and women in the Zoetermeer study,[81] men and women in NHES and NHANES I for combined hand/foot OA,[76] and in men only of the Goteborg population,[79] but not in men[84] or women[85] in the BLSA. In the Michigan Bone Health Study, no association was detected between the presence of hand OA and BMI; relationship between BMI and hand radiographic scores did not persist after adjusting for age and bone mineral density (BMD).[57]

Cross-sectional studies examining the relationship between specific hand joint groups and weight have had conflicting results. In the Zoetermeer survey, obesity was associated with DIP and PIP OA but not with CMC OA,[81] while in the Chingford population, BMI was associated with CMC OA but not with DIP or PIP OA.[86]

Age

Aged cartilage has altered chondrocyte function and material properties and responds differently to cytokines and growth factors. In addition, joint-protective neural and mechanical factors may become impaired with age, such as proprioception, varus-valgus laxity,[87] and muscle strength.[88]

In a longitudinal study of the Chingford population (women, mean age 54 years), belonging to the highest of three age groups was associated with an increased risk of knee OA (OR 2.41, 95% CI 1.11-5.24), adjusting for hysterectomy, estrogen replacement therapy, smoking, physical activity, pain, social class, height, and weight.[74] Knee osteophyte development increased by 20% per 5-year age increase. The magnitude of risk associated with aging appears to decrease as older ages are reached. Age did not affect the risk of knee OA in a longitudinal Framingham study in which the mean subject age at baseline was 70.5 years.[73] Several cross-sectional studies have demonstrated a higher prevalence of knee OA with increasing age, including those of Lawrence et al.,[53] the Framingham study,[54] NHANES I,[12,55] and the Zoetermeer survey.[19]

Hip OA is more prevalent at older ages. A relationship between age and hip OA is supported by two Scandinavian studies,[21,23] the Zoetermeer survey,[19] and NHANES I.[61] In the NHANES I data, age increased the risk of hip OA (OR 2.38 for ages 70 to 74 years versus 55 to 59 years, 95% CI 1.15-4.92), adjusting for gender, race, marital status, education, and family income.[61]

Age is closely associated with the development of hand OA[11] as shown in the reports of Lawrence,[53] the BLSA,[52,84] the Zoetermeer survey,[19] and the Michigan Bone Health Study.[57] In a longitudinal BLSA study, Kallman et al. found that age increased the risk of OA for almost every radiographic feature in every hand joint group.[52] In pre- and perimenopausal women, age was more strongly linked to hand than knee OA.[57]

Gender

Gender may influence knee OA via multiple routes including hormonal influences on cartilage metabolism, gender variation in injury risk, and gender differences in the mechanical environment of the knee (e.g., varus-valgus laxity,[87] strength relative to body weight[88]).

Women develop knee OA more frequently than men. In a longitudinal Framingham study, women had a greater risk of developing OA than men (OR 1.8, 95% CI 1.1-3.1), adjusting for age, BMI, smoking, injury, chondrocalcinosis, hand OA, and physical activity.[73] Cross-sectional studies have demonstrated that knee OA is more prevalent in women.[12,19,55] In NHANES I, bilateral OA was twice as prevalent in women than in men.[12] No gender difference was seen in the prevalence of unilateral OA. Anderson et al. found that, among NHANES I subjects aged 35 to 74 years, knee OA increased with age in both sexes and, beginning in those 45 to 54 years, was greater in women than in men.[55] In the Zoetermeer survey, severe OA was much more prevalent in women.[19]

In a cross-sectional study involving a convenience sample, in which 15% of men and 19% of women had radiographic OA, men had greater patellar and tibial cartilage volume than women. Differences were reduced (though some difference remained) after adjusting for gender differences in height, weight, and bone size.[89] In a small study of young persons with healthy knees, Faber et al. found that a gender difference in cartilage volume was primarily due to difference in joint surface area (epiphyseal bone size) and not to difference in cartilage thickness.[90]

Hip OA may be more common in women than men at older ages, but the gender difference is less pronounced than at the knee. Danielsson et al. found no difference between men and women in the prevalence of hip OA.[21] Jorring reported a female to male ratio of 3:2.[23] In those over 60 years, severe hip OA was more common in women. In the Zoetermeer survey, between ages 55 and 64 years, hip OA was more common in men; in those aged 65 and older, hip OA was more common in women.[19] Analyses of NHANES I data revealed no association between hip OA and gender.[61] Parity, age at menarche, and age at menopause were not linked to the presence of hip OA.

In the Tecumseh study, women had 2.6 (95% CI 1.65-4.18) times the risk than men of developing hand OA, adjusting for baseline age, weight, and cigarettes per day.[51] In the Zoetermeer survey, DIP OA was more common in women than men.[19] Cauley et al, examining white women mean age 74 years, found no association between serum sex hormones (estrone, estradiol, testosterone, and androstenedione) and severity of hand OA.[91] In the Michigan Bone Health Study, estradiol levels were not associated with hand OA scores.[57]

Occupational Activity

The health of cartilage and other joint tissues requires regular joint loading. However, if loading is extreme in frequency or intensity, it could exceed the tolerance of a joint and contribute to OA development. The role of occupational activity is better understood in men than in women, in part because previous studies assessed paid labor, did not include homemaking or child-rearing activities, and occurred when most women did not work outside the home. In a longitudinal Framingham study, risk of later radiographic knee OA was highest in men whose jobs, ascertained 20 years earlier, were classified as having at least medium physical demands and as likely to involve knee bending (OR. 2.2, 95% CI 1.4-3.6) versus a job with sedentary demands and no knee bending.[92] Analyses were adjusted for age, BMI, history of knee injury, education, and smoking. Analyses of NHANES I data revealed that radiographic knee OA was more common in 55- to 64-year-old men and women whose current job by title included much knee-bending versus some knee bending

(OR 2.45 for men and 3.49 for women), adjusting for race, education level, and BMI.[55] In women, job title associated with high versus moderate strength demands was associated with knee OA. Kivimaki et al. found an association between duration of knee bending activities and knee OA in male carpenters, floor layers, and painters.[93]

In a case-control study, an increased risk of knee OA was found in those whose main job entailed more than 30 minutes/day squatting or kneeling, or climbing more than 10 flights of stairs, adjusting for BMI and the presence of Heberden's nodes.[94] Regularly lifting >25 kg, as well as kneeling, squatting, or climbing stairs was associated with a fivefold increase in risk of knee OA, versus no exposure to these activities. No association was found between knee OA and prolonged walking, standing, sitting, or driving. Other studies have suggested an increase in knee OA in miners[95] and dockworkers.[96]

As summarized by Maetzel et al.,[97] a consistent though weak relationship between work-related exposure (especially farming) and hip OA in men has been reported. Farming for 10 or more years (vs. <1 year) was associated with hip OA in men (OR 2.0, 95% CI 0.9-4.4), adjusting for age, height, and weight.[82,98] Analyses of NHANES I data revealed a nonsignificant 40% to 50% increase in the odds of radiographic hip OA among men in rural areas, after adjusting for age, race, and BMI.[99] Male veterans administration clinic patients with hip OA and controls were surveyed about lifetime occupational and recreational activities and grouped based on estimates of joint compression forces produced.[100] Participants in the intermediate and heavy work groups had, respectively, 2.0 and 2.4 times the odds of having hip OA.

Certain occupations predispose toward hand OA. Lawrence et al. found that British cotton mill workers had more hand OA than did age matched controls.[101] Hadler et al. found in textile workers that burlers and spinners (tasks involving precision grip) had significantly more DIP OA than did winders (task involving a power grip).[102] Winders did not have more OA in the CMC joint by radiographic score but did have decreased CMC range of motion as compared to burlers and spinners. The likelihood of more severe OA (grade 3 or more) in the right-hand thumb and the index and middle fingers was elevated in dentists compared to teachers.[103]

Nonoccupational Physical Activity

The role of nonoccupational physical activity has been evaluated in epidemiologic studies in a variety of ways, e.g., OA prevalence in ex-elite athlete groups (competed at the national or international levels), the relationship between running and OA development, and the relationship between composite physical activity and OA.

In a study of men who were formerly elite athletes, the highest prevalence of tibiofemoral OA was found in soccer players (26%), and the highest prevalence of patellofemoral OA was found in weight-lifters (28%).[104] Previous knee injury, higher BMI at age 20, and hours of participation in team sports predicted tibiofemoral OA; previous knee injury, higher BMI at age 20, years spent in heavy work, and work involving kneeling or squatting predicted patellofemoral OA. Of note, unlike Framingham participants,[72] elevations in BMI within the non-obese range were linked to knee OA in these athletes, introducing the possibility that the pathogenic role of excess weight in knee OA may be modified by the nature and intensity of physical activity. Women who were formerly elite athletes (67 runners and 14 tennis players) had a threefold increase in the risk of tibiofemoral and patellofemoral OA versus age-matched women, adjusting for height and weight differences.[105] Results were unaffected by further adjustment for injury, smoking, menopause, hysterectomy, BMI, or age.

Recreational runners do not appear to have an increased risk of knee OA. In a study of runners versus controls matched for age, sex, education, and occupation, Lane et al. found that, of 73 participants, 9 developed knee OA over a 5-year period by ACR criteria: 5 were controls and 4 were runners.[106] Panush et al. also found no difference in rate of OA development between 17 male runners (53% marathon runners) and age- and weight-matched controls.[107]

In the Framingham study, habitual physical activity (a weighted and summed measure of hours/day at various activities), assessed at two previous exams, did not predict the presence of knee OA.[108] In a case-control study, there was no association between knee OA and lifetime leisure activities including walking, cycling, gardening, dancing, and outdoor sports in subjects aged 55 years and older.[109] In participants with a mean age of 79 years, Bagge et al. found no association between occupational or leisure activity and knee OA.[79] In longitudinal studies of the Chingford cohort, physical activity was not linked to incident OA in the uninvolved knee in those with unilateral knee OA[12], nor was it linked to incident OA in the full cohort.[74] As the authors note,[74,79] only a small number of participants were involved in heavy activity.

There are two caveats to note. First, it is believed, although not based upon formal investigation, that an anatomic abnormality in a joint or periarticular structure may increase the physical activity-associated risk of OA.[110] Second, one longitudinal study introduces the possibility that the combination of very heavy physical activity and age may be linked to an increased risk of knee OA.[73,111] In elderly persons (mean age of 70 years), the odds of developing radiographic knee OA between two exams 8 years apart were increased by heavy physical activity (e.g., OR 7.2, 95% CI 2.5-20.0 for >4 hours per day of heavy activity) assessed by a questionnaire at mid-study, adjusting for age, gender, BMI, weight loss, injury, health status, calorie intake, and smoking.[111] Risk was greatest in the top tertile of BMI. No relationship was detected with moderate or light physical activity, number of blocks walked, or number of flights of stairs climbed daily.

Based on a small number of studies, high intensity, nonoccupational activity may be linked to hip OA. A case control study of men up to age 49 with total hip replacements versus men from the general population revealed that high exposure to any sport increased the risk of hip OA (RR 3.5 to 4.5), adjusting for age, BMI, smoking, and occupational physical activity.[112] Puranen et al. found that hip OA prevalence was not greater in former champion dis-

tance runners than individuals who were not runners.[113] However, Marti et al. found that hip OA was more prevalent in former national team long-distance runners than in bobsled competitors or controls.[114] Age and mileage run in 1973 predicted radiographic hip OA in 1988.

Bone Mineral Density

The relationship between BMD and knee OA has been examined in longitudinal studies including those of the Framingham, Rotterdam, and Chingford cohorts. As reported by Zhang et al., over 8 years of follow-up of the Framingham cohort, risk of incident OA was lowest in the lowest femoral neck BMD quartile (5.6%) and was higher in the higher 3 BMD quartiles (14.2%, 10.3%, and 11.8%).[115] Similarly, in the Rotterdam study, the incidence of radiographic knee OA was higher in those in the highest femoral neck (10.5%) and spine BMD (14.3%) quartiles than in those in the lower quartiles (3.4% and 3.3%).[116] Women in the Chingford study with incident knee osteophytes had significantly higher baseline spine and hip BMD than those without incident disease.[117]

In the Rotterdam population, those with knee and/or hip OA had 3% to 8% higher femoral neck BMD versus those without OA, a difference that was significant in women only.[118] Repeat BMD measurements 2 years later revealed that the rate of bone loss was higher in participants with OA. In theory, a decline in BMD might be cytokine mediated or a consequence of reduced physical activity.[118]

Both the Framingham and Chingford studies revealed that participants with knee OA had a 5% to 10% higher BMD than those without knee OA.[56,119] In the Framingham study, women with K/L 1 and 2 knees had a 5% to 9% higher femoral neck BMD than those with K/L 0 knees, adjusting for age, BMI, and smoking, and men with K/L 1 knees had a higher femoral neck BMD than men with K/L 0 knees.[119] Women in the Chingford study with knee OA had a 7.6% and 6.2% higher BMD at lumbar spine and femoral neck sites, respectively, versus controls, adjusting for age and BMI.[56] Results were unaffected by further adjustment for smoking, alcohol use, exercise, estrogen replacement therapy, social class, and spine osteophytes. In the BLSA, lumbar spine BMD was 4% higher in men and 3.7% higher in women with knee osteophytes, adjusting for age, BMI, and smoking.[120] Knee OA was not linked to BMD assessed at upper extremity sites.[119,121]

Several studies support that those with hip OA have a higher bone mass at both axial and appendicular sites (reviewed in Lane and Nevitt[122]). In cross-sectional analyses in the SOF, women with K/L grade 3–4 hip OA had higher age-adjusted BMD at the femoral neck and Ward's triangle, trochanter, lumbar spine, distal radius, and calcaneus versus those with K/L grade 0–1 in the worse hip.[123] Elevations in BMD were greatest in the femoral neck of hips with OA, in women with bilateral hip OA, and in women with hip osteophytes.

In the longitudinal Tecumseh study, women who developed OA were more likely to have had higher baseline bone mass (metacarpal bone cortical area) than women who did not develop OA; these women also had a greater likelihood of bone loss over time.[124] In men[84] and women[125] in the BLSA, upper extremity BMD, adjusted for age and BMI, was not correlated with radiographic grade of hand OA. Women in the Chingford study with OA had higher BMD than controls, adjusting for age and BMI: those with DIP OA had 5.8% greater BMD at the lumbar spine only; those with CMC OA had 2.5% to 3% greater BMD at the femoral neck and lumbar spine.[56] Results were not altered by adjustment for smoking, alcohol use, exercise, estrogen replacement therapy, social class, and spine osteophytes.

Postmenopausal Hormone Replacement Therapy

Estrogen may have direct effects on articular cartilage, or may influence OA development via effects on bone or other joint tissues. Postmenopausal estrogen replacement therapy may protect against the development of knee OA. In many studies, the relationship does not achieve significance. However, results are consistent in the direction and magnitude of the relationship, and suggest a gradient of protection (i.e., greater protection conferred with current estrogen replacement therapy vs. past use).[126] In a longitudinal Framingham study, the odds ratio for incident OA associated with past estrogen replacement therapy use versus never use was 0.8 (95% CI 0.5-1.4) and associated with current use versus never use was 0.4 (95% CI 0.1-3.0), adjusting for age, BMI, femoral neck BMD, physical activity, weight change, knee injury, smoking, and baseline K/L grade.[127] Similarly, a nonsignificant protective effect for incident knee osteophytes was seen with current estrogen replacement therapy in a longitudinal Chingford study (OR 0.41, 95% CI 0.12-1.42), adjusted for hysterectomy, smoking, physical activity, knee pain, and social class.[74] In a case control study, Samanta et al. also found a nonsignificant association between estrogen replacement therapy and reduced likelihood of large joint OA (OR 0.31, 95% CI 0.07–1.35).[128]

An MRI-based study suggests that women using estrogen replacement therapy may have greater articular cartilage volume than non-users.[129] Total tibial cartilage volume was 7.7% (0.23 mL) greater in the group of estrogen users than in the non-users. The difference persisted after adjusting for years since menopause, BMI, age at menopause, and smoking (adjusted difference 0.30 mL, 95% CI 0.08-0.52), and findings were very similar after excluding women with established knee OA.

In a cross-sectional study of white women 65 years and older in the SOF, current users of estrogen replacement therapy had a reduced risk of any hip OA (OR 0.62, 95% CI 0.49-0.86), and of moderate-severe hip OA.[130] Current users for 10 or more years had a greater reduction in risk of any hip OA versus users of less than 10 years. Current use for 10 or more years was also associated with a nonsignificant trend for a reduced risk of moderate to severe symptomatic hip OA. In the Chingford population, for current users there was a hint of protective effect, though not significant, of hormone replacement therapy for DIP OA (OR 0.48 95% CI 0.17-1.42) and no clear effect for CMC OA, adjusting for age, height and weight, menopausal age, and femoral neck BMD.[131]

Injury

OA may result after an injury, either as a primary effect (i.e., direct damage to articular cartilage) or secondarily, due to the greater stress to cartilage resulting from damage to load-attenuating knee tissues. Apparent in several cross-sectional studies, the link between knee injury and OA has been more difficult to demonstrate in longitudinal studies,[73,74] perhaps due to the possibility that injured individuals developed OA before the baseline evaluation of a given study and would therefore not be included in analyses of incident OA.[73] In a study by Gelber and colleagues, over a median follow-up of 36 years, the cumulative incidence of knee OA by age 65 was 13.9% in persons who had a knee injury during adolescence and young adulthood and 6.0% in those who did not.[132] Joint injury at cohort entry or during follow-up substantially increased the risk for subsequent osteoarthritis specific to site (RR 5.17, 95% CI 3.07-8.71 and 3.50, 95% CI 0.84-14.69 for knee and hip, respectively).

Cross-sectional studies have shown a link between knee injury and knee OA.[12,57,109] Though linked to both unilateral and bilateral knee OA, knee injury was more closely associated with unilateral OA.[12] Knee injury (OR 16.3, 95% CI 6.50-40.89) was a stronger predictor than obesity (OR 3.4) of unilateral knee OA. Injury increased OA risk at both tibiofemoral and patellofemoral sites.[109]

In analyses of NHANES I data, hip trauma was associated with hip OA (OR 7.84, 95% CI 2.11-29.10), adjusting for sex, age, race, and education.[61] When men and women were examined separately, the relationship remained significant for men but not for women. Hip trauma was significantly associated with unilateral hip OA; no hip trauma was reported among those with bilateral hip OA. In women in the Michigan Bone Health Study, hand injury was associated with hand OA (OR 2.98, 95% CI 1.05-8.46).[57]

Genetic Factors

A large literature dealing with genetic factors has been produced since Stecher's observation that Heberden's nodes were three times more common than expected in the sisters of affected individuals,[133] and Kellgren observed that the first-degree relatives of patients with generalized OA were more likely to have OA.[134] Twin, sibling-risk, and segregation studies make up much of this literature. The original approach, a focus on generalized OA, fed by the belief that this subset had a major genetic component, did not have anticipated yields; it is increasingly believed that a more joint-specific approach will be superior.[135] It is only feasible to provide a few examples of studies in the space available here. Outstanding overviews have recently been published.[135-137]

The correlations of specific features of hand and knee OA were higher in monozygotic twins than in dizygotic twins; adjusting for age and weight, 39% to 65% of the variance of hand and knee OA was attributed to genetic factors.[138] Further adjustment for estrogen replacement therapy, smoking, exercise, menopause, and height had little effect on the results.

The heritability of OA involving hand and knee was assessed in a large sample of randomly ascertained families.[139] The correlation of OA joint count was higher between siblings (r = 0.12 to r = 0.31) and between mothers and offspring than between fathers and offspring. The models that best fit were those postulating a mixed model, i.e., a mendelian gene in the context of multifactorial transmission. The familial aggregation of hand and knee OA was also evaluated by Hirsch et al. in the BLSA cohort.[140] After adjustment for age, sex, and BMI, sib-sib correlations were found for OA of the DIP, PIP, CMC-1 joints, for OA at two or three hand sites, and for polyarticular OA (r = 0.33 to 0.81).

Studies have described a greater frequency in subjects with generalized OA of HLA-A1B8 and MZ alpha-1 antitrypsin phenotypes,[141] particular estrogen receptor genotypes,[142] and in those with hip, hand, spine, or knee OA, an association of IGF-1 genotype.[143] In a study using affected sib pair analysis, an association between nodal OA and two loci on the short arm of chromosome 2 was detected (candidate genes include fibronectin, alpha-2 chain of collagen type V, IL-8 receptor).[144] A specific CRTM allele appeared to protect against the presence of hip OA (OR 0.51, 95% CI 0.26-0.99), adjusting for age and BMI.[1] The Rotterdam Study revealed a predisposition for radiographic OA of the hip in heterozygous and homozygous carriers of the IL1B-511T and of the IL1RN VNTR allele 2.[145] An additive effect was observed with carriers for risk alleles of both polymorphisms.

Two population-based studies have described an association between the VDR locus and knee osteophytes, adjusting for age, BMI, and BMD.[146,147] In the Framingham study, no linkage of OA with VDR/COL2A1 locus was found.[148] Using affected sib pair analyses, with control allele frequencies calculated from an unrelated group of unknown OA status, no linkage was demonstrated between generalized OA and three cartilage matrix genes, COL2A1, CRTL1 (encodes cartilage link protein), or CRTM.[149] In another study, an association between hip OA and polymorphisms of candidate genes, VDR, COL1A1, and COL2A1, were not seen in postmenopausal women.[150]

Findings from the Framingham study revealed eight chromosome regions—1, 2, 7, 9, 11–13, 19—with suggestive linkages for at least one phenotype for hand OA, none clearly coinciding with areas previously linked with OA.[151] A linkage study by Gillaspy et al. using fine mapping did not demonstrate any clear linkage at chromosome 2q for hand or knee OA.[152] These studies in aggregate suggest that hand OA, globally considered, have not consistently shown strong linkage to any chromosome sites. The Framingham Study revealed four sites showing evidence of linkage when a more joint-specific approach was undertaken. A linkage region for DIP OA was found on chromosome 7, for first CMC OA on chromosome 15, and, in women only, for DIP OA on chromosome 1 and first CMC OA on chromosome 20.[153]

As summarized by Loughlin,[135] genes that are believed to play some role in susceptibility include the IL-1 cluster,[145] the matrilin 3 gene (MATN3), the IL-4 receptor [alpha]-chain gene (IL4R), the secreted frizzled-related protein 3 gene (FRZB),[154,155] the metalloproteinase gene ADAM12, and the asporin gene (ASPN).[156,157]

An area of recent interest has been heritability of cartilage volume and other articular and periarticular features. A twin study revealed heritability estimates of 61%, 76%, 66%, and 73% for femoral, tibial, patellar, and total cartilage volume.[158] In a longitudinal study of sibling offspring of patients who had undergone total knee replacement for OA, heritability estimates (for change) were 73% and 40% for medial and lateral cartilage volume, 20% and 62% for medial and lateral tibial bone size, 98% for medial chondral defects, and 64% for muscle strength; adjusting for other change parameters and what was predominantly mild OA had little impact.[159]

Congenital Abnormalities

Local factors that affect the shape of the joint may increase local stress on cartilage and contribute to the development of OA, especially in the hip joint. Blatant examples of such abnormalities include congenital hip dislocation, Legg-Perthes disease, and slipped capital femoral epiphysis. However, more subtle and asymptomatic anatomic variations have also been associated with hip OA. Lane et al., examining baseline and 8-year follow-up x-rays in the SOF, found that an abnormal center-edge angle and acetabular dysplasia were each associated with increased risk of incident hip OA, adjusting for age, current weight, BMI, affected side, and investigational site (adjusted OR 3.3, 95% CI 1.1-10.1, and 2.8, 95% CI 1.0-7.9, respectively).[160] In this study population with a mean +/− SD age of 65.6 +/− 6.5 years, 9.3% developed incident radiographic hip OA. In the Rotterdam study, individuals with acetabular dysplasia (center-edge angle <25 degrees) had a 4.3-fold increased risk for incident radiographic OA of the hip (95% CI 2.2-8.7) compared with individuals without acetabular dysplasia.[161]

Meniscectomy

Cooper et al. demonstrated that meniscectomy increased the risk of knee OA, controlling for BMI, Heberden's nodes, and a family history of OA.[109] The prevalence of knee OA 21 years after open meniscectomy was 48% versus 7% in age and gender matched control.[162] A series of studies by Englund et al. have shown that: the risk of tibiofemoral OA was increased more than threefold by a history of total meniscectomy and doubled by partial meniscectomy;[163] obesity substantially increased the likelihood of OA in the those with a history of meniscectomy;[163] and the likelihood of patellofemoral OA (either isolated or, more often, with tibiofemoral OA) was greater in those who had undergone medial or lateral meniscectomy than controls matched on age, sex, and postal code who had not undergone meniscectomy.[164]

Other Factors

In a longitudinal Framingham study, smokers had a lower risk of knee OA than nonsmokers, which persisted after adjusting for age, sex, BMI, knee injury, chondrocalcinosis, hand OA, and physical activity.[73] However, smoking was not linked to incident knee OA in a longitudinal Chingford study.[165] Cross-sectional studies have had mixed results.

Analyses of NHANES I data including those aged 35 to 74 revealed that African-American women had an increased risk of knee OA versus white women (OR 2.12, 95% CI 1.39-3.23), adjusting for age, BMI, skinfold thickness, income, education, marital status, uric acid level, and smoking.[55] The risk of knee OA was not greater in African-American men than in white men. In women, knee extensor strength was 18% lower at baseline among those who developed incident knee OA than among controls, adjusting for body weight.[88] Reduced quadricep strength relative to body weight may be a risk factor for knee OA.

In a longitudinal Framingham study, greater grip strength in men was associated with increased risk of OA at the PIP joints, MCP joints, and thumb base, and in women at the MCP joints (OR 2.7 to 2.9).[166] Maximal grip is a global measure of the muscle force that can be generated during a common activity. Forces at the DIP during grip are less than those at the other hand joints. These findings support the concept that OA development relates not only to the frequency of certain tasks, but also to the magnitude of force generated during the task. In cross-sectional analyses of BLSA men, associations between increasing grade of DIP OA and lower grip strength and forearm circumference did not persist after adjusting for age.[84]

A modest association between the presence of chondrocalcinosis and knee OA, accounting for age, was present in a cross-sectional Framingham study.[167] In a longitudinal study, chondrocalcinosis was not a risk factor for incident knee OA; analyses were limited by the small number of participants with chondrocalcinosis.[73] Doherty et al. reported that, in 100 patients 25 years after unilateral meniscectomy, chondrocalcinosis was detected in 20% of operated knees versus only 4% of unoperated knees.[168] Severe radiographic changes were more common when chondrocalcinosis was present.

The prevalence of hand OA in patients with CVA and hemiparalysis was significantly lower than in elderly persons without stroke.[169] The differences between paretic and nonparetic hand radiographs were greater when only those with moderate to severe paralysis were considered, and greatest when severe paralysis of over 3 years was considered.

PROGRESSION OF OSTEOARTHRITIS

Gaps in knowledge of the natural history of human OA are due in part to difficulty dealing with heterogeneous presentations, the inability to pinpoint disease onset, slow course, intra- and intersubject variation in progression rate, and variation in how progression is assessed especially as the technology of image acquisition evolves. Efforts to consolidate the information provided by published studies are frustrated by methodologic variations, especially regarding how images were obtained, how measurements were made off the image, and how progression was defined. Efforts to develop consensus and standardized approaches have clearly improved studies to assess OA progression.[37,170-172]

Knee Osteoarthritis

Most epidemiologic studies are using both x-ray and MRI, with a gradual shift toward MR based outcomes as a primary approach.

Application of X-ray

Historically, most epidemiologic studies relied on conventional, extended knee radiography. Acquisition protocols have been developed over the past several years to enhance the quality of medial tibiofemoral joint space measurement by improving superimposition of the anterior and posterior medial tibial rims. Generally accepted protocols include two with fluoroscopic confirmation, the Buckland-Wright protocol[173] and the Lyon-Schuss protocol,[174] and two not using fluoroscopy, the MTP protocol[175] and the fixed-flexion protocol.[176] A discussion of the strengths and weaknesses of these protocols has been published.[172,177]

It is recommended that individual radiographic features as well as a global score be recorded.[37] Recommendations to treat joint space width as the primary outcome in tibiofemoral OA progression studies are supported by joint space width reflects cartilage loss; with adherence to protocol, joint space width can reliably reflect medial compartment cartilage thickness;[178] joint space narrowing was the best single variable for assessing progression;[179] and sensitivity to change was higher for joint space measurements than for K/L grade.[180] Rates of progression vary widely between studies. Different sources of subjects may explain some of this variation; progression may be faster in clinic-based samples.

Application of MRI

The advantages of MRI over plain radiography—e.g., direct three-dimensional visualization of cartilage, ability to detect focal and diffuse cartilage changes, less vulnerability to joint positioning and technique, and opportunity to visualize other tissues affected by OA—have led to a dramatic increase in its use in epidemiologic studies, especially as longitudinal MRI data have become available. Both the validity and the reliability (in persons with and without knee OA, short- and long-term) of image acquisition and processing for cartilage volume have been demonstrated in several studies, summarized in recent reviews.[181,182] MRI allows shorter duration studies with fewer participants than if x-ray is used. Longitudinal data on changes in cartilage volume suggest that 4% to 6% of cartilage volume is lost per year in knees with OA.[183-186] MRI may be able to detect change in knee OA cartilage volume as early as 6 months.[181] Cartilage volume loss was modestly associated with worsening of pain (R = 0.21) and function (R = 0.28) in one study.[187] As there have been no head-to-head comparisons of cartilage volume assessment and cartilage integrity grading,[188] it is unclear which approach is more sensitive to change and which is more closely related to person-relevant outcomes.

Much effort is being directed toward identifying imaging parameters that could ultimately serve as early indicators of disease progression and outcome measures of treatment response, i.e., even before anatomic damage. One approach, delayed gadolinium enhanced MRI of cartilage, or dGEMRIC, has been used to examine the relative distribution of glycosaminoglycan (GAG) in cartilage.[189] Longitudinal studies applying dGEMRIC are underway.

Ultimately, how progression is assessed impacts not only issues of the necessary sample size and study duration, but also potentially the profile of factors linked to progression. Current beliefs about the natural history of knee OA are based on less than optimal radiographic techniques, and may undergo some revision as we evolve in our ability to assess disease progression.

Table 1–6 shows several knee OA progression studies and the risk factors they have identified.[15,16,190–207]

Malalignment

Alignment at the knee (the hip-knee-ankle angle as measured by full-limb radiography) can either be varus (bow-legged), valgus (knock-knee), or neutral. In the MAK study mechanical factors in arthritis of the knee study (MAK), the presence of varus malalignment was associated with a fourfold increase in the risk of medial tibiofemoral OA progression (4.1, 95% CI 2.2-7.6), while valgus malalignment increased the risk of lateral tibiofemoral disease progression (4.9, 95% CI 2.1-11.2).[198,199] Varus-valgus alignment also influenced the likelihood of patellofemoral OA progression in a compartment-specific manner at 18 month follow-up.[203] Varus alignment increased the odds of patellofemoral OA progression isolated to the medial patellofemoral compartment (adjusted OR 1.85, 95% CI 1.00-3.44). Valgus alignment increased the odds of PF OA progression isolated to the lateral compartment (adjusted OR 1.64, 95% CI 1.01-2.66).

In a longitudinal MRI-based study, Cicuttini et al. found that for every 1 degree increase in baseline varus angulation, there was an average annual loss of medial femoral cartilage of 17.7 μl (95% CI 6.5-28.8), with a trend toward a similar relationship with medial tibial cartilage volume loss.[204] For every 1 degree increase in valgus angle, there was an average loss of lateral tibial cartilage volume of 8.0 μl (95% CI 0.0-16.0).

Alignment and BMI in Osteoarthritis Progression

Recent evidence suggests that alignment, in addition to its effect on load distribution, may also amplify or mediate the effect of other factors associated with knee OA progression. Load distribution between the compartments is more equitable in valgus knees (until severe valgus is reached) than in varus knees. In keeping with this, the relationship between BMI and disease severity in the MAK study had a significantly steeper slope in varus than in valgus knees.[208] Also, the BMI/medial OA severity relationship was substantially attenuated after adjusting for varus severity. That alignment modifies the BMI effect is also supported by a recent longitudinal study, in which some effect of BMI on progression was found in knees with moderate malalign-

ment (OR 1.23/2-unit increase in BMI, 95% CI 1.05-1.45) but not in knees with neutral alignment.[209] Collectively, these findings are most likely related to the malalignment-associated alteration in distribution of body weight forces between the two tibiofemoral compartments.

Nutritional Factors

As reported by McAlindon et al., in the Framingham cohort, risk for knee OA progression was greater in those with lower vitamin D intake (OR for lower compared with upper tertile 4.0, 95% CI 1.4-11.6) and in those with lower serum levels of vitamin D (OR for the lower compared with the upper tertile 2.9, 95% CI 1.0-8.2).[195] Low serum levels of vitamin D specifically predicted loss of joint space as well as osteophyte growth. A randomized clinical trial of vitamin D, including assessment of potential disease-modifying effect, is underway at Tufts University.

A threefold reduction in risk of OA progression was found for both the middle and highest tertiles of vitamin C intake, primarily related to a reduced risk of joint space loss.[196] Those with high vitamin C intake also had a reduced risk of developing knee pain (adjusted OR 0.3, 95% CI 0.1-0.8). No significant association of incident OA was found with any nutrient.

Quadriceps Strength

Several cross-sectional studies and short-term trials suggest strength is a correlate of physical function and that increasing quadriceps strength reduces pain and improves function. In women without knee OA, those who went on to develop disease were 18% weaker at baseline than those who did not develop knee OA, suggesting that quadriceps strength may protect against knee OA in women.[88] However, the two studies examining the relationship of quadriceps strength and subsequent tibiofemoral OA progression found no evidence of a protective effect.[210,211] In a study in which the strength/progression relationship was examined within knee subsets, in malaligned knees and in lax knees, greater strength at baseline was associated with a greater risk of OA.[211] This finding suggests that a generic muscle strengthening intervention may not be appropriate for all persons with knee OA and that strength programs tailored to knee subsets need to be developed.

The Role of Bone

Dieppe and others have emphasized the important role of subchondral bone in OA progression.[212] Baseline subchondral bone activity as reflected by scintigraphy was strongly related to knee OA progression: 88% of knees with severe scan abnormalities progressed, while none of the knees with normal scans at entry progressed.[192]

Bone Mineral Density. As reported by Zhang et al., over 8 years of follow-up of the Framingham cohort, risk of incident OA was lowest in the lowest 4-year BMD quartile (5.6%) and was higher in the higher 3 BMD quartiles (14.2%, 10.3%, and 11.8%).[115] Among those with OA, however, with greater BMD at baseline, risk of progressive OA decreased from 34.4% in the lowest BMD quartile to 19% in the

TABLE 1–6
STUDIES OF KNEE OSTEOARTHRITIS PROGRESSION*

Study	Duration (years)	Source of Participants	Imaging Approach	Risk Factors (at Baseline) for Progression Identified
Schouten,[190] 1992	12	Population-based	Conventional x-ray	BMI, weight, age, Heberden's nodes, generalized OA, self-report past bow-leg or knock-knee
Dougados,[191] 1992	1	Clinic	Conventional x-ray	NSAID intake, synovial effusion, weight, number of OA joints
Spector,[16] 1992	11	Clinic	Conventional x-ray	Baseline knee pain, contralateral knee OA
Dieppe,[192] 1993	5	Clinic	Conventional x-ray	Bone scintigraphic abnormality, joint swelling, crepitus, instability
Spector,[15] 1994	2	Population-based	Conventional x-ray	BMI (for contralateral emergence incident definite osteophytes)
Sharif,[193] 1995	5	Clinic	Conventional x-ray	Weight to height ratio, number of OA joints
Ledingham,[194] 1995	2	Clinic	Conventional x-ray	Multiple joint OA, synovial fluid volume, nodal OA, knee warmth, BMI, female gender, knee OA severity, CPPD
McAlindon,[195] 1996	8	Population-based	Conventional x-ray	Intake and serum level vitamin D (protective)
McAlindon,[196] 1996	8	Population-based	Conventional x-ray	Vitamin C and beta carotene (protective)
Cooper,[197] 2000	5	Population-based	Conventional x-ray	Knee pain, Heberden's nodes
Sharma,[198] 2001	1.5	Community-recruited	Fluoro-based, semiflexed x-ray	Varus-valgus alignment
Miyazaki,[199] 2002	6	Clinic	x-ray, posterior tilt of the medial tibial plateau used to determine beam angle	Knee adduction moment during gait
Cicuttini,[200] 2002	2	Community-recruited	MRI patellar cartilage volume	Female gender, BMI, pain severity
Wluka,[201] 2002	2	Community-recruited	MRI tibial cartilage volume	Cartilage volume
Felson,[202] 2003	2.5	VA clinic + community recruited	Fluoro-based, semiflexed x-ray	Bone marrow edema lesions
Cahue,[203] 2004	1.5	Community-recruited	Axial, 30° flexion (patellofemoral)	Varus-valgus alignment
Cicuttini,[204] 2004	2	Community-recruited	MRI, cartilage volume	Varus-valgus alignment
Chang,[205] 2004	1.5	Community-recruited	Fluoro-based, semiflexed x-ray	Varus thrust during gait
Berthiaume,[206] 2005	2	Clinic	MRI cartilage volume	Medial meniscal tear, medial meniscal extrusion
Chang,[207] 2005	1.5	Community-recruited	Fluoro-based, semiflexed x-ray	Internal hip abduction moment (protective)

*All participants in each of these studies had radiographic knee OA at baseline, and all studies were longitudinal.
All x-rays in each study were weight-bearing. The progression was assessed in the tibiofemoral compartment unless noted otherwise.

highest quartile. While the Rotterdam study also found a protective effect of high femoral neck BMD (at baseline) on progression of OA, this effect was lost after accounting for mobility.[116] Persons with progressive knee OA were more disabled and more often were using a walking aid. This may be the source of an apparent link between low BMD and knee OA progression.

Hurwitz et al.[213] and Wada et al.[214] demonstrated a relationship between the adduction moment and medial to lateral ratio of proximal tibial BMD. As noted by Hurwitz, while it is a long held belief that the adduction moment is the chief determinant of medial/lateral tibiofemoral load distribution, these studies represent the first evidence of its relationship to underlying bone,[213] recently Lo et al. found that medial bone marrow lesions were associated with a higher medial to lateral BMD ratio, and lateral bone lesions to a lower ratio.[215]

Bone Marrow Edema. Investigators are increasingly using the phrase "bone marrow abnormality" to describe the increased focal signal in the subchondral marrow of the knee of fat-suppressed T2-weighted MR images, rather than bone marrow edema, because of the abundance of other histopathologic findings in these lesions (fibrosis, osteonecrosis, bony remodeling[216]). Presence of these lesions was strongly associated with subsequent knee OA progression.[202] There was a greater than sixfold increase in the likelihood of medial tibiofemoral OA progression in knees with medial bone marrow abnormality (OR 6.5, 95% CI 3.0-14.0), and in the odds of lateral progression in knees with lateral bone marrow abnormality, with some attenuation after adjustment for severity of malalignment. Varus-aligned limbs had a higher prevalence of medial lesions than neutral or valgus limbs (74.3% vs. 16.4%). Similarly, the prevalence of lateral bone marrow abnormality was higher in valgus than in neutral or varus knees.

Varus Thrust and Knee Adduction Moment

A varus thrust is the dynamic worsening or abrupt onset of varus alignment while the limb is bearing weight during ambulation, with return to less varus alignment during non-weight-bearing conditions. In an 18-month study, Chang and colleagues found that the presence of a varus thrust visualized during gait was associated with a fourfold increase (95% CI 2.11-7.43) in the likelihood of medial OA progression.[205] In varus-aligned knees examined separately, a thrust was associated with a threefold increase in the likelihood of progression, suggesting that a thrust further increases the risk of progression over and above the risk conferred by static varus alignment. In theory, the impact of a varus thrust on progression of knee OA may be mediated through the associated dynamic instability of the knee and/or an acute increase in load across the medial tibiofemoral compartment, the most common site of OA disease at the knee. Having a thrust in both versus neither knee was associated with a twofold increase in the OR for poor physical function outcome (not achieving significance).[213]

The moment that adducts the knee during the stance phase of gait and assessed during quantitative gait analysis is widely believed to be a correlate of medial tibiofemoral load. Miyazaki et al. found that baseline adduction moment magnitude was strongly associated with risk of medial OA progression (OR 6.46, 95% CI 2.40-17.45), adjusting for age, gender, BMI, pain, mechanical axis, and joint space width.[199]

Meniscus Tears and Extrusion

In patients with knee osteoarthritis, MR images every 6 months for 2 years revealed that knees with severe medial meniscal tear at baseline lost on average 10% of global cartilage volume and 14% of medial compartment cartilage volume (vs. 5% and 6%, respectively, in knees without a tear).[206] Knees with medial meniscal extrusion experienced a 15.4% loss of medial cartilage volume versus 4.5% in knees with no extrusion.

Hip Abduction Moment

Recently, a greater hip internal abduction moment at baseline was identified as a factor protecting against ipsilateral medial OA progression over 18 months.[207] The odds of medial OA progression were reduced by 50% with every additional one unit of hip abduction moment. This protective effect persisted after adjustment for potential confounders (OR 0.43, 95% CI 0.22-0.81). The magnitude of hip muscle torque generated during ambulation can be measured in quantitative gait analysis. Weakness of hip abductor muscles in the stance limb may cause excessive pelvic drop in the contralateral swing limb, thereby shifting the body's center of mass toward the swing limb and increasing forces across the medial tibiofemoral compartment of the stance limb. Hip muscle strength is the major source of hip abduction moment magnitude with the hip joint ligaments and capsule also making a small contribution to the moment. These results suggest the need for future studies to examine the effect of interventions targeting hip abductor strengthening.

Hip Osteoarthritis

More information about risk factors for progression of hip OA is emerging. In the Rotterdam study, age, female sex (OR 1.8, 95% CI 1.4-2.4), presence of hip pain (OR 2.4, 95% CI 1.7-3.5), joint space width at baseline 2.5 mm or less (OR 1.9, 95% CI 1.2-2.9), and a K/L score of 2 or more at baseline (OR 5.8, 95% CI 4.0-8.4) independently predicted hip OA progression.[217] Similarly, in the SOF, progression was greater by all measures in those with both radiographic OA and hip pain at baseline (OR 1.9, 95% CI 1.4-2.6); femoral osteophytes, superolateral joint space narrowing, and subchondral bone changes independently predicted progression.[218] Of note, Seifert et al. had also observed that radiographic cysts at baseline were linked to worse 5-year outcome.[219] In another study, rapid structural progression, i.e., loss of more than 50% of hip joint space, was more common in women.[220]

In hospital patients, Ledingham et al found that hips with rapid radiographic progression more often had superior migration or an atrophic bone response; those with no progression more often had an indeterminate, medial or axial migration, protrusio or mild OA at presentation.[221] Higher rates of progression were seen in women, and were linked to older age at symptom onset and higher K/L grade at entry. BMI, symptom duration, chondrocalcinosis, hand OA/Heberden's nodes, or Forestiers disease had no effect on progression. Functional status decline was more common in those with radiographic progression.

In the SOF, over 8 years, 64.6% of hips with OA showed radiographic progression or were replaced, 12.9% of women with baseline radiographic OA underwent THR, and 22.8% had substantial worsening of lower extremity disability.[218] As reported by Danielsson et al from another study, among 121 osteoarthritic hips (identified in 4000 individuals), 7% had radiographic improvement, 28% had no change, and 65% had deterioration over 10 years.[21] In a study of hospital hip OA patients (followed for a median of 27 months), about 15% of hips progressed by one K/L grade, 47% progressed using another global scoring system, and 64% progressed in at least one radiographic feature.[221] Ten % experienced functional deterioration by Steinbrocker index.

Based on clinical observation and some data,[21] radiographic improvement is believed to be more common at the hip than at other joint sites. Perry et al. described 14 hips in which definite or probable joint space recovery occurred, possibly linked to the formation of upper and lower pole osteophytes that developed after early joint space loss.[222]

Hand Osteoarthritis

Over half of BLSA men with DIP OA had radiographic progression over 10 years.[52] Progression was most rapid in the DIP joints. The median time for 50% of the cohort to progress one K/L grade was 8.9 years for older subjects, 12.4 years for middle-aged subjects, and 15.8 years for young subjects. In a clinic-based study, progression at DIP, PIP, and CMC-1 sites was similar, with 47% to 50% progressing, 45% to 46% unchanged, and 6% to 8% improving over a 10 years, using the highest K/L grade.[223] Using the sum of grades for all sites, 96% of subjects deteriorated using K/L, 90% using osteophytes, and 74% using joint space narrowing. Age, gender, and BMI did not differ between "severe" and "minor" progressors.

RISK FACTORS FOR PAIN AND DISABILITY IN OSTEOARTHRITIS

Risk factor profiles for each of the three domains—structural disease, pain, and disability—overlap but are not identical. For example, analyses of NHANES I and NHES data demonstrated that known or suspected correlates of radiographic OA (age, gender, race, obesity, physical activity, Heberden's nodes) were not associated with knee pain.[224] Pain is complex to study longitudinally; it does not inexorably worsen and may not follow a pattern. Current knowledge of determinants of pain and disability in OA is based on a small number of longitudinal studies and several cross-sectional studies, examples of which are provided here.

Correlates of Pain

More severe radiographic disease has been associated with increased reports of knee pain in most but not all studies.

In the Framingham cohort, 8% with K/L 0 knees had pain on most days in the previous month, 11% with K/L 1, 19% with K/L 2, and 40% with K/L 3–4.[54] Though there was a relationship between pain and K/L, the proportion at K/L 3–4 without pain is noteworthy. Lethbridge-Cejku et al. found in BLSA participants that 56% of those with K/L 3–4 knee OA had current pain.[225] The presence of radiographic knee OA was associated with ever pain (OR 4.0, 95% CI 2.3–6.4) and current pain (OR 4.8), adjusting for age, sex, and BMI. Odds ratios increased with increasing radiographic severity.

Recent studies have attempted to identify specific features of OA that are responsible not only for pain presence but also for severity. Bone and synovium[226] are emerging as potential sources of pain. In BOKS, bone marrow lesions were more common in OA knees with symptoms (defined as pain, aching, or stiffness on most days) than in knees without symptoms.[227] Also, knees in which bone marrow lesions were present had higher pain scores on average than knees without such lesions, though the difference was not significant.

Sowers et al. found that bone marrow lesions 1 cm or larger in size were more frequent in OA knees with pain than in OA knees without pain.[228] In their study, a primary difference between painful and painless OA knees was whether or not bone was intact under full-thickness cartilage defects. They termed this feature bone ulceration, defined as any defect of the subchondral cortex beneath a cartilage defect. Most full-thickness cartilage defects in persons with painful OA were accompanied by bone ulceration. They questioned whether a bone marrow lesion has to be accompanied by other changes in bone to cause pain.

Among subjects with knee and/or hip OA, an association has been reported between joint pain and psychological factors, including poor psychological well being,[224] "feeling in low spirits,"[229] depression, anxiety or coping style,[230-232] and hypochondriasis.[233] Quadriceps weakness and pain have been associated[232,234] although the studies of Slemenda et al.[235] provide evidence that the relationship between pain and weakness may not be as strong prior to OA or in prodromal stages as in more advanced stages.

Function Limitation

Most studies of OA have emphasized physical function limitation, assessed by self-report and/or specific task performance, and have less often examined disability, i.e., performance within a typical physical, social, and cultural context. Like pain, physical function is predicted by radiographic disease severity in some studies and not others. More recent studies have dealt with specific pathoanatomic/pathophysiologic aspects of disease (i.e., beyond radiographic aspects) and how they contribute to impaired function.

In the longitudinal organization to assess strategies for ischemic syndromes (OASIS) and MAK studies, self-efficacy predicted both self-reported and performance outcomes, after adjusting for pain, strength, and other potential confounders or mediators.[237,238] In both studies, greater baseline knee pain intensity predicted function decline. In OASIS, the relationship between pain intensity and function decline was reduced after accounting for self-efficacy and the self-efficacy-strength interaction.[236] In the MAK study, the strength/function outcome relationship was lost after adjustment for self-efficacy.[238] Together, these results suggest a close relationship between strength, knee pain intensity, and self-efficacy in their effect on physical function in knee OA. Pain may acutely reduce the maximal voluntary contraction and lead to chronic activity revision or avoidance. A downward spiral of pain, weakness, and reduced self-efficacy may lead to substantial reduction in activity.

Other factors linked to physical function in knee OA from longitudinal analyses of the MAK study were age, medial-lateral laxity, varus-valgus alignment, social support, and SF36 mental health score.[238] A relationship between depressive symptoms and physical function has also been described in longitudinal studies not limited to individuals with arthritis, as summarized by Ormel et al.[239]

The association between baseline radiographic knee OA and physical functioning 10 years later was evaluated in NHANES I participants.[240] For women with knee OA, difficulty was most often identified with heavy chores, and, for men, walking 1/4 mile. In women, moderate to severe arthritis was associated with worse scores than seen with mild disease for 14 activities. The added presence of knee OA substantially increased the likelihood of disability in those with heart disease, pulmonary disease, hypertension, or obesity.[241] In the Framingham study, persons with infrequent symptoms but severe radiographic disease were more likely to have lower extremity functional limitations than those with symptoms and less severe disease.[241] Radiographic knee OA increased the odds of dependence in stair climbing, walking one mile, light housekeeping, and carrying bundles.[4] Radiographic OA of the hand, wrist, foot, or ankle was associated with disability in women.[243] In another study, radiographic hand/wrist OA was linked to health assessment questionnare (HAQ) score.[244]

Pain is a key correlate of physical functioning in OA.[58, 240–242,245–247] Ettinger et al. found that of men with symptomatic knee OA, 50% reported difficulty with ambulation and 43.8% with transfer; only 19% of men with OA and without symptoms reported difficulty with each activity.[241] In women with symptomatic OA, 70.5% reported difficulty with ambulation and 67.2% with transfer versus 24.8% and 27.5%, respectively, of those without pain. The odds of functional impairment among those with radiographic knee OA were increased by the presence of symptoms, adjusting for age, race, and education.

A number of studies demonstrate a link between impaired physical function and psychological factors including pain coping,[247] psychological well-being,[247] depression, and anxiety.[230–232,249] Bivariate correlations between self-efficacy and task performance were similar in magnitude to those seen for aerobic capacity and for strength. Several studies have linked quadriceps strength and function in knee OA.[234,245–247,250]

CONCLUSION

As the most common arthritis and a leading cause of chronic disability, osteoarthritis (OA) is associated with substantial cost to the individual and to society. Epidemiologic studies have supplied, in addition to incidence, prevalence, and risk factor data, much of what is known about the natural history of OA. Especially given the anticipated increase in OA prevalence, the need to identify risk factors for incident OA, OA progression, OA associated physical function decline, and disability is a high priority. In recent years, emphasis has shifted toward the identification of risk factors for OA progression. Several risk factors for progression are emerging, many of which originate or relate to the local joint organ environment. This shift in focus relates in part to the concept that risk factors for progression might ultimately be targeted to delay OA progression or to enhance the effect of a potentially disease-modifying drug. As additional studies are completed and more is learned about these and other factors, opportunities will very likely arise for intervention and prevention strategy development.

REFERENCES

1. Meulenbelt I, Bijkerk C, de Wildt SCM, et al. Investigation of the association of the CRTM and CRTL-1 genes with radiographically evident osteoarthritis in subjects from the Rotterdam study. Arthritis Rheum 40:1760–1765, 1997.
2. Global Economic and Health Care Burden of Musculoskeletal Disease. 2001, World Health Organization. *www.boneandjoint-decade.org.*
3. Lawrence RC, Helmick CG, Arnett FC, et al. Estimates of the prevalence of arthritis and selected musculoskeletal disorders in the United States. Arthritis Rheum 41:778–799, 1998.
4. Guccione AA, Felson DT, Anderson JJ, et al. The effects of specific medical conditions on the functional limitations of elders in the Framingham Study. Am J Public Health 84:351–357, 1994.
5. Kuettner KE, Goldberg VM. Introduction. In: Kuettner KE, Goldberg VM, editors. Osteoarthritic disorders. Rosemont: American Academy of Orthopaedic Surgeons; 1995, pp xxi–xxv.
6. Altman R, Asch E, Bloch D, et al. Development of criteria for the classification and reporting of osteoarthritis. Classification of osteoarthritis of the knee. Arthritis Rheum 29:1039–1049, 1986.
7. Altman R, Alarcon G, Appelrouth D, et al. Criteria for classification and reporting of osteoarthritis of the hip. Arthritis Rheum 1991;34:505–514, 1991.
8. Altman R, Alarcon G, Appelrouth D, et al. Criteria for classification and reporting of osteoarthritis of the hand. Arthritis Rheum 33:1601–1610, 1990.
9. Nevitt MC. Definition of hip osteoarthritis for epidemiological studies. Ann Rheum Dis 55:652–655, 1996.
10. Croft P, Cooper C, Coggon D. Case definition of hip osteoarthritis in epidemiologic studies. J Rheumatol 21:591–592, 1994.
11. Cicuttini FM, Spector TD. The epidemiology of osteoarthritis of the hand. Rev. Rhum. [Engl. Ed.] 62 (suppl):3S–8S, 1995.
12. Davis MA, Ettinger WH, Neuhaus JM, et al. The association of knee injury and obesity with unilateral and bilateral osteoarthritis of the knee. Am J Epidemiol 130:278–288, 1989.
13. Felson DT, Zhang Y, Hannan MT, et al. The incidence and natural history of knee osteoarthritis in the elderly: the Framingham osteoarthritis study. Arthritis Rheum 38:1500–1505, 1995.
14. Cooper C, Egger P, Coggon D, et al. Generalized osteoarthritis in women: pattern of joint involvement and approaches to definition for epidemiological studies. J Rheumatol 23:1938–1942, 1996.

15. Spector TD, Hart DJ, Doyle DV. Incidence and progression of osteoarthritis in women with unilateral knee disease in the general population: the effect of obesity. Ann Rheum Dis 53:565–568, 1994.

16. Spector TD, Dacre JE, Harris RA, et al. Radiological progression of osteoarthritis: an 11 year follow up study of the knee. Ann Rheum Dis 51:1107–1110, 1992.

17. McAlindon T, Zhang Y, Hannan M, et al. Are risk factors for patellofemoral and tibiofemoral knee osteoarthritis different? J Rheumatol 23:332–337, 1996.

18. McAlindon TE, Snow S, Cooper C, et al. Radiographic patterns of osteoarthritis of the knee joint in the community: the importance of the patellofemoral joint. Ann Rheum Dis 51:844–849, 1992.

19. Van Saase JL, Van Romunde LK, Cats A, et al. Epidemiology of osteoarthritis: Zoetermeer survey. Comparison of radiographical osteoarthritis in a Dutch population with that in 10 other populations. Ann Rheum Dis 48:271–280, 1989.

20. Neame R, Zhang W, Deighton C, et al. Distribution of Radiographic osteoarthritis between the right and left hands, hips, and knees. Arthritis Rheum 50:1487–1490, 2004.

21. Danielsson L, Lindberg H, Nilsson B. Prevalence of coxarthrosis. Clin Orthop 191:110–115, 1984.

22. Ledingham J, Dawson S, Preston B. Radiographic patterns and associations of osteoarthritis of the hip. Ann Rheum Dis 51:1111–1116, 1992.

23. Jorring K. Osteoarthritis of the hip, epidemiology and clinical role. Acta Orthop Scand 51:523–530, 1980.

24. Chaisson CE, Zhang Y, McAlindon TE, et al. Radiographic hand osteoarthritis: incidence, patterns, and influence of pre-existing disease in a population based sample. J Rheumatol 24:1337–1343, 1997.

25. Egger P, Cooper C, Hart DJ, et al. Patterns of joint involvement in osteoarthritis of the hand: the Chingford study. J Rheumatol 22:1509–1513, 1995.

26. Lane NE, Bloch DA, Jones HH, et al. Osteoarthritis of the hand: a comparison of handedness and hand use. J Rheumatol 16:637–642, 1989.

27. Poole J, Sayer A, Hardy R, et al. Patterns of interphalangeal hand joint involvement of osteoarthritis among men and women: a British cohort study. Arthritis Rheum 48:3371–3376, 2003.

28. Hirsch R, Lethbridge-Cejku M, Scott WW, et al. Association of hand and knee osteoarthritis: evidence for a polyarticular disease subset. Ann Rheum Dis 55:25–29, 1996.

29. Croft P, Cooper C, Wickham C, et al. Is the hip involved in generalized osteoarthritis? Br J Rheumatol 31:325–328, 1992.

30. Hochberg MC, Lane NE, Pressman AR, et al. The association of radiographic changes of osteoarthritis of the hand and hip in elderly women. J Rheumatol 22:2291–2294, 1995.

31. Cushnaghan J, Dieppe P. Study of 500 patients with limb joint osteoarthritis. I. Analysis by age, sex, and distribution of symptomatic joint sites. Ann Rheum Dis 50:8–13, 1991.

32. Doherty M, Watt I, Dieppe P. Influence of primary generalised osteoarthritis on development of secondary osteoarthritis. Lancet ii:8–11, 1983.

33. Englund M, Paradowski PT, Lohmander LS. Association of radiographic hand osteoarthritis with radiographic knee osteoarthritis after meniscectomy. Arthritis Rheum 50:469–475, 2004.

34. Kellgren JH, Lawrence JS. Atlas of standard radiographs, Department.

35. Buckland-Wright JC, Macfarlane DG. Radioanatomic assessment of therapeutic outcome in osteoarthritis. In: Kuettner KE, Goldberg VM, editors. Osteoarthritic disorders. Rosemont: American Academy of Orthopaedic Surgeons, 1995, pp 51–65.

36. Spector TD, Hart DJ, Byrne J, et al. Definition of osteoarthritis of the knee for epidemiological studies. Ann Rheum Dis 52:790–794, 1993.

37. Dieppe P, Altman RD, Buckwalter JA, et al. Standardization of methods used to assess the progression of osteoarthritis of the hip or knee joints. In: Kuettner KE, Goldberg VM, editors. Osteoarthritic disorders. Rosemont: American Academy of Orthopaedic Surgeons, 1995, pp 481–496.

38. Boegard T, Rudling O, Petersson IF, et al. Correlation between radiographically diagnosed osteophytes and magnetic resonance detected cartilage defects in the tibiofemoral joint. Ann Rheum Dis 57:401–407, 1998.

39. Boegard T, Rudling O, Petersson IF, et al. Correlation between radiographically diagnosed osteophytes and magnetic resonance detected cartilage defects in the patellofemoral femoral joint. Ann Rheum Dis 57:395–400, 1998.

40. Croft P, Cooper C, Wickham C, et al. Defining osteoarthritis of the hip for epidemiologic studies. Am J Epidemiol 132:514–522, 1990.

41. Jacobsen S, Sonne-Holm S, Soballe K, et al. Factors influencing hip joint space in asymptomatic subjects. A survey of 4151 subjects of the Copenhagen City Heart Study: The Osteoarthritis Substudy. Osteoarthritis and Cartilage 12:698–703, 2004.

42. Hirsch R, Fernandes RJ, Pillemer SR, et al. Hip osteoarthritis prevalence estimates by three radiographic scoring systems. Arthritis Rheum 41:361–368, 1998.

43. Kallman DA, Wigley FM, Scott WW, et al. New radiographic grading scales for osteoarthritis of the hand: reliability for determining prevalence and progression. Arthritis Rheum 32:1584–1591, 1989.

44. Jacobsson LTH. Definitions of osteoarthritis in the knee and hand. Ann Rheum Dis 55: 656–658, 1996.

45. Cicuttini FM, Baker J, Hart DJ, et al. Relation between Heberden's nodes and distal interphalangeal joint osteophytes and their role as markers of generalised disease. Ann Rheum Dis 57:246–248, 1998.

46. Schouten JSAG. A 12-year follow-up study on osteoarthritis of the knee in the general population. An epidemiological study of classification criteria, risk factors and prognostic factors. Dissertation, Erasmus University Medical School, Rotterdam, 1991.

47. Bagge E, Bjelle A, Svandorg A. Radiographic osteoarthritis in the elderly. A cohort comparison and a longitudinal study of the 70-year old people in Goteborg. Clin Rheumatol 11:486–491, 1992.

48. Oliveria SA, Felson DT, Reed JI, et al. Incidence of symptomatic hand, hip, and knee osteoarthritis among patients in a health maintenance organization. Arthritis Rheum 38:1134–1141, 1995.

49. Wilson MG, Michet CJ, Ilstrup DM, et al. Idiopathic symptomatic osteoarthritis of the hip and knee: a population-based incidence study. Mayo Clin Proc 65:1214–1221, 1990.

50. Nevitt MC, Arden NK, Lane NE, et al. Incidence of radiographic changes of hip OA in elderly white women. Arthritis Rheum 41:S181, 1998.

51. Carman WJ, Sowers M, Hawthorne VM, et al. Obesity as a risk factor for osteoarthritis of the hand and wrist: a prospective study. Am J Epidemiol 139:119–129, 1994.

52. Kallman DA, Wigley FM, Scott WW, et al. The longitudinal course of hand osteoarthritis in a male population. Arthritis Rheum 33:1323–1331, 1990.

53. Lawrence JS, Bremner JM, Bier F. Osteo-arthrosis, prevalence in the population and relationship between symptoms and x-ray changes. Ann Rheum Dis 25:1–23, 1966.

54. Felson DT, Naimark A, Anderson J, et al. The prevalence of knee osteoarthritis in the elderly. Arthritis Rheum 30:914–918, 1987.

55. Anderson JJ, Felson DT. Factors associated with osteoarthritis of the knee in the first National Health and Nutrition Examination Survey (HANES I), evidence for an association with overweight, race, and physical demands of work. Am J Epidemiol 128: 179–189, 1988.

56. Hart DJ, Mootoosamy I, Doyle DV, et al. The relationship between osteoarthritis and osteoporosis in the general population: the Chingford Study. Ann Rheum Dis 53:158–162, 1994.

57. Sowers M, Hochberg M, Crabbe JP, et al. Association of bone mineral density and sex hormone levels with osteoarthritis of the hand and knee in premenopausal women. Am J Epidemiol 143:38–47, 1996.

58. Odding E, Valkenburg HA, Algra D, et al. Associations of radiological osteoarthritis of the hip and knee with locomotor disability in the Rotterdam study. Ann Rheum Dis 57:203–208, 1998.

59. Zhang Y, Xu L, Nevitt MC, et al. Comparison of the prevalence of knee osteoarthritis between elderly Chinese population in Beijing

and whites in the United States: The Beijing Osteoarthritis Study. Arthritis Rheum 44:2065–2071, 2001.

60. Maurer K. Basic data on arthritis: knee, hip, and sacroiliac joints, in adults aged 25–74 years: United States, 1971–1975. National Center for Health Statistics. Vital and Health Statistics Series 11-Number 213, 1979.

61. Tepper S, Hochberg MC. Factors associated with hip osteoarthritis: data from the First National Health and Nutrition Examination Survey (NHANES-I). Am J Epidemiol 137:1081–1088, 1993.

62. Hoaglund FT, Yau ACMC, Wong WL. Osteoarthritis of the hip and other joints in southern Chinese in Hong Kong. J Bone Joint Surg 55-A:545–557, 1973.

63. Lau EMC, Lin F, Lam D, et al. Hip osteoarthritis and dysplasia in Chinese men. Ann Rheum Dis 54:965–969, 1995.

64. Nevitt MC, Xu L, Zhang Y, et al. Very low prevalence of hip osteoarthritis among Chinese elderly in Beijing China, compared with whites in the United States: The Beijing Osteoarthritis Study. Arthritis Rheum 46:1773–1779, 2002.

65. Lawrence JS, Molyneux M. Degenerative joint disease among populations in Wensleydale, England and Jamaica. Int J Biometeorol 12:163–175, 1968.

66. Mukhopadhaya B, Barooah B. Osteoarthritis of the hip in Indians: an anatomical and clinical study. Ind J Orthop 1:55–63, 1967.

67. Ali-Gombe A, Croft PR, Silman AJ. Osteoarthritis of the hip and acetabular dysplasia in Nigerian men. J Rheumatol 23:512–515, 1996.

68. Plato CC, Norris AH. Osteoarthritis of the hand: age specific joint-digit prevalence rates. Am J Epidemiol 109:169–180, 1979.

69. Engle A. Osteoarthritis in adults by selected demographic characteristics, United States—1960–1962. Vital Health Stat 11:20, 1966.

70. Felson DT, Nevitt MC. Epidemiologic studies for osteoarthritis: new versus conventional study design approaches. Rheum Dis Clin North Am 30:783–797, 2004.

71. Felson DT, Anderson JJ, Naimark A, et al. Obesity and knee osteoarthritis, the Framingham study. Ann Intern Med 109:18–24, 1988.

72. Felson DT, Zhang Y, Anthony JM, et al. Weight loss reduces the risk for symptomatic knee osteoarthritis in women: the Framingham study. Ann Intern Med 116:535–539, 1992.

73. Felson DT, Zhang Y, Hannan MT, et al. Risk factors for incident radiographic knee osteoarthritis in the elderly. Arthritis Rheum 40:728–733, 1997.

74. Hart DJ, Doyle DV, Spector TD. Incidence and risk factors for radiographic knee osteoarthritis in middle-aged women, the Chingford Study. Arthritis Rheum 42:17–24, 1999.

75. Hart DJ, Doyle DV, Spector TD. Association between metabolic factors and knee osteoarthritis in women: the Chingford Study. J Rheumatol 22:1118–112, 1995.

76. Davis MA, Neuhaus JM, Ettinger WH, et al. Body fat distribution and osteoarthritis. Am J Epidemiol 132:701–707, 1990.

77. Davis MA, Ettinger WH, Neuhaus JM. The role of metabolic factors and blood pressure in the association of obesity with osteoarthritis of the knee. J Rheumatol 15:1827–1832, 1988.

78. Hochberg MC, Lethbridge-Cejku M, Scott WW, et al. The association of body weight, body fatness and body fat distribution with osteoarthritis of the knee: data from the Baltimore Longitudinal Study of Aging. J Rheumatol 22:488–493, 1995.

79. Bagge E, Bjelle A, Eden S, et al. Factors associated with radiographic osteoarthritis: results from the population study 70-year-old people in Goteborg. J Rheumatol 18:1218–1222, 1991.

80. Cicuttini FM, Spector T, Baker J. Risk factors for osteoarthritis in the tibiofemoral and patellofemoral joints of the knee. J Rheumatol 24:1164–1167, 1997.

81. Van Saase JLCM, Vandenbroucke JP, van Romunde LKJ, et al. Osteoarthritis and obesity in the general population. A relationship calling for an explanation. J Rheumatol 15:1152–1158, 1988.

82. Croft P, Coggon D, Cruddas M, et al. Osteoarthritis of the hip: an occupational disease in farmers. BMJ 304:1269–1272, 1992.

83. Reijman M, Belo JN, Lievense AM, et al. Is BMI associated with the onset and progression of osteoarthritis of the knee and hip?

The Rotterdam Study. Osteoarthritis Cartilage 13 (supplement A):S28, 2005.

84. Hochberg MC, Lethbridge-Cejku M, Plato CC, et al. Factors associated with osteoarthritis of the hand in males: data from the Baltimore Longitudinal Study of Aging. Am J Epidemiol 134:1121–1127, 1991.

85. Hochberg MC, Lethbridge-Cejku M, Scott WW, et al. Obesity and osteoarthritis of the hands in women. Osteoarthritis Cartilage 1:129–135, 1993.

86. Hart DJ, Spector TD. The relationship of obesity, fat distribution and osteoarthritis in women in the general population: the Chingford Study. J Rheumatol 20:331–335, 1993.

87. Sharma L, Lou C, Felson DT, et al. Laxity in healthy and osteoarthritic knees. Arthritis Rheum, in press.

88. Slemenda C, Heilman DK, Brandt KD, et al. Reduced quadriceps strength relative to body weight: a risk factor for knee osteoarthritis in women? Arthritis Rheum 41:1951–1959, 1998.

89. Ding C, Cicuttini F, Scott F, et al. Sex differences in knee cartilage volume in adults: role of body and bone size, age and physical activity. Rheumatology 42:1317–1323, 2003.

90. Faber SC, Eckstein F, Lukasz S, et al. Sex differences in knee joint cartilage thickness, volume, and articular surface areas: assessment with quantitative three-dimensional MR imaging. Skeletal Radiol 30:144–150, 2001.

91. Cauley JA, Kwoh CK, Egeland G, et al. Serum sex hormones and severity of osteoarthritis of the hand. J Rheumatol 20:1170–1175, 1993.

92. Felson DT, Hannan MT, Naimark A, et al. Occupational physical demands, knee bending, and knee osteoarthritis: results from the Framingham study. J Rheumatol 18:1587–1592, 1991.

93. Kivimaki J, Riihimaki H, Hanninen K. Knee disorders in carpet and floor layers and painters. Scand J Work Environ Health 18:310–316, 1992.

94. Cooper C, McAlindon T, Coggon D, et al. Occupational activity and osteoarthritis of the knee. Ann Rheum Dis 53:90–93, 1994.

95. Kellgren JH, Lawrence JS. Rheumatism in miners: part II. X-ray study. Br J Indust Med 9:197–207, 1952.

96. Partridge REH, Duthie JJR. Rheumatism in dockers and civil servants: a comparison of heavy manual and sedentary workers. Ann Rheum Dis 27:559–569, 1968.

97. Maetzel A, Makela M, Hawker G, et al. Osteoarthritis of the hip and knee and mechanical occupational exposure—a systematic overview of the evidence. J Rheumatol 24:1599–1607, 1997.

98. Croft P, Cooper C, Wickham C, et al. Osteoarthritis of the hip and occupational activity. Scand J Work Environ Health. 18:59–63, 1992.

99. Grubber JM, Callahan LF, Helmick CG, et al. Prevalence of radiographic hip and knee osteoarthritis by place of residence. J Rheumatol 25:959–963, 1998.

100. Roach KR, Persky V, Miles T, et al. Biomechanical aspects of occupation and osteoarthritis of the hip: a case-control study. J Rheumatol 21:2334–2340, 1994.

101. Lawrence JS. Rheumatism in cotton operatives. Br J Ind Med 18:270–276, 1961.

102. Hadler NM, Gillings DB, Imbus HR, et al. Hand structure and function in an industrial setting. Arthritis Rheum 21:210–220, 1978.

103. Soloviewa S, Vehmas T, Rlinimaki H, et al. Measurement of structural progression in osteoarthritis of the hip: The Barcelona Consensus Group. Osteoarthritis Cartilage 12:515–524, 2004.

104. Kujala UM, Kettunen J, Paananen H, et al. Knee osteoarthritis in former runners, soccer players, weight lifters and shooters. Arthritis Rheum 38:539–546, 1995.

105. Spector TD, Harris PA, Hart DJ, et al. Risk of osteoarthritis associated with long-term weight-bearing sports. Arthritis Rheum 39:988–995, 1996.

106. Lane NE, Michel B, Bjorkengren A, et al. The risk of osteoarthritis with running and aging: a 5-year longitudinal study. J Rheumatol 20:461–468, 1993.

107. Panush RS, Schmidt C, Caldwell JR, et al. Is running associated with degenerative joint disease? JAMA. 255:1152–1154, 1986.

108. Hannan MT, Felson DT, Anderson JJ, et al. Habitual physical activity is not associated with knee osteoarthritis: the Framingham Study. J Rheumatol 20:704–709, 1993.

109. Cooper C, McAlindon T, Snow S, et al. Mechanical and constitutional risk factors for symptomatic knee osteoarthritis: differences between medial tibiofemoral and patellofemoral disease. J Rheumatol 21:307–313, 1994.

110. Buckwalter JA, Lane NE. Athletics and osteoarthritis. Am J Sports Med 25:873–881, 1997.

111. McAlindon TE, Wilson PW, Aliabadi P, et al. Level of physical activity and risk of radiographic and symptomatic knee osteoarthritis in the elderly: the Framingham Study. Am J Med 106:151–157, 1999.

112. Vingard E, Alfredsson L, Goldie I, et al. Sports and osteoarthosis of the hip, an epidemiologic study. Am J Sports Med 21:195–200, 1993.

113. Puranen J, Ala-Ketola L, Peltokallio P, et al. Running and primary osteoarthritis of the hip. Br Med J 285:424–425, 1975.

114. Marti B, Knobloch M, Tschopp A, et al. Is excessive running predictive of degenerative hip disease? Br Med J 299:91–93, 1989.

115. Zhang Y, Hannan MT, Chaisson CE, et al. Bone mineral density and risk of incident and progressive radiographic knee osteoarthritis in women: the Framingham Study. J Rheumatol 27:1032–1039, 2000.

116. Berginsk AP, Uitterlinden AG, Van Leeuwen JP, et al. Bone mineral density and vertebral fracture history are associated with incident and progressive radiographic knee osteoarthritis in elderly men and women: the Rotterdam Study. Bone 37:446–456, 2005.

117. Hart D, Cronin C, Daniels M, et al. The relationship of bone density and fracture to incident and progressive radiographic osteoarthritis of the knee. Arthritis Rheum 46:92–99, 2002.

118. Burger H, van Daele PLA, Odding E, et al. Association of radiographically evident osteoarthritis with higher bone mineral density and increased bone loss with age. Arthritis Rheum 39:81–86, 1996.

119. Hannan MT, Anderson JJ, Zhang Y, et al. Bone mineral density and knee osteoarthritis in elderly men and women, the Framingham Study. Arthritis Rheum 36:1671–1680, 1993.

120. Lethbridge-Cejku M, Tobin JD, Scott WW, et al. Axial and hip bone mineral density and radiographic changes of osteoarthritis of the knee: data from the Baltimore Longitudinal Study of Aging. J Rheumatol 23:1943–1947, 1996.

121. Hochberg MC, Lethbridge-Cejku M, Scott WW, et al. Upper extremity bone mass and osteoarthritis of the knees: data from the Baltimore Longitudinal Study of Aging. J Bone Miner Res 10:432–438, 1995.

122. Lane NE, Nevitt MC. Osteoarthritis, bone mass, and fractures: how are they related? Arthritis Rheum 46:1–4, 2002.

123. Nevitt MC, Lane NE, Scott JC, et al. Radiographic osteoarthritis of the hip and bone mineral density. Arthritis Rheum 38:907–916, 1995.

124. Sowers M, Zobel D, Weissfeld L, et al. Progression of osteoarthritis of the hand and metacarpal bone loss. Arthritis Rheum 34:36–42, 1991.

125. Hochberg MC, Lethbridge-Cejku M, Scott WW, et al. Appendicular bone mass and osteoarthritis of the hands in women: data from the Baltimore Longitudinal Study of Aging. J Rheumatol 21:1532–1536, 1994.

126. Felson DT, Zhang Y. An update on the epidemiology of knee and hip osteoarthritis with a view to prevention. Arthritis Rheum 41:1343–1355, 1998.

127. Zhang, Y, McAlindon TE, Hannan MT, et al. Estrogen replacement therapy and worsening of radiographic knee osteoarthritis, the Framingham Study. Arthritis Rheum 41:1867–1873, 1998.

128. Samanta A, Jones A, Regan M, et al. Is osteoarthritis in women affected by hormonal changes or smoking? Br J Rheumatol 32:366–370, 1993.

129. Wluka AE, Davis SR, Bailey M, et al. Users of oestrogen replacement therapy have more knee cartilage than non-users. Ann Rheum Dis 60:332–336, 2001.

130. Nevitt MC, Cummings SR, Lane NE, et al. Association of estrogen replacement therapy with the risk of osteoarthritis of the hip in elderly white women. Arch Intern Med 156:2073–2080, 1996.

131. Spector TD, Nandra D, Hart DJ, et al. Is hormone replacement therapy protective for hand and knee osteoarthritis in women?: the Chingford study. Ann Rheum Dis 56:432–434, 1997.

132. Gelber AC, Hochberg MC, Mead LA, et al. Joint injury in young adults and risk for subsequent knee and hip osteoarthritis. Ann Int Med. 133:321–328, 2000.

133. Stecher RM. Heberden's nodes. Heredity in hypertrophic arthritis of the finger joints. Am J Med Sci 201:801, 1941.

134. Kellgren JH, Lawrence JS, Bier F. Genetic factors in generalised osteoarthritis. Ann Rheum Dis 22:237–255, 1963.

135. Loughlin J. Polymorphism in signal transduction is a major route through which osteoarthritis susceptibility is acting. Curr Opin Rheumatol 17:629–633, 2005.

136. Loughlin J. The genetic epidemiology of human primary OA: current status. Expert Rev Mol Med 7:1–12, 2005.

137. Zhang W, Doherty M. How important are genetic factors in osteoarthritis? Contributions from family studies. J Rheumatol 32:1139–1142, 2005.

138. Spector TD, Cicuttini F, Baker J, et al. Genetic influences on osteoarthritis in women: a twin study. BMJ 312:940–943, 1996.

139. Felson DT, Couropmitree NN, Chaisson CE, et al. Evidence for a mendelian gene in a segregation analysis of generalized radiographic osteoarthritis. Arthritis Rheum 41:1064–1071, 1998.

140. Hirsch R, Lethbridge-Cejku M, Hanson R, et al. Familial aggregation of osteoarthritis, data from the Baltimore Longitudinal Study on Aging. Arthritis Rheum 41:1227–1232, 1998.

141. Pattrick M, Manhire A, Ward AM, et al. HLA-A, B antigens and alpha1-antitrypsin phenotypes in nodal generalised osteoarthritis and erosive osteoarthritis. Ann Rheum Dis 48:470–475, 1989.

142. Ushiyama T, Ueyama H, Inoue K, et al. Estrogen receptor gene polymorphism and generalized osteoarthritis. J Rheumatol 25:134–137, 1998.

143. Meulenbelt I, Bijkerk C, Miedema HS, et al. A genetic association study of the Igf-1 gene and radiological osteoarthritis in a population-based cohort study (the Rotterdam study). Ann Rheum Dis 57:371–374, 1998.

144. Wright GD, Hughes AE, Regan M, et al. Association of two loci on chromosome 2q with nodal osteoarthritis. Ann Rheum Dis 55:317–331, 1996.

145. Meulenbelt I, Seymour AB, Nieuwland M, et al. Association of interleukin-1 gene cluster with radiographic signs of osteoarthritis of the hip. Arthritis Rheum 50:1179–1186, 2004.

146. Keen RW, Hart DJ, Lanchbury JS, et al. Association of early osteoarthritis of the knee with a Taq I polymorphism of the vitamin D receptor gene. Arthritis Rheum 40:1444–1449, 1997.

147. Uitterlinden AG, Burger H, Huang Q, et al. Vitamin D receptor genotype is associated with radiographic osteoarthritis at the knee. J Clin Invest 100:259–263, 1997.

148. Baldwin CT, Cupples LA, Joost O, et al. Absence of linkage or associations for osteoarthritis with vitamin D receptor/type II collagen: The Framingham Osteoarthritis Study. J Rheum 29:161–165, 2002.

149. Loughlin J, Irven C, Ferfusson C, et al. Sibling pair analysis shows no linkage of generalized osteoarthritis to the loci encoding type II collagen, cartilage link protein or cartilage matrix protein. Br J Rheumatol 33:1103–1106, 1994.

150. Aerssens J, Dequeker J, Peeters J, et al. Lack of association between osteoarthritis of the hip and gene polymorphisms of VDR, col1a1, and col2a1 in postmenopausal women. Arthritis Rheum 41:1946–1950, 1998.

151. Demissie S, Cupples LA, Myers R, et al. Genome scan for Quantity of hand osteoarthritis: The Framingham Study. Arthritis Rheum 46:946–952, 2002.

152. Gillaspy E, Sprekley K, Wallis G, et al. Investigation of linkage on chromosome 2 q and hand and knee osteoarthritis. Arthritis Rheum 46:3386–3387, 2002.

153. Hunter DJ, Denussue S, Cupples LA, et al. A genome scan for joint specific hand osteoarthritis susceptibility: The Framingham Study. Arthritis Rheum 50:2489–2496, 2004.

154. Loughlin J, Dowling B, Chapman K, et al. Functional variants within the secreted frizzled-related protein 3 gene are associated with hip osteoarthritis in females. Proc Natl Acad Sci USA 101:9757–9762, 2004.

155. Min JL, Meulenbelt I, Riyazi N, et al. Association of the frizzled-related protein gene with symptomatic osteoarthritis at multiple sites. Arthritis Rheum 52:1077–1080, 2005.

156. Kizawa H, Kou I, Iida A, et al. An aspartic acid repeat polymorphism in asporin inhibits chondrogenesis and increases susceptibility to osteoarthritis. Nat Genet 37:138–144, 2005.

157. Mustafa Z, Dowling B, Chapman K, et al. Investigating the aspartic acid (D) repeat of asporin as a risk factor for osteoarthritis in a U.K. Caucasian population. Arthritis Rheum 52:3502–3506, 2005.

158. Hunter DJ, Snieder H, March L, et al. Genetic contribution to cartilage volume in women, a classical twin study. Rheumatology 42:1495–1500, 2003.

159. Zhai G, Ding C, Stankovich J, et al. The genetic contribution to longitudinal changes in knee structure and muscle strength: a sibpair study. Arthritis Rheum 52:2830–2834, 2005.

160. Lane NE, Lin P, Christiansen L, et al. Association of mild acetabular dysplasia an increased risk of incident hip OA in eldely white women: the Study of Osteoperotic Fractures. Arthritis Rheum 43:400–404, 2000.

161. Reijman M, Hazes JM, Pols HA, et al. Acetabular dysplasia predicts incident osteoarthritis of the hip: the Rotterdam study. Arthritis Rheum 52:787–793, 2005.

162. Roos H, Lauren M, Adalberth T, et al. Knee osteoarthritis after meniscectomy. Arthritis Rheum 41:687–693, 1998.

163. Englund M, Lohmander LS. Risk factors for symptomatic knee osteoarthritis fifteen to twenty-two years after meniscectomy. Arthritis Rheum 50:2811–2819, 2004.

164. Englund M, Lohmander L. Patellofemoral osteoarthritis coexistent with tibiofemoral osteoarthritis in a meniscectomy population. Ann Rheum Dis 64:1721–1726, 2005.

165. Hart DJ, Spector TD. Cigarette smoking and risk of osteoarthritis in women in the general population: the Chingford Study. Ann Rheum Dis 52:93–96, 1993.

166. Chaisson CE, Zhang Y, Sharma L, et al. Grip strength and the risk of developing radiographic hand osteoarthritis, results from the Framingham Study. Arthritis Rheum 42:33–38, 1999.

167. Felson DT, Anderson JJ, Naimark A, et al. The prevalence of chondrocalcinosis in the elderly and its association with knee osteoarthritis: the Framingham Study. J Rheumatol 16:1241–1245, 1989.

168. Doherty M, Watt I, Dieppe PA. Localised chondrocalcinosis in post-meniscectomy knees. Lancet ii:1207–1210, 1982.

169. Segal R, Avrahami E, Lebdinski E, et al. The impact of hemiparalysis on the expression of osteoarthritis. Arthritis Rheum 41:2249–2256, 1998.

170. Altman RD, Hochberg M, Murphy WA, et al. Atlas of individual radiographic features in osteoarthritis. Osteoarthritis Cartilage 3:3–70, 1995.

171. Altman RD, Bloch DA, Dougados M, et al. Measurement of structural progression in osteoarthritis of the hip: the Barcelona consensus group. Osteoarthritis Cartilage 12:515–524, 2004.

172. Nevitt M, Sharma L. OMERACT Workshop Radiography Session 1. Osteoarthritis Cartilage 14 (Supplement 1):4–9, 2006 (Epub January 6, 2006)

173. Buckland-Wright CB. Protocols for precise radio-anatomical positioning of the tibiofemoral and patellofemoral compartments of the knee. Osteoarthritis Cartilage 3 (suppl A):71–80, 1995.

174. Vignon E, Piperno M, Le Graverand MP, et al. Measurement of radiographic joint space width in the tibiofemoral compartment of the osteoarthritic knee: comparison of standing anteroposterior and Lyon-Schuss views. Arthritis Rheum 48:378–384, 2003.

175. Buckland-Wright JC, Wolfe F, Ward RJ, et al. Substantial superiority of semiflexed (MTP) views in knee osteoarthritis: a comparative radiographic study, without fluoroscopy, of standing extended, semiflexed (MTP), and schuss views. J Rheumatol 26:2664–2674, 1999.

176. Peterfy C, Li J, Zaim S, et al. Comparison of fixed-flexion positioning with fluoroscopic semi-flexed positioning for quantifying radiographic joint-space width in the knee: test-retest reproducibility. Skeletal Radiol 32:128–132, 2003.

177. Brandt KD, Mazzuca SA, Conrozier T, et al. Which is the best radiographic protocol for a clinical trial of a structure modifying drug in patients with knee osteoarthritis? J Rheumatol 29:1308–1320, 2002.

178. Buckland-Wright JC, Macfarlane DG, Lynch JA, et al. Joint space width measures cartilage thickness in osteoarthritis of the knee: high resolution plain film and double contrast macroradiographic investigation. Ann Rheum Dis 54:263–268, 1995.

179. Altman RD, Fries JF, Bloch DA, et al. Radiographic assessment of progression in osteoarthritis. Arthritis Rheum 30:1214–1225, 1987.

180. Ravaud P, Giraudeau B, Auleley G-R, et al. Variability in knee radiographing: implication for definition of radiological progression in medial knee osteoarthritis. Ann Rheum Dis 57:624–629, 1998.

181. Raynauld JP. Quantitative magnetic resonance imaging of articular cartilage in knee osteoarthritis. Curr Opin Rheum. 12:647–650, 2003.

182. Eckstein F, Glaser C. Measuring cartilage morphology with quantitative magnetic resonance imaging. Semin Musculoskelet Radiol 8:329–353, 2004.

183. Raynauld JP, Martel-Pelletier J, Berthiaume MJ, et al. Quantitative magnetic resonance imaging evaluation of knee osteoarthritis progression over two years and correlation with clinical symptoms and radiologic changes. Arthritis Rheum 50:476–487, 2004.

184. Cicuttini FM, Wluka AE, Wang Y, et al. Longitudinal study of changes in tibial and femoral cartilage in knee osteoarthritis. Arthritis Rheum 50:94–97, 2004.

185. Glaser C, Draeger M, Englmeier KH, et al. Cartilage loss over two years in femorotibial osteoarthritis. Radiology 225 (Supppl):330 [abstract], 2002.

186. Peterfy CG, White DL, Zhao J, et al. Longitudinal measurement of knee articular cartilage volume inosteoarthritis. Arthritis Rheum 41:S361, 1998.

187. Wluka AE, Wolfe R, Stuckey S, et al. How does tibial cartilage volume relate to symptoms in subjects with knee osteoarthritis? Ann Rheum Dis 63:264–268, 2004.

188. Peterfy CG, Guermazi A, Zaim S, et al. Whole-organ magnetic resonance imaging score (WORMS) of the knee in osteoarthritis. Osteoarthritis Cartilage 12:177–190, 2004.

189. Burstein D, Gray M. New MRI techniques for imaging cartilage. J Bone Joint Surg Am 85-A Suppl 2:70–77, 2003.

190. Schouten JSAG, van den Ouweland FA, Valkenburg HA. A 12 year follow up study in the general population on prognostic factors of cartilage loss in osteoarthritis of the knee. Ann Rheum Dis 51:932–937, 1992.

191. Dougados M, Gueguen A, Nguyen M, et al. Longitudinal radiologic evaluation of osteoarthritis of the knee. J Rheumatol 19:378–384, 1992.

192. Dieppe PA, Cushnaghan J, Young P, et al. Prediction of the progression of joint space narrowing in osteoarthritis of the knee by bone scintigraphy. Ann Rheum Dis 52:557–563, 1993.

193. Sharif M, George E, Shepstone L, et al. Serum hyaluronic acid level as a predictor of disease progression in osteoarthritis of the knee. Arthritis Rheum 38:760–767, 1995.

194. Ledingham J, Regan M, Jones A, et al. Factors affecting radiographic progression of knee osteoarthritis. Ann Rheum Dis 54:53–58, 1995.

195. McAlindon TE, Felson DT, Zhang Y, et al. Relation of dietary intake and serum levels of vitamin D to progression of osteoarthritis of the knee among participants in the Framingham study. Ann Intern Med 125:353–359, 1996.

196. McAlindon TE, Jacques P, Zhang Y, et al. Do antioxidant micronutrients protect against the development and progression of knee osteoarthritis? Arthritis Rheum 39:648–656, 1996.

197. Cooper C, Snow S, McAlindon TE, et al. Risk factors for the incidence and progression of radiographic knee osteoarthritis. Arthritis Rheum 2000;43:995–1000.

198. Sharma L, Song J, Felson DT, et al. The role of knee alignment in disease progression and functional decline in knee osteoarthritis. JAMA 286:188–195, 2001.

199. Miyazaki T, Wada M, Kawahara H, et al. Dynamic load at baseline can predict radiographic disease progression in medial compartment knee osteoarthritis. Ann Rheum Dis 61:617–622, 2002.

200. Cicuttini F, Wluka A, Wang Y, et al. The determinants of change in patella cartilage volume in osteoarthritic knees. J Rheumatol 2002;29:2615–2619.

201. Wluka AE, Stuckey S, Snaddon J, et al. The determinants of change in tibial cartilage volume in osteoarthritic knees. Arthritis Rheum 2002;46:2065–2072.

202. Felson D, McLaughlin S, Goggins J, et al. Bone marrow edema and its relation to progression of knee osteoarthritis. Ann Intern Med 139:330–336, 2003.

203. Cahue S, Dunlop D, Hayes K, et al. Varus-valgus alignment in the progression of patellofemoral osteoarthritis. Arthritis Rheum. 50:2184–2190, 2004.

204. Cicuttini F, Wluka A, Hankin J, et al. Longitudinal study of the relationship between knee angle and tibiofemoral cartilage volume in subjects with knee osteoarthritis. Rheumatology (Oxford) 43:321–324, 2004.

205. Chang A, Hayes K, Dunlop D, et al. Thrust during ambulation and progression of knee osteoarthritis. Arthritis Rheum 50:3897–3903, 2004.

206. Berthiaume MJ, Raynauld JP, Martel-Pelletier J, et al. Meniscal tear and extrusion are strongly associated with progression of symptomatic knee osteoarthritis as assessed by quantitative magnetic resonance imaging. Ann Rheum Dis 64:556–563, 2005. Epub 2004 Sep 16.

207. Chang A, Hayes K, Dunlop D, et al. Hip abduction moment and protection against medial tibiofemoral osteoarthritis progression. Arthritis Rheum 52:3515–3519, 2005.

208. Sharma L, Lou C, Cahue S, et al. The mechanism of effect of obesity in knee osteoarthritis: the mediating role of malalignment. Arthritis Rheum 43:568–575, 2000.

209. Felson DT, Goggins J, Niu J, et al. The effect of body weight on progression of knee osteoarthrtis is dependent on alignment. Arthritis Rheum 50:3904–3909, 2004.

210. Brandt KD, Heilman DK, Slemenda C, et al. Quadriceps strength in women with radiographically progressive osteoarthritis of the knee and those with stable radiographic changes. J Rheumatol 26:2431–2437, 1999.

211. Sharma L, Dunlop DD, Cahue S, et al. Quadriceps strength and osteoarthritis progression in malaligned and lax knees. Ann Int Med 138:613–619, 2003.

212. Dieppe P. Subchondral bone should be the main target for the treatment of pain and disease progression in osteoarthritis. Osteoarthritis Cartilage 7:325–326, 1999.

213. Hurwitz DE, Sumner DR, Andriacchi TP, et al. Dynamic knee loads during gait predict proximal tibial bone distribution. J Biomech 31:423–430, 1998.

214. Wada M, Maezawa Y, Baba H, et al. Relationships among bone mineral densities, static alignment and dynamic load in patients with medial compartment knee osteoarthritis. Rheumatology 40:499–505, 2001.

215. Lo G, Hunter D, Zhang Y, et al. Bone marrow lesions in the knee are associated with increased local bone density. Arthritis Rheum. 52:2814–2821, 2005.

216. Zanetti M, Bruder E, Romero J, et al. Bone marrow edema pattern in osteoarthritic knees: correlation between MR imaging and histologic findings. Radiology 215:835–840, 2000.

217. Reijman M, Hazes JM, Pols HA, et al. Role of radiography in predicting progression of osteoarthritis of the hip: prospective cohort study. BMJ 330(7501):1183, 2005. Epub 2005 May 13.

218. Lane NE, Nevitt MC, Hochberg MC, et al. Progression of radiographic hip osteoarthritis over eight years in a community sample of elderly white women. Arthritis Rheum 50:1477–1486, 2004.

219. Seifert MH, Whiteside CG, Savage O. A 5-year follow-up of fifty cases of idiopathic osteoarthritis of the hip. Ann Rheum Dis 28:325–326, 1969.

220. Maillefert JF, Gueguen A, Monreal M, et al. Sex differences in hip osteoarthritis: results of a longitudinal study in 508 patients. Ann Rheum Dis 62:931–993, 2003.

221. Ledingham J, Dawson S, Preston B, et al. Radiographic progression of hospital referred osteoarthritis of the hip. Ann Rheum Dis 52:263–267, 1993.

222. Perry GH, Smith MJG, Whiteside CG. Spontaneous recovery of the joint space in degenerative hip disease. Ann Rheum Dis 31:440–448, 1972.

223. Harris PA, Hart DJ, Dacre JE, et al. The progression of radiological hand osteoarthritis over ten years: a clinical follow-up study. Osteoarthritis Cartilage 2:247–252, 1994.

224. Davis MA, Ettinger WH, Neuhaus JM, et al. Correlates of knee pain among U.S. adults with and without radiographic knee osteoarthritis. J Rheumatol 19:1943–1949, 1992.

225. Lethbridge-Cejku M, Scott WW, Reichle R, et al. Association of radiographic features of osteoarthritis of the knee with knee pain: Data from the Baltimore Longitudinal Study of Aging. Arthritis Care Res 8:182–188, 1995.

226. Hill CL, Gale DG, Chaisson CE, et al. Knee effusions, popliteal cysts, and synovial thickening: association with knee pain in osteoarthritis. J Rheumatol 28:1330–1337, 2001.

227. Felson DT, Chaisson CE, Hill CL, et al. The association of bone marrow lesions with pain in knee osteoarthritis. Ann Intern Med 134:541–549, 2001.

228. Sowers MF, Hayes C, Jamadar D, et al. Magnetic resonance-detected subchondral bone marrow and cartilage defect characteristics associated with pain and x-ray defined knee osteoarthritis. Osteoarthritis Cartilage 11:387–393, 2003.

229. Hochberg MC, Lawrence RC, Everett DF, et al. Epidemiologic associations of pain in osteoarthritis of the knee: data from the National Health and Nutrition Examination Survey and the National Health and Nutrition Examination-I Epidemiologic Follow-up Survey. Semin Arthritis Rheum 18:4–9, 1989.

230. Summers MN, Haley WE, Reveille JD, et al. Radiographic assessment and psychologic variables as predictors of pain and functional impairment in osteoarthritis of the knee or hip. Arthritis Rheum 31:204–209, 1988.

231. Lunghi ME, Miller PM, McQuillan WM. Psychological factors in osteoarthritis of the hip. J Psychosom Res 22:57–63, 1978.

232. O'Reilly SC, Jones A, Muir KR, et al. Quadriceps weakness in knee osteoarthritis: the effect on pain and disability. Ann Rheum Dis 57:588–594, 1998.

233. Lichtenberg PA, Skehan MW, Swensen CH. The role of personality, recent life stress and arthritic severity in predicting pain. J Psychosom Res 28:231–236, 1984.

234. Lankhorst GJ, van de Stadt RJ, van der Korst JK. The relationships of functional capacity, pain, and isometric and isokinetic torque in osteoarthrosis of the knee. Scand J Rehabil Med 17:167–172, 1985.

235. Slemenda C, Brandt KD, Heilman DK, et al. Quadriceps weakness and osteoarthritis of the knee. Ann Intern Med 127:97–104, 1997.

236. Rejeski WJ, Miller ME, Foy C, et al. Self-efficacy and the progression of functional limitations and self-reported disability in adults with knee pain. J Gerontol 56B:S261–265, 2001.

237. Miller ME, Rejeski WJ, Messier SP, et al. Modifiers of change in physical functioning in older adults with knee pain: the Observational Arthritis Study in Seniors (OASIS). Arthritis Care Res 2001;45:331–339.

238. Sharma L, Cahue S, Song J, et al. Physical functioning over 3 years in knee osteoarthritis. Arthritis Rheum 48:3359–3370, 2003.

239. Ormel J, Rijsdijk FV, Sullivan M, et al. Temporal and reciprocal relationship between IADL/ADL disability and depressive symptoms in late life. J Gerontol B Psychol Sci Soc Sci 57:P338–347, 2002.

240. Davis MA, Ettinger WH, Neuhaus JM, et al. Knee osteoarthritis and physical functioning: Evidence from the NHANES I Epidemiologic Followup Study. J Rheumatol 18:591–599, 1991.

241. Ettinger WH, Davis MA, Neuhaus JM, et al. Long-term physical functioning in persons with knee osteoarthritis from NHANES I: effects of comorbid medical conditions. J Clin Epidemiol 47:809–815, 1994.

242. Guccione AA, Felson DT, Anderson JJ. Defining arthritis and measuring functional status in elders: methodological issues in the study of disease and physical disability. Am J Public Health 80:945–949, 1990.

243. Acheson RM, Ginsburg GN. New Haven survey of joint diseases. XVI. Impairment, disability and arthritis. Br J Prev Soc Med 27:168–176, 1973.

244. Baron M, Dutil E, Berkson L, et al. Hand function in the elderly: relation to osteoarthritis. Arthritis Rheum 14:815–819, 1987.

245. Rejeski WJ, Craven T, Ettinger WH, et al. Self-efficacy and pain in disability with osteoarthritis of the knee. J Geront: Psychol Sci 51B:P24–P2, 1996.

246. Van Baar ME, Dekker J, Lemmens JAM, et al. Pain and disability in patients with osteoarthritis of hip or knee: the relationship with articular, kinesiological, and psychological characteristics. J Rheumatol 25:125–133, 1998.

247. McAlindon TE, Cooper C, Kirwan JR, et al. Determinants of disability in osteoarthritis of the knee. Ann Rheum Dis 52:258–262, 1993.

248. Jordan J, Luta G, Renner J, et al. Knee pain and knee osteoarthritis severity in self-reported task specific disability: the Johnston County osteoarthritis project. J Rheumatol 24:1344–1349, 1997.

249. Salaffi F, Cavalieri F, Nolli M, et al. Analysis of disability in knee osteoarthritis. Relationship with age, psychological variables, but not with radiographic score. J Rheumatol 18:1581–1586, 1991.

250. Fisher NM, Pendergast DR, Gresham GE, et al. Muscle rehabilitation: its effect on muscular and functional performance of patients with knee osteoarthritis. Arch Phys Med Rehabil 72:367–370, 1991.

Etiopathogenesis of Osteoarthritis

2

A. Robin Poole   Farshid Guilak   Steven B. Abramson

Osteoarthritis (OA) is a condition that represents a pathological imbalance of degradative and reparative processes involving the whole joint and its component parts, with secondary inflammatory changes, particularly in the synovium, but also in the articular cartilage itself (Fig. 2–1). Idiopathic primary OA may involve one particular joint, or it may be generalized or involve multiple joints in erosive inflammatory forms[1,2] (Table 2–1). The presentation of this pathological condition in joints may be a consequence of the biomechanics within the joint which reveal otherwise masked systemic genetically determined changes. The mechanical pressures within the joint may therefore reveal weaknesses in tissue maintenance that are more widespread than previously considered.

Most forms of OA fall into two categories, depending on the predominant background: those that are primary, and often idiopathic, with abnormalities of joint biomaterial and biomechanically faulty joint structure that may result from a recognizable mutation, and those that are secondary and result from superimposed risk factors affecting distribution and severity of loading forces acting on specific joints, such as joint injury.

RISK FACTORS FOR OSTEOARTHRITIS

Risk Factors Associated with Abnormalities in Joint Biomaterial and Biomechanical Properties, Chemical Injury, or Endocrine Disorders

Familial OA (Table 2–1) may result from abnormal cartilage structure and properties such as a consequence of a mutation in the type II collagen COL2A1 gene (localized on chromosome 12), which causes not only cartilage dysplasia but also a severe form of OA with defective collagen.[3,4]

Onset is usually soon after cessation of growth. (See Chapter 6 for other gene defects relevant to OA associated with dysplasias and joint laxity.) Chronic abnormalities of growth plate development and bone growth leading to altered congruity of articulating surfaces can also cause OA. OA can develop in patients after traumatic injury or damage to chondrocytes associated with abnormal deposits in the cartilage matrix found in metabolic diseases such as hemochromatosis, ochronosis or alkaptonuria, Wilson disease, and Gaucher disease. OA can also result from disturbances in cartilage metabolism caused by endocrine disorders, such as acromegaly[5] (see Chapter 13).

Risk Factors Related to Abnormalities in the Quality and Distribution of Loading Forces on a Joint

Cartilage damage due to trauma, impact injuries, abnormal joint loading, and excessive wear, or as part of an aging process, can lead to changes in the composition, structure, and material properties of the tissue (Fig. 2–2). These alterations can compromise the ability of cartilage to function and survive in the strenuous mechanical environment normally found in load-bearing joints. Joint injury and subsequent joint instability, from loss of ligamental or meniscal support, are significant risk factors for OA.[6] Injury and abnormal loading, due to overexercise or abnormal joint use, are a risk for OA.[7,8] In regard to underloading, disuse immobilization from chronic inanition, neurologic disorders, or postoperative casting can lead to cartilage disuse atrophy, with increased vulnerability to cartilage injury, unless exercise programs for rehabilitation are carefully controlled. Evidence for this is available from studies of casted animals and those subsequently subjected to controlled or excessive treadmill exercise. Immobilized joint cartilage exhibits arrest of cartilage proteoglycan aggrecan

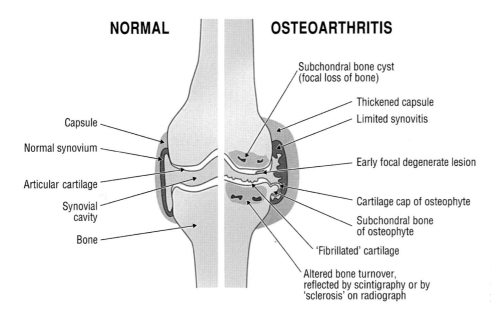

NORMAL   OSTEOARTHRITIS

Subchondral bone cyst
(focal loss of bone)

Thickened capsule

Limited synovitis

Capsule

Normal synovium

Early focal degenerate lesion

Articular cartilage

Synovial
cavity

Cartilage cap of osteophyte

Subchondral bone
of osteophyte

Bone

'Fibrillated' cartilage

Altered bone turnover,
reflected by scintigraphy or by
'sclerosis' on radiograph

Figure 2–1 Gross pathologic changes observed in OA joints during many years of degenerative change.

synthesis,[8,9] altered biomechanical properties,[10–12] and associated elevated metalloproteinases that may contribute to cartilage damage[13] (reviewed in Helminen et al.[14]). Deep ulcerative lesions with elevated protease activity can result from treadmill overexercise after disuse immobilization.[15] Standard levels of exercise may cause site-specific changes in proteoglycan content and cartilage stiffness, although these changes are not believed to be deleterious[16] and may potentially have a beneficial effect in the normal joint.[17–19] Altered joint loading due to instability or injury of the joint is now well known to be a significant risk factor for the onset and progression of OA.[8,20,21] Alterations in joint loading, brought about through ligament transection[22] or meniscectomy,[23] may lead to profound and repeatable changes in joint tissues which mimic changes seen in early human OA, including increased hydration and proteoglycan turnover, and decreased tissue stiffness in tension, compression, and shear.[11,24–28] Obesity is a well-defined risk factor involving excessive joint loading[29] as well as systemic metabolic changes that include low-grade chronic inflammation.[30] In this respect, obesity is regarded as the number one preventable risk factor for OA.[19,31] Evolutionary adaptations to the upright posture by humans have redistributed preponderant loading forces to new sites, predisposing to an increased risk for development of OA in hips, knees, bunion joints, and the lumbar spine.[32]

Age-related changes in the magnitude and pattern of stresses on joint cartilage may arise from a number of factors, including altered gait, muscle weakness, changes in proprioception, and changes in body weight. A neuromuscular control deficit is likely to contribute to the loss of normal attenuation of body weight-bearing forces during walking. This is manifested in OA patients as the "digging of the heels" on forceplate analysis.[7] The development of experimental canine OA can be accelerated by posterior nerve root section at the spinal cord, which affects the afferent signals governing stereognostic control of the affected arthritic limb;[33] this provides important insights

into the pathophysiologic process of the Charcot joint. The mechanism of impact loading, in which energy is normally predominantly absorbed or attenuated by strong muscle groups in the thigh and leg, is also significantly impaired in OA patients,[34] who exhibit decreased muscle strength. Quadriceps weakness is associated with knee pain, especially in OA.[35] Biomechanical changes in the joint capsule as a consequence of genetic or post-translational changes, such as those affecting collagen fibers, may also influence joint loading.

Examination of nutritional factors in the etiopathology of OA has provided evidence for an increased risk of development of OA of the knee with vitamin E and C deficiencies,[36] no doubt influencing matrix assembly and function. In Asia, Kashin-Beck disease, a form of OA, may be caused by dietary exposure to an endemic fungus.[37] Hypothyroidism afflicts many of these patients because of a dietary selenium deficiency.[38]

ARTICULAR CARTILAGE

Composition

Normal articular cartilage consists of an extensive, hydrated extracellular matrix that is synthesized and maintained by a sparse population of specialized cells, the chondrocytes (Fig. 2–3). In the adult human, these cells may occupy as little as 2% of the total volume. The matrix consists mainly of collagen (mostly type II with lesser amounts of other collagen types) and proteoglycans, principally aggrecan, which is large and aggregates with hyaluronic acid (HA).[39] Types II, IX, and XI collagens of cartilage combine to form a fibrillar network that provides a structural framework of the matrix in the form of an inhomogeneous and anisotropic meshwork of fibers, which is surrounded by a highly concentrated solution of the proteoglycan aggrecan. A secondary microfibrillar

TABLE 2–1
CLASSIFICATION OF OSTEOARTHRITIS

PRIMARY (IDIOPATHIC)
Peripheral joints (single vs. multiple joints)
Interphalangeal joints (nodal) (e.g., distal interphalangeal, proximal interphalangeal)
Other small joints (e.g., first carpometacarpal, first metacarpophalangeal)
Large joints (e.g., hip, knee)

SPINE
Apophyseal joints
Intervertebral joints

VARIANT SUBSETS
Erosive inflammatory osteoarthritis
Generalized osteoarthritis
Chondromalacia patellae
Diffuse idiopathic skeletal hyperostosis (DISH, ankylosing hyperostosis)

SECONDARY
Trauma
Acute
Chronic (occupational, sports, obesity)

OTHER JOINT DISORDERS
Local (fracture, avascular necrosis, infection)
Diffuse (rheumatoid arthritis, hypermobility syndrome, hemorrhagic diatheses)

SYSTEMIC METABOLIC DISEASE
Ochronosis (alkaptonuria)
Hemochromatosis
Wilson disease
Kashin-Beck disease

ENDOCRINE DISORDERS
Acromegaly
Hyperparathyroidism
Diabetes mellitus

CALCIUM CRYSTAL DEPOSITION DISEASES
Calcium pyrophosphate dihydrate
Calcium apatite

NEUROPATHIC DISORDERS (CHARCOT JOINTS)
(e.g., tabes dorsalis, diabetes mellitus, intra-articular steroid overuse)

FAMILIAL OSTEOARTHRITIS (associated with skeletal dysplasias such as multiple epiphyseal dysplasia, spondyloepiphyseal dysplasia)

MISCELLANEOUS
Frostbite
Long-leg arthropathy

network involving type VI collagen is concentrated in the pericellular matrix between the cell surface and the territorial matrix.

Proteoglycans are complex macromolecules with a protein core to which are attached glycosaminoglycan chains, primarily of chondroitin sulfate and keratan sulfate. These glycosaminoglycans, which are negatively charged in solution, are responsible for the hydration and large swelling pressure of this tissue.[40,41] Many other smaller proteoglycans and other molecules are present within the tissue, some of which may be directly associated with the collagen fibrils. For more details, please see Chapter 4.

Biomechanics of Articular Cartilage

Articular cartilage serves as a low-friction, wear-resistant surface for load support, load transfer, and motion between the bones of the diarthrodial joint. Under normal circumstances, this tissue, bathed in synovial fluid, is able to withstand millions of cycles of loading each year at stresses that may reach 18 MPa,[42] while exhibiting little or no wear. These unique properties are endowed by the composition and structure of the major constituents of articular cartilage, and their associated spatial variations provide a complex and inhomogeneous set of material properties.

From a biomechanical standpoint, articular cartilage can be viewed as a fiber-reinforced, porous, and permeable composite material that is saturated with an interstitial fluid, water.[43] These characteristics provide for mechanical properties that are viscoelastic (time- or rate-dependent), anisotropic (dependent on direction), and nonlinear (dependent on magnitude of strain). Accordingly, the biomechanical properties of cartilage have been widely studied using models that take into account the multiple phases (collagen solid matrix, interstitial fluid, and mobile and "fixed" ionic groups) and the interactions among these phases.[43-45]

The largest constituent, water, provides load support through fluid pressurization and energy dissipation by fluid flow in response to applied loading.[43] The second largest constituent, the collagen fibril, provides articular cartilage with its nonlinear properties in tension,[46,47] which are inhomogeneously distributed with depth from the tissue surface. However, these tensile properties decrease progressively with increasing age after 30 years in articular cartilages, such as of the hip, that most commonly develop OA.[48] Age-related changes in cartilage tensile properties are believed to arise in part from the accumulation of advanced glycation end products (AGE) which increase the "brittleness" of the cartilage, increasing the potential for tissue fracture and aging-associated biomechanical dysfunction.[49]

The high concentration of negative charges associated with the proteoglycans in cartilage has a significant effect on the mechanical behavior of the tissue. The negatively charged nature of cartilage arises primarily from the glycosaminoglycans, namely, the many chondroitin sulfate and keratan sulfate chains that are present on aggrecan molecules.[50] The large size of aggrecan and its interactions with HA to form macromolecular aggregates serve to retain aggrecan molecules in the extracellular matrix so that their negative charges are "fixed." These fixed charges are responsible for the physicochemical and electrokinetic properties of this tissue, such as a large osmotic pressure and associated propensity to swell and exhibit streaming potentials, streaming currents, and electro-osmotic effects.[41,45] As a result, the mechanical behavior of articular cartilage exhibits an interdependence on physicochemical factors, such as the structural organization and properties

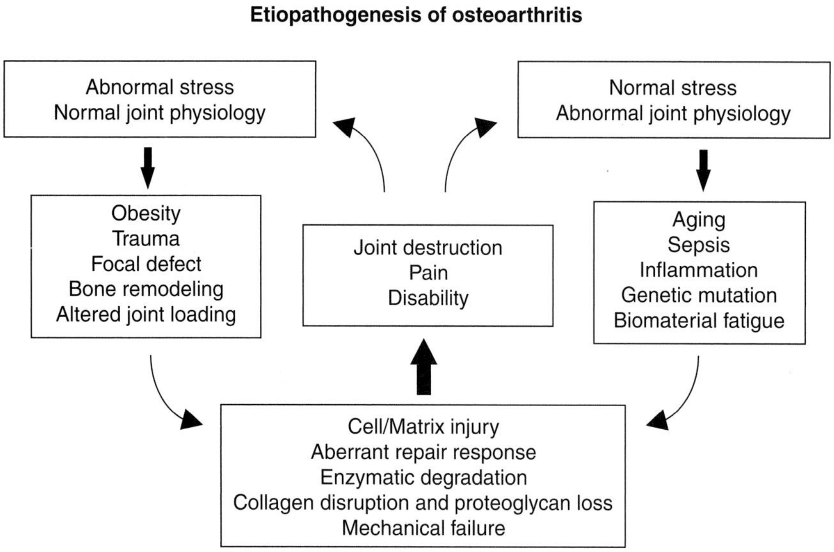
Etiopathogenesis of osteoarthritis
Abnormal stress
Normal joint physiology
Normal stress
Abnormal joint physiology
Obesity
Trauma
Focal defect
Bone remodeling
Altered joint loading
Joint destruction
Pain
Disability
Aging
Sepsis
Inflammation
Genetic mutation
Biomaterial fatigue
Cell/Matrix injury
Aberrant repair response
Enzymatic degradation
Collagen disruption and proteoglycan loss
Mechanical failure

Figure 2–2 Potential mechanisms involved in the etiopathogenesis of OA.

of the collagen fibrillar network, the proteoglycan aggrecan concentration, and the type or distribution of counterions.[44] These physicochemical properties significantly contribute to the function of articular cartilage.[45] The swelling pressure is believed to largely contribute to residual stresses in the cartilage matrix that enhance the support and distribution of applied loads.[51,52] The loss of tensile properties and swelling pressure as collagen and proteoglycans are degraded and lost in OA results in mechanical decompensation and an ensuing increase in the magnitude of tissue strains under similar magnitudes of physiologic loading,[10,28,53] particularly at the cellular level.[54]

Articular cartilage endows the synovial joint with frictional properties that remain unmatched by man-made joints. The coefficient of friction (ratio of frictional force to compressive force) of cartilage gliding on cartilage has been reported to be as low as 0.002.[55] The mechanisms by which the synovial joint achieves these properties involve a combination of biomechanical and biomolecular factors.[56]

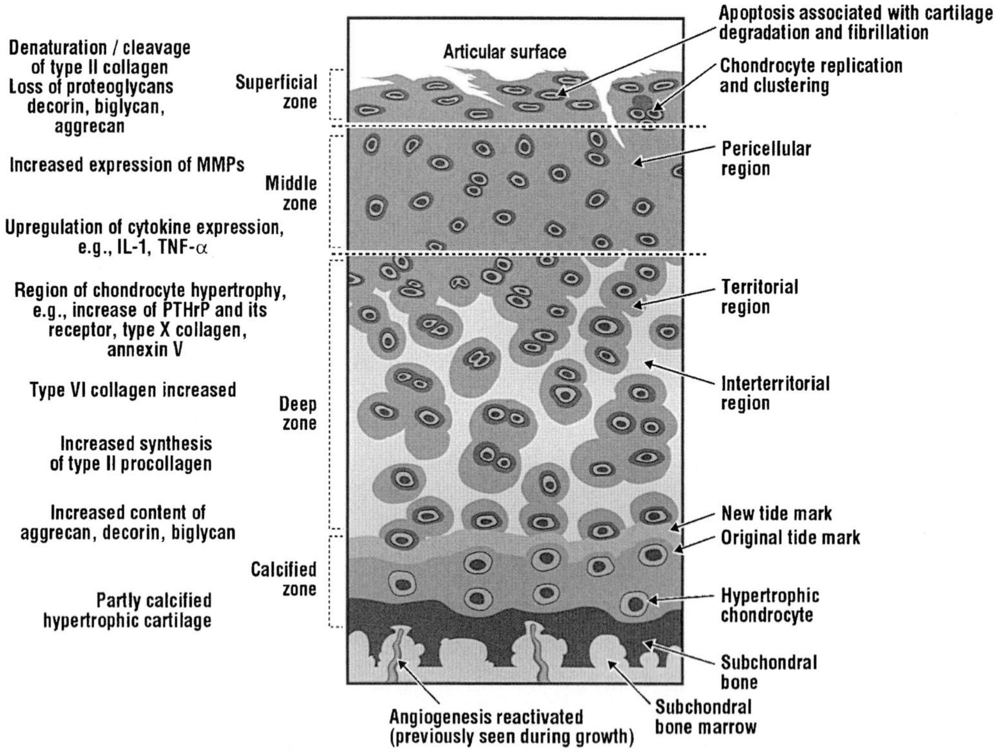
Denaturation / cleavage of type II collagen
Loss of proteoglycans decorin, biglycan, aggrecan
Superficial zone
Increased expression of MMPs
Middle zone
Upregulation of cytokine expression, e.g., IL-1, TNF-α
Region of chondrocyte hypertrophy, e.g., increase of PTHrP and its receptor, type X collagen, annexin V
Type VI collagen increased
Deep zone
Increased synthesis of type II procollagen
Increased content of aggrecan, decorin, biglycan
Calcified zone
Partly calcified hypertrophic cartilage
Articular surface
Apoptosis associated with cartilage degradation and fibrillation
Chondrocyte replication and clustering
Pericellular region
Territorial region
Interterritorial region
New tide mark
Original tide mark
Hypertrophic chondrocyte
Subchondral bone
Subchondral bone marrow
Angiogenesis reactivated (previously seen during growth)

Figure 2–3 Changes observed in articular cartilage in OA involving chondrocytes and extracellular matrix.

For example, joint congruity and cartilage deformation serve to distribute loads over a larger contact area, thereby minimizing contact stresses. The high water content and low hydraulic permeability of the cartilage extracellular matrix provide a unique mechanism of supporting loads whereby fluid pressurization within the tissue can bear nearly 90% of the load and thus minimize stresses on the solid extracellular matrix.[57,58] Synovial fluid plays multiple roles in joint lubrication by providing a high viscosity "squeeze film" layer that delays cartilage-to-cartilage contact under compression[59] but also serves as a source of boundary lubricant molecules within the joint.

Boundary lubricants are molecules that may be adsorbed or bound to the cartilage surface and decrease friction in cases when the tissue surfaces actually contact one another. In the past two decades, there have been significant advances in our understanding of the composition, structure, and properties of biomolecular components of the synovial fluid that serve as the primary boundary lubricants for the joint. "Lubricin," a ~227 kDa glycoprotein, was first identified from bovine synovial fluid by density gradient sedimentation and gel-permeation chromatography.[60] This molecule was first identified as a product of synovial fibroblasts expressing the gene for megakaryocyte stimulating factor (MSF, also termed *PRG4*). Subsequent investigations have identified a 345 kDa protein, termed "superficial zone protein" (SZP), as an additional product of the MSF gene.[61,62] The importance of these molecules in the health of the joint have been demonstrated by the rare autosomal recessive disorder, camptodactyly-arthropathy-coxa vara-pericarditis (CACP) syndrome, which has been attributed to mutations in the *PRG4* gene.[63] The loss of SZP function in CACP is associated with a severe juvenile-onset joint failure that is noninflammatory in nature.

Biomechanical Regulation of Cartilage Metabolism

A number of in vivo studies have emphasized the relationship between mechanical loading and the health of the joint, and suggest that a critical level and pattern of mechanical stress is required to maintain the normal balance of cartilage synthesis and breakdown. Under normal physiological conditions, the components of the extracellular matrix are in a state of slow turnover, retained in a homeostatic balance between the catabolic and anabolic events of the chondrocytes. These activities are controlled through the processing of both genetic and environmental information, which includes the action of soluble mediators (e.g., growth factors and cytokines), extracellular matrix composition, and physical factors such as mechanical stress. Indeed, many studies have shown that the mechanical stress environment of the joint is an important factor that influences (and presumably regulates) the activity of the chondrocytes in vivo.[14,64]

Considerable research effort has been directed toward understanding the processes by which physical signals are converted to a biochemical signal by the chondrocyte population. Clarification of the specific signaling mechanisms

in normal and inflamed cartilage would not only provide a better understanding of the processes which regulate the physiology of cartilage, but would also be expected to yield new insights on the pathogenesis of OA. In this respect, in vitro explant models of mechanical loading provide a model system in which the biomechanical and biochemical environments can be better controlled as compared to the in vivo situation. Explant models of cartilage loading have been utilized in a number of different loading configurations, including unconfined compression, indentation, tension, shear, and osmotic and hydrostatic pressure (reviewed in Guilak et al.[64]). The general consensus of these studies is that static compression suppresses matrix biosynthesis, and cyclic and intermittent loading stimulate chondrocyte metabolism (e.g., Gray et al.,[65] Sah et al.,[66] Guilak et al.,[67] Torzilli et al.[68]). These responses have been reported over a wide range of loading magnitudes, and exhibit a stress-dose dependency. Excessive loading (e.g., high magnitude, long duration) seems to have a deleterious effect, resulting in cell death, tissue disruption, and swelling.[69-71]

The cellular transduction mechanisms responsible for converting mechanical stress into a biochemical response are the subject of much study but are not fully understood. Currently, there is significant evidence that chondrocytes may transduce mechanical signals into biochemical responses through various intracellular and intercellular signaling pathways, including activation of the traditional second messenger pathways such as cyclic AMP (cAMP), inositol trisphosphate, or calcium ion (see Guilak et al.[64] and Stockwell[72] for reviews).

The Degeneration of Articular Cartilage in Osteoarthritis

The classic loss of articular cartilage observed in OA may be initiated as a focal process that first appears to manifest at the articular cartilage surface. These lesions, which are commonly observed in aging human populations, have all the biochemical features of OA cartilages at arthroplasty.[73] They may progressively enlarge to involve specific compartments, inducing alterations in other articulating surfaces by producing changes in loading. Some of the clues as to whether these focal lesions enlarge may have been revealed by recent studies on these lesions in the ankle versus the knee joint. In knee lesions, the emphasis in the cartilage is on matrix degradation, whereas in the ankle it is on matrix synthesis.[39] Moreover, in the ankle the response involving increased matrix turnover is more generalized, whereas in the knee it is associated with the lesion.[39,73] These fundamental differences in the response and in the lesions could help explain why knee OA is much more common. More widespread changes in loading after traumatic injury may involve the whole joint cartilage, in which alterations in cartilage matrix turnover are detectable within days, weeks, or months after damage to the anterior cruciate ligament or meniscus.[74,75] In particular, joint injuries that involve fracture of the articular surface tend to accelerate more rapidly to a degenerative state of post-traumatic arthritis.[76]

Cartilage degeneration is first observed at the articular surface in the form of fibrillation (Fig. 2–3). Splits are initially parallel to the articular surface; later, they vertically penetrate the damaged cartilage, eventually reaching subchondral bone. Cell cloning is observed early around the splits but is confined to more superficial sites. Many of these cells have become hypertrophic. Progressive loss of cartilage thickness, starting at the surface, is observed.

In large joints, idiopathic OA is ordinarily believed to be a slow process that may take as long as 20 to 30 years, but it is accelerated in cases of joint injury[75,77–79] or may present clinically on cessation of growth as in familial OA.[80] Degeneration is often more pronounced in the tibial cartilage, particularly in the medial compartment. This characteristic is observed in both human and in experimental OA.

Other examples of long-term development of OA come from experimental studies of anterior cruciate ligament transection in dogs, in which bone, ligament, and synovial changes are also observed early[28,81,82] (see Chapter 5), presenting as an advanced lesion after a period of only 3 or more years. The earliest changes in the unstable knee that can be seen in articular cartilage in injured joints in animals and humans feature cartilage swelling (also called a hypertrophic reaction), with enhanced synthesis of matrix with an increased content of aggrecan.[24] This is followed by a phase of increased matrix turnover, with net depletion of principal matrix components. Finally, severe damage to and loss of the collagen network is observed.[11,28,75,83,84] The hypertrophic stage, not to be confused with chondrocyte hypertrophy, clearly precedes the occurrence of the lesional stage with its characteristic deep focal loss of cartilage. In the dog, the biomechanical properties correlate well with a reduction in proteoglycan aggregation and the loss of hyaluronan and link protein.[84,85] The presence of smaller proteoglycan aggregates in uncovered or unprotected areas of tibial plateau cartilage in normal control subjects, coupled with the presence of elevated protease activity after surgery, may result in part from a shift of load-bearing sites during the development of OA in this model.[86,87]

Proteinases of Osteoarthritis Cartilage

Metalloproteinases (MMPs) are generally considered to play a principal role in the cleavage of matrix macromolecules, including type II collagen and the cartilage proteoglycan aggrecan. Collagenases cleave type II collagen, which contains a long triple-helical domain, at a specific site approximately three quarters from the amino terminus. This results in unwinding (denaturation) of the α-chains, which are then susceptible to secondary cleavage by collagenases and other MMPs such as stromelysin 1(MMP-3) and the gelatinases MMP-2 and MMP-9. Aggrecan is cleaved by different MMPs and by the aggrecanases (adamolysins) ADAMTS-4 and -5.

Four collagenases may be active in articular cartilage, namely, MMP-1, -8, -13, and -14 (Table 2–2). MMP-13 is the most efficient at cleaving type II collagen.[88] It may be involved in type II collagen cleavage in articular cartilage more than any other collagenase.[89,90] Overexpression of constitutively active MMP-13 in cartilage induces the early onset of OA in mice.[91] MMP-2 and -9 have also been reported to have collagenase activity. Most MMPs are secreted as latent proenzymes and are then activated. MMP-1 and -13, for example, can bind to collagen fibrils where they can be activated. MMP-3 and MMP-14 are involved in activating other MMPs. Like other MMPs, these activators may themselves be activated by plasmin generated from plasminogen by urokinase-type activator produced by chondrocytes or by cysteine proteinases such as cathepsin B,[92] or by MT1-MMP (MMP-14), which possesses a furin cleavage site, which means that it is usually activated within the cell before secretion. Cathepsin K, a cysteine proteinase, can also cleave triple-helical collagen but in primary sites different from the primary cleavage produced by collagenases.[93] It is expressed by superficial chondrocytes in increased amounts in OA cartilage.[94] There is unpublished evidence that this proteinase is involved in collagen cleavage in OA articular cartilage in culture (V. Dejica, J.S. Mort, and A.R. Poole, unpublished data).

In OA, there is increased expression and content of various MMPs, including MMP-1, MMP-3, MMP-13, and MMP-28 (epilysin), but not ADAMTS-4 (a disintegrin and metalloproteinase with thrombospondin motifs) or ADAMTS-5, the latter being downregulated.[95] Others have observed that increased MMP-13 expression is the most dominant of the collagenases, being stronger in late stage disease when MMP-3 is downregulated; of the aggrecanases, only ADAMTS-5 was clearly expressed.[96] This increased expression is first observed at or close to the articular surface very early in the degenerative process.[97,98] Similarly there is increased expression of MMP-2, MMP-9, MMP-8,[99,100] MMP-11,[101] MMP-14,[102,103] and matrilysin.[104] Plasminogen activator[105] and cathepsin B[106,107] are also upregulated in human and experimental OA cartilage.

Cleavage and denaturation of type II collagen by collagenases are first observed around chondrocytes in these superficial sites where MMP-1 and -13 are present in increased amounts.[97,108,109] This change is also seen with aging but more so in OA. It extends into the territorial and interterritorial matrix and then progressively extends into the mid and deep zones with lesion development.[97] Collagenase activity, the denaturation of type II collagen, and the associated loss of type II collagen[73,110] are much increased in OA cartilages.[73,89,108] These changes in articular cartilage are seen within months of anterior cruciate ligament rupture, which is a major risk factor for OA development in a joint.[75,111]

In established OA of the knee, the synthesis of type II collagen is simultaneously increased markedly.[39,112–114] However, these new molecules, as well as resident preexisting collagen, are the subject of excessive proteolysis.[90] The same applies to aggrecan.[115]

The core protein of aggrecan is cleaved by different proteinases.[50] Cleavage sites are common in the interglobular domain between the G1 and G2 domains as well as in the chondroitin sulfate–rich region. In the interglobular domain, two principal cleavage sites have been identified: the aggrecanase site, where proteinases such as cell surface–associated

TABLE 2–2

EARLY CHANGES IN THE STRUCTURE AND COMPOSITION OF ARTICULAR CARTILAGE IN HUMAN OSTEOARTHRITIS

Molecule	Synthesis, Content, and Activity	Reference
COLLAGENS		
Type IIB		
Content and expression	−	108, 112
Denaturation	+	108, 109
Cleavage by collagenase	+	89, 90
Synthesis	+	114
Type IIA	+ (mid zone)	161*, 162
Type III		
mRNA and content	+ (surface zone)	112
Type VI	+ (pericellular)	164*, 165, 166
Type X	+	195
PROTEOGLYCANS		
Aggrecan	− Surface zone; + (mid and deep zones)	50, 92
Decorin	+ (mid and deep zones);	160
Biglycan	− (surface zone)	160
OTHER PROTEINS		
Cartilage oligomeric protein	Altered distribution	176
Tenascin	+	178
Fibronectin	+	131
Cartilage matrix protein	+	177
Osteonectin	+	143
PROTEINASES		
Metalloproteinases		
Collagenases 1, 2, 3	+	88, 206, 207
Stromelysin 1	+	50, 92
Gelatinase A	+	102
Gelatinase B	+	314
Matrilysin	+	104
MT–MMP-1	+	102, 103
Proteinases, other		
Plasmin, plasminogen	+	105, 155
Cathepsin B	+	106, 107*
INHIBITORS		
TIMP	−	154, 155
CYTOKINES, NITRIC OXIDE, GROWTH FACTORS		
IL-1α and IL-1β receptor	+	135, 136
TNF-α receptor	+	136, 137
Inducible nitric oxide synthase	+	136, 140
IGF-1	+	173, 174
CHONDROCYTE HYPERTROPHY		
Annexin V	+	201
Type X	+	195
Mineralization	+	212, 213
Apoptosis	+	112, 197
Parathyroid hormone–related peptide	+	202, 203

These changes are typical of early degeneration with limited fibrillation at the articular surface and are mainly observed in the superficial and mid zones unless otherwise indicated. Increases (+) and decreases (−) are indicated. Experimental studies (*) are shown. These changes are reflective primarily of large joint disease.

aggrecanases or ADAMTS-4 and -5 can cleave;[116] the MMP cleavage site is a target for multiple MMPs.[92] There is evidence for enhanced degradation of aggrecan at both these cleavage sites in cartilage matrix in OA.[117]

Of the aggrecanases, ADAMTS-5 has been shown to be the major enzyme responsible for aggrecan loss in experimental murine OA[118] and inflammatory joint disease.[119] These proteinases are also activated outside the cell, probably at the cell surface.[119,120]

A variety of cleavage products of aggrecan accumulate in OA cartilages. Early in cartilage degeneration (Mankin score of 1 to 6), the excessive proteolysis leads to a reduction in molecular size of aggrecan fragments that have accumulated with aging as a result of degradation, probably during a period of many years.[115] With increased degeneration, the sizes of aggrecan fragments increase.[115] This may reflect altered proteolysis, but is more likely the partial degradation of more recently synthesized larger molecules. That new aggrecan synthesis and incorporation occur is reflected by the appearance of epitopes on chondroitin sulfate that are normally only commonly found in actively biosynthetic fetal cartilages.[115,121–123] Some of these epitopes that increase in OA in synovial fluid, such as the 846 epitope,[124,125] are thought to present on newly synthesized molecules that have been released by matrix degradation.[126]

The Causes and Regulation of Cartilage Matrix Degradation

The reasons for this increased proteolysis have been widely studied. Degradation products of matrix molecules may themselves stimulate degradation through chondrocyte and synovial cell receptor-mediated activation, forming a chronic cycle (Fig. 2–4). Different fragments of fibronectin can stimulate chondrocyte-mediated cartilage resorption by cell surface receptor activation[127–129] just as in synovial fibroblasts, where RGD–integrin receptor activation is involved.[130] Fibronectin is produced in increased amounts in OA cartilage.[131] Its degradation may therefore play an important role in establishing positive feedback generation of proteolysis. Cellular responses in OA cartilage involve the production of cytokines such as interleukin (IL)–1, which are known to stimulate degradation[50] and also play an essential autocrine and paracrine role[132] in fibronectin fragment–mediated degradation (Fig. 2–4). Fragments of type II collagen can, when present in sufficient concentration, also induce matrix resorption.[133,134]

In OA, there is increased expression on chondrocytes of the receptors for IL-1[135] and of IL-1 itself, even more than in rheumatoid arthritis,[136] as well as the receptor for tumor necrosis factor α (TNF-α)[99,137] (Table 2–2). The

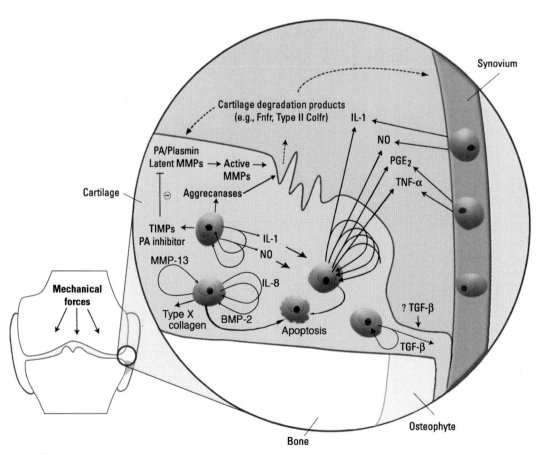

Figure 2–4 Responses of chondrocytes to mechanical forces, cytokines, and matrix degradation products generated by MMPs.

presence of the TNF-α p55 receptor (but not the p75) on OA chondrocytes correlates with the susceptibility of cartilage explants to TNF-α–induced proteoglycan loss.[137]

IL-1 and TNF-α are potent activators of cartilage degradation in vitro.[50] In combination with oncostatin M, IL-1 is even more potent in causing cartilage resorption, but levels of oncostatin M, a member of the IL-6 family, are not usually elevated in synovial fluid in OA.[138] Inhibition of IL-1 or TNF-α by biologic antagonists can suppress cartilage matrix resorption in articular cartilage in culture. It can also stimulate an increase in aggrecan content,[139] probably by inhibiting degradation of newly synthesized molecules.

Inducible nitric oxide synthase (iNOS, or NOS2) is upregulated in OA chondrocytes[140] more so than in rheumatoid articular cartilage,[136] leading to an increased generation of nitric oxide. IL-1α, IL-1β, and TNF-α are potent stimulators of nitric oxide production in cartilage[141] in a manner that can be arrested by osteopontin,[142] which is also upregulated in OA cartilages.[143] The expression by chondrocytes of iNOS, TNF-α, IL-1α, and IL-1β are correlated in arthritis[136] (Fig. 2–4). Nitric oxide mediates the inhibition of aggrecan synthesis induced by IL-1.[144] However, protease activity and proteoglycan degradation are enhanced when nitric oxide production is blocked,[145,146] suggesting that nitric oxide may also play a protective role. Nitric oxide can also induce apoptosis in chondrocytes,[147] but only in the presence of other reactive oxygen species. Inhibition of iNOS reduces the progression of experimental OA.[148] Nonexpression of IL-1β or IL-1 converting enzyme or iNOS can also accelerate the development of surgically-induced murine OA. These observations together point to the importance of physiological

amounts of these molecules to maintain a healthy joint,[146] and suggest that complete suppression of activity could be detrimental from a therapeutic dosing standpoint.

Changes in matrix loading can also induce the production of a variety of pro-inflammatory mediators and promote matrix degradation as well as alter the synthesis of matrix molecules[50,78] (Fig. 2–4). Mechanical compression causes a dose-dependent increase in the synthesis of nitric oxide and prostaglandin E2 through the activation of NOS2 and cyclooxygenase 2 (COX2), respectively, with significant interaction between the NOS2 and COX2 pathways.[149,150] Injurious mechanical compression of cartilage explants at high loading rates and magnitudes results in significant upregulation of MMPs and aggrecanases[151,152] that are also associated with increased loss of proteoglycans as well as other biomarkers of OA.[153]

The pathologic changes in cartilage matrix structure in OA are likely to cause fundamental disturbances in the normal balance resulting from controlled mechanical loading and cytokine and growth factor signaling, which leads to changing gene expression of matrix macromolecules, signaling molecules, and enzymes (Fig. 2–5). Activities of these MMPs are regulated not only at the levels of transcriptional activation, translation, and extracellular proenzyme activation, but also extracellularly at the level of inhibition by tissue inhibitors of metalloproteinases (TIMPs). Four such inhibitors have been described, namely, TIMP-1, -2, -3, and -4. These react with the active MMP in a 1:1 molar ratio. In OA, there is a deficiency of TIMP activity[154,155] favoring excessive proteolysis (Table 2–2). TIMP-3, which is the only TIMP that can bind to extracellular matrix, is capable of inhibiting aggrecan degradation in hyaline cartilage.[156]

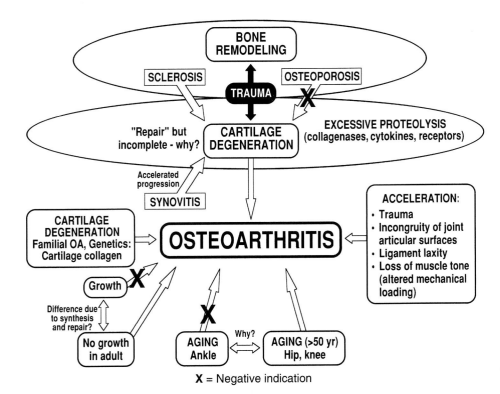

Figure 2–5 Changes observed in cartilage and bone in OA and factors that protect against, accelerate, or are associated with the OA process.

Its expression is upregulated in OA cartilage whereas TIMP-1 and -4 are downregulated.[95]

TGF-β1 can downregulate MMP-1 and -13 as well as IL-1 and TNF receptors on OA chondrocytes.[99] Yet, it can stimulate ADAMTS-4 expression and aggrecan degradation.[157] TGF-β2 can rather selectively suppress the cleavage of type II collagen by collagenases in OA cartilage in culture and reduce the expression of MMPs and proinflammatory cytokines: this also involves suppression of hypertrophy associated genes.[158] The Chitinase 3-like protein glycoprotein 39 (GP39), which is upregulated in OA cartilage, can suppress chondrocyte induction of proinflammatory cytokines, chemokines, and collagenases by IL-1 and TNF-α.[159]

General Changes in Cartilage Matrix Protein Content and Gene Expression

The early damage to the more superficial matrix in early OA is accompanied by an increased content of biglycan and decorin[160] and aggrecan (A.R. Poole and A. Reiner, unpublished data) in the mid and deep zones, no doubt to compensate for the increased loading on the chondrocytes and the damage to and loss of these molecules from the more superficial cartilage. This accompanies the marked increase in the synthesis of type II procollagen in these deeper sites,[114] mainly type IIB as revealed by experimental studies[113] but also some type IIA,[161,162] which is normally observed only before chondroblast differentiation early in development.[163] Overall there is a loss of type II collagen, starting in the more superficial cartilage.[108] There is limited expression and synthesis of type III collagen.[112] Type VI content is, however, increased[164-166] and its filamentous structure is altered,[167] presumably as a result of pericellular remodeling which frequently results in an enlargement of the pericellular matrix.[168] These changes are also reflected as a loss of mechanical properties of the pericellular matrix,[169,170] which results in significant alterations in the biomechanical environment of the chondrocytes.[54]

Aggrecan and link protein synthesis or expression are upregulated in response to the increased damage.[50,115,121,171] There is a general increased expression and synthesis of the proteoglycans versican, fibromodulin, lumican, decorin, and biglycan.[171,172] This is associated with an increase in insulin-like growth factor 1 (IGF-1)[173] and its receptor.[174] IGF-1 is a potent stimulant of aggrecan synthesis and may be responsible for this increase. This increased synthesis is often seen in the same sites where degradation is enhanced. Although bone morphogenetic proteins play key roles in promoting matrix synthesis, BMP-3 is markedly downregulated in OA.[175]

There are changes in the distributions and contents of many other matrix molecules in OA.[50] Cartilage oligomeric protein (COMP) is altered in distribution.[176] Contents of cartilage matrix protein,[177] tenascin,[178] osteonectin,[143] and fibronectin[131] and other molecules are increased with the result that the cartilage reverts in part to a more fetal tissue. These changes are summarized in Table 2–2 and Figure 2–3.

The Chitinase 3-like protein GP 39 (YKL-39), but not YKL-40, is also markedly upregulated in OA cartilage. This protein can modulate IL-1 activity as well as suppress apoptosis and stimulate cell division. It therefore seems to offer protection against degeneration.[159,179] The significance of a variety of early changes in gene expression in OA detected in articular cartilage and of genes that are expressed in cartilage which change in expression in peripheral blood cells in early OA remains to be determined.[180]

The Regulation of Cartilage Matrix Assembly in Osteoarthritis

Throughout the development of OA, synthetic processes are probably much influenced by the degradative cytokines IL-1 and TNF-α, the major anabolic growth factors IGF-1, the transforming growth factor-β (TGF-β) family,[181] the bone morphogenetic proteins (particularly BMP-2 and -7), and the anti-inflammatory or modulatory cytokines of the synovium, cartilage, and other tissues, including platelet-derived growth factor, fibroblast growth factor-2, IL-4, IL-6, IL-10, and IL-13. These and other regulatory molecules contribute in many different ways to anabolism.[50,181,182] Cytokines such as IL-1 can inhibit matrix synthesis whereas IGF-1 can suppress this inhibition.[183] IGF-1 and mRNA levels are increased in OA articular tissue.[184] IGF-1 can decrease the degradation and inhibition of synthesis induced by IL-1.[185] IGF-1 release from chondrocytes is in fact stimulated by IL-1 and TNF-α.[186] In spite of the increase in IGF-1 in OA, OA chondrocytes are hyporesponsive to this growth factor. This may be because IGF-1 activity is excessively restricted by IGFBPs, which are also upregulated[174,187] by cytokines such as IL-1. Proteases can also cleave these binding proteins, regulating their activity.[186,188] Fibroblast growth factor-2 stimulates cell proliferation in articular chondrocytes but does not stimulate synthesis of glycosaminoglycans.[189,190] Synergistic relationships have been demonstrated between growth factors and cytokines in articular cartilage, which help regulate important cellular processes. Chondrocyte proliferation can be amplified by combinations of IL-6 and TGF-β or of fibroblast growth factor and IGF.[186]

Moreover, TGF-β stimulates type II collagen and aggrecan gene expression and inhibits metalloproteinase mRNA expression in synovial fibroblasts and chondrocytes.[181,182] It can suppress IL-1 expression and type collagen cleavage in cartilage,[158] stimulate production of plasminogen activator inhibitor protein 1,[191] and also TIMP synthesis,[50] thereby regulating proteolysis and enhancing synthesis. However, injection of TGF-β in the knee joint of mice results in increased osteoarthritic degeneration, possibly due to increased bone formation and remodeling.[192,193] The balance between these pro-proliferative, anabolic, and catabolic molecules is very complex and clearly fundamentally perturbed in OA and by injury that leads to an altered mechanical environment of the chondrocytes, affecting the biosynthesis of these molecules. Studies of Guinea pig strains with different rates of natural OA development have revealed from serum measurements of cartilage molecular markers of type II collagen synthesis and degradation that the ratio of the markers favors degradation over synthesis in more rapid progressors[194] (N. Gerwin, K. Rudolphi, A.R. Poole, et al., unpublished data).

CHANGES IN THE CHONDROCYTE PHENOTYPE IN RELATIONSHIP TO CELL DEATH, MATRIX DEGRADATION, AND CALCIFICATION IN OSTEOARTHRITIS

In previously uncalcified articular cartilage in OA, there is induction of type X collagen expression and synthesis.[195] Expression of this and other hypertrophy-related genes including MMP-13 is seen very early in micro-lesion development.[98] Hypertrophy is normally only seen in the growth plate when the extracellular collagen network is partially resorbed by MMP-13[50,97,196] and then calcified as cells die as a result of apoptosis. In OA, these events including apoptosis[197,198] reappear in degenerate OA cartilage although some expression data argue against this.[199] The increase in apoptosis corresponds to a reduced cell density and expression of caspase 3.[200] These changes are in association with expression of the cell surface type II collagen receptor annexin V,[201] also highly expressed by early hypertrophic chondrocytes. Parathyroid hormone–related peptide (PTHrP), which is also produced by prehypertrophic cells in the growth plate and suppresses hypertrophy, is also upregulated in OA cartilage.[202,203] The calcium-sensing receptor, expressed by hypertrophic cells, is upregulated with the onset of OA in the guinea pig together with PTHrP.[204]

These changes are initially observed in OA cartilage mainly in the more superficial and mid zones where damage to collagen is most pronounced[205] (Fig. 2–3), and may represent a chondrocyte response to a damaged extracellular matrix with the reversion to a more fetal phenotype. There is also a marked increase in expression of type II collagen[112-114] and MMP-13,[88,206,207] which are also a feature of the shift to hypertrophy in the growth plate.[208] An inhibitor of MMP-13 can suppress hypertrophy,[97] suggesting that MMP-13 is a key proteinase in this process and that excessive collagen cleavage is a trigger for further chondrocyte differentiation.

In the partially calcified OA cartilage delimited by the tidemark and bordered by the subchondral bone, there is a reactivation of endochondral ossification characterized by upregulation of type X collagen expression and duplication or replication of the tidemark, separating this zone from uncalcified cartilage. Vascular invasion from subchondral bone is reinitiated, resembling that seen in endochondral ossification. Moreover, osteophyte formation, an endochondral process, is initiated peripheral to the articular cartilages, leading to bone spurs capped with articular cartilage (Fig. 2–1). Thus, there is a major shift in the physiology of the articular cartilage characteristic of a superimposition of endochondral changes within and associated with articular cartilages. We know that TGF-β signaling is essential to prevent hypertrophy since mice with a functionless type II receptor[209] or a deletion in a Smad signaling component[210] develop a rapid degeneration of articular cartilage associated with extensive chondrocyte hypertrophy and the formation of large osteophytes. PGE$_2$, generated when TGF-β2 is added to OA cartilage, suppresses hypertrophy and collagenase activity.[158] A transcription factor, early growth response protein-1 (Egr-1), which can stimulate TGF-β expression and suppress apoptosis, is very down-regulated in OA, favoring a drop in TGF-β content.[211]

Hypertrophy is accompanied by calcification of the normally uncalcified extracellular matrix of articular cartilage. More than 90% of OA subjects show evidence for limited calcification of articular cartilages;[212] there is also a high incidence of hydroxyapatite crystals in joint fluids.[213,214] In calcium pyrophosphate deposition (CPPD) disease, joints affected by mineral deposition, such as the shoulders, wrists, and metacarpophalangeal joints, are different from those affected in idiopathic OA[215] (see Chapter 13).

Although CPPD and hydroxyapatite crystal aggregates can, under some conditions, be markedly phlogistic in both animal models and cell culture, there is equivocal evidence in cartilage that crystals can injure chondrocytes directly.[216-218] As in growth cartilage matrix, matrix vesicles have been detected in OA articular cartilages, often with associated minerals as well as cellular generation of pyrophosphate.[219] Apoptotic cell particles may also generate minerals in the presence of adenosine triphosphate.[220] These changes in OA cartilage are summarized in Table 2–2 and Figure 2–3.

Physiologic concentrations of extracellular pyrophosphate (PP$_i$) regulate calcification that results in basic calcium phosphate crystal deposition. Hydrolysis of excess PP$_i$ promotes crystal formation in OA via elevated inorganic phosphate generation.[221] PP$_i$ is generated from nucleoside triphosphates by nucleotide pyrophosphatase phosphodiesterase PC-1. The extracellular concentration of PP$_i$ is regulated via the trans-membrane protein ANK. In OA cartilage, ANK is upregulated.[222] This would this favor the elevation of extracellular PP$_i$. Interestingly, increased ANK expression promotes MMP-13 expression,[222] providing a link between calcification and increased MMP-13 expression, both of which are features of chondrocyte hypertrophy.[50]

THE REMODELLING OF SUBCHONDRAL BONE IN OSTEOARTHRITIS

Pronounced changes in subchondral bone occur in OA, and may even occur in sites remote from the affected joints. Femoral neck bone is less stiff and less dense in hip OA, but not as reduced in density as in osteoporosis.[223] Bone mineral density remote from degenerate joints in arms and spine is elevated.[224,225] Bone loss is elevated in men with hip OA.[225] Women with incident knee OA have a higher bone mineral density in the spine and hip than those without disease.[226] In generalized OA, there is also hypermineralization;[227] yet in hand OA in women, there is evidence that with increasing grade of OA, bone mass is decreased.[228] Subchondral bone in hip OA is less mineralized and has more osteoid indicative of incomplete mineralization.[229,230] The elevated content of osteoid is accompanied by increased synthesis and content of type I collagen and increased alkaline phosphatase content.[230] Together, these changes are indicative of increased turnover of bone in hip OA. TGF-β, a bone growth factor, is also increased in content.[230] Such changes are also seen in remote sites, such as in the iliac crest, where osteocalcin, IGF-1, IGF-2, and TGF-β contents are increased.[227]

These observations raise the possibility that bone turnover may be different in people before the development of OA and that these changes may vary according to the type of OA. They may clearly contribute to or even cause the onset of OA. Analyses of type II procollagen production in OA articular cartilages reveal increased synthesis reflected by elevated C-propeptide concentration. Yet in the peripheral blood of OA patients, there is a significant reduction of the C-propeptide. This also suggests a systemic alteration in cartilage type II collagen synthesis, which again may be a risk factor for the onset of OA.[114] Observations of this kind raise questions as to whether idiopathic OA may result more from specific fundamental differences wherein local factors (such as biomechanical) precipitate joint disease via interactions with systemic metabolic factors in any given individual. Thus systemic bone or cartilage changes alone may predispose people to these degenerative changes in joints where the mechanical environment may reveal such abnormalities. It is interesting to note that peak bone mass is increased in the hips of daughters of women with hand OA.[231] Clearly there would appear to be genetic linkages in the etiology of this disease.

The degeneration of articular cartilage may be accompanied or possibly preceded by increased subchondral bone turnover, as suggested by bone scintigraphy. In the absence of MRI, it is not possible to be clear as to whether the bone changes preceded those in articular cartilages. Such bone changes are predictive of the development of hand OA,[232] the progression of knee OA,[233] and generalized nodal OA.[234] Studies in humans and animals, such as the aging guinea pig, using histologic analyses and magnetic resonance imaging, suggest that degenerative changes in articular cartilages are accompanied by local changes in subchondral bone that involve cyst formation and altered trabecular and osteoid thickness and bone formation and turnover.[235-238]

The development of osteophytes so often seen peripherally in an OA joint involves the formation of a cap of new articular cartilage as well as new bone formation as part of an endochondral process. Experimentally, it has been shown to be correlated with articular cartilage loss elsewhere in the joint.[239] These changes and relationships are often compartmental, suggesting localized events. The overall increase in bone turnover in OA and resultant changes are reflected by increases in bone-specific deoxypyridinoline cross-links in urine as a result of enhanced osteoclastic resorption of bone.[126,240] These changes in urine may also result from more extensive systemic change.

Changes in both the articular cartilages and the subchondral bone of a degenerate joint no doubt reflect the interdependence of these tissues within the joint. Changes in one tissue would influence mechanical loading of the other and alter tissue turnover. Thus, it is not surprising that such changes may occur simultaneously. The presence of bone marrow abnormalities on MRI has been reported to be associated with cartilage remodeling based on a type II collagen biomarker assay.[241] Whether this marker reflects changes in uncalcified cartilage or in the calcified cartilage adjacent to subchondral bone or both is not known. It is noteworthy that in the ankle, where OA is much less common than in the hip or knee, cartilage degeneration of the talar is not associated with an increase in subchondral bone density,[242] indicating different responses in ankle joints that may influence OA development. Studies of bone changes in familial OA (caused by a cartilage collagen mutation, for example) compared with idiopathic OA may be of use in determining whether these cartilage changes occur together with or independently of those in bone.

In osteoporosis, a condition that results in excessive resorption and a net loss of bone mineral density, it is uncommon to observe OA (Fig. 2–5), and vice versa.[243-245] The structure, turnover, and density of bone would therefore appear to influence articular cartilage turnover and play a significant role in the pathogenesis of OA. Thus, a controlled reduction in bone density may help in controlling joint degeneration.

The interrelationships between bone and cartilage changes in OA may also result from the molecular effects of the products of one tissue on another. Bone cell cultures from OA subchondral bone, but not from nonarthritic bone, can stimulate proteoglycan release from nonarthritic human articular cartilage.[246] Further studies of this kind are needed.

Calcitonin suppresses osteoclastic resorption of bone, a key component of the remodeling of bone. It can also reduce both cartilage pathology[85] and suppress bone changes[247] in experimental dog OA. Whether this effect is achieved through the control of bone changes or also involves a more direct stimulation of proteoglycan synthesis by chondrocytes[248] is unclear. Alendronate, another potent inhibitor of bone resorption, can also reduce cartilage degeneration and osteophyte formation in experimental OA in the rat,[249] again suggesting that bone remodeling in OA plays an important role in the degenerative process.

SYNOVITIS AND INFLAMMATION IN OSTEOARTHRITIS

OA is not considered an inflammatory arthritis, and the synovial fluid leukocyte count is characteristically less than 3000 cells/mL. To the extent that acute synovial fluid leukocytic inflammation does occur in OA, it is often the result of secondary crystal-induced synovitis (either calcium apatite or calcium pyrophosphate dihydrate). However, low-grade inflammatory processes nevertheless occur in osteoarthritic synovial tissues that contribute to disease pathogenesis, and many of the clinical symptoms and signs seen in OA joints clearly reflect synovial inflammation (e.g., joint swelling and effusion, stiffness, occasionally redness). Synovial histological changes include synovial hypertrophy and hyperplasia with an increased number of lining cells, often accompanied by infiltration of the sublining tissue with scattered foci of lymphocytes. Cartilage breakdown products, derived from the articular surface as a result of mechanical or enzymatic destruction of the cartilage, can provoke the release of collagenase and other hydrolytic enzymes from synovial cells and macrophages.[250]

Cartilage breakdown products are also believed to result in mononuclear cell infiltration and vascular hyperplasia in the synovial membrane in OA.[251] A consequence of these low-grade inflammatory processes is the induction of synovial IL-1β and TNF-α, which are likely contributors to the degradative cascade.

Recent studies have also demonstrated that, even in the absence of clinical signs of synovitis, there is frequently localized synovitis in patients with OA, which may be most pronounced immediately adjacent to the OA lesion of the articular cartilage. For example, arthroscopy has demonstrated localized synovial proliferative and inflammatory changes in up to 50% of patients with knee OA.[252,253] Proteases and cytokines produced by activated synovium have been suggested to accelerate deterioration of contiguous cartilage lesions.[253] Areas of increased radionuclide uptake ("hot spots") on bone scintigraphy have also been reported to identify joints more likely to progress by radiographic criteria—or to require surgical intervention—over a 5-year period.[233]

Synovial tissues and cartilage also synthesize anti-inflammatory cytokines, including IL-13, IL-4, and IL-10. Indeed, synovial fluid of OA patients contains increased levels of these factors, which can decrease PGE$_2$ release, IL-β, TNF-α, and MMPs while upregulating TIMP.[254,255] Another anti-inflammatory molecule produced by joint tissues is the IL-1 receptor antagonist (IL-1Ra), which, like soluble IL-1 receptors discussed above, competes with cell surface receptors for IL-1 and thereby reduces nitric oxide production, PGE2 synthesis, or protease secretion. Although the production of IL-1Ra is increased in OA, increased production is insufficient to reverse the catabolic effects of augmented IL-β.

A number of investigations have revealed that serum HA is upregulated in patients with rheumatoid arthritis and is related to joint inflammation and radiologic progression.[256] HA is also often increased in OA patients.[257] Those with persistently elevated serum HA levels exhibit more rapid disease progression.[258] HA levels also indirectly correlate with minimal joint space.[258,259] COMP is synthesized by synovial cells as well as by chondrocytes. COMP synthesis is stimulated by TGF-β1, which is produced in inflammation.[260] Patients who show serum elevations of COMP often exhibit progression of joint damage.[261-263] Serum/plasma levels appear to be closely associated with hip synovitis[241] and knee OA.[264] Elevation of both HA and COMP is associated with a greater risk of progression in hip OA.[265]

A glycosylated derivative of the pyridinoline collagen cross-link is enriched in human synovium and present in low levels in cartilage and other soft tissues.[266] It can be detected in urine. Its close association with the presence of knee OA and severity[267] suggests the presence of synovitis, a feature of which is increased content of type I and III collagens and their turnover.

MMP-3 and MMP-9, which are elevated in synovial cells from patients with rapidly destructive hip OA, are also elevated in synovial fluid, plasma, and sera in these patients.[268,269] The elevation of MMP-9 is markedly reduced a year after arthroplasty, pointing to the joint carti-

lages and/or bone as the cause of this elevation, probably by triggering a synovitis. This may involve an immune reaction since T lymphocyte immunity to cartilage aggrecan and link protein is enhanced in OA.[270] In experimental OA, T cell immunity to fibrillar collagens also develops.[271]

Chemokines are also elevated. Macrophage inflammatory protein-1 is elevated in OA synovial fluid over serum as in RA.[272] Eotaxin-1, RANTES, and MCP-1$_α$ are elevated in plasma of OA patients.[273]

Fas ligand, which induces apoptosis, is also present in synovial fluid in OA[274] and may account in part for the enhanced apoptosis in articular cartilage in OA by engagement of the receptor for this ligand on chondrocytes and synovial cells. The presence of systemic inflammation in OA, albeit limited, is also revealed by the small but significant increase in the serum acute-phase molecule C-reactive protein,[275] which is predictive of progression in early onset disease.[276] These are but some examples of evidence for an inflammatory process in OA that in some cases may be more pronounced within a joint and may accelerate joint degeneration by the release of cytokines, chemokines, proteinases, and other mediators that cause joint degeneration.

Pain in Osteoarthritis

Arthritis pain is the most common cause of pain in aged populations[277] and arguably the most debilitating aspect of OA. Although the presence of knee pain increases with radiographic disease severity in most studies, it is apparent that the severity of abnormalities by routine radiography does not correlate with pain severity in the individual patient. MRI studies have indicated that in patients with knee OA, knee pain severity was associated with subarticular bone attrition, bone marrow lesions, synovitis/effusion, and meniscal tears.[278]

Pain severity in persons with OA is not a simple phenomenon, and can arise from any of several innervated tissues. The joints of the appendicular skeleton are innervated by the peripheral nervous system in every tissue except cartilage where innervation is peripheral in the periosteum, synovium, capsule, ligaments, and subchondral bone. Here nociceptors monitor the environment. Neuro-innervation can determine disease onset. Limbs paralyzed by hemiplegia or poliomyelitis are often spared in the development of OA or RA.[279,280] Patients with different joint involvement in OA can exhibit pronounced hyperalgesia to thermal and mechanical stimuli including uninvolved joints.[281-283] Following total hip arthroplasty, there is a return to normal pain thresholds in the contralateral hip.[284] The association of movement with pain suggests the contribution of central mechanisms.[285] Nerve growth factor plays a major role in inflammatory hyperalgesia: IL-1 contributes to the upregulation of this neurotrophin and hyperalgesia.[286] There is evidence for an association between pain, synovitis, and changes in subchondral bone.[287] Neuropeptides generated by nerve fibers are messengers that link the peripheral nervous system and inflammation. C-fiber stimulation causes Substance P release, which in turn induces mast cell and platelet degranulation with histamine, serotonin, bradykinin, and platelet activating factor release, capable of not only causing vasodilation and vasopermiabilisation but of stimulating nociceptors and amplifying and prolonging afferent discharge into the central nervous system.[288] Prostaglandins can also contribute to painful afferent sensory responses.[289,290] Substance P can directly activate synovial cells to induce collagenase and PGE$_2$ release[291] and stimulate monocytes/macrophages and other inflammatory cells to produce IL-1, TNF-α, and IL-6.[292]

Neuropeptides can also perform various regulatory functions. Calcitonin gene-related peptide and vasoactive intestinal peptide (VIP) can each inhibit synovial cell proliferation and the expression of proinflammatory cytokines and MMP-2.[293] Somatostatin can modulate the production of MMP-1 and MMP-9.[294] The parasympathetic vagus nerve, which innervates all major organs, can control TNF-α synthesis. It has sensory (input) and motor (output) fibers to sense and suppress inflammation. The sensory nerve can detect IL-1 and respond by releasing acetylcholine which suppresses TNF-α and IL-1 generation by macrophages. Electrical stimulation of this nerve prevents TNF release from macrophages. Surgical section removes this protection.[295] This is because the acetylcholine normally released by the nerve activates α7 nicotinic acid receptors on macrophages which suppress the release of these proinflammatory cytokines.[296] The sympathetic nervous system mediates unloading-induced bone loss through the suppression of bone formation by osteoblasts and enhanced resorption by osteoclasts.[297] Leptin has an anti-osteogenic function that is mediated by sympathetic neural pathways that control bone remodeling. This occurs by sympathetic signaling of β2 adrenergic receptors on osteoblasts. In mice deficient in the receptor Adrb2, the sympathetic system favors bone resorption; this occurs by an increase in Rankl expression on osteoblast progenitor cells. Leptin controls the expression of the neuropeptide cocaine amphetamine regulated transcript 9CART, which inhibits bone resorption by modulating Rankl expression. Thus leptin regulated neural pathways control both aspects of bone remodeling.[298]

Neuropeptides can also help explain some of the effects of the nervous system on the skeleton. VIP potentiates IL-6 production by osteoblasts induced by proinflammatory osteotropic cytokines, including IL-1.[299] Substance P stimulates osteoclast formation.[300] Chondrocytes express functional μ-opioid receptors that can be activated with β-endorphin[301] causing increased IL-1 and TNF-α generation.[302]

Ipsilateral and contralateral joint involvement whereby joint inflammation in a single joint can induce distal bilateral degeneration of articular cartilage has also been ascribed to neurogenic mechanisms and neuropeptides by using an antagonist of neurokinin-1 and spinal compression to inhibit the involvement of the other joint.[280]

Thus it can be seen with these examples that neurological mechanisms influence not only the perception of pain that is altered in OA but also regulate skeletal turnover and

inflammation. There is still much to be learned of this much neglected area of research in our understanding of the pathogenesis of OA.

THERAPEUTIC TARGETS FOR THE MANAGEMENT OF OSTEOARTHRITIS

Cartilage is clearly a principal target because of its paramount importance in joint articulation. Despite the tremendous impact of this disease, however, current therapies are palliative and there are no disease-modifying OA drugs (DMOADs) currently available for clinical use. Nonetheless, a number of promising molecular targets exist in the development of pharmacologic therapies for OA, and useful and comprehensive review of such therapeutic approaches has recently been published.[303]

For example, there has been significant emphasis on targeting MMPs that cleave collagen because collagen degradation is clearly indicated in OA pathogenesis. The collagenase MMP-13 is thought to be an important target for the control of collagen fibril damage in articular cartilage. To date, doxycycline is the only molecule that can regulate collagenase activities in vitro,[304] control the progression of experimental OA,[305] and be used without serious side effects in the treatment of knee OA.[306]

Cartilage proteoglycan aggrecan degradation by aggrecanases is also of very much interest as a target. Although the aggrecanase ADAMTS-5 may be rate limiting in the degradation of this molecule in animals (see section on Proteinases of OA Cartilage), it remains to be seen whether it is in humans. This is because aggrecan, unlike type II collagen, is susceptible to cleavage by many proteinases such as those of the ADAMTS family. Based upon experiments in knockout mice, ADAMTS-5 has been reported to be the "primary" aggrecanase responsible for aggrecan degradation in a murine model of OA, and could be a potential target for therapeutic intervention in human OA.[119]

Another approach is to restore the balance between synthesis and degradation by enhancing cartilage matrix synthesis. A clearer identification of the key growth factors involved in matrix assembly is a priority, particularly since some of these can suppress degradation. IGF-1 is of obvious importance in view of its potency and upregulation in OA,[173] but there may be more potent growth factors or combinations thereof that can be used to renew matrix assembly and control degradation. A combination of MMP inhibitors and enhanced stimulation of matrix synthesis may prove most effective.

Work with bone morphogenetic protein 7 has revealed its capacity to promote matrix assembly in articular cartilage and to inhibit the degradative effects of IL-1.[307] We have already discussed how TGF-β2 is a potent stimulant of matrix synthesis,[50] and can suppress the cleavage of collagen by collagenases and chondrocyte hypertrophy in OA cartilage in culture.[158] Still other approaches have targeted the pro-inflammatory mediators such as nitric oxide through selective inhibition of NOS2 and animal models of OA.[148] These studies have shown significant promise for inhibiting disease progression by decreasing chondrocyte apoptosis as well as cartilage catabolism via inhibition of NOS2. While the mechanisms for these findings are not fully understood, they may involve the local suppression of other inflammatory cytokines such as IL-1 or TNF-α.

Brandt et al. recently reported that doxycyline slows joint space narrowing (JSN) in patients with OA of the medial tibiofemoral compartment.[306] In this placebo-controlled trial, 431 obese women (ages 45 to 64 years) with unilateral radiographic knee OA were randomly assigned to receive 30 months of treatment with doxycycline 100 mg or placebo twice daily. Doxycycline reduced JSN in the OA knee by approximately 30% at 30 months; however, the mean progression of JSN in both groups was limited (0.30 ± 0.60 mm vs. 0.45 ± 0.70 mm).

IL-1β has attracted significant interest as a target for disease modification in OA. The intra-articular injection of recombinant human IL-1Ra attenuates the development of cartilage lesions and the expression of MMPs in the canine experimental OA model.[308] Two groups have also demonstrated that in vivo transfer of the IL-1Ra gene prevents disease progression in the meniscectomy rabbit model of knee OA.[309,310] In human OA, the benefit of intra-articular IL-1Ra injection for symptomatic knee OA has been reported in an open-label 12-week study;[311] however, in a follow-up controlled trial by these authors, intra-articular injection of IL1-Ra reduced knee pain at day 4, but was not more effective than placebo at 1 month. In addition to biological IL-1 antagonists, small molecule drugs are in development that interfere with the conversion of intracellular precursor IL-1β to active IL-1β by inhibiting caspase-1, the iNOS. Fundamental changes in bone in OA and the relative absence of OA in patients with osteoporosis (and vice versa) raise issues as to the possibility of controlling cartilage degeneration by modifying bone turnover and density. This has also been reviewed in the section on bone changes. Would controlled loss of bone density slow the process of degeneration? To date, DMOAD trials using the bisphosphonate to slow progression of knee OA have had mixed results.[312]

Regulation of synovitis is another target. About 10% of the OA population is thought to have a pronounced synovitis, comparable in numbers to the total rheumatoid population. We know that the incidence of much of the hip and knee OA is greater in women than in men, but we know almost nothing of the reasons for this. Clearly, much needs to be done to determine whether sex hormones regulate cartilage turnover.

None of these treatments will be effective if we rely on existing clinical assessments for the degenerative process. When most patients present with an OA joint, the disease is usually advanced and much damage has been done. For the future, it is important to detect and treat the disease early by employing new detection systems such as new imaging and biomarker modalities be they protein or gene based. Only then will therapy be most likely to succeed. Inevitably, this will mean the introduction of screening programs to identify these early changes. Otherwise, we must be content for now with halting further degeneration and slowing OA development elsewhere. We must also not forget the opportunities to treat single large joints such as the knee. This is an attractive consideration in view of the experience gained with intra-articular therapy with HA preparations and steroid usage. It also offers an opportunity to avoid or minimize possible side effects.

If we can effectively control the pain of OA, we will have already made a great stride forward. Much research has pinpointed new targets to control the pain of arthritis. Pharmacologic stimulation of the vagus nerve cholinergic anti-inflammatory pathway offers new therapeutic opportunities.[313] These discoveries are being very actively pursued. We will probably find that many disease modifying drugs lack symptomatic relief for the patient. Inevitably, combination therapy will be needed in such cases.

CONCLUSIONS

In the last two decades, we have made significant progress in our understanding of the pathophysiology of OA. This has revealed a complex series of molecular changes at the cell, matrix, and tissue levels and complex interactions between tissues that make up the joint. Some of these are summarized in Figure 2–2 and Figure 2–5. We can now better understand how these changes develop and progress, as well as the fact that tissues other than cartilage are involved in the disease process. Opportunities for the management of disease progression and targets for therapeutic intervention have been identified and can now be tested for the first time. The future of OA research is extremely promising, and some real opportunities for the effective therapeutic management of OA are now available.

ACKNOWLEDGMENTS

The authors' work has been funded by Shriners Hospitals for Children; the Canadian Institutes of Health Research and the Canadian Arthritis Network (A.R.P.); and the National Institutes of Health (A.R.P., F.G., S.B.A.).

REFERENCES

1. Altman R, Asch E, Bloch D, et al. Development of criteria for the classification and reporting of osteoarthritis. Classification of osteoarthritis of the knee. Diagnostic and Therapeutic Criteria Committee of the American Rheumatism Association. Arthritis Rheum 29:1039–1049, 1986.
2. Brandt KD, Mankin HJ, Shulman LE. Workshop on etiopathogenesis of osteoarthritis. J Rheumatol 13:1126–1160, 1986.
3. Holderbaum D, Haqqi TM, Moskowitz RW. Genetics and osteoarthritis: exposing the iceberg. Arthritis Rheum 42:397–405, 1999.
4. Olsen BR. Role of cartilage collagens in formation of the skeleton. Ann N Y Acad Sci 785:124–130, 1996.
5. Lieberman SA, Bjorkengren AG, Hoffman AR. Rheumatologic and skeletal changes in acromegaly. Endocrinol Metab Clin North Am 21:615–631, 1992.
6. Evans CH, Brown TD. Role of physical and mechanical agents in degrading the matrix. In: Woessner JFJ, Howell DS, eds. Joint Cartilage Degradation; Basic and Clinical Aspects. New York: Marcel Dekker; 1993:187–208.
7. Radin EL, Burr DB, Caterson B, et al. Mechanical determinants of osteoarthrosis. Semin Arthritis Rheum 21:12–21, 1991.

8. Buckwalter JA. Osteoarthritis and articular cartilage use, disuse, and abuse: experimental studies. J Rheumatol Suppl 43:13–15, 1995.

9. Palmoski MJ, Brandt KD. Running inhibits the reversal of atrophic changes in canine knee cartilage after removal of a leg cast. Arthritis Rheum 24:1329–1337, 1981.

10. Setton LA, Elliott DM, Mow VC. Altered mechanics of cartilage with osteoarthritis: human osteoarthritis and an experimental model of joint degeneration. Osteoarthritis Cartilage 7:2–14, 1999.

11. Setton LA, Mow VC, Muller FJ, et al. Mechanical properties of canine articular cartilage are significantly altered following transection of the anterior cruciate ligament. J Orthop Res 12:451–463, 1994.

12. Setton LA, Mow VC, Muller FJ, et al. Mechanical behavior and biochemical composition of canine knee cartilage following periods of joint disuse and disuse with remobilization. Osteoarthritis Cartilage 5:1–16, 1997.

13. Grumbles RM, Howell DS, Howard GA, et al. Cartilage metalloproteases in disuse atrophy. J Rheumatol Suppl 43:146–148, 1995.

14. Helminen HJ, Jurvelin J, Kiviranta I, et al. Joint loading effects on articular cartilage: A historical review. In: Helminen HJ, Kiviranta I, Tammi M, et al., eds. Joint Loading: Biology and Health of Articular Structures. Bristol: Wright and Sons; 1–46, 1987.

15. Cheung HS, Setton LA, Guilak F, et al. Upregulation of metalloproteinases in articular cartilage resultant from disuse immobilization, as well as subsequent vigorous exercise. Trans Orthop Res Soc 24:40, 1999.

16. Lammi MJ, Hakkinen TP, Parkkinen JJ, et al. Effects of long-term running exercise on canine femoral head articular cartilage. Agents & Actions—Supplements 39:95–99, 1993.

17. Lane NE, Buckwalter JA. Exercise: a cause of osteoarthritis? Rheum Dis Clin North Am 19:617–633, 1993.

18. Kraus VB. Pathogenesis and treatment of osteoarthritis. Med Clin North Am 81:85–112, 1997.

19. Griffin TM, Guilak F. The role of mechanical loading in the onset and progression of osteoarthritis. Exerc Sport Sci Rev 33:195–200, 2005.

20. Lane JM, Chisena E, Black J. Experimental knee instability: Early mechanical property changes in articular cartilage in a rabbit model. Clin Orthop Rel Res 140:262–265, 1979.

21. Howell DS, Treadwell BV, Trippel SB. Etiopathogenesis of osteoarthritis. In: Moskowitz RW, Howell DS, Goldberg VM, et al., eds. Osteoarthritis, Diagnosis and Medical/Surgical Management. 2nd ed. Philadelphia: W.B. Saunders; pp 233–252, 1992.

22. Pond MJ, Nuki G. Experimentally induced osteoarthritis in the dog. Ann Rheum Dis 32:387–388, 1973.

23. Moskowitz RW, Davis W, Sammarco J. Experimentally induced degenerative joint lesions following partial meniscectomy in the rabbit. Arthritis Rheum 16:397–405, 1973.

24. McDevitt C, Gilbertson E, Muir H. An experimental model of osteoarthritis; early morphological and biochemical changes. J Bone Joint Surg 59B:24–35, 1977.

25. Eyre DR, McDevitt CA, Billingham ME, et al. Biosynthesis of collagen and other matrix proteins by articular cartilage in experimental osteoarthrosis. Biochem J 188:823–837, 1980.

26. Altman RD, Tenenbaum J, Latta L, et al. Biomechanical and biochemical properties of dog cartilage in experimentally induced osteoarthritis. Ann Rheum Dis 43:83–90, 1984.

27. Sandy JD, Adams ME, Billingham ME, et al. In vivo and in vitro stimulation of chondrocyte biosynthetic activity in early experimental osteoarthritis. Arthritis Rheum 27:388–397, 1984.

28. Guilak F, Ratcliffe A, Lane N, et al. Mechanical and biochemical changes in the superficial zone of articular cartilage in canine experimental osteoarthritis. J Orthop Res 12:474–484, 1994.

29. Messier SP. Osteoarthritis of the knee and associated factors of age and obesity: effects on gait. Med Sci Sports Exerc 26:1446–1452, 1994.

30. Das UN. Obesity, metabolic syndrome X, and inflammation. Nutrition 18:430–432, 2002.

31. Powell A, Teichtahl AJ, Wluka AE, et al. Obesity: a preventable risk factor for large joint osteoarthritis which may act through biomechanical factors. Br J Sports Med 39:4–5, 2005.

32. Hutton CW. Generalised osteoarthritis: an evolutionary problem? Lancet 1:1463–1465, 1987.

33. O'Connor BL, Palmoski MJ, Brandt KD. Neurogenic acceleration of degenerative joint lesions. J Bone Joint Surg Am 67:562–572, 1985.

34. Yang KH, Riegger CL, Rodgers MM. Diminished lower limb deceleration as a factor in early stage osteoarthrosis. Trans Orthop Res Soc 14:52, 1989.

35. O'Reilly SC, Jones A, Muir KR, et al. Quadriceps weakness in knee osteoarthritis: the effect on pain and disability. Ann Rheum Dis 57:588–594, 1998.

36. McAlindon T, Felson DT. Nutrition: risk factors for osteoarthritis. Ann Rheum Dis 56:397–400, 1997.

37. Sokoloff L. The history of Kashin-Beck disease. N Y State J Med 89:343–351, 1989.

38. Utiger RD. Kashin-Beck disease—expanding the spectrum of iodine-deficiency disorders. N Engl J Med 339:1156–1158, 1998.

39. Aurich M, Squires GR, Reiner A, et al. Differential matrix degradation and turnover in early cartilage lesions of human knee and ankle joints. Arthritis Rheum 52:112–119, 2005.

40. Hardingham TE, Fosang AJ, Dudhia J. The structure, function and turnover of aggrecan, the large aggregating proteoglycan from cartilage. Eur J Clin Chem Clin Biochem 32:249–257, 1994.

41. Maroudas A. Physicochemical properties of articular cartilage. In: Freeman M, ed. Adult Articular Cartilage. Tunbridge Wells: Pitman Medical; 1979, pp 215–290.

42. Hodge W, Fijan R, Carlson K, et al. Contact pressures in the human hip joint measured in vivo. Proc Natl Acad Sci USA 83:2879–2883, 1986.

43. Mow VC, Kuei SC, Lai WM, et al. Biphasic creep and stress relaxation of articular cartilage in compression: Theory and experiments. J Biomech Eng 102:73–84, 1980.

44. Frank EH, Grodzinsky AJ. Cartilage electromechanics—I. Electrokinetic transduction and the effects of electrolyte pH and ionic strength. J Biomech Eng 20:615–627, 1987.

45. Lai WM, Hou JS, Mow VC. A triphasic theory for the swelling and deformation behaviors of articular cartilage. J Biomech Eng 113:245–258, 1991.

46. Kempson GE, Muir H, Pollard C, et al. The tensile properties of the cartilage of human femoral condyles related to the content of collagen and glycosaminoglycans. Biochim Biophys Acta 297:456–472, 1973.

47. Roth V, Mow VC. The intrinsic tensile behavior of the matrix of bovine articular cartilage and its variation with age. J Bone Joint Surg 62:1102–1117, 1980.

48. Kempson GE. Age-related changes in the tensile properties of human articular cartilage: a comparative study between the femoral head of the hip joint and the talus of the ankle joint. Biochim Biophys Acta 1075:223–230, 1991.

49. Chen AC, Temple MM, Ng DM, et al. Induction of advanced glycation end products and alterations of the tensile properties of articular cartilage. Arthritis Rheum 46:3212–3217, 2002.

50. Poole AR. Cartilage in health and disease. In: Koopman WJ, Moreland LW, eds. Arthritis and Allied Conditions. A Textbook of Rheumatology. 15th ed. Baltimore: Williams & Wilkins; 2005, pp 223–269.

51. Setton LA, Tohyama H, Mow VC. Swelling and curling behaviors of articular cartilage. J Biomech Eng 120:355–361, 1998.

52. Narmoneva DA, Wang JY, Setton LA. Nonuniform swelling-induced residual strains in articular cartilage. J Biomech 32:401–408, 1999.

53. Flahiff CM, Kraus VB, Huebner JL, et al. Cartilage mechanics in the guinea pig model of osteoarthritis studied with an osmotic loading method. Osteoarthritis Cartilage 12:383–388, 2004.

54. Alexopoulos LG, Setton LA, Guilak F. The biomechanical role of the chondrocyte pericellular matrix in articular cartilage. Acta Biomater 1:317–325, 2005.

55. Malcom LL. An experimental investigation of the frictional and deformational responses of articular cartilage interfaces to static and dynamic loading [dissertation]. San Diego, University of California, San Diego, 1976.

56. Mow VC, Ateshian GA. Lubrication and wear of diarthrodial joints. In: Mow VC, Hayes WC, eds. Basic Orthopaedic Biomechanics, 2nd Ed. Philadelphia: Lippincott-Raven; 1997, pp 275–315.

57. Park S, Krishnan R, Nicoll SB, et al. Cartilage interstitial fluid load support in unconfined compression. J Biomech 36: 1785–1796, 2003.
58. McCutchen CW. Joint lubrication. Bull Hosp Jt Dis Orthop Inst 43:118–129, 1983.
59. Hou JS, Mow VC, Lai WM, et al. An analysis of the squeeze-film lubrication mechanism for articular cartilage. J Biomech 25: 247–259, 1992.
60. Swann DA, Slayter HS, Silver FH. The molecular structure of lubricating glycoprotein-I, the boundary lubricant for articular cartilage. J Biol Chem 256:5921–5925, 1981.
61. Flannery CR, Hughes CE, Schumacher BL, et al. Articular cartilage superficial zone protein (SZP) is homologous to megakaryocyte stimulating factor precursor and is a multifunctional proteoglycan with potential growth-promoting, cytoprotective, and lubricating properties in cartilage metabolism. Biochem Biophys Res Commun 254:535–541, 1999.
62. Jay GD, Tantravahi U, Britt DE, et al. Homology of lubricin and superficial zone protein (SZP): products of megakaryocyte stimulating factor (MSF) gene expression by human synovial fibroblasts and articular chondrocytes localized to chromosome 1q25. J Orthop Res 19:677–687, 2001.
63. Marcelino J, Carpten JD, Suwairi WM, et al. CACP, encoding a secreted proteoglycan, is mutated in camptodactyly-arthropathy-coxa vara-pericarditis syndrome. Nat Genet 23:319–322, 1999.
64. Guilak F, Sah RL, Setton LA. Physical regulation of cartilage metabolism. In: Mow VC, Hayes WC, eds. Basic Orthopaedic Biomechanics. 2nd ed. Philadelphia: Lippincott-Raven, 1997, 179–207.
65. Gray ML, Pizzanelli AM, Grodzinsky AJ, et al. Mechanical and physiochemical determinants of the chondrocyte biosynthetic response. J Orthop Res 6:777–792, 1988.
66. Sah RL, Doong JY, Grodzinsky AJ, et al. Effects of compression on the loss of newly synthesized proteoglycans and proteins from cartilage explants. Arch Biochem Biophys 286:20–29, 1991.
67. Guilak F, Meyer BC, Ratcliffe A, et al. The effects of matrix compression on proteoglycan metabolism in articular cartilage explants. Osteoarthritis Cartilage 2:91–101, 1994.
68. Torzilli PA, Grigiene R, Huang C, et al. Characterization of cartilage metabolic response to static and dynamic stress using a mechanical explant test system. J Biomech 30:1–9, 1997.
69. Farquhar T, Xia Y, Mann K, et al. Swelling and fibronectin accumulation in articular cartilage explants after cyclical impact. J Orthop Res 14:417–423, 1996.
70. Chen C-T, Burton-Wurster N, Borden C, et al. Chondrocyte necrosis and apoptosis in impact damaged articular cartilage. J Orthop Res 19:703–711, 2001.
71. Loening AM, James IE, Levenston ME, et al. Injurious mechanical compression of bovine articular cartilage induces chondrocyte apoptosis. Arch Biochem Biophys 381:205–212, 2000.
72. Stockwell RA. Structure and function of the chondrocyte under mechanical stress. In: Helminen HJ, Kiviranta I, Tammi M, et al., eds. Joint Loading: Biology and Health of Articular Structures. Bristol: Wright and Sons, 1987, pp 126–148.
73. Squires GR, Okouneff S, Ionescu M, et al. The pathobiology of focal lesion development in aging human articular cartilage and molecular matrix changes characteristic of osteoarthritis. Arthritis Rheum 48:1261–1270, 2003.
74. Lohmander LS. Markers of cartilage metabolism in arthrosis. A review. Acta Orthop Scand 62:623–632, 1991.
75. Nelson F, Billinghurst RC, Pidoux I, et al. Early post-traumatic osteoarthritis-like changes in human articular cartilage following rupture of the anterior cruciate ligament. Osteoarthritis Cartilage 14:114–119, 2006.
76. Harris AM, Patterson BM, Sontich JK, et al. Results and outcomes after operative treatment of high-energy tibial plafond fractures. Foot Ankle Int 27:256–265, 2006.
77. Buckwalter JA, Brown TD. Joint injury, repair, and remodeling: roles in post-traumatic osteoarthritis. Clin Orthop Relat Res 7–16, 2004.
78. Guilak F, Fermor B, Keefe FJ, et al. The role of biomechanics and inflammation in cartilage injury and repair. Clin Orthop Relat Res 17–26, 2004.
79. Olson SA, Marsh JL. Posttraumatic osteoarthritis. Clin Orthop Relat Res 2, 2004.
80. Bleasel JF, Poole AR, Heinegard D, et al. Changes in serum cartilage marker levels indicate altered cartilage metabolism in families with the osteoarthritis-related type II collagen gene COL2A1 mutation. Arthritis Rheum 42:39–45, 1999.
81. Matyas JR, Atley L, Ionescu M, et al. Analysis of cartilage biomarkers in the early phases of canine experimental osteoarthritis. Arthritis Rheum 50:543–552, 2004.
82. Tiraloche G, Girard C, Chouinard L, et al. Effect of oral glucosamine on cartilage degradation in a rabbit model of osteoarthritis. Arthritis Rheum 52:1118–1128, 2005.
83. Adams ME, Brandt KD. Hypertrophic repair of canine articular cartilage in osteoarthritis after anterior cruciate ligament transection. J Rheumatol 18:428–435, 1991.
84. Brandt KD, Braunstein EM, Visco DM, et al. Anterior (cranial) cruciate ligament transection in the dog: a bona fide model of osteoarthritis, not merely of cartilage injury and repair. J Rheumatol 18:436–446, 1991.
85. Manicourt DH, Altman RD, Williams JM, et al. Treatment with calcitonin suppresses the responses of bone, cartilage, and synovium in the early stages of canine experimental osteoarthritis and significantly reduces the severity of the cartilage lesions. Arthritis Rheum 42:1159–1167, 1999.
86. Manicourt DH, Thonar EJ, Pita JC, et al. Changes in the sedimentation profile of proteoglycan aggregates in early experimental canine osteoarthritis. Connect Tissue Res 23:33–50, 1989.
87. Pelletier JP, Martel-Pelletier J, Altman RD, et al. Collagenolytic activity and collagen matrix breakdown of the articular cartilage in the Pond-Nuki dog model of osteoarthritis. Arthritis Rheum 26:866–874, 1983.
88. Mitchell PG, Magna HA, Reeves LM, et al. Cloning, expression, and type II collagenolytic activity of matrix metalloproteinase-13 from human osteoarthritic cartilage. J Clin Invest 97:761–768, 1996.
89. Billinghurst RC, Dahlberg L, Ionescu M, et al. Enhanced cleavage of type II collagen by collagenases in osteoarthritic articular cartilage. J Clin Invest 99:1534–1545, 1997.
90. Dahlberg L, Billinghurst RC, Manner P, et al. Selective enhancement of collagenase-mediated cleavage of resident type II collagen in cultured osteoarthritic cartilage and arrest with a synthetic inhibitor that spares collagenase 1 (matrix metalloproteinase 1). Arthritis Rheum 43:673–682, 2000.
91. Neuhold LA, Killar L, Zhao W, et al. Postnatal expression in hyaline cartilage of constitutively active human collagenase-3 (MMP-13) induces osteoarthritis in mice. J Clin Invest 107: 35–44, 2001.
92. Poole AR, Alini M, Hollander AP. Cellular biology of cartilage degradation. In: Henderson B, Edwards JCW, Pettipher ER, eds. Mechanisms and Models in Rheumatoid Arthritis. London: Academic Press, 1995, pp 163–204.
93. Kafienah W, Bromme D, Buttle DJ, et al. Human cathepsin K cleaves native type I and II collagens at the N-terminal end of the triple helix. Biochem J 331 (Pt 3):727–732, 1998.
94. Konttinen YT, Mandelin J, Li TF, et al. Acidic cysteine endoproteinase cathepsin K in the degeneration of the superficial articular hyaline cartilage in osteoarthritis. Arthritis Rheum 46: 953–960, 2002.
95. Kevorkian L, Young DA, Darrah C, et al. Expression profiling of metalloproteinases and their inhibitors in cartilage. Arthritis Rheum 50:131–141, 2004.
96. Bau B, Gebhard PM, Haag J, et al. Relative messenger RNA expression profiling of collagenases and aggrecanases in human articular chondrocytes in vivo and in vitro. Arthritis Rheum 46: 2648–2657, 2002.
97. Wu CW, Tchetina EV, Mwale F, et al. Proteolysis involving matrix metalloproteinase 13 (collagenase-3) is required for chondrocyte differentiation that is associated with matrix mineralization. J Bone Miner Res 17:639–651, 2002.
98. Tchetina EV, Squires G, Poole AR. Increased type II collagen degradation and very early focal cartilage degeneration is associated with upregulation of chondrocyte differentiation related genes in early human articular cartilage lesions. J Rheumatol 32:876–886, 2005.
99. Shlopov BV, Gumanovskaya ML, Hasty KA. Autocrine regulation of collagenase 3 (matrix metalloproteinase 13) during osteoarthritis. Arthritis Rheum 43:195–205, 2000.

100. Cole AA, Kuettner KE. MMP-8 (neutrophil collagenase) mRNA and aggrecanase cleavage products are present in normal and osteoarthritic human articular cartilage. Acta Orthop Scand Suppl 266:98–102, 1995.
101. Aigner T, Zien A, Gehrsitz A, et al. Anabolic and catabolic gene expression pattern analysis in normal versus osteoarthritic cartilage using complementary DNA-array technology. Arthritis Rheum 44:2777–2789, 2001.
102. Imai K, Ohta S, Matsumoto T, et al. Expression of membrane-type 1 matrix metalloproteinase and activation of progelatinase A in human osteoarthritic cartilage. Am J Pathol 151:245–256, 1997.
103. Buttner FH, Chubinskaya S, Margerie D, et al. Expression of membrane type 1 matrix metalloproteinase in human articular cartilage. Arthritis Rheum 40:704–709, 1997.
104. Ohta S, Imai K, Yamashita K, et al. Expression of matrix metalloproteinase 7 (matrilysin) in human osteoarthritic cartilage. Lab Invest 78:79–87, 1998.
105. Martel-Pelletier J, Faure MP, McCollum R, et al. Plasmin, plasminogen activators and inhibitor in human osteoarthritic cartilage. J Rheumatol 18:1863–1871, 1991.
106. Baici A, Horler D, Lang A, et al. Cathepsin B in osteoarthritis: zonal variation of enzyme activity in human femoral head cartilage. Ann Rheum Dis 54:281–288, 1995.
107. Mehraban F, Tindal MH, Proffitt MM, et al. Temporal pattern of cysteine endopeptidase (cathepsin B) expression in cartilage and synovium from rabbit knees with experimental osteoarthritis: gene expression in chondrocytes in response to interleukin-1 and matrix depletion. Ann Rheum Dis 56:108–115, 1997.
108. Hollander AP, Heathfield TF, Webber C, et al. Increased damage to type II collagen in osteoarthritic articular cartilage detected by a new immunoassay. J Clin Invest 93:1722–1732, 1994.
109. Hollander AP, Pidoux I, Reiner A, et al. Damage to type II collagen in aging and osteoarthritis starts at the articular surface, originates around chondrocytes, and extends into the cartilage with progressive degeneration. J Clin Invest 96:2859–2869, 1995.
110. Poole AR. Biochemical/immunochemical biomarkers of osteoarthritis: utility for prediction of incident or progressive osteoarthritis. Rheum Dis Clin North Am 29:803–818, 2003.
111. Price JS, Till SH, Bickerstaff DR, et al. Degradation of cartilage type II collagen precedes the onset of osteoarthritis following anterior cruciate ligament rupture. Arthritis Rheum 42:2390–2398, 1999.
112. Aigner T, Bertling W, Stoss H, et al. Independent expression of fibril-forming collagens I, II, and III in chondrocytes of human osteoarthritic cartilage. J Clin Invest 91:829–837, 1993.
113. Matyas JR, Adams ME, Huang D, et al. Major role of collagen IIB in the elevation of total type II procollagen messenger RNA in the hypertrophic phase of experimental osteoarthritis. Arthritis Rheum 40:1046–1049, 1997.
114. Nelson F, Dahlberg L, Laverty S, et al. Evidence for altered synthesis of type II collagen in patients with osteoarthritis. J Clin Invest 102:2115–2125, 1998.
115. Rizkalla G, Reiner A, Bogoch E, et al. Studies of the articular cartilage proteoglycan aggrecan in health and osteoarthritis. Evidence for molecular heterogeneity and extensive molecular changes in disease. J Clin Invest 90:2268–2277, 1992.
116. Tortorella MD, Burn TC, Pratta MA, et al. Purification and cloning of aggrecanase-1: a member of the ADAMTS family of proteins. Science 284:1664–1666, 1999.
117. Lark MW, Bayne EK, Flanagan J, et al. Aggrecan degradation in human cartilage. Evidence for both matrix metalloproteinase and aggrecanase activity in normal, osteoarthritic, and rheumatoid joints. J Clin Invest 100:93–106, 1997.
118. Glasson SS, Askew R, Sheppard B, et al. Deletion of active ADAMTS5 prevents cartilage degradation in a murine model of osteoarthritis. Nature 434:644–648, 2005.
119. Stanton H, Rogerson FM, East CJ, et al. ADAMTS5 is the major aggrecanase in mouse cartilage in vivo and in vitro. Nature 434:648–652, 2005.
120. Gao G, Plaas A, Thompson VP, et al. ADAMTS4 (aggrecanase-1) activation on the cell surface involves C-terminal cleavage by glycosylphosphatidyl inositol-anchored membrane type 4-matrix metalloproteinase and binding of the activated proteinase to chondroitin sulfate and heparan sulfate on syndecan-1. J Biol Chem 279:10042–10051, 2004.
121. Cs-Szabo G, Roughley PJ, Plaas AH, et al. Large and small proteoglycans of osteoarthritic and rheumatoid articular cartilage. Arthritis Rheum 38:660–668, 1995.
122. Visco DM, Johnstone B, Hill MA, et al. Immunohistochemical analysis of 3-B-(-) and 7-D-4 epitope expression in canine osteoarthritis. Arthritis Rheum 36:1718–1725, 1993.
123. Carlson CS, Loeser RF, Johnstone B, et al. Osteoarthritis in cynomolgus macaques. II. Detection of modulated proteoglycan epitopes in cartilage and synovial fluid. J Orthop Res 13:399–409, 1995.
124. Lohmander LS, Ionescu M, Jugessur H, et al. Changes in joint cartilage aggrecan after knee injury and in osteoarthritis. Arthritis Rheum 42:534–544, 1999.
125. Poole AR, Ionescu M, Swan A, et al. Changes in cartilage metabolism in arthritis are reflected by altered serum and synovial fluid levels of the cartilage proteoglycan aggrecan. Implications for pathogenesis. J Clin Invest 94:25–33, 1994.
126. Poole AR. Skeletal and inflammation markers in aging and osteoarthritis. In: Hamerman D, ed. Osteoarthritis and the Ageing Population. Baltimore: Johns Hopkins University Press, 1997, pp 187–214.
127. Homandberg GA, Meyers R, Xie DL. Fibronectin fragments cause chondrolysis of bovine articular cartilage slices in culture. J Biol Chem 267:3597–3604, 1992.
128. Yasuda T, Poole AR. A fibronectin fragment induces type II collagen degradation by collagenase through an interleukin-1-mediated pathway. Arthritis Rheum 46:138–148, 2002.
129. Yasuda T, Poole AR, Shimizu M, et al. Involvement of CD44 in induction of matrix metalloproteinases by a COOH-terminal heparin-binding fragment of fibronectin in human articular cartilage in culture. Arthritis Rheum 48:1271–1280, 2003.
130. Werb Z, Tremble PM, Behrendtsen O, et al. Signal transduction through the fibronectin receptor induces collagenase and stromelysin gene expression. J Cell Biol 109:877–889, 1989.
131. Chevalier X, Claudepierre P, Groult N, et al. Presence of ED-A containing fibronectin in human articular cartilage from patients with osteoarthritis and rheumatoid arthritis. J Rheumatol 23:1022–1030, 1996.
132. Arner EC, Tortorella MD. Signal transduction through chondrocyte integrin receptors induces matrix metalloproteinase synthesis and synergizes with interleukin-1. Arthritis Rheum 38:1304–1314, 1995.
133. Yasuda T, Tchetina E, Ohsawa K, et al. Peptides of type II collagen can induce the cleavage of type II collagen and aggrecan in articular cartilage. Matrix Biol, In press, 2006.
134. Fichter M, Korner U, Schomburg J, et al. Collagen degradation products modulate matrix metalloproteinase expression in cultured articular chondrocytes. J Orthop Res 24:63–70, 2006.
135. Martel-Pelletier J, McCollum R, DiBattista J, et al. The interleukin-1 receptor in normal and osteoarthritic human articular chondrocytes. Identification as the type I receptor and analysis of binding kinetics and biologic function. Arthritis Rheum 35:530–540, 1992.
136. Melchiorri C, Meliconi R, Frizziero L, et al. Enhanced and coordinated in vivo expression of inflammatory cytokines and nitric oxide synthase by chondrocytes from patients with osteoarthritis. Arthritis Rheum 41:2165–2174, 1998.
137. Webb GR, Westacott CI, Elson CJ. Chondrocyte tumor necrosis factor receptors and focal loss of cartilage in osteoarthritis. Osteoarthritis Cartilage 5:427–437, 1997.
138. Cawston TE, Curry VA, Summers CA, et al. The role of oncostatin M in animal and human connective tissue collagen turnover and its localization within the rheumatoid joint. Arthritis Rheum 41:1760–1771, 1998.
139. Kobayashi M, Squires GR, Mousa A, et al. Role of interleukin-1 and tumor necrosis factor alpha in matrix degradation of human osteoarthritic cartilage. Arthritis Rheum 52:128–135, 2005.
140. Amin AR, Di Cesare PE, Vyas P, et al. The expression and regulation of nitric oxide synthase in human osteoarthritis-affected chondrocytes: evidence for up-regulated neuronal nitric oxide synthase. J Exp Med 182:2097–2102, 1995.

141. Palmer RM, Hickery MS, Charles IG, et al. Induction of nitric oxide synthase in human chondrocytes. Biochem Biophys Res Commun 193:398–405, 1993.

142. Attur MG, Dave MN, Stuchin S, et al. Osteopontin: an intrinsic inhibitor of inflammation in cartilage. Arthritis Rheum 44: 578–584, 2001.

143. Nakamura S, Kamihagi K, Satakeda H, et al. Enhancement of SPARC (osteonectin) synthesis in arthritic cartilage. Increased levels in synovial fluids from patients with rheumatoid arthritis and regulation by growth factors and cytokines in chondrocyte cultures. Arthritis Rheum 39:539–551, 1996.

144. Taskiran D, Stefanovic-Racic M, Georgescu H, et al. Nitric oxide mediates suppression of cartilage proteoglycan synthesis by interleukin-1. Biochem Biophys Res Commun 200:142–148, 1994.

145. Stefanovic-Racic M, Morales TI, Taskiran D, et al. The role of nitric oxide in proteoglycan turnover by bovine articular cartilage organ cultures. J Immunol 156:1213–1220, 1996.

146. Clements KM, Price JS, Chambers MG, et al. Gene deletion of either interleukin-1beta, interleukin-1beta-converting enzyme, inducible nitric oxide synthase, or stromelysin 1 accelerates the development of knee osteoarthritis in mice after surgical transection of the medial collateral ligament and partial medial meniscectomy. Arthritis Rheum 48:3452–3463, 2003.

147. Blanco FJ, Ochs RL, Schwarz H, et al. Chondrocyte apoptosis induced by nitric oxide. Am J Pathol 146:75–85, 1995.

148. Pelletier JP, Jovanovic DV, Lascau-Coman V, et al. Selective inhibition of inducible nitric oxide synthase reduces progression of experimental osteoarthritis in vivo: possible link with the reduction in chondrocyte apoptosis and caspase 3 level. Arthritis Rheum 43:1290–1299, 2000.

149. Fermor B, Weinberg JB, Pisetsky DS, et al. The influence of oxygen tension on the induction of nitric oxide and prostaglandin E2 by mechanical stress in articular cartilage. Osteoarthritis Cartilage 13:935–941, 2005.

150. Fermor B, Weinberg JB, Pisetsky DS, et al. Induction of cyclooxygenase-2 by mechanical stress through a nitric oxide-regulated pathway. Osteoarthritis Cartilage 10:792–798, 2002.

151. Lee JH, Fitzgerald JB, Dimicco MA, et al. Mechanical injury of cartilage explants causes specific time-dependent changes in chondrocyte gene expression. Arthritis Rheum 52:2386–2395, 2005.

152. Patwari P, Cook MN, DiMicco MA, et al. Proteoglycan degradation after injurious compression of bovine and human articular cartilage in vitro: interaction with exogenous cytokines. Arthritis Rheum 48:1292–1301, 2003.

153. Piscoya JL, Fermor B, Kraus VB, et al. The influence of mechanical compression on the induction of osteoarthritis-related biomarkers in articular cartilage explants. Osteoarthritis Cartilage 13: 1092–1099, 2005.

154. Dean DD, Martel-Pelletier J, Pelletier JP, et al. Evidence for metalloproteinase and metalloproteinase inhibitor imbalance in human osteoarthritic cartilage. J Clin Invest 84:678–685, 1989.

155. Yamada H, Nakagawa T, Stephens RW, et al. Proteinases and their inhibitors in normal and osteoarthritic articular cartilage. Biomed Res 8:289–300, 1987.

156. Gendron C, Kashiwagi M, Hughes C, et al. TIMP-3 inhibits aggrecanase-mediated glycosaminoglycan release from cartilage explants stimulated by catabolic factors. FEBS Lett 555:431–436, 2003.

157. Moulharat N, Lesur C, Thomas M, et al. Effects of transforming growth factor-beta on aggrecanase production and proteoglycan degradation by human chondrocytes in vitro. Osteoarthritis Cartilage 12:296–305, 2004.

158. Tchetina EV, Antoniou J, Tanzer M, et al. Transforming growth factor-beta2 suppresses collagen cleavage in cultured human osteoarthritic cartilage, reduces expression of genes associated with chondrocyte hypertrophy and degradation, and increases prostaglandin E(2) production. Am J Pathol 168:131–140, 2006.

159. Ling H, Recklies AD. The Chitinase 3-like protein human cartilage glycoprotein 39 inhibits cellular responses to the inflammatory cytokines interleukin-1 and tumour necrosis factor-alpha. Biochem J 380:651–659, 2004.

160. Poole AR, Rosenberg LC, Reiner A, et al. Contents and distributions of the proteoglycans decorin and biglycan in normal and

osteoarthritic human articular cartilage. J Orthop Res 14: 681–689, 1996.

161. Lefkoe TP, Nalin AM, Clark JM, et al. Gene expression of collagen types IIA and IX correlates with ultrastructural events in early osteoarthrosis: new applications of the rabbit meniscectomy model. J Rheumatol 24:1155–1163, 1997.

162. Aigner T, Zhu Y, Chansky HH, et al. Reexpression of type IIA procollagen by adult articular chondrocytes in osteoarthritic cartilage. Arthritis Rheum 42:1443–1450, 1999.

163. Sandell LJ, Morris N, Robbins JR, et al. Alternatively spliced type II procollagen mRNAs define distinct populations of cells during vertebral development: differential expression of the amino-propeptide. J Cell Biol 114:1307–1319, 1991.

164. McDevitt CA, Pahl JA, Ayad S, et al. Experimental osteoarthritic articular cartilage is enriched in guanidine soluble type VI collagen. Biochem Biophys Res Commun 157:250–255, 1988.

165. Ronziere MC, Ricard-Blum S, Tiollier J, et al. Comparative analysis of collagens solubilized from human foetal, and normal and osteoarthritic adult articular cartilage, with emphasis on type VI collagen. Biochim Biophys Acta. 1038:222–230, 1990.

166. Hambach L, Neureiter D, Zeiler G, et al. Severe disturbance of the distribution and expression of type VI collagen chains in osteoarthritic articular cartilage. Arthritis Rheum 41:986–996, 1998.

167. Soder S, Hambach L, Lissner R, et al. Ultrastructural localization of type VI collagen in normal adult and osteoarthritic human articular cartilage. Osteoarthritis Cartilage 10:464–470, 2002.

168. Lee GM, Paul TA, Slabaugh M, et al. The pericellular matrix is enlarged in osteoarthritic cartilage. Trans Orthop Res Soc 22:495, 1997.

169. Alexopoulos LG, Williams GM, Upton ML, et al. Osteoarthritic changes in the biphasic mechanical properties of the chondrocyte pericellular matrix in articular cartilage. J Biomech 38: 509–517, 2005.

170. Alexopoulos LG, Haider MA, Vail TP, et al. Alterations in the mechanical properties of the human chondrocyte pericellular matrix with osteoarthritis. J Biomech Eng 125:323–333, 2003.

171. Cs-Szabo G, Melching LI, Roughley PJ, et al. Changes in messenger RNA and protein levels of proteoglycans and link protein in human osteoarthritic cartilage samples. Arthritis Rheum 40: 1037–1045, 1997.

172. Nishida Y, Shinomura T, Iwata H, et al. Abnormal occurrence of a large chondroitin sulfate proteoglycan, PG-M/versican in osteoarthritic cartilage. Osteoarthritis Cartilage 2:43–49, 1994.

173. Schneiderman R, Rosenberg N, Hiss J, et al. Concentration and size distribution of insulin-like growth factor-I in human normal and osteoarthritic synovial fluid and cartilage. Arch Biochem Biophys 324:173–188, 1995.

174. Dore S, Pelletier JP, DiBattista JA, et al. Human osteoarthritic chondrocytes possess an increased number of insulin-like growth factor 1 binding sites but are unresponsive to its stimulation. Possible role of IGF-1-binding proteins. Arthritis Rheum 37: 253–263, 1994.

175. Chen AL, Fang C, Liu C, et al. Expression of bone morphogenetic proteins, receptors, and tissue inhibitors in human fetal, adult, and osteoarthritic articular cartilage. J Orthop Res 22:1188–1192, 2004.

176. Di Cesare PE, Carlson CS, Stolerman ES, et al. Increased degradation and altered tissue distribution of cartilage oligomeric matrix protein in human rheumatoid and osteoarthritic cartilage. J Orthop Res 14:946–955, 1996.

177. Okimura A, Okada Y, Makihira S, et al. Enhancement of cartilage matrix protein synthesis in arthritic cartilage. Arthritis Rheum 40:1029–1036, 1997.

178. Chevalier X, Groult N, Larget-Piet B, et al. Tenascin distribution in articular cartilage from normal subjects and from patients with osteoarthritis and rheumatoid arthritis. Arthritis Rheum 37:1013–1022, 1994.

179. Recklies AD, White C, Ling H. The Chitinase 3-like protein human cartilage glycoprotein 39 (HC-gp39) stimulates proliferation of human connective-tissue cells and activates both extracellular signal-regulated kinase- and protein kinase B-mediated signalling pathways. Biochem J 365:119–126, 2002.

180. Marshall KW, Zhang H, Yager TD, et al. Blood-based biomarkers for detecting mild osteoarthritis in the human knee. Osteoarthritis Cartilage 13:861–871, 2005.

181. van den Berg WB, van der Kraan PM, van Beuningen HM. Synovial mediators of cartilage damage and repair in OA. In: Brandt KD, Doherty M, Lohmander LS, eds. Osteoarthritis. Oxford: Oxford University Press, 1998.

182. Goldring MB. Osteoarthritis and cartilage: the role of cytokines. Curr Rheumatol Rep 2:459–465, 2000.

183. Morales T, I. The role of signaling factors in articular cartilage homeostasis and osteoarthritis. In: Kuettner KE, Goldberg VM, eds. Osteoarthritic Disorders. Rosemont, IL: American Academy of Orthopaedic Surgeons, 1995, pp 261–270.

184. Middleton JF, Tyler JA. Upregulation of insulin-like growth factor I gene expression in the lesions of osteoarthritic human articular cartilage. Ann Rheum Dis 51:440–447, 1992.

185. Tyler JA. Insulin-like growth factor 1 can decrease degradation and promote synthesis of proteoglycan in cartilage exposed to cytokines. Biochem J 260:543–548, 1989.

186. Trippel SB, Corvol MT, Dumontier MF, et al. Effect of somatomedin-C/insulin-like growth factor I and growth hormone on cultured growth plate and articular chondrocytes. Pediatr Res 25:76–82, 1989.

187. Martel-Pelletier J, Di Battista JA, Lajeunesse D, et al. IGF/IGFBP axis in cartilage and bone in osteoarthritis pathogenesis. Inflamm Res 47:90–100, 1998.

188. Fowlkes JL, Serra DM, Rosenberg CK, et al. Insulin-like growth factor (IGF)-binding protein-3 (IGFBP-3) functions as an IGF-reversible inhibitor of IGFBP-4 proteolysis. J Biol Chem 270:27481–27488, 1995.

189. Sachs BL, Goldberg VM, Moskowitz RW, et al. Response of articular chondrocytes to pituitary fibroblast growth factor (FGF). J Cell Physiol 112:51–59, 1982.

190. Kato Y, Gospodarowicz D. Sulfated proteoglycan synthesis by confluent cultures of rabbit costal chondrocytes grown in the presence of fibroblast growth factor. J Cell Biol 100:477–485, 1985.

191. Campbell IK, Wojta J, Novak U, et al. Cytokine modulation of plasminogen activator inhibitor-1 (PAI-1) production by human articular cartilage and chondrocytes. Down-regulation by tumor necrosis factor alpha and up-regulation by transforming growth factor-B basic fibroblast growth factor. Biochim Biophys Acta 1226:277–285, 1994.

192. Bakker AC, van de Loo FA, van Beuningen HM, et al. Overexpression of active TGF-beta-1 in the murine knee joint: evidence for synovial-layer-dependent chondro-osteophyte formation. Osteoarthritis Cartilage 9:128–136, 2001.

193. van Beuningen HM, Glansbeek HL, van der Kraan PM, et al. Osteoarthritis-like changes in the murine knee joint resulting from intra-articular transforming growth factor-beta injections. Osteoarthritis Cartilage 8:25–33, 2000.

194. Huebner JL, Kraus VB. Assessment of the utility of biomarkers of osteoarthritis in the guinea pig. Osteoarthritis Cartilage 2006.

195. von der Mark K, Kirsch T, Nerlich A, et al. Type X collagen synthesis in human osteoarthritic cartilage. Indication of chondrocyte hypertrophy. Arthritis Rheum 35:806–811, 1992.

196. Mwale F, Tchetina E, Wu CW, et al. The assembly and remodeling of the extracellular matrix in the growth plate in relationship to mineral deposition and cellular hypertrophy: an in situ study of collagens II and IX and proteoglycan. J Bone Miner Res 17:275–283, 2002.

197. Hashimoto S, Ochs RL, Komiya S, et al. Linkage of chondrocyte apoptosis and cartilage degradation in human osteoarthritis. Arthritis Rheum 41:1632–1638, 1998.

198. Blanco FJ, Guitian R, Vazquez-Martul E, et al. Osteoarthritis chondrocytes die by apoptosis. A possible pathway for osteoarthritis pathology. Arthritis Rheum 41:284–289, 1998.

199. Gebhard PM, Gehrsitz A, Bau B, et al. Quantification of expression levels of cellular differentiation markers does not support a general shift in the cellular phenotype of osteoarthritic chondrocytes. J Orthop Res 21:96–101, 2003.

200. Sharif M, Whitehouse A, Sharman P, et al. Increased apoptosis in human osteoarthritic cartilage corresponds to reduced cell density and expression of caspase-3. Arthritis Rheum 50:507–515, 2004.

201. Mollenhauer J, Mok MT, King KB, et al. Expression of anchorin CII (cartilage annexin V) in human young, normal adult, and osteoarthritic cartilage. J Histochem Cytochem 47:209–220, 1999.

202. Terkeltaub R, Lotz M, Johnson K, et al. Parathyroid hormone-related protein is abundant in osteoarthritic cartilage, and the parathyroid hormone-related protein 1-173 isoform is selectively induced by transforming growth factor beta in articular chondrocytes and suppresses generation of extracellular inorganic pyrophosphate. Arthritis Rheum 41:2152–2164, 1998.

203. Okano K, Tsukazaki T, Ohtsuru A, et al. Expression of parathyroid hormone-related peptide in human osteoarthritis. J Orthop Res 15:175–180, 1997.

204. Burton DW, Foster M, Johnson KA, et al. Chondrocyte calcium-sensing receptor expression is up-regulated in early guinea pig knee osteoarthritis and modulates PTHrP, MMP-13, and TIMP-3 expression. Osteoarthritis Cartilage 13:395–404, 2005.

205. Wu W, Billinghurst RC, Pidoux I, et al. Sites of collagenase cleavage and denaturation of type II collagen in aging and osteoarthritic articular cartilage and their relationship to the distribution of matrix metalloproteinase 1 and matrix metalloproteinase 13. Arthritis Rheum 46:2087–2094, 2002.

206. Shlopov BV, Lie WR, Mainardi CL, et al. Osteoarthritic lesions: involvement of three different collagenases. Arthritis Rheum 40:2065–2074, 1997.

207. Reboul P, Pelletier JP, Tardif G, et al. The new collagenase, collagenase-3, is expressed and synthesized by human chondrocytes but not by synoviocytes. A role in osteoarthritis. J Clin Invest 97:2011–2019, 1996.

208. Poole AR, Laverty S, Mwale F. Endochondral bone formation and development in the axial and appendicular skeleton. In: Henderson JE, Goltzman D, eds. The Osteoporosis Primer. Cambridge: Cambridge University Press, 2000, pp 3–17.

209. Serra R, Johnson M, Filvaroff EH, et al. Expression of a truncated, kinase-defective TGF-beta type II receptor in mouse skeletal tissue promotes terminal chondrocyte differentiation and osteoarthritis. J Cell Biol 139:541–552, 1997.

210. Yang X, Chen L, Xu X, et al. TGF-beta/Smad3 signals repress chondrocyte hypertrophic differentiation and are required for maintaining articular cartilage. J Cell Biol 153:35–46, 2001.

211. Wang FL, Connor JR, Dodds RA, et al. Differential expression of egr-1 in osteoarthritic compared to normal adult human articular cartilage. Osteoarthritis Cartilage 8:161–169, 2000.

212. Gordon GV, Villanueva T, Schumacher HR, et al. Autopsy study correlating degree of osteoarthritis, synovitis and evidence of articular calcification. J Rheumatol 11:681–686, 1984.

213. Ali SY, Rees JA, Scotchford CA. Microcrystal deposition in cartilage and in osteoarthritis. Bone Miner 17:115–118, 1992.

214. Swan A, Chapman B, Heap P, et al. Submicroscopic crystals in osteoarthritic synovial fluids. Ann Rheum Dis 53:467–470, 1994.

215. McCarty DJ. Calcium pyrophosphate dihydrate crystals deposition disease (pseudogout syndrome)—clinical aspects. Clin Rheum Dis 3:61–89, 1977.

216. Schumacher HR, Jr. Synovial inflammation, crystals, and osteoarthritis. J Rheumatol Suppl 43:101–103, 1995.

217. Watanabe W, Baker DG, Schumacher HR, Jr. Comparison of the acute inflammation induced by calcium pyrophosphate dihydrate, apatite and mixed crystals in the rat air pouch model of a synovial space. J Rheumatol 19:1453–1457, 1992.

218. Fam AG, Morava-Protzner I, Purcell C, et al. Acceleration of experimental lapine osteoarthritis by calcium pyrophosphate microcrystalline synovitis. Arthritis Rheum 38:201–210, 1995.

219. Derfus B, Steinberg M, Mandel N, et al. Characterization of an additional articular cartilage vesicle fraction that generates calcium pyrophosphate dihydrate crystals in vitro. J Rheumatol 22:1514–1519, 1995.

220. Hashimoto S, Ochs RL, Rosen F, et al. Chondrocyte-derived apoptotic bodies and calcification of articular cartilage. Proc Natl Acad Sci USA 95:3094–3099, 1998.

221. Terkeltaub RA. What does cartilage calcification tell us about osteoarthritis? J Rheumatol 29:411–415, 2002.

222. Johnson K, Terkeltaub R. Upregulated ank expression in osteoarthritis can promote both chondrocyte MMP-13 expression and calcification via chondrocyte extracellular PPi excess. Osteoarthritis Cartilage 12:321–335, 2004.

223. Li B, Aspden RM. Mechanical and material properties of the subchondral bone plate from the femoral head of patients with osteoarthritis or osteoporosis. Ann Rheum Dis 56:247–254, 1997.

224. Nevitt MC, Lane NE, Scott JC, et al. Radiographic osteoarthritis of the hip and bone mineral density. The Study of Osteoporotic Fractures Research Group. Arthritis Rheum 38:907–916, 1995.

225. Burger H, van Daele PL, Odding E, et al. Association of radiographically evident osteoarthritis with higher bone mineral density and increased bone loss with age. The Rotterdam Study. Arthritis Rheum 39:81–86, 1996.

226. Hart DJ, Cronin C, Daniels M, et al. The relationship of bone density and fracture to incident and progressive radiographic osteoarthritis of the knee: the Chingford Study. Arthritis Rheum 46:92–99, 2002.

227. Dequeker J, Mokassa L, Aerssens J, et al. Bone density and local growth factors in generalized osteoarthritis. Microsc Res Tech 37:358–371, 1997.

228. Hochberg MC, Lethbridge-Cejku M, Scott WW, Jr., et al. Appendicular bone mass and osteoarthritis of the hands in women: data from the Baltimore Longitudinal Study of Aging. J Rheumatol 21:1532–1536, 1994.

229. Grynpas MD, Alpert B, Katz I, et al. Subchondral bone in osteoarthritis. Calcif Tissue Int 49:20–26, 1991.

230. Mansell JP, Bailey AJ. Abnormal cancellous bone collagen metabolism in osteoarthritis. J Clin Invest 101:1596–1603, 1998.

231. Naganathan V, Zochling J, March L, et al. Peak bone mass is increased in the hip in daughters of women with osteoarthritis. Bone 30:287–292, 2002.

232. McCarthy C, Cushnaghan J, Dieppe P. The predictive role of scintigraphy in radiographic osteoarthritis of the hand. Osteoarthritis Cartilage 2:25–28, 1994.

233. Dieppe P, Cushnaghan J, Young P, et al. Prediction of the progression of joint space narrowing in osteoarthritis of the knee by bone scintigraphy. Ann Rheum Dis 52:557–563, 1993.

234. Hutton CW, Higgs ER, Jackson PC, et al. 99mTc HMDP bone scanning in generalised nodal osteoarthritis. II. The four hour bone scan image predicts radiographic change. Ann Rheum Dis 45:622–626, 1986.

235. Huebner JL, Hanes MA, Beekman B, et al. A comparative analysis of bone and cartilage metabolism in two strains of guinea-pig with varying degrees of naturally occurring osteoarthritis. Osteoarthritis Cartilage 10:758–767, 2002.

236. Matsui H, Shimizu M, Tsuji H. Cartilage and subchondral bone interaction in osteoarthrosis of human knee joint: a histological and histomorphometric study. Microsc Res Tech 37:333–342, 1997.

237. Burr DB, Schaffler MB. The involvement of subchondral mineralized tissues in osteoarthrosis: quantitative microscopic evidence. Microsc Res Tech 37:343–357, 1997.

238. Watson PJ, Hall LD, Malcolm A, et al. Degenerative joint disease in the guinea pig. Use of magnetic resonance imaging to monitor progression of bone pathology. Arthritis Rheum 39:1327–1337, 1996.

239. van Osch GJ, van der Kraan PM, van Valburg AA, et al. The relation between cartilage damage and osteophyte size in a murine model for osteoarthritis in the knee. Rheumatol Int 16:115–119, 1996.

240. Seibel MJ, Duncan A, Robins SP. Urinary hydroxy-pyridinium crosslinks provide indices of cartilage and bone involvement in arthritic diseases. J Rheumatol 16:964–970, 1989.

241. Garnero P, Mazieres B, Gueguen A, et al. Cross-sectional association of 10 molecular markers of bone, cartilage, and synovium with disease activity and radiological joint damage in patients with hip osteoarthritis: the ECHODIAH cohort. J Rheumatol 32:697–703, 2005.

242. Muehleman C, Berzins A, Koepp H, et al. Bone density of the human talus does not increase with the cartilage degeneration score. Anat Rec 266:81–86, 2002.

243. Marcelli C, Favier F, Kotzki PO, et al. The relationship between osteoarthritis of the hands, bone mineral density, and osteoporotic fractures in elderly women. Osteoporos Int 5:382–388, 1995.

244. Hart DJ, Mootoosamy I, Doyle DV, et al. The relationship between osteoarthritis and osteoporosis in the general population: the Chingford Study. Ann Rheum Dis 53:158–162, 1994.

245. Dequeker J. Inverse relationship of interface between osteoporosis and osteoarthritis. J Rheumatol 24:795–798, 1997.

246. Westacott CI, Webb GR, Warnock MG, et al. Alteration of cartilage metabolism by cells from osteoarthritic bone. Arthritis Rheum 40:1282–1291, 1997.

247. Behets C, Williams JM, Chappard D, et al. Effects of calcitonin on subchondral trabecular bone changes and on osteoarthritic cartilage lesions after acute anterior cruciate ligament deficiency. J Bone Miner Res 19:1821–1826, 2004.

248. Franchimont P, Bassleer C, Henrotin Y, et al. Effects of human and salmon calcitonin on human articular chondrocytes cultivated in clusters. J Clin Endocrinol Metab 69:259–266, 1989.

249. Hayami T, Pickarski M, Wesolowski GA, et al. The role of subchondral bone remodeling in osteoarthritis: reduction of cartilage degeneration and prevention of osteophyte formation by alendronate in the rat anterior cruciate ligament transection model. Arthritis Rheum 50:1193–1206, 2004.

250. Smith MD, Triantafillou S, Parker A, et al. Synovial membrane inflammation and cytokine production in patients with early osteoarthritis. J Rheumatol 24:365–371, 1997.

251. Pelletier JP, Martel-Pelletier J, Abramson SB. Osteoarthritis, an inflammatory disease: potential implication for the selection of new therapeutic targets. Arthritis Rheum 44:1237–1247, 2001.

252. Lindblad S, Hedfors E. Arthroscopic and immunohistologic characterization of knee joint synovitis in osteoarthritis. Arthritis Rheum 30:1081–1088, 1987.

253. Ayral X, Pickering EH, Woodworth TG, et al. Synovitis: a potential predictive factor of structural progression of medial tibiofemoral knee osteoarthritis—results of a 1 year longitudinal arthroscopic study in 422 patients. Osteoarthritis Cartilage 13:361–367, 2005.

254. Martel-Pelletier J, Alaaeddine N, Pelletier JP. Cytokines and their role in the pathophysiology of osteoarthritis. Front Biosci 4: D694–703, 1999.

255. Alaaeddine N, Di Battista JA, Pelletier JP, et al. Inhibition of tumor necrosis factor alpha-induced prostaglandin E2 production by the antiinflammatory cytokines interleukin-4, interleukin-10, and interleukin-13 in osteoarthritic synovial fibroblasts: distinct targeting in the signaling pathways. Arthritis Rheum 42:710–718, 1999.

256. Poole AR, Dieppe P. Biological markers in rheumatoid arthritis. Semin Arthritis Rheum 23:17–31, 1994.

257. Goldberg RL, Huff JP, Lenz ME, et al. Elevated plasma levels of hyaluronate in patients with osteoarthritis and rheumatoid arthritis. Arthritis Rheum 34:799–807, 1991.

258. Sharif M, George E, Shepstone L, et al. Serum hyaluronic acid level as a predictor of disease progression in osteoarthritis of the knee. Arthritis Rheum 38:760–767, 1995.

259. Sharma L, Hurwitz DE, Thonar EJ, et al. Knee adduction moment, serum hyaluronan level, and disease severity in medial tibiofemoral osteoarthritis. Arthritis Rheum 41:1233–1240, 1998.

260. Recklies AD, Baillargeon L, White C. Regulation of cartilage oligomeric matrix protein synthesis in human synovial cells and articular chondrocytes. Arthritis Rheum 41:997–1006, 1998.

261. Sharif M, Saxne T, Shepstone L, et al. Relationship between serum cartilage oligomeric matrix protein levels and disease progression in osteoarthritis of the knee joint. Br J Rheumatol 34:306–310, 1995.

262. Petersson IF, Boegard T, Svensson B, et al. Changes in cartilage and bone metabolism identified by serum markers in early osteoarthritis of the knee joint. Br J Rheumatol 37:46–50, 1998.

263. Conrozier T, Saxne T, Fan CS, et al. Serum concentrations of cartilage oligomeric matrix protein and bone sialoprotein in hip osteoarthritis: a one year prospective study. Ann Rheum Dis 57:527–532, 1998.

264. Vilim V, Olejarova M, Machacek S, et al. Serum levels of cartilage oligomericl matrix protein (COMP) correlate with radiographic progression of knee osteoarthritis. Osteoarthritis Cartilage 10:707–713, 2002.

265. Mazieres B, Garnero P, Gueguen A, et al. Molecular markers of cartilage breakdown and synovitis at baseline as predictors of structural progression of hip osteoarthritis. The ECHODIAH Cohort. Ann Rheum Dis 65:354–359, 2006.

266. Gineyts E, Garnero P, Delmas PD. Urinary excretion of glucosyl-galactosyl pyridinoline: a specific biochemical marker of synovium degradation. Rheumatology (Oxford) 40:315–323, 2001.

267. Jordan KM, Syddall HE, Garnero P, et al. Urinary CTX-II and glucosyl-galactosyl-pyridinoline are associated with the presence and severity of radiographic knee osteoarthritis in men. Ann Rheum Dis 65:871–877, 2006.

268. Masuhara K, Nakai T, Yamaguchi K, et al. Significant increases in serum and plasma concentrations of matrix metalloproteinases 3 and 9 in patients with rapidly destructive osteoarthritis of the hip. Arthritis Rheum 46:2625–2631, 2002.

269. Tchetverikov I, Lohmander LS, Verzijl N, et al. MMP protein and activity levels in synovial fluid from patients with joint injury, inflammatory arthritis, and osteoarthritis. Ann Rheum Dis 64:694–698, 2005.

270. Guerassimov A, Zhang Y, Cartman A, et al. Immune responses to cartilage link protein and the G1 domain of proteoglycan aggrecan in patients with osteoarthritis. Arthritis Rheum 42:527–533, 1999.

271. Champion BR, Poole AR. Immunity to homologous type III collagen after partial meniscectomy and sham surgery in rabbits. Arthritis Rheum 25:274–287, 1982.

272. Koch AE, Kunkel SL, Shah MR, et al. Macrophage inflammatory protein-1 beta: a C-C chemokine in osteoarthritis. Clin Immunol Immunopathol 77:307–314, 1995.

273. Hsu YH, Hsieh MS, Liang YC, et al. Production of the chemokine eotaxin-1 in osteoarthritis and its role in cartilage degradation. J Cell Biochem 93:929–939, 2004.

274. Hashimoto H, Tanaka M, Suda T, et al. Soluble Fas ligand in the joints of patients with rheumatoid arthritis and osteoarthritis. Arthritis Rheum 41:657–662, 1998.

275. Sharif M, Elson CJ, Dieppe PA, et al. Elevated serum C-reactive protein levels in osteoarthritis. Br J Rheumatol 36:140–141, 1997.

276. Spector TD, Hart DJ, Nandra D, et al. Low-level increases in serum C-reactive protein are present in early osteoarthritis of the knee and predict progressive disease. Arthritis Rheum 40:723–727, 1997.

277. Linaker CH, Walker-Bone K, Palmer K, et al. Frequency and impact of regional musculoskeletal disorders. Baillieres Clin Rheumatol 13:197–215, 1999.

278. Torres L, Dunlop DD, Peterfy C, et al. The relationship between specific tissue lesions and pain severity in persons with knee osteoarthritis. Osteoarthritis Cartilage 2006.

279. Segal R, Avrahami E, Lebdinski E, et al. The impact of hemiparalysis on the expression of osteoarthritis. Arthritis Rheum 41:2249–2256, 1998.

280. Decaris E, Guingamp C, Chat M, et al. Evidence for neurogenic transmission inducing degenerative cartilage damage distant from local inflammation. Arthritis Rheum 42:1951–1960, 1999.

281. Farrell M, Gibson S, McMeeken J, et al. Pain and hyperalgesia in osteoarthritis of the hands. J Rheumatol 27:441–447, 2000.

282. Ordeberg G. Characterization of joint pain in human OA. Novartis Found Symp 260:105–115; discussion 115–121, 277–109, 2004.

283. Kosek E, Ordeberg G. Lack of pressure pain modulation by heterotopic noxious conditioning stimulation in patients with painful osteoarthritis before, but not following, surgical pain relief. Pain 88:69–78, 2000.

284. Kosek E, Ordeberg G. Abnormalities of somatosensory perception in patients with painful osteoarthritis normalize following successful treatment. Eur J Pain 4:229–238, 2000.

285. Farrell MJ, Gibson SJ, McMeeken JM, et al. Increased movement pain in osteoarthritis of the hands is associated with A beta-mediated cutaneous mechanical sensitivity. J Pain 1:229–242, 2000.

286. Garabedian BV, Lemaigre-Dubreuil Y, Mariani J. Central origin of IL-1beta produced during peripheral inflammation: role of meninges. Brain Res Mol Brain Res 75:259–263, 2000.

287. Dieppe PA, Lohmander LS. Pathogenesis and management of pain in osteoarthritis. Lancet 365:965–973, 2005.

288. Richardson JD, Vasko MR. Cellular mechanisms of neurogenic inflammation. J Pharmacol Exp Ther 302:839–845, 2002.

289. Heppelmann B, Pfeffer A, Schaible HG, et al. Effects of acetyl-salicylic acid and indomethacin on single groups III and IV sensory units from acutely inflamed joints. Pain 26:337–351, 1986.

290. Dubois RN, Abramson SB, Crofford L, et al. Cyclooxygenase in biology and disease. FASEB J 12:1063–1073, 1998.

291. Lotz M, Carson DA, Vaughan JH. Substance P activation of rheumatoid synoviocytes: neural pathway in pathogenesis of arthritis. Science 235:893–895, 1987.

292. Kimball ES. Substance P, cytokines, and arthritis. Ann N Y Acad Sci 594:293–308, 1990.

293. Takeba Y, Suzuki N, Kaneko A, et al. Evidence for neural regulation of inflammatory synovial cell functions by secreting calcitonin gene-related peptide and vasoactive intestinal peptide in patients with rheumatoid arthritis. Arthritis Rheum 42:2418–2429, 1999.

294. Takeba Y, Suzuki N, Takeno M, et al. Modulation of synovial cell function by somatostatin in patients with rheumatoid arthritis. Arthritis Rheum 40:2128–2138, 1997.

295. Borovikova LV, Ivanova S, Zhang M, et al. Vagus nerve stimulation attenuates the systemic inflammatory response to endotoxin. Nature 405:458–462, 2000.

296. Wang H, Yu M, Ochani M, et al. Nicotinic acetylcholine receptor alpha7 subunit is an essential regulator of inflammation. Nature 421:384–388, 2003.

297. Kondo H, Nifuji A, Takeda S, et al. Unloading induces osteoblastic cell suppression and osteoclastic cell activation to lead to bone loss via sympathetic nervous system. J Biol Chem 280:30192–30200, 2005.

298. Elefteriou F, Ahn JD, Takeda S, et al. Leptin regulation of bone resorption by the sympathetic nervous system and CART. Nature 434:514–520, 2005.

299. Persson E, Lerner UH. The neuropeptide VIP potentiates IL-6 production induced by proinflammatory osteotropic cytokines in calvarial osteoblasts and the osteoblastic cell line MC3T3-E1. Biochem Biophys Res Commun 335:705–711, 2005.

300. Matayoshi T, Goto T, Fukuhara E, et al. Neuropeptide substance P stimulates the formation of osteoclasts via synovial fibroblastic cells. Biochem Biophys Res Commun 327:756–764, 2005.

301. Elvenes J, Andjelkov N, Figenschau Y, et al. Expression of functional mu-opioid receptors in human osteoarthritic cartilage and chondrocytes. Biochem Biophys Res Commun 311:202–207, 2003.

302. Andjelkov N, Elvenes J, Martin J, et al. Opiate regulation of IL-1beta and TNF-alpha in cultured human articular chondrocytes. Biochem Biophys Res Commun 333:1295–1299, 2005.

303. Wieland HA, Michaelis M, Kirschbaum BJ, et al. Osteoarthritis-an untreatable disease? Nat Rev Drug Discov 4:331–344, 2005.

304. Smith GN, Jr., Mickler EA, Hasty KA, et al. Specificity of inhibition of matrix metalloproteinase activity by doxycycline: relationship to structure of the enzyme. Arthritis Rheum 42:1140–1146, 1999.

305. Yu LP, Jr., Smith GN, Jr., Brandt KD, et al. Reduction of the severity of canine osteoarthritis by prophylactic treatment with oral doxycycline. Arthritis Rheum 35:1150–1159, 1992.

306. Brandt KD, Mazzuca SA, Katz BP, et al. Effects of doxycycline on progression of osteoarthritis: results of a randomized, placebo-controlled, double-blind trial. Arthritis Rheum 52:2015–2025, 2005.

307. Flechtenmacher J, Huch K, Thonar EJ, et al. Recombinant human osteogenic protein 1 is a potent stimulator of the synthesis of cartilage proteoglycans and collagens by human articular chondrocytes. Arthritis Rheum 39:1896–1904, 1996.

308. Caron JP, Fernandes JC, Martel-Pelletier J, et al. Chondroprotective effect of intraarticular injections of interleukin-1 receptor antagonist in experimental osteoarthritis. Suppression of collagenase-1 expression. Arthritis Rheum 39:1535–1544, 1996.

309. Zhang X, Mao Z, Yu C. Suppression of early experimental osteoarthritis by gene transfer of interleukin-1 receptor antagonist and interleukin-10. J Orthop Res 22:742–750, 2004.

310. Fernandes J, Tardif G, Martel-Pelletier J, et al. In vivo transfer of interleukin-1 receptor antagonist gene in osteoarthritic rabbit knee joints: prevention of osteoarthritis progression. Am J Pathol 154:1159–1169, 1999.

311. Chevalier X, Giraudeau B, Conrozier T, et al. Safety study of intraarticular injection of interleukin 1 receptor antagonist in patients with painful knee osteoarthritis: a multicenter study. J Rheumatol 32:1317–1323, 2005.

312. Spector TD, Conaghan PG, Buckland-Wright JC, et al. Effect of risedronate on joint structure and symptoms of knee osteoarthritis: results of the BRISK randomized, controlled trial [ISRCTN01928173]. Arthritis Res Ther 7:R625–633, 2005.

313. Bernik TR, Friedman SG, Ochani M, et al. Pharmacological stimulation of the cholinergic antiinflammatory pathway. J Exp Med 195:781–788, 2002.

314. Mohtai M, Smith RL, Schurman DJ, et al. Expression of 92-kD type IV collagenase/gelatinase (gelatinase B) in osteoarthritic cartilage and its induction in normal human articular cartilage by interleukin 1β. J Clin Invest 92:179–185, 1993.

Pathology of Osteoarthritis

3

Aubrey J. Hough, Jr.

HISTORICAL CONCEPTS OF OSTEOARTHRITIS

Medical science is to a degree inseparable from its ancient origins in so-called natural philosophy. Disease itself was originally regarded as the visitation of evil recompense, often for specific sins of omission or commission. Thus, the naming of diseases took on a semantic basis reflecting primitive ideas about causation as well as symptoms. In some ways, the naming of diseases was originally analogous to the naming of other perceived manifestations of evil, such as demons, before exorcism. In other words, the name of the disease must necessarily precede its cure. Hence, the Latin noun rheuma, denoting a fluid exudation, became the linguistic source for rheumatism. This illustrated both a principal external sign of joint disease, swelling, and the theoretical consideration of imbalance in fluid (phlegm) derived from the galenic humoral theory of disease.

It was not until the period of the enlightenment (1600–1760) that serious scientific attempts were made to subclassify accurately the various forms of arthritis known to us today. In the nineteenth century, subsequent accumulation of scientific and clinical evidence led to the first delineations of specific arthritic disorders,[1] such as gout and rheumatoid arthritis (Alfred B. Garrod, circa 1858–1876) and ankylosing spondylitis (Adolph Strumpell, 1897; Pierre Marie, 1898). Morbid anatomy played an important part in these discoveries. Perhaps owing to the lack of systemic symptoms in most cases, the entity now known as osteoarthritis emerged fairly late as a distinct disorder, although specific manifestations, such as Heberden (1802) and Bouchard (1884) nodes, were described before recognition that they were associated with a specific disease state. Although several individuals had earlier observed localized erosion of cartilage, especially in relation to deforming lesions of the hip,

Archibald E. Garrod (1907) was the first to clearly distinguish rheumatoid arthritis from osteoarthritis. The twentieth century emergence of more unitary concepts of osteoarthritis has been reviewed in detail by Sokoloff.[2] Understanding of the significance of the pathologic events on a molecular basis has amplified, rather than reduced the apparent complexity of the disorder and increased the need for careful consideration of sequential pathologic changes in its evolution.

DEFINITIONS AND TERMINOLOGY

The definition and terminology of osteoarthritis have long been the subject of conjecture, debate, and, at times, some degree of polemics. Even before the impact of molecular biology on medicine, Tarnopolsky[3] identified 54 different names for the entity, and the intervening half-century has produced more. The term osteoarthritis has gained primacy through long use in the English-speaking medical community, but it is less than satisfactory because of the implicit connotation that inflammation is the root cause of the disorder. Interestingly, osteoarthritis was the term originally proposed by John Spender in 1886 as a more suitable name for rheumatoid arthritis.[1] The terms osteoarthrosis and degenerative joint disease have a certain appeal but are nonspecific. Furthermore, they give no information about the pathologic processes that characterize the disorder. Arthritis deformans, as proposed by Heine[4] in 1926, was for many years considered a synonym for osteoarthritis in the European medical community. However, this usage primarily reflects the gross proliferative changes seen in advanced cases of primary osteoarthritis, particularly of the hip joint, and neglects the contributions of early destabilizing events that occur in either the articular cartilage or underlying subchondral bone. Articular cartilage changes did not come to the forefront until in the investigations of

51

Bennett, Waine, and Bauer[5] in 1942. In a far-reaching career, based almost entirely on pathologic examination, Johnson[6] promulgated the concept that osteoarthritis represents a decompensated remodeling of the joint in response to chronic biomechanical stress. That view persists, in at least modified form, to this day.

One current definition of osteoarthritis[7] takes into account "morphologic, biochemical, molecular and biomechanical changes of both cells and matrix which lead to softening, fibrillation, ulceration and loss of articular cartilage, sclerosis and eburnation of subchondral bone, osteophytes, and subchondral cysts." This chapter lays out the pathologic basis of osteoarthritis and current concepts of the role of pathology in understanding its pathogenesis.

MICROSCOPIC ANATOMY OF NORMAL JOINTS

The typical diarthrodial synovial joint has two opposing surfaces composed of hyaline articular cartilage. The cartilage is composed of four distinct zones. These are a superficial tangential zone characterized by chondrocytes and collagen fibers aligned roughly parallel to the surface, an intermediate zone, a deep radial zone with chondrocytes and collagen fibers aligned perpendicular to the surface, and a zone of calcified cartilage firmly joined to the underlying subchondral bone (Fig. 3–1A). The arrangement of the collagen fibers can be clearly appreciated when a section is illuminated with plane-polarized light (Fig. 3–1B). The junction of the zone of calcified cartilage with the deep radial zone is marked by an undulating hematoxyphilic line that is visible even in decalcified sections. The junction of this zone with subchondral bone is abruptly demarcated by a cement line into which fibers insert. This is seen clearly in electron micrographs (Fig. 3–2). Under normal conditions, the zone of calcified cartilage is slowly replaced by bone surrounding vascular ingrowths penetrating from the underlying subchondral bone marrow, but remodeling of this zone is an early feature of osteoarthritis.[8]

The viscoelastic behavior of cartilage is dependent on the water-binding properties of the matrix protein-polysaccharide moieties, which are in turn contained within a meshwork of collagen as illustrated in Figure 3–1b. The meshwork is predominantly the unique monomeric type II collagen that is enriched with hydroxylysine, but other minor collagens, such as type VI and type IX, are also present. Type IX collagen has been postulated to act as a link between proteoglycans and type II collagen. Type X collagen, itself more characteristic of epiphyseal cartilage, is found in calcified zones containing hypertrophic chondrocytes. Specific immunocytochemical procedures can demonstrate these collagens both in the normal state and in pathologic changes accompanying osteoarthritis. The marginal tissues of normal diarthrodial joints contain some areas of fibrocartilage, easily detectable because of the larger diameter of the collagen fibers contained therein and the reduced content of metachromatic proteoglycans compared with hyaline cartilage. Proliferative cartilage

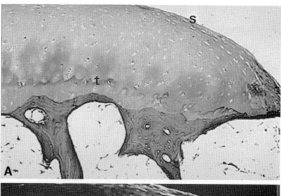
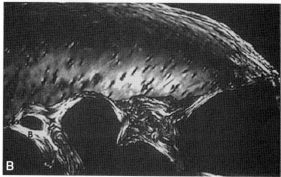

Figure 3–1 Normal proximal interphalangeal joint. *A,* Zone of calcified cartilage is delimited from deep radial zone by undulating tidemark (t). Tangential zone at surface (S) is clearly visible. Chondrocytes are small and disposed singly in lacunae. *B,* Same section viewed in plane-polarized light. Arrangements of the collagen fibers in the superficial tangential and deep radial zones and in the lamellar subchondral bone are clearly seen. (*A* and *B,* magnification ×40.)

associated with osteoarthritis is frequently overtly fibrocartilaginous in appearance, adding to the heterogeneity that exists even in the normal state.

CURRENT HYPOTHESES REGARDING PATHOLOGIC LESIONS

Most current ideas devolve from the concept that osteoarthritis arises from a chain of events leading to abnormal remodeling. Remodeling in this sense results in gradual removal of "old bone" at some sites and simultaneous production of "new bone" at others. This goes on normally with aging, but that which occurs in osteoarthritis is both qualitatively and quantitatively different from the normal situation in that it is both aberrant and progressive.

The maintenance of homeostasis in cartilage is analogous to that in bone; experimental models demonstrate loss of cartilage matrix in areas of decreased pressure and necrosis of chondrocytes in areas of increased pressure.[9] Similar loss of matrix with resultant thinning of articular cartilage is observed in humans in hip joints of patients with spastic cerebral palsy. Both chondrocyte[10] and osteocyte[11] death have been described in human osteoarthritis. Likewise, the view that fibrillation or denudation of cartilage always precedes bone remodeling is problematic. Fibrillation and remodeling of the basal calcified cartilage

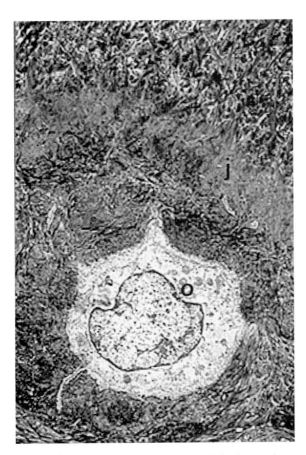

Figure 3–2 Electron micrograph of decalcified normal osteo-chondral junction of adult femoral head. Collagen fibers of zone of calcified cartilage insert into osteochondral junction (j). Osteocyte (o) is seen below. This arrangement creates an extremely strong bond between the two tissues. (Magnification ×6000.)

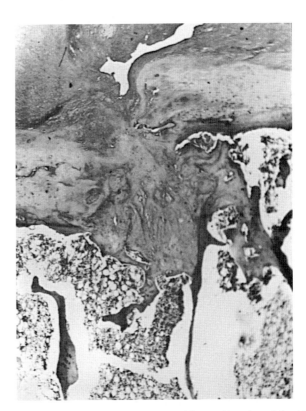

Figure 3–3 Osteochondral junction of femoral head in adult with early osteoarthritis. Microfracture of zone of calcified cartilage has extended through subchondral bony plate. Enchondral ossification is transpiring at that point. (Magnification ×50.)

often coexist but in different portions of the articular surface. Remodeling is prominent in non–weight-bearing areas with fibrillation occurring in the weight-bearing zones.[12] Microfractures[13] of the calcified cartilage (Fig. 3–3) themselves contribute to cartilage destruction by allowing vascularized marrow elements to penetrate the articular cartilage[8] thereby promoting dissolution or ossification in the cartilage. Subchondral bone remodeling of microfracture[14] may in itself promote cartilage destruction by increasing the stiffness of the underlying bone. In this view, repair of microfractures may cause the cartilage to absorb a greater portion of the energy impacting the joint.[15] The situation is clearly complex. However, disordered remodeling is the source of much of the pathology seen in progressive osteoarthritis.

Articular Cartilage in Osteoarthritis

Any consideration of the pathologic process of osteoarthritis begins with articular cartilage. As a nonvascularized tissue, articular cartilage displays a limited number of response patterns to injury. Fibrillation, characterized by vertically oriented superficial dehiscence of the extracellular matrix, is apparent in most cases of early osteoarthritis

examined at autopsy. This gives the cartilage the gross appearance of velvet rather than the normal glistening smooth appearance. Many of these examples of fibrillation apparently do not progress to clinically significant osteoarthritis. However, fibrillation is frequently seen in association with osteoarthritis, albeit in a pattern different from that described previously (Fig. 3–4). On microscopic examination, the fibrillation in osteoarthritis is usually associated with deeper clefts, more obvious dissolution of matrix, and chondrocyte proliferation in response to injury. A more pronounced stage of cartilage injury, less common than fibrillation, is known as cracking. Here, the vertical dehiscences are deeper, often extending into the zone of calcified cartilage, and are accompanied by a horizontal component as well (Fig. 3–5). Similar changes have been described in degenerating meniscal fibrocartilage.[16] This type of cracking can be seen macroscopically and is associated with erosion of cartilage from the loaded or weight-bearing areas that is characteristic of progressive osteoarthritis (Fig. 3–6).

Chondromalacia or softening of articular cartilage has been associated with fibrillation and has been described as an early change in progressive osteoarthritis. It is particularly prominent in precocious patellofemoral osteoarthritis (chondromalacia patellae) of younger individuals. However, differences in the histologic findings exist between chondromalacia of young adults and progressive osteoarthritis.[17] In addition, chondromalacia patellae without malalignment often does not progress to clinically

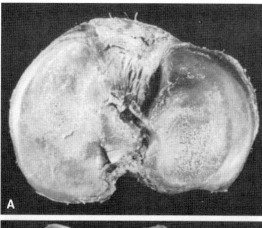

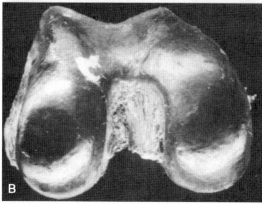

Figure 3–4 *A,* Gross photograph of the tibial side of a knee joint obtained at necropsy from a 55-year-old man. This photograph was made with use of ultraviolet light, which provides much more surface detail. Note the fibrillation on both the medial and lateral sides, especially prominent in the areas not covered by the meniscus. *B,* Corresponding femoral surfaces, also photographed with ultraviolet light. Note the lack of fibrillation on this joint surface. In the early stages of degenerative joint disease, more often than not, fibrillation is seen on only one of the opposed articular surfaces. This is in marked contrast to eburnation, in which both of the opposed surfaces are affected.

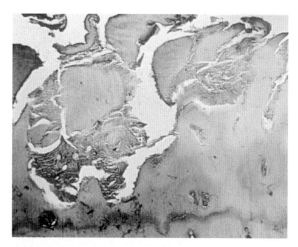

Figure 3–5 Femoral head of adult demonstrates severe fibrillation leading to cracking that extends into tidemark zone. Lateral extension has produced a poorly attached fragment. Resulting defect will be filled by either repair fibrocartilage or ossifying granulation tissue penetrating from the subchondral bone. (Magnification ×50.)

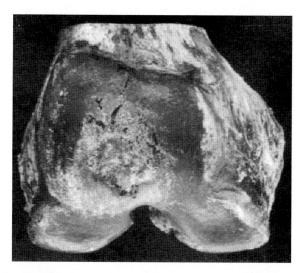

Figure 3–6 Gross photograph made with ultraviolet light demonstrates an erosion on the femoral side of the patellofemoral joint. Such lesions are common in older individuals. Note that there is not only fibrillation but also some cracking of the cartilage.

significant osteoarthritis[18] and the disorder is related more strongly to injury than osteoarthritis.[19] Chondromalacia is also associated with changes in the type and content of proteoglycans.[20] This predisposes the cartilage to erosion with exposure of underlying bone in severe examples. The loss of matrix proteoglycans also exposes the collagen fibrils so that they may undergo disaggregation[21] and release type II collagen fragments.[22]

Early accounts[5] noted the increased numbers of chondrocytes adjacent to areas of chondromalacia and the increased affinity of the perilacunar matrix for hematoxylin. More recent studies have confirmed an increase in the synthetic activities of chondrocytes, including collagens[23] and degradative enzymes,[24] in these zones. Although apoptosis of chondrocytes in osteoarthritis has been documented,[25] there is an obvious increase in numbers of chondrocytes characterized by multiple cells per lacuna adjacent to zones of fibrillation and chondromalacia (Fig. 3–7). Notwithstanding that metaplastic chondrocytes in osteoarthritis might be capable of migration to produce this appearance,[26] the preponderance of evidence supports focal mitotic activity as the basis of the "clones."[27] The proliferating chondrocytes associated with erosive lesions have been demonstrated to contain unstable DNA with tetraploidy.[28] Other studies have identified trisomy 7 as a characteristic acquired somatic mutation in osteoarthritic synovia and cartilage.[29] Enlarged, phenotypically altered chondrocytes are also seen, particularly in the deeper zones (Fig. 3–8). These cells have been shown to produce type X collagen, normally associated with the hypertrophic zone of epiphyseal cartilage.[30]

The proliferation of chondrocytes has long been associated with the perilacunar dissolution phenomenon known as Weichselbaum lacunar resorption. This change (Fig. 3–9) was once identified as relatively specific for early osteoarthritis but is also seen in rheumatoid arthritis. It is best regarded as a histologic expression of degrading of cartilage matrix by chondrocytes responding to cytokines, recently described quanitatively.[31]

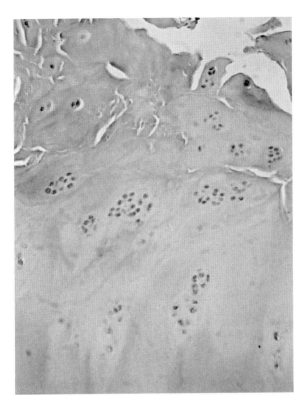

Figure 3–7 Photomicrograph from osteoarthritic proximal tibial articular surface demonstrates chondrocyte proliferation adjacent to area of fibrillation. (Magnification ×50.)

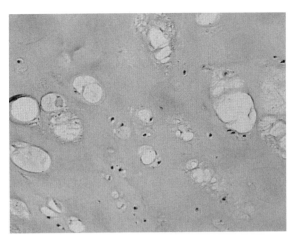

Figure 3–9 Chondrocytic resorption of surrounding matrix in osteoarthritis, which is occurring even at a distance from any zones of fibrillation or repair. This is evidence of cytokine stimulation of degradative enzyme release. (Magnification ×50.)

Suppression of anabolic activities, particularly those of matrix protein synthesis, has been demonstrated in upper zones of osteoarthritic cartilage.[32] Secretion of several matrix metalloproteinases is increased over that in normal cartilage,[33] particularly in response to tumor necrosis factor-α (TNF-α)[33] or interleukin-1α.[33] Consequent release of type II collagen fragments correlates with the progression of osteoarthritis.[34,35]

In osteoarthritis the original hyaline articular cartilage is partially replaced in progressive disease by a repair cartilage (Fig. 3–10). This cartilage often overlies a deeper zone of original articular cartilage (Fig. 3–11). Frequently, this repair cartilage has the histologic and histochemical characteristics of fibrocartilage, containing obvious broad collagen fibers and reduced amounts of matrix proteoglycans compared with native hyaline articular cartilage. In advanced osteoarthritis, none of the original hyaline cartilage may remain (Fig. 3–12). Although type II collagen continues to be produced[36] in osteoarthritic repair cartilage, a class switch to type I collagen[23] has been demonstrated in more advanced osteoarthritis[37] as well as marked loss of type VI collagen from the perilanucunar matrix.[38]

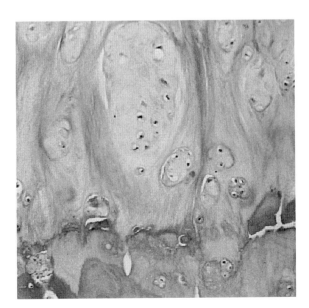

Figure 3–8 Enlarged chondrocytes in deep radial zone have proliferated and are undergoing hypertrophy followed by enchondral ossification in the zone of calcified cartilage. This contributes to thinning of the articular cartilage. (Magnification ×50.)

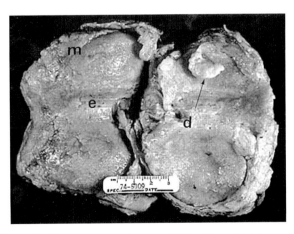

Figure 3–10 Gross view of osteoarthritis of knee joint in an elderly man. Menisci have been removed to enhance visibility. Femoral condyles demonstrate roughened surface composed of repair fibrocartilage. This is especially prominent at joint margins (m). Intercondylar groove and corresponding area on tibia demonstrate some eburnation (e). Joint mouse (arrow) corresponds to defect (d) in tibial surface.

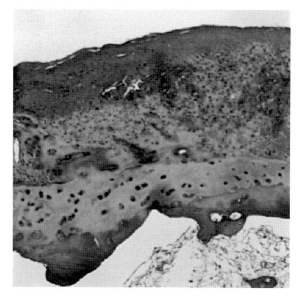

Figure 3–11 Cellular repair fibrocartilage on surface of joint. Note underlying residual hyaline articular cartilage. (Magnification ×50.)

The cartilaginous surface of osteophytes is covered by a mixture of fibrocartilage and fibrous tissue, at times overlying a residual area of hyaline cartilage and original subchondral bone (Fig. 3–13). For these reasons, biochemical and molecular studies of osteoarthritic cartilage frequently produce heterogeneous results, depending on the admixture of native cartilage, repair cartilage, and fibrocartilage in the specimens examined.

The tidemark, as seen in Fig. 3–1, is defined as an undulating hematoxyphilic line marking the boundary of the zone of calcified cartilage with the deep radial zone of articular

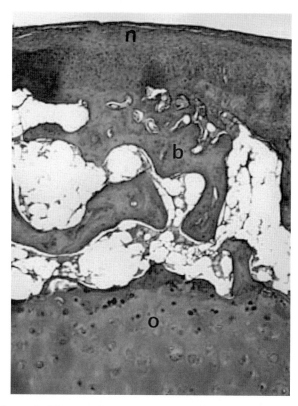

Figure 3–13 Formation of an osteophyte. New cartilaginous surface composed of cellular repair cartilage (n) and subchondral bone (b) lies over old hyaline cartilaginous surface (o), which will eventually be eliminated by bidirectional enchondral ossification. (Magnification ×50.)

cartilage. In osteoarthritis, this line becomes extensively reduplicated, often with irregular projections of calcified cartilage into the basal articular cartilage (Fig. 3–14). Several types of degenerative change in the zone of calcified cartilage have been reported[39] in association with osteoarthritis.

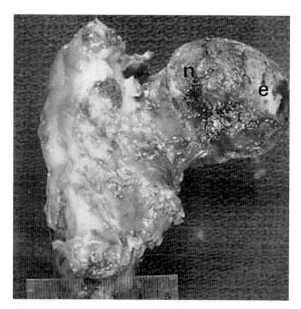

Figure 3–12 Gross view of femoral head and neck removed at autopsy in 62-year-old man with severe bilateral hip osteoarthritis. No residual hyaline articular cartilage remains. Margins of joint demonstrate bosselated nodules of fibrocartilage (n) overlying marginal buttress osteophytes. An area of eburnation (e) is present on the superolateral weight-bearing surface.

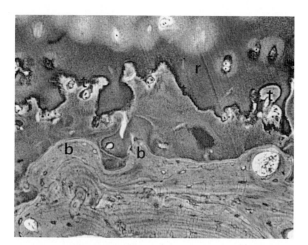

Figure 3–14 Remodeling changes of calcified cartilage and osteochondral junction in osteoarthritis as shown by a Bodian protargol impregnation stain. Tidemark (t) is tortuous with extensions of calcified cartilage into deep radial zone (r). Chondrocytes of calcified cartilage are hypertrophic. Tongues of bone (b) extend into the calcified cartilage. (Magnification ×50.)

Degenerative changes in the zone of calcified cartilage, including reduplication and advancement into the basal noncalcified articular cartilage, occur early in the course of osteoarthritis, often apparent in underlying areas with only minimal fibrillation. As a result, considerable speculation remains as to the possible role of changes in the calcified cartilage in initiating or promoting osteoarthritis.[40,41] Advancement of the vascularized subchondral ossification front could contribute to thinning of the articular cartilage, thereby leading to progression of osteoarthritis. It may also be related to the re-expression of vascular endothelial growth factor by chondrocytes noted in an experimental model.[42]

Subchondral Bone in Osteoarthritis

As heretofore discussed, remodeling of the bone-cartilage interface occurs early in the course of osteoarthritis, often in areas underlying fibrillated articular cartilage. Several other forms of remodeling also occur in the subchondral bone, either directly beneath the weight-bearing surface or at the margins of the joint. The latter constitute the osteophytes so characteristic of primary osteoarthritis.

Proliferation of bone in the subchondral areas leads to remodeling of the bone–calcified cartilage interface with vascular incursion into the articular cartilage.[8,43] Eventually, spikes of granulation and fibrous tissue reach the joint surface. Enchondral ossification, together with intramembranous ossification of fibrovascular tissue penetrating the cartilaginous surface (Fig. 3–15), produces thinning of cartilage[44] and eventual exposure of smooth, dense bone on the articular surface (Fig. 3–16). This phenomenon, known as eburnation, is characterized not only by dense bone at the articular surface, but also by marked sclerosis of the subchondral cancellous bone. This change can be observed while some cartilage remains on the joint surface but is most marked when cartilage is totally absent as suggested by quantitative studies.[45] At times, the resulting dense bone demonstrates secondary osteonecrosis characterized by small zones of devitalized bone with empty lacunae devoid of viable osteocytes. Although usually appreciated only on microscopic examination, the zones are large enough at times to be visible grossly (Fig. 3–17). The appearance is distinctly different from primary osteonecrosis (avascular necrosis), in which a subchondral bony sequestrum underlies viable articular cartilage. The

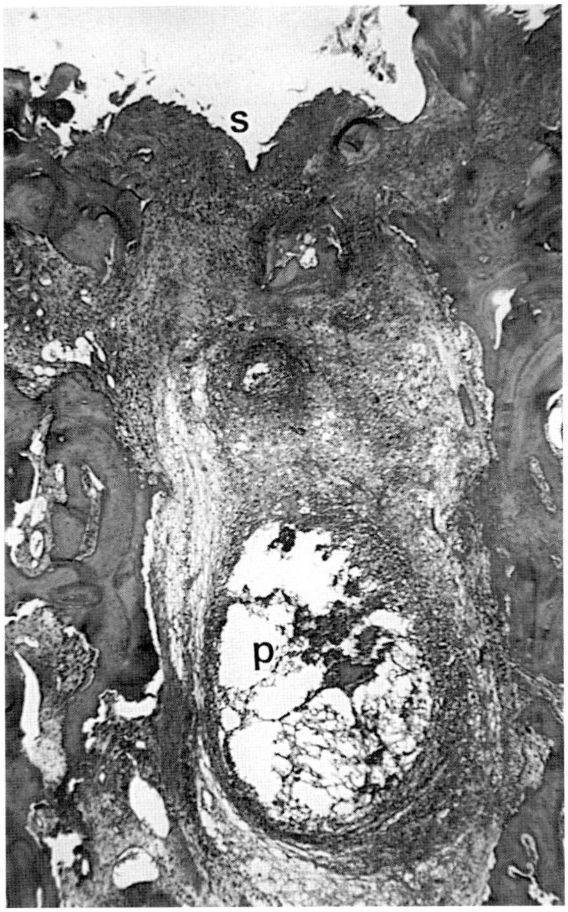

Figure 3–15 Established osteoarthritis of femoral head. Fibrocartilaginous surface (s) is breached by a column of granulation tissue extending from underlying subchondral marrow. This is a stage in the eburnation of the joint surface. A small pseudocyst (p) is present. (Magnification ×60.)

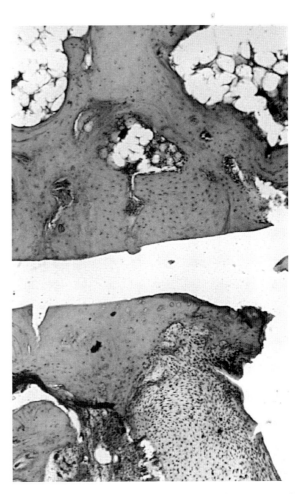

Figure 3–16 Eburnation of opposing joint surfaces in interphalangeal joint of elderly woman with generalized osteoarthritis of the nodal type. Articular cartilage has been replaced by sclerotic bone. (Magnification ×50.)

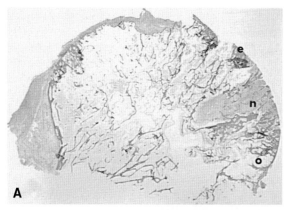

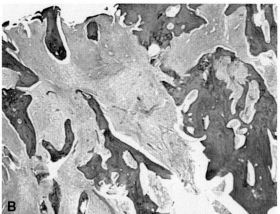

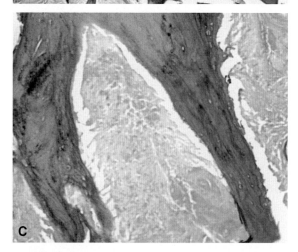

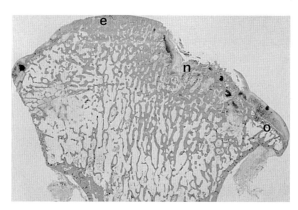

Figure 3–18 Whole mount coronal section of femoral head from adult man with long-standing osteoarthritis. Eburnation of weight-bearing surface (e) borders zone of superficial secondary osteonecrosis (n) that has collapsed. Rapid progression can occur under these conditions. Note osteophyte (o) adjacent to collapse. (Magnification ×2.)

patients with osteoarthritis develop sterile subchondral inflammatory microabscess-like accumulations.[47] The pathogenesis of these zones is uncertain, but they may contribute to collapse associated with rapidly progressive variants of osteoarthritis.

Microfractures of subchondral bone trabeculae also have a potential role in the provocation and progression of osteoarthritis. Subchondral trabecular fractures must be distinguished from microfractures of the calcified cartilage (Fig. 3–3) and bony plate.[48] These allow vascularization of the cartilage, and when communicating with the surface, provoke intra-oseous pseudocyst formation (Fig. 3–19). Vascular invasion of the basal calcified cartilage may lead to ossification and resulting thinning of the cartilage, increasing shear stresses.[49] Microfractures are easily demonstrated in load-bearing zones of subchondral bone,[50] but they are decreased in osteoarthritis.[49,51] This suggests the remodeling of bone into thicker, less compliant trabeculae[52] may be the primary event in producing

Figure 3–17 Osteoarthritic femoral head with secondary osteonecrosis. *A*, Whole mount coronal section shows area of eburnation (e), adjacent superficial subchondral bone necrosis (n), and osteophyte (o). (Magnification ×2.) *B*, Medium-power photomicrograph of same slide clearly shows devitalized bone and bone marrow. (Magnification ×50.) *C*, Higher power view shows absence of nuclei in bone and bone marrow. This type of superficial necrosis must be distinguished from primary avascular necrosis. (Magnification ×300.)

role of this secondary osteonecrosis in promoting collapse of the articular surface (Fig. 3–18) in advanced osteoarthritis has been the subject of discussion for years. The pathogenesis of this condition is presumably related to occlusion of minute intramedullary arteries. At any rate, it is common, occurring in up to14% of femoral heads resected for severe osteoarthritis.[46] In addition, some

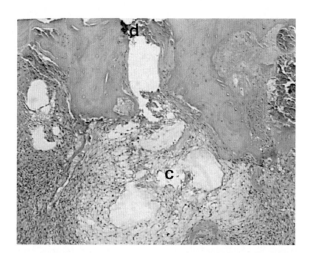

Figure 3–19 Photomicrograph from femoral head with osteoarthritis. Low-power view shows defect (d) in surface that has penetrated into subchondral bone marrow. Pseudocyst (c) filled with myxoid material lies beneath defect. (Magnification ×50.)

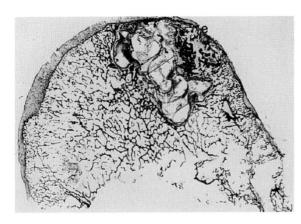

Figure 3–20 Whole mount coronal section of femoral head with established osteoarthritis. Eburnation (e) borders large pseudocyst (arrows) surrounded by reactive bone. Marginal osteophytes increase apparent diameter of femoral head. (Magnification ×1.5.)

cartilage damage rather than microfractures themselves. Remodeling of bone in osteoarthritis has been confirmed by both direct observation and fractal analysis.[53]

Another characteristic of progressive osteoarthritis is the formation of subchondral pseudocysts (Fig. 3–20). These are especially prominent in both the acetabular and femoral components of the hip joint. These spaces usually contain fluid and fibromyxoid material with occasional fragments of nonviable bone or cartilage. When mature, the pseudocyst is surrounded by a thin rim of reactive bone (Fig. 3–20). Minute gaps penetrating through the subchondral plate and articular cartilage are commonly seen at the apex of these pseudocysts, especially if serial sections are obtained (Fig. 3–19). The most attractive theory regarding pseudocysts is that the intrusion of intra-articular pressure through osteocartilaginous discontinuities produces local necrosis leading to the rarefied zones.[54] This is also supported by the observation that the pseudocysts tend to

disappear as osteoarthritis progresses to an advanced state with the joint surface being replaced by either a solid layer of eburnated bone (Fig. 3–16) or repair fibrocartilage (Fig. 3–21). Enchondral bone formation is characteristic of progressive osteoarthritis. This may take the form of enchondral bone formation at the base of articular cartilage (Fig. 3–13) or at the margins of the joint.[55] The latter type, when fully developed, leads to osteophytes (Fig. 3–22). These bony outgrowths characteristically appear in areas away from the major weight-bearing zones. Large osteophytes are particularly characteristic of primary osteoarthritis of the hip joint; their absence suggests that osteoarthritis, if it is present, has resulted from prior inflammatory lysis of cartilage resulting in secondary rather than primary osteoarthritis (Fig. 3–23). Another characteristic phenomenon is the presence of osteochondral loose bodies known as joint mice. These fragments are composed of proliferative cartilage surrounding devitalized bone (Fig. 3–24). Their origin from the disordered joint surface is proved by the presence of corresponding defects left by their avulsion (Fig. 3–4). Whether the primary factor in their genesis is underlying subchondral necrosis, disordered enchondral ossification, or mechanical avulsion is difficult to prove. The primacy of cartilage versus bone alterations in the provocation of osteoarthritis remains debatable. However, there can be no doubt that the latter stages are characterized by marked proliferative and degenerative changes of subchondral and marginal bone.

Periarticular Soft Tissues in Osteoarthritis

Current theories focus on osteoarthritis as a disorder resulting from aberrant responses of articular cartilage and subchondral bone to cytokines produced both systemically and locally.[56,57] Inflammatory aspects of osteoarthritis have, until recently, attracted less interest.[58,59] This should not obscure the fact that some degree of synovial villous

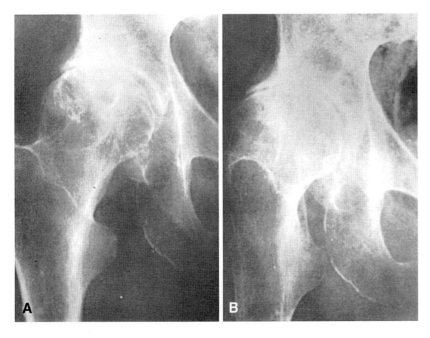

Figure 3–21 A, Clinical radiograph of a patient with advanced osteoarthritis is characterized by loss of the joint space and extensive cyst formation both on the acetabular side of the joint and in the femoral head. This patient was observed without treatment for 3½ years after this radiograph was taken. At that time, another radiograph of the hip was taken B, in which it can be appreciated that there is a diminution of the cysts in both the acetabulum and the femoral head, an apparent decrease in the sclerosis, and an increase in the joint space.

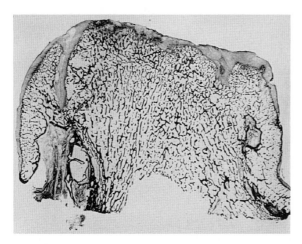

Figure 3–22 Whole mount coronal section of femoral head of adult woman with advanced osteoarthritis. Weight-bearing portion of joint is deformed, flattened, and covered with repair cartilage. Large bilateral osteophytes are present. (Magnification ×1.5.)

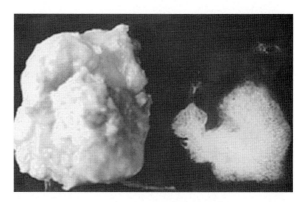

Figure 3–24 Gross appearance and matching radiograph of osteocartilaginous loose body (joint mouse). Nodular proliferative cartilage on surface is characteristic, as is the faint calcification seen in the cartilage at upper right of radiograph.

hypertrophy accompanied by fibrosis (Fig. 3–25) is common in osteoarthritis.[60] It is important to distinguish the stage of any particular case of osteoarthritis before ascribing causation to the synovial inflammation. This is one reason that autopsy hip joints with comparatively mild osteoarthritis do not reflect the synovial pathology of surgical specimens from hip replacement.[2] The synovial response in osteoarthritis has been postulated to evolve from an early exudative stage characterized by intimal hyperplasia to a late fibrotic stage.[60] Most studies of synovium in early osteoarthritis have shown that the synovitis is characterized histologically by a mild infiltrate composed primarily of lymphocytes and mononuclear cells[61] and that the infiltrates differ both qualitatively and quantitatively from those associated with rheumatoid arthritis.[62] Differences include greater overall cellularity[61] and

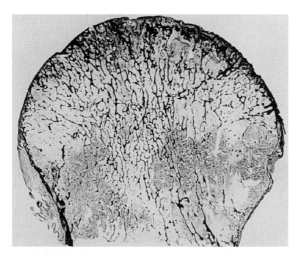

Figure 3–23 Whole mount coronal section of femoral head of adult woman with advanced secondary osteoarthritis after rheumatoid arthritis. Surface shows eburnation accompanied by underlying bony sclerosis. Note absence of osteophytes. (Magnification ×2.)

numbers of macrophages,[63] plasma cells, and CD4 T cells[64] in rheumatoid arthritis as opposed to osteoarthritis. Although the cellular and molecular character of the infiltrate in osteoarthritis clearly differs from that in rheumatoid arthritis, the presence of inflammation is undeniable. In one study, higher levels of the inflammatory marker C-reactive protein in serum of women predicted progression of early knee osteoarthritis.[65] Although cells with CD4 phenotype are more plentiful in rheumatoid arthritis,[64,66] cells with CD16+/56 phenotype indicative of natural killer cell activity are actually more numerous in osteoarthritis synovium.[66] Mast cells, with possible roles in mediating inflammation and bone destruction, are increased in the synovium in osteoarthritis and in one study were significantly more numerous than in rheumatoid synovium.[67] Other studies have examined the relationship of low-grade synovial inflammation in osteoarthritis to cytokine production.[68] Chondrocytes responding to chronic cytokine stimulation may well produce the degradation of matrix macromolecules, including type II collagen, so characteristic of progressive osteoarthritis.[34,35]

Many cases of advanced osteoarthritis are characterized by joint detritus consisting of cartilaginous or osteocartilaginous fragments embedded in the synovium.[69] This resulting detritic synovitis (Fig. 3–26) not only induces inflammation but stimulates production of degradative enzymes and cytokines by synovial macrophages. Detritic synovitis also creates the possibility that autosensitization to cartilage structural proteins may generate an immune response in osteoarthritis. In this regard, circulating proteoglycans have been demonstrated in the sera of patients with osteoarthritis.[70]

The immunopathology of osteoarthritis is equally complex. Deposits of immunoglobulin are definitely present in the superficial zone of cartilage in osteoarthritis.[71] Although the possibility exists that antibody formation is a response to matrix damage or detritic synovitis, autoantibodies are also seen in early osteoarthritis suggesting a role in provocation.[72]

Synovial inflammation in osteoarthritis cannot be separated from the role of crystal-induced inflammation. In osteoarthritis, both calcium pyrophosphate dihydrate

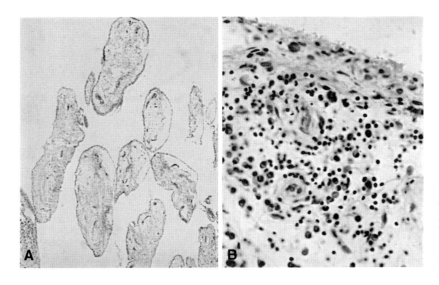

Figure 3–25 Photomicrographs of synovial tissue obtained from an osteoarthritic joint. *A,* Typical villous synovitis is characterized by fibrous projections lined by hyperplastic synovial cells. (Magnification ×30.) *B,* Higher magnification shows scattered lymphocytes and plasma cells in subsynovial tissue. (Magnification ×500.)

(CPPD) and basic calcium phosphate (BCP) have been identified in synovium, cartilage, and synovial fluid.[73] Crystals stimulate synthesis of interleukin-1, which causes synovial cells to release proteases capable of destroying cartilage matrix. Studies implicate TNF-α in this process[74] as well. The role of crystals in the genesis of inflammation in osteoarthritis is part of the larger question of the overall contribution of chondrocalcinosis to osteoarthritis.[73] The relationship of chondrocalcinosis in general to osteoarthritis has been the subject of continuing debate. It has been proposed that BCP crystals are correlated with osteoarthritis,[75] whereas CPPD crystals are associated with aging. Nevertheless, about half of the knees treated surgically for osteoarthritis after the age of 68 years have meniscal chondrocalcinosis, a sixfold increase above that of an age- and sex-adjusted postmortem population.[76] Chondrocalcinosis is much less frequent, however, in femoral heads removed for fracture. Deposition of CPPD in the menisci ordinarily does not generate an inflammatory reaction,[16] unlike synovial crystal deposition.

Periarticular soft tissues other than synovium are also involved, either directly or indirectly, in osteoarthritis. Barely visible or microscopic tears in capsular tissues are commonly seen. The ligaments and menisci of the knee joint develop fraying and cracking not unlike that of lesions of articular cartilage.[16] Substantial clinical evidence associates prior meniscectomy with subsequent osteoarthritis,[77] but there is a strong correlation between osteoarthritis of the knee and generalized osteoarthritis.[78] This would suggest that meniscectomy accentuates osteoarthritis in a genetically predisposed population.

Joint capsular tissues are also the site of other degenerative phenomena in osteoarthritis. These include lipochondral degeneration in capsular tissues of the hip that have undergone previous nodular chondroid metaplasia.[79] This change was not associated with CPPD deposition. However, calcific degeneration of the ligamentum teres is common in osteoarthritis of the hip. Deposits of the amyloid-associated protein type are also common (Fig. 3–27) in joint capsule and articular cartilage in osteoarthritis,[80]

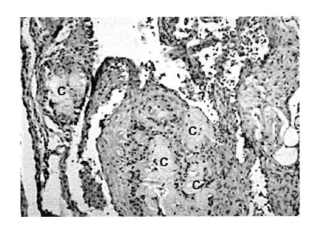

Figure 3–26 Detritic synovitis resulting from shards of abraded articular cartilage (C) impacted in the synovium. This is a feature of destructive, advanced osteoarthritis. (Magnification ×200.)

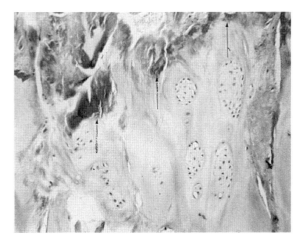

Figure 3–27 Congo red stain of elderly male patient with osteoarthritis demonstrates darkly stained deposits of amyloid (arrows) in cartilage. Note proliferation of chondrocytes. (Magnification ×50.)

but they also occur in joints of normal older individuals, and are strongly associated with concomitant deposition of CPPD crystals.[81] Periarticular fibrosis is also common and is especially marked in the subsynovial retinaculum in advanced osteoarthritis.[60] In the reverse of the situations described before, numerous connective tissue disorders including osteogenesis imperfecta types I and III,[82] Ehlers-Danlos syndrome (EDS) type VII,[83] and Larsen syndrome (osteochondrodysplasia with joint laxity) are associated with premature secondary osteoarthritis related to joint hypermobility. These are but one of several forms of heritable generalized osteoarthritis.

VARIANTS OF OSTEOARTHRITIS

The pathologic lesions more or less common to the induction and progression of osteoarthritis give ample evidence for the complexity of the disorder. This problem is exacerbated by the numerous variations on the central themes of the disease. These variations may be classified by one of several nosologic arrangements, such as generalized versus localized, primary versus secondary, and heritable versus acquired, or by some combination of such systems. For purposes of this discussion, secondary osteoarthritis is defined as that which develops in the setting of a known antecedent condition, which may be one of any number of disease states. Regardless of the classification employed, several distinct varieties have emerged on the basis of characteristic clinical and pathologic findings.

Primary Generalized Osteoarthritis

Primary generalized osteoarthritis is a variant of osteoarthritis characterized by a preponderance in middle-aged or older women and by Heberden node formation as well as carpometacarpal and knee involvement. Most cases have clinical signs of articular inflammation. Proliferation of adjacent bone to form osteophytes is the most conspicuous pathologic finding, and this apparently begins prior to destruction of the surface cartilage.[84] Progression of articular cartilage erosion to eburnation is not as common as in weight-bearing joints. Heberden and Bouchard nodes are actually osteophytes in a characteristic location (Fig. 3–28) and are not a unique pathologic process. For many years, debate has continued as to whether osteoarthritis of the hip and knee joints is more frequent in patients with generalized osteoarthritis than in those without it. Notwithstanding the obvious differing contributions that occupation and obesity might bring to the hands versus the hips,[85] most epidemiologic studies have affirmed a positive relationship,[86] as with bilateral knee involvement.[78,87] However, no unique pathologic features distinguish primary hip and knee osteoarthritis in patients with hand disease from those without it.

The familial tendency of generalized osteoarthritis has been recognized for decades, although workload on the hands may contribute to the full expression of the disorder.[88] More recent investigations have linked a region of

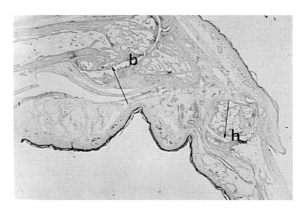

Figure 3–28 Whole mount coronal section of finger of elderly woman with generalized osteoarthritis. Heberden (h) and Bouchard (b) nodes are seen as osteophytes (arrows). (Magnification ×2.)

chromosome 2q23–35[89] to osteoarthritis of the hand. Familial aggregation with evidence for a mendelian recessive inheritance with a residual multifactorial component has been recently reconfirmed.[90]

Osteoarthritis with Heritable Collagen Defects

During the past decade, several kindreds have been reported with precocious osteoarthritis associated with various defects in type II collagen synthesis. In some instances, mild spondylodysplasia is associated with osteoarthritis.[91,92] Some families have point mutations,[91,92] whereas others suggest aberrancies in a promoter or intron region.[93] Another condition, Stickler syndrome (hereditary arthro-ophthalmopathy), is likewise associated with structural abnormalities in type II collagen.[94] The peripheral joints in these kindreds show marked erosion of cartilage. Electron microscopy in one spondylodysplasia kindred demonstrated parallel lamellar arrays of fine collagen fibrils in a case involving an arginine-cysteine point mutation.[95] Linkage analysis in families with early onset osteoarthritis demonstrates locus and allelic heterogeneity in three different collagen genes.[96] Thus, the genetic predisposition to the much more common types of primary osteoarthritis, although definite, appears to reside in several genetic loci.[97]

Endemic Osteoarthritis

Unlike some primary generalized or hereditary collagen defect–associated osteoarthritis variants, these are composed of cohorts primarily united by geography. At this time, several distinct types have been described clinically and pathologically. These include Kashin-Beck disease (endemic osteoarthrosis deformans) found in certain zones of northern China, Tibet, North Korea, and Siberia;[98] Mseleni disease found in South Africa's Zululand region;[99] and Handigodu disease found in southern India.[100] These share features in common that distinguish them from generalized osteoarthritis of the usual sort. These include occurrence in young people of both sexes and marked proliferative tendencies of bone and cartilage. In Kashin-Beck disease, the early changes consist of zonal necrosis of both articular and epiphyseal chondrocytes,[101] beginning in childhood and progressing to profound deformity, especially in the distal extremities. One study described decreased vascularization of the proximal cartilage end plate,[102] and increased apoptosis of chondrocytes has also been described.[103] Although selenium deficiency has been proposed as the agent in the disorder,[104] concomitant iodine deficiency may well be the evocative factor.[105] In addition, mold toxins have also been implicated,[106] and one, fulvic acid, has been shown to produce a Kashin-Beck–type picture in selenium-deficient mice[107] and to disturb oxidative metabolism of cultured chondrocytes.[108] Mseleni disease, like Kashin-Beck disease, is polyarticular, but the hip is particularly severely affected. Pathologic studies[109] of resected femoral heads have demonstrated a rough articular surface composed of degenerated and regenerated articular cartilage rather than eburnated bone. Interestingly, the disorder is also associated with pathologically demonstrated osteomalacia.[110]

Although familial aggregation of Mseleni osteoarthropathy is present, molecular studies have shown no relationship to the histocompatibility complex (HLA) system; however, a mutation in type II collagen might be involved in some cases.[99] Heterogeneity is further suggested by the observation that some patients with Mseleni disease also have a dwarfing spondylodysplasia.[111] Handigodu disease[100] shows many pathologic similarities to Mseleni osteoarthropathy but demonstrates an autosomal dominant pattern of inheritance. These relatively obscure diseases may yet offer information applicable to more common types of joint disease.

Secondary Osteoarthritis Variants

Numerous antecedent conditions result in secondary osteoarthritis of polyarticular, oligoarticular, or monoarticular patterns. These conditions are summarized in Table 3–1. A variety of mechanisms are involved, but all eventually lead to cartilage erosion and bone remodeling characteristic of osteoarthritis. Generally speaking, the more tendency to inflammation shown by the evocative disorder, the less prominent will be the bone remodeling manifested as osteophytes. In other circumstances, specific infiltrates, such as urate in gout or hemosiderin in hemophilic arthropathy, may give mute testimony to the origin of the secondary osteoarthritis. In others, the profoundly degenerated "end-stage" joint may pose a diagnostic dilemma as to the antecedent condition. In some circumstances, such as CPPD deposition disease, distinguishing primary osteoarthritis associated with CPPD deposition from secondary osteoarthritis can be almost impossible, especially in the knee joint.[112]

Osteoarthritis with Joint Hypermobility

A number of heritable disorders of connective tissue result in abnormal joint laxity, often with recurrent dislocations. Precocious osteoarthritis associated with erosion

TABLE 3–1
PATHOGENETIC CLASSIFICATION OF SECONDARY OSTEOARTHRITIS

HERITABLE STRUCTURAL ABNORMALITIES
Abnormal joint laxity
  Ehlers-Danlos (type VII) and tenascin-x def.
  Osteogenesis imperfecta (types I and III)
  Marfan syndrome
  Larsen syndrome
Abnormal cartilage structure
  Achondroplasia
  Spondyloepiphyseal dysplasias
  Multiple epiphyseal dysplasias
  Diastrophic dysplasia
  Metaphyseal chondrodysplasias
  Ochronosis
  Mucopolysaccharidoses
  Hemophilia

ACQUIRED STRUCTURAL ABNORMALITIES
Avascular necrosis
Steroid arthropathy
Paget disease
Post-traumatic incongruity
Legg-Perthes disease
Slipped capital femoral epiphysis
Neuropathic degeneration
Acromegaly
Diabetes mellitus*

CRYSTAL DEPOSITION DISEASES
Calcium pyrophosphate
  Primary: including 8q (ANKH) and 5p associated
  Secondary: hyperparathyroidism, hemochromatosis, hepatolenticular degeneration, ochronosis, others
Basic calcium phosphate
Urate (gout)
  Primary: including heritable forms
  Secondary: chemotherapy, diuretics, alcoholism, others
Oxalate
  Primary: heritable forms
  Secondary: renal failure, intestinal bypass, chronic inflammatory bowel disease

SYNOVIUM-MEDIATED STRUCTURAL ALTERATIONS
Postinflammatory
  Rheumatoid arthritis
  Seronegative spondyloarthritis
  Miscellaneous
Infectious and postinfectious

*Heritable component also.

of articular cartilage customarily results. EDS is a heterogenous disorder frequently involving joint hypermobility. Two types are definitely associated with osteoarthritis. These include EDS type VII due to mutations in the type I collagen α2 chain[113] and EDS due to mutations in the gene for tenascin-X.[114] Although osteoarthritis of multiple major joints is the rule, congenital hip dislocation is also encountered,[115] potentially leading to severe deformity in that joint resembling that seen in cerebral palsy. Osteogenesis imperfecta types I and III are associated with mutations in the $\alpha1(I)$ and $\alpha2(I)$ collagen chains, respectively.[116] In addition to osteoarticular deformity due to recurrent fractures, there is also ligamentous laxity. The combination results in early onset osteoarthritis. Ligamentous laxity is also the cause of the precocious osteoarthritis in Marfan syndrome. In Larsen syndrome (osteochondrodysplasia with joint laxity), multiple congenital dislocations also lead to premature osteoarthritis.[117] Major weight-bearing joints are particularly affected.

Osteoarthritis with Heritable Structural Abnormalities of Cartilage

A number of heritable conditions result in structurally abnormal articular cartilage or overall joint morphologic features. Osteoarthritis with variable degrees of generalization results. Achondroplasia, the most common form of short-limbed dwarfism, eventuates in severe osteoarthritis of the hips by early middle age with other joints variably affected. Numerous types of spondylodysplasias eventuate in osteoarthritis as well. The existence of kindreds with spondylodysplasias and specific mutations in type II collagen has been discussed previously. Stickler syndrome, an infantile presentation of spondylodysplasia with ocular abnormalities, is also associated with type II collagen mutations. Multiple epiphyseal dysplasias are forms of dwarfism not associated with spinal involvement that also culminate in severe osteoarthritis in weight-bearing joints in early adult life. Several forms of autosomal dominant multiple epiphyseal dysplasia have been described,[118] although less than half have an identified mutation.[119] The femoral head is the specimen most often available for pathologic study, and these specimens usually demonstrate marked eburnation and sclerosis without conspicuous osteophytes. Diastrophic dwarfism is another form of dwarfing chondrodysplasia resulting in a twisted appearance of the long bones. Because patients survive for normal life spans, severe degeneration of major joints occurs. Bilateral osteoarthritis of the hips requiring joint replacement is the rule. In cases of chondrodystrophic epiphyseal dysplasia, the small size of the femoral head should suggest that some variant of secondary osteoarthritis involving such a syndrome may be involved. Caution in diagnosis is required because similar small size coupled with severe osteoarthritis can also be seen in congenital hip dysplasia and Still disease.

Ochronotic Arthropathy. Another variant of osteoarthritis develops in patients with alkaptonuria, an autosomal recessive disorder resulting in a deficiency of homogentisic acid oxidase. Polymers of homogentisic acid accumulate in connective tissues, particularly cartilage, producing a bluish black discoloration and altering the water-binding properties of the matrix protein-polysaccharides. The resulting fragility of articular and intervertebral cartilage leads to precocious erosion[120] and, in the case of the diarthrodial joints, severe detritic synovitis. A type of generalized secondary osteoarthritis is the result. Unlike primary osteoarthritis, remodeling and osteophyte formation are not prominent. The pathogenesis of the disorder is complex. Calcium pyrophosphate crystals are frequently identified in ochronotic synovium, and homogentisic acid itself induces chondrocyte DNA damage through an oxidative process.[121] Unlike many forms of secondary osteoarthritis due to structurally abnormal cartilage, synovial inflammation due to joint detritus (and perhaps CPPD deposition) is a prominent feature.

Hemophilic Arthropathy. Hemophilic joint disease shares many common pathologic features with osteoarthritis.[122] These include early erosion of articular cartilage with accompanying bone remodeling leading to eburnation, subchondral sclerosis, and marginal osteophyte formation. Several additional distinctive findings are characteristic of hemophilic arthropathy. One such feature is the large quantity of hemosiderin pigment deposited in synovium in both intracellular and extracellular sites. Synovium is often brownish red but does not display the marked hyperplasia seen in pigmented villonodular synovitis, although invasive pannus may extend from the synovium during early stages of the hemophilic arthropathy (Fig. 3–29). Subchondral pseudocysts are usually prominent and, unlike those in primary osteoarthritis, contain hemosiderin pigment deposited in macrophages. Ankylosis, extremely rare in osteoarthritis, is not uncommon in late cases of hemophilic arthropathy. Joint contractures are also common and may be related to concomitant muscle injury from the hematomas. Interestingly, a single hemarthrosis of a traumatic origin does not ordinarily result in subsequent secondary osteoarthritis unless the joint surface or neighboring bone is fractured. Thus, recurrent exposure of synovium and cartilage to hemorrhage, perhaps under pressure, is necessary to produce chronic degenerative disease of hemophilic type.[123]

Osteoarthritis with Acquired Structural Abnormalities

Numerous acquired structural abnormalities result in severe secondary osteoarthritis. Among the more common are avascular necrosis,[124] trauma (especially that involving

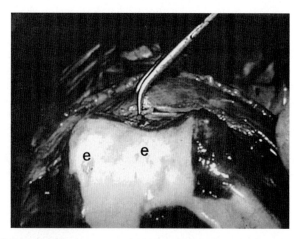

Figure 3–29 Gross photograph of knee joint with early hemophilic arthropathy. Vascularized pannus has extended over articular cartilage of femoral condyle. Erosions of cartilage (e) are already present.

the articular surface),[125] developmental dysplasia of the hip (formerly congential hip dysplasia),[126] and Paget disease.[127] Although diabetes mellitus is associated with a wide variety of connective tissue disorders, many of which affect the joints,[128] it is more difficult to demonstrate a direct causal relationship to osteoarthritis. Although some older studies have shown an increased prevalence of osteoarthritis among adult diabetics,[129] others have not linked osteoarthritis with impaired glucose tolerance.[130] Any association of osteoarthritis with diabetes mellitus would be extremely complex owing to confounding variables, including serum insulin and growth hormone levels, possible neurogenic acceleration, direct cartilage damage from glycosylation,[131] and the contribution of associated obesity.[132] Even if diabetes is removed as a comorbid factor, women with full-body radiographically defined osteoarthritis show decreased survival,[133] indicating that viewing any variant of generalized osteoarthritis as a joint disease devoid of serious systemic relationships is questionable.

Although uncommon, acromegaly uniformly results in severe generalized osteoarthritis.[134] Overgrowth of the ends of long bones in the disorder involves a combination of factors, including thickening of articular cartilage, enhanced enchondral bone formation in the osteochondral junction, and exuberant osteophyte formation. The terminal phalanges develop an "arrowhead" configuration because of these processes, but the appearance is dissimilar to generalized nodal osteoarthritis. The major weight-bearing joints are affected as well. In contrast to primary osteoarthritis, the cartilage is increased rather than decreased in thickness with marked fibrillation and cracking. Cellularity of the cartilage is increased, and enchondral ossification is usually prominent (Fig. 3–30). The possible relationship of acromegalic arthropathy to osteoarthritis in adult-onset diabetes mellitus is interesting because both groups of patients have elevated serum growth hormone levels,[135] as do patients with diffuse interstitial skeletal hyperostosis, a disorder that is definitely related to type II diabetes.

Some forms of secondary osteoarthritis related to acquired structural abnormalities tend to be localized to a joint or group of joints. The hip joint is the most common site for several such conditions, such as avascular necrosis. Others are entirely limited to the hips. This group includes congenital hip dysplasia, Legg-Perthes disease, and slipped capital femoral epiphysis. Although congenital hip dysplasia in canines is strongly heritable, the situation is far less clear in humans. Some evidence favors a generalized inherited connective tissue defect[136,137] but other findings support environmental influences[138] in the pathogenesis. Even when repaired early in childhood, severe precocious osteoarthritis often develops (Fig. 3–31). The femoral heads are small, in contrast to those of primary osteoarthritis, and characterized by exuberant repair cartilage. The gross deformation and osteoporosis seen in recurrent hip dislocation associated with cerebral palsy (Fig. 3–32) are even more severe. Some have suggested that subclinical childhood hip dysplasia is responsible for a significant proportion of localized coxarthrosis in mature adults.[139] However, one study in women failed to support this concept.[140]

Another cause of severe secondary osteoarthritis in the hip joints is Legg-Perthes disease. This disorder is manifested as necrosis of the growth center of the femoral head, usually occurring between 6 and 12 years of age, more commonly in boys; about one in seven cases is bilateral.[141] The resulting deformity is a characteristic small, flattened femoral head with bilateral beak-like osteophytes. Similar pathologic change is seen in secondary osteoarthritis due to aseptic necrosis of the hip in childhood from steroid administration, probably because of similar damage to the growth center. Eburnation can occur but is not characteristic. Although the cause of the disorder is obscure, synovitis is a characteristic feature of the early stages.[142] Studies have shown an increased prevalence of inherited factor V (Leiden) mutations in Legg-Perthes disease, but this still appears to be comparatively rare[143] as a fraction of those affected by the disorder.

The third type of childhood hip disease resulting in localized precocious osteoarthritis is slipped capital

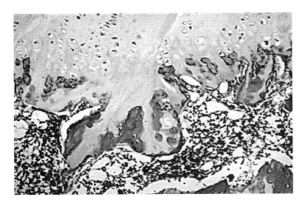

Figure 3–30 Photomicrograph of osteochondral junction from femoral head of adult male patient with acromegalic arthropathy and secondary osteoarthritis. Active enchondral ossification is present. Note resemblance of basal cartilage to a growing epiphysis. (Magnification ×75.)

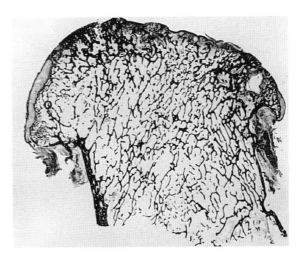

Figure 3–31 Whole mount coronal section of femoral head from 28-year-old woman with congenital hip dysplasia (dislocation). Large inferomedial osteophyte (o) is characteristic, as is small size of head compared with diameter of femoral neck. (Magnification ×2.0.)

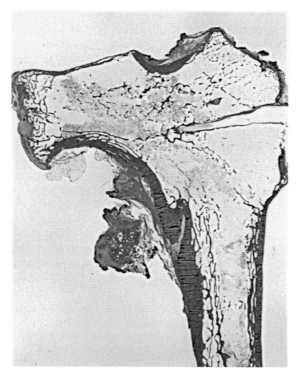

Figure 3–32 Whole mount macrosection of proximal femur from patient with spastic cerebral palsy and recurrent hip dislocation. Femoral head is small compared with greater trochanter and has a characteristic cuboid appearance. Cartilage is thin and degenerated, but eburnation is absent. (Magnification ×0.9.)

femoral epiphysis.[144] Affected patients are most commonly older male children who are likely to be obese. The disorder results from a fracture through the growth plate. The femoral head then slips inferiorly and posteriorly by variable amounts. Bilaterality is 25% to 40% and is predicted by greater physiologic age of the patient at the time of presentation.[145] Complete or total detachment is associated with osteonecrosis and more severe subsequent osteoarthritis. In such cases, the femoral head may be found reattached to the femoral neck at a lower position than normal. In addition to acromegaly, treatment with growth hormone for any of several indications, including chronic renal failure, is a risk factor for this condition.[146] One study of a large number of archived adult human skeletons suggested that 8% were involved by some degree of slipped capital femoral epiphysis and that severe osteoarthritis was likely to accompany it.[147] This degree of frequency remains to be established in clinical practice.

Osteoarthritis with Crystal Deposition Diseases

The complex biology of the crystal deposition diseases offers insights into the relationship of osteoarthritis to the deleterious effects of chronic low-grade synovial inflammation. All of the major crystal deposition diseases (CPPD, BCP, urate, and oxalate) occur in both primary and secondary forms. Some are clearly heritable.[148] The first two are largely diseases of the joints and supporting structures, whereas urate and oxalate arthropathies are systemic

diseases that affect the joints, oxalate inconstantly and usually in the setting of chronic renal failure.

Osteoarthritis with Calcium Pyrophosphate Dihydrate Deposition Disease. Osteoarthritis is clearly associated with the primary form of this disorder,[73] especially in the elderly, although it is difficult to prove a causal relationship absolutely because both diseases are common in that age group.[149] Although hereditary variants of primary chondrocalcinosis due to CPPD deposition certainly exist,[150] one family study failed to show an increased risk in siblings of chondrocalcinosis patients.[151] However, the condition may be underdiagnosed as serum nucleotide pyrophosphohydrolase activity was significantly elevated in patients with osteoarthritis whether CPPD crystals were demonstrated or not.[152] In one study, apoptotic chondrocytes induced by nitric oxide produced pyrophosphate,[153] providing a possible common mechanism between osteoarthritis and calcium pyrophosphate deposition disease. In addition, some cases of osteoarthritis clearly have CPPD crystals that are too small to be detected by conventional polarizing microscopy.[154] Thus, the association of CPPD crystals with osteoarthritis and their possible role in its pathogenesis may well be underestimated. In addition, secondary CPPD deposition disease occurs in association with several predisposing disease states, including hemochromatosis,[155] hyperparathyroidism, ochronosis, Wilson disease,[156] acromegaly,[134] neuropathic arthropathy,[157] and hemophilic arthropathy.[122]

The CPPD deposition disease associated with hemochromatosis is particularly likely to present as a generalized clinical arthropathy,[158] which may imitate rheumatoid arthritis. Genetic analyses have shown increased frequency of hemochromatosis genetic mutations in both apparently ordinary CPPD disposition disease[159] and undifferentiated arthritis.[160] The extent of CPPD deposition in Wilson disease is less severe. The contribution of CPPD deposition to neuropathic arthropathy can be particularly difficult to discern.[157] Calcific deposits in the synovium due to the severe detritic synovitis that results from joint disintegration are one of the hallmarks of the disorder. However, rapidly destructive neuropathic-like changes have been described with both BCP and CPPD deposition.[161]

Osteoarthritis with Basic Calcium Phosphate Deposition Disease. BCP deposition disease also occurs in both primary and secondary forms. Both extra-articular and intra-articular deposition are recognized and are associated with radiologic chondrocalcinosis. Periarthritis, tendinitis, erosive polyarthritis, or destructive monoarthritis (usually of the shoulder or knee) can be seen in any individual patient.[162] Severe local joint destruction may occur. Accurate diagnosis requires specialized techniques because the crystals are less than 100 nm in length and cannot be detected by conventional polarizing microscopy.[154] Alizarin red S staining of synovial fluid sediment is a customary method of screening.[161] Unlike uncomplicated primary osteoarthritis, increased granulocytes are present in both synovium and synovial fluid in acute BCP deposition disease. The destructive nature of BCP deposition disease may be derived not only from synovial release of enzymes and cytokines, but also by chrondocyte production of nitric oxidize synthase.[163] This may play a more general role in osteoarthritis as well.[164] BCP crystal shedding has also been demonstrated in cases that are clearly primary osteoarthritis.[161] Thus, potentiating effects of BCP crystal deposition may well be more common than is customarily realized.

Osteoarthritis with Urate Arthropathy (Gout). As in generalized osteoarthritis, strong hereditary tendencies are present in gout, even in the absence of defined enzymatic defects. However, the increasing incidence is principally related to dietary changes and obesity.[165]

In susceptible individuals, urate crystals deposited in and around joints evoke periodic attacks of severe acute inflammation, often in the small joints of the toes. Recurrent acute episodes usually lead to severe secondary osteoarthritis in the affected joints similar to that following infections. Such patients have clinical and pathologic features that allow ready separation from localized primary osteoarthritis. These include overwhelming male preponderance; small osteophytes; unusual articular distribution; and presence of urate deposits in synovial fluid, articular cartilage, synovium, joint capsule, and subchondral bone (Fig. 3–33). Deposits within articular cartilage are surrounded by necrotic chondrocytes. Eburnation and subchondral sclerosis are characteristic of advanced lesions, but the osteophytes, unlike those seen in primary osteoarthritis, are usually not prominent. Urate crystals are soluble in neutral buffered 4% formaldehyde, the customary fixative for surgical specimens. Hence, 95% alcohol should be employed for that purpose when urate arthropathy is suspected.[166] Viewing of sections from undecalcified tissues under plane-polarized light can then distinguish the leading contenders in the differential diagnosis [calcium pyrophosphate deposition disease (pseudogout), avascular necrosis, and infectious or postinfectious arthropathy] from chronic urate arthropathy. Secondary osteoarthritis from recurrent attacks of acute gout may affect any of the peripheral joints. However, for some unexplained reason, the first metatarsal joint is characteristically involved (podagra). The disease may be diagnosed during the intercritical period between acute attacks by the continuing presence of monosodium urate crystals in the synovial fluid.[167] This is more sensitive than aspiration of tophi because most patients with intercritical gout do not manifest them. Urate arthropathy has become a recognized phenomenon in elderly women, often in association with prolonged diuretic therapy.[165] These patients are more likely to have gout superimposed on generalized osteoarthritis even to the point of having tophi coexisting with and even deposited in Heberden nodes.[168] It is also prudent to remember that CPPD[169] and BCP crystals can coexist with those of urate and that patients with gout are more likely than their normal counterparts to have joint infections.[170] Tophaceous presentations of CPPD deposition disease can also imitate gout clinically.[171] Thus, pathologic examination of synovial fluid and joint tissues should be carried forth in such a manner as to exclude concurrent processes, even if a diagnosis of gout has previously been established.

Calcium Oxalate Deposition Disease. This heterogeneous group of disorders is composed of heritable primary oxalosis[172] and the much more common secondary variants associated with renal failure, intestinal bypass surgery, and chronic inflammatory bowel disease.[173] Articular manifestations of oxalosis in chronic renal failure, the most common antecedent, are usually less prominent than the bone lesions and often must be distinguished from dialysis osteoarthropathy due to either secondary hyperparathyroidism or β_2-microglobulin amyloid. Intracellular oxalate crystals are readily demonstrated by polarizing microscopy, but they are easily confused with CPPD crystals. Although large joints may be involved and the condition may be superimposed on existing osteoarthritis, involvement of the finger joints is characteristic.[173] The condition is unlikely to be confused with uncomplicated generalized nodal osteoarthritis, however, because of the antecedent historical information and the associated multifocal lytic bone lesions.

Osteoarthritis with Synovium-Mediated Structural Alterations

Several types of acute or chronic synovial inflammatory diseases produce structural damage to bone and cartilage by means of inflammatory vascularized pannus formation. This ultimately results in cartilage erosion and bone remodeling often leading to secondary osteoarthritis. Rheumatoid arthritis is the most common disorder of this group, but the seronegative spondyloarthropathies[174] as well as other miscellaneous disorders can create the destabilizing osteoarticular conditions that result in the superimposition of osteoarthritis on the preexisting inflammatory arthritis. This is particularly apparent when large weight-bearing joints such as femoral heads are removed for long-standing rheumatoid arthritis (Fig. 3–23). Eburnated bone with areas of fibrocartilage occupies the articular surface, and marked subchondral sclerosis may be present. Large osteophytes are absent. Similar changes may be seen in the large joints in other forms of chronic inflammatory arthritis if ankylosis does not supervene. Infectious arthropathies of several types also culminate in severe secondary osteoarthritis. Depending on the degree of residual bone and cartilage

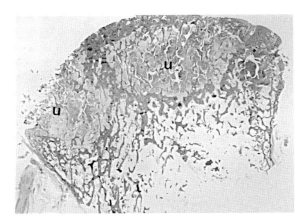

Figure 3–33 Whole mount coronal section of femoral head from adult man with severe secondary osteoarthritis due to recurrent gout. Large subchondral deposits of urate (u) and associated lipid are present. The joint surface shows marked eburnation, but osteophytes are inconspicuous. (Magnification ×2.)

deformity resulting from the infection, the affected joint or joints can assume bizarre configurations. In such cases, confusion with Charcot neuropathic arthropathy or destructive arthropathy associated with BCP or urate deposition is a possibility. Careful radiologic and pathologic studies can usually resolve the differential diagnosis.

SUMMARY CONCEPTS

The pathology of osteoarthritis gives insight into the pathogenesis of the disorder, as do several other fields of study. However, pathology in the clinical setting customarily views the morphologic changes only at one fixed point in time. Thus, the order in which events occurred, their dependency on one another, and their relative contributions to the final outcome can be difficult to discern. Nevertheless, the available pathologic evidence points to a multifactorial causation. Osteoarthritic cartilage lesions may result from heritable or acquired deficiencies in cartilage structural proteins, abnormal loading patterns, injury by inflammatory mediators, or changes in the underlying bone that result in decreased plasticity. Changes in the bone-cartilage interface and tidemark zones may also alter the metabolic state of the basal articular cartilage and result in ingress of cytokines and other mediators. Much of the obvious pathologic change of advanced osteoarthritis, such as eburnation, osteophytes, subchondral pseudocysts, secondary osteonecrosis, and detritic synovitis, is clearly reactive rather than etiologic. In some sites, such as the hands and possibly others as well, the genetic contribution to osteoarthritis may be dominant[86, 89,90] although not exclusive.[88,175] In others, such as the hips[85,176] and the knees,[177] strong environmental influences engendered by body weight [132] or occupation[178] are clearly operative as well. Conflicting evidence regarding similar dichotomous theories accompanies experimentally induced arthritis in animals. The true impact of genetic predisposition to osteoarthritis is only beginning to become manifest through the application of molecular biology. Pathology has its limits because it deals primarily with the realm of that which has already happened. From this, one infers what would have transpired had the process continued. Thus, the pathologist is only a pundit who relies on personal or collective experience to predict relationships from a finite body of information. This is why rational explanation of the etiopathogenesis of osteoarthritis requires contributions from other fields to supplement pathologic findings.

REFERENCES

1. Benedek TG. History of the rheumatic diseases. In: Klippel JH, ed. Primer on the Rheumatic Diseases. 11th ed. Atlanta, Arthritis Foundation, 1997, pp 1–5.
2. Sokoloff L. Some highlights in the emergence of modern concepts of osteoarthritis. Semin Arthritis Rheum 31:71–107, 2001.
3. Tarnopolsky S. Revision de la nomenclature rheumatologique. I. Les noms de Parthrose. Rev Rhum 17:497–500, 1950.
4. Heine J. Über die Arthritis deformans. Virchows Arch Pathol Anat 260:521–535, 1926.
5. Bennett GA, Waine H, Bauer W. Changes in the Knee Joint at Various Ages. New York, Commonwealth Fund, 1942.
6. Johnson LC, Kinetics of Osteoarthritis. Lab Invest 8:1223–1238, 1959.
7. Keuttner KE, Goldberg V, eds. Osteoarthritic Disorders. Rosemont, IL, American Academy of Orthopaedic Surgeons, 1995, pp 21–25.
8. Bonde HV, Talman MLM, Kofoed H. The area of the tidemark in osteoarthritis—a three dimensional sterelogical study in 21 patients. APMIS 113:349–352, 2005.
9. Martin JA, Brown TD, Heiner AD, et al. Chrondrocyte senescence, joint loading and osteoarthritis. Clin Orthop Relat Res 427; Suppl: S96–103, 2004.
10. Sharif M, Whitehouse A, Sharan P, et al. Increased apoptosis in human osteoarthritic cartilage corresponds to reduced cell density and expression of caspase-3. Arthritis Rheum 50: 507–515, 2004.
11. Mitrovic DR, Riera H. Synovial, articular cartilage and bone changes in rapidly destructive arthropathy (osteoarthritis) of the hip. Rheumatol Int 12:17–22, 1992.
12. Gelse K, Soder S, Eger W, et al. Osteophyte development-molecular characterization of differentiation stages. Osteoarthritis Cartilage 11:141–148, 2003.
13. Mori S, Haruff R, Burr DB. Microcracks in the articular cartilage of human femoral heads. Arch Pathol Lab Med 117:196–198, 1993.
14. Fazzalari NL, Kuliwaba JS, Forword MR. Cancellous bone microdamage in the proximal femur: influence of age and osteoarthritis on damage morphology and regional distribution. Bone 31:697–702, 2002.
15. Dequeker J, Aerssens SJ, Luyten FP. Ostseoarthritis and ostseoporosis: Clinical and research evidence of inverse relationship. Aging Clin Exp Res 15: 426–439, 2003.
16. Hough AJ, Webber RJ. The pathology of the meniscus. Clin Orthop 252:32–40, 1990.
17. Mori Y, Kubo M, Okumo H, et al. Histological comparison of patellar cartilage degeneration between chondromalacia in youth and osteoarthritis in aging. Knee Surg Sports Traumatol Arthrosc 3:167–172, 1995.
18. Jensen DB, Albrektsen SB. The natural history of chondromalacia patellae. A 12-year follow-up. Acta Orthop Belg 56:503–506, 1990.
19. Zhang H, Kong XQ, Cheng C, et al. A correlative study between prevalence of chondromalacia patellae and sports injury in 4068 students. Clin J. Traumatol 6:370–374, 2004.
20. Lorenzo P, Bayliss MT, Heiṅegard D. Altered patterns and synthesis of extracellular matrix macromolecules in early osteoarthritis. Matrix Biol 23:381–391, 2004.
21. Curtin WA, Reville WJ. Ultrastructural observations on fibril profiles in normal and degenerative human articular cartilage. Clin Orthop 313:224–230, 1995.
22. Tchetina EV, Squires G, Poole AR. Increased type II collagen degradation and very early focal cartilage degeneration is associated with upregulation of chondrocyte differentiation related genes in early human articular cartilage lesions. J Rheumatol 32:876–886, 2005.
23. Misoge N, Hartmann M, Maelicke C, et al. Expression of collagen type I and type II in consecutive stages of human osteoarthritis. Histochem Cell Biol 122:229–236, 2004.
24. Walter H, Kawashima A, Nebelung W, et al. Immunohistochemical analysis of several proteolytic enzymes as parameters of cartilage degradation. Pathol Res Pract 194:73–81, 1998.
25. Chen MN, Wang JL, Wong CY, et al. Relationship of chondrocyte apoptosis to matrix degradation and swelling potential of osteoarthritis cartilage. J Formos Med Assoc 104:264–272, 2005.
26. Kouri JB, Jimenes SA, Quintero M, et al. Ultrastructural study of chondrocytes from fibrillated and non-fibrillated human osteoarthritic cartilage. Osteoarthritis Cartilage 4:111–125, 1996.
27. Rotzer A, Mohr W: ^{3}H-thymidine incorporation into chondrocytes of arthritic cartilage [in German]. Z Rheumatol 51:172–176, 1992.
28. Macha N, Older J, Bitensky L, et al. Abnormalities of DNA in human osteoarthritic cartilage. Cell Biochem Funct 11:63–69, 1993.
29. Broberg K, Limon J, Palsson E, et al. Clonal chromosome aberrations are present in vivo in synovia and osteophytes from patients with osteoarthritis. Hum Genet 101:295–298, 1997.

30. Boos N, Nerlich AG, Wiest I, et al. Immunohistochemical analysis of type-X-collagen expression in osteoarthritis of the hip joint. J Orthop Res 17:495–502, 1999.

31. Konttinen YT, Ma J, Ruuttilal P, et al. Chrondrocyte-mediated collagenolysis correlates with cartilage destruction grades in osteoarthritis. Clin Exp Rheumatol 23:19–26, 2005.

32. Aigner T, Vornehm SI, Zeiler G, et al. Suppression of cartilage matrix gene expression in upper zone chondrocytes of osteoarthritic cartilage. Arthritis Rheum 40:562–569, 1997.

33. Imai K, Ohta S, Matsumoto T, et al. Expression of membrane–type I matrix metalloproteinase and activation of progelatinase A in human osteoarthritic cartilage. Am J Pathol 151:245–256, 1997.

34. Poole AR, Kobayashi M, Yasuda T, et al. Type II collagen degradation and its regulation in articular cartilage in osteoarthritis. Ann Rheum Dis 61:78–81, 2002.

35. Henrotin Y, Debert M, Dubuc JE, et al. Type II collagen peptides for measuring cartilage degradation. Biorheology 41:543–547, 2004.

36. Gebhard PM, Gehrsitz A, Bau B, et al. Quantification of expression levels of cellular differentiation markers does not support a general shift in the cellular phenotype of osteoarthritic chondrocytes. J Orthop Res 21:96–101, 2003.

37. Misoge N, Waletzko K, Bode C, et al. Light and electron microscopic in-situ hybridization of collagen type I and type II mRNA in the fibrocartilaginous tissue of late-stage osteoarthritis. Osteoarthritis Cartilage 6:278–285, 1998.

38. Soder S, Hambach L, Lissner R, et al. Ultrastructural localization of type VI collagen in normal adult and osteoarthritic human articular cartilage. Osteoarthritis Cartilage 10:464–470, 2002.

39. Amir G, Pirie CJ, Rashad S, et al. Remodeling of subchondral bone in osteoarthritis: a histomorphometric study. J Clin Pathol 45:990–992, 1992.

40. Oegema TR, Carpenter RJ, Hofmeister F, et al. The interaction of the zone of calcified cartilage and subchondral bone in osteoarthritis. Microsc Res Tech 37:324–332, 1997.

41. Burr DB. Anatomy and physiology of the mineralized tissues: role in the pathogenesis of osteoarthrosis. Osteoarthritis Cartilage 12; Supp A: 520–530, 2004.

42. Tanaka E, Aoyama J, Miyauchi M., et al. Vascular endothelial growth factor plays an important autocrine/paracrine role in the progression of osteoarthritis. Histochem Cell Biol 123: 275–281, 2005.

43. Shibakawa A, Yudoh K, Masuko-Hongo K, et al. The role of subchondral resorption pits in osteoarthritis: MMP production by cells derived from bone marrow. Osteoarthritis Cartilage 13: 679–687, 2005.

44. Dequeker J, Mokassa L, Aerssens J, et al. Bone density and local growth factors in generalized osteoarthritis. Microsc Res Tech 37:358–371, 1997.

45. Bobinac D, Spanjol J, Zoricic S, et al. Changes in articular cartilage and subchondral bone histomorphometry in osteoarthritic knee joints in humans. Bone 32:284–290, 2003.

46. Franchi A, Bullough PG. Secondary avascular necrosis in coxarthrosis: a morphologic study. J Rheumatol 19:1263–1268, 1992.

47. O'Connell JX, Nielsen GP, Rosenberg AE. Subchondral acute inflammation in severe arthritis: a sterile osteomyelitis? Am J Surg Pathol 23:192–197, 1999.

48. Sokoloff L. Microcracks in the calcified layer of articular cartilage. Arch Pathol Lab Med 117:191–195, 1993.

49. Burr DB, Radin EL. Microfractures and mircocracks in subchondral bone: are they relevant to osteoarthrosis? Rheum Dis Clin North Am 29:675–685, 2003.

50. Fassalari NL. Trabecular microfracture. Calcified Tissue Int 53 Suppl 1: 5143–5146, 1993.

51. Koszyca B, Fazzalari NL, Vernon-Roberts B. Microfractures in coxarthrosis. Acta Orthop Scand 61:307–310, 1990.

52. Ding M, Odgaarda A, Hvid I. Changes in the three-dimensional microstructure of human tibial cancellous bone in early osteoarthritis. J Bone Joint Surg Br. 85:906–912, 2003.

53. Fazzalari NL, Parkinson IH. Fractal properties of subchondral cancellous bone in severe osteoarthritis of the hip. J Bone Miner Res 12:632–640, 1997.

54. Dorr HD, Martin H, Pellengahr C, et al. The cause of subchondral bone cysts in osteoarthrosis: a finite element analysis. Acta Orthop Scand. 75:554–558, 2004.

55. Neuman P, Hulth A, Linden B, et al. The role of osteophytic growth in hip osteoarthritis. Int Orthop 27:262–266, 2003.

56. Martel-Pelletier J, DiBattista JA, Lejeunesse D, et al. IGF/IGFBP axis in cartilage and bone in osteoarthritis pathogenesis. Inflamm Res 47:90–100, 1998.

57. Fernandes JC, Martel-Pelletier J, Pelletier JP. The role of cytokines in osteoarthritis pathophysiology. Biorheology 39:237–246, 2002.

58. Haywood L, McWilliams DF, Pearson CI, et al. Inflammation and angiogenesis in osteoarthritis. Arthritis Rheum 48: 2173–2177, 2003.

59. Ayral X, Pickering EH, Woodworth TG, et al. Synovitis: a potential predictive factor of structural progression of medial tibiofemoral knee osteoarthritis—results of a 1 year longitudinal arthroscopic study in 422 patients. Osteoarthritis Cartilage 13:361–367, 2005.

60. Dijkgraaf LC, Liem RS, de Bont LG. Ultrastructural characteristics of the synovial membrane in osteoarthritic temporomandibular joints. J Oral Maxillofac Surg 55:1269–1279, 1997.

61. Goldenberg DL, Egan MS, Cohen AS. Inflammatory synovitis in degenerative joint disease. J Rheumatol 9:204–209, 1982.

62. Schulte E, Fisseler-Eckhoff A, Muller KM. Differential diagnosis of synovitis. Correlation of arthroscopic-biopsy to clinical findings [in German]. Pathologie 15:22–27, 1994.

63. Demarziere A. Macrophages in rheumatoid synovial membrane: an update [in French]. Rev Rhum Ed Fran 60:568–579, 1993.

64. Ezawa K, Yamamura M, Matsui H, et al. Comparative analysis of CD45RA- and CD45RO-positive CD4 T cells in peripheral blood, synovial fluid, and synovial tissue in patients with rheumatoid arthritis and osteoarthritis. Acta Med Okayama 51:25–31, 1997.

65. Spector TD, Hart DJ, Nandra D, et al. Low-level increases in serum C-reactive protein are present in early osteoarthritis of the knee and predict progressive disease. Arthritis Rheum 40:723–733, 1997.

66. Fort JG, Flanigan M, Smith JB. Mononuclear cell (MNC) subtypes in osteoarthritis synovial fluid. J Rheumatol 22:1335–1337, 1995.

67. Pu J, Nishida K, Inoue H, et al. Mast cells in osteoarthritic and rheumatoid arthritic synovial tissues of the human knee. Acta Med Okayama 52:35–39, 1998.

68. Smith MD, Triantafillou S, Parker A, et al. Synovial membrane inflammation and cytokine production in patients with early osteoarthritis. J Rheumatol 24:365–371, 1997.

69. Myers SL, Flusser D, Brandt KD, et al. Prevalence of cartilage shards and their association with synovitis in patients with early and endstage osteoarthritis. J Rheumatol 19:1247–1251, 1992.

70. Garnero P, Mazieres B, Gueguen A, et al. Cross-sectional association of 10 molecular markers of bone, cartilage, and synovium with disease activity and radiological joint damage in patients with hip osteoarthritis: ECHODIAH cohort. J Rheumatol 32: 697–703, 2005.

71. Vetto AA, Mannik M, Zatarain-Rios E, et al. Immune deposits in articular cartilage of patients with rheumatoid arthritis have a granular pattern not seen in osteoarthritis. Rheumatol Int 10: 13–20, 1990.

72. Du H, Masuko-Hongo K, Nakamura H, et al. The prevalence of autoantibodies against cartilage intermediate layer protein, YKL-39, osteopontin, and cyclic citrullinated peptide in patients with early-stage knee osteoarthritis: evidence of a variety of autoimmune processes. Rheumatol Int 26:35–41, 2004.

73. Cheung HS. Role of calcium-containing crystals in osteoarthritis. Front Biosci 10:1336–1340, 2005.

74. Webb GR, Westacott CI, Elson CJ. Chondrocyte tumor necrosis factor receptors and focal loss of cartilage in osteoarthritis. Osteoarthritis Cartilage 5:427–437, 1997.

75. Van Linthoudt D, Beutler A, Clayburne G, et al. Morphometric studies on synovium in advanced osteoarthritis: Is there an association between apatite-like material and collagen deposits? Clin Exp Rheum 15:493–497, 1997.

76. Sokoloff L, Varma AA. Chondrocalcinosis in surgically resected joints. Arthritis Rheum 31:750–756, 1988.

77. Lanzer WL, Komenda G. Changes in articular cartilage after meniscectomy. Clin Orthop 252:41–48, 1990.

78. Abe M, Takahashi M, Naitou K, et al. Investigation of generalized osteoarthritis by combining x-ray grading of the knee, spine, and hand using biochemical markers for arthritis in patients with knee ostseoarthritis. Clin Rheumatol 22:425–431, 2003.

79. Sokoloff L, DiFrancesco L. Lipochondral degeneration of capsular tissue in osteoarthritic hips. Am J Surg Pathol 19:278–283, 1995.

80. Ladefoged C, Merrild V, Jorgensen B. Amyloid deposits in surgically removed articular and periarticular tissue. Histopathology 15:289–296, 1989.

81. Athanasou NA, Sallie B. Localized deposition of amyloid in articular cartilage. Histopathology 20:41–46, 1992.

82. Beighton PM, De Paepe A, Hall JG, et al. Molecular nosology of heritable disorders of connective tissue. Am J Med Genet 42:431–438, 1992.

83. De Paepe A. Heritable collagen disorders: from phenotype to genotype. Verh K Acad Geneeskd Belg 60:463–482, 1998.

84. Irlenbusch U, Dominic G. [Examination of Heberden arthrosis with a histological-histochemical score]. Z Orthop Ihre Grenzgeb 137:355–361, 1999.

85. Vingard E, Alfredsson L, Malchau H. Osteoarthrosis of the hip in women and its relation to physical load at work and in the home. Ann Rheum Dis 56:293–298, 1997.

86. Hirsch R, Lethbridge-Cejku M, Hanson R, et al. Familial aggregation of osteoarthritis: data from the Baltimore Longitudinal Study on Aging. Arthritis Rheum 41:1227–1232, 1998.

87. Englund M, Paradowski PT, Lohmander LS. Association of radiographic hand osteoarthritis with radiographic knee osteoarthritis after meniscectomy. Arthritis Rheum 50: 469–475, 2004.

88. Solovieva S, Vehmas T, Riihimaki H, et al. Hand use and patterns of joint involvement in osteoarthritis. A comparison of female dentists and teachers. Rheumatol (Oxford) 44:521–528, 2005.

89. Doherty M. Genetics of hand osteoarthritis. Osteoarthritis Cartilage 8, Suppl A: 508–510, 2000.

90. Felson DT, Couropmitree NN, Chaisson CE, et al. Evidence for a Mendelian gene in a segregation analysis of generalized radiographic osteoarthritis: the Framingham study. Arthritis Rheum 41:1064–1071, 1998.

91. Reginato AJ, Passolno GM, Neumann G, et al. Familial spondyloepiphyseal dysplasia tarda, brachydactyly, and precocious osteoarthritis associated with an arginine 75 → cysteine mutation in the procollagen type II gene in a kindred of Chiloe Islanders. I. Clinical, radiographic, and pathologic findings. Arthritis Rheum 37:1078–1086, 1994.

92. Pun YL, Moskowitz RW, Lie S, et al. Clinical correlations of osteoarthritis associated with a single-base mutation (arginine 519 to cysteine) in type II procollagen gene. A newly defined pathogenesis. Arthritis Rheum 37:264–269, 1994.

93. Vikkula M, Palotie A, Rituaniemi P, et al. Early onset osteoarthritis linked to the type II procollagen gene. Detailed clinical phenotype and further analyses of the gene. Arthritis Rheum 36:401–409, 1993.

94. Lieberfarb RM, Levy HP, Rose PS, et al. The Stickler syndrome: genotype/phenotype correlation in 10 families with Stickler syndrome resulting from seven mutations in the type II collagen gene locus COL2A1. Genet Med 5:21–27, 2003.

95. Bleasel JF, Bisagni-Faure A, Holderbaum D, et al. Type II procollagen gene (COL2A1) mutation in exon 11 associated with spondyloepiphyseal dysplasia, short stature, and precocious osteoarthritis. J Rheumatol 22:255–261, 1995.

96. Jakkula E, Melkoniemi M, Kiuinanta I. et al. The role of sequence variations within the genes encoding collagen II, IX, and XI in non-syndromic, early-onset osteoarthritis. Osteoarthritis Cartilage 13:497–507, 2005.

97. Loughlin J. The genetic epidemiology of human primary osteoarthritis: current status. Expert Rev Mol Med 7:1–12, 2005.

98. Mathieu F, Begaux F, Lan ZY, et al. Clinical manifestations of Kashin-Beck disease in Nyemo Valley, Tibet. Int Orthop 21: 151–156, 1997.

99. Ballo R, Viljoen D, Machado M. et al. Mseleni joint disease—a molecular genetic approach to defining the etiology. S Afr Med J 86: 956–958. 1996.

100. Agarwal SS, Phadke SR, Fredlund V, et al. Mseleni and Handigodu familial osteoarthropathies: syndromic identity? Am J Med Genet 72:435–439, 1997.

101. Sokoloff L. Endemic forms of osteoarthritis. Clin Rheum Dis 11:187–202, 1985.

102. Pasteels JL, Liu FD, Hinsenhamp M, et al. Histology of Kashin-Beck lesions. Int Orthop 25:151–153, 2001.

103. Wang SJ, Guo X, Zuo H, et al. [Chondrocyte apoptosis and the expression of Bcl-2, Bax, Fas and Inos in articular cartilage in Kashin-Beck disease]. Di YI, Jun YI, Da Xue, Xue Bao. 25: 643–646, 2005.

104. Yang GQ, Xia YM. Studies on human dietary requirements and safe range of dietary intakes of selenium in China and their application in the prevention of related endemic diseases. Biomed Environ Sci 8:187–201, 1995.

105. Moreno-Reyes R, Mathieu F, Boelaert M, et al. Selenium and iodine supplementation of rural Tibetan children affected by Kashin-Beck osteoarthropathy. Am J Clin Nutr 78:137–144, 2003.

106. Zhang WH, Neve J, Xu JP, et al. Selenium, iodine, and fungal contamination in Yulin District (People's Republic of China) endemic for Kashin-Beck disease. Int Orthop 25:188–190, 2001.

107. Yang C, Niu C, Bodo M, et al. Fulvic acid supplementation and selenium deficiency disturb the structural integrity of mouse skeletal tissue. An animal model to study the molecular effects of Kashin-Beck disease. Biochem J 289:829–835, 1993.

108. Liang HJ, Tsai CL, Lu FJ. Oxidative stress induced by humic acid solvent extraction fraction in cultured rabbit articular chondrocytes. J Toxicol Environ Health 54:477–489, 1998.

109. Sokoloff L, Fincham JE, du Toit GT. Pathological features of the femoral head in Mseleni disease. Hum Pathol 16:117–120, 1985.

110. Schnitzler CM, Pieczkowski WM, Fredlund V, et al. Histomorphometric analysis of osteopenia associated with endemic osteoarthritis (Mseleni joint diease). Bone 9:21–27, 1988.

111. Viljoen D, Fredlund V, Ramesar R, et al. Brachydactylous dwarfs of Mseleni. Am J Med Genet 46:636–640, 1993.

112. Derfus BA, Kurian JB, Butler JJ, et al. The high prevalence of pathologic calcium crystals in preoperative knees. J Rheumatol 29:570–574, 2002.

113. Giunta C, Superti-Furga A, Spranger S, et al. Ehlers-Danlos syndrome type VII: clinical features and molecular defects. J Bone Joint Surg Am 81:225–238, 1999.

114. Zweers MC, Dean WB, Van Kuppevelt TH, et al. Elastic fiber abnormalities in hypermobility type Ehler-Danlos syndrome patients with tenascin-x mutations. Clin Genet 67:330–334, 2005.

115. Badelon O, Bensahel H, Csukonyi Z, et al. Congenital dislocation of the hip in Ehlers-Danlos syndrome. Clin Orthop 255: 138–143, 1990.

116. Roughley PJ, Rauch F, Glorieux FH. Osteogenesis imperfecta—clinical and molecular diversity. Eur Cell Mater 30: 41–47, 2003.

117. Vujic M, Hallstensson, Wahlstrom J, et al. Localization of a gene for autosomal dominant Larsen syndrome to chromosome region 3p 21.1–14.1 in the proximity of, but distinct from, the COL7A1 locus. Am J Hum Genet 57:1104–1113, 1995.

118. Meabuchi A, Haga N, Maeda K, et al. Novel and recurrent mutations clustered in von Willebrand factor A domain of MA7N3 in multiple epiphyseal dysplasia. Human Mutat 24:439–440, 2004.

119. Jakkula E, Makitie O, Czarny-Ratacjzak M, et al. Mutations in the known genes are not the major cause of MED; distinctive phenotypic entities among patients with no identified mutations. Eur J Hum Genet 13:292–301, 2005.

120. Melis M, Onori P, Aliberti G, et al. Ochronotic arthropathy: structural and ultrastructural features. Ultrastruct Pathol 18:467–471, 1994.

121. Hiraku Y, Yamasaki M, Kawanishi S. Oxidative DNA damage induced by homogentisic acid, a tyrosine metabolite. FEBS Lett 432:13–16, 1998.

122. Roosendaal G, van Rinsum AC, Vianen ME, et al. Haemophilic arthropathy resembles degenerative rather than inflammatory joint disease. Histopathology 34:144–153, 1999.

123. Roosendaal G, Lafeber FP. Blood-induced joint damage in hemophilia. Semin Thromb Hemost 29:37–42, 2003.

124. Ito H, Matsuno T, Kaneda K. Prognosis of early stage avascular necrosis of the femoral head. Clin Orthop 358:149–157, 1999.

125. Van der Schoot DK, den Outer AJ, Bode PJ, et al. Degenerative changes at the knee and ankle related to malunion of tibial fractures: 15-Year follow-up of 88 patients. J Bone Joint Surg Br 78:722–725, 1996.

126. Jacobsen S, Sonne-holm S. Hip dysplasia; a significant risk factor for development of hip osteoarthritis. A cross-sectional survey. Rheumatology (Oxford) 44:211–218, 2005.

127. Helliwell PS. Osteoarthritis and Paget's disease. Br J Rheumatol 34:1061–1063, 1995.

128. Crispin JC, Alcocer-Varela J. Rheumatologic manifestations of diabetes mellitus. Am J Med 114: 753–757, 2003.

129. Cimmino MA, Cutolo M. Plasma glucose concentration in symptomatic osteoarthritis: a clinical and epidemiological survey. Clin Exp Rheumatol 8:251–257, 1990.

130. Frey MI, Barrett-Connor E, Sledge PA, et al. The effect of noninsulin dependent diabetes mellitus on the prevalence of clinical osteoarthritis. A population based study. J Rheumatol 23: 716–722, 1996.

131. Senolt L, Braun M, Olejarova M, et al. Increased pentosidine, an advanced glycation end product in serum and synovial fluid from patients with knee osteoarthritis and its relation with cartilage oligomeric matrix protein. Ann Rheum Dis 64:886–890, 2005.

132. Holmberg S, Thelin A, Thelin N. Knee osteoarthritis and body mass index: a population-based case-control study. Scand J. Rheumatol 34:59–64, 2005.

133. Cerhan JR, Wallace RB, el-Khoury GY, et al. Decreased survival with increasing prevalence of full-body radiographically defined osteoarthritis in women. Am J Epidemiol 141:225–234, 1995.

134. Lieberman SA, Bjorkengren AG, Hoffman AR. Rheumatologic and skeletal changes in acromegaly. Endocrinol Metab Clin North Am 21:615–631, 1992.

135. Denko CW, Boja B, Moskowitz RW. Growth promoting peptides in osteoarthritis and diffuse idiopathic skeletal hyperostosis—insulin, insulin-like growth factor I, growth hormone. J Rheumatol 21:1725–1730, 1994.

136. Wikinson JA. Etiologic factors in congenital displacement of the hip and myelodysplasia. Clin Orthop 281:75–83, 1992.

137. Uden A, Lindhagen T. Inguinal hernia in patients with congenital hip dislocation. Acta Orthop Scand 59:667–668, 1988.

138. Hoaglund FT, Healey JH. Osteoarthrosis and congenital dysplasia of the hip in family members of children who have congenital dysplasia of the hip. J Bone Joint Surg Am 72:1510–1518, 1990.

139. Jacobsen S, Sonne-Holm S, Soballe K, et al. Hip dysplasia and osteoarthrosis: a survey of 4151 subjects from the Osteoarthrosis Substudy of the Copenhagen City Heart Study. Acta Orthop 76:149–158, 2005.

140. Lane NE, Neuitt MC, Cooper C, et al. Acetabular dysplasia and osteoarthritis of the hip in elderly white women. Ann Rheum Dis 56:627–630, 1997.

141. Guille JT, Lipton GE, Szoke G, et al. Legg-Calvé-Perthes disease in girls. A comparison of the results with those seen in boys. J Bone Joint Surg Am 80:1256–1263, 1998.

142. Hochbergs P, Eckerwall G, Egund N, et al. Synovitis in Legg-Calvé-Perthes disease. Evaluation with MR imaging in 84 hips. Acta Radiol 39:532–537, 1998.

143. Arruda VR, Belangero WD, Ozelo MC, et al. Inherited risk factors for thrombophilia among children with Legg-Calvé-Perthes disease. J Pediatr Orthop 19:84–87, 1999.

144. Poussa M, Schlenzka D, Yrjonen T. Body mass index and slipped capital femoral epiphysis. J Pediatr Orthop B 12:369–371, 2003.

145. Stasikelis PJ, Sullivan CM, Phillips WA, et al. Slipped capital femoral epiphysis. Prediction of contralateral involvement. J Bone Joint Surg Am 78:1149–1155, 1996.

146. Docquier PL, Mousny M, Jouret M, et al. Orthopedic concerns in children with growth hormone therapy. Acta Orthop Belg 70:299–305, 2004.

147. Goodman DA, Feighan JE, Smith AD, et al. Subclinical slipped capital femoral epiphysis. Relationship to osteoarthrosis of the hip. J Bone Joint Surg Am 79:1489–1497, 1997.

148. Baldwin CT, Farrer LA, Adair R, et al. Linkage of early-onset osteoarthritis and chondrocalcinosis to human chromosome 8q. Am J Hum Genet 56:692–697, 1995.

149. Pereira ER, Brown RR, Resnick D. Prevalence and patterns of tendon calcifications in patients with chondrocalcinosis of the knee: radiographic study of 156 patients. Clin Imaging 22:371–375, 1998.

150. Zhang Y, Johnson K, Russell RG, et al. Association of sporadic chondrocalcinosis with a 4-basepair G-to-A transition in the 5-untranslated region of ANKH that promotes enhanced expression of ANKH protein and excess generation of extracellular inorganic pyrophosphate. Arthritis Rheum 52:1110–1117, 2005.

151. Zhang W, Neame R, Doherty S, et al. Relative risk of knee chondrocalcinosis in siblings of index cases with pyrophosphate arthropathy. Ann Rheum Dis 63:969–973, 2004.

152. Cardenal A, Masuda I, Ono W, et al. Serum nucleotide pyrophosphatase activity; elevated levels in osteoarthritis, calcium pyrophosphate crystal deposition disease, scleroderma, and fibromyalgia. J Rheumatol 25:2175–2180, 1998.

153. Hashimoto S, Ochs RL, Rosen F, et al. Chondrocyte-derived apoptotic bodies and calcification of articular cartilage. Proc Natl Acad Sci USA 95:3094–3099, 1998.

154. Swan A, Chapman B, Heap P, et al. Submicroscopic crystals in osteoarthritic synovial fluids. Ann Rheum Dis 53:467–470, 1994.

155. Axford JS, Bomford A, Revell P, et al. Hip arthropathy in genetic hemochromatosis. Radiographic and histologic features. Arthritis Rheum 34:357–361, 1991.

156. Kramer U, Weinberger A, Yarom R, et al. Synovial copper deposition as a possible explanation of arthropathy in Wilson's disease. Bull Hosp Jt Dis 52:46–49, 1993.

157. Sequeira W. The neuropathic joint. Clin Exp Rheumatol 12: 325–327, 1994.

158. Ines LS, Da Silva JA, Mealcata AB, et al. Arthropathy of genetic hemochromatosis: a major and distinctive manifestation of the disease. Clin Exp Rheumatol 19:98–102, 2001.

159. Timms AE, Sathananthan R, Bradbury L, et al. Genetic testing for haemochromatosis in patients with chondrocalcinosis. Ann Rheum Dis. 61: 745–747, 2002.

160. Cauza E, Hanusch-Enserer U, Etemad M, et al. HFE genotyping demonstrates a significant indcidence of hemochromatosis in undifferentiated arthritis. Clin Exp Rheumatol 23:7–12, 2005.

161. Halverson PB, McCarty DJ. Patterns of radiographic abnormalities associated with basic calcium phosphate and calcium pyrophosphate dihydrate crystal deposition in the knee. Ann Rheum Dis 45:603–605, 1986.

162. Molloy ES, McCarthy GM. Hydroxyapatite deposition disease of the joint. Curr Rheumatol Rep 5:215–221, 2003.

163. Ea HK, Uzan B, Rey C, et al. Octacalcium phosphate crystals directly stimulate expression of inducible nitric oxide synthase through p38 and JNK mitogen-activated protein kinases in articular chondrocytes. Arthritis Res Ther 7:R915–R926, 2005.

164. Vignon E, Balblanc JC, Mathieu P, et al. Metalloprotease activity, phospholipase A_2 activity and cytokine concentration in osteoarthritis synovial fluids. Osteoarthritis Cartilage 1:115–120, 1993.

165. Choi HK, Mount DB, Reginato AM. Pathogenesis of gout. Ann Int Med 143: 499–518, 2005.

166. Brancroft JD, Stevens A. Theory and Practice of Histological Techniques. 3rd ed. Edinburgh, Churchill Livingstone, 1990, pp 262–263.

167. Pascual E. Persistence of monosodium urate crystals and low grade inflammation in the synovial fluid of patients with untreated gout. Arthritis Rheum 34:141–145, 1991.

168. Fam AG, Stein J, Rubenstein J. Gouty Arthritis in nodal osteoarthritis. J Rheumatol 23:684–689, 1996.

169. Jaccard YB, Gerster JC, Calame L. Mixed monosodium urate and calcium pyrophosphate crystal-induced arthropathy. A review of seventeen cases. Rev Rhum Engl Ed 63:331–335, 1996.

170. Yu KH, Luo SF, Liou LB, et al. Concomitant septic and gouty arthritis—an analysis of 30 cases. Rheumatology (Oxford) 42:1062–1066, 2003.

171. Ishida T, Dorfman HD, Bullough PG. Tophaceous pseudogout (tumoral calcium pyrophosphate dihydrate crystal deposition disease). Hum Pathol 26:587–593, 1995.

172. Milliner S. The primary hyperoxalurias: an algorithm for diagnosis. Am J Nephrol 25:154–160, 2005.

173. Maldonado I, Prasad V, Reginato AJ. Oxalate crystal deposition disease. Current Rheumatol Rep 4:257–264, 2002.

174. Torii H, Nakagawa H, Ishibashi Y. Osteoarthritis in 84 Japanese patients with palmoplantar pustulosis. J Am Acad Dermatol 31:732–735, 1994.

175. Verrouil E, Mazieres B. Etiologic factors in finger osteoarthritis. Rev Rhum Engl Ed 62(suppl):95–135, 1995.

176. Roach KE, Persky V, Miles T, et al. Biomechanical aspects of occupation and osteoarthritis of the hip: a case-control study. J Rheumatol 21:2334–2340, 1994.

177. Spector TD, Hart DJ, Doyle DV. Incidence and progression of osteoarthritis in women with unilateral knee disease in the general population: the effect of obesity. Ann Rheum Dis 53:565–568, 1994.

178. Maetzel A, Makela M, Hawker G, et al. Osteoarthritis of the hip and knee and mechanical occupational exposure—a systematic overview of the evidence. J Rheumatol 24:1599–1607, 1997.

Cell Biology, Biochemistry, and Molecular Biology of Articular Cartilage in Osteoarthritis

4

Linda J. Sandell   Dick Heinegard   Thomas M. Hering

CARTILAGE: TISSUE ORGANIZATION

Articular cartilage is comprised largely of an extracellular matrix synthesized by chondrocytes.[1] In synovial joints, the layer of hyaline articular cartilage tissue faces the joint cavity (i.e., the synovial fluid space) on one side and is linked to the subchondral bone plate via a narrow layer of calcified cartilage tissue on the other. The medial femoral articular cartilage of humans is about 2 to 3 mm thick. The organization of the extracellular matrix and the distribution of zones is slightly different in immature versus mature cartilage. In young individuals, the layer of articular cartilage is generally much thicker and unstratified, with chondrocytes being distributed in a more random, isotropic pattern. As the tissue matures, there is a much higher degree of anisotropy with the cells and matrix being arranged into the clearly defined zones. These changes are accompanied by a significant increase in the mechanical competence of the cartilage with improvement in its stiffness and resistance to shearing and compressive forces.[2] The zones of articular cartilage (Fig. 4–1) are the superficial (tangential), the middle (transitional), the deep (radial), and calcified cartilage. The material properties of the cartilage at different depths also change because they are determined by the biochemical nature, content, and organization of the matrix macromolecules. The zonal variations in the extracellular matrix must result from metabolic differences among the cells. In experiments where the different zones are isolated and cultured, striking differences are found in terms of their morphology, metabolism, phenotypic stability, and responsiveness to interleukin-1α (IL-1).[3]

CHONDROCYTE CELL BIOLOGY

Unlike many other tissues in the body, the only cell type found in cartilage is the chondrocyte.[4] Chondrocyte morphology varies from rounded or polygonal, to the flattened, discoid shaped cells at the articular surface of joints. The chondrocyte has intracellular features characteristic of a metabolically active cell (Fig. 4–2), due to its role in synthesis and turnover of extracellular matrix components. Generally, chondrocytes occupy about 10% of the tissue volume in articular cartilage. Embyologically, chondrocytes of limb elements are derived from the mesoderm, and those of the facial skeleton from the neural crest. The earliest differentiated chondrocytes arise following mesenchymal condensation at sites of future skeletal elements, a process involving the expression of tissue specific genes, including Sox9, L-Sox5, Sox6, and collagen

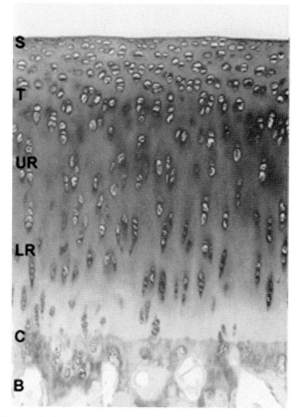

Figure 4–1 Articular cartilage from adult rabbit showing the superficial (S); middle, composed of the transitional (T) and upper radia zones (UR); and deep or lower radial zone (LR).

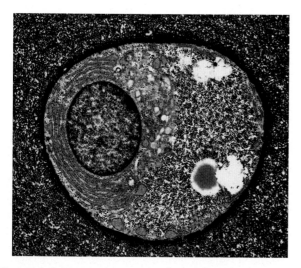

Figure 4–2 Electron micrograph of articular chondrocyte. Cell shape can vary from flattened or discoid near the articular surface, to a more rounded morphology in the middle and deep cartilage regions. Evident in the cytoplasm are cytoplasmic organelles including rough endoplasmic reticulum and Golgi apparatus, as well as glycogen and lipid droplets. Note the high ratio of extracellular matrix to cell volume. (Reprinted from Archer and Francis-West, Int. J. Biochem. Cell Biol 35:401–404, 2003.)

type IIA.[5] Whereas chondrocytes in articular cartilage persist, those in the epiphyseal growth plates proceed to become terminally differentiated hypertrophic chondrocytes, a cell that facilitates endochondral ossification. One function of chondrocytes is in growth. Chondrocytes within the epiphysial plates achieve tissue growth through proliferation to increase cell number, through matrix production, and through increased cell volume during terminal differentiation. The major function of chondrocytes within supporting cartilages is to maintain the extracellular matrix. A proteomic reference map of human chondrocytes has been published,[6] leading to the identification of 93 different intracellular chondrocyte proteins. Of these, 26% are involved in cell organization, 16% in energy, 14% in protein fate, 12% in metabolism, and 12% in cell stress.[6]

BIOCHEMICAL COMPOSITION OF THE CARTILAGE EXTRACELLULAR MATRIX

Cartilage is composed of an extracellular matrix that has been biosynthesized by chondrocytes. Compared to other tissues, the ratio of matrix to cell volume is very high. It is a hyperhydrated tissue, with values for water ranging from 60% to almost 80% of the total wet weight. The remaining 20% to 30% of the wet weight of the tissue is principally accounted for by two macromolecular materials: type II collagen, which composes up to 60% of the dry weight, and the large proteoglycan, aggrecan, which accounts for a large part of the remainder. "Minor" amounts of other collagens, including collagen types IX, XI, III, V, VI, X, XII, and XIV, are found in the matrix. Other structural proteins, glycoproteins, proteoglycans, and enzymic molecules make up a small percentage of the tissue, but may be of critical importance in the structure and function of the tissue. Minor amounts of other "large" proteoglycans are found in cartilage including versican, perlecan, and SZP/Lubricin. Among small proteoglycans of the small leucine-rich repeat proteoglycan (SLRP) family, those localized to cartilage include biglycan (DS-PGI), decorin (DS-PGII), epiphycan (DS-PGIII), fibromodulin, and lumican. Additional structural, regulatory, and enzymic proteins of the cartilage extracellular matrix are described below. Figure 4–3 is a schematic representation of many of the molecules of cartilage showing some of their interactions.

The Cartilage Proteoglycan Aggregate

The cartilage proteoglycan aggregate is a unique assembly of macromolecules that, along with type II collagen and a number of accessory molecules, confers upon cartilage its special biomechanical properties. The cartilage proteoglycan aggregate is composed of chondroitin sulfate proteoglycan (aggrecan) monomers bound into very large aggregates with hyaluronan. This interaction is stabilized by the binding of a third component, the link protein, a 45- to 50-kDa glycoprotein which is bivalent, in that it has binding sites

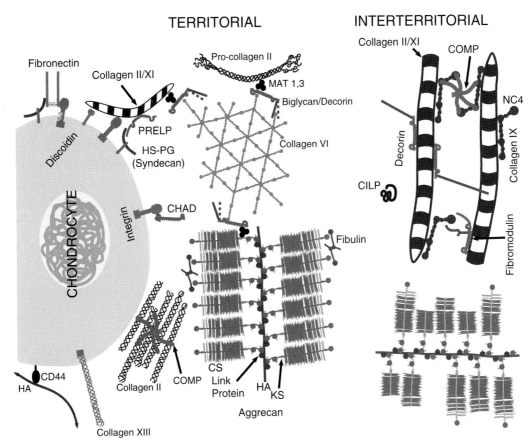

TERRITORIAL   INTERTERRITORIAL

Figure 4–3 Schematic representation of the cartilage matrix. Matrix closest to the chondrocyte is indicated as territorial and between chondrocytes is interterritorial. Note the fibrils of collagen coated with the small proteoglycans decorin and fibromodulin as well as with the collagen IX. The proteoglycans bind by their protein core, leaving their side chains free to self-interact or to interact with other collagen fibers or with the NC4 domain of collagen IX or with fibulin. Proteins and protein interactions are discussed in the text.

for both the aggrecan amino terminal globular (G1) region and for hyaluronan (Fig. 4–4).

Aggrecan Core Protein Structure

Aggrecan is a large, complex, hybrid proteoglycan having a 220- to 250-kDa multiple-domain core protein which is substituted with both chondroitin sulfate (CS) and keratan sulfate (KS) chains in addition to N- and O-linked oligosaccharides (reviewed in Kiani et al.[7]). The core protein possesses two globular regions near the amino-terminus, referred to as G1 and G2, separated by an interglobular domain (IGD). A third globular region, G3, is found at the carboxyl terminal end of the core protein. An extended region containing KS- and CS-attachment sites is found between the G2 and G3 domains.

The globular region G1 of aggrecan is composed of three domains referred to as A, B, and B', and the G2 region is subdivided into B and B' domains similar to those in G1. The A domain has also been referred to as the "Ig fold" domain due to its sequence homology to immunoglobulin-like proteins[8] and has been suggested to mediate the interaction of aggrecan with link protein in the proteoglycan

aggregate.[9,10] The B and B' domains of the aggrecan G1 region are believed to mediate interaction with hyaluronan. These domains have also been referred to as proteoglycan tandem repeat (PTR) domains. The related B and B' (or PTR) domains in the G2 region apparently do not interact with hyaluronan[11] and their function is unknown at present.

Between the G2 region and the G3 region of the molecule are found the KS and CS attachment regions. This extended region of the molecule is heavily substituted with KS and CS chains, with KS chains concentrated in the amino-terminal portion of this extended region.[12] The KS domain consists mainly of hexapeptide repeats, the number of which is variable between species.[13] The CS attachment region is generally subdivided into CS-1, and CS-2 subdomains, which differ in terms of the repeated sequence comprising each subdomain, and in the length and sulfation of the CS chains. Each of these subdomains has been found to be variably conserved between species.[14] The number of CS-1 repeats in human aggrecan has been found to be structurally polymorphic, with the number of repeats varying from 13 to 33 between individuals.[15,16]

(a) Proteoglycan aggregates

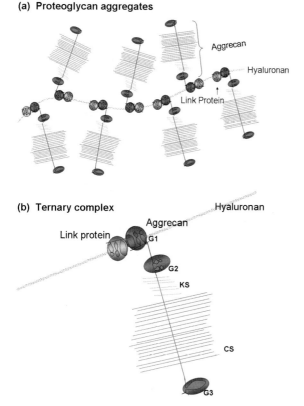

(b) Ternary complex

Figure 4–4 The cartilage proteoglycan aggregate is a complex of hyaluronan, aggrecan monomers, and link proteins. (a) Multiple aggrecan monomers bind to a single hyaluronan filament. This interaction is stabilized by link protein. (b) Aggrecan binds to HA and link protein through its G1 domain to form a ternary complex. Highly charged KS and CS polysaccharides are located in the extended region between the G2 and G3 domains of aggrecan. (Reprinted from Miwa HE. A recombinant system to model proteoglycan aggregate interactions and aggrecan degradation. Doctoral dissertation, Case Western Reserve University, Cleveland, OH, 2006.)

The G3 domain at the C-terminus of aggrecan is made up of three modules, including an Epidermal growth factor (EGF) like region, a C-type lectin-like domain (also termed carbohydrate-recognition domain [CRD]), and a complement binding protein (CBP)-like domain. The EGF-like region is alternatively spliced in humans and may contain an EGF-1, EGF-2, or both modules.[17] The C-type lectin-like module of aggrecan can bind to fucose and galactose.[18] In addition, this module is able to bind tenascin-C,[18] sulfated glycolipids,[19] and fibulin-1[20] and -2.[21]

A functionally null mutation of the aggrecan gene has been identified in mice, termed cartilage matrix deficiency (*cmd*). This is a natural aggrecan gene knockout and was the first example of a proteoglycan gene mutation observed in mammals.[22] The cmd aggrecan gene contains a 7 bp deletion in exon 5, which codes for the B loop of the G1 domain, which causes a frame shift and premature termination in exon 6. Homozygotes (cmd/cmd) exhibited dwarfism, a cleft palate, and a short snout and die soon after birth due to respiratory failure. The cartilage of homozygous mice contains tightly packed chondrocytes with little apparent matrix. Heterozygous mice (cmd/+) are born normal. Although cmd mice produce no aggrecan, link protein and collagen type II are produced normally.[23]

Link Protein

The link protein bears sequence homology and a parallel domain structure to the G1 domain of aggrecan.[24] Link protein stabilizes the binding interaction between the hyaluronic acid binding region (HABR) of aggrecan and hyaluronan. Link protein is capable of binding independently to either hyaluronan or the aggrecan G1 domain, and there is evidence that this binding occurs through separate functional domains within the link protein molecule.[9] Link protein contains one copy of an immunoglobulin (Ig) fold-like sequence at the N-terminus and also contains two homologous sequences known as PTR domains between the N-terminal Ig fold domain and the carboxyl terminus (Fig. 4–5). The vertebrate hyaluronan and proteoglycan-binding link protein gene family (HAPLN) consists of four members, including cartilage link protein (HAPLN1), two forms that are expressed in the brain and CNS (HAPLN2 and HAPLN4), and a form that is widely expressed (HAPLN3).[25]

Homozygous link protein knockout mice ($LP^{-/-}$)[26] exhibit dwarfism and a flat face. As with *cmd* mice, most homozygotes die shortly after birth due to respiratory failure. Heterozygous mice show no apparent phenotype.

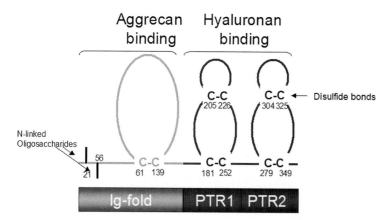

Figure 4–5 Domain structure of cartilage link protein. The N-terminal Ig-fold domain is involved in aggrecan binding and the PTR domains are involved in HA binding. Link protein is a glycoprotein containing N-linked oligosaccharides and multiple disulfide bonds. The structure of the aggrecan G1 domain is closely related to that of link protein. (Reprinted from Miwa HE. A recombinant system to model proteoglycan aggregate interactions and aggrecan degradation. Doctoral dissertation, Case Western Reserve University, Cleveland, OH, 2006.)

In heterozygotes, long bones are shortened and skulls are small with a shortened anterior-posterior axis. Growth plate in $LP^{-/-}$ mice shows disorganization of the chondrocytes, suggesting that the lack of link protein affects chondrocyte differentiation. As might be expected, the level of aggrecan in $LP^{-/-}$ cartilage is significantly reduced, confirming a role for link protein in aggregate stabilization.

Hyaluronan

Hyaluronan (reviewed in Laurent et al.[27]) is a polysaccharide having the repeating disaccharide structure poly [(1/3)-β-DGlcNAc-(1/4)-β-D-GlcA-]. Hyaluronan is predominantly localized to the extracellular and pericellular matrix, although it may occur intracellularly.[28] Functionally, it contributes to the elastoviscosity of fluid connective tissues[29] including synovial fluid and vitreous humor, it modulates hydration and transport of water through tissues, and functions in receptor-mediated cell detachment, mitosis, and migration,[30] inflammation,[28] tumor development, and metastasis.[31] In cartilage, hyaluronan functions in the supramolecular assembly of proteoglycans and link protein into aggregates.[1]

Collagens

Type II Collagen

Mature collagen fibers provide the capacity to withstand tensile and shear forces, while proteoglycans are generally responsible for solute flow and deformation of the tissue. The collagens of cartilage are listed in Table 4–1. The predominant collagen in the mature articular cartilage is the fibrillar collagen, type II. Type II collagen is a triple helix composed of three identical alpha chains synthesized from the COL2A1 gene. Type II procollagen is synthesized in two splice forms: type IIA contains an additional cysteine-rich exon in the N-propeptide and is found in chondroprogenitor cells and other embryonic tissues (Fig. 4–6); type IIB lacks this cysteine-rich domain of the N-propeptide and is

TABLE 4–1
THE GENETICALLY DISTINCT COLLAGENS IN ARTICULAR CARTILAGE

Class	Type	Molecules	α-Chain $M_r \times 10^{-3}$	Concentrations	Biosynthetic Changes in OA
Fibrillar	II	Two splice forms, IIA and IIB	95	IIA characteristic of chondroprogenitors, perichondrium; IIB characteristic of cartilage	Increase IIA re-expressed IIB increased
	III	[α1(III)]₃	95	40%	Degradation
	V/XI	[α1(V)]₂ α2(V) [α1(V) α2(V) α3(V)] [α1(XI) α2(XI) α3(XI)] Mixed molecules of V and XI α1(XI) and α2(XI) have alternative splice form	120–145	Cartilage-heterotypic fibrils of V with I and XI with II, but mixed molecules of V/XI with I and/or II possible <10%	Not known
Microfibrillar	VI	[α1(VI) α2(VI) α3(IX)]	α1/α2 = 140 α3 = 200–280	Chondrocyte Pericellular <40%	Increased expression
Fibril-associated (FACITs)	IX	[α(IX) α2(IX) α3(IX)] Different forms due to use of different gene promoters	α1 = 66 (short form) or 84 (long form) α2 = 66 (non-glycanated) or 66–115 (glycanated) α3 – 72	<10%	Increased synthesis Cleaved proteins
	XII	[α1(XII)]₃	220 (short form) 340 (long form) Long form can be glycanated	<1%	Not known
	XIV	[α1(XIV)]₃	220 Can be glycanated	<1%	Not known
Short-chain	X	[α1(X)]₃	59	45% in hypertrophic chondrocytes	Increased and present in articular cartilage

Type IIA procollagen

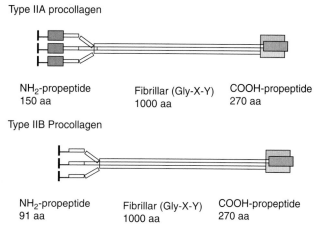

NH₂-propeptide
150 aa

Fibrillar (Gly-X-Y)
1000 aa

COOH-propeptide
270 aa

Type IIB Procollagen

NH₂-propeptide
91 aa

Fibrillar (Gly-X-Y)
1000 aa

COOH-propeptide
270 aa

Figure 4–6 Type II collagen. Type IIA procollagen contains an additional cysteine-rich protein domain in the NH₂-propeptide (shaded box) that binds to bone morphogenetic proteins during skeletal development. Type IIA procollagen is synthesized by chondroprogenitor cells. Type IIB procollagen is made by chondrocytes and lacks the cysteine rich domain of the NH₂-propeptide. In chondroprogenitor cells, Type IIA procollagen is deposited into the matrix with the NH₂-propeptide intact. It is subsequently removed by matrix enzymes. In chondrocytes, both propeptides are removed with the mature collagen molecule deposited in the extracellular matrix. This molecule forms associates laterally into the fibrils indicated in Table 4–2. The black box is the signal peptide (removed during translation into protein).

the predominant collagen in all cartilaginous tissues. These alpha chains form the characteristic collagen triple helical structure when three chains are wound around each other during biosynthesis to form collagen molecules. The collagen molecules then associate in a lateral staggered array to form collagen fibrils. These fibrils are not necessarily one single type of collagen, even in cartilage, and often contain, within the fibril or surrounding it, other types of collagens. These other collagens are considered "minor" in amount but have important functional roles. Mutations in the predominant collagen, type II, can weaken the cartilage matrix and predispose the tissue to osteoarthritis. The diameter of the collagen fibril in cartilage is shown in Table 4–2. In articular cartilage of mammals, the content and interaction of predominant and minor collagens as well as other collagen-binding molecules contributes to the differences in collagen fibril diameters observed in the different zones of the tissue.

Type II collagen is biosynthesized as a procollagen molecule containing N- and C-terminal propeptides. In cartilage, the propeptides are removed prior to assembly of the mature collagen. The C-terminal propeptide has been isolated from cartilage (called chondrocalcin) and at one time was thought to be an independent molecule. Although synthesized in all cartilages, chondrocalcin appears to be associated with extracellular matrix undergoing mineralization.[32] In chondroprogenitor tissues, type IIA procollagen containing cysteine-rich amino propeptide is secreted into the extracellular matrix and functions to bind bone morphogenetic proteins.[33]

TABLE 4–2
COLLAGEN FIBRIL DIAMETERS IN CARTILAGE

Zone/Region	Diameter (nm) Mean ± SD	(n)
Superficial zone		
1. Pericellular	15.4 ± 8.3	(18)
2. Territorial	29.2 ± 5.4	(22)
Middle zone		
3. Pericellular	21.5 ± 12.7	(18)
4. Territorial	31.8 ± 5.0	(23)
Deep zone		
5. Pericellular	19.0 ± 4.4	(23)
6. Territorial	48.5 ± 7.0	(23)
7. Interterritorial	57.5 ± 7.6	(25

All measurements were made from one experiment (BC14). Student's test analyses revealed that the following were significantly different from each other ($P < 0.001$): 1 and 2, 3 and 4, 5 and 6, 6 and 7, 4 and 6, 4 and 7.
From Poole AR, et al. J Cell Biol., 1982:93:921–937.

Minor Collagens

Type IX Collagen. Type IX collagen can represent up to 10% of the articular collagen in the immature animal and 1% to 5% in the adult.[34] Type IX collagen is classified as a FACIT collagen (fibril associated collagen with an interrupted triple-helix) forming heterotypic fibrils with types II and XI collagen. It is a heterotrimer [α1(IX) α2(IX) α3(IX)] composed of three chains being products of three distinct genes.[35] Type IX collagen is different from type II collagen in that it has three triple-helical collagenous domains (COL1, 2, and 3) and four noncollagenous domains (NC1, 2, 3, and 4). These noncollagenous regions are more susceptible to proteolysis than collagenous domains. Overall, type IX is shorter than the fibrillar interstitial collagens and is stabilized by interchain disulfide bonds. There are long and short forms depending on the presence or absence of a large globular domain (NC4) at the amino terminal of the α1 chain. Most unusual for a collagen molecule, it has a CS chain, leading to its additional classification as a proteoglycan. The type IX molecule is shown in Figure 4–7. A schematic representation of the type II collagen fibril with type IX associated is shown in Figure 4–8.

While the exact function of type IX collagen is not known, it is thought to function to limit the fibril diameter of the fibrillar collagen and is attached to the type II collagen by covalent hydroxylysyl pyridinoline and lysyl pyridinoline crosslinks. The possession of a large globular N-terminal domain and a CS chain are characteristics that suggest a potential to interact with other matrix components. Transgenic mice have been produced with a defective col9A1 gene that expresses a truncated α1(IX) chain.[36,37] These animals develop pathological changes in the articular condyle of the knee joint which resembled those seen in osteoarthritis. Furthermore, mice that were homozygous for the mutation were found to have a mild chondrodysplasia. Another transgenic mouse

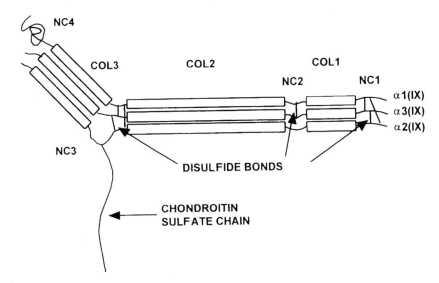

Figure 4–7 Diagram of a heterotypic fibril consisting of types II, IX and XI collagen.

has been generated that lacks the α1(IX) chain.[38] Surprisingly, even the homozygous mutants appear normal at birth, but later they develop a severe degenerative joint disease with similarities to human osteoarthritis. These findings suggest that changes in or lack of type IX collagen chains do not directly affect the gross appearance of the cartilage or its overall development. However, they may affect the organization of cartilage components on a molecular level leading to conditions such as chondrodysplasia or osteoarthritis, perhaps due to a loss of cartilage integrity which only becomes apparent when the cartilage is exposed to conditions of loading after birth. In humans where the cartilage must be maintained for a longer time, small defects in this collagen could contribute to early osteoarthritis, although no direct evidence for type IX defects leading to OA have been reported.

Collagen. Like type IX collagen, type XI is more abundant in immature cartilage from which it was originally isolated.[40] It consists of three distinct polypeptide chains, α1(XI), α2(XI), and α3(XI), that form predominantly heterotrimeric molecules containing one of each chain. The α1(XI) and α2(XI) chains are products of separate genes, COL11A1 and COL11A2, respectively, and the proα3(XI) chain is a product of the COL2A1 gene, which codes for

the α1(II) chain. The difference between the two chains is due to post-translational hydroxylation and glycosylation.[41] Type XI is usually found in association with type II collagen in cartilaginous matrices (Fig. 4–7). In common with other fibrillar collagens, the α-chains of type XI collagen are synthesized as precursor procollagen chains consisting of a triple helical domain of more than 1,000 amino acids, with globular extensions at the amino and carboxy-termini. Type XI collagen has five major domains: NC1 (C-terminal, noncollagenous "hinge"-like region), NC2 (C-terminus), COL1 (major collagenous domain), COL2 (minor collagenous domain), and NC3 (N-terminal noncollagenous domain).

Processing of type XI collagen has been studied in embryonic chick sterna in vitro and is slower and more complex than that of collagen types I and II. All three chains of type XI collagen are initially processed at the C-terminal domains, which are linked through cysteines. α3(XI) undergoes one processing step at the N-terminal domain (removal of the signal peptide), which results in the fully processed matrix form of this chain.[35] The other two chains undergo a two-step processing that result in portions remaining in the extracellular matrix. The matrix form of type XI is approximately 315 nm in length. The COL1 triple helical domain has binding sites which may be involved in interacting with other extracellular matrix components. α2(XI) and α2(XI) both have heparin binding sites and can also bind to aggrecan, the major cartilage proteoglycan, through these sites. It has been suggested that heparan sulfate–type XI collagen interactions may be of importance on the chondrocyte surface. Along the COL1 domain of α2(XI) there are three Arg-Gly-Asp (RGD) motifs which could contribute to chondrocyte surface interaction by binding to cellular integrins.

The NC3 noncollagenous globular domain of type XI collagen differs from those of collagen types I, II, and III in length and structure. The NC3 domains of proα1(XI) and proα2(XI) may be divided into two main subdomains. The N-terminal is a module rich in acidic residues, isolated originally from cartilage as a disulfide-bonded molecule called PARP (proline/arginine rich protein).[42]

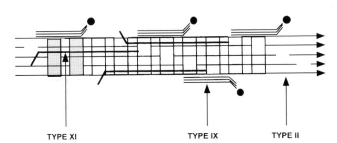

Figure 4–8 Diagram of a heterotopic fibril consisting of types II (COL2), IX (COL3) and XI (COL1) collagen.
Boxes are triple helical domains and lines are globular protein domains. *NC* = noncollagenous domain; *COL* = Collagenous domain

C-terminal of PARP is a variable region (VR). Variations of this region occur as a result of alternative exon usage, conferring acidic or basic properties on the protein domain. The function of different domains is not presently known. The $\alpha 3(XI)$ is the type IIB splice form of type II collagen.[43,44] These N-terminal domains that are retained in the mature type XI molecule likely contribute to lateral aggregation of collagen molecules.

The function of type XI collagen is thought to primarily lie in its role in fibril formation with type II collagen and interactions with components of cartilage proteoglycans and chondrocytes. Identification of mutations that cause specific chondrodysplasias have provided further evidence of the biological role of type XI collagen in cartilage and in skeletal morphogenesis. Mice homozygous for the autosomal recessive chondrodysplasia (cho) mutation have abnormalities in cartilage, notably large collagen fibrils and loss of cohesion with increased ease of proteoglycan extraction. Both the COL11A1 and COL11A2 genes have also been implicated in forms of Stickler syndrome.[45]

Types III and V Collagens. Small amounts of type III collagen are seen in cartilage, primarily associated with type II collagen.[46] In cell culture, human articular chondrocytes synthesize type III collagen.[47] Type V collagen has been found in cartilage, particularly in older tissue[48] where it replaces the $\alpha 1(XI)$ collagen chain in the type XI molecule.

Type VI Collagen. Type VI collagen is not considered to be characteristic of cartilage, but is present in articular cartilage and located largely in the pericellular capsule around the chondrocytes. It may play a role in cell adhesion. Type VI collagen is not a fibrillar collagen, but contains a short triple-helical domain (105 nm) and N- and C-terminal globular domains that are very large and account for more than two thirds of the mass of the molecule. There are three α-chains ($\alpha 1$, $\alpha 2$, and $\alpha 3$), all with a multidomain structure: their globular domains contain modules homologous to von Willebrand factor A (vWFA). The type VI molecules assemble into dimers in an antiparallel fashion that aggregate laterally to form disulfide bonded tetramers. These associate noncovalently to form networks of microfibrils. The type VI microfibrils have a beaded appearance and are found in most connective tissues including articular cartilage where they are stabilized by interaction of the large globular domain of the $\alpha 1(VI)$ chain with hyaluranon.[49] In addition type VI collagen is rich in RGD sequences and has been shown to bind to the surface of many cells including chondrocytes.[50] Type VI is distributed widely throughout the ECM in fetal cartilage but becomes restricted to the pericellular domain during growth.[51] Type VI collagen is enriched in human OA cartilage and in cartilage from surgically induced OA in dogs.[52] The role played by type VI collagen in normal tissue and in OA tissue is unknown.

Type X Collagen. Type X collagen is characteristic of hypertrophic chondrocytes in growth plate and is expressed primarily in this tissue with some localized in the calcified articular cartilage. Type X collagen is a homotrimer comprised of three identical $\alpha 1(X)$ chains (M_r 59kDa) with 45 kDa of triple-helical collagenous domain flanked by two noncollagenous regions.[53] The triple helix contains eight imperfections of the Gly-X-Y triplet structure allowing cleavage by MMP-1 at two sites.[54] The accumulation of type X collagen mRNA and protein deposition in hypertrophic cartilage was found always to precede vascular invasion and mineralization of the matrix. It has generally been accepted that type X collagen is a product of chondrocytes undergoing hypertrophy, and collagen X expression is frequently used as a marker for chondrocyte hypertrophy. However, Ekanayake and Hall[55] demonstrated that chondrocytes derived from chick mandibular ectomesenchyme, a normally permanent cartilage, can be induced to undergo maturation in culture, indicating that chondrocyte hypertrophy is not a prerequisite for collagen X expression. Also type X collagen has been immunolocalized in normal porcine, neonatal, and human articular cartilage, and in the mineralized fibrocartilage at the femoral insertion of the bovine medial collateral ligament where cell hypertrophy does not normally occur.[56]

Type X collagen may serve primarily as a structural element, either alone or in conjunction with other matrix components. The hypertrophic zone of the growth plate is structurally the weakest point within the growth plate by virtue of the increase in chondrocyte size and the decrease in the amount of type II collagen fibrils. It is generally accepted that collagen X provides a permissive matrix for chondrocyte hypertrophy, mineralization, and vascular invasion to occur during endochondral ossification. Type X collagen has been shown to have calcium binding properties[57], to be associated with alkaline phosphatase[58] and with matrix vesicles[59] considered by some to be the initial site of mineral deposition in cartilage. However, it is safe to say that the exact role played by this collagen is not known.

Synthesis of type X collagen primarily by hypertrophic chondrocytes suggests that there must be a unique program of differentiation that is expressed only during the later stages of cartilage development. Due to the restricted expression of the gene, its regulation is of considerable interest. Lu Valle and associates have shown that the gene actually is driven by a very strong promoter and is regulated by multiple negative regulatory elements that aid in restricting expression in nonhypertrophic chondrocytes and other cells.[60]

Types XII and XIV Collagens. Types XII and XIV collagen have features in common with type IX collagen, but also have a very large noncollagenous amino-terminal domain.[61] These collagens are closely associated with type I fibrillar collagen and are speculated to be located on the surface of type I collagen in a similar manner to the association of type IX with type II. The direct interaction of types XII and XIV and fibrillar type II has not been reported, although it is likely.

Other Molecules in Cartilage

Cartilage contains a large number of extracellular matrix proteins in addition to collagens and proteoglycans (Fig. 4–3). These have a wide range of roles, e.g., in facilitating matrix assembly, in maintaining the mechanical properties of the tissue, in sequestering growth factors and proteinases to specific compartments of the matrix, and in interacting with the cells important in the regulation of cellular activities. In several instances the functions of the proteins are becoming known, while in many cases functional properties remain to be elucidated. The following description is focused on proteins where functional properties are becoming known.

Thrombospondins (TSPs)

One of the major proteins in cartilage is cartilage oligomeric matrix protein (COMP), a member of the thrombospondin family as TSP-5.[62,63,64] The thrombospondins are proteins built from a number of similar modules that share a number of functional properties. The proteins contain three (TSP 1 and 2) or five (TSP 3, 4, and 5) identical subunits. The subunits share a typical structure of their C-terminal part with a conserved globular domain, followed by a domain with seven calcium binding T3 repeats and a domain of three or four EGF-like T2 repeats. The 3D-structure of thrombospondin 1 has been resolved[65] and shows that the T3 repeats contain the DxDxDGxxDxxD motif that binds two calcium ions. The repeats wrap around a core of central calcium ions. The T3 domain appears to form the C-terminal globular domain together with the very C-terminal cartilage oligomeric protein (CTD). The folding and structure of the chains of the thrombospondin proteins to a large extent depend on the large number of calcium ions bound with high affinity, particularly in the T3 domain. The total number of bound calcium ions is estimated to be 26 for the whole chain of thrombospondin 1.[65]

Another feature common to all the thrombospondins is the heptad repeat domain forming a coiled coil uniting the chains in the molecule.[66] Disulfide bonds making the association covalent stabilize this structure. In COMP or thrombospondin 5, this domain is localized very close to the N-terminus of the protein. Different from COMP, the other thrombospondins contain a domain on the N-terminal side of the coiled coil linking the chains, with an overall folding similar to the G-domain of laminins.[62] Thrombospondin 1 and 2 contain additional domains in the form of a von Willebrand factor C domain and a repeat T1 (properdin-like). These domains contribute cell binding to these proteins. Additional functions involve heparin binding which could also influence cell surface molecules in the form of syndecans. These domains also have roles in modulating cell behavior and particularly angiogenesis. One structure particularly relevant appears to be the heparin-binding motif present in the T1-domain. This may engage cell surface proteoglycans carrying heparan sulfate side chains.

The thrombospondins identified in cartilage are primarily TSP-1, TSP-3, and TSP-5/COMP, where COMP is predominant.[67] The functions of this protein, most likely shared by the other two thrombospondins in the tissue, are being unraveled. The examples provided primarily make use of COMP as an example but are likely to apply to the other members of the TSP family, although in some cases when the multivalency of the protein is important there may be a difference between those with five and three chains, respectively.

The C-terminal globular domain mediates very tight $K_D = 10^{-9}$ binding to collagen type I or type II molecules with the ability to bind each of four sites with the same affinity.[68] A role for this binding appears to be to accelerate and enhance collagen fibrillogenesis, where the COMP molecule appears to simultaneously bind several collagen molecules and arrange them in close proximity and facilitate their association upon forming fibrils.

COMP has been shown to also interact with collagen type IX, bound into collagen fibers such that particularly the col3 and NC4 domains protrude out from the fiber. In this case, the binding appears to be directed primarily to the noncollagenous domains, perhaps allowing the molecule to cross-bridge neighboring fibers. The COMP also binds to fibronectin.[69] It is not known whether this interaction occurs in vivo and will modulate functions such as interactions of the fibronectin at the cell surface.

The thrombospondins have been shown to bind cells via an RGD-motif present in the T3-domain.[70] However, this motif appears to be primarily exposed in low calcium concentrations and a physiological role needs to be established. Indeed it appears that COMP from rat does not contain the RGD-sequence found in the human and bovine protein.[63]

A number of mutations, often point mutations, primarily in the T3 and some in the C-terminal domain of COMP have been shown to lead to pseudoachondroplasia and multiple epiphyseal dysplasia[71] with growth disturbances. It appears that an important part of the defect is that the mutated molecule is retained in the endoplasmic reticulum (ER) of the chondrocytes thereby creating major deposits[72] apparently affecting cell function possibly via dilation of the ER or by retaining other molecules via interactions. The total absence of the molecule in the extracellular matrix has apparently no or very limited effects on the tissue since the mouse where the COMP gene has been inactivated shows no detectable alterations in phenotype[73] despite the absence of the protein.

COMP production and abundance in the matrix is markedly increased in early osteoarthritis, both at very early, preclinical stages and at late stages.[67] The distribution of the protein is shifted from the interterritorial matrix of the normal adult cartilage to a pericellular environment, implying concomitant degradation and new deposition in a different compartment.

A novel observation that adds complexity to the understanding of thrombospondin functions is the finding in tendon samples of hetero-oligomers where a molecule contains subunits of both TSP-4 and TSP-5.[74] This may not represent a form present in cartilage in view of the apparent lack of the protein in this tissue.

Matrilins

A family of proteins present in various tissues is the four matrilins, 1 to 4,[75] which represent different gene products. They have in common that they are multimeric proteins, with three of four chains held together by a coiled coil domain. They contain four vWFA that are often seen in proteins involved in interactions. In cartilage, matrilins 1 and 3 are primarily found.[76] They contain two and one such domains per chain, respectively. Interestingly, there are also matrilin molecules that contain a mixture of chains of type 1 and 3.[77]

The vWFA domain contributes binding properties to the matrilins, involving the fibrillar collagens as well as a number of other molecules.[78,79] In proof of the relevance of some of these interactions, it has been possible to use tissue homogenization of cartilaginous tissues such as the Swarm rat chondrosarcoma to isolate complexes of collagen type VI with other sets of molecules still attached. Thus biglycan or decorin were bound at the C-terminal globular domains of the collagen and were in turn binding a molecule of the matrilin family, where matrilins-1, -2, and -3 were identified, binding with one of the subunits.[80] The matrilin in turn binds other molecules such as a collagen fiber or the proteoglycan aggrecan.[80,81] It thus appears that the combination of a small proteoglycan in the form of decorin or biglycan and a matrilin can act as a linker molecule between the collagen VI beaded filaments to other major structural assemblies in the tissue. The finding of bound procollagen type II at the linker module[80] may indicate that there is also a function in regulating assembly of the collagen fibers.

The matrilins also appear to be able to associate into networks on their own,[82] probably involving their vWFA domains. The exact relevance of these interactions to tissue function is not known. The genes for the various matrilins have been inactivated, without providing a major phenotype.[83,84,85] However, patients with mutations of the matrilins show multiple epiphyseal dysplasia (MED) with skeletal growth abnormalities,[86] perhaps via mechanisms similar to those of COMP mutations.

Matrilin 3 is present in most cartilages, while matrilin-1 shows a very restricted distribution. Thus the protein is present in young growing tissue and also very abundant in cartilage like that in the trachea. At the same time the protein is not detected in articular cartilage, not even at a level of 1000-fold lower, neither in the intervertebral disc structures.[87] When mice or rats with certain genetic backgrounds are immunized with the protein, they develop severe respiratory failure due to autoimmune reaction and inflammation in the trachea.[88] The animals also have engagement of other tissues where the protein is found, such as the nasal cartilage. However, they show no joint disease.

CILP

CILP is the acronym for cartilage intermediate layer protein, which was first identified as a component in articular cartilage that is upregulated in early osteoarthritis.[67] The protein was found to be primarily present in the interterritorial matrix in the middle of articular cartilage from adult individuals.[89] The cloned and sequenced protein was shown to represent a larger molecule.[90] This precursor form was cleaved to two parts upon secretion from the cells. The N-terminal portion represents the previously isolated CILP protein with a molecular mass of 78.5 kDa, while the C-terminal part shows a very different structure, homologous to the NTPPHase enzyme, molecular mass 51.8 kDa, not including posttranslational modifications. Whether this putative enzyme actually has activity is not clear, although found data indicate that it is not active.[91] There is a related protein referred to as CILP-2, initially as a genomic sequence. It is homologous to CILP (now CILP-1) and shares about 50% of the structure. CILP-2 has an N-terminal part related to CILP and a C-terminal part related in sequence to

NTPPHase. To avoid confusion, the N-terminal parts are now referred to as CILP 1-1 and CILP 2-1 while the C-terminal parts are CILP 1-2 and CILP 2-2. To date we know very little about the role of CILP in cartilage. It has, however, been shown that it increases in OA and may serve as an antigen in joint disease.[92] It has been suggested that CILP may have a role in regulating the activity of insulin-like growth factor on cells.[91]

Leucine-Rich Repeat Proteins

The leucine-rich repeat (LRR) proteins in the extracellular matrix can be divided into families with sets of members that differ in gene organization and structural features. They share a common feature with a central domain of 10 or 11 (in decorin, biglycan, and asporin 12) repeats, each with some 25 amino acids and with leucine residues at conserved locations.[93,94,95] This central repeat region is surrounded by disulfide loop structures, where there are two disulfide bridges on the N-terminal side and one on the C-terminal side. Three of the LRR proteins regularly possess one or two glycosaminoglycan (GAG) chains and are therefore proteoglycans. Many of the others contain one or several N-glycosidically linked KS chains, but this is a variable between species, tissues, and age of the animal. Those with GAG chains have been termed small leucine-rich repeat proteoglycans (SLRPs).

It is likely that the 3D structure of this leucine rich domain shares the features of the one determined for decorin[96] and verified for biglycan.[97] The curved core of the repeat region exposes a parallel β-sheet surface on the concave side. This face is involved in interactions between two molecules that results in the formation of dimers where the N-terminal end of one molecule is located close to the middle of the concave face of the other, thus exhibiting a very large interacting surface. If all the LRR molecules are involved in such a dimer formation, this will influence how these proteins interact with other molecules. The LRR portion of all the proteins appears to bind with high affinity to fiber-forming collagens (DEC, BIGN, FM, LUMICAN, PRELP, CHAD), although for most of the proteins, the exact binding sites have not been identified. The sites along the collagen molecule appear from preliminary data to be different for many of the proteins, with the possible exception of fibromodulin and lumican.[98] In several cases, it appears that there is more than one site along the collagen (PRELP, CHAD).[99,100] It also appears that other interactions involve the LRR-repeat domain, including binding of growth factors within the TGF-β family.[101,102] It also appears that interactions with, for example, the matrilins and collagen type VI described involve the LRR-region,[80,103] but the exact specificity is not known. The major differences between the molecules are found in the N-terminal and C-terminal portions outside the disulfide loops flanking the LRR-repeats. There are some characteristic differences between each family of molecules, described below. At the same time, there are distinct differences between individuals in a given family.

Four distinct classes of SLRPs have been described (Fig. 4–9) (LLR), based upon general structural[103] class I SLRPs decorin[93] and biglycan,[104] and LRR protein Asporin[95]

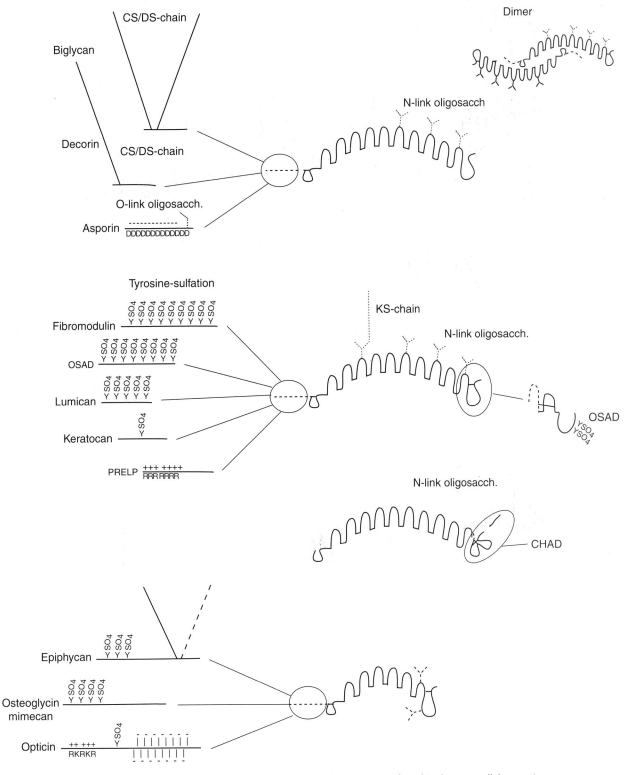

Figure 4–9 Schematic depiction of the four groups of LRR proteins found in the extracellular matrix. The curved shape of the core protein and dimer formation observed by x-ray crystallography for biglycan and decorin are indicated. The variable N-terminal region (to the left) of the molecules in each group are indicated separately with glycosaminoglycan chains as filaments (black), tyrosine sulfate as a SO_4, and N-linked oligosaccharides as a Y-structure (black). In some cases the N-linked oligosaccharide may exist in the form of a KS chain, with a longer arm representing the disaccharide repeat. Clusters of basic (e.g., PRELP) amino acids are denoted by R and a plus (+) sign, while arrays of acidic amino acids (in asporin) are denoted by a D and a minus (–) sign. The mucin like cluster of O-linked oligosaccharides in opticin are denoted as fat rods with a minus (–) sign. In the cases of osteoadherin (OSAD) and chondroadherin (CHAD), the C-terminal part is different as is indicated.

show high structural similarity. Class II includes fibromodulin,[105] lumican,[106] keratocan,[107] PRELP,[108] and osteoadherin.[109] Class II can be subdivided into subclasses, with fibromodulin and lumican showing greater relatedness, as well as keratocan and PRELP. Osteoadherin may represent a member of a third subclass within Class II.[109] Class III contains epiphican[110,111] (also known as PG-Lb) and osteoglycin.[112] PRELP should most likely be considered an LRR glycoprotein as little evidence exists that it is substituted with GAG chains. Another LRR protein, chondroadherin, particularly prominent in cartilage, has a distinct gene arrangement distinguishing this protein to a separate class. It contains neither GAG chains nor N-glycosidically linked oligosaccharides.

Decorin, Biglycan, and Asporin. The members of the first family are decorin, biglycan, and asporin. Decorin has a single N-terminal site for addition of a CS or DS GAG chain, and three potential sites for N-linked oligosaccharide substitution.[114] Decorin (as well as biglycan and asporin) is synthesized with amino terminal propeptides that apparently may be removed intracellularly during biosynthesis[114] or extracellularly[115] (as both processed and proforms can be detected in culture medium and cartilage extracellular matrix.[115] A role for decorin in collagen fibrillogenesis is supported by the observation that decorin-null animals demonstrate skin fragility.[115a] The reduction in tensile strength could be associated with abnormal collagen fiber formation in the skin. Decorin has also been shown to have a high affinity for TGF-β, which may permit decorin to sequester these growth factors in the extracellular matrix.[101] Independent of the interaction of decorin with TGF-ß, decorin may function to inhibit cellular proliferation by acting directly upon a signal-transduction pathway leading to activation of cyclin-dependent kinase inhibitors.[116]

Biglycan has two N-terminal sites for CS or DS GAG substitution, and two potential N-linked oligosaccharide sites. Biglycan, unlike decorin, has been shown to be present in cartilage as intact and N-terminally degraded forms with increasing age.[116b] Biglycan-deficient mice[117] show diminished bone mass with increasing age, and are deficient in their capacity to form bone. This is likely due to a diminished capacity to produce marrow stromal cells (bone cell precursors). These cells also have reduced response to TGF-β, reduced collagen synthesis, and increased apoptosis.

Asporin differs from decorin and biglycan in that it contains an array of aspartates in its N-terminal that show a polymorphism with a variable number from 11 up to 15 such residues.[96] Studies of individuals with osteoarthritis indicate that in some populations there is a correlation of a higher risk for the disease with 13 aspartates[118] while in other cohorts this relation has not been verified.[101,119,120] Like other LRR-proteins, asporin is expected to bind to fibril-forming collagens type I and II. This has not been verified although some preliminary data indicate that this is true. It has been suggested that asporin can bind TGF-β[118] similarly to decorin, biglycan, and fibromodulin.[101] Such an interaction could contribute to sequestering the growth factor to certain structures in the matrix to be released, for example, upon

degradation of these structures in pathology. The released factor can then activate the cells to an adequate repair response.

Fibromodulin, Lumican, Keratocan, Osteoadherin, and PRELP. Most members of this family of proteins contain tyrosine sulfate residues in the N-terminal extension. Fibromodulin is the most prominent example with up to nine such tyrosine sulfates over a short domain[121] providing the molecule with an extremely anionic domain. Because fibromodulin is present bound at the collagen fiber surface in the tissue,[122] it is likely that this N-terminal extension is available for interactions with more cationic motifs on surrounding structures. Indeed the availability of this domain is indicated by the fact that upon stimulation of degradation processes in cartilage by IL-1, a specific cleavage accomplished by MMP-13 will release almost the entire tyrosine sulfate domain[123] and leave the rest of the protein bound to collagen. The large variability in the number of tyrosine sulfate residues within a given preparation provides for variable potential functions. Fibromodulin contains additional anionic structures in the form of KS chains,[124,125] but this is not obligatory and varies between species and age of the individual.

Osteoadherin[109,126] contains up to eight tyrosine sulfates that show a different clustering compared to fibromodulin.[121] Much less is known about this protein that is restricted to bone but also made by hypertrophic chondrocytes. It does bind cells via their $\alpha_v\beta_3$ integrins,[126] but the details of this interaction are not known. Osteoadherin differs from the other members of this family by having an extensive C-terminal portion containing two tyrosine sulfates.[121] Also osteoadherin contains KS chains depending on tissue.[126] Lumican[127] contains a maximum of four tyrosine sulfates in the N-terminus,[121] and contains KS in some tissues it appears to bind to the same site on collagen fibers as fibromodulin although with somewhat lower affinity.[98]

In support of the collagen binding of these molecules, the fibromodulin- and lumican-null mice show distinct alterations of the collagen fiber assembly.[128,129,130]

Keratocan[107] has only one potential site for tyrosine sulfation, but shares many other features with the other molecules in the family.

PRELP[131] is distinct in containing an N-terminal extension with clusters of basic amino acids forming a domain that binds heparin with high affinity. Its affinity is highest for heparin with three O-sulfates per disaccharide. This protein was originally found in cartilage,[132] but later studies have revealed its presence at basement membranes where it appears to bind to the heparan sulfate chains of, for example, perlecan via the specific N-terminal binding domain. At the same time the protein can bind to collagen serving to provide anchorage of basement membranes to underlying tissues. The protein is relatively abundant in cartilage, but its exact role is not known. Cartilage indeed contains perlecan as one potential interaction partner[133] and a role in network formation by simultaneous binding to the collagen fibers is likely.

Chondroadherin. Chondroadherin[113] forms its own family and differs from the other LRR proteins by having a double disulfide loop on the C-terminal side of the repeat domain. Another difference is that this protein has no N-terminal extension, while a short basic extension in the C-terminal should contribute functional properties, possibly involving interactions with anionic constituents like the GAG chains. The protein is also unique among the LRR-proteins in having no post-translational modifications.[134] The protein has been shown to bind to the integrin $\alpha_2\beta_1$, but not to any of the other collagen binding integrins.[135] Upon binding, the cells do not spread, but signals are induced, e.g., ERK-phosphorylation. Interestingly, the protein can also bind to fibril-forming collagen types I and II.[100] Indeed, complexes with chondroadherin bound at two sites along the collagen II molecule could be isolated from cartilage after induction of endogenous proteinases. It is possible that chondroadherin can provide a bridging from the cell to collagen in the surrounding matrix. At this time little is know of the exact function of the protein in cartilage and the role of the interactions with the integrin has not been elucidated. Chondroadherin is quite restricted to cartilage. The protein is found particularly enriched in the growth plate and particularly in a zone corresponding to the prehypertrophic area.[136] Novel findings have identified expression of the protein in several structures of the eye and in other tissues including some neurological.[137]

Proteins with a Shorter LRR-repeat region (opticin, mimecan/osteoglycin, and epiphycan). There is also a family of proteins/proteoglycans with only six or seven LRR repeats. This family consists of epiphycan, mimecan, and opticin. Available data indicate that these proteins also bind to fibril-forming collagens.[138] This seems to be a feature of the LRR proteins. Also these proteins have N-terminal extensions with different properties. Opticin[139,140] originally isolated from the vitreous of the eye is present in cartilage and is quite unique in that it contains a mucin stretch with O-glycosidically linked oligosaccharides. Further to the N-terminus, the protein contains a stretch rich in basic amino acids and apparently having the ability to bind to heparin and other GAG.[141] This molecule may add to the network and quality of the cartilage matrix.

Mimecan[142] contains an N-terminal domain with putative substitution with tyrosine sulfate. In addition to this anionic domain, the molecule when present in cornea contains KS. A smaller version of mimecan, osteoglycin, lacks the tyrosine sulfate domain. Epiphycan[111] contains both a short stretch of tyrosine sulfate and up to two CS/dermatan sulfate chains in its N-terminal extension.

Tenascin-C

Tenascin-C is a member of the tenascin family with four members (C, R, W, X)[143] having different tissue distributions. Tenascin-C is the one of these molecules with a significant presence in cartilage, particularly during growth and in pathology.[144,145] The protein is also produced by fibroblasts including those in tumor stroma, smooth muscle cells, and in the nervous system.[143] Tenascin-C forms a homo-hexamer, originally referred to as hexabrachion, where the chains are linked via a heptad repeat close to the N-terminus. Tenascin-C is present in several differently spliced forms, where the overall structure is similar. The C-terminal end of the chain contains a fibrinogen globe followed by a variable number (at least 8) of fibronectin type III repeats and some 15 EGF-like repeats.

One function of the tenascins is to modulate cell behavior. Thus it appears that the protein can bind to fibronectin and block its binding to syndecan,[143] important in cell spreading and migration (see section fibronectin discussed later). This may be an important factor in the role of the protein in wound healing and tumor growth, but also of potential relevance to the cell multiplication seen in osteoarthritis and to events in the growth plate.

Tenascins have been shown to bind to the C-type lectin domain[146] of the hyalectins, where aggrecan is the abundant representative in cartilage. The binding of the lectin is to the fibronectin type III repeat domain.[146] This interaction may serve to crossbridge this end of the aggrecan to other molecular networks in the cartilage as is supported by in vitro studies demonstrating complex formation by electron microscopy.[147]

Tenascin expression is upregulated upon mechanical stress, particularly studied in fibroblasts.[148] The role in cartilage pathology, where the mechanical environment is an important factor, is underscored by the increased production in cartilage from patients with osteoarthritis.[145]

Fibulin

The fibulins represent a family of six members, where fibulins-6 or hemicentin-1 may represent a different family.[149,150] The fibulins often show differently spliced forms. For instance, fibulin-1s occur in four forms showing minor differences.[149]

The overall composition of fibulin-1 includes three anaphylatoxin (AT) domains in the N-terminus followed by nine EGF-homology repeats and the Domain III in the C-terminus. Fibulin-2 contains an additional two EGF repeats and has a unique additional N-terminal domain of some 400 amino acids.

Fibulins interact with a number of macromolecules in the extracellular matrix. Fibulin-1 and -2 thus bind components of the elastic fiber[151] and are important in the development of major blood vessels where elastic fibers are important. The fibulins also bind to a number of basement membrane components, including laminins, nidogen-1, and perlecan.[149,151] All these proteins have been found in cartilage. An interaction particularly important for cartilage super-molecular structure is the one between fibulins-1 and -2 and the C-terminal lectin homology domain of the lecticans,[21,147] particularly aggrecan. This Ca-dependant binding involves portions of the EGF domain, where the two most C-terminal appear to be essential. In view of the other interactions of the fibulins, it is apparent that the molecule has the potential to crossbridge to other molecules being part of the supramolecular networks in cartilage.

Fibulin-1–null mice primarily suffer from defective functions of the basement membrane. There is, however, a genetic defect lacking the fibulin-1D variant, where patients show polydactyly demonstrating a role in limb formation.

Fibrillin

Fibrillins have been extensively studied, partly because a number of mutations lead to Marfan syndrome (for a comprehensive review on fibrillins and Marfan syndrome, see Robinson et al.[152]). There are three variants of fibrillins and an additional four variants of the closely related family of latent TGF-β binding proteins (LTBPs). The fibrillins are large, e.g., almost 1,100 amino acids for fibrillin-1. The major motif seen in the fibrillins are a large number of EGF-motifs (47 in fibrillin-1). There is also a repeat domain unique with eight cysteine residues.[153,154] Some of these domains mediate binding of LTBP[152] and thereby TGF-β important in the regulation of tissue homeostasis. The protein also contains a number of other motifs, where the C-terminal domain is homologous to that of the fibulins. This may be involved in interactions with other such domains.

Fibrillins form microfibrils showing a beaded appearance and are particularly abundant where tissues are exposed to mechanical stress.[154] The exact molecular organization of the microfibers is not known although a head to tail organization is important. It appears that crosslinks formed by transglutaminase are important for the stability of the fiber. One set of molecules interacting with the fibrillin fiber is the microfibril-associated glycoprotein-1 and -2 (MAGP-1 and -2).[153,155] MAGP-1 has been shown to also bind to the collagen type VI α3-chain,[156] potentially mediating networking in the matrix. Fibrillin can bind to heparin, an interaction that may mediate binding to cell surface proteoglycans such as syndecan and glypican with a potential role in the assembly of fibrillin.[157] Fibrillin in early development is expressed in limbs, primarily in the perichondrium, but not in the cartilage. At a later stage and through growth, fibrillin forms a network of thin fibrils in the cartilage matrix. Later the fibrils are reorganized into more coarse fibers in the matrix surrounding the chondrocyte.[158]

There is in excess of 500 mutations described for fibrillin-1 occurring in various parts of the molecule,[152] resulting in a wide range of phenotypes in, for example, Marfan syndrome. One component important to the phenotypes observed may be an altered binding of LTBP and therefore an altered sequestering of TGF-β in the matrix.[159,160]

Fibronectin

Fibronectin is a homodimer found in most tissues and also abundantly in the general circulation. However, a splice variant is found in cartilage.[161] Each subunit has an apparent dimension of 220 kDa and the two units are linked close to the C-terminal end. The protein contains a number of modules[162,163] referred to as FN type I (twelve), II (two), and III (fifteen to seventeen depending on splicing). The N-terminal five type I repeats form a heparin and fibrin binding domain followed by a collagen/gelatin binding domain. The two domains altogether constitute about one third of the protein containing nine type I repeats and two type 2 repeats. The following type III modules contain the classical domain binding the $\alpha_5\beta_1$, but also the $\alpha_V\beta_3$ integrin, where the RGD sequence in module 10 and a synergy sequence in module 9 are involved.[164] Toward the C-terminus there is another heparin binding domain that also serves in binding to other fibronectin molecules. Close to the C-terminus there is a fibrin-binding domain. There is also a variable sequence containing structures binding to a different set of integrins $\alpha_4\beta_1$ and $\alpha_4\beta_7$.

Fibronectin has important roles in regulating cell proliferation and migration. Key elements are the integrin binding RGD sequence and the heparin binding sequence promoting binding to cell surface syndecans. The combined engagement of these two cell surface molecules is necessary to accomplish the arrangement of the cytoskeleton elements required for migration, i.e., the focal adhesion complex.[165,166] Fibronectin forms fibrils[163,167,168] in a process where β_1 integrins are required for the assembly process.[169] These fibrils appear to have roles in directing cell movements and may serve as a scaffold for the organization of the many other matrix molecules that interact with fibronectin.[170]

Fibronectin thus appears to have a central role in providing signals to the cells and in providing one of the tools that the cell can use to organize the matrix.

Fibronectin production is markedly upregulated in cartilage in osteoarthritis[67,171] and also the level of the protein in the matrix is increased. This appears to be an early event but is maintained throughout the disease development.[67] It is likely to represent an attempted repair.

Other Proteins Present in the Cartilage Extracellular Matrix

Chitinase 3-like (CHI3L) Proteins. There are two members of this family. Chitinase 3-like protein 1 (CHI3L-1) was initially described under different names (gp-39/YKL-40).[172-174] The protein has 383 amino acids and an apparent molecular weight of 39 kDa. It is related to YKL-39 or Chitinase 3-like protein 2 (CHI3L-2) with 311 amino acids.[173] The proteins are expressed in and present in many tissues, particularly in pathology. According to one report, the Chitinase 3-like protein 2 (YKL-39) is upregulated while Chitinase 3-like protein 1 does not appear to change in osteoarthritis.[173,175] According to another study, the Chitinase 3-like protein 1 is upregulated in osteoarthritis contrasting to low levels in the normal cartilage from old individuals. The protein is also produced in the synovial membrane in joints with an inflammatory response, and the higher levels observed in joint fluid from patients with joint disease described for CHI3L-1 (YKL-40) may result from alterations in the synovium as well as in the cartilage.[176,177]

CHI3L-1 protein is upregulated in chondrocytes stimulated with cyokines, e.g., TNF-α.[178] Thus the inflammatory component often observed in joint disease may effectuate the higher levels observed. The functional roles of the proteins are not known, but they show affinity for chitin structures[179] although not expressing any Chitinase activity. No endogenous carbohydrate ligand has been identified.

Matrix Gla Protein/MGP. This 103 amino acid protein contains vitamin K-dependent modification of specific glutamic acid residues to γ-carboxyglutamic acid. The protein is present in many tissues and has an apparent role in mineralization by acting as an inhibitor. The null mouse shows major arterial calcification.[181,182] The γ-carboxylated glutamates are essential for the inhibition.[182] Furthermore, abnormal cartilage calcification in the Keutel syndrome results from mutations in the matrix Gla protein.[182]

Pleiotrophin. This 18-kDa protein shows binding to heparin and also to CS D. This GAG is recognized by having disaccharides sulfated both at the 2-position of the uronic acid and at the 6-position of the hexosamine. Binding was also shown for CS E with a 4,6-disulfated disaccharide unit.[184] It is likely that cartilage contains putative binding structures of both heparan sulfate and oversulfated CS chains, albeit the latter is a very minor constituent in the tissue.

The protein is abundant in young growing cartilage but present only in very low amounts in the adult individual.[185] Whether it will interact with the heparan sulfate chains of cell surface syndecans involved in cell spreading and migration is not known.

Chondromodulin. Chondromodulin is produced as a 334 amino acid precursor with a transmembrane domain.[186,187] This precursor is cleaved to form the active protein, represented by the C-terminal 121 amino acids.[186] A major property of the protein is to inhibit angiogenesis and it is found in tissues where angiogenesis is important such as normal articular cartilage and cornea.[186,187] It is more abundant in the proliferative and prehypertrophic zones of the growth plate, while the concentration is much lower in the hypertrophic zone where blood vessel invasion is imminent.[188] Interestingly, the level of the protein is decreased in osteoarthritis.[189] A related protein named tenomodulin is abundant in tendon.[187,190] The tenomodulin null mouse shows increased collagen fiber dimensions, although the synthesis of collagen appears not to change. Also ablation of the protein leads to a decreased proliferation of the tenocytes.

Chondrocalcin. Chondrocalcin represents the released C-terminal propeptide of collagen type II. The protein is retained in the cartilage and appears to have roles in regulating mineralization.[32,191] A role in normal articular cartilage is not known.

PARP. This protein was originally isolated as a low molecular weight protein from cartilage.[42] Subsequent work indicates that it represents the amino-terminal domain of the collagen XI α2 chain,[192] and may be a product of collagen processing, similar to chondrocalcin, the type II collagen C-terminal peptide.[191] The function of PARP is as yet unknown.

NUTRITION OF ARTICULAR CARTILAGE

Cartilage from mature animals is totally avascular, aneural, and alymphatic.[193] The surface is not covered by a perichondrium, nor has a synovial layer been observed. The source of nutritive material for the cartilaginous surfaces has long been a puzzle. Because the tissue is avascular in adult life, the earliest investigators thought that the nutritive materials diffuse through the matrix either from the synovial fluid that bathes the surface of the cartilage or from the underlying bone. In 1920, Strangeways reported an experiment suggesting that the synovial route is the only source of nutrients for adult cartilage.[194] Subsequent dye diffusion studies by Brower and colleagues[195] and studies using other substrates or hydrogen gas have confirmed this. Since 1950, experimental evidence has suggested that in immature animals, at least a portion of the substrates enter the articular cartilage by diffusion from the underlying bony end plate; in the adult, with the appearance of the tidemark and heavy disposition of apatite in the calcified zone, this type of diffusion disappears or becomes severely limited.

Synovial fluid, then, appears to serve as the primary source of nutrition for the chondrocytes in adult articular cartilage. The fluid itself arises by diffusion from the synovial vascular network and represents a diffusate of plasma (without fibrinogen and with the somewhat diminished levels of urea, glucose, and plasma protein) to which the synoviocytes have added hyaluronate and some additional proteins.[196] Only a small volume of synovial fluid is present in normal joints, but sufficient quantities of nutrients and oxygen reach the chondrocytes, presumably by diffusion through the cartilage matrix. Extensive studies performed by Maroudas[197] have shown that the diffusion of nutrients through the matrix of the cartilage is not unrestricted but is limited by the size and charge of the molecule and perhaps also by steric configuration. The "pore size" was originally thought to be 6.8 nm (large enough to admit a hemoglobin molecule), but a study by Maroudas suggests that larger molecules (such as albumin) may enter the cartilage under special circumstances. Because synovial inflammation may play an important role in the pathogenesis of oesteoarthritis (OA), it should be noted that cytokines, such as interleukin-1 and tumor necrosis factor, and prostaglandins derived from the synovium have been shown to reach the chondrocytes and have profound effects on the metabolism of these cells.

Nutritional factors such as glucose and glucose-derived sugars (such as glucosamine sulfate) have been the subject of increased interest in recent years (reviewed in Mobasheri et al.[198]). Chondrocytes consume glucose as the primary substrate for glycolysis and ATP production and use glucosamine sulfate and other sulfated sugars in the biosynthesis of GAG. Utilization of these sugars is dependent on hexose uptake and transport to metabolic pools. Chondrocytes have been shown to express several isoforms of the GLUT/SLC2A family of glucose/polyol transporters. Recent studies have suggested that cartilage degeneration may be related to metabolic disorders of glucose balance, and that OA may be coincident with metabolic disease, endocrine dysfunction, and diabetes mellitus.

The dietary supplements glucosamine and CS have been the subject of intense popular interest, as options for symptomatic management of osteoarthritis. An NIH sponsored, multicenter, double blind, placebo- and celecoxib-controlled clinical trial of glucosamine and CS (Glucosamine/chondroitin Arthritis Intervention Trial [GAIT]) was published in 2006.[199]) It was concluded that glucosamine and CS alone or in combination did not reduce pain effectively in the overall group of patients with osteoarthritis of the knee. Although ineffective individually, combination treatment of a subgroup of patients with moderate to severe pain showed significant knee pain reduction, a result awaiting further confirmation. A number of other studies have been done to evaluate the efficacy of glucosamine[199-203] and CS.[204,205] Although some showed positive results, possible flaws included the participation of insufficient numbers of patients, possible bias in studies sponsored by nutriceutical manufacturers, and insufficient masking of the tested agent. Furthermore, these studies generally recruited patients having low levels of knee pain[200-203] and demonstrated no improvement in Western Ontario and McMaster Universities Osteoarthritis Index (WOMAC) pain scores.[206] Using other outcome measures,[200,201] however, glucosamine has shown some benefits.

EXTRACELLULAR MATRIX BIOSYNTHESIS AND ASSEMBLY

The cartilage extracellular matrix is an interconnected complex of collagens, proteoglycans, and glycoproteins that are synthesized, secreted, maintained, and degraded by chondrocytes. OA pathology may arise as a consequence of qualitative changes in matrix collagens or proteoglycans resulting from altered biosynthesis. Proteoglycans in OA cartilage typically are extensively degraded, but also show additional molecular heterogeneity due to new biosynthesis during an intrinsic repair process.[207-209] Monoclonal antibodies have been used to reveal subtle biochemical changes in proteoglycans in a canine model of OA[210] and in human OA.[211] Unique epitopes reactive with these antibodies are likely to be markers of newly synthesized proteoglycans in OA cartilage and may reflect OA specific differences related to post-translational modification of aggrecan.

It has been observed that inflammation or pain-relieving medication such as aspirin, Nonsteroidal anti-inflammatory drugs (NSAIDs), and steroid drugs can alter cartilage metabolism. NSAIDS have been found to suppress proteoglycan synthesis.[212] In other studies, some NSAIDS appeared to block or stimulate proteoglycan synthesis depending on the concentration.[213,214] Aspirin has been found to block CS synthesis.[215] Details of the biosynthesis of individual components of these matrix macromolecules are beyond the scope of this discussion, but in the following sections we describe general aspects of the normal biosynthesis of collagens and proteoglycans.

Collagen Biosynthesis

Collagens contain very specific post-translational modifications. The first of these is hydroxylation of proline and lysine to produce the amino acids hydroxyproline and hydroxylysine, which are almost unique to collagen.[216] This process requires specific enzymes, i.e., proline hydroxylase and lysine hydroxylase, and, as cofactors, molecular oxygen, ferrous iron, ketoglutarate, and a reducing agent, ascorbic acid. The second process, the synthesis of hydroxylysyl glycosides, is dependent on the presence of galactose and glucose in the form of uridine diphosphate (UDP) derivatives and two specific transfer enzymes. Once assembled, the procollagen molecule undergoes enzymic conversion to native collagen during or following export when the amino and carboxyl propeptides are removed. To date, the exact site and nature of both this conversion and the method by which the molecule is secreted from the cell are not clearly understood. The remaining processes affecting collagen occur in the extracellular matrix and consist of cross-link formation, which provides intramolecular links between the chains of the collagen molecules, intrafilament cross-links between the tropocollagen, molecules composing the primary unit, and interfilament cross-links between the primary filaments making up the fibril and to other collagens that are part of the fibril. For more detailed description of collagen synthesis, please see Olsen.[217]

Proteoglycan Biosynthesis

Proteoglycan core proteins are variably substituted with GAG chains. GAGs are linear polysaccharides having repeating disaccharide subunits (Fig. 4–10). Almost 90% of the mass of aggrecan is due to GAG chain substitution of the core protein, including CS and KS, as well as numerous N- and O-linked oligosaccharides. Many enzymes are involved in GAG and oligosaccharide biosynthesis, and the abundance and type of glycosyltransferases and sulfotransferases expressed may be regulated to contribute to developmental stage-specific or age-specific glycosylation.

Chondroitin Sulfate Biosynthesis

Biosynthesis of CS is initiated by the xylosyltransferase-catalyzed addition of xylose at Ser, usually within a Ser-Gly dipeptide motif.[218] Next, the so-called "linkage region" (Gal-Gal-GlcA) is constructed by the action of Gal I, Gal II, and GluA transferases (Fig. 4–11). Finally, CS chains elongation is accomplished by CS synthases that catalyze the alternating addition of GalNAc and GluA. During chain elongation, GalNAc residues are sulfated either at the 4-O-position, the 6-O-position, or at both, by CS sulfotransferases. Evidence from previous studies using fragmentation with proteolytic enzymes or direct visualization by electron microscopy also suggests that not all Ser-Gly sequences are substituted with GAG chains.

Keratan Sulfate Biosynthesis

Biosynthesis, structure, and function of KS has been reviewed by Funderburgh.[219] KS is an oligomer of sulfated N-acetyllactosamine disaccharide (Gal and GlcNac) repeats. KS is synthesized in the Golgi apparatus by the action of glycosyltransferases and sulfotransferases. Additionally, KS chains may be fucosylated and capped with sialic acid. KS displays a great deal of heterogeneity in

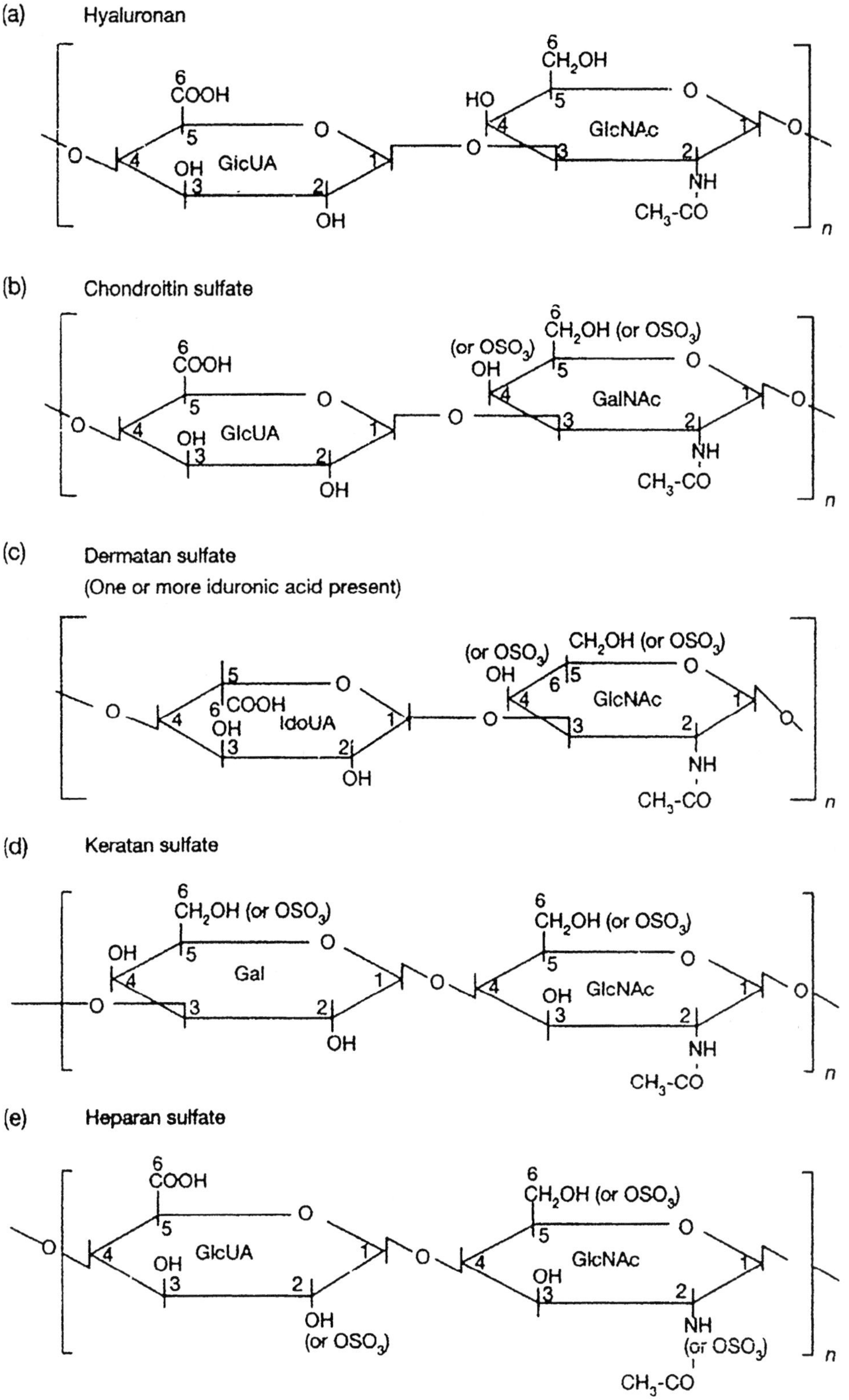

Figure 4–10 Structure of glycosaminoglycans (GAGs). Brackets enclose repeating disaccharide units. Except for hyaluronan, all are modified with sulfate groups and are covalently attached to protein. GlcUA, glucuronic acid; GlcNAc, D-N-acetylgluosamine; GalNAc, D-N-acetylgalactosamine; IdoUA, iduronic acid; Gal, galactose. (Reprinted from Dudhia J.Cell. Mol Life Sci. 62:2241–2256, 2005.)

the degree of KS sulfation, fucosylation, and sialylation. The number of disaccharide repeats can be tissue-specific or proteoglycan-specific, and may even vary between the sites of substitution on a proteoglycan. KS chains can be attached to Asn (N-link) or Ser/Thr (O-link) structures.

Both N-linked and O-linked KS are found on aggrecan expressed in cartilage. N-linked KS is attached to Asn in the core protein via a complex-type N-linked branched oligosaccharide, whereas O-linked KS is attached to Thr/Ser in the core protein.

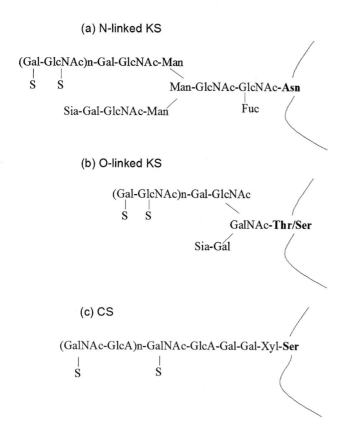

(a) N-linked KS

(Gal-GlcNAc)n-Gal-GlcNAc-Man

    | |

    S   S   Man-GlcNAc-GlcNAc-**Asn**

Sia-Gal-GlcNAc-Man   Fuc

(b) O-linked KS

    (Gal-GlcNAc)n-Gal-GlcNAc

        | |

        S   S   GalNAc-**Thr/Ser**

         Sia-Gal

(c) CS

(GalNAc-GlcA)n-GalNAc-GlcA-Gal-Gal-Xyl-**Ser**

 | |

 S   S

Figure 4–11 Keratan sulfate and chondroitin sulfate polysaccharide structures and glycosylation linkages. (a) N-linked KS, (b) O-linked KS, and (c) O-linked CS. Monosaccharide abbreviations, GlcA, glucuronic acid; GalNAc-S, N-acetylgalactosamine 4 (or 6) sulfate; Gal, galactose; Xyl, xylose; GlcNAc, N-acetylglucosamine; Man, mannose; Sia, sialic acid; Fuc, fucose; GalNac, N-acetylgalactosamine. (Reprinted from Miwa HE. A recombinant system to model proteoglycan aggregate interactions and aggrecan degradation. Doctoral dissertation, Case Western Reserve University, Cleveland, OH, 2006.)

N-linked and O-linked Glycosylation

Asparagine-linked (N-linked) glycosylation is a cotranslational protein modification that occurs in the endoplasmic reticulum (ER). The mechanism for addition of N-linked oligosaccharides (reviewed by Yan and Lennarz[220]) involves the transfer by oligosaccharyltransferase (OT) of an oligosaccharyl moiety (Glc3Man9GlcNAc2) from the dolichol-linked pyrophosphate donor to Asn residues occurring within a consensus sequence of Asn-X-Thr/Ser, where X can be any amino acid residue except for Pro. This modification functions as a primary determinant for specific molecular recognition as well as protein folding and stability. It has been demonstrated that only selective -Asn-X-Thr/Ser- motifs in a glycoprotein are glycosylated. A likely explanation is that in addition to the consensus sequence, adjacent amino acids may play a role in substrate-enzyme recognition. The biosynthesis of different N-linked oligosaccharide structures involves two series of reactions: first, the formation of Glc3Man9(GlcNAc)2-pyrophosphoryl-dolichol, by the sequential addition of GlcNAc, mannose, and glucose to dolichol-P, and secondly, the removal of glucose and

mannose by membrane-bound glycosidases and the subsequent addition of GlcNAc, galactose, sialic acid, and fucose by Golgi-localized glycosyltransferases to produce different complex oligosaccharide structures.

O-glycosylation of proteins and proteoglycans is a complex, post-translational event (reviewed in Van den Steen et al.[221]). The first step in synthesis of O-glycans is the transfer of GalNAc to Ser or Thr residues by UDP-GalNAc:polypeptide a-GalNAc transferase (ppGalNac transferase). At present, ten ppGalNac transferase isoforms have been described. Among these, peptide substrate specificities are variable; many show sensitivity to prior glycosylation, and others require prior addition of GalNac for activity. The expression of particular ppGalNac transferase isoforms is therefore the first step in the determination of O-glycan structure by peptide sequence. Elongation of O-glycans proceeds by the stepwise addition of single sugars via a series of substrate-specific Golgi transferases. The major dictates of O-glycan structure and elongation are therefore Golgi localization, nucleotide sugar concentration, and competition among transferases.

Hyaluronan Biosynthesis

Hyaluronan biosynthesis differs from the synthesis of other GAGs[222] in that it occurs at the plasma membrane and does not require a core protein to initiate synthesis. Polymer growth occurs from the reducing end of the chain.[223,224] During synthesis, the elongating carbohydrate chain is pushed from within the plasma membrane into the extracellular space, leading with the nonreducing end of the chain. Three mammalian hyaluronan synthase genes, termed HAS1, HAS2, and HAS3, have been described (reviewed in Itano and Kimata[225]). These isoforms differ in their kinetic properties and the size of hyaluronan produced. When cells are stimulated with cytokines, these enzymes are regulated independently. Hyaluronan is critical during mammalian embryogenesis,[226] functions to expand the extracellular space, plays a role in stimulation of intracellular signaling pathways resulting in cell migration and invasion in the developing heart, and plays a role in epithelial-mesenchymal transformation. Specific biological functions of hyaluronan may be regulated by temporally regulated and spatially restricted expression of particular HAS isoforms.

PROTEINASES INVOLVED IN CARTILAGE MATRIX DEGRADATION

A great deal of attention has been paid to mechanisms by which the major components of the cartilage extracellular matrix, specifically collagen and proteoglycans, are degraded in OA. Although nonproteolytic mechanisms have been proposed, such as degradation by free radicals produced by neutrophils,[227] it has become more likely that specific proteinases are involved. These proteinases may originate from the chondrocytes themselves, or from cells infiltrating inflamed synovium, as occurs in rheumatoid arthritis. There is evidence for sequential degradation of matrix molecules by multiple proteinases. If these enzymes could be identified, it may be possible to develop drugs to inhibit their activity. There are four distinct types of proteolytic enzymes, classified according to their catalytic mechanism. These groups are termed cysteine, aspartic, serine, and metalloproteinases.

Cysteine Proteinases

Cysteine proteinases, including cathepsins B, H, K, L, and S, have been shown to function in matrix degradation during development, growth, remodeling, aging, and in pathologic process. These genes are expressed in most tissues, and show tissue-specific patterns of expression. Cysteine cathepsins, and in particular cathepsin K, are highly expressed in bone and cartilage.[228] The combined endopeptidase and exopeptidase activities of cathepsin B can degrade aggrecan to generate a cleavage site also ascribed to aggrecanases.[229] In experimental OA in rabbits, cathepsin B was upregulated in synovial tissue in the early degenerative phase, and progression of OA was accompanied by upregulation of cathepsin B in cartilage.[230] The quantitative topographic distribution of cathepsin B in human femoral head cartilage, when comparing specimens from various regions of normal and OA tissue, revealed uniform and low activity throughout, as was also observed in apparently intact OA cartilage and severely degraded tissue. Sites of active disease, however, showed much greater activity, with the activity profile displaying an irregular zonal distribution, correlating with tissue degeneration, hypercellularity, or cloning of chondrocytes. Regenerating cartilage displayed some zonal peaks with 20-fold greater activity than controls.[231] A specific inactivator of cathepsin B was shown to prevent IL-1 mediated proteoglycan release from cartilage.[232] Cathepsins K and L have been immunolocalized to both osteoclasts and chondroclasts. Cathepsin L has been immunostained in both proliferating and hypertrophic chondrocytes.[233]

Cysteine proteases of the papain family have emerged as potential drug targets for musculoskeletal diseases. Of most interest are cathepsins S and K, which are selectively expressed in immune system cells and cells which can efficiently degrade collagens and other ECM proteins.[234]

The calpains, a family of calcium-dependent neutral cysteine proteinases, are intracellular cytoplasmic or membrane associated enzymes.[235] Calpain 1 (μ-calpain) and calpain 2 (m-calpain) are so named because they are activated at micro- and millimolar concentrations of $Ca2+$, respectively. M-calpain has been detected in articular chondrocytes,[236–238] growth plate cartilage chondrocytes,[239] and synoviocytes.[240] Oshita et al.[241] demonstrated that m-calpain, or a proteinase with the same substrate specificity, may be responsible for the production of a major proportion of the C-terminally truncated forms of aggrecan found in mature articular cartilages in vivo. Although primarily a cytosolic protein, m-calpain can translocate to both focal complexes/adhesions or the plasma membrane.[237,242,243] There is evidence that it may function at the ER/Golgi apparatus interface and in membrane lipid rafts.[244] These interesting results suggest that calpain-mediated aggrecanolysis might occur during aggrecan biosynthesis and/or secretion. Additional support for this concept is provided

by biosynthetic studies in which large and small populations of aggregating proteoglycan are produced over short labeling periods.[245,246]

Aspartate Proteinases

Lysosomal cathepsins have long been implicated in matrix degradation of cartilage. A cathepsin D-type enzyme activity was detected in two to three times greater amounts in yellowish or ulcerated articular cartilage from patients with primary osteoarthritis than in control "normal" human cartilages.[247] Subsequently, cathepsin D was purified from human patellar cartilage, and positive identification was made on the basis of substrate specificity.[248] Cathepsin D has been immunolocalized in chondroclasts attached to cartilage matrix during endochondral ossification in the human, and has also been immunostained in hypertrophic chondrocytes adjacent to the osteochondral junction.[233] In a recent proteomic analysis of normal human chondrocytes, cathepsin D has been shown to be the most abundant intracellular chondrocyte protease.[6]

Serine Proteinases

Serine proteinases are structurally related to trypsin, active at a neutral pH, and possess an essential serine residue at their catalytic site. Serine proteinases with trypsin-like specificity have been implicated in chondrocyte-mediated cartilage proteoglycan breakdown occurring as a result of stimulation with proinflammatory cytokines. These enzymes may act indirectly, by activation of other proteinases, or may directly degrade ECM macromolecules.

Serine proteinases may be import activators of proMMPs. Plasmin can activate matrix metalloproteinases by cleaving propeptides of the latent proenzyme. Plasmin is converted from the precursor plasminogen by plasminogen activators, which include tissue-type plasminogen activator (tPA) and urokinase-type plasminogen activator (uPA). A selective proteinase inactivator of urokinase-type plasminogen activator has been shown to inhibit IL-1 and TNF-stimulated proteoglycan release from cartilage. This trypsin-like activity, possibly urokinase-type plasminogen activator, was chondrocyte-associated.[249] In another study, human urinary trypsin inhibitor (UTI), a multipotent inhibitor of serine proteases including plasmin, was found to inhibit the activation of proMMP-1, proMMP-3, and proMMP-9 when added to cultures of rabbit articular cartilage chondrocytes together with IL-1 alpha and plasminogen[250] and could inhibit the release of proteoglycans induced by IL-1 alpha and plasminogen from rabbit articular cartilage explants.

The serine proteinases, PMN elastase and cathepsin G, have been suspected to play a role in articular cartilage degradation, and compounds have been studied for their potential to inhibit these enzymes.[251] Polymorphonuclear leukocyte (PMN) elastase, the enzyme responsible for degradation of highly cross-linked elastin, is able to degrade other extracellular matrix components including fibronectin, laminins, proteoglycans, and collagen type IV. Elastase activity in OA cartilage extracts as well as synovial fluid from patients with rheumatoid arthritis has been reported, but appears to be due primarily to metalloenzymes rather than PMN elastase.[252] Cathepsin G is a serine proteinase of PMN. It may play a direct and an indirect role in extracellular matrix degradation in the annulus fibrosis, contributing to intervertebral disk degeneration.[253] Its role during articular cartilage degeneration of OA has not been thoroughly explored.

Metalloproteinases

In OA cartilage, the major extracellular matrix components, namely, type II collagen and aggrecan, are degraded extracellularly by metalloproteinases, the identity of which has been the subject of numerous investigations in recent years. Although members of other proteinase families (cysteine, aspartic, and serine) may be involved in normal turnover and pathological degradation of cartilage matrix, metalloproteinases have been found to interact with collagen II and aggrecan at very specific sites (Fig. 4–12) which have likely co-evolved with these enzymes to permit normal turnover to occur. Metalloproteinases are enzymes with an active site containing a metal ion (generally zinc) that is necessary for proteolytic activity. Two families of metalloproteinases are believed to degrade cartilage collagen and aggrecan, which are the matrix metalloproteinases (MMPs) and ADAMTS (a disintegrin and a metalloproteinase with thrombospondin motifs) proteinases.

Matrix Metalloproteinases (MMPs)

A number of different matrix metalloproteinases, including MMP-1 (interstitial collagenase), MMP-2 (72 kDa gelatinase), MMP-3 (stromelysin), MMP-7 (PUMP), MMP-8 (neutrophil collagenase), MMP-9 (95-kDa gelatinase), and MMP-13 (collagenase-3), have been shown capable of cleaving at the Asn^{341}-Phe^{342} site of the aggrecan core protein.[254–258] Neoepitopes have been detected in the growth plate as evidence of MMP activity.[259] MMP-13 (collagenase-3) and MMP-1 (interstitial collagenase) are major secreted MMPs expressed by chondrocytes, which are induced by cytokines and growth factors in arthritic joints.[260]

Although it is less abundant than MMP-1, MMP-13 efficiently hydrolyzes type II collagen.[261] During skeletal development, MMP-13 is present in cartilaginous growth plates and primary centers of ossification.[262] Its expression in both terminal hypertrophic chondrocytes of the growth plate and osteoblasts[263] suggests that MMP-13 may play an essential role in skeletogenesis. A number of MMPs are known to cleave aggrecan at a site within the IGD, which results in a neoepitope detectible in growth plate cartilage.[259] Degradation of growth plate aggrecan may be required to permit collagen cleavage.[264] MMPs are suspected to participate in aggrecan degradation in OA as well, and evidence suggests that this may occur in later stages of cartilage degradation concomitant with collagen cleavage.[265]

Tissue inhibitors of metalloproteinases (TIMP) specifically inhibit matrix metalloproteinase activity. Fine regulation of extracellular matrix turnover in cartilage depends on a balance between MMP and TIMP activity, alterations of which are associated with excessive connective tissue deposition, as in fibrotic diseases, or matrix destruction, as occurs in OA and RA. At present, the sequences of four human TIMPs (TIMP-1, -2, -3, and -4) have been determined.[266–274] TIMP proteins function to modulate MMP activity by binding to either the active site of MMP or to the precursor form of the protease. TIMP genes are differentially regulated.[275] The structure of the TIMP-2 and -3 gene promoters have been described, revealing features characteristic of "housekeeping genes" including the lack of a classic TATA box, an abundance of CG, and the presence of multiple SP1 sites.[273,276] The TIMP-1 promoter, on the other hand, has elements characteristic of inducible promoters, such as c-Fos, c-Jun, phorbol ester-responsive elements, and Ets binding motifs.[277,278] Catabolic cytokines including interleukin-1 (IL-1) and tumor necrosis factor-α promote MMP synthesis and matrix catabolism, but inhibit the expression of TIMP-1 by chondrocytes. IL-6, on the other hand, does not induce the synthesis of MMPs, but can induce TIMP synthesis by human articular chondrocytes and fibroblasts.[279] Since IL-6 is synthesized in response to IL-1 or TNF-α stimulation, the upregulation of TIMP-1 by IL-6 could be a protective mechanism preventing excessive matrix destruction.

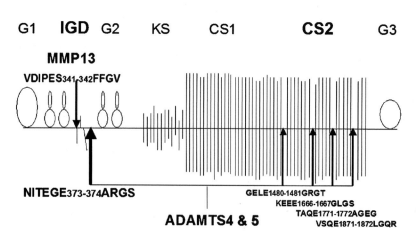

Figure 4–12 Sites of cleavage by MMPs and aggrecanases. Amino acids are numbered for bovine aggrecan (Hering, et al. Arch. Biochem. Biophys. 345, 259-270, 1997). Cleavage site for MMP13 (and other MMPs), and for ADAMTS4 and 5 (and other aggrecanases) are indicated by arrows. Amino acid residues flanking each cleavage site can be recognized by anti-"neoepitope" antisera. (Modified from Miwa HE. A recombinant system to model proteoglycan aggregate interactions and aggrecan degradation. Doctoral dissertation, Case Western Reserve University, Cleveland, OH, 2006.)

ADAMTS Proteases

ADAMTS-1, -4, -5, -9, and -15 have all been shown to be aggrecan-degrading enzymes, among which ADAMTS-4 and -5 appear to be the most active.[280,281] ADAMTS-4 and ADAMTS-5 were initially isolated from cartilage cultures stimulated with interleukin-1.[282] These enzymes are also known as aggrecanase-1 and -2, respectively.

ADAMTS proteinases are multiple domain enzymes having features that are variably conserved among family members (reviewed in Apte.[283]). Following a signal peptide and prodomain, the catalytic domain contains a zinc-binding active-site motif. This is followed by a disintegrin-like region, a thrombospondin type 1 repeat (TSR), a cysteine-rich domain, and a cysteine-free spacer domain, which in most family members is followed by additional TSRs and distinctive C-terminal domains (Fig. 4–13).

Recent studies have revealed that ADAMTS-4 is processed from a 100-kDa proform by a proprotein convertase[284] and secreted as a 68-kDa active enzyme. Further proteolytic processing converts the 68-kDa enzyme to smaller 53- and 40-kDa forms, via C-terminal truncation which occurs either autoproteolytically[285] or more likely through an interaction with MT4-MMP (MMP-17) and the CS and heparan sulfate (HS) chains of syndecan-1.[286] There is evidence that substrate recognition is mediated, at least in part, by binding of the thrombospondin motifs and additional sites in the C-terminal cysteine-rich and/or spacer domains to GAGs.[285,287] The p68 isoform of ADAMTS-4 has been found to have negligble catalytic activity at E373-A374 within the IGD of aggrecan[286,288] whereas the p53 and p40 isoforms cleave efficiently within the IGD.[285,286] When C-terminally processed, ADAMTS-4 is less specific, and is active against carboxymethylated transferrin, fibromodulin, and decorin.[288] Based on the most current observations,[285,286,289] the model shown in Figure 4–14 can be proposed, which describes the ADAMTS-4 activation pathway.

Knockout mouse experiments have shown that ADAMTS-5 may be the major aggrecanase of articular cartilage.[290,291] ADAMTS-4 knockout mice, however, show no gross or histological abnormalities. Although ADAMTS-4 is expressed in the growth plates of wild-type mice, there were no abnormalities in skeletal development, growth, or remodeling in the knockout. Neither was there an effect of the ADAMTS-4 knockout on severity of OA after surgical induction of joint instability.

Some ADAMTS genes are induced by growth factors, inflammatory cytokines, and hormones. TGF-β can induce ADAMTS-4, but not ADAMTS-5 in fibroblast-like synoviocytes.[292] Increased ADAMTS-4 protein was apparent in IL-1 treated pig cartilage explants.[288] ADAMTS-1, -4, and -5 were regulated in TC28a4 cells by IL-1α and oncostatin M.[293] The proinflammatory cytokine IL-17 produced by synovial membranes in RA upregulates ADAMTS-4 in bovine articular chondrocytes via phosphorylation of ERK, p38, and JNK mitogen-activated protein kinases.[294] IL-1 stimulation of chondrocytes or cartilage explants results in an increase in aggrecanase activity without an increase in ADAMTS-4 protein.[264] IL-1 has been shown to modulate the ability of ADAMTS-4 to cleave aggrecan within the IGD by promoting C-terminal truncation through the action of MT4-MMP.[289] Hormonal stimuli may regulate some ADAMTS genes. In growth plate cartilage during endochondral ossification, triiodothyronine (T3) upregulates *ADAMTS-5* mRNA expression, but not *ADAMTS-4*, resulting in subsequent aggrecan degradation.[295]

In OA cartilage, eight ADAMTS genes were shown to be dysregulated: *ADAMTS-1, -5, -9,* and *-15,* which are all aggrecanases, were downregulated, while *ADAMTS-2, -12, -14,* and *-16* were upregulated in OA cartilage compared to normal cartilage.[296] The consistent downregulation of aggrecanase mRNAs in OA cartilage was unexpected. Cartilage examined in this study was from end-stage disease, however, and may not reflect the regulation of these enzymes in earlier stages of OA matrix degradation.

Although TIMPs are relatively broad-spectrum inhibitors of MMPs, they are much more selective inhibitors of the ADAMTS proteinases. ADAMTS-4 and ADAMTS-5 are inhibited by TIMP-3, but are insensitive to TIMP-1, -2, and -4.[282,297,298] ADAMTS-1 is also inhibited by TIMP-3, as well as TIMP-2, but not by TIMP-1 or -4.[299] Based on these inhibition profiles, it is likely that TIMP-3 functions as the physiological inhibitor of aggrecanases in cartilage.[300] Certain nonphysiological inhibitors of ADAMTS proteases may prove to be useful therapeutically. ADAMTS-1, -4, and -5 are inhibited by catechin gallate esters, a component of green tea. Both epigallocatechin gallate and epicatechin gallate were found to be potent inhibitors of these three ADAMTSs, with IC50 values in the nanomolar range.[301]

There has been a lively debate concerning the relative roles of MMPs and aggrecanases in normal turnover and pathological degradation of aggrecan. Aggrecanase appears to be the primary degradative enzyme in short-term experiments, in

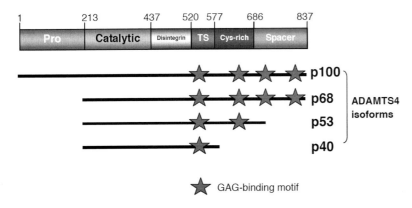

Figure 4–13 ADAMTS4 isoforms and GAG binding motifs. ADAMTS4 consists of six functional domains and motifs. The prodomain is removed before ADAMTS4 is secreted. Three major isoforms, p68, p53, and p40, have proteolytic activity that cleaves aggrecan. (Modified from Miwa HE. A recombinant system to model proteoglycan aggregate interactions and aggrecan degradation. Doctoral dissertation, Case Western Reserve University, Cleveland, OH, 2006.)

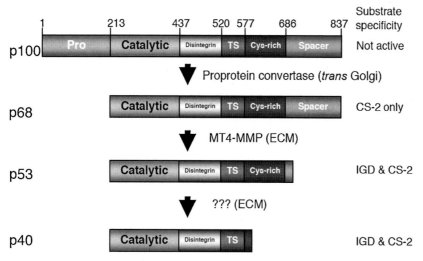

Figure 4–14 ADAMTS4 activation pathway and substrate specificity of each isoform. The N-terminal prodomain of full-length ADAMTS4 (p100) is removed by proprotein convertase in the *trans* Golgi network. Secreted p68 binds to MT4-MMP on the cell surface where C-terminal truncation takes place to obtain p53 by removal of the spacer domain. The p53 remains on the cell surface by binding to GAGs on membrane-anchored syndecan-1. By an unknown mechanism, a cysteine-rich domain can be removed and p40 is released into the medium. (Reprinted from Miwa HE. A recombinant system to model proteoglycan aggregate interactions and aggrecan degradation. Doctoral dissertation, Case Western Reserve University, Cleveland, OH, 2006.)

which cartilage explants are treated with IL-1, TNF-α, or retinoic acid.[265,302] In this model system, MMP-mediated cleavage occurs only at later stages of tissue degeneration.[265] The response of cartilage to catabolic agents appears to be tissue specific. Stimulation of bovine nasal cartilage with IL-1 or retinoic acid results in aggrecanase-mediated degradation. Human cartilage, however, will respond to retinoic acid, but not IL-1.[303] Intriguingly, through an as yet unknown mechanism, fetal bovine epiphseal cartilage stimulated with retinoic acid, but not with IL-1, will release GAGs without any apparent core protein cleavage.[303] In normal human cartilage, neoepitopes resulting from both MMP and aggrecanase-mediated cleavage increase with age and attain a steady state between 20 and 30 years of age.[304] It appears that 15% to 20% of resident aggrecan monomers show evidence of MMP mediated cleavage (VDIPEN neoepitope). Although higher levels of staining are observed in areas of damage, the proportion of the VDIPEN neoepitope does not appear to be increased in OA and rheumatoid arthritic (RA) cartilage. The NITEGE and VDIPEN reactivity was not always colocalized, suggesting that each activity may be site specific.[304] Normal human cartilage contains multiple variably truncated aggrecan species likely to be the result of MMP-mediated cleavage. OA synovial fluid contains abundant aggrecanase-generated fragments of aggrecan, however, suggesting that OA is the result of excessive aggrecanase activity, while MMP activity is restricted to C-terminal trimming of aggrecan monomers, leaving most of the molecule intact.[305] MMPs may participate in cartilage destruction in certain instances, however. STR/ort mice spontaneously develop OA closely resembling the human disease.[306] Although MMP and aggrecanase neoepitopes localize to different regions of normal cartilage in these mice, their distribution becomes similar during disease progression.[307]

CHANGES IN OSTEOARTHRITIS

It is well established that cartilage has a poor intrinsic reparative potential. There is also some provision for turnover of the extracellular matrix, although this is very slow. However, during degenerative change or upon wounding, cartilage displays responses that may be interpreted as reparative. These include elevated matrix synthesis and renewed chondrocyte proliferation. Indeed, it has recently been shown that the proinflammatory cytokines IL-1β and TNF-α stimulate production of BMP-2 in adult articular chondrocytes,[308,309] and that BMP-2 is elevated in OA.[308] While the mechanism of mild inflammation could very likely lead to repair in normal and early OA cartilage, it is evident that these responses are insufficient to heal even limited lesions particularly under functional loading. Interesting hypotheses have arisen from studies using cell and molecular biology. Some investigators believe that the cells are randomly metabolically stimulated and all molecules are increased. However, studies looking for mRNA expression in OA chondrocytes have failed to detect the expression of type I collagen, a molecular hallmark of "dedifferentiated" chondrocytes. Other investigators have proposed that the chondrocytes of OA tissue are undergoing further differentiation to a phenotype similar to the hypertrophic expression of growth plate chondrocytes. The characteristic events of hypertrophic chondrocytes are synthesis of type X collagen, alkaline phosphatase, osteocalcin, and eventually apoptosis (programmed cell death). On the other hand, other investigators have proposed that the cells revert to a chondroprogenitor phenotype in an effort to recapitulate the development of the chondrocytes. A unifying hypothesis to account for all of the current data on OA cartilage does not exist. Overall, biosynthesis and activation of degradative enzymes provides activity that overwhelms the biosynthesis of proper extracellular matrix. Figure 4–15 shows a schematic representation of the possible phenotypes of OA chondrocytes.

The primary metabolic response of chondrocytes in osteoarthritis and in models of osteoarthritis is an increase in the rate of synthesis of type II collagen by the articular chondrocytes. As will be seen in detail below, most extracellular matrix molecules are increased, as well as increased in the synthesis of degradative enzymes. Techniques of molecular biology combined with immunohistochemistry and biochemistry have provided an accurate profile of the metabolic changes that occur in OA. In addition, cells are

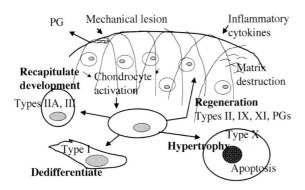

Figure 4–15 Hypothetical pathways of phenotypic alterations of articular chondrocytes in osteoarthritis. (Based on von der Mark et al., 1992.)

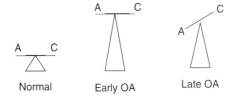

Figure 4–16 Diagram of cell metabolism in normal and OA cartilage. A, anabolism; C, catabolism; height of the triangle represents cell activity.

also stimulated to divide, forming clusters of chondrocytes. Recently, apoptosis or programmed cell death has become an area of intense study. A single regulatory molecule or even group of molecules responsible for the induction of osteoarthritis has not come to light. There is no known single event, or gene regulatory factor, that could trigger the magnitude and variety of changes observed.

Regulatory Molecules

In normal cartilage, the chondrocytes synthesize matrix components at a very slow rate. During development, however, a variety of anabolic cytokines and growth factors such as TGF-β, bone morphogenetic proteins, and IGF I stimulate biosynthesis. In OA, many of these factors, as well as others such as inflammatory cytokines tumor necrosis factor-alpha (TNF-α) and interkeukin-1 (IL-1), are produced by the synovium and the chondrocytes. Normally, there is strict regulation of matrix turnover: a careful balance between synthesis and degradation. In OA, however, this balance is disturbed (Fig. 4–6), with both degradation and usually enhanced synthesis. It is believed that the production of the catabolic and anabolic cytokines activates the chondrocytes. Interestingly, no single cytokine can stimulate all the metabolic reactions observed in OA. TNF-α and IL-1 can potently enhance expression of matrix metalloproteinases leading to increased proteolysis in vitro and in vivo. These factors also can inhibit cartilage matrix biosynthesis.[47]

To investigate the possible role of candidate regulators of cartilage metabolism in OA, Clements et al.[310] investigated the development of osteoarthritis induced by transection of the medial collateral ligament and partial medial meniscectomy in mice in which genes coding for either IL-1ß, IL-1ß-converting enzyme (ICE), stromelysin 1, or inducible nitric oxide synthase (iNOS) were deleted. They observed that all knockout mice exhibited accelerated development of OA lesions compared to wild-type mice. This unexpected result suggested that deletion of these genes changed homeostatic controls regulating the balance between anabolism and catabolism, resulting in accelerated cartilage breakdown (Fig. 4–16). It is apparent that inhibiting normal catabolism had deleterious effects, and caused increased susceptibility to lesion formation.

Nitric oxide (NO) is a free radical formed by combination of a guanidino nitrogen from arginine with molecular oxygen in a reaction catalyzed by NO synthase (NOS). Although NO was only identified as a biologic mediator in 1987, its ubiquity and importance are such that, by 1992, it had become Science Magazine's "Molecule of the Year". While three isoforms of NOS have been identified, only the macrophage form was thought to be inducible and expressed only in injury and disease. It came as some surprise, then, when inducible NOS (iNOS) was found in chondrocytes. NO is now implicated in OA as activated chondrocytes produce levels of NO and NOS. In this case, a single cytokine, IL-1, can induce the production of as much NO per cell as macrophages. The role of NO in OA is not completely known, but it can inhibit proteoglycan synthesis and may play a role in apoptosis of chondrocytes. Some reports have appeared indicating that NO plays a role in the stimulation of apoptosis of chondrocytes,[311,312] although this area is controversial.[313]

Aggrecan Metabolism in Aging and Osteoarthritis

Aggrecan residing within cartilage has been shown to show changes with age. Some of the changes are related to cleavage within the CS-containing regions of the aggrecan monomer, resulting in the accumulation in the tissue of G1-containing, KS-rich, and CS-poor fragments of aggrecan.[314-317] This may not be true of all cartilages, as degraded aggrecan does not appear to be as predominant in bovine nasal or tracheal cartilage.[318] Aggrecan degradation was found to be a feature of intervertebral disk tissue with age, in which both metalloproteinase and aggrecanase-derived cleavage products have been observed.[303] Changes in the GAG chains have been demonstrated, with an increase in 6-sulfation relative to 4-sulfation of CS.[314,315,319] In older cartilage, aggrecan monomers are shorter and more variable in length, have shorter CS chain clusters, and have a shorter thin segment that may result from an increase in KS content. With age, aggregates are shorter with fewer KS monomers per aggregate. The proportion of monomers that aggregate decreases, perhaps due to a decreasing concentration of link protein, or from the accumulation of G1-containing aggrecan core protein fragments.[320] In osteoarthritis, aggrecan is lost from cartilage, and appears to be degraded by aggrecanases[281] produced by the chondrocytes themselves. Numerous earlier studies on aggrecan in OA cartilage have generated conflicting data, however, showing either no change,[321] a reduction,[322,323] or and increase[324] in aggrecan monomer size. In OA cartilage, in contrast to aggrecan in aging cartilage, a high ratio of CS to KS has been observed[322] as is typical of immature cartilage. These inconsistencies appear to be due to differences between specimens and a failure to relate molecular changes to different stages of cartilage degeneration. These differences can be resolved by considering that there may be two phases in the disease process[207] which relate to pathological degradation and attempted repair. In the first phase, there appears to be a general reduction in the size of aggrecan relative to normal, resulting from the loss of G3 and CS-2 domains. In the second phase, where fibrillation is extensive and the cartilage is degenerate in appearance, aggrecan monomers were found to be larger than normal, indicating the presence of newly synthesized intact aggrecan monomers. Altered reactivity of CS chains to antibodies has indicated that changes in the environment of the chondrocyte in OA cartilage may cause changes in CS synthesis.[207,325]

Collagen Metabolism in Osteoarthritis

Type II Collagen Synthesis. In a classic study, Lippiello and colleagues showed that collagen synthesis in osteoarthritic human cartilage, as measured by incorporation of ^{3}H-proline

into hydroxyproline, was five times greater than normal and the rate of collagen synthesis seemed to vary with the severity of the disease.[326] In a canine model system where earlier events of osteoarthritis progression could be studied, Floman and co-workers demonstrated a similar increment in the rate of collagen synthesis when compared to normal controls.[327] Using techniques of *in situ* hybridization to localiz the expression of mRNA and hence gene activity in cells, Matyas and colleagues[328] demonstrated that collagen synthesis is greatly increased compared to normal and that there is a disregulation between collagen and aggrecan synthesis with the collagen eightfold higher than aggrecan. These interesting results indicate that there may be an imbalance in the production of extracellular matrix. Distinct cellular phenotypes have been observed in OA cartilage. Attempts to characterize the phenotype of chondrocytes from OA cartilage have been made by analyzing their collagen synthesis or mRNA expression (Fig. 4–17); the major type of collagen synthesized in OA is type II.[329,330] Chondrocytes from OA samples were found to express type III collagen mRNA, as determined by *in situ* hybridization using a specific probe and by immunohistochemical analysis of the protein.[331] This later observation suggests that chondrocytes can undergo dedifferentiation to a fibroblast-like phenotype. On the other hand, the expression of type I collagen mRNA, another marker for dedifferentiation, was absent in chondrocytes, arguing against the

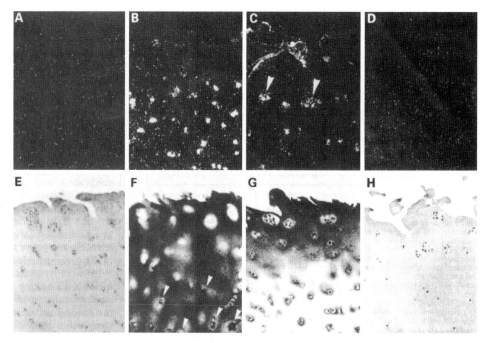

Figure 4–17 Phenotyping of osteoarthritic chondrocytes: in situ hybridization analysis of chondrocytes revealed in all osteoarthritic specimens collagen type II mRNA expression in the middle zones (B), where intracellular staining for type II collagen was also found immunohistochemically (F; arrow heads). In chondrocytes of the upper zone the expression of collagen type I ceased. Interestingly, in the upper middle zone, an onset of type III collagen mRNA expression was observed in most samples (C). This was confirmed by immunohistochemical staining for collagen type III (G). Neither collagen type I (A, E) nor collagen type X (D, H) expression or deposition, as marker collagens of dedifferentiated and hypertrophic chondrocytes, respectively, was observed in the upper and middle zones of osteoarthritic cartilage samples. (A-D: dark field microscopy; femoral head, 69 years old, female; Mankin's grade 5). (Taken from Aigner and Dudhia, 1997.)

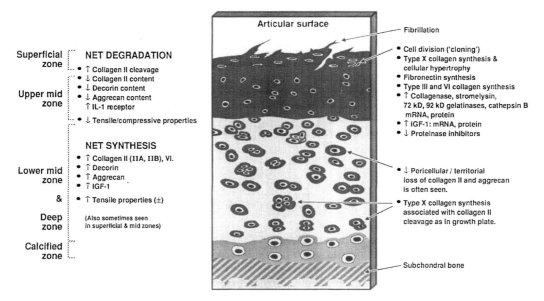

Figure 4–18 General changes in articular cartilage in OA (Mankin grade 2-7). Increases and decreases in content, synthesis, or mRNA, and mechanical properties are indicated. (Taken from Poole, AR. Imbalances of anabolism and catabolism of cartilage matrix components in osteoarthritis. In: Kuettner, KI, Goldberg, VM, eds. Osteoarthritic Disorders. Rosemeont, IL, American Academy of Orthopaedic Surgeons, 1995, pp 247–260.)

assumption of the fibroblastic phenotype.[330] Although type I collagen was reported in human OA cartilage[332] and in rabbit cartilage after mechanical trauma,[332] the bulk of evidence demonstrates that chondrocytes, instead of dedifferentiating to a fibroblastic cell, favor the repair of cartilage matrix by expressing chondrocyte-characteristic collagens. A summary of many of the known metabolic changes is presented in Figure 4–18.

Girkontait and colleagues demonstrated the onset of chondrocyte hypertrophy in the deep zone of OA cartilage as represented by the synthesis of type X collagen.[333] Recently, type X collagen mRNA and protein have also been localized in certain cell populations of OA cartilage and correlated with clinical and radiological alterations.[334] In this study of femoral heads obtained from following the hip joint replacement for femoral neck fractures, osteoarthritis or without hip-joint pathology, they showed that type X collagen is consistently found in osteoarthritic cartilage and is absent from normal adult cartilage. The collagen was primarily in the middle zone cells in advanced stages of OA, but only up to 20% of the cartilage was positive. Therefore, these authors suggest that type X collagen may not play a direct biomechanical role in the weakening of osteoarthritic cartilage, but may indicate a change in chondrocyte phenotype that consistently coincides with the formation of chondrocyte clusters, one of the first alterations in osteoarthritis visible on histologic examination.

Apoptosis is believe to be the means by which hypertrophic cells are removed from the growth plate cartilage[335] so that the hypertrophic cartilage can be removed by osteoclasts and new bone laid down. To examine the occurrence of apoptosis in human osteoarthritis cartilage, and to determine its relationship to cartilage degradation, osteoarthritic samples have been analyzed by flow cytometry, terrminal deoxynucleotidyl transferase–mediated dUTP nick end labeling (TUNEL) assay, and electron microscopy. All of these techniques can detect specific changes in DNA indicative of the fragmentation that occurs in apoptosis. In one study, flow cytometry on cell suspensions showed that approximately 22% of OA chondrocytes and 5% of normal chondrocytes were undergoing apoptosis. Staining of cartilage sections demonstrated the presence of apoptotic cells in the superficial and middle zones. Cartilage areas that contained apoptotic cells showed proteoglycan depletion, and the number of apoptotic cells were significantly correlated with the OA grade.[312] A second study found significant agreement with 51% of cells of OA chondrocytes and 11% of normal cells were apoptotic,[336] primarily in the superficial and middle zones. Other studies have explored various mechanisms of apoptosis including involvement of NO and the Fas ligand, but these results are controversial. Because apoptotic cells are not removed effectively from cartilage, the products of cell death such as pyrophosphate and precipitated calcium may contribute to the pathologic cartilage degradation.

Apoptosis and Osteoarthritis

Programmed cell death (apoptosis) is a mechanism by which cells are intentionally removed from tissue and is most evident during embryonic tissue remodeling.

Osteophyte Formation

One of the most remarkable and consistent features of joints affected with osteoarthritis, whether naturally occurring or experimentally induced, is the development of prominent osteochondral nodules known as osteophytes, osteochondrophytes, and chondro-osteophytes. Indeed, the presence of chondro-osteophytes in a joint, more than any other pathological feature, distinguishes osteoarthritis from other arthritides.[337] It seems likely that both mechanical and humoral factors are involve in stimulating the formation of osteophytes, though the exact functional significance of osteophyte growth remains unclear. There is, however, direct evidence that osteophytes help stabilize osteoarthritic joints.[338] Notwithstanding uncertainties of how and why they form, osteophytes are an example of

new cartilage and bone development in osteoarthritic joints, which are ultimately characterized by articular cartilage degeneration. Close examination of the biosynthetic activity of developing chondro-osteophyte in the Pond-Nuki dog model of osteoarthritis revealed that the cells arise from tissue associated with the chondro-synovial junction, indicating that there is a population of pluripotential cells in the periosteum that is responsive to the mechanical and humoral sequelae of joint injury.[339] The formation of chondro-osteophytes in OA joints is a unique example of adult neochondrogenesis that bears some similarities to growth plate elongation and fracture callus formation. Studies using *in situ* hybridization histochemistry to define the molecular phenotype of cells in active chondro-osteophytes have been performed in a dog model of early OA.[340] Chondro-osteophytes are composed of fibrocytes and osteoblasts that express type I procollagen mRNA, mesenchymal prechondrocytes that express type IIA procollagen mRNA, and maturing chondrocytes that express type IIB procollagen mRNA. Based on the spatial pattern of gene expression and cytomorphology, the neochondrogenesis associated with chondro-osteophyte formation closely resembles that of the healing fracture callus and recapitulates events of endochondral bone formation (Fig. 4–19). The fact that BMP-2 is a morphogenetic factor stimulated by pro-inflammatory cytokines, strongly suggests that this factor could stimulate differentiation in multipotent cells into osteophyte in the joint tissues.[308,309]

SUMMARY

Osteoarthritis is characterized by active cells that divide and synthesize many types of molecules from NO to cytokines to extracellular matrix to enzymes. Clearly, the tissue repairs for some unknown time, then the process is tipped toward degeneration. While a great deal of information has been accumulated recently, over the next 10 years rapid progress in understanding the molecular defects in osteoarthritis will be made. It is expected that drugs will be available to inhibit cartilage degeneration and that repair will be stimulated in situ. Alternatively, our new knowledge can be applied to the tissue engineering of cartilage for use in repair, resurfacing, and replacement.

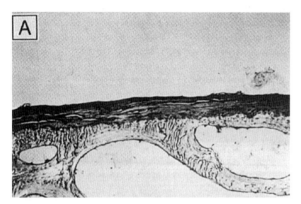
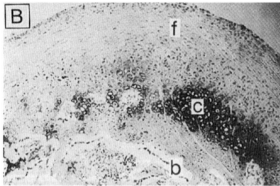
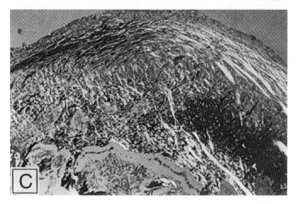

Figure 4–19 Microscopic anatomy of chondro-osteophytes, low-magnification photomicrographs. *A,* Control site. (Brightfield, original magnification X1.) *B,* Chondro-osteophyte showing superficial fibrous layer (*f*), chondroid area (*C*), and bone (*b*). (Brightfield, original magnification ×5.) *C,* Polarized light illumination of B to highlight collagen bundles. (Hematoxylin and eosin stain.) (From Matyas JR, Adams ME, Huang D, et al. Discoordinate gene expression of aggrecan and type II collagen in experimental osteoarthritis. Arthritis Rheum 38:410–425, 1995.)

REFERENCES

1. Poole AR, Kojima T, Yasuda T, et al. Composition and structure of articular cartilage: a template for tissue repair. Clin Orthop Relat Res. 391 (Suppl):S26–33, 2001.
2. Mow V, Rosenwasser MP. Articular cartilage biomechanics. In: Buckwalter JA, ed. Injury and Repair of Musculoskeletal Soft Tissues. Park Ridge, IL, AAOS, 1987, pp 427–463.
3. Aydelotte MB, Schumacher BL, Kuettner KE. Heterogeneity of articular chondrocytes in articular cartilage. In: Hascall VC, ed. Osteoarthritis. New York, Raven Press, 1992.
4. Archer CW, Francis-West P. The chondrocyte. Int J Biochem Cell Biol. 35(4):401–404, 2003.
5. Hall BK, Miyake T. All for one and one for all: condensations and the initiation of skeletal development. Bioessays. 22(2): 138–147, 2000.

6. Ruiz-Romero C, Lopez-Armada MJ, Blanco FJ. Proteomic characterization of human normal articular chondrocytes: a novel tool for the study of osteoarthritis and other rheumatic diseases. Proteomics. 5(12):3048–3059, 2005.

7. Kiani C, Chen L, Wu YJ, et al. Structure and function of aggrecan. Cell Res. 12(1):19–32, 2002.

8. Bonnet F, Perin JP, Lorenzo F, et al. An unexpected sequence homology between link proteins of the proteoglycan complex and immunoglobulin-like proteins. Biochim Biophys Acta. 873:152–155, 1986.

9. Perin J-P, Bonnet F, Thurieau C, et al. Link protein interactions with hyaluronate and proteoglycans. Characterization of two distinct domains in bovine cartilage link proteins. J Biol Chem. 262:13269–13272, 1987.

10. Perkins SJ, Miller A. Physical properties of the hyaluronate binding region of proteoglycan from pid laryngeal cartilage. J Mol Biol. 150:69–95, 1981.

11. Morgelin M, Paulsson M, Hardingham TE, et al. Cartilage proteoglycans. Assembly with hyaluronate and link protein as studied by electron microscopy. Biochem J. 253:175–185, 1988.

12. Heinegard D, Axelsson I. Distribution of keratan sulfate in cartilage proteoglycans. J Biol Chem. 252(6):1971–1979, 1977.

13. Barry FP, Neame PJ, Sasse J, et al. Length variation in the keratan sulfate domain of mammalian aggrecan. Matrix Biol. 14(4):323–328, 1994.

14. Upholt WB, Chandrasekaran L, Tanzer ML. Molecular cloning and analysis of the protein modules of aggrecans. Experientia. 49:384–392, 1993.

15. Doege KJ, Coulter SM, Meek L, et al. A human-specific polymorphism in the coding region of the aggrecan gene. Variable number of tandem repeats produce a range of core protein sizes in the general population. J Biol Chem. 272:13974–13979, 1997.

16. Roughley P, Martens D, Rantakokko J, et al. The involvement of aggrecan polymorphism in degeneration of human intervertebral disc and articular cartilage. Eur Cell Mater. 11:1–7, 2006.

17. Fulop C, Walcz E, Valyon M, et al. Expression of alternatively spliced epidermal growth factor-like domains in aggrecans of different species. Evidence for a novel module. J Biol Chem. 268:17377–17383, 1993.

18. Halberg DF, Proulx G, Doege K, et al. A segment of the cartilage proteoglycan has lectin-like activity. J Biol Chem. 263:9486–9490, 1988.

19. Miura R, Aspberg A, Ethell IM, et al. The proteoglycan lectin domain binds sulfated cell surface glycolipids and promotes cell adhesion. J Biol Chem. 274(16):11431–11438, 1999.

20. Aspberg A, Adam S, Kostka G, et al. Fibulin-1 is a ligand for the C-type lectin domains of aggrecan and versican. J Biol Chem. 274(29):20444–20449, 1999.

21. Olin AI, Morgelin M, Sasaki T, et al. The proteoglycans aggrecan and Versican form networks with fibulin-2 through their lectin domain binding. J Biol Chem. 12: 276(2):1253–1261, 2001.

22. Watanabe H, Kimata K, Line S, et al. Mouse cartilage matrix deficiency (cmd) caused by a 7 bp deletion in the aggrecan gene. Nat Genet. 7(2):154–157, 1994.

23. Kimata K, Barrach HJ, Brown KS, et al. Absence of proteoglycan core protein in cartilage from the cmd/cmd (cartilage matrix deficiency) mouse. J Biol Chem. 256(13):6961–6968, 1981.

24. Hering TM, Kollar J, Huynh TD, et al. Bovine chondrocyte link protein cDNA sequence: interspecies conservation of primary structure and mRNA untranslated regions. Comp Biochem Physiol Part B, Biochem Mol Biol. 112(2):197–203, 1995.

25. Spicer AP, Joo A, Bowling RA, Jr. A hyaluronan binding link protein gene family whose members are physically linked adjacent to chondroitin sulfate proteoglycan core protein genes: the missing links. J Biol Chem. 278(23):21083–21091, 2003.

26. Watanabe H, Yamada Y. Mice lacking link protein develop dwarfism and craniofacial abnormalities [see comments]. Nat Genet. 21(2):225–229, 1999.

27. Laurent TC, Laurent UB, Fraser JR. The structure and function of hyaluronan: An overview. Immunol Cell Biol. 74(2):A1–7, 1996.

28. Hascall VC, Majors AK, De La Motte CA, et al. Intracellular hyaluronan: a new frontier for inflammation? Biochim Biophys Acta. 1673(1-2):3–12, 2004.

29. Balazs EA. Viscoelastic properties of hyaluronic acid and biological lubrication. Univ Mich Med Cent J.:255–259, 1968.

30. Turley EA, Noble PW, Bourguignon LY. Signaling properties of hyaluronan receptors. J Biol Chem. 277(7):4589–4592, 2002.

31. Toole BP, Wight TN, Tammi MI. Hyaluronan-cell interactions in cancer and vascular disease. J Biol Chem. 277(7):4593–4596, 2002.

32. Poole AR, Pidoux I, Reiner A, et al. The association of a newly discovered protein, called chondrocalcin, with cartilage calcification. Acta Biol Hung. 35:143–149, 1984.

33. Zhu Y, Oganesian A, Keene DR, et al. Type IIA procollagen containing the cysteine-rich amino propeptide is deposited in the extracellular matrix of prechondrogenic tissue and binds to TGF-beta1 and BMP-2. J Cell Biol. 144(5):1069–1080, 1999.

34. Duance V, Wotton S. Changes in the distribution of mammalian cartilage collagens with age. Biochem Soc Trans. 19: 376S, 1991.

35. Eyre D. Collagen structure and function in articular cartilage: Metabolic changes in the development of osteoarthritis. In: Kuettner K, Goldberg V, eds. Osteoarthritis Disorders. Rosemont, IL: AAOS 1995, pp 219–228.

36. Nakata K, Ono K, Miyazaki J-I, et al. Osteoarthritis associated with mild chondrodysplasia in transgenic mice expressing a1(IX) collagen chains with a central deletion. Proc Natl Acad Sci USA. 90:2870–2874, 1993.

37. Olsen B. New insights into the function of collagens from genetic analysis. Curr Opin Biol. 7:720–727, 1995.

38. Fassler R, Schnegelsberg P, Dausman J, et al. Mice lacking alpha 1 (IX) collagen develop noninflammatory degenerative joint disease. Proc Natl Acad Sci USA. 91:5070–5074, 1994.

39. Alizadeh BZ, Njajou OT, Bijkerk C, et al. Evidence for a role of the genomic region of the gene encoding for the alpha1 chain of type IX collagen (COL9A1) in hip osteoarthritis: A population-based study. Arthritis Rheum. 52(5):1437–1442, 2005.

40. Burgeson RE, Hollister DW. Collagen heterogeneity in human cartilage: identification of several new collagen chains. Biochem Biophys Res Commun. 87:1124–1131, 1979.

41. Burgeson R, Hebda P, Morris N, et al. Human cartilage collagens. Comparison of cartilage collagens with human type V collagen. J Biol Chem. 257:7852–7856, 1982.

42. Neame P, Young C, Treep J. Isolation and primary structure of PARP, a 24-kDa proline- and arginine-rich protein from bovine cartilage closely related to the NH2-terminal domain in collagen alpha 1 (XI). J Biol Chem. 265:20401–20408, 1990.

43. Wu J-J, Eyre DR. Structural anaylsis of cross-linking domains in cartilage type XI collagen: Insights on polymeric assembly. J Biol Chem. 270:18865–18870, 1995.

44. Sandell LJ, Morris N, Robbins JR, et al. Alternatively spliced type II procollagen mRNAs define distinct populations of cells during vertebral development: differential expression of the amino-propeptide. J Cell Biol. 114:1307–1319, 1991.

45. Vikkula M, Mariman E, Lui V, et al. Autosomal dominant and recessive osteochondrodhysplasias associated with the COL11A2 locus. Cell. 80:431–437, 1995.

46. Young R, Lawrence P, Duance V, et al. Immunolocalization of type III collagen in human articular cartilage prepared by high-pressure cryofixation, freeze-substitution, and low- temperature embedding. J Histochem Cytochem. 43(4):421–427, 1995.

47. Goldring MB, Sandell LJ, Stephenson ML, et al. Immune interferon suppresses levels of procollagen mRNA and type II collagen synthesis in cultured human articular and costal chondrocytes. J Biol Chem. 261:9049–9056, 1986.

48. Niyibizi C, Eyre DR. Structural analysis of the extension peptides on matrix forms of type V collagen in fetal calf bone and skin. Biochim Biophys Acta. 1203:304–309, 1993.

49. Kielty C, Whittaker S, Grant ME, et al. Type VI collagen microfibrils: evidence for a structural association with hyaluronan. J Cell Biol. 118:979–990, 1992.

50. Marcelino J, McDevitt C. Attachment of articular cartilage chondrocytes to the tissue form of type VI collagen. Biochim Biophys Acta. 1249:180–188, 1995.

51. Morrison E, Ferguson M, Bayliss M, et al. The development of articular cartilage: I. The spatial and temporal patterns of collagen types. J Anat. 189:9–22, 1996.

52. McDevitt CA, Pahl JA, Ayad S, et al. Experimental osteoarthritic articular cartilage is enriched in guanidine-soluble type VI collagen. Biochem Biophys Res Commun. 157:250–255, 1988.

53. Schmid TM, Conrad HE. A unique low molecular weight collagen secreted by cultured chick embryro chondrocytes. J Biol Chem. 257:12444–12450, 1982.

54. Apte SS, Seldin MF, Hayashi M, et al. Cloning of the human and mouse type X collagen genes and mapping of the mouse type X collagen gene to chromosome 10. Eur J Biochem. 206:217–224, 1992.

55. Ekanayake S, Hall BK. Hypertrophy is not a prerequisite for type X collagen expression or mineralization of chondrocytes derived from cultured chick mandibular ectomesenchyme. Int J Dev Biol. 38:683–694, 1994.

56. Niyibizi C, Visconti C, Gibson GJ, et al. Identification and immunolocalization of type X collagen at the ligament-bone interface. Biochem Biophys Res Commun. 222:584–589, 1996.

57. Kirsch T, von der Mark K. Ca2+ binding properties of type X collagen. FEBS Lett. 294:149–152, 1991.

58. Habuchi H, Kimata K, Suzuki S. Changes in proteoglycan composition during development of rat skin. The occurence in fetal skin of a chondroitin sulfate proteoglycan with high turnover rate. J Biol Chem. 261:1031–1040, 1986.

59. Wu L, Genge B, Lloyd G, et al. Collagen-binding proteins in collagenase-released matrix vesicles from cartilage. Interaction between matrix vesicle proteins and different types of collagen. J Biol Chem. 266:1195–1203, 1991.

60. Lu Valle P, Iwamoto M, Fanning P, et al. Multiple negative elements in a gene that codes for an extracellular matrix protein, collagen X, restrict expression to hypertrophic chondrocytes. J Cell Biol. 121:1173–1179, 1993.

61. Lunstrum GP, Morris NP, McDonough AM, et al. Identification and partial characterization of two type XII-like collagen molecules. J Cell Biol. 113:963–969, 1991.

62. Adams JC, Lawler J. The thrombospondins. Int J Biochem Cell Biol. 36:961–968, 2004.

63. Oldberg A, Antonsson P, Lindblom K, et al. COMP (cartilage oligomeric matrix protein) is structurally related to the thrombospondins. J Biol Chem. 267(31):22346–22350, 1992.

64. Hankenson KD, Hormuzdi SG, Meganck JA, et al. Mice with a disruption of the thrombospondin 3 gene differ in geometric and biomechanical properties of bone and have accelerated development of the femoral head. Mol Cell Biol. 25(13): 5599–5606, 2005.

65. Kvansakul M, Adams JC, Hohenester E. Structure of a thrombospondin C-terminal fragment reveals a novel calcium core in the type 3 repeats. EMBO. 23:1223–1233, 2004.

66. Malashkevich VN, Kammerer RA, Efimov VP, et al. The crystal structure of a five-stranded coiled coil in COMP: A prototype ion channel? Science. 274(5288):761–765, 1996.

67. Lorenzo P, Bayliss M, Heinegard D. Altered patterns and synthesis of extracellular matrix macromolecules in early osteoarthritis. Matrix Biol. 23(6):381–391, 2004.

68. Rosenberg K, Olsson H, Morgelin M, et al. Cartilage oligomeric matrix protein shows high affinity zinc-dependent interaction with triple helical collagen. J Biol Chem. 273(32):20397–20403, 1998.

69. Di Cesare PE, Chen FS, Moergelin M, et al. Matrix-matrix interaction of cartilage oligomeric matrix protein and fibronectin. Matrix Biol. 21(5):461–470, 2002.

70. Chen FH, Thomas AO, Hecht JT, et al. Cartilage oligomeric matrix protein/thrombospondin 5 supports chondrocyte attachment through interaction with integrins. J Biol Chem. 280(38):32655–32661, 2005.

71. Hecht JT, Hayes E, Haynes R, et al. COMP mutations, chondrocyte function and cartilage matrix. Matrix Biol. 23(8): 525–533, 2005.

72. Hecht JT, Makitie O, Hayes E, et al. Chondrocyte cell death and intracellular distribution of COMP and type IX collagen in the pseudoachondroplasia growth plate. J Orthop Res. 22(4): 759–767, 2004.

73. Svensson L, Aszodi A, Heinegard D, et al. Cartilage oligomeric matrix protein-deficient mice have normal skeletal development. Mol Cell Biol. 22(12):4366–4371, 2002.

74. Sodersten F, Ekman S, Schmitz M, et al. Thrombospondin-4 and cartilage oligomeric matrix protein form heterooligomers in equine tendon. Connect Tissue Res. 47(2):85–91, 2006.

75. Deak F, Wagener R, Kiss I, et al. The matrilins: a novel family of oligomeric extracellular matrix proteins. Matrix Biol. 18(1):55–64, 1999.

76. Segat D, Frie C, Nitsche PD, et al. Expression of matrilin-1, -2 and -3 in developing mouse limbs and heart. Matrix Biol. 19(7): 649–655, 2000.

77. Wu J-J, Eyre DR. Matrilin-3 forms disulfide-linked oligomers with matrilin-1 in bovine epiphyseal cartilage. J Biol Chem. 273(28):17433–17438, 1998.

78. Tondravi MM, Winterbottom N, Haudenschild DR, et al. Cartilage matrix protein binds to collagen and plays a role in collagen fibrillogenesis. Prog Clin Biol Res. 383B:515–522, 1993.

79. Paulsson M, Piecha D, Segat D, et al. The matrilins: a growing family of A-domain-containing proteins. Biochem Soc Trans. 27(6):824–826, 1999.

80. Wiberg C, Klatt AR, Wagener R, et al. Complexes of matrilin-1 and biglycan or decorin connect collagen VI microfibrils to both collagen II and aggrecan. J Biol Chem. 278(39): 37698–37704, 2003.

81. Hauser N, Paulsson M, Heinegard D, et al. Interaction of cartilage matrix protein with aggrecan. Increased covalent cross-linking with tissue maturation. J Biol Chem. 271(50):32247–32252, 1996.

82. Chen C, Xu N, Shyu A. mRNA decay mediated by two distinct AU-rich elements from c-fos and granulocyte-macrophage colony-stimulating factor transcripts: different deadenylation kinetics and uncoupling from translation. Mol Cell Biol. 15(10):5777–5788, 1995.

83. Ko Y, Kobbe B, Nicolae C, et al. Matrilin-3 is dispensable for mouse skeletal growth and development. Mol Cell Biol. 24(4): 1691–1699, 2004.

84. Mates L, Nicolae C, Morgelin M, et al. Mice lacking the extracellular matrix adaptor protein matrilin-2 develop without obvious abnormalities. Matrix Biol. 23(3):195–204, 2004.

85. Aszodi A, Bateman JF, Hirsch E, et al. Normal skeletal development of mice lacking matrilin 1: redundant function of matrilins in cartilage? Mol Cell Biol. 19(11):7841–7845, 1999.

86. Cotterill SL, Jackson GC, Leighton MP, et al. Multiple epiphyseal dysplasia mutations in MATN3 cause misfolding of the A-domain and prevent secretion of mutant matrilin-3. Hum Mutat. 26(6):557–565, 2005.

87. Paulsson M, Inerot S, Heinegard D. Variation in quantity and extractability of the 148-kilodalton cartilage protein with age. Biochem J. 221(3):623–630, 1984.

88. Hansson A-S, Heinegard D, Holmdahl R. A new animal model for relapsing polychondritis, induced by cartilage matrix protein (matrilin-1). J Clin Invest. 104(5):589–598, 1999.

89. Lorenzo P, Bayliss MT, Heinegard D. A novel cartilage protein (CILP) present in the mid-zone of human articular cartilage increases with age. J Biol Chem. 273(36):23463–23468, 1998.

90. Lorenzo P, Neame P, Sommarin Y, et al. Cloning and deduced amino acid sequence of a novel cartilage protein (CILP) identifies a proform including a nucleotide pyrophosphohydrolase. J Biol Chem. 273(36):23469–23475, 1998.

91. Johnson K, Farley D, Hu SI, et al. One of two chondrocyte-expressed isoforms of cartilage intermediate-layer protein functions as an insulin-like growth factor 1 antagonist. Arthritis Rheum. 48(5):1302–1314, 2003.

92. Yao Z, Nakamura H, Masuko-Hongo K, et al. Characterisation of cartilage intermediate layer protein (CILP)-induced arthropathy in mice. Ann Rheum Dis. 63(3):252–258, 2004.

93. Krusius T, Ruoslahti E. Primary structure of an extracellular matrix proteoglycan core protein deduced from cloned cDNA. Proc Natl Acad Sci USA. 83:7683–7687, 1986.

94. Fisher LW, Termine JD, Young MF. Deduced protein sequence of bone small proteoglycan I (biglycan) shows homology with proteoglycan II (decorin) and several nonconnective tissue proteins in a variety of species. J Biol Chem. 264:4571–4576, 1989.

95. Lorenzo P, Aspberg A, Onnerfjord P, et al. Identification and characterization of asporin. A novel member of the leucine-rich repeat protein family closely related to decorin and biglycan. J Biol Chem. 276(15):12201–12211, 2001.

96. Scott PG, McEwan PA, Dodd CM, et al. Crystal structure of the dimeric protein core of decorin, the archetypal small leucine-rich repeat proteoglycan. Proc Natl Acad Sci. 101(44):15633–15638, 2004.

97. Scott PG, Dodd CM, Bergmann EM, et al. Crystal structure of the biglycan dimer and evidence that dimerization is essential for folding and stability of Class I small leucine-rich repeat proteoglycans. J Biol Chem. 281(19): 13324–13332, 2006.

98. Svensson L, Narlid I, Oldberg A. Fibromodulin and lumican bind to the same region on collagen type I fibrils. FEBS Lett. 470(2): 178–182, 2000.

99. Bengtsson E, Morgelin M, Sasaki T, et al. The leucine-rich repeat protein PRELP binds perlecan and collagens and may function as a basement membrane anchor. J Biol Chem. 277(17): 15061–15068, 2002.

100. Mansson B, Wenglen C, Morgelin M, et al. Association of chondroadherin with collagen type II. J Biol Chem. 276(35): 32883–32888, 2001.

101. Hildebrand A, Romaris M, Rasmussen LM, et al. Interaction of the small interstitial proteoglycans biglycan, decorin and fibromodulin with transforming growth factor beta. Biochem J. 302 (Pt 2): 527–534, 1994.

102. Schonherr E, Broszat M, Brandan E, et al. Decorin core protein fragment Leu155-Val260 interacts with TGF-beta but does not compete for decorin binding to type I collagen. Arch Biochem Biophys. 355(2):241–248, 1998.

103. Wiberg C, Hedbom E, Khairullina A, et al. Biglycan and decorin bind close to the N-terminal region of the collagen VI triple helix. J Biol Chem. 276(22):18947–18952, 2001.

104. Fisher LW, Termine JD, Young MF. Deduced protein sequence of bone small proteoglycan I (Biglycan) shows homology with proteoglycan II (Decorin) and several nonconnective tissue proteins in a variety of species. J Biol Chem. 264:4571–4576, 1989.

105. Antonsson P, Heinegard D, Oldberg A. The keratan sulfate-enriched region of bovine cartilage proteoglycan consists of a consecutively repeated hexapeptide motif. J Biol Chem. 264:16170–16173, 1989.

106. Blochberger TC, Vergnes J-P, Hempel J, et al. cDNA to chick lumican (corneal keratan sulfate proteoglycan) reveals homology to the small interstitial proteoglycan gene family and expression in muscle and intestine. J Biol Chem. 267:347–352, 1992.

107. Corpuz LM, Funderburgh JL, Funderburgh ML, et al. Molecular cloning and tissue distribution of keratocan. Bovine corneal keratan sulfate proteoglycan 37A. J Biol Chem. 271(16):9759–9763, 1996.

108. Bengtsson E, Neame PJ, Heinegard D, et al. The primary structure of a basic leucine-rich repeat protein, PRELP, found in connective tissues. J Biol Chem. 270(43):25639–25644, 1995.

109. Sommarin Y, Wendel M, Shen Z, et al. Osteoadherin, a cell-binding keratan sulfate proteoglycan in bone, belongs to the family of leucine-rich repeat proteins of the extracellular matrix. J Biol Chem. 273(27):16723–16729, 1998.

110. Deere M, Johnson J, Garza S, et al. Characterization of human DSPG3, a small dermatan sulfate proteoglycan. Genomics. 38(3): 399–404, 1996.

111. Johnson HJ, Rosenberg L, Choi HU, et al. Characterization of epiphycan, a small proteoglycan with a leucine-rich repeat core protein. J Biol Chem. 272(30):18709–18717, 1997.

112. Bentz H, Nathan RM, Rosen DM, et al. Purification and characterization of a unique osteoinductive factor from bovine bone. J Biol Chem. 264(34):20805–20810, 1989.

113. Neame PJ, Sommarin Y, Boynton RE, et al. The structure of a 38-kDa leucine-rich protein (chondroadherin) isolated from bovine cartilage. J Biol Chem. 269(34):21547–21554, 1994.

114. Oldberg et al. FEBS Lett. 386,29–32, 1996.

115. Roughley et al. Biochem J. Presence of pro-forms of decorin and biglycan in human articular cartilage. 318:779–784, 1996.

115a. Danielson KG, Baribault H, Holmes DF, et al. Targeted disruption of decorin leads to abnormal collagen fibril morphology and skin fragility. J Cell Biol. 136(3):729–743, 1997.

116a. De Luca A, Santra M, Baldi A, et al. Decorin-induced growth suppression is associated with up-regulation of p21, an inhibitor of cyclin-dependent kinases. J Biol Chem. 271(31):18961–18965, 1996.

116b. Roughley et al. Biochem J. 295:421–426, 1993.

117. Young MF, Bi Y, Ameye L, et al. Biglycan knockout mice: new models for musculoskeletal diseases. Glycoconj J. 19(4-5):257–262, 2002.

118. Kizawa H, Kou I, Iida A, et al. An aspartic acid repeat polymorphism in asporin inhibits chondrogenesis and increases susceptibility to osteoarthritis. Nat Genet. 37(2):138–144, 2005.

119. Rodriguez-Lopez J, Pombo-Suarez M, Liz M, et al. Lack of association of a variable number of aspartic acid residues in the asporin gene with osteoarthritis susceptibility: case-control studies in Spanish Caucasians. Arthritis Res Ther. 8(3):R55, 2006.

120. Mustafa Z, Dowling B, Chapman K, et al. Investigating the aspartic acid (D) repeat of asporin as a risk factor for osteoarthritis in a U.K. Caucasian population. Arthritis Rheum. 52(11):3502–3506, 2005.

121. Onnerfjord P, Heathfield TF, Heinegard D. Identification of tyrosine sulfation in extracellular leucine-rich repeat proteins using mass spectrometry. J Biol Chem. 279(1):26–33, 2004.

122. Hedlund H, Mengarelli-Widhol S, Heinegard D. Fibromodulin distribution and association with collagen. Matrix Biol. 14(3): 227–232, 1994.

123. Heathfield TF, Onnerfjord P, Dahlberg L, et al. Cleavage of fibromodulin in cartilage explants involves removal of the N-terminal tyrosine sulfate-rich region by proteolysis at a site that is sensitive to matrix metalloproteinase-13. J Biol Chem. 279(8):6286–6295, 2004.

124. Oldberg A, Antonsson P, Lindblom K, et al. A collagen-binding 59-kd protein (fibromodulin) is stucturally related to the small interstitial proteoglycans PG-S1 and PG-S2 (decorin). Embo J. 8:2601–2604, 1989.

125. Plaas AH, Neame PJ, Niven CM, et al. Identification of the keratan sulfate attachment sites on bovine fibromodulin. J Biol Chem. 265:20634–20646, 1990.

126. Wendel M, Sommarin Y, Heinegard D. Bone matrix proteins: isolation and characterization of a novel cell-binding keratan sulfate proteoglycan (osteoadherin) from bovine bone. J Cell Biol. 141(3):839–847, 1998.

127. Funderburgh JL, Funderburgh ML, Brown SJ, et al. Sequence and structural implications of a bovine corneal keratan sulfate proteoglycan core protein. Protein 37B represents bovine lumican and proteins 37A and 25 are unique. J Biol Chem. 268(16): 11874–11880, 1993.

128. Svensson L, Aszodi A, Reinholt FP, et al. fibromodulin-null mice have abnormal collagen fibrils, tissue organization, and altered lumican deposition in tendon. J Biol Chem. 274(14):9636–9647, 1999.

129. Ezura Y, Chakravarti S, Oldberg A, et al. Differential expression of lumican and fibromodulin regulate collagen fibrillogenesis in developing mouse tendons. J Cell Biol. 151(4):779–788, 2000.

130. Jepsen KJ, Wu F, Peragallo JH, et al. A syndrome of joint laxity and impaired tendon integrity in lumican- and fibromodulin-deficient mice. J Biol Chem. 277(38):35532–35540, 2002.

131. Bengtsson E, Aspberg A, Heinegard D, et al. The amino-terminal part of PRELP binds to heparin and heparan sulfate. J Biol Chem. 275(52):40695–40702, 2000.

132. Heinegard D, Larsson T, Sommarin Y, et al. Two novel matrix proteins isolated from articular cartilage show wide distributions among connective tissues. J Biol Chem,. 261:13866–13872, 1986.

133. Costell M, Gustafsson E, Aszodi A, et al. Perlecan maintains the integrity of cartilage and some basement membranes. J Cell Biol. 147(5):1109–1122, 1999.

134. Larsson T, Sommarin Y, Paulsson M, et al. Cartilage matrix proteins. A basic 36 kDa protein with a restricted distribution to cartilage and bone. J Biol Chem. 266:20428–20433, 1991.

135. Camper L, Heinegard D, Lundgren-Akerlund E. Integrin alpha 2beta 1 is a receptor for the cartilage matrix protein chondroadherin. J Cell Biol. 138(5):1159–1167, 1997.

136. Shen Z, Gantcheva S, Mansson B, et al. Chondroadherin expression changes in skeletal development. Biochem J. 330 (Pt 1): 549–557, 1998.

137. Tasheva ES, Ke A, Conrad GW. Analysis of the expression of chondroadherin in mouse ocular and non-ocular tissues. Mol Vis. 10:544–554, 2004.

138. Tasheva ES, Koester A, Paulsen AQ, et al. Mimecan/osteoglycin-deficient mice have collagen fibril abnormalities. Mol Vis. 8:407–415, 2002.
139. Reardon A, Sandell L, Jones CJ, et al. Localization of pN-type IIA procollagen on adult bovine vitreous collagen fibrils. Matrix Biol. 19(2):169–173, 2000.
140. Pellegrini B, Acland GM, Ray J. Cloning and characterization of opticin cDNA: evaluation as a candidate for canine oculo-skeletal dysplasia. Gene. 282(1-2):121–131, 2002.
141. Hindson VJ, Gallagher JT, Halfter W, et al. Opticin binds to heparan and chondroitin sulfate proteoglycans. Invest Ophthalmol Vis Sci. 46(12):4417–4423, 2005.
142. Tasheva ES, Funderburgh ML, McReynolds J, et al. The Bovine Mimecan Gene. Molecular cloning and characterization of two major RNA transcripts generated by alternative use of two splice acceptor sites in the third exon. J Biol Chem. 274(26):18693–18701, 1999.
143. Chiquet-Ehrismann R, Tucker RP. Connective tissues: signalling by tenascins. Int J Biochem Cell Biol. 36(6):1085–1089, 2004.
144. Mackie EJ, Ramsey S. Expression of tenascin in joint-associated tissues during development and postnatal growth. J Anat. 188 (Pt 1):157–165, 1996.
145. Salter DM. Tenascin is increased in cartilage and synovium from arthritic knees. Rheumatology. 32(9):780–786, 1993.
146. Aspberg A, Miura R, Bourdoulous S, et al. The C-type lectin domains of lecticans, a family of aggregating chondroitin sulfate proteoglycans, bind tenascin-R by protein- protein interactions independent of carbohydrate moiety. Prorc Natl Acad Sci. 94(19):10116–10121, 1997.
147. Lundell A, Olin AI, Morgelin M, et al. Structural basis for interactions between tenascins and lectican C-type lectin domains: evidence for a crosslinking role for tenascins. Structure. 12(8):1495–1506, 2004.
148. Chiquet-Ehrismann R, Chiquet M. Tenascins: regulation and putative functions during pathological stress. J Pathol. 200(4):488–499, 2003.
149. Chu ML, Tsuda T. Fibulins in development and heritable disease. Birth Defects Res C Embryo Today. 72(1):25–36, 2004.
150. Gallagher WM, Currid CA, Whelan LC. Fibulins and cancer: friend or foe? Trends Mol Med. 11(7):336–340, 2005.
151. Sasaki T, Gohring W, Pan TC, et al. Binding of mouse and human fibulin-2 to extracellular matrix ligands. J Mol Biol. 254(5):892–899, 1995.
152. Robinson PN, Arteaga-Solis E, Baldock C, et al. The molecular genetics of Marfan syndrome and related disorders. J Med Genet. 2006.
153. Kielty CM, Sherratt MJ, Marson A, et al. Fibrillin microfibrils. Adv Protein Chem. 70:405–436, 2005.
154. Kielty CM, Baldock C, Lee D, et al. Fibrillin: from microfibril assembly to biomechanical function. Philos Trans R Soc Lond B Biol Sci. 357(1418):207–217, 2002.
155. Penner AS, Rock MJ, Kielty CM, et al. Microfibril-associated glycoprotein-2 interacts with fibrillin-1 and fibrillin-2 suggesting a role for MAGP-2 in elastic fiber assembly. J Biol Chem. 277(38):35044–35049, 2002.
156. Cain SA, Morgan A, Sherratt MJ, et al. Proteomic analysis of fibrillin-rich microfibrils. Proteomics. 6(1):111–122, 2006.
157. Tiedemann K, Batge B, Muller PK, et al. Interactions of fibrillin-1 with heparin/heparan sulfate, implications for microfibrillar assembly. J Biol Chem. 276(38):36035–36042, 2001.
158. Keene DR, Jordan CD, Reinhardt DP, et al. Fibrillin-1 in human cartilage: developmental expression and formation of special banded fibers. J Histochem Cytochem. 45(8):1069–1082, 1997.
159. Sinha S, Heagerty AM, Shuttleworth CA, et al. Expression of latent TGF-beta binding proteins and association with TGF-beta 1 and fibrillin-1 following arterial injury. Cardiovasc Res. 53(4):971–983, 2002.
160. Dietz HC, Loeys B, Carta L, et al. Recent progress towards a molecular understanding of Marfan syndrome. Am J Med Genet C Semin Med Genet. 139(1):4–9, 2005.
161. Burton-Wurster N, Borden C, Lust G, et al. Expression of the (V + C)- fibronectin isoform is tightly linked to the presence of a cartilaginous matrix. Matrix Biol. 17(3):193–203, 1998.
162. Pankov R, Yamada KM. Fibronectin at a glance. J Cell Sci. 115(20):3861–3863, 2002.
163. Magnusson MK, Mosher DF. Fibronectin: Structure, assembly, and cardiovascular implications. Arterioscler Thromb Vasc Biol. 18(9):1363–1370, 1998.
164. Komoriya A, Green LJ, Mervic M, et al. The minimal essential sequence for a major cell type-specific adhesion site (CS1) within the alternatively spliced type III connecting segment domain of fibronectin is leucine-aspartic acid-valine. J Biol Chem. 266(23):15075–15079, 1991.
165. Couchman JR, Chen L, Woods A. Syndecans and cell adhesion. Int Rev Cytol. 207:113–150, 2001.
166. Woods A, Longley RL, Tumova S, et al. Syndecan-4 binding to the high affinity heparin-binding domain of fibronectin drives focal adhesion formation in fibroblasts. Arch Biochem Biophys. 374(1):66–72, 2000.
167. Tomasini-Johansso BR, Annis DS, Mosher DF. The N-terminal 70-kDa fragment of fibronectin binds to cell surface fibronectin assembly sites in the absence of intact fibronectin. Matrix Biol. 25(5):282–293, 2006.
168. Mao Y, Schwarzbauer JE. Fibronectin fibrillogenesis, a cell-mediated matrix assembly process. Matrix Biol. 24(6):389–399, 2005.
169. Wennerberg K, Lohikangas L, Gullberg D, et al. Beta 1 integrin-dependent and -independent polymerization of fibronectin. J Cell Biol. 132(1):227–238, 1996.
170. Velling T, Risteli J, Wennerberg K, et al. Polymerization of type I and III collagens is dependent on fibronectin and enhanced by integrins alpha 11beta 1 and alpha 2beta 1. J Biol Chem. 277(40):37377–37381, 2002.
171. Lust G, Burton-Wurster N, Leipold H. Fibronectin as a marker for osteoarthritis. J Rheumatol. 14 (Spec No):28–29, 1987.
172. Hakala BE, White C, Recklies AD. Human cartilage gp-39, a major secretory product of articular chondrocytes and synovial cells, is a mammalian member of a Chitinase protein family. J Biol Chem. 268(34):25803–25810, 1993.
173. Steck E, Breit S, Breusch SJ, et al. Enhanced expression of the human Chitinase 3-like 2 gene (YKL-39) but not Chitinase 3-like 1 gene (YKL-40) in osteoarthritic cartilage. Biochem Biophys Res Commun. 299(1):109–115, 2002.
174. Volck B, Price PA, Johansen JS, et al. YKL-40, a mammalian member of the Chitinase family, is a matrix protein of specific granules in human neutrophils. Proc Assoc Am Physicians. 110(4):351–360, 1998.
175. Knorr T, Obermayr F, Bartnik E, et al. YKL-39 (Chitinase 3-like protein 2), but not YKL-40 (Chitinase 3-like protein 1), is up regulated in osteoarthritic chondrocytes. Ann Rheum Dis. 2003 62(10):995–998.
176. Johansen JS, Kirwan JR, Price PA, et al. Serum YKL-40 concentrations in patients with early rheumatoid arthritis: relation to joint destruction. Scand J Rheumatol. 30(5):297–304, 2001.
177. Nordenbaek C, Johansen JS, Junker P, et al. YKL-40, a matrix protein of specific granules in neutrophils, is elevated in serum of patients with community-acquired pneumonia requiring hospitalization. J Infect Dis. 180(5):1722–1726, 1999.
178. Recklies AD, Ling H, White C, et al. Inflammatory cytokines induce production of CHI3L1 by articular chondrocytes. J Biol Chem. 280(50):41213–41221, 2005.
179. Houston DR, Recklies AD, Krupa JC, et al. Structure and ligand-induced conformational change of the 39-kDa glycoprotein from human articular chondrocytes. J Biol Chem. 278(32):30206–30212, 2003.
180. Price PA, Fraser JD, Metz-Virca G. Molecular cloning of matrix Gla protein: implications for substrate recognition by the vitamin K-dependent gamma -carboxylase. Proc Natl Acad Sci. 84(23):8335–8339, 1987.
181. Yagami K, Suh J-Y, Enomoto-Iwamoto M, et al. Matrix GLA protein is a developmental regulator of chondrocyte mineralization and, when constitutively expressed, blocks endochondral and iIntramembranous ossification in the limb. J Cell Biol. 147(5):1097–1108, 1999.
182. Luo G, Ducy P, McKee MD, et al. Spontaneous calcification of arteries and cartilage in mice lacking matrix GLA protein. Nature. 386(6620):78–81, 1997.

183. Hur DJ, Raymond GV, Kahler SG, et al. A novel MGP mutation in a consanguineous family: review of the clinical and molecular characteristics of Keutel syndrome. Am J Med Genet A 135(1): 36–40, 2005.

184. Maeda N, Fukazawa N, Hata T. The binding of chondroitin sulfate to pleiotrophin/heparin-binding growth-associated molecule is regulated by chain length and oversulfated structures. J Biol Chem. 281(8):4894–4902, 2006.

185. Neame PJ, Barry FP. The link proteins. Experientia. 49:393–402, 1993.

186. Hiraki Y, Tanaka H, Inoue H, et al. Molecular cloning of a new class of cartilage-specific matrix, chondromodulin-I, which stimulates growth of cultured chondrocytes. Biochem Biophys Res Commun. 175(3):971–977, 1991.

187. Shukunami C, Oshima Y, Hiraki Y. Chondromodulin-I and tenomodulin: a new class of tissue-specific angiogenesis inhibitors found in hypovascular connective tissues. Biochem Biophys Res Commun. 333(2):299–307, 2005.

188. Azizan A, Gaw JU, Govindraj P, et al. Chondromodulin I and pleiotrophin gene expression in bovine cartilage and epiphysis. Matrix Biol. 19(6):521–531, 2000.

189. Hayami T, Funaki H, Yaoeda K, et al. Expression of the cartilage derived anti-angiogenic factor chondromodulin-I decreases in the early stage of experimental osteoarthritis. J Rheumatol. 30(10):2207–2217, 2003.

190. Docheva D, Hunziker EB, Fassler R, et al. Tenomodulin is necessary for tenocyte proliferation and tendon maturation. Mol Cell Biol. 25(2):699–705, 2005.

191. Van der Rest M, Rosenberg LC, Olsen BR, et al. Chondrocalcin is identical with the C-propeptide of type II procollagen. Biochem J. 237(3):923–925, 1986.

192. Zhidkova NI, Brewton RG, Mayne R. Molecular cloning of PARP (proline/arginine-rich protein) from human cartilage and subsequent demonstration that PARP is a fragment of the NH2-terminal domain of the collagen alpha 2(XI) chain. FEBS Lett. 326(1-3): 25–28, 1993.

193. Barnett CH, Davies DV, MacConnaill MS. Synovial Joints: Their Structure and Mechanics. Springfield, IL, Charles C Thomas, 1961.

194. Strangeways TSP. Observations in the nutrition of articular cartilage. Br Med J. 1:661–663, 1920.

195. Brower TD, Akahoshi Y, Orlic P. The diffusion of dyes through articular cartialge in vivo. J Bone Joint Surg Am. 44-A(3):456–463, 1962.

196. Swann DA, Mintz G. The isolation and properties of a second glycoprotein (LGP-II) from the articular lubricating fraction from bovine synovial fluid. Biochem J. 1179(3):465–471,1979.

197. Maroudas A. Physiochemical properties of articular cartilage. In: Freeman MAR, ed. Adult Articular Cartilage. New York, Grune & Stratton, 1973, pp 131–170.

198. Mobasheri A, Vannucci SJ, Bondy CA, et al. Glucose transport and metabolism in chondrocytes: a key to understanding chondrogenesis, skeletal development and cartilage degradation in osteoarthritis. Histol Histopathol. 17(4):1239–1267, 2002.

199. Clegg DO, Reda DJ, Harris CL, et al. Glucosamine, chondroitin sulfate, and the two in combination for painful knee osteoarthritis. N Engl J Med. 23 354(8): 795–808, 2006.

200. Reginster JY, Deroisy R, Rovati LC, et al. Long-term effects of glucosamine sulphate on osteoarthritis progression: a randomised, placebo-controlled clinical trial. [see comments]. Lancet. 357(9252):251–256, 2001.

201. Pavelka K, Gatterova J, Olejarova M, et al. Glucosamine sulfate use and delay of progression of knee osteoarthritis: a 3-year, randomized, placebo-controlled, double-blind study. Arch Intern Med. 162(18):2113–2123, 2002.

202. Cibere J, Kopec JA, Thorne A, et al. Randomized, double-blind, placebo-controlled glucosamine discontinuation trial in knee osteoarthritis. Arthritis Rheum. 51(5):738–745, 2004.

203. McAlindon T, Formica M, LaValley M, et al. Effectiveness of glucosamine for symptoms of knee osteoarthritis: results from an internet-based randomized double-blind controlled trial. Am J Med. 117(9):643–649, 2004.

204. Mazieres B, Loyau G, Menkes CJ, et al. [Chondroitin sulfate in the treatment of gonarthrosis and coxarthrosis. 5-months result of a multicenter double-blind controlled prospective study using placebo]. Rev Rhum Mal Osteoartic. 59(7–8):466–472, 1992.

205. Conrozier T. [Anti-arthrosis treatments: efficacy and tolerance of chondroitin sulfates (CS 4&6)]. Presse Med. 27(36):1862–1865, 1998.

206. Towheed TE, Maxwell L, Anastassiades TP, et al. Glucosamine therapy for treating osteoarthritis. Cochrane Database Syst Rev. 2:CD002946, 2005.

207. Rizkalla G, Reiner A, Bogoch E., et al. Studies of the articular cartilage aggrecan in health and osteoarthritis. J Clin Invest. 90:2268–2277, 1992.

208. Cs-Szabo G, Roughley PJ, Plaas AH, et al. Large and small proteoglycans of osteoarthritic and rheumatoid articular cartilage. Arthritis Rheum. 38(5):660–668, 1995.

209. Cs-Szabo G, Melching LI, Roughley PJ, et al. Changes in messenger RNA and protein levels of proteoglycans and link protein in human osteoarthritic cartilage samples. Arthritis Rheum. 40(6):1037–1045, 1997.

210. Visco DM, Johnstone B, Hill MA, et al. Immunohistochemical analysis of 3-B-3 (-) and 7-D-4 epitope expression in canine osteoarthritis. Arthritis Rheum. 36:1718–1725, 1993.

211. Caterson B, Buckwalter J. Articular cartilage repair and remodeling. In: Maroudas A, Kuettner K, eds. Methods In Cartilage Research. San Diego, Academic Press, 1990, pp 313–318.

212. Brandt KD. Effects of nonsteroidal anti-inflammatory drugs on chondrocyte metabolism in vitro and in vivo. Am J Med. 83(Suppl):29–34, 1987.

213. Redini F, Mauviel A, Loyau G, et al. Modulation of extracellular matrix metabolism in rabbit articular chondrocytes and human rheumatoid synovial cells by the non-steroidal anti-inflammatory drug etodolac. II: Glycosaminoglycan synthesis. Agents Actions. 31(3-4):358–367, 1990.

214. Dekel S, Falconer J, Francis MJ. The effect of anti-inflammatory drugs on glycosaminoglycan sulphation in pig cartilage. Prostaglandins Med. 4(3):133–140, 1980.

215. Hugenberg ST, Brandt KD, Cole CA. Effect of sodium salicylate, aspirin, and ibuprofen on enzymes required by the chondrocyte for synthesis of chondroitin sulfate. J Rheumatol. 20(12): 2128–2133, 1993.

216. Dehm P, Prockop DJ. Biosynthesis of cartilage procollagen. Eur J Biochem. 35(1):159–166, 1973.

217. Olsen BR. Collagen biosynthesis. In: Hay ED, ed. Cell Biology of Extracellular Matrix. 2nd ed. New York, Plenum, 1991, pp 177–220.

218. Silbert JE, Sugumaran G. Biosynthesis of chondroitin/dermatan sulfate. IUBMB Life. 54(4):177–186, 2002.

219. Funderburgh JL. Keratan sulfate: structure, biosynthesis, and function. Glycobiology. 10(10):951–958, 2000.

220. Yan A, Lennarz WJ. Unraveling the mechanism of protein N-glycosylation. J Biol Chem. 280(5):3121–3124, 2005.

221. Van den Steen P, Rudd PM, Dwek RA, et al. Concepts and principles of O-linked glycosylation. Crit Rev Biochem Mol Biol. 33(3):151–208, 1998.

222. Prehm P. Hyaluronate is synthesized at plasma membranes. Biochem J. 220(2):597–600, 1984.

223. Prehm P. Synthesis of hyaluronate in differentiated teratocarcinoma cells. Mechanism of chain growth. Biochem J. 211(1):191–198, 1983.

224. Prehm P. Biosynthesis of hyaluronan: direction of chain elongation. Biochem J. 398(3):469–473, 2006.

225. Itano N, Kimata K. Mammalian hyaluronan synthases. IUBMB Life. 54(4):195–199, 2002.

226. McDonald JA, Camenisch TD. Hyaluronan: genetic insights into the complex biology of a simple polysaccharide. Glycoconj J. 19(4–5):331–339, 2002.

227. Roberts CR, Mort JS, Roughley PJ. Treatment of cartilage proteoglycan aggregate with hydrogen peroxide. Relationship between observed degradation products and those that occur naturally during aging. Biochem J. 247(2):349–357, 1987.

228. Soderstrom M, Salminen H, Glumoff V, et al. Cathepsin expression during skeletal development. Biochim Biophys Acta. 1446(1-2):35–46, 1999.

229. Mort JS, Magny MC, Lee ER. Cathepsin B: an alternative protease for the generation of an aggrecan 'metalloproteinase' cleavage neoepitope. Biochem J. 335(Pt 3):491–494, 1998.

230. Mehraban F, Tindal MH, Proffitt MM, et al. Temporal pattern of cysteine endopeptidase (cathepsin B) expression in cartilage and

synovium from rabbit knees with experimental osteoarthritis: gene expression in chondrocytes in response to interleukin-1 and matrix depletion. Ann Rheum Dis. 56(2):108–115, 1997.

231. Baici A, Horler D, Lang A, et al. Cathepsin B in osteoarthritis: zonal variation of enzyme activity in human femoral head cartilage. Ann Rheum Dis. 54(4):281–288, 1995.

232. Buttle DJ, Handley CJ, Ilic MZ, et al. Inhibition of cartilage proteoglycan release by a specific inactivator of cathepsin B and an inhibitor of matrix metalloproteinases. Evidence for two converging pathways of chondrocyte-mediated proteoglycan degradation. Arthritis Rheum. 36(12):1709–1717, 1993.

233. Nakase T, Kaneko M, Tomita T, et al. Immunohistochemical detection of cathepsin D, K, and L in the process of endochondral ossification in the human. Histochem Cell Biol. 114(1): 21–27, 2000.

234. Yasuda Y, Kaleta J, Bromme D. The role of cathepsins in osteoporosis and arthritis: rationale for the design of new therapeutics. Adv Drug Deliv Rev. 57(7):973–993, 2005.

235. Gafni J, Hermel E, Young JE, et al. Inhibition of calpain cleavage of huntingtin reduces toxicity: accumulation of calpain/caspase fragments in the nucleus. J Biol Chem. 279(19):20211–20220, 2004.

236. Fujimori Y, Shimizu K, Suzuki K, et al. Immunohistochemical demonstration of calcium-dependent cysteine proteinase (calpain) in collagen-induced arthritis in mice. Z Rheumatol. 53(2):72–75, 1994.

237. Szomor Z, Shimizu K, Fujimori Y, et al. Appearance of calpain correlates with arthritis and cartilage destruction in collagen induced arthritic knee joints of mice. Ann Rheum Dis. 54(6):477–483, 1995.

238. Szomor Z, Shimizu K, Yamamoto S, et al. Externalization of calpain (calcium-dependent neutral cysteine proteinase) in human arthritic cartilage. Clin Exp Rheumatol. 17(5):569–574, 1999.

239. Yasuda T, Shimizu K, Nakagawa Y, et al. m-Calpain in rat growth plate chondrocyte cultures: its involvement in the matrix mineralization process. Dev Biol. 170(1):159–168, 1995.

240. Yamamoto S, Shimizu K, Suzuki K, et al. Calcium-dependent cysteine proteinase (calpain) in human arthritic synovial joints. Arthritis Rheum. 35(11):1309–1317, 1992.

241. Oshita H, Sandy JD, Suzuki K, et al. Mature bovine articular cartilage contains abundant aggrecan that is C-terminally truncated at Ala719-Ala720, a site which is readily cleaved by m-calpain. Biochem J. 382(Pt 1):253–259, 2004.

242. Cuevas BD, Abell AN, Witowsky JA, et al. MEKK1 regulates calpain-dependent proteolysis of focal adhesion proteins for rear-end detachment of migrating fibroblasts. Embo J. 22(13):3346–3355, 2003.

243. Pontremoli S, Melloni E, Salamino F, et al. Activation of neutrophil calpain following its translocation to the plasma membrane induced by phorbol ester or fMet-Leu-Phe. Biochem Biophys Res Commun. 160(2):737–743, 1989.

244. Hood JL, Logan BB, Sinai AP, et al. Association of the calpain/calpastatin network with subcellular organelles. Biochem Biophys Res Commun. 310(4):1200–1212, 2003.

245. Sandy JD, Plaas AH. Studies on the hyaluronate binding properties of newly synthesized proteoglycans purified from articular chondrocyte cultures. Arch Biochem Biophys. 271(2):300–314, 1989.

246. Carney SL, Bayliss MT, Collier JM, et al. Electrophoresis of 35S-labeled proteoglycans on polyacrylamide-agarose composite gels and their visualization by fluorography. Anal Biochem. 156(1): 38–44, 1986.

247. Sapolsky AI, Altman RD, Woessner JF, et al. The action of cathepsin D in human articular cartilage on proteoglycans. J Clin Invest. 52(3):624–633, 1973.

248. Sapolsky AI, Howell DS, Woessner JF, Jr. Neutral proteases and cathepsin D in human articular cartilage. J Clin Invest. 53(4):1044–1053, 1974.

249. Bryson H, Bunning RA, Feltell R, et al. A serine proteinase inactivator inhibits chondrocyte-mediated cartilage proteoglycan breakdown occurring in response to proinflammatory cytokines. Arch Biochem Biophys. 355(1):15–25, 1998.

250. Hashimoto K, Nagao Y, Kato K, et al. Human urinary trypsin inhibitor inhibits the activation of pro-matrix metalloproteinases and proteoglycans release in rabbit articular cartilage. Life Sci. 63(3):205–213, 1998.

251. Steinmeyer J, Kalbhen DA. The inhibitory effects of antirheumatic drugs on the activity of human leukocyte elastase and cathepsin G. Inflamm Res. 45(7):324–329, 1996.

252. Chevalier X, Groult N, Texier JM, et al. Elastase activity in cartilage extracts and synovial fluids from subjects with osteoarthritis or rheumatoid arthritis: the prominent role of metalloproteinases. Clin Exp Rheumatol. 14(3):235–241, 1996.

253. Konttinen YT, Kaapa E, Hukkanen M, et al. Cathepsin G in degenerating and healthy discal tissue. Clin Exp Rheumatol. 17(2): 197–204, 1999.

254. Fosang AJ, Neame PJ, Hardingham TE, et al. Cleavage of cartilage proteoglycan between G1 and G2 domains by stromelysins. J Biol Chem. 266:15579–15582, 1991.

255. Fosang AJ, Neame PJ, Last K, et al. The interglobular domain of cartilage aggrecan is cleaved by PUMP, gelatinases and cathepsin B. J Biol Chem. 267:19470–19474, 1992.

256. Flannery CR, Lark MW, Sandy JD. Identification of a stromelysin cleavage site within the interglobular domain of human aggrecan. Evidence for proteolysis at this site in vivo in human articular cartilage. J Biol Chem. 267:1008–1014, 1992.

257. Fosang AJ, Last K, Knauper V, et al. Fibroblast and neutrophil collagenases cleave at two sites in the cartilage aggrecan interglobular domain. Biochem J. 295:273–276, 1993.

258. Fosang AJ, Last K, Knauper V, et al. Degradation of cartilage aggrecan by collagenase-3 (MMP-13). FEBS Lett. 380:17–20, 1996.

259. Lee ER, Lamplugh L, Leblond CP, et al. Immunolocalization of the cleavage of the aggrecan core protein at the Asn341-Phe342 bond, as an indicator of the location of the metalloproteinases active in the lysis of the rat growth plate. Anat Rec. 252(1): 117–132, 1998.

260. Vincenti MP, Brinckerhoff CE. Transcriptional regulation of collagenase (MMP-1, MMP-13) genes in arthritis: integration of complex signaling pathways for the recruitment of gene-specific transcription factors. Arthritis Res. 4(3):157–164, 2002.

261. Mitchell PG, Magna HA, Reeves LM, et al. Cloning, expression, and type II collagenolytic activity of matrix metalloproteinase-13 from human osteoarthritic cartilage. J Clin Invest. 97(3): 761–768, 1996.

262. Inada M, Wang Y, Byrne MH, et al. Critical roles for collagenase-3 (Mmp13) in development of growth plate cartilage and in endochondral ossification. Proc NatL Acad Sci USA. 101(49):17192–17197, 2004.

263. Ortega N, Behonick D, Stickens D, et al. How proteases regulate bone morphogenesis. Ann N Y Acad Sci. 995:109–116, 2003.

264. Pratta MA, Scherle PA, Yang G, et al. Induction of aggrecanase 1 (ADAM-TS4) by interleukin-1 occurs through activation of constitutively produced protein. Arthritis Rheum. 48(1):119–133, 2003.

265. Little CB, Hughes CE, Curtis CL, et al. Matrix metalloproteinases are involved in C-terminal and interglobular domain processing of cartilage aggrecan in late stage cartilage degradation. Matrix Biol. 21(3):271–288, 2002.

266. Apte SS, Mattei MG, Olsen BR. Cloning of the cDNA encoding human tissue inhibitor of metalloproteinases-3 (TIMP-3) and mapping of the TIMP3 gene to chromosome 22. Genomics. 19(1):86–90, 1994.

267. Carmichael DF, Sommer A, Thompson RC, et al. Primary structure and cDNA cloning of human fibroblast collagenase inhibitor. Proc Natl Acad Sci USA. 83(8):2407–2411, 1986.

268. Denhardt DT, Rajan S, Walther SE. Structure-function studies of mouse tissue inhibitor of metalloproteinases-1. Ann NY Acad Sci. 732:65–74, 1994.

269. Gasson JC, Golde DW, Kaufman SE, et al. Molecular characterization and expression of the gene encoding human erythroid-potentiating activity. Nature. 315(6022):768–771, 1985.

270. Greene J, Wang M, Liu YE, et al. Molecular cloning and characterization of human tissue inhibitor of metalloproteinase 4. J Biol Chem. 271(48):30375–30380, 1996.

271. Pavloff N, Staskus PW, Kishnani NS, et al. A new inhibitor of metalloproteinases from chicken: ChIMP-3. A third member of the TIMP family. J Biol Chem. 267(24):17321–17326, 1992.

272. Stetler-Stevenson WG, Krutzsch HC, Liotta LA. Tissue inhibitor of metalloproteinase (TIMP-2). A new member of the metalloproteinase inhibitor family. J Biol Chem. 264(29):17374–17378, 1989.

273. Wick M, Haronen R, Mumberg D, et al. Structure of the human TIMP-3 gene and its cell cycle-regulated promoter. Biochem J. 311(Pt 2):549–554, 1995.

274. Wilde CG, Hawkins PR, Coleman RT, et al. Cloning and characterization of human tissue inhibitor of metalloproteinases-3. DNA Cell Biol. 13(7):711–718, 1994.

275. Sato H, Kida Y, Mai M, et al. Expression of genes encoding type IV collagen-degrading metalloproteinases and tissue inhibitors of metalloproteinases in various human tumor cells. Oncogene. 7(1):77–83, 1992.

276. De Clerck YA, Darville MI, Eeckhout Y, et al. Characterization of the promoter of the gene encoding human tissue inhibitor of metalloproteinases-2 (TIMP-2). Gene. 139(2):185–191, 1994.

277. Logan SK, Garabedian MJ, Campbell CE, et al. Synergistic transcriptional activation of the tissue inhibitor of metalloproteinases-1 promoter via functional interaction of AP-1 and Ets-1 transcription factors. J Biol Chem. 271(2):774–782, 1996.

278. Uchijima M, Sato H, Fujii M, et al. Tax proteins of human T-cell leukemia virus type 1 and 2 induce expression of the gene encoding erythroid-potentiating activity (tissue inhibitor of metalloproteinases-1, TIMP-1). J Biol Chem. 269(21):14946–14950, 1994.

279. Lotz M, Guerne PA. Interleukin-6 induces the synthesis of tissue inhibitor of metalloproteinases-1/erythroid potentiating activity (TIMP-1/EPA). J Biol Chem. 266(4):2017–2020, 1991.

280. Nagase H, Kashiwagi M. Aggrecanases and cartilage matrix degradation. Arthritis Res Ther. 5(2):94–103, 2003.

281. Porter S, Clark IM, Kevorkian L, et al. The ADAMTS metalloproteinases. Biochem J. 15 386(Pt 1):15–27, 2005.

282. Arner EC, Pratta MA, Trzaskos JM, et al. Generation and characterization of aggrecanase. A soluble, cartilage-derived aggrecan-degrading activity. J Biol Chem. 274(10):6594–6601, 1999.

283. Apte SS. A disintegrin-like and metalloprotease (reprolysin type) with thrombospondin type 1 motifs: the ADAMTS family. Int J Biochem Cell Biol. 36(6):981–985, 2004.

284. Wang P, Tortorella M, England K, et al. Proprotein convertase furin interacts with and cleaves pro-ADAMTS4 (Aggrecanase-1) in the trans-Golgi network. J Biol Chem. 279(15):15434–15440, 2004.

285. Flannery CR, Zeng W, Corcoran C, et al. Autocatalytic cleavage of ADAMTS-4 (Aggrecanase-1) reveals multiple glycosaminoglycan-binding sites. J Biol Chem. 277(45):42775–42780, 2002.

286. Gao G, Plaas A, Thompson VP, et al. ADAMTS4 (aggrecanase-1) activation on the cell surface involves C-terminal cleavage by glycosylphosphatidyl inositol-anchored membrane type 4-matrix metalloproteinase and binding of the activated proteinase to chondroitin sulfate and heparan sulfate on syndecan-1. J Biol Chem. 279(11):10042–10051, 2004.

287. Tortorella M, Pratta M, Liu RQ, et al. The thrombospondin motif of aggrecanase-1 (ADAMTS-4) is critical for aggrecan substrate recognition and cleavage. J Biol Chem. 275(33):25791–25797, 2000.

288. Kashiwagi M, Enghild JJ, Gendron C, et al. Altered proteolytic activities of ADAMTS-4 expressed by C-terminal processing. J Biol Chem. 279(11):10109–10119, 2004.

289. Patwari P, Gao G, Lee JH, et al. Analysis of ADAMTS4 and MT4-MMP indicates that both are involved in aggrecanolysis in interleukin-1-treated bovine cartilage. Osteoarthritis Cartilage. 13(4):269–277, 2005.

290. Glasson SS, Askew R, Sheppard B, et al. Deletion of active ADAMTS5 prevents cartilage degradation in a murine model of osteoarthritis. Nature. 434(7033):644–648, 2005.

291. Stanton H, Rogerson FM, East CJ, et al. ADAMTS5 is the major aggrecanase in mouse cartilage in vivo and in vitro. Nature. 434(7033):648–652, 2005.

292. Yamanishi Y, Boyle DL, Clark M, et al. Expression and regulation of aggrecanase in arthritis: the role of TGF-beta. J Immunol. 168(3):1405–1412, 2002.

293. Koshy PJ, Lundy CJ, Rowan AD, et al. The modulation of matrix metalloproteinase and ADAM gene expression in human chondrocytes by interleukin-1 and oncostatin M: a time-course study using real-time quantitative reverse transcription-polymerase chain reaction. Arthritis Rheum. 46(4):961–967, 2002.

294. Sylvester J, Liacini A, Li WQ, et al. Interleukin-17 signal transduction pathways implicated in inducing matrix metalloproteinase-3, -13 and aggrecanase-1 genes in articular chondrocytes. Cell Signal. 16(4):469–476, 2004.

295. Makihira S, Yan W, Murakami H, et al. Thyroid hormone enhances aggrecanase-2/ADAM-TS5 expression and proteoglycan degradation in growth plate cartilage. Endocrinology. 144(6):2480–2488, 2003.

296. Kevorkian L, Young DA, Darrah C, et al. Expression profiling of metalloproteinases and their inhibitors in cartilage. Arthritis Rheum. 50(1):131–141, 2004.

297. Hashimoto T, Wen G, Lawton MT, et al. Abnormal expression of matrix metalloproteinases and tissue inhibitors of metalloproteinases in brain arteriovenous malformations. Stroke. 34(4):925–931, 2003.

298. Kashiwagi M, Tortorella M, Nagase H, et al. TIMP-3 is a potent inhibitor of aggrecanase 1 (ADAM-TS4) and aggrecanase 2 (ADAM-TS5). J Biol Chem. 276(16):12501–12504, 2001.

299. Rodriguez-Manzaneque JC, Westling J, Thai SN, et al. ADAMTS1 cleaves aggrecan at multiple sites and is differentially inhibited by metalloproteinase inhibitors. Biochem Biophys Res Commun. 293(1):501–508, 2002.

300. Gendron C, Kashiwagi M, Hughes C, et al. TIMP-3 inhibits aggrecanase-mediated glycosaminoglycan release from cartilage explants stimulated by catabolic factors. FEBS Lett. 555(3):431–436, 2003.

301. Vankemmelbeke MN, Jones GC, Fowles C, et al. Selective inhibition of ADAMTS-1, -4 and -5 by catechin gallate esters. Eur J Biochem. 270(11):2394–2403, 2003.

302. Little CB, Flannery CR, Hughes CE, et al. Aggrecanase versus matrix metalloproteinases in the catabolism of the interglobular domain of aggrecan in vitro. Biochem J. 344 Pt 1:61–68, 1999.

303. Sztrolovics R, White RJ, Roughley PJ, et al. The mechanism of aggrecan release from cartilage differs with tissue origin and the agent used to stimulate catabolism. Biochem J. 362(Pt 2): 465–472, 2002.

304. Lark MW, Bayne EK, Flanagan J, et al. Aggrecan degradation in human cartilage. Evidence for both matrix metalloproteinase and aggrecanase activity in normal, osteoarthritic, and rheumatoid joints. J Clin Invest. 100(1):93–106, 1997.

305. Sandy JD, Verscharen C. Analysis of aggrecan in human knee cartilage and synovial fluid indicates that aggrecanase (ADAMTS) activity is responsible for the catabolic turnover and loss of whole aggrecan whereas other protease activity is required for C-terminal processing in vivo. Biochem J. 358(Pt 3):615–626, 2001.

306. Mason RM, Chambers MG, Flannelly J, et al. The STR/ort mouse and its use as a model of osteoarthritis. Osteoarthritis Cartilage. 9(2):85–91, 2001.

307. Chambers MG, Cox L, Chong L, et al. Matrix metalloproteinases and aggrecanases cleave aggrecan in different zones of normal cartilage but colocalize in the development of osteoarthritic lesions in STR/ort mice. Arthritis Rheum. 44(6):1455–1465, 2001.

308. Fukui N, Zhu Y, Maloney WJ, et al. Stimulation of BMP-2 expression by pro-inflammatory cytokines IL-1 and TNF-alpha in normal and osteoarthritic chondrocytes. J Bone Joint Surg Am. 85-A(Suppl 3):59–66, 2003.

309. Fukui N, Ikeda Y, Ohnuki T, et al. Pro-inflammatory cytokine TNF-alpha induces BMP-2 in chondrocytes via mRNA stabilization and transcriptional up-regulation. J Biol Chem. 281: 27229–27241, 2006.

310. Clements K, Price J, Chambers M, et al. Gene deletion of either interleukin-1beta, interleukin-1beta-converting enzyme, inducible nitric oxide synthase, or stromelysin 1 accelerates the development of knee osteoarthritis in mice after surgical transection of the medial collateral ligament and partial medial meniscectomy. Arthritis Rheum. 48(12):3452–3463, 2003.

311. Amin A, Abramson S. The role of nitric oxide in articular cartilage breakdown in osteoarthritis. Curr Opin Rheumatol. 10(3): 263–268, 1998.

312. Hashimoto S, Ochs RL, Rosen F, et al. Chondrocyte-derived apoptotic bodies and calcification of articular cartilage. Proc Natl Acad Sci USA. 95(6):3094–3099, 1998.

313. Studer R, Jaffurs D, Stefanovic-Racic M, et al. Nitric oxide in osteoarthritis. Osteoarthritis Cartilage. 7(4):377–379, 1999.

314. Bayliss MT, Ali SY. Age-related changes in the composition and structure of human articular-cartilage proteoglycans. Biochem J. 176(3):683–693, 1978.

315. Roughley PJ, White RJ. Age-related changes in the structure of the proteoglycan subunits from human articular cartilage. J Biol Chem. 255(1):217–224, 1980.

316. Webber C, Glant T, Roughley P, et al. The identification and characterization of two populations of aggregating proteoglycans of high buoyant density isolated from post-natal human articular cartilages of different ages. Biochem J. 248(3): 735–740, 1987.

317. Roughley PJ, White RJ, Poole AR. Identification of a hyaluronic acid-binding protein that interferes with the preparation of high-buoyant-density proteoglycan aggregates from adult human articular cartilage. Biochem J. 231:129–138, 1985.

318. Franzen A, Inerot S, Hejderup, et al. Variations in the composition of bovine hip articular cartilage with distance from the articular surface. 195(3):535–543, 1981.

319. Lauder RM, Huckerby TN, Brown GM, et al. Age-related changes in the sulphation of the chondroitin sulfate linkage region from human articular cartilage aggrecan. Biochem J. 358(Pt 2): 523–528, 2001.

320. Buckwalter JA, Rosenberg LC. Electron microscopic studies of cartilage proteoglycans. Electron Microsc Rev. 1(1):87–112, 1988.

321. Brocklehurst R, Bayliss MT, Maroudas A, et al. The composition of normal and osteoarthritic articular cartilage from human knee joints. J Bone Joint Surg. 66(1):95–106, 1984.

322. Sweet MB, Thonar EJ, Immelman AR, et al. Biochemical changes in progressive osteoarthrosis. Ann Rheum Dis. 36(5):387–398, 1977.

323. Vasan N. Proteoglycans in normal and severely osteoarthritic human cartilage. Biochem J. 187(3):781–787, 1980.

324. Bayliss MT, Ali SY. Isolation of proteoglycans from human articular cartilage. Biochem J. 169(1):123–132, 1978.

325. Caterson B, Mahmoodian F, Sorrell JM, et al. Modulation of native chondroitin sulfate structures in tissue development and in disease. J Cell Sci. 97: 411–417, 1990.

326. Lippiello L, Kaye C, Neumata T, et al. In vitro metabolic response of articular cartilage segments to low levels of hydrostatic pressure. Connect Tissue Res. 13:99, 1985.

327. Floman Y, Eyre DR, Glimcher MJ. Induction of osteoarthrosis in the rabbit knee joint: Biochemical studies on the articular cartilage. Clin Orthop Relat Res. 147:278–286, 1980.

328. Matyas JR, Adams ME, Huang D, et al. Discoordinate gene expression of aggrecan and type II collagen in experimental osteoarthritis. Arthritis Rheum. 38:420–425, 1995.

329. Eyre D, McDevitt CA, Billingham MEJ, et al. Biosynthesis of collagen and other matrix proteins by articular cartilage in experimental osteoarthritis. Biochem J. 188:823–837, 1980.

330. Aigner T, Bertling W, Stoss H, et al. Independent expression of fibril-forming collagens I, II, and III in chondrocytes of human osteoarthritic cartilage. J Clin Invest. 91:829–837, 1993.

331. Aigner T, Zhu Y, Chansky HH, et al. Reexpression of type IIA procollagen by adult articular chondrocytes in osteoarthritic cartilage. Arthritis Rheuma. 42(7):1443–1450, 1999.

332. Nimni M, Deshmukh K. Differences in collagen metabolism between normal and osteoarthritic human articular cartilage. Science. 181:751–752, 1973.

333. Girkontaite I, Frischholz S, Lammi P, et al. Immunolocalization of type X collagen in normal fetal and adult osteoarthritic cartilage with monoclonal antibodies. Matrix Biol. 15(4):231–238, 1996.

334. Boos N, Nerlich A, Wiest I, et al. Immunohistochemical analysis of type X-collagen expression in osteoarthritis of the hip joint. J Orthop Res. 17:495–502, 1999.

335. Farnum CE, Wilsman NJ. Cellular turnover at the chondro-osseous junction of growth plate cartilage: Analysis by serial sections at the light microscopical level. J Orthop Res. 7:654–666, 1989.

336. Blanco FJ, Guitian R, Vazquez-Martul E, et al. Osteoarthritis chondrocytes die by apoptosis. A possible pathway for osteoarthritis pathology. Arthritis Rheumat. 41(2):284–289, 1998.

337. Altman R, Asch E, Bloch D, et al. Development of criteria for the classification and reporting of osteoarthritis. Arthritis Rheum. 29:1039–1049, 1986.

338. Pottenger LA, Phillips FM, Draganich L. The effect of marginal osteophytes on reduction of varus-valgus instability in osteoarthritic knees. Arthritis Rheum. 33:853–858, 1990.

339. Aigner T, Dietz U, Stob H, et al. Differential expression of collagen types I, II, III, and X in human osteophytes. Lab Invest. 73:236–243, 1995.

340. Matyas JR, Sandell LJ, Adams ME. Gene expression of type II collagens in chondro-osteophytes in experimental osteoarthritis. Osteoarthritis Cartilage. 5:99–105, 1997.

Experimental Models of Osteoarthritis

5

Margaret M. Smith   Christopher B. Little

Although the etiopathogenesis of osteoarthritis (OA) is still the subject of intense debate and research, its pathology is well established.[1] The pathologic process of the OA joint is characterized by extensive fibrillation of articular cartilage in those regions subjected to high contact stress accompanied by sclerosis of subchondral bone. At the joint margins, osteophytosis and bone remodeling generally occur, the synovial capsule becomes fibrotic, and the lining is usually inflamed.[2,3] As a consequence of the synovitis, the metabolism of type B lining cells, the synoviocytes, is disturbed, resulting in the biosynthesis of hyaluronan with a reduced molecular weight.[4] Because the rheologic properties of hyaluronan depend on its molecular size and its concentration,[5] a decrease in either leads to a decline of the viscoelastic and lubricating ability of synovial fluid, imposing additional mechanical stresses on articular cartilage and subchondral bone. There is also evidence that blood flow in the intraosseous vasculature of OA joints may be impaired owing to the presence of lipid emboli and fibrin thrombi.[6,7] The ischemia so arising may compromise osteocyte viability, leading to necrosis and bone remodeling.[6]

The complex pathobiologic changes of human OA normally take several decades to develop and may be influenced by a multitude of factors, such as genetic predisposition, hormonal status, occupation, and body mass index, among others. The need to clarify the molecular events that occur in the various joint tissues at the onset and during the progression of OA has necessitated the use of models, which, although imperfect, can exhibit many of the pathologic features that characterize the human disease. In vitro studies using cell and tissue culture models have proven invaluable in defining specific molecular and cellular events in degradation of joint tissues such as cartilage. However, to fully understand the complex inter-relationship between the different disease mechanisms, joint tissues, and body systems, studying OA in animal models is necessary. The realization by workers in the field that OA is not a normal physiologic

consequence of the aging process and that it might be amenable to therapeutic intervention provided a major stimulus to the development and use of animal models to test hypotheses concerning the pathogenesis of this disorder. This experimental approach represents one of the cornerstones for the discovery of new anti-OA drugs, and agents have emerged from such animal model studies that are now the subject of clinical evaluation. This chapter will concentrate on the in vivo animal models used to study OA.

Animal models of inflammatory arthropathies (rheumatoid arthritis [RA]), such as collagen-induced arthritis (CIA) in mice, have proven predictive of clinical efficacy, as therapies that are beneficial in CIA have moved into clinical use with proven benefit in RA treatment in humans (e.g., anti-TNF and anti-IL-1treatments).[8,9] To date, however, none of the available animal models of OA can truly be said to be similarly "predictive," as no anti-OA therapies have yet been proven in human trials. In this chapter, we review the literature on the most frequently used animal models of OA, particularly with regard to their use for determining the pathophysiology of the disease process. Many of these models have been used to evaluate various forms of treatment, but the vast amount of literature relating to this will not be exhaustively reviewed in this chapter. We have included reports on OA models that have appeared since the previous edition was published either if they describe a novel pathophysiological mechanism or method for evaluation of a previously published model, or they include an entirely new model. In the interests of brevity, many of the older citations have been deleted and readers are referred to previous editions for details.[10] We have confined our review to models of OA in weight-bearing appendicular joints and thus have not included the temporomandibular or spinal facet joints although the disease processes are likely to be similar. The models are divided by the method of induction rather than the animal used. It is important to keep in mind inherent physiological differences that may exist between species that could influence the comparison with human disease. For example, adult rodents (rats, mice) do not express MMP-1, a major collagenase implicated in human disease,[11,12] and their aggrecan core protein lacks the extended keratan sulfate binding region of other species including humans.[13]

INDUCTION OF OSTEOARTHRITIS BY INJECTION OF COMPOUNDS INTO JOINTS

A variety of agents, when they are injected intra-articularly into animal joints, elicit pathologic changes that show some resemblance to those seen in OA. Whereas two or three daily injections of physiologic saline into rabbit joints produced a decrease in the aggregation of cartilage proteoglycans,[14] five daily injections of 10% saline provoked synovial hyperplasia, cartilage hypertrophy, and osteophyte formation after 2 months.[15] Corticosteroids are known to have detrimental effects on the metabolism of human cartilage,[16] and when high doses of these agents are administered intra-articularly to mice[17] or rabbits,[18,19] experimental arthropathies generally result. In hydrocortisone-injected rabbit joints, cartilage was depleted of hyaluronan, which may lead to a reduction in the ability of proteoglycans to aggregate and subsequent diffusion out of the cartilage matrix.[20] Studies in horses have further demonstrated the potential detrimental effect of intra-articular corticosteroids on long-term cartilage metabolism and biomechanical properties.[21–23] This chondrodestructive effect of some corticosteroids in animal models has raised the question of their indiscriminate use in clinical practice; however, these studies using normal joints do not mimic the disease situation, where the benefit of modulating the inflammatory process may outweigh the detrimental effects. Co-administration of hyaluronan with corticosteroids was found to decrease proteoglycan degradation and loss from equine cartilage.[24]

Postmenopausal women receiving estrogen replacement therapy have a decreased OA incidence,[25] radiologic progression of their disease[26] particularly in large joints,[27] and decreased levels of cartilage and bone collagen breakdown biomarkers.[28] This is consistent with the observation that ovariectomy increased cartilage collagen breakdown and erosion in rats,[29,30] inflammatory arthritis severity in DBA/1 mice,[31] and surgically induced OA in sheep.[32] However, intra-articular administration of estrogen induced degenerative changes in cartilage that resembled human knee OA when it was given at 0.3 mg/kg/day in mice[33] and rabbits.[18,33] It was noted in subsequent studies[34] that estrogen receptors were upregulated in the femoral but not in the tibial cartilages of rabbit knees with estradiol-induced OA.

Models of OA directed toward selective degradation of the cartilage extracellular matrix have been developed by the use of intra-articular injections of proteolytic enzymes such as papain, trypsin, hyaluronidase, and collagenase in mice, rats, and rabbits (see review by Pritzker[35]). The mechanisms responsible for cartilage degradation in these models,

particularly those in which papain or trypsin was injected, may deviate significantly from those that normally occur in the human disease because these proteins elicit an acute inflammatory reaction that may also contribute to cartilage destruction. Intra-articular injection of collagenase has been acknowledged to provoke additional joint instability by degrading the surrounding capsule and ligaments as well as by directly cleaving the cartilage collagen.[36] Studies with $C57Bl_{10}$ mice injected intra-articularly with bacterial collagenase demonstrated correlations between the degree of instability of the joint, the amount of cartilage damage, and the size of the osteophytes formed.[37–39] Activation of the synovial macrophages also plays a pivotal role in osteophyte formation and fibrosis in this model.[40]

Intra-articular monosodium iodoacetate, an inhibitor of cellular glycolysis, has been used to induce OA-like cartilage changes in joints of hens, mice, guinea pigs, rats, rabbits, and horses.[10] Cartilage lesions appeared in all species with marked loss of safranin O staining, indicating depletion of proteoglycans that is associated with an increase in aggrecan proteolysis by aggrecanases (ADAMTS) and matrix metalloproteinases (MMPs).[41–43] This model was used to show that cartilage lesions in rat joints could be detected by scanning acoustic microscopy[44] and ultrasonography[45] and that the lesions could be ameliorated by MMP-inhibitors[46] or by exercise in guinea pigs.[42]

Models of cartilage degeneration have been induced by intra-articular injection of specific cytokines, such as interleukin-1 (IL-1)[47,48] and transforming growth factor-β,[39,49,50] in both rabbits[48,50] and mice.[39,47,49,51] Intra-articular IL-1 injection in mice following immunization with methylated bovine serum albumin induces a transient inflammatory arthropathy more characteristic of RA rather than OA.[52,53] Many other compounds, such as carrageenan and zymosan, when they are given by intra-articular injection, elicit degenerative changes in joint tissues; however, these substances also elicit an early acute synovitis and hence are relevant to inflammatory arthropathies more than to OA. In both rabbits[54] and horses,[55] intra-articular injection of autogenous cartilage particles led to cartilage degeneration over time. The interaction of these immunogenic particles with the synovial macrophages was considered to be responsible for the ensuing synovitis and subsequent joint disease. Oral quinolones induce cartilage lesions in young animals of a number of species, including rats,[56] guinea pigs,[57] dogs,[58] and rabbits.[59] The pathologic change in cartilage may be associated with chelation of magnesium[60,61] and the changes are reported to be similar to human OA except that osteophytes do not develop in this model.[59]

IMMOBILIZATION MODELS OF OSTEOARTHRITIS

That articular cartilage requires joint motion and loading to maintain its normal composition, structure, and function is now widely accepted.[62–64] Immobilization of a limb has been shown to induce atrophic changes within the articular cartilage of the joint, which include thinning,[63,64] increased hydration,[62,63,65,66] reduced proteoglycan content,[62–70] altered proteoglycan structure,[62,63,65,68] decreased proteoglycan synthesis,[62,64,66,67,71] and increased collagen content and synthesis.[65,68,72,73] Increased synthesis of prothrombin by chondrocytes may contribute to the cartilage remodeling and thinning observed in immobilized rat joints.[74] Because many of these cartilage changes are similar to those described for human OA joints, limb immobilization has been used as a model particularly for studying the process of cartilage degeneration and more recently evaluation of potential biomarkers[75] and anti-arthritic therapies such as chondroitin sulfate.[76] However, fundamental morphologic differences in cartilage have been noted that may diminish the usefulness of the immobilization models. In OA cartilage, chondrocytes proliferate into clones or nests, often remaining active into the late stages of the disease. In contrast, chondrocytes within cartilage of immobilized joints do not form clones but undergo necrosis, particularly if there is no residual movement within the splint.[77] This response of cartilage most likely results from impaired nutrition of the chondrocytes in the immobilized joint because of the absence of movement and loading.[78] If a limited range of motion is allowed in the immobilized limb, however, the extent of cartilage degeneration is markedly reduced.[66] Early work with immobilization models of OA in various species including rat, rabbit, and dog has been reviewed by Troyer[79] and in the previous edition of this chapter.[10]

MODELS OF SPONTANEOUS OSTEOARTHRITIS

Naturally occurring OA is known to manifest spontaneously in a number of animal species. Selected studies using mice, rats, guinea pigs, and macaques are summarized in Table 5–1. Some breeds of dogs, including Labradors, German shepherds, and beagles, also develop OA with age, but this is generally secondary to hip dysplasia.[107] In the spontaneously developing OA in dogs, a common pathologic feature of the early disease is a greater degree of synovitis and fibrosis of the joint capsule than is reported for human OA.[108,109] A spontaneous decrease in afferent joint nerves with aging in Fisher 344 rats, and worsening of age-related OA with joint denervation in this species, suggested that loss of neuromuscular control and subsequent aberrant loading may be associated with spontaneous OA.[110]

Many inbred strains of mice develop spontaneous OA with age, including STR/ORT, BALB/c, DBA/1, and C57BL/6 (see Table 5–1). The incidence of the disease varies with strain and sex but can be as high as 90% in aged mice. Characteristic features of OA progression in these models include joint space narrowing, osteophyte formation, focal cartilage lesions, and decreased staining for cartilage proteoglycan. Although aging is a high-risk factor for OA in these models, the morphologic changes arising from the aging process alone have not been satisfactorily addressed. As with age-related OA in rats, loss of joint innervation has been implicated in spontaneous OA in C57BL6Nia mice.[111] In some strains of mice such as DBA/1 and STR/ORT, OA is largely confined to the male gender and has been shown to depend on the presence of testosterone and aggressive behavior.[80] The development of refined immunohistochemical techniques, computer-

assisted digital image analysis, and advances in molecular biology investigation methodologies (in situ hybridization, genome wide microarray, etc.) has allowed the small amount of joint tissue from mice to be thoroughly investigated. Upregulation of chondrocyte expression of different matrix molecules, cytokines and MMPs, and proteolysis of collagen and aggrecan by MMPs and ADAMTS enzymes in a similar manner to human OA has been demonstrated in spontaneous OA in STR/ort mice.[82–84,112,113]

Research with spontaneous OA in guinea pigs has mostly been confined to the Hartley or Dunkin-Hartley strain (see Table 5–1), which has been widely used as an OA model in recent years. These animals have visible cartilage lesions by 3 months of age and a high incidence of bilateral knee OA by 12 months with subchondral bone sclerosis.[90] Magnetic resonance imaging (MRI) has been successfully used to study this species,[94] and there is enough joint tissue available for mRNA expression studies.[11] Disease progression has been slowed by diet restriction[91] and exercise modification[114] demonstrating the role of mechanical factors in the disease process. It has been suggested that altered subchondral bone remodeling[97] and abnormalities in the cruciate ligament[115] may precede and lead to cartilage erosion in this animal model. However, changes in chondrocyte metabolism with ATP depletion and increased NO production have also been found preceding and in association with OA onset.[116] This naturally occurring model has proven useful for evaluating potential therapies.[117,118]

Both rhesus (*Macaca mulatta*) and cynomolgus (*Macaca fascicularis*) macaques show a high incidence of spontaneous OA (see Table 5–1); its epidemiology and joint pathology resemble those of OA in humans.[100] OA changes have been noted separately from those due to aging[98] and, like the guinea pig (see above), both cartilage metabolic changes[105,119] and subchondral bone mineralization abnormalities[106] are implicated in the disease. In female macaques ovariectomy worsens the cartilage lesions and this can be inhibited by estrogen replacement therapy.[120] The joints are also of a sufficient size for radiologic, histologic, and biochemical studies, and the prevalence allows the use of age-matched non-OA controls.[99] However, because these animals are free ranging and have an extended life span (18 to 30 years), studies may require years for completion and may be influenced by uncontrollable environmental factors. Ethical and financial considerations make widespread use of this model unlikely.

OSTEOARTHRITIS IN GENETICALLY MODIFIED MICE

The mouse is a convenient species for genetic modification (GM), and a number of spontaneous and engineered mutants have been studied that have, among their phenotypic abnormalities, an increased incidence of spontaneous OA (recently reviewed by Helminen et al.[121]). A selection of GM mice that have an increased incidence of OA or OA-like joint disease is given in Table 5–2. Homozygous deficiency in the major structural components of cartilage such as collagen II and its associated

TABLE 5–1
SELECTED STUDIES OF SPONTANEOUS OA IN ANIMALS

Species	Age	Findings	Reference
DBA/1 mice	0–6 months old	OA development at 4 months old only in males	80
STR/ORT mice	5–50 weeks	OA in 85% of all male mice; MMP and aggrecanase activity increase and colocalize with advancing OA; MMP-2, -3, -7, -9, -13, and -14 gene expression upregulated in AC at all ages but only MMP-3 and -14 protein detected by immunolocalization; collagen cleavage evident only where AC surface fibrillation occurred; chondrocyte apoptosis by TUNEL correlated with severity of OA lesions	81–86
C57BL/6 mice	18 months old ± running	Increased incidence and severity of OA changes in mice run 1 km/day, therefore running accelerated OA development; collagen degradation absent in areas of chondrocyte death	87, 88
C57 mice	6 and 8–12 months old	Some heat shock proteins, interleukin-6, and interferon expression were upregulated; expression of other heat shock proteins and interleukin-1 was unchanged in AC	89
Hartley guinea pigs	2–30 months old	OA AC lesions visible by 3 months increasing to >50% of medial tibial AC bilaterally by 1 year old, with subchondral sclerosis; severity of OA lesions was reduced by 40% at 9 months, 56% at 18 months on restricted diet. At 12 months OA on unprotected medial tibial plateau, lateral not affected; increased volume of AC and subchondral bone. Despite gross OA changes only moderate and focal collagen ultrastructure network disruption; no fibre thickening. MRI showed AC thickness increased over first 6 months then decreased, T2 relaxation times increased with time so more predictable AC OA indicator. At onset of OA, AC PG and collagen decreased, AC small and large PG synthesis decreased, water increased and AC PG degradation was unchanged. Collagenase 1 and 3 mRNA expression varied with age and compartment; focal areas of collagenase 1 and 3 proteins in matrix in AC at OA lesions; initial bone density higher	11, 90–97
Rhesus macaque	5–25 years old	Young animals with OA had increased PG levels whereas old had decreased; collagen correlated with age in both normal and OA but lower in OA AC. OA changes progressive through life with high prevalence. OA frequency increased with age and parity (in females); epidemiology and histology resembled OA in man. Increased OA by histology correlated with increased collagen extractability	98–101
Cynomolgus macaque	5–30 years old	High prevalence of OA lesions, subchondral bone changes common and severe, showing before AC changes; subchondral bone thickness of medial tibia correlated with severity of OA lesions and increasing weight; prevalence and severity of OA lesions increased with age. All chondrocytes in OA lesions stained positive for α1, α3 and α5β1 integrins; in normal cells only α5β1. Increasing OA associated with reduced response to IGF-1 by chondrocytes. The mineralized plate beneath the AC thickened, overmineralized calcified AC and subchondral bone worse with age and OA	102–106

AC = articular cartilage; IGF = insulin growth factor; MMP = matrix metalloproteinase; PG = proteoglycan.

"minor" collagens IX and XI, or components of the proteoglycan aggregates (aggrecan and link protein), are usually lethal during embryogenesis or in the early postnatal period. However, it is noteworthy that while heterozygous deficiencies in the collagen network result in spontaneous OA-like changes in cartilage with aging, haplo-insufficiency of aggrecan or link protein does not cause joint cartilage abnormalities although intervertebral disc degeneration may be seen.[157–161] Conversely, GM mice may also have a reduced incidence of spontaneous OA, or show protection in models of induced arthritis, and these animals are invaluable for advancing our

TABLE 5–2
TRANSGENIC MODELS OF OA IN MICE

Genetic Modification	Resulting Phenotype	Reference
Spontaneous deletion in Col2a1 gene giving defect in the C-propeptide (Dmm)	Chondrodysplasia and early onset OA	122, 123
150-bp deletion mutation in the Col2a1 gene (Del1)	Develop OA in knee joints; cathepsin K upregulated at lesion sites; knee OA increased with exercise	124–127
A large internal deletion in the Col2a1 gene	Chondrodysplasia and increased incidence of OA in 15-month-old animals	128
Heterozygous deletion of Col2a1	Normal cartilage PG content and thickness, increased superficial zone fibrillation (73% v 21%) in 15-month-olds, reduced with running	127, 129
Arg519Cys mutation in Col2a1	Chondrodysplasia and generalized OA by 2 months of age	130, 131
Truncated Col9a1	Mild chondrodysplasia, with increased incidence of OA; loss of PG by 4–6 months and progressive fibrillation and erosion of AC by 12–18 months	132, 133
Deletion of Col9a1	AC fibrillation, chondrocyte proliferation, and osteophytosis by 9 months	134
1-bp deletion in Col11a1 resulting in effective deletion (Cho)	Heterozygous mice have loss of AC PG, increased type II collagen degradation and AC fibrillation with increased MMP-13 in knee by 3–6 months	135–137
Single or double knockout of biglycan and fibromodulin (fdn); double knockout of lumican and fdn	Tendon mineralization, gait abnormality, increased joint laxity, and increased OA evident by 6 months of age	138–142
ADAM-15 knockout	Increased loss of proteoglycan and AC erosion with synovial hyperplasia in knee joints at 12–14 months of age in male mice	143
MMP-14 knockout	Bone development and growth abnormalities with early onset of marked synovial hyperplasia and arthritis at 1–2 months of age	144
Interleukin-6 knockout	Increased knee OA in males but not females associated with decreased aggrecan synthesis and bone mineral density	145
Mig-6 knockout	Abnormal gait by 1 month, early onset osteophytes and AC degradation	146
Unknown spontaneous mutation (B6C3F1)	Ankylosing OA—tiptoe walking, swelling of ankle joints, and radiographic and histologic findings of OA AC changes by 9 months old in 80% of males	147
Unknown spontaneous mutation mapping to chromosome 10 (twy)	Autosomal recessive trait, tip-toe walking mouse with multiple osteochondral lesions and longitudinal ligament calcification; decreased AC PG staining and presence of degenerated collagen fibers by 4–8 weeks	148, 149
Defect in a copper transporting gene (Blotchy)	Affects elastin and collagen cross-linking resulting in spontaneous OA	150
Tissue specific BMP receptor type 1a deficiency	Under Gdf5 control no BMP receptor in developing joints—retention of webbing, failure of joint formation, and premature AC proteoglycan loss and erosion	151, 152
alpha-1 integrin knockout	Earlier onset of OA with increased PG loss, AC degradation and synovial hyperplasia from 4–10 months but not different from wildtype at 12–15 months	153
Postnatal overexpression of MMP-13	Aggrecan depletion, collagen proteolysis, fibrillation, and erosion of articular cartilage along with synovial hyperplasia after 5 months	154
Transgenic overexpression of bovine growth hormone	Chondrocyte and synovial hypertrophy with cartilage fibrillation at 6 months	155
Truncated kinase-deficient TGF-β type II receptor	Musculoskeletal developmental abnormalities and progressive chondrocyte hypertrophy with cartilage fibrillation by 6 months of age	156

AC = articular cartilage; BMP = bone morphogenic protein; mig-6 = mitogen inducible gene 6; PG = proteoglycan; TGF-β = transforming growth factor β.

understanding of the pathways involved in arthritis development and defining novel targets for disease therapy.[162-164] While GM mice with increased spontaneous OA are extremely useful for investigating the role of specific proteins or mutations in the pathophysiology of OA, their utility as more universal models for evaluating therapy of OA in general, as opposed to the disease induced by the specific genetic abnormality they carry, must be questioned.

SURGICALLY INDUCED DESTABILIZATION MODELS OF OSTEOARTHRITIS

Anterior Cruciate Ligament Transection

Traumatic rupture of the anterior cruciate ligament (ACL) is a relatively common event in dogs, particularly in the larger breeds. As is the case for human ACL rupture, canine joints may become osteoarthritic unless they are stabilized surgically. Pond and Nuki[165] and Gilbertson[166] described a method of reproducing this injury experimentally in normal dogs by transection of the ACL with a 2-mm stab (blind) incision through the capsule without damaging the adjacent periarticular ligaments or tendons. This closed surgical procedure was employed by McDevitt and Muir[167] to observe the biochemical changes that occurred in cartilage 3, 6, 9, and 48 weeks after surgery. Histologic studies confirmed the progression of cartilage damage with time, as assessed by loss of staining for proteoglycans, chondrocyte cloning, and increased surface fibrillation.[168] These experimentally induced biochemical and histologic changes in joints of mongrel dogs were analogous to those observed in the naturally occurring disorder resulting from spontaneous rupture of the ACL.

In the years after the initial reports of McDevitt and Muir,[167,168] a plethora of publications appeared using the canine Anterior Cruciate Ligament Transection (ACLT) model to generate data on cartilage metabolism, its composition and structure, the production of cytokines and inflammatory mediators by synovial tissues, and structural changes in subchondral bone (reviewed in Smith and Ghosh[10]). This model was also used to evaluate the effects of nonsteroidal anti-inflammatory drugs, corticosteroids, and potential disease-modifying OA drugs on cartilage and synovial tissue metabolism in OA (reviewed in Smith and Ghosh[10]). More recent studies using the ACLT model in dogs are summarized in Table 5–3, which also notes important criteria that can influence the rate of progression of OA with use of this surgical procedure. Of particular relevance are the weights of the animals used, their ages, and the post-ACLT duration and treatment. There are no reports of comparative studies on the outcomes of ACLT in different canine breeds. Because ACLT destabilizes the joint and increases the shearing (plowing) stresses on cartilage, joints of heavy breeds subjected to post-surgical exercise would be expected to incur more damage than joints of the smaller, lighter breeds, but again, this has not been confirmed experimentally. It is also clear from the biomechanical studies that weight bearing on the ACLT joint is diminished postoperatively, the contralateral and forelimbs carrying more of the body load than before surgery. This reduced mechanical loading of the ACLT joint retards the

progression of cartilage and bone injuries. However, dorsal root ganglionectomy of the destabilized limb can bypass the physiologic protection of the injured joint, and O'Connor and coworkers[206] have shown that rapid joint destruction occurs when dorsal root ganglionectomy is combined with ACLT.

Open Versus Closed Anterior Cruciate Ligament Transection

In the original procedure described by Gilbertson,[166] Pond and Nuki,[165] and McDevitt and Muir,[167,168] the ACL was transected by the blind insertion of a scalpel blade through the joint capsule. It was apparent, however, that synovial inflammation generally accompanied this technique.[207-209] Intra-articular bleeding, largely from the vessels serving the ACL itself, was thought to contribute to the synovitis. When electrocautery and irrigation were applied during ACLT in an open procedure, synovitis was reduced to 24% compared with 69% in open surgery in which precautions to prevent bleeding were not observed.[210] Moreover, cartilage hypertrophy, chondrocyte cloning, and fibrillation 10 weeks after surgery were less prominent in the surgically cauterized group than in the noncauterized group. It may be concluded from these and other studies cited in Table 5–3 that open ACLT, when care was taken to minimize intra-articular bleeding and inflammation, resulted in a model of hypertrophic OA that progressed only slowly, possibly because of lateral stabilization of the transected joint by osteophyte formation as well as reduced weight bearing on the limb. This early hypertrophic phase of cartilage response after open ACLT evolved into the classic joint disease of OA, including full-depth cartilage erosion, after 4 to 5 years.[211]

Anterior Cruciate Ligament Transection in Small Animals

ACLT has also been undertaken in cats, rats, guinea pigs, rabbits, and mice. These studies are summarized in Table 5–3. In small animals, frank cartilage lesions and synovitis develop much more rapidly than in larger animals. Whereas this offers potential advantages for experimental evaluation of antiarthritic preparations, the relevance of these rapidly progressive changes to the human disease may be diminished. Nevertheless, it is evident that OA resulting from ACLT in rats and rabbits involves changes in both the cartilage and subchondral bone, which in rabbits can be monitored using MRI.[194,195] ACLT induces biochemical changes in cartilage that mimic those observed in humans, including altered expression of collagens and MMPs, increased loss of aggrecan (although the proteinases responsible for this in rats and rabbits have not been defined), and cleavage of type II collagen by MMPs.[197,200,212]

Meniscectomy and Meniscal Injury/ Destabilization Models of Osteoarthritis

The medial and lateral menisci are crescent-shaped fibro-cartilaginous wedges interposed between the femoral condyles and tibial plateau of diarthrodial joints. These structures perform important mechanical functions because

TABLE 5–3

SELECTED STUDIES USING ANTERIOR CRUCIATE LIGAMENT TRANSECTION (ACLT)

Species	Post-ACLT Duration and Treatment	Age or Body Weight	Findings	Reference
Dog			**Open Unilateral**	
Mongrel dog	4, 10, and 32 weeks	17–27 kg	Aggrecan mRNA up at 10 and 32 weeks; collagen type II mRNA up at all time points–signals for transcription must be different	169
	3 and 12 weeks	17–27 kg	Decreased bone mineral density and structural changes in trabecular architecture of cancellous bone observed 3 weeks post-ACLT, worse at 12 weeks	170, 171
	3 and 12 weeks	17–27 kg	ACLT induced increased collagen type I and VI expression by menisci at 3 and 12 weeks; increases greater in medial than lateral	172
	3 and 12 weeks	29–32 kg	Aggrecan gene expression greater than collagen type II in control AC, reversed in OA AC at both timepoints	173
	10 and 39 weeks	16–28 kg	Micro MRI and polarised light microscopy can detect changes in AC collagen fiber orientation at 12 weeks	174
	3 and 12 weeks	16–34 kg	AC hypertropy worse at 12 weeks than 3 weeks; synovial fluid collagen type II markers, serum aggrecan and collagen II markers up at both timepoints	175
	36 and 72 weeks	Adult	Significant trabecular bone loss with architectural adaptation by 36 weeks, less obvious at 72 weeks	176
Fox-hound	2 years	2 years old	AC changes in expression of decorin and fibromodulin different in ACLT dogs to dogs with spontaneous OA	177
	2–24 months	2–3 years old	Some kinematic parameters were worse immediately after ACLT and did not improve with time, others worsened at 6–12 months post ACLT	178
	2–24 months ± running	2–3 years old	AC changes occurred early; decreased severity in longterm AC damage is associated with increased osteophyte formation and less severe medial meniscus damage	179
Dog			**Closed Unilateral**	
Dog	1–26 weeks	Not published	OA-like changes in AC included fibrillation, acellular zones in superficial layer synovial inflammation subsides within 1 week	165
	1–48 weeks	15–30 kg	Development of periarticular osteophytes at synovial margin commenced as early as 3 days and still progressed at 48 weeks	166
Mongrel dog	12 weeks	2–3 years old (20–25 kg)	Chondrocyte apoptosis, caspase 3 and Bcl-2 markedly increased in OA AC	180
	8 and 12 weeks	2–3 years old (22–27 kg)	Osteocalcin increased at 8 weeks; increased alkaline phosphatase and prostaglandin-E_2 at 12 weeks in subchondral and trabecular bone	181
	12 weeks	20–25 kg	Interleukin(IL)-1 converting enzyme and IL-18 levels increased in OA cartilage	182
	8 weeks	20–25 kg	Expression of MMP-13, cathepsin K, ADAMTS-4, ADAMTS-5, and 5-lipoxygenase increased in OA cartilage; decreased bone thickness with increased osteoclast staining of MMP-13 and cathepsin K	183, 184
Fox-hound	2, 10, and 18 weeks	19.0–28.5 kg	Synovial fluid prostaglandin E_2 correlated with clinical gait changes and may indicate lameness	185
Beagle	6, 12, 24, and 48 weeks	15–22 kg	Early stable elevation of collagen I and II expression by chondrocytes; MMP-13 not elevated until 24 weeks and aggrecan and tenascin C until 48 weeks	186
	6, 12, 24, and 48 weeks	15–22 kg	MRI revealed subchondral bone edema in posteromedial tibia after 6 weeks, followed by erosion of AC after 12 weeks	187

(continued)

TABLE 5-3

SELECTED STUDIES USING ANTERIOR CRUCIATE LIGAMENT TRANSECTION (ACLT) (continued)

Species	Post-ACLT Duration and Treatment	Age or Body Weight	Findings	Reference
Rabbit			**Open Unilateral**	
Rabbit	9 weeks	1 year old	Menisci from ACLT knees contained high numbers of apoptotic cells and nitrotyrosine immunoreactivity	188
	9 weeks	Adult	In transected knees, the compression modulus of the AC was reduced by 18%, while the permeability and electrokinetic coefficient were not detectably altered	189
	3 and 8 weeks	12 months old	ACLT caused matrix deterioration, cell cloning, clustering, and depletion in menisci; collagen type I and III were increased in medial and lateral; type II increased in medial	190
	2, 4, and 9 weeks	9–10 months old	MMP-1, -3, and -13 gene expression in AC and meniscus increased rapidly in OA, whereas expression of aggrecanases remained stable	191
	4, 9, and 12 weeks	12 months old	Osteophyte formation associated with expression of vascular endothelial growth factor (VEGF) in chondrocytes	192
	2, 4, and 8 weeks	4.5–5.8 kg	Micro-MRI reliably detects synovial effusion and osteophyte formation but not contour abnormalities of AC	193
	4, 8, and 12 weeks	2.5 years old (4.6 ± 0.4 kg)	3-D MRI and micro-computed tomography used to quantify AC damage, joint space, bone mineral density and calcified tissue changes	194, 195
	9 weeks	Adult	Chondrocyte apoptosis increases with ACLT	196
	11 weeks	3.7 ± 1.4 kg	Differing rates of regional AC proteoglycan loss detected	197
	3, 6, and 12 weeks	4 kg	Increased expression of hyaluronan receptor CD44v6 over time course of OA development	198
Other			**Open Unilateral**	
Rat	2–70 days	220–240 g	Early proteoglycan depletion and collagen disruption at margins of AC after 4 weeks central regions showed surface fibrillation	199
	2, 4, and 8 weeks	220–240 g	AC degeneration starts at the AC surface and is associated with localized expression of collagen type II degradation products	200
	2 and 4 weeks ± exercise	8 weeks old	Beneficial effect of slight and moderate but not intense exercise on AC lesions, heat shock protein 70 expression, and chondrocyte apoptosis	201
	2 and 10 weeks	20 weeks old	ACLT increased serum cartilage oligomeric matrix protein (COMP) levels, urinary C-telopeptide, and deoxypyridinoline	202
	1, 2, 4, 6, and 10 weeks	10 weeks old	Subchondral bone resorption by 2 weeks before AC thinning; osteophytes by 10 weeks	203
Guinea pig	1–8 months	40 days old	ACLT progressively increases OA histopathological changes; osteophytes first visible at 3 months	204
Cat	16 weeks and 5 years	2–22 years	Age related decrease in cancellous bone mass and subchondral plate thickness by 5 years exacerbated by ACLT	205

AC = articular cartilage; ADAMTS—A disintegrin and metalloproteinase with thrombospondin motifs.

they distribute up to 50% of the load applied to the joint; they increase its stability and congruence and enhance articular cartilage lubrication and nutrition by moving synovial fluid over the joint surfaces.[213–217] It is not unexpected, therefore, that mechanical failure or excision of these structures results in the imposition of abnormally high focal stresses on articular cartilage leading to premature degeneration and OA. This has been demonstrated both in long-term follow-up studies of patients after meniscectomy[218–220] and in experimental animals[10] (Table 5–4).

Small Animal Meniscectomy Models

Partial excision of the anterior portion of the medial meniscus was used by Moskowitz and coworkers[251] to induce degenerative changes in rabbit joints. A rapid (2 to 3 weeks)

TABLE 5–4
STUDIES IN MENISCECTOMY (MX) AND MENISCAL DESTABILIZATION (MD) MODELS OF OA

Species	Mx Method	Post-Mx Duration	Age or Body Weight	Findings	Reference
Rabbit	Unilateral partial medial Mx	2, 4, 8, and 10 weeks	8 weeks (2.0–2.5 kg)	Increase in AC thickness from 4 weeks; AC eburnation, erosion, and osteophytes from 6 weeks	221
		8 and 52 weeks	2.5–3.5 kg	Parathyroid hormone-related protein increased in late OA AC in proliferating chondrocyte clones	222
	Unilateral total medial Mx	2–52 weeks	Various	Mx caused decreased tibial bone mineral density as well as typical AC OA lesions. Swelling of AC (increase in height) detected by MRI was due to PG and cell loss in early OA. Micro-MRI reliably detects synovial effusion and osteophyte formation but not contour abnormalities of AC. Macroscopic and histologic AC degeneration at 2 weeks that correlated with collagen type II epitope in synovial fluid.	193, 223–225
Guinea pig	Unilateral partial medial Mx	1–42 weeks	0.6–0.8 kg	Moderate to severe AC focal lesions by week 1; the contralateral joint was affected by 12 weeks. AC lesions first on medial tibial plateau then medial femoral condyle then lateral compartment. MMP inhibitor prevented loss of AC thickness but not PG loss. PPAR-γ agonist reduced AC lesions and chondrocyte staining of MMP-13 and interleukin-1	226–229
Rat	Partial Mx	20 and 45 days	150 g	Disruption of Golgi complex in chondrocytes increases with time and OA	230
	Medial meniscal transection	Up to 32 days	Adult	Pain assessment over 28 days showed little hyperalgesia but increasing tactile allodynia	231
Mouse	Medial MD	4 and 8 weeks	10 weeks	No reduction of severity of AC destruction in ADAMTS-4 knockout mice compared to wild type but significant reduction of severity of AC destruction in ADAMTS-5 knockout mice	163, 232
Grey hounds	Bilateral total medial Mx	6 months ± exercise	Adult	AC degeneration in all Mx joints; lower glycosaminoglycan levels and more extractable PGs in AC from mobile contralateral Mx joints than in Mx or control joints. Femoral head AC from Mx group had decreased hyaluronan levels and increased PG extractability; no change in collagen or uronic acid levels compared to non-Mx	233, 234
Mongrel dogs	Unilateral total medial Mx	12 weeks	25–35 kg	AC tensile modulus decreased with no change in water or PG content. Reliable degenerative changes occurred Synovial fluid biomarkers altered with different acute and medium-term responses eg cartilage oligomeric matrix protein (COMP)	235, 236
Sheep	Unilateral total medial Mx	6 months ± exercise	2 years old	PG content down at 6 months in passive and active Mx group; low salt extract of PGs; PG aggregation and water remained high. Still early OA features (AC fibrillation, chondrocyte hypertrophy, matrix proliferation, marginal osteophytes) more marked in exercised group	237–239
	Unilateral total lateral Mx			Lateral Mx induced higher PG loss from AC and lower PG synthesis rates than medial Mx. Mx increased ostoid volume and surfaces with increased labelling of subchondral bone; AC has higher Mankin score after Mx. Mx animals reduced loading of operated limb. PG synthesis lower in lateral than in medial compartment. Keratan sulphate-peptide levels in synovial fluid	240–246

(continued)

TABLE 5–4

STUDIES IN MENISCECTOMY (MX) AND MENISCAL DESTABILIZATION (MD) MODELS OF OA (continued)

Species	Mx Method	Post-Mx Duration	Age or Body Weight	Findings	Reference
				increase progressively after Mx. Lower PG synthesis and more PGs released in high stress areas of AC; AC had increased synthesis of decorin and biglycan and increased aggrecan breakdown and release	
	Bilateral total lateral Mx	3 months	8–10 years	Higher AC lesion scores and lower AC PG content; bone mineral density unchanged	247
		2 and 16 weeks	12–15 months	AC biomechanical changes throughout joint; collagen organization more important to dynamic shear modulus than PG content; not important for phase lag	248
		6 months	7 years	Mx increased thickness and density of subchondral bone and serum osteocalcin levels	249
Grivet monkey	Unilateral total medial Mx	21–252 days	Young	Loss of cells from superficial layer, decrease in PG content of AC, cloning of deep layer cells	250

AC = articular cartilage; ADAMTS—A disintegrin and metalloproteinase with thrombospondin motifs; PPARγ = peroxisome proliferators activated receptor gamma; PG = proteoglycan.

loss of proteoglycans from cartilage, fibrillation, and erosion with osteophytosis at the inner prominence of the medial tibial plateau were the outcomes of meniscectomy in this species.[252–254] This model was subsequently used to identify the disturbance in cartilage metabolism and composition during the development of OA and provided a means of assessing the effects of hormones and antiarthritic drugs on these changes.[10,221,222] More recently, total medial meniscectomy in rabbits has been reported to induce OA changes in cartilage and bone which can be reliably detected by micro-MRI.[193,223–225]

Meniscal surgery has been used to induce OA in other small animal species including guinea pigs, rats, and mice. Partial medial meniscectomy in guinea pigs induces focal cartilage erosion within 1 week and by 12 weeks the contralateral (nonoperated) joint was also affected.[227] Erosion of cartilage, but not proteoglycan loss, in the guinea pig meniscectomy model is abrogated by inhibition of MMPs.[226] In the rat, meniscal transection has been shown to be a useful model to study the pain and hyperalgesia associated with joint destabilization.[231] In mice, destabilization of the medial meniscus has recently been used to identify ADAMTS-5 and not ADAMTS-4, as the primary aggrecan-degrading enzyme in this species.[163,232]

Negating the weight-bearing function of the meniscus through the various surgical procedures consistently induces OA in small animals. However, the limited joint tissue available restricts the analyses that are possible, e.g., topographical differences in cartilage metabolism and biomechanics.[255] Use of large animal models of meniscal surgery would overcome these deficiencies.

Large Animal Meniscectomy Models

In 1936, King[256] demonstrated that medial meniscectomy in dogs caused early degenerative changes in articular cartilage,

the extent of which was proportional to the amount of tissue excised. Cox and associates[257] confirmed the findings of King[256] but also compared the outcome of total unilateral meniscectomy with partial meniscectomy in which the outer rim was preserved. Animals were sacrificed at postoperative intervals of 3 to 10 months, and the results showed that the extent of joint damage, which included increased synovial fluid volume, synovitis, and focal erosion of cartilage, was proportional to the amount of meniscus removed. Ghosh and coworkers[233,234] undertook unilateral medial meniscectomy in greyhounds and noted that postoperative immobilization of the joint decreased the extent of cartilage degeneration[234] and meniscal regrowth[233] (Table 5–4). Despite the advantages of using purebred dogs, economic and public antivivisection considerations associated with the use of these animals prompted the search for alternatives. Merino sheep, widely used wool- and food-producing animals, were therefore subjected to meniscectomy, and the joints were examined to determine whether the animal was a suitable model of OA. Initial investigations showed that unilateral medial meniscectomy produced hypertrophy of cartilage and only moderate fibrillation 3 months after surgery. However, marginal osteophytes, cell cloning, and subchondral bone changes were more evident after 6 months.[237–240,258] As with the canine ACL model, progression of the hypertrophic phase to the stage when full cartilage lesions occurred was a slow process and was consistently observed only after 24 months.[259] The rate of progression could be accelerated, however, by maintaining the animals on a regular weight-bearing exercise program.[239]

In human joints, the lateral meniscus protects a larger area of the tibial plateau articular cartilage than does the medial meniscus in its compartment.[260] Because the anatomic features of human and ovine joints are essentially the same and the menisci perform similar functions,[261] it was reasoned that removal of the lateral meniscus of ovine joints would impose higher focal stresses on cartilage than occurred after medial meniscectomy. Consistent with this, cartilage explant cultures derived from the laterally meniscectomized animals displayed a greater loss of proteoglycans and a lower synthesis rate than in the corresponding cartilage cultures from joints of animals who were subjected to medial meniscectomy.[240]

In both unilateral medial and lateral meniscectomy models, gait analysis[243,258] and metabolic studies of cartilage of the nonoperated contralateral limb[242] showed that weight bearing on this joint was different from that in control animals not undergoing meniscectomy. This disparity most likely arose from the innate protective mechanisms that would prompt the animal to favor weight bearing on the side that was not operated on as well as on the forelimbs. From these observations, it was deduced that the contralateral joints of unilaterally meniscectomized sheep could not be used as control joints. This view was consistent with reports of others who used the canine ACLT model.[262] Collectively, these observations have led to a further modification of the ovine model whereby bilateral lateral meniscectomy was undertaken to compel the animals to distribute their body weight equally on both hind limbs. This procedure also provides two experimental joints from each animal, thereby enlarging the scope for histopathologic, biochemical, and biomechanical investigations of cartilage, synovium, and subchondral bone.

Other Surgical Models of Osteoarthritis

Numerous studies have used combinations of joint ligament transections with and without meniscal surgery to induce OA in rabbits, rats, guinea pigs, and mice (Table 5–5). Hulth and

TABLE 5–5
SELECTED STUDIES USING OTHER SURGICAL MODELS OF OA

Species	OA Induction Method	Post-surgery Duration	Age or Body Weight	Findings	Reference
Rabbit	Resection of ACL and MCL	4–12 weeks	3.0–3.5 kg	OA changes by 4 weeks persisting through to 12 weeks; friction coefficient of joint significantly increased	263, 264
	Partial medial Mx; resection of MCL	4 and 16 weeks	3 kg	Proteoglycan content of AC decreased at 4 weeks, increased at 6 weeks	265
Guinea pig	Resection of ACL, PCL, and MCL	21 weeks	0.5–0.6 kg	Less OA pathology (AC pitting, ulceration, eburnation) with vitamin C supplementation; ACLT caused higher AC acid phosphatase	266
Rat	Resection of ACL, PCL, and MCL	2, 4, and 6 weeks	150–200 g	Changes in distribution of protein kinase C isoenzymes in cells of subchondral bone in OA joints	267
	Resection of ACL, MCL, and Mx	1–10 weeks	10 weeks	Bone loss and dull AC surface within 2 weeks; osteophyte formation by 6 weeks; bone eburnation by 10 weeks	203
	MD; resection of MCL	1, 2, 3, and 6 weeks	300–350 g	Increased depth of AC lesion over time, less increase in extent of lesion; early OA lesions detected by optical coherence tomography (OCT)	268, 269
		0–42 days	7–9 weeks	Progressive pattern of cartilage damage resembling human OA lesions	270
		6 weeks ± FGF-18	300–375 g	Fibroblast growth factor-18 (FGF-18) induced dose-dependent increases in AC thickness and reduced AC OA scores	271
Mouse	Partial medial Mx; resection of MCL	4 days–4 weeks	25–30 g	Gene deletion of either interleukin (IL)-1β, IL-1β-converting enzyme, iNOS, or MMP-3 accelerated development of OA	162
	Combinations of Mx and ligament transection	2, 4, and 8 weeks	18–22 g	Increasing OA scores with increasing instability. Bilateral Mx plus all ligaments transacted gave AC destruction by 2 weeks and osteophytes by 4 weeks. ACLT only gave partial AC destruction by 8 weeks. Collagen type X and MMP-13 induced early in OA.	272
Beagle	Grooved AC and limb loading	3–40 weeks	10–15 kg	Characteristic OA progression in AC observed at 10 weeks not evident at 3 weeks; mild synovial inflammation present; model has no permanent joint instability	273, 274

AC = articular cartilage; iNOS = inducible nitric oxide synthase; MD = meniscal destabilization; Mx = meniscectomy.

coworkers[275] employed medial meniscectomy in rabbits but further destabilized the joint by severing the medial collateral ligament (MCL), ACL, and posterior cruciate ligament (PCL). The joint disease that developed was characterized by extensive osteophytosis and full-depth cartilage lesions. Columbo and associates[276] undertook partial lateral meniscectomy in rabbits but also sectioned the sesamoid and fibular collateral ligaments. The procedure produced more consistent OA changes in rabbit joints[276] and was subsequently used to evaluate the effects of a plethora of antiarthritic drugs on the development of cartilage lesions.[10] The severity and speed of onset of OA following combination destabilization procedures in rabbit joints does not parallel the human disease, however, and may limit the relevance of such models.

In the rat and mouse, MCL transection has been combined with meniscal transection/destabilization.[162,268-271] It is likely that the OA changes induced in this model (at least in the rat) are due solely to the meniscal surgery; as in a limited comparison, MCL transection alone did not cause any disease.[270] Combining ACLT and medial meniscectomy in rats resulted in more extensive and earlier osteophytosis than ACLT alone.[203] With increasing combinations of ligament transection and subsequent joint instability in mice, a similar worsening pattern of OA progression and bone remodeling was observed.[272] In line with earlier comments in the rabbit, the severity and speed of joint destruction in mouse joints with multiple destabilizations limits their comparison with human disease, and to date no studies have demonstrated genetic or therapeutic modulation of such severe OA.

Tibial osteotomy[277-279] and paw amputation[64] in dogs confirmed the importance of weight bearing for the maintenance of cartilage integrity. Lameness induced by gluteal myectomy in Hartley guinea pigs[280] also caused OA changes in the knee joints; however, because these animals are predisposed to spontaneous OA (see earlier), other factors may have contributed to disease progression. Cartilage defects have been surgically produced in rabbit,[281,282] dog,[273,274,283] sheep,[284] and horse[285] knee joints, resulting in post-traumatic OA-like changes in joint tissues.

MISCELLANEOUS MODELS OF OSTEOARTHRITIS

A number of other techniques have been used to induce OA-like changes in joint tissues. Because the incidence of OA in humans is known to be associated with certain occupations that require repetitive mechanical activities,[286] animals have been subjected to a variety of protocols in an attempt to reproduce stress-related changes in their joints. Rabbits running uphill on a treadmill for 5 days showed changes in cartilage proteoglycan content and synthesis.[287] Similar experiments have been undertaken with beagles,[70,288] but long-term moderate running exercise (4 km/day) failed to cause cartilage degeneration; the tissue remained essentially normal except in joint regions of high weight bearing, where it showed signs of hypertrophic change. Horses maintained on treadmill running demonstrated overload arthrosis in fetlock joints;[289] high-stress treadmill

training of standardbred horses for 8 weeks increased the degradation of aggrecan but increased the synthesis of decorin in cartilage explants sampled from the radial facet of the carpal joint.[290] Changes in weight bearing have also been induced by repetitive impulse loading to rabbit joints[291-293] and transarticular loading of dog joints.[294] These techniques appear to cause excessive macrostructural damage to cartilage, such as the formation of deep clefts and fissures into the superficial and radial zone, but OA-like changes appear only after 6 months.[294]

SUMMARY AND CONCLUSIONS

Osteoarthritic changes have been induced in the joints of a large number of animal species by use of a wide range of experimental techniques. The rate of progression of OA lesions in these models is highly variable, being dependent on the species of animal and its age, sex, weight, and the type of housing and care used after the arthropathy has been induced. Moreover, the ostensibly same animal model may produce different outcomes in the hands of different investigators (e.g., ACLT in dogs, in which open and closed surgical methods are both widely employed). Using undefined or diverse genetic backgrounds of animals (e.g., mongrel compared with a single species of dog) not only increases the variability within experiments but makes comparisons between research facilities more difficult. Because animal models are now routinely used to evaluate potential therapeutic modalities for treatment of OA, it is clearly important to standardize the techniques and species employed to induce the arthropathy. Moreover, disease- or structure-modifying OA drugs are now under active development, but there is as yet no consensus on the most appropriate models to be used to identify such agents or indeed what pharmacologic activities the agents should possess to qualify them for inclusion under this classification. A great deal can be learned from OA models in small animal species, particularly with the use of powerful GM techniques in mice. However, in large animals, the increased load bearing more closely mimics human joints and, along with the potential to evaluate regional differences within a single joint, may make these species more physiologically relevant as models. Although we are of the opinion that large animal models of OA offer distinct advantages over rodent models, we recognize that economic and other considerations may preclude their use in many laboratories. A likely and logical approach is that promising compounds identified from in vitro and genetic (mouse) studies will be tested in "high throughput" small animal models. Those that prove useful in such preliminary studies can then be manufactured in sufficient quantities to be tested and validated in a large animal model.

REFERENCES

1. Hough (Jr) AJ. The pathology of osteoarthritis. In: Moskowitz RW, Goldberg V, Howell DS, eds. Osteoarthritis: Diagnosis and Medical/Surgical Management. 3rd ed. Philadelphia: WB Saunders Co, 1999, pp 69–99.

2. Smith MD, Triantafillou S, Parker A, et al. Synovial membrane inflammation and cytokine production in patients with early osteoarthritis. J Rheumatol 24:365–371, 1997.

3. Lindblad S, Hedfors E. Arthroscopic and immunohistologic characterization of knee joint synovitis in osteoarthritis. Arthritis Rheum 30:1081–1088, 1987.

4. Dahl LB, Dahl IM, Engstrom-Laurent A, et al. Concentration and molecular weight of sodium hyaluronate in synovial fluid from patients with rheumatoid arthritis and other arthropathies. Ann Rheum Dis 44:817–822, 1985.

5. Balazs E. The physical properties of synovial fluid and the special role of hyaluronic acid. In: Helfet AJ, ed. Disorders of the Knee. Philadelphia: JB Lippincott, 1982, pp 61–74.

6. Kiaer T, Gronlund J, Sorensen KH. Intraosseous pressure and partial pressures of oxygen and carbon dioxide in osteoarthritis. Semin Arthritis Rheum 18:57–60, 1989.

7. Starklint H, Lausten GS, Arnoldi CC. Microvascular obstruction in avascular necrosis. Immunohistochemistry of 14 femoral heads. Acta Orthop Scand 66:9–12, 1995.

8. Ross SE, Williams RO, Mason LJ, et al. Suppression of TNF-alpha expression, inhibition of Th1 activity, and amelioration of collagen-induced arthritis by rolipram. J Immunol 159:6253–6259, 1997.

9. Joosten LA, Helsen MM, van de Loo FA, et al. Anticytokine treatment of established type II collagen-induced arthritis in DBA/1 mice. A comparative study using anti-TNF alpha, anti-IL-1 alpha/beta, and IL-1Ra. Arthritis Rheum 39:797–809, 1996.

10. Smith M, Ghosh P. Experimental Models of Osteoarthritis. In: Moskowitz R, Howell D, Altman R, Buckwalter J, Goldberg V, eds. Osteoarthritis. 3rd ed. Philadelphia: WB Saunders, 2001, 171–199.

11. Huebner JL, Otterness IG, Freund EM, et al. Collagenase 1 and collagenase 3 expression in a guinea pig model of osteoarthritis. Arthritis Rheum 41:877–890, 1998.

12. Balbin M, Fueyo A, Knauper V, et al. Identification and enzymatic characterization of two diverging murine counterparts of human interstitial collagenase (MMP-1) expressed at sites of embryo implantation. J Biol Chem 276:10253–10262, 2001.

13. Barry FP, Neame PJ, Sasse J, et al. Length variation in the keratan sulfate domain of mammalian aggrecan. Matrix Biol 14: 323–328, 1994.

14. Frost L, Ghosh P. Microinjury to the synovial membrane may cause disaggregation of proteoglycans in rabbit knee joint articular cartilage. J Orthop Res 2:207–220, 1984.

15. Vasilev V, Merker HJ, Vidinov N. Ultrastructural changes in the synovial membrane in experimentally-induced osteoarthritis of rabbit knee joint. Histol Histopath 7:119–127, 1992.

16. Alarcon-Segovia D, Ward LE. Marked destructive changes occurring in osteoarthric finger joints after intra-articular injection of corticosteroids. Arthritis Rheum 9:443–463, 1966.

17. Silberberg M, Silberberg R, Hasler M. Fine structure of articular cartilage on mice receiving cortisone acetate. Arch Path 82: 569–582, 1966.

18. Tsai CL, Liu TK. Estradiol-induced knee osteoarthrosis in ovariectomized rabbits. Clin Orthop Relat Res: 295–302, 1993.

19. Moskowitz RW, Davis W, Sammarco J, et al. Experimentally induced corticosteroid arthropathy. Arthritis Rheum 13:236–243, 1970.

20. Kongtawelert P, Brooks PM, Ghosh P. Pentosan polysulfate (Cartrophen) prevents the hydrocortisone induced loss of hyaluronic acid and proteoglycans from cartilage of rabbit joints as well as normalizes the keratan sulfate levels in their serum. J Rheumatol 16:1454–1459, 1989.

21. Celeste C, Ionescu M, Robin Poole A, et al. Repeated intraarticular injections of triamcinolone acetonide alter cartilage matrix metabolism measured by biomarkers in synovial fluid. J Orthop Res 23:602–610, 2005.

22. Robion FC, Doize B, Boure L, et al. Use of synovial fluid markers of cartilage synthesis and turnover to study effects of repeated intra-articular administration of methylprednisolone acetate on articular cartilage in vivo. J Orthop Res 19:250–258, 2001.

23. Murray RC, DeBowes RM, Gaughan EM, et al. The effects of intra-articular methylprednisolone and exercise on the mechanical properties of articular cartilage in the horse. Osteoarthritis Cartilage 6:106–114, 1998.

24. Roneus B, Lindblad A, Lindholm A, et al. Effects of intraarticular corticosteroid and sodium hyaluronate injections on synovial fluid production and synovial fluid content of sodium hyaluronate and proteoglycans in normal equine joints. Zentralbl Veterinarmed A 40:10–16, 1993.

25. Zhang Y, McAlindon TE, Hannan MT, et al. Estrogen replacement therapy and worsening of radiographic knee osteoarthritis: the Framingham Study. Arthritis Rheum 41:1867–1873, 1998.

26. Felson DT. Preventing knee and hip osteoarthritis. Bull Rheum Dis 47:1–4, 1998.

27. Hanna FS, Wluka AE, Bell RJ, et al. Osteoarthritis and the postmenopausal woman: Epidemiological, magnetic resonance imaging, and radiological findings. Semin Arthritis Rheum 34:631–636, 2004.

28. Ravn P, Warming L, Christgau S, et al. The effect on cartilage of different forms of application of postmenopausal estrogen therapy: comparison of oral and transdermal therapy. Bone 35:1216–1221, 2004.

29. Hoegh-Andersen P, Tanko LB, Andersen TL, et al. Ovariectomized rats as a model of postmenopausal osteoarthritis: validation and application. Arthritis Res Ther 6:R169–180, 2004.

30. Christgau S, Tanko LB, Cloos PA, et al. Suppression of elevated cartilage turnover in postmenopausal women and in ovariectomized rats by estrogen and a selective estrogen-receptor modulator (SERM). Menopause 11:508–518, 2004.

31. Jochems C, Islander U, Erlandsson M, et al. Osteoporosis in experimental postmenopausal polyarthritis: the relative contributions of estrogen deficiency and inflammation. Arthritis Res Ther 7:R837–843, 2005.

32. Cake MA, Appleyard RC, Read RA, et al. Ovariectomy alters the structural and biomechanical properties of ovine femoro-tibial articular cartilage and increases cartilage iNOS. Osteoarthritis Cartilage 13:1066–1075, 2005.

33. Silberberg M, Silberberg R. Modifying action of estrogen on the evolution of osteoarthritis in mice of different ages. Endocrinol 72:449–457, 1963b.

34. Tsai CL, Liu TK. Up-regulation of estrogen receptors in rabbit osteoarthritic cartilage. Life Sci 50:1727–1735, 1992.

35. Pritzker KP. Animal models for osteoarthritis: processes, problems and prospects. Ann Rheum Dis 53:406–420, 1994.

36. van der Kraan PM, Vitters EL, van de Putte LBA, et al. Development of osteoarthritis lesions in mice by "metabolic" and "mechanical" alterations in knee joints. Am J Pathol 135:1001–1014, 1989.

37. van Osch GJ, van der Kraan PM, van Valburg AA, et al. The relation between cartilage damage and osteophyte size in a murine model for osteoarthritis in the knee. Rheumatol Int 16:115–119, 1996.

38. van Valburg AA, van Osch GJ, van der Kraan PM, et al. Quantification of morphometric changes in murine experimental osteoarthritis using image analysis. Rheumatol Int 15:181–187, 1996.

39. van den Berg WB, van Osch GJ, van der Kraan PM, et al. Cartilage destruction and osteophytes in instability-induced murine osteoarthritis: role of TGF beta in osteophyte formation? Agents Actions 40:215–219, 1993.

40. Blom AB, van Lent PL, Holthuysen AE, et al. Synovial lining macrophages mediate osteophyte formation during experimental osteoarthritis. Osteoarthritis Cartilage 12:627–635, 2004.

41. Gustafson SB, Trotter GW, Norrdin RW, et al. Evaluation of intra-articularly administered sodium monoiodoacetate-induced chemical injury to articular cartilage of horses. Am J Vet Res 53:1193–1202, 1992.

42. Williams JM, Brandt KD. Exercise increases osteophyte formation and diminishes fibrillation following chemically induced articular cartilage injury. J Anat 139 (Pt 4):599–611, 1984.

43. Janusz MJ, Little CB, King LE, et al. Detection of aggrecanase- and MMP-generated catabolic neoepitopes in the rat iodoacetate model of cartilage degeneration. Osteoarthritis Cartilage 12: 720–728, 2004.

44. Saied A, Cherin E, Gaucher H, et al. Assessment of articular cartilage and subchondral bone: subtle and progressive changes in experimental osteoarthritis using 50 MHz echography in vitro. J Bone Miner Res 12:1378–1386, 1997.

45. Cherin E, Saied A, Laugier P, et al. Evaluation of acoustical parameter sensitivity to age-related and osteoarthritic changes in articular cartilage using 50-MHz ultrasound. Ultrasound Med Biol 24:341–354, 1998.

46. Janusz MJ, Hookfin EB, Heitmeyer SA, et al. Moderation of iodoacetate-induced experimental osteoarthritis in rats by matrix metalloproteinase inhibitors. Osteoarthritis Cartilage 9:751–760, 2001.

47. van de Loo AA, Arntz OJ, Otterness IG, et al. Proteoglycan loss and subsequent replenishment in articular cartilage after a mild arthritic insult by IL-1 in mice: impaired proteoglycan turnover in the recovery phase. Agents Actions 41:200–208, 1994.

48. Borella L, Eng CP, DiJoseph J, et al. Rapid induction of early osteoarthritic-like lesions in the rabbit knee by continuous intra-articular infusion of mammalian collagenase or interleukin-1. Agents Actions 34:220–222, 1991.

49. van den Berg WB. Growth factors in experimental osteoarthritis: transforming growth factor beta pathologic? J Rheumatol 22:143–145, 1995.

50. Elford PR, Graeber M, Ohtsu H, et al. Induction of swelling, synovial hyperplasia and cartilage proteoglyan loss upon intra-articular injection of transforming growth factor-beta-2 in the rabbit. Cytokine 4:232–238, 1992.

51. van Beuningen HM, Glansbeek HL, van der Kraan PM, et al. Osteoarthritis-like changes in the murine knee joint resulting from intra-articular transforming growth factor-beta injections. Osteoarthritis Cartilage 8:25–33, 2000.

52. Lawlor KE, Campbell IK, Metcalf D, et al. Critical role for granulocyte colony-stimulating factor in inflammatory arthritis. Proc Natl Acad Sci USA 101:11398–11403, 2004.

53. Lawlor KE, Campbell IK, O'Donnell K, et al. Molecular and cellular mediators of interleukin-1-dependent acute inflammatory arthritis. Arthritis Rheum 44:442–450, 2001.

54. Evans CH, Mazzocchi RA, Nelson DD, et al. Experimental arthritis induced by intraarticular injection of allogenic cartilaginous particles into rabbit knees. Arthritis Rheum 27:200–207, 1984.

55. Hurtig MB. Use of autogenous cartilage particles to create a model of naturally occurring degenerative joint disease in the horse. Equine Vet J Suppl:19–22, 1988.

56. Kato M, Onodera T. Morphological investigation of cavity formation in articular cartilage induced by ofloxacin in rats. Fundam Appl Toxicol 11:110–119, 1988.

57. Bendele AM, Bean JS, Hulman JF. Passive role of articular chondrocytes in the pathogenesis of acute meniscectomy-induced cartilage degeneration. Vet Path 28:207–215, 1991.

58. Burkhardt JE, Hill MA, Carlton WW. Morphologic and biochemical changes in articular cartilages of immature beagle dogs dosed with difloxacin. Toxicol Pathol 20:246–252, 1992.

59. Sharpnack DD, Mastin JP, Childress CP, et al. Quinolone arthropathy in juvenile New Zealand white rabbits. Lab Anim Sci 44:436–442, 1994.

60. Egerbacher M, Wolfesberger B, Gabler C. In vitro evidence for effects of magnesium supplementation on quinolone-treated horse and dog chondrocytes. Vet Pathol 2001 38:143–148, 1994.

61. Stahlmann R, Lode H. Toxicity of quinolones. Drugs 58 Suppl 2:37–42, 1999.

62. Palmoski M, Perricone E, Brandt KD. Development and reversal of a proteoglycan aggregation defect in normal canine knee cartilage after immobilization. Arthritis Rheum 22:508–517, 1979.

63. Palmoski MJ, Brandt KD. Running inhibits the reversal of atrophic changes in canine knee cartilage after removal of a leg cast. Arthritis Rheum 24:1329–1337, 1981.

64. Palmoski MJ, Colyer RA, Brandt KD. Joint motion in the absence of normal loading does not maintain normal articular cartilage. Arthritis Rheum 23:325–334, 1980.

65. Tammi M, Saamanen AM, Jauhiainen A, et al. Proteoglycan alterations in rabbit knee articular cartilage following physical exercise and immobilization. Connect Tissue Res 11:45–55, 1983.

66. Behrens F, Kraft EL, Oegema TR. Biochemical changes in articular cartilage after joint immobilization by casting or external fixation. J Orthop Res 7:335–343, 1989.

67. Eronen I, Videman T, Friman C, et al. Glycosaminoglycan metabolism in experimental osteoarthritis caused by immobilization. Acta Orthop Scand 49:329–334, 1978.

68. Saamanen AM, Tammi M, Kiviranta I, et al. Maturation of proteoglycan matrix in articular cartilage under increased and decreased joint loading. A study in young rabbits. Connect Tissue Res 16:163–175, 1987.

69. Paukkonen K, Jurvelin J, Helminen HJ. Effects of immobilization on the articular cartilage in young rabbits. A quantitative light microscopic stereological study. Clin Orthop Relat Res 270–280, 1986.

70. Kiviranta I, Jurvelin J, Tammi M, et al. Weight bearing controls glycosaminoglycan concentration and articular cartilage thickness in the knee joints of young beagle dogs. Arthritis Rheum 30:801–809, 1987.

71. Videman T, Michelsson JE, Rauhamaki R, et al. Changes in 35S-sulfate uptake in different tissues in the knee and hip regions of rabbits during immobilization, remobilization the development of osteoarthritis. Acta Orthop Scand 47:290–298, 1976.

72. Videman T, Eronen I, Candolin T. [3H]proline incorporation and hydroxyproline concentration in articular cartilage during the development of osteoarthritis caused by immobilization. A study in vivo with rabbits. Biochem J 200:435–440, 1981.

73. Tammi M, Kiviranta I, Peltonen L, et al. Effects of joint loading on articular cartilage collagen metabolism: assay of procollagen prolyl 4-hydroxylase and galactosylhydroxylysyl glucosyltransferase. Connect Tissue Res 17:199–206, 1988.

74. Trudel G, Uhthoff HK, Laneuville O. Prothrombin gene expression in articular cartilage with a putative role in cartilage degeneration secondary to joint immobility. J Rheumatol 32:1547–1555, 2005.

75. Haapala J, Arokoski JP, Ronkko S, et al. Decline after immobilisation and recovery after remobilisation of synovial fluid IL1, TIMP, and chondroitin sulfate levels in young beagle dogs. Ann Rheum Dis 60:55–60, 2001.

76. Torelli SR, Rahal SC, Volpi RS, et al. Histopathological evaluation of treatment with chondroitin sulfate for osteoarthritis induced by continuous immobilization in rabbits. J Vet Med A Physiol Pathol Clin Med 52:45–51, 2005.

77. Troyer H. The effect of short-term immobilization on the rabbit knee joint cartilage: A histochemical study. Clin Orthop 107:249–257, 1975.

78. Maroudas A, Bullough P, Swanson SA, et al. The permeability of articular cartilage. J Bone Joint Surg Br 50:166–177, 1968.

79. Troyer H. Experimental models of osteoarthritis: a review. Semin Arthritis Rheum 11:362–374, 1982.

80. Holmdahl R, Jansson L, Andersson M, et al. Genetic, hormonal and behavioural influence on spontaneously developing arthritis in normal mice. Clin Exp Immunol 88:467–472, 1992.

81. Mason R, Chambers M, Flannelly J, et al. The STR/ort mouse and its use as a model of osteoarthritis. Osteoarthritis Cartilage 9:85–91, 2001.

82. Chambers MG, Cox L, Chong L, et al. Matrix metalloproteinases and aggrecanases cleave aggrecan in different zones of normal cartilage but colocalize in the development of osteoarthritic lesions in STR/ort mice. Arthritis Rheum 44:1455–1465, 2001.

83. Flannelly J, Chambers M, Dudhia J, et al. Metalloproteinase and tissue inhibitor of metalloproteinase expression in the murine STR/ort model of osteoarthritis. Osteoarthritis Cartilage 10:722–733, 2002.

84. Price JS, Chambers MG, Poole AR, et al. Comparison of collagenase-cleaved articular cartilage collagen in mice in the naturally occurring STR/ort model of osteoarthritis and in collagen-induced arthritis. Osteoarthritis Cartilage 10:172–179, 2002.

85. Mistry D, Oue Y, Chambers MG, et al. Chondrocyte death during murine osteoarthritis. Osteoarthritis Cartilage 12:131–141, 2004.

86. Regan E, Flannelly J, Bowler R, et al. Extracellular superoxide dismutase and oxidant damage in osteoarthritis. Arthritis Rheum 52:3479–3491, 2005.

87. Lapvetelainen T, Nevalainen T, Parkkinen JJ, et al. Lifelong moderate running training increases the incidence and severity of osteoarthritis in the knee joint of C57BL mice. Anat Rec 242:159–165, 1995.

88. Stoop R, van der Kraan PM, Buma P, et al. Type II collagen degradation in spontaneous osteoarthritis in C57Bl/6 and BALB/c mice. Arthritis Rheum 42:2381–2389, 1999.

89. Takahashi K, Kubo T, Goomer RS, et al. Analysis of heat shock proteins and cytokines expressed during early stages of

osteoarthritis in a mouse model. Osteoarthritis Cartilage 5:321–329, 1997.

90. Bendele AM, White SL, Hulman JF. Osteoarthrosis in guinea pigs—Histopathologic and scanning electron microscopic features. Lab Animal Sci 39:115–121, 1989.

91. Bendele AM, Hulman JF. Effects of body weight restriction on the development and progression of spontaneous osteoarthritis in guinea pigs. Arthritis Rheum 34:1180–1184, 1991.

92. de Bri E, Reinholt FP, Svensson O. Primary osteoarthrosis in guinea pigs: a stereological study. J Orthop Res 13:769–776, 1995.

93. Hedlund H, de Bri E, Mengarelli-Widholm S, et al. Ultrastructural changes in primary guinea pig osteoarthritis with special reference to collagen. APMIS 104:374–382, 1996.

94. Watson PJ, Carpenter TA, Hall LD, et al. Cartilage swelling and loss in a spontaneous model of osteoarthritis visualized by magnetic resonance imaging. Osteoarthritis Cartilage 4:197–207, 1996.

95. Wei L, Svensson O, Hjerpe A. Proteoglycan turnover during development of spontaneous osteoarthrosis in guinea pigs. Osteoarthritis Cartilage 6:410–416, 1998.

96. Wei L, Svensson O, Hjerpe A. Correlation of morphologic and biochemical changes in the natural history of spontaneous osteoarthrosis in guinea pigs. Arthritis Rheum 40:2075–2083, 1997.

97. Anderson-MacKenzie JM, Quasnichka HL, Starr RL, et al. Fundamental subchondral bone changes in spontaneous knee osteoarthritis. Int J Biochem Cell Biol 37:224–236, 2005.

98. Chateauvert JM, Pritzker KP, Kessler MJ, et al. Spontaneous osteoarthritis in rhesus macaques 1 chemical and biochemical-studies. J Rheumatol 16:1098–1104, 1989.

99. Pritzker KPH, Chateauvert J, Grynpas MD, et al. Rhesus macaques as an experimental model for degenerative arthritis. Puerto Rico J Health Sci 8:99–102, 1989.

100. Chateauvert JMD, Grynpas MD, Kessler MJ, et al. Spontaneous osteoarthritis in rhesus macaques II Characterization of disease and morphometric studies. J Rheumatol 17:73–83, 1990.

101. Grynpas MD, Gahunia HK, Yuan J, et al. Analysis of collagens solubilized from cartilage of normal and spontaneously osteoarthritic rhesus monkeys. Osteoarthritis Cartilage 2:227–234, 1994.

102. Carlson CS, Loeser RF, Jayo MJ, et al. Osteoarthritis in cynomolgus macaques: a primate model of naturally occurring disease. J Orthop Res 12:331–339, 1994.

103. Loeser RF, Carlson CS, McGee MP. Expression of beta 1 integrins by cultured articular chondrocytes and in osteoarthritic cartilage. Exp Cell Res 217:248–257, 1995.

104. Carlson CS, Loeser RF, Purser CB, et al. Osteoarthritis in cynomolgus macaques. III: Effects of age, gender, and subchondral bone thickness on the severity of disease. J Bone Miner Res 11:1209–1217, 1996.

105. Loeser RF, Shanker G, Carlson CS, et al. Reduction in the chondrocyte response to insulin-like growth factor 1 in aging and osteoarthritis: studies in a non-human primate model of naturally occurring disease. Arthritis Rheum 43:2110–2120, 2000.

106. Miller LM, Novatt JT, Hamerman D, et al. Alterations in mineral composition observed in osteoarthritic joints of cynomolgus monkeys. Bone 35:498–506, 2004.

107. Olsewski JM, Lust G, Rendano VT, et al. Degenerative joint disease: multiple joint involvement in young and mature dogs. Am J Vet Res 44:1300–1308, 1983.

108. Greisen HA, Summers BA, Lust G. Ultrastructure of the articular cartilage and synovium in the early stages of degenerative joint disease in canine hip joints. Am J Vet Res 43:1963–1971, 1982.

109. Lust G, Summers BA. Early, asymptomatic stage of degenerative joint disease in canine hip joints. Am J Vet Res 42:1849–1855, 1981.

110. Salo PT, Hogervorst T, Seerattan RA, et al. Selective joint denervation promotes knee osteoarthritis in the aging rat. J Orthop Res 20:1256–1264, 2002.

111. Salo PT, Seeratten RA, Erwin WM, et al. Evidence for a neuropathic contribution to the development of spontaneous knee osteoarthrosis in a mouse model. Acta Orthop Scand 73:77–84, 2002.

112. Chambers MG, Kuffner T, Cowan SK, et al. Expression of collagen and aggrecan genes in normal and osteoarthritic murine knee joints. Osteoarthritis Cartilage 10:51–61, 2002.

113. Chambers MG, Bayliss MT, Mason RM. Chondrocyte cytokine and growth factor expression in murine osteoarthritis. Osteoarthritis Cartilage 5:301–308, 1997.

114. Brismar BH, Lei W, Hjerpe A, et al. The effect of body mass and physical activity on the development of guinea pig osteoarthrosis. Acta Orthop Scand 74:442–448, 2003.

115. Young RD, Vaughan-Thomas A, Wardale RJ, et al. Type II collagen deposition in cruciate ligament precedes osteoarthritis in the guinea pig knee. Osteoarthritis Cartilage 10:420–428, 2002.

116. Johnson K, Svensson CI, Etten DV, et al. Mediation of spontaneous knee osteoarthritis by progressive chondrocyte ATP depletion in Hartley guinea pigs. Arthritis Rheum 50:1216–1225, 2004.

117. Greenwald RA. Treatment of destructive arthritic disorders with MMP inhibitors. Potential role of tetracyclines. Ann N Y Acad Sci 732:181–198, 1994.

118. Ding M, Christian Danielsen C, Hvid I. Effects of hyaluronan on three-dimensional microarchitecture of subchondral bone tissues in guinea pig primary osteoarthrosis. Bone 36:489–501, 2005.

119. Loeser RF, Carlson CS, Del Carlo M, et al. Detection of nitrotyrosine in aging and osteoarthritic cartilage: Correlation of oxidative damage with the presence of interleukin-1beta and with chondrocyte resistance to insulin-like growth factor 1. Arthritis Rheum 46:2349–2357, 2002.

120. Ham KD, Loeser RF, Lindgren BR, et al. Effects of long-term estrogen replacement therapy on osteoarthritis severity in cynomolgus monkeys. Arthritis Rheum 46:1956–1964, 2002.

121. Helminen HJ, Saamanen AM, Salminen H, et al. Transgenic mouse models for studying the role of cartilage macromolecules in osteoarthritis. Rheumatology (Oxford) 41:848–856, 2002.

122. Pace JM, Li Y, Seegmiller RE, et al. Disproportionate micromelia (Dmm) in mice caused by a mutation in the C-propeptide coding region of Col2a1. Dev Dyn 208:25–33, 1997.

123. Seegmiller RE, Brown K, Chandrasekhar S. Histochemical, immunofluorescence, and ultrastructural differences in fetal cartilage among three genetically distinct chondrodystrophic mice. Teratology 38:579–592, 1988.

124. Saamanen AK, Salminen HJ, Dean PB, et al. Osteoarthritis-like lesions in transgenic mice harboring a small deletion mutation in type II collagen gene. Osteoarthritis Cartilage 8:248–257, 2000.

125. Rintala M, Metsaranta M, Saamanen AM, et al. Abnormal craniofacial growth and early mandibular osteoarthritis in mice harbouring a mutant type II collagen transgene. J Anat 190 (Pt 2):201–208, 1997.

126. Morko JP, Soderstrom M, Saamanen AM, et al. Up regulation of cathepsin K expression in articular chondrocytes in a transgenic mouse model for osteoarthritis. Ann Rheum Dis 63:649–655, 2004.

127. Lapvetelainen T, Hyttinen MM, Saamanen AM, et al. Lifelong voluntary joint loading increases osteoarthritis in mice housing a deletion mutation in type II procollagen gene, and slightly also in non-transgenic mice. Ann Rheum Dis 61:810–817, 2002.

128. Helminen HJ, Kiraly K, Pelttari A, et al. An inbred line of transgenic mice expressing an internally deleted gene for type II procollagen (COL2A1). Young mice have a variable phenotype of a chondrodysplasia and older mice have osteoarthritic changes in joints. J Clin Invest 92:582–595, 1993.

129. Hyttinen MM, Toyras J, Lapvetelainen T, et al. Inactivation of one allele of the type II collagen gene alters the collagen network in murine articular cartilage and makes cartilage softer. Ann Rheum Dis 60:262–268, 2001.

130. Sahlman J, Pitkanen MT, Prockop DJ, et al. A human COL2A1 gene with an Arg519Cys mutation causes osteochondrodysplasia in transgenic mice. Arthritis Rheum 50:3153–3160, 2004.

131. Arita M, Li SW, Kopen G, et al. Skeletal abnormalities and ultrastructural changes of cartilage in transgenic mice expressing a collagen II gene (COL2A1) with a Cys for Arg-alpha1-519 substitution. Osteoarthritis Cartilage 10:808–815, 2002.

132. Kimura T, Nakata K, Tsumaki N, et al. Progressive degeneration of articular cartilage and intervertebral discs. An experimental study in transgenic mice bearing a type IX collagen mutation. Int Orthop 20:177–181, 1996.

133. Nakata K, Ono K, Miyazaki J, et al. Osteoarthritis associated with mild chondrodysplasia in transgenic mice expressing alpha 1(IX) collagen chains with a central deletion. Proc Natl Acad Sci USA 90:2870–2874, 1993.

134. Fassler R, Schnegelsberg PN, Dausman J, et al. Mice lacking alpha 1 (IX) collagen develop noninflammatory degenerative joint disease. Proc Natl Acad Sci USA 91:5070–5074, 1994.

135. Rodriguez RR, Seegmiller RE, Stark MR, et al. A type XI collagen mutation leads to increased degradation of type II collagen in articular cartilage. Osteoarthritis Cartilage 12:314–320, 2004.

136. Xu L, Flahiff CM, Waldman BA, et al. Osteoarthritis-like changes and decreased mechanical function of articular cartilage in the joints of mice with the chondrodysplasia gene (cho). Arthritis Rheum 48:2509–2518, 2003.

137. Xu L, Peng H, Wu D, et al. Activation of the discoidin domain receptor 2 induces expression of matrix metalloproteinase 13 associated with osteoarthritis in mice. J Biol Chem 280:548–555, 2005.

138. Wadhwa S, Embree MC, Kilts T, et al. Accelerated osteoarthritis in the temporomandibular joint of biglycan/fibromodulin double-deficient mice. Osteoarthritis Cartilage 13:817–827, 2005.

139. Young MF, Bi Y, Ameye L, et al. Biglycan knockout mice: new models for musculoskeletal diseases. Glycoconj J 19:257–262, 2002.

140. Ameye L, Young MF. Mice deficient in small leucine-rich proteoglycans: novel in vivo models for osteoporosis, osteoarthritis, Ehlers-Danlos syndrome, muscular dystrophy, and corneal diseases. Glycobiology 12:107R–116R, 2002.

141. Ameye L, Aria D, Jepsen K, et al. Abnormal collagen fibrils in tendons of biglycan/fibromodulin-deficient mice lead to gait impairment, ectopic ossification, and osteoarthritis. FASEB J 16:673–680, 2002.

142. Jepsen KJ, Wu F, Peragallo JH, et al. A syndrome of joint laxity and impaired tendon integrity in lumican- and fibromodulin-deficient mice. J Biol Chem 277:35532–35540, 2002.

143. Bohm BB, Aigner T, Roy B, et al. Homeostatic effects of the metalloproteinase disintegrin ADAM15 in degenerative cartilage remodeling. Arthritis Rheum 52:1100–1109, 2005.

144. Holmbeck K, Bianco P, Caterina J, et al. MT1-MMP-deficient mice develop dwarfism, osteopenia, arthritis, and connective tissue disease due to inadequate collagen turnover. Cell 99:81–92, 1999.

145. de Hooge AS, van de Loo FA, Bennink MB, et al. Male IL-6 gene knock out mice developed more advanced osteoarthritis upon aging. Osteoarthritis Cartilage 13:66–73, 2005.

146. Zhang YW, Su Y, Lanning N, et al. Targeted disruption of Mig-6 in the mouse genome leads to early onset degenerative joint disease. Proc Natl Acad Sci USA 102:11740–11745, 2005.

147. Yamamoto H, Iwase N. Spontaneous osteoarthritic lesions in a new mutant strain of the mouse. Exp Anim 47:131–135, 1998.

148. Sakamoto M, Hosoda Y, Kojimahara K, et al. Arthritis and ankylosis in twy mice with hereditary multiple osteochondral lesions: with special reference to calcium deposition. Pathol Int 44:420–427, 1994.

149. Okawa A, Ikegawa S, Nakamura I, et al. Mapping of a gene responsible for twy (tip-toe walking Yoshimura), a mouse model of ossification of the posterior longitudinal ligament of the spine (OPLL). Mamm Genome 9:155–156, 1998.

150. Glasson SS, Trubetskoy OV, Harlan PM, et al. Blotchy mice: a model of osteoarthritis associated with a metabolic defect. Osteoarthritis Cartilage 4:209–212, 1996.

151. Rountree RB, Schoor M, Chen H, et al. BMP receptor signaling is required for postnatal maintenance of articular cartilage. PLoS Biol 2:1815–1827, 2004.

152. Young MF. Mouse models of osteoarthritis provide new research tools. Trends Pharmacol Sci 26:333–335, 2005.

153. Zemmyo M, Meharra EJ, Kuhn K, et al. Accelerated, aging-dependent development of osteoarthritis in alpha1 integrin-deficient mice. Arthritis Rheum 48:2873–2880, 2003.

154. Neuhold LA, Killar L, Zhao W, et al. Postnatal expression in hyaline cartilage of constitutively active human collagenase-3 (MMP-13) induces osteoarthritis in mice. J Clin Invest 107:35–44, 2001.

155. Ogueta S, Olazabal I, Santos I, et al. Transgenic mice expressing bovine GH develop arthritic disorder and self-antibodies. J Endocrinol 165:321–328, 2000.

156. Serra R, Johnson M, Filvaroff EH, et al. Expression of a truncated, kinase-defective TGF-beta type II receptor in mouse skeletal tissue promotes terminal chondrocyte differentiation and osteoarthritis. J Cell Biol 139:541–552, 1997.

157. Watanabe H, Yamada Y. Chondrodysplasia of gene knockout mice for aggrecan and link protein. Glycoconj J 19:269–273, 2002.

158. Krueger RC, Jr., Kurima K, Schwartz NB. Completion of the mouse aggrecan gene structure and identification of the defect in the cmd-Bc mouse as a near complete deletion of the murine aggrecan gene. Mamm Genome 10:1119–1125, 1999.

159. Wai AW, Ng LJ, Watanabe H, et al. Disrupted expression of matrix genes in the growth plate of the mouse cartilage matrix deficiency (cmd) mutant. Dev Genet 22:349–358, v.

160. Watanabe H, Nakata K, Kimata K, et al. Dwarfism and age-associated spinal degeneration of heterozygote cmd mice defective in aggrecan. Proc Natl Acad Sci USA 94:6943–6947, 1997.

161. Watanabe H, Kimata K, Line S, et al. Mouse cartilage matrix deficiency (cmd) caused by a 7 bp deletion in the aggrecan gene. Nat Genet 7:154–157, 1994.

162. Clements KM, Price JS, Chambers MG, et al. Gene deletion of either interleukin-1beta, interleukin-1beta-converting enzyme, inducible nitric oxide synthase, or stromelysin 1 accelerates the development of knee osteoarthritis in mice after surgical transection of the medial collateral ligament and partial medial meniscectomy. Arthritis Rheum 48:3452–3463, 2003.

163. Glasson SS, Askew R, Sheppard B, et al. Deletion of active ADAMTS5 prevents cartilage degradation in a murine model of osteoarthritis. Nature 434:644–648, 2005.

164. Stanton H, Rogerson FM, East CJ, et al. ADAMTS5 is the major aggrecanase in mouse cartilage in vivo and in vitro. Nature 434:648–652, 2005.

165. Pond MJ, Nuki G. Experimentally induced osteoarthritis in the dog. Ann Rheum Dis 32:387–388, 1973.

166. Gilbertson EMM. The development of periarticular osteophyte in experimently induced OA in the dog. A study using microradiographic, microangiographic, and fluorescent bone-labelling techniques. Ann Rheum Dis 34:12–25, 1975.

167. McDevitt CA, Muir H. Biochemical changes in the cartilage of the knee in experimental and natural osteoarthritis in the dog. J Bone Joint Surg 58-B:94–101, 1976.

168. McDevitt CA, Gilbertson EM, Muir H. An experimental model of osteoarthritis: Early morphological and biochemical changes. J Bone Joint Surg 59-B:24–35, 1977.

169. Matyas JR, Ehlers PF, Huang D, et al. The early molecular natural history of experimental osteoarthritis. I. Progressive discoordinate expression of aggrecan and type II procollagen messenger RNA in the articular cartilage of adult animals. Arthritis Rheum 42:993–1002, 1999.

170. Boyd SK, Muller R, Matyas JR, et al. Early morphometric and anisotropic change in periarticular cancellous bone in a model of experimental knee osteoarthritis quantified using microcomputed tomography. Clin Biomech (Bristol, Avon) 15:624–631, 2000.

171. Boyd SK, Matyas JR, Wohl GR, et al. Early regional adaptation of periarticular bone mineral density after anterior cruciate ligament injury. J Appl Physiol 89:2359–2364, 2000.

172. Wildey GM, Billetz AC, Matyas JR, et al. Absolute concentrations of mRNA for type I and type VI collagen in the canine meniscus in normal and ACL-deficient knee joints obtained by RNase protection assay. J Orthop Res 19:650–658, 2001.

173. Matyas JR, Huang D, Chung M, et al. Regional quantification of cartilage type II collagen and aggrecan messenger RNA in joints with early experimental osteoarthritis. Arthritis Rheum 46:1536–1543, 2002.

174. Alhadlaq HA, Xia Y, Moody JB, et al. Detecting structural changes in early experimental osteoarthritis of tibial cartilage by microscopic magnetic resonance imaging and polarised light microscopy. Ann Rheum Dis 63:709–717, 2004.

175. Matyas JR, Atley L, Ionescu M, et al. Analysis of cartilage biomarkers in the early phases of canine experimental osteoarthritis. Arthritis Rheum 50:543–552, 2004.

176. Pardy CK, Matyas JR, Zernicke RF. Doxycycline effects on mechanical and morphometrical properties of early- and late-stage osteoarthritic bone following anterior cruciate ligament injury. J Appl Physiol 97:1254–1260, 2004.

177. Liu W, Burton-Wurster N, Glant T, et al. Spontaneous and experimental osteoarthritis in dog: similarities and differences in proteoglycan levels. J Orthop Res 21:730–737, 2003.

178. Tashman S, Anderst W, Kolowich P, et al. Kinematics of the ACL-deficient canine knee during gait: serial changes over two years. J Orthop Res 22:931–941, 2004.

179. Anderst WJ, Les C, Tashman S. In vivo serial joint space measurements during dynamic loading in a canine model of osteoarthritis. Osteoarthritis Cartilage 13:808–816, 2005.

180. Pelletier JP, Jovanovic DV, Lascau-Coman V, et al. Selective inhibition of inducible nitric oxide synthase reduces progression of experimental osteoarthritis in vivo: possible link with the reduction in chondrocyte apoptosis and caspase 3 level. Arthritis Rheum 43:1290–1299, 2000.

181. Lavigne P, Benderdour M, Lajeunesse D, et al. Subchondral and trabecular bone metabolism regulation in canine experimental knee osteoarthritis. Osteoarthritis Cartilage 13:310–317, 2005.

182. Boileau C, Martel-Pelletier J, Moldovan F, et al. The in situ up-regulation of chondrocyte interleukin-1-converting enzyme and interleukin-18 levels in experimental osteoarthritis is mediated by nitric oxide. Arthritis Rheum 46:2637–2647, 2002.

183. Pelletier JP, Boileau C, Boily M, et al. The protective effect of licofelone on experimental osteoarthritis is correlated with the downregulation of gene expression and protein synthesis of several major cartilage catabolic factors: MMP-13, cathepsin K and aggrecanases. Arthritis Res Ther 7:R1091–1102, 2005.

184. Pelletier JP, Boileau C, Brunet J, et al. The inhibition of subchondral bone resorption in the early phase of experimental dog osteoarthritis by licofelone is associated with a reduction in the synthesis of MMP-13 and cathepsin K. Bone 34:527–538, 2004.

185. Trumble TN, Billinghurst RC, McIlwraith CW. Correlation of prostaglandin E2 concentrations in synovial fluid with ground reaction forces and clinical variables for pain or inflammation in dogs with osteoarthritis induced by transection of the cranial cruciate ligament. Am J Vet Res 65:1269–1275, 2004.

186. Lorenz H, Wenz W, Ivancic M, et al. Early and stable upregulation of collagen type II, collagen type I and YKL40 expression levels in cartilage during early experimental osteoarthritis occurs independent of joint location and histological grading. Arthritis Res Ther 7:R156–165, 2005.

187. Libicher M, Ivancic M, Höffmann M, et al. Early changes in experimental osteoarthritis using the Pond-Nuki dog model: technical procedure and initial results of in vivo MR imaging. Eur Radiol 15:390–394, 2005.

188. Hashimoto S, Takahashi K, Ochs RL, et al. Nitric oxide production and apoptosis in cells of the meniscus during experimental osteoarthritis. Arthritis Rheum 42:2123–2131, 1999.

189. Sah RL, Yang AS, Chen AC, et al. Physical properties of rabbit articular cartilage after transection of the anterior cruciate ligament. J Orthop Res 15:197–203, 1997.

190. Hellio Le Graverand MP, Vignon E, Otterness IG, et al. Early changes in lapine menisci during osteoarthritis development: Part I: cellular and matrix alterations. Osteoarthritis Cartilage 9:56–64, 2001.

191. Bluteau G, Conrozier T, Mathieu P, et al. Matrix metalloproteinase-1, -3, -13 and aggrecanase-1 and -2 are differentially expressed in experimental osteoarthritis. Biochim Biophys Acta 1526:147–158, 2001.

192. Hashimoto S, Creighton-Achermann L, Takahashi K, et al. Development and regulation of osteophyte formation during experimental osteoarthritis. Osteoarthritis Cartilage 10:180–187, 2002.

193. Wachsmuth L, Keiffer R, Juretschke HP, et al. In vivo contrast-enhanced micro MR-imaging of experimental osteoarthritis in the rabbit knee joint at 7.1T1. Osteoarthritis Cartilage 11:891–902, 2003.

194. Batiste DL, Kirkley A, Laverty S, et al. High-resolution MRI and micro-CT in an ex vivo rabbit anterior cruciate ligament transection model of osteoarthritis. Osteoarthritis Cartilage 12:614–626, 2004.

195. Batiste DL, Kirkley A, Laverty S, et al. Ex vivo characterization of articular cartilage and bone lesions in a rabbit ACL transection model of osteoarthritis using MRI and micro-CT. Osteoarthritis Cartilage 12:986–996, 2004.

196. Diaz-Gallego L, Prieto JG, Coronel P, et al. Apoptosis and nitric oxide in an experimental model of osteoarthritis in rabbit after hyaluronic acid treatment. J Orthop Res 23:1370–1376, 2005.

197. Tiraloche G, Girard C, Chouinard L, et al. Effect of oral glucosamine on cartilage degradation in a rabbit model of osteoarthritis. Arthritis Rheum 52:1118–1128, 2005.

198. Tibesku CO, Szuwart T, Ocken SA, et al. Increase in the expression of the transmembrane surface receptor CD44v6 on chondrocytes in animals with osteoarthritis. Arthritis Rheum 52:810–817, 2005.

199. Stoop R, Buma P, van der Kraan PM, et al. Differences in type II collagen degradation between peripheral and central cartilage of rat stifle joints after cranial cruciate ligament transection. Arthritis Rheum 43:2121–2131, 2000.

200. Stoop R, Buma P, van der Kraan P, et al. Type II collagen degradation in articular cartilage fibrillation after anterior cruciate ligament transection in rats. Osteoarthritis Cartilage 9:308–315, 2001.

201. Galois L, Etienne S, Grossin L, et al. Dose-response relationship for exercise on severity of experimental osteoarthritis in rats: a pilot study. Osteoarthritis Cartilage 12:779–786, 2004.

202. Hayami T, Pickarski M, Wesolowski GA, et al. The role of subchondral bone remodeling in osteoarthritis: reduction of cartilage degeneration and prevention of osteophyte formation by alendronate in the rat anterior cruciate ligament transection model. Arthritis Rheum 50:1193–1206, 2004.

203. Hayami T, Pickarski M, Zhuo Y, et al. Characterization of articular cartilage and subchondral bone changes in the rat anterior cruciate ligament transection and meniscectomized models of osteoarthritis. Bone 38:234–243, 2006.

204. Jimenez PA, Harlan PM, Chavarria AE, et al. Induction of osteoarthritis in guinea pigs by transection of the anterior cruciate ligament: radiographic and histopathological changes. Inflamm Res 44 Suppl 2:S129–130, 1995.

205. Boyd SK, Muller R, Leonard T, et al. Long-term periarticular bone adaptation in a feline knee injury model for post-traumatic experimental osteoarthritis. Osteoarthritis Cartilage 13:235–242, 2005.

206. O'Connor BL, Visco DM, Brandt KD, et al. Sensory nerves only temporarily protect the unstable canine knee joint from osteoarthritis. Evidence that sensory nerves reprogram the central nervous system after cruciate ligament transection. Arthritis Rheum 36:1154–1163, 1993.

207. Schiavinato A, Lini E, Guidolin D, et al. Intraarticular sodium hyaluronate injections in the Pond-Nuki experimental model of osteoarthritis in dogs. II. Morphological findings. Clin Orthop Relat Res:286–299, 1989.

208. Abatangelo G, Botti P, Del Bue M, et al. Intraarticular sodium hyaluronate injections in the Pond-Nuki experimental-model of osteoarthritis in dogs. 1: Biochemical results. Clin Orthop 241:278–285, 1989.

209. Gardner DL, Bradley WA, O'Connor P, et al. Synovitis after surgical division of the anterior cruciate ligament of the dog. Clin Exp Rheumatol 2:11–15, 1984.

210. Myers SL, Brandt KD, O'Connor BL, et al. Synovitis and osteoarthritic changes in canine articular cartilage after anterior cruciate ligament transection—effect of surgical hemostasis. Arthritis Rheum 33:1406–1415, 1990.

211. Brandt KD, Braunstein EM, Visco DM, et al. Anterior (cranial) cruciate ligament transection in the dog—A bona-fide model of osteoarthritis, not merely of cartilage injury and repair. J Rheumatol 18:436–446, 1991.

212. Bluteau G, Gouttenoire J, Conrozier T, et al. Differential gene expression analysis in a rabbit model of osteoarthritis induced by anterior cruciate ligament (ACL) section. Biorheology 39:247–258, 2002.

213. MacConaill MA. The function of intra-articular fibrocartilages, with special reference to the knee and inferior radioulnar joints. J Anat 66:210–217, 1931.

214. Levy IM, Torzilli PA, Gould JD, et al. The effect of lateral meniscectomy on motion of the knee. J Bone Joint Surg Am 71:401–406, 1989.

215. Seedhom BB. Loadbearing function of the menisci. Physiotherapy 62:223–226, 1976.

216. Krause WR, Pope MH, Johnson RJ, et al. Mechanical changes in the knee after meniscectomy. J Bone Joint Surg Am 58:599–604, 1976.

217. Walker PS, Erkman MJ. The role of the menisci in force transmission across the knee. Clin Orthop Relat Res:184–192, 1975.

218. Cargill AO, Jackson JP. Bucket-handle tear of the medial meniscus. A case for conservative surgery. J Bone Joint Surg Am 58:248–251, 1976.

219. Tapper EM, Hoover NW. Late results after meniscectomy. J Bone Joint Surg Am 51:517–526, 1969.

220. Fairbank TJ. Knee joint changes after meniscectomy. J Bone Joint Surg (Br) 30:664–670, 1948.

221. Calvo E, Palacios I, Delgado E, et al. High-resolution MRI detects cartilage swelling at the early stages of experimental osteoarthritis. Osteoarthritis Cartilage 9:463–472, 2001.

222. Gomez-Barrena E, Sanchez-Pernaute O, Largo R, et al. Sequential changes of parathyroid hormone related protein (PTHrP) in articular cartilage during progression of inflammatory and degenerative arthritis. Ann Rheum Dis 63:917–922, 2004.

223. Messner K, Fahlgren A, Ross I, et al. Simultaneous changes in bone mineral density and articular cartilage in a rabbit meniscectomy model of knee osteoarthrosis. Osteoarthritis Cartilage 8:197–206, 2000.

224. Calvo E, Palacios I, Delgado E, et al. Histopathological correlation of cartilage swelling detected by magnetic resonance imaging in early experimental osteoarthritis. Osteoarthritis Cartilage 12:878–886, 2004.

225. Lindhorst E, Wachsmuth L, Kimmig N, et al. Increase in degraded collagen type II in synovial fluid early in the rabbit meniscectomy model of osteoarthritis. Osteoarthritis Cartilage 13:139–145, 2005.

226. Sabatini M, Lesur C, Thomas M, et al. Effect of inhibition of matrix metalloproteinases on cartilage loss in vitro and in a guinea pig model of osteoarthritis. Arthritis Rheum 52:171–180, 2005.

227. Bendele AM. Progressive chronic osteoarthritis in femorotibial joints of partial medial meniscectomized guinea pigs. Vet Pathol 24:444–448, 1987.

228. Meacock SC, Bodmer JL, Billingham ME. Experimental osteoarthritis in guinea-pigs. J Exp Pathol (Oxford) 71:279–293, 1990.

229. Kobayashi T, Notoya K, Naito T, et al. Pioglitazone, a peroxisome proliferator-activated receptor gamma agonist, reduces the progression of experimental osteoarthritis in guinea pigs. Arthritis Rheum 52:479–487, 2005.

230. Kouri JB, Rojas L, Perez E, et al. Modifications of Golgi complex in chondrocytes from osteoarthrotic (OA) rat cartilage. J Histochem Cytochem 50:1333–1340, 2002.

231. Fernihough J, Gentry C, Malcangio M, et al. Pain related behaviour in two models of osteoarthritis in the rat knee. Pain 112:83–93, 2004.

232. Glasson S, Askew R, Sheppard B, et al. Characterization of and osteoarthritis susceptibility in ADAMTS-4-knockout mice. Arthritis Rheum. 50:2547–2558, 2004.

233. Ghosh P, Sutherland JM, Taylor TK, et al. The effects of postoperative joint immobilization on articular cartilage degeneration following meniscectomy. J Surg Res 35:461–473, 1983.

234. Ghosh P, Sutherland JM, Taylor TK, et al. The effect of bilateral medial meniscectomy on articular cartilage of the hip joint. J Rheumatol 11:197–201, 1984.

235. Elliott DM, Guilak F, Vail TP, et al. Tensile properties of articular cartilage are altered by meniscectomy in a canine model of osteoarthritis. J Orthop Res 17:503–508, 1999.

236. Lindhorst E, Vail TP, Guilak F, et al. Longitudinal characterization of synovial fluid biomarkers in the canine meniscectomy model of osteoarthritis. J Orthop Res 18:269–280, 2000.

237. Ghosh P, Sutherland J, Bellenger C, et al. The influence of weight-bearing exercise on articular cartilage of meniscectomized joints. An experimental study in sheep. Clin Orthop Relat Res:101–113, 1990.

238. Ghosh P, Burkhardt D, Read R, et al. Recent advances in animal models for evaluating chondroprotective drugs. J Rheumatol Suppl 27:143–146, 1991.

239. Armstrong SJ, Read RA, Ghosh P, et al. Moderate exercise exacerbates the osteoarthritic lesions produced in cartilage by menis-

240. Ghosh P, Numata Y, Smith S, et al. The metabolic response of articular cartilage to abnormal mechanical loading induced by medial or lateral meniscectomy. In: van den Berg WB, van der Kraan PM, van Lent P, eds. Joint Destruction on Arthritis and Osteoarthritis. Basel: Birkhauser Verlag, 89, 1993.

241. Armstrong S, Read R, Ghosh P. The effects of intraarticular hyaluronan on cartilage and subchondral bone changes in an ovine model of early osteoarthritis. J Rheumatol 21:680–688, 1994.

242. Ghosh P, Read R, Numata Y, et al. The effects of intraarticular administration of hyaluronan in a model of early osteoarthritis in sheep. II. Cartilage composition and proteoglycan metabolism. Semin Arthritis Rheum 22:31–42, 1993.

243. Ghosh P, Read R, Armstrong S, et al. The effects of intraarticular administration of hyaluronan in a model of early osteoarthritis in sheep. I. Gait analysis and radiological and morphological studies. Semin Arthritis Rheum 22:18–30, 1993.

244. Ghosh P, Holbert C, Read R, et al. Hyaluronic acid (hyaluronan) in experimental osteoarthritis. J Rheumatol Suppl 43:155–157, 1995.

245. Little CB, Ghosh P, Bellenger CR. Topographic variation in biglycan and decorin synthesis by articular cartilage in the early stages of osteoarthritis: an experimental study in sheep. J Orthop Res 14:433–444, 1996.

246. Little C, Smith S, Ghosh P, et al. Histomorphological and immunohistochemical evaluation of joint changes in a model of osteoarthritis induced by lateral meniscectomy in sheep. J Rheumatol 24:2199–2209, 1997.

247. Parker D, Hwa S-Y, Sambrook P, et al. Estrogen replacement therapy mitigates the loss of joint cartilage proteoglycans and bone mineral density induced by ovariectomy and osteoarthritis. APLAR J Rheumatol 6:116–127, 2003.

248. Oakley SP, Lassere MN, Portek I, et al. Biomechanical, histologic and macroscopic assessment of articular cartilage in a sheep model of osteoarthritis. Osteoarthritis Cartilage 12:667–679, 2004.

249. Cake MA, Read RA, Appleyard RC, et al. The nitric oxide donor glyceryl trinitrate increases subchondral bone sclerosis and cartilage degeneration following ovine meniscectomy. Osteoarthritis Cartilage 12:974–981, 2004.

250. Lufti AM. Morphological changes in the articular cartilage after meniscectomy. J Bone Joint Surg (Br) 57:525–528, 1975.

251. Moskowitz RW, Davis W, Sammarco J. Experimentally induced degenerative joint lesions following partial meniscectomy in the rabbit. Arthritis Rheum 16:397–405, 1973.

252. Moskowitz RW, Goldberg VM, Malemud CJ. Metabolic responses of cartilage in experimentally induced osteoarthritis. Ann Rheum Dis 40:584–592, 1981.

253. Moskowitz RW, Howell DS, Goldberg VM, et al. Cartilage proteoglycan alterations in an experimentally induced model of rabbit osteoarthritis. Arthritis Rheum 22:155–163, 1979.

254. Mayor MB, Moskowitz RW. Metabolic studies in experimentally-induced degenerative joint disease in the rabbit. J Rheumatol 1:17–23, 1974.

255. Appleyard RC, Burkhardt D, Ghosh P, et al. Topographical analysis of the structural, biochemical and dynamic biomechanical properties of cartilage in an ovine model of osteoarthritis. Osteoarthritis Cartilage 11:65–77, 2003.

256. King D. The healing of semilunar cartilages. J Bone Joint Surg (Br) 18:333–342, 1936.

257. Cox JS, Nye CE, Schaeffer WW, et al. The degenerative effects of partial and total resection of the medial meniscus in dogs' knees. Clin Orthop 109:178–183, 1975.

258. Ghosh P, Armstrong S, Read R, et al. Animal models of early osteoarthritis: Their use for the evaluation of potential chondroprotective agents. Agents Actions Suppl 39:195–206, 1993.

259. Ghosh P, Read R, Armstrong S, et al. High contact stress induced by meniscectomy results in cartilage and synovial fluid changes consistent with early osteoarthritis. Trans Comb Orthop Res:57, 1995.

260. Fukubayashi T, Kurosawa H. The contact area and pressure distribution pattern of the knee. A study of normal and osteoarthrotic knee joints. Acta Orthop Scand 51:871–879, 1980.

261. Bellenger CR, Pickles DM. Loadbearing in the ovine medial tibial condyle: effect of meniscectomy. Vet Comp Orthop Traumatol 6:100–104, 1993.

262. Rumph PF, Kincaid SA, Visco DM, et al. Redistribution of vertical ground reaction force in dogs with experimentally induced chronic hindlimb lameness. Vet Surg 24:384–389, 1995.

263. Kuo SY, Chu SJ, Hsu CM, et al. An experimental model of osteoarthritis in rabbit. Zhonghua Yi Xue Za Zhi (Taipei) 54:377–381, 1994.

264. Kawano T, Miura H, Mawatari T, et al. Mechanical effects of the intraarticular administration of high molecular weight hyaluronic acid plus phospholipid on synovial joint lubrication and prevention of articular cartilage degeneration in experimental osteoarthritis. Arthritis Rheum 48:1923–1929, 2003.

265. Hulmes DJ, Marsden ME, Strachan RK, et al. Intra-articular hyaluronate in experimental rabbit osteoarthritis can prevent changes in cartilage proteoglycan content. Osteoarthritis Cartilage 12:232–238, 2004.

266. Schwartz ER, Oh WH, Leveille CR. Experimentally induced osteoarthritis in guinea pigs—metabolic responses in articular cartilage to developing pathology. Arthritis Rheum 24:1345–1355, 1981.

267. Satsuma H, Saito N, Hamanishi C, et al. Alpha and epsilon isozymes of protein kinase C in the chondrocytes in normal and early osteoarthritic articular cartilage. Calcif Tissue Int 58:192–194, 1996.

268. Janusz MJ, Bendele AM, Brown KK, et al. Induction of osteoarthritis in the rat by surgical tear of the meniscus: Inhibition of joint damage by a matrix metalloproteinase inhibitor. Osteoarthritis Cartilage 10:785–791, 2002.

269. Roberts MJ, Adams SB, Jr., Patel NA, et al. A new approach for assessing early osteoarthritis in the rat. Anal Bioanal Chem 377:1003–1006, 2003.

270. Wancket LM, Baragi V, Bove S, et al. Anatomical localization of cartilage degradation markers in a surgically induced rat osteoarthritis model. Toxicol Pathol 33:484–489, 2005.

271. Moore EE, Bendele AM, Thompson DL, et al. Fibroblast growth factor-18 stimulates chondrogenesis and cartilage repair in a rat model of injury-induced osteoarthritis. Osteoarthritis Cartilage 13:623–631, 2005.

272. Kamekura S, Hoshi K, Shimoaka T, et al. Osteoarthritis development in novel experimental mouse models induced by knee joint instability. Osteoarthritis Cartilage 13:632–641, 2005.

273. Marijnissen AC, van Roermund PM, Verzijl N, et al. Steady progression of osteoarthritic features in the canine groove model. Osteoarthritis Cartilage 10:282–289, 2002.

274. Mastbergen SC, Marijnissen AC, Vianen ME, et al. The canine 'groove' model of osteoarthritis is more than simply the expression of surgically applied damage. Osteoarthritis Cartilage. 14:39–46, 2006.

275. Hulth A, Lindberg L, Telhag H. Experimental osteoarthritis in rabbits: preliminary report. Acta Orthop Scand 41:522–530, 1970.

276. Colombo C, Butler M, O'Byrne E, et al. A new model of osteoarthritis in rabbits. I. Development of knee joint pathology following lateral meniscectomy and section of the fibular collateral and sesamoid ligaments. Arthritis Rheum 26:875–886, 1983.

277. Panula HE, Hyttinen MM, Arokoski JP, et al. Articular cartilage superficial zone collagen birefringence reduced and cartilage thickness increased before surface fibrillation in experimental osteoarthritis. Ann Rheum Dis 57:237–245, 1998.

278. Panula HE, Helminen HJ, Kiviranta I. Slowly progressive osteoarthritis after tibial valgus osteotomy in young beagle dogs. Clin Orthop Relat Res 343:192–202, 1997.

279. Olah EH, Kostenszky KS. Effect of loading and prednisolone treatment on the glycosaminoglycan content of articular cartilage in dogs. Scand J Rheumatol 5:49–52, 1976.

280. Arsever CL, Bole GG. Experimental osteoarthritis induced by selective myectomy and tendotomy. Arthritis Rheum 29:251–261, 1986.

281. Lefkoe TP, Walsh WR, Anastasatos J, et al. Remodeling of articular step-offs. Is osteoarthrosis dependent on defect size? Clin Orthop Relat Res 253–265, 1995.

282. Lefkoe TP, Trafton PG, Ehrlich MG, et al. An experimental model of femoral condylar defect leading to osteoarthrosis. J Orthop Trauma 7:458–467, 1993.

283. Altman RD, Kates J, Chun LE, et al. Preliminary observations of chondral abrasion in a canine model. Ann Rheum Dis 51:1056–1062, 1992.

284. Ogi N, Ishimaru J, Kurita K, et al. Comparison of different methods of temporomandibular joint disc reconstruction—an animal model. Aust Dent J 42:121–124, 1997.

285. Collier MA, Burba DA, DeBault LE, et al. In vivo kinetic study of intramuscular tritium-labeled polysulphated glycosaminoglycan in equine body fluid compartments and articular cartilage in an arthritis model. Acta Vet Scand Suppl 87:266–267, 1992.

286. Ghosh P. Role of biomechanical factors in osteoarthritis. In: Reginster J-Y, Pelletier JP, Martel-Pelletier J, al. e, eds. Osteoarthritis: clinical and experimental. Heidelberg: Springer-Verlag, 1999, p 111.

287. Videman T, Eronen I, Candolin T. Effects of motion load changes on tendon tissues and articular cartilage. A biochemical and scanning electron microscopic study on rabbits. Scand J Work Environ Health 5(suppl 3):56–67, 1979.

288. Kiviranta I, Tammi M, Jurvelin J, et al. Moderate running exercise augments glycosaminoglycans and thickness of articular cartilage in the knee joint of young beagle dogs. J Orthop Res 6:188–195, 1988.

289. Norrdin R, Kawcak C, Capwell B, et al. Subchondral bone failure in an equine model of overload arthrosis. Bone 22:133–139, 1998.

290. Little C, Ghosh P, Rose R. The effect of strenuous versus moderate exercise on the metabolism of proteoglycans in articular cartilage from different weight-bearing regions of the equine third carpal bone. Osteoarthritis Cartilage 5:161–172, 1997.

291. Haut RC, Ide TM, De Camp CE. Mechanical responses of the rabbit patello-femoral joint to blunt impact. J Biomech Eng 117:402–408, 1995.

292. Lukoschek M, Boyd RD, Schaffler MB, et al. Comparison of joint degeneration models - surgical instability and repetitive impulsive loading. Acta Orthop Scand 57:349–353, 1986.

293. Radin EL, Martin RB, Burr DB, et al. Effects of mechanical loading on the tissues of the rabbit knee. J Orthopaedic Res 2:221–234, 1984.

294. Thompson RC, Oegema TR, Lewis JL, et al. Osteoarthrotic changes after acute transarticular loa—An animal model. J Bone Joint Surg [Am] 73:990–1001, 1991.

Molecular Genetics of Osteoarthritis

6

John Loughlin   Kay Chapman

OUTLINE

There has long been a suspicion that genes play a role in the development of osteoarthritis (OA). However, it is only in the last 10 years that comprehensive epidemiological studies have enabled scientists to construct a reasonably clear picture of the extent and likely nature of the OA genetic component. We now know that OA is a multifactorial disease with a major polygenic element. This genetic susceptibility shows heterogeneity between different skeletal sites and, possibly, between the two sexes. Genes harboring common OA risk alleles are now being reported in reasonably powerful, and therefore robust, linkage and association studies. Several of these genes code for proteins that regulate cartilage homeostasis, but effects on other tissues of the synovial joint cannot be ruled out. Identifying OA susceptibility genes will enhance our understanding of this common arthritis and will assist in the development of new treatments. It will also help in the identification of individuals at increased risk and will aid the characterization of the environmental factors that can also influence OA aetiology. This chapter will focus on the most compelling findings from the numerous linkage and association studies that have been performed. It will bring the reader up-to-date on the molecular genetics of this common disease.

OA can exist in two main forms: primary OA and secondary OA. Primary, or idiopathic, OA is the common late-onset form of the disease with radiographic evidence first detectable in the fifth decade. It has no obvious cause and is either localized to a particular joint group or more generalized. Secondary OA arises in response to clearly identifiable factors such as trauma, or a congenital or a developmental abnormality. In a small number of cases, secondary OA is associated with developmental abnormalities that are transmitted as mendelian traits. These diseases are members of the osteochondrodysplasia class of skeletal dysplasias and the OA in these familial cases is often early

onset, precocious, and severe. Linkage and positional cloning has identified the disease genes and causal mutations in several of the osteochondrodysplasias. Because primary OA is the form of OA that impacts most significantly in the population, it is the form that we will concentrate on in this chapter.

Geneticists studying OA have used several strategies to try and identify susceptibility genes. These include candidate gene studies based solely on biological clues, systematic and model-free genome-wide linkage and association scans, and gene expression studies. These investigations are beginning to yield compelling data. They will each be discussed in turn.

Candidate Gene Studies

Without any prior linkage data to guide them toward particular chromosomal locations, a number of investigators have used their biological understanding of OA to select candidate genes for association studies. The initial candidate gene studies focused on genes that code for cartilage extracellular matrix (ECM) structural proteins. These included *COL2A1*, which codes for the α1 polypeptide chain of type II collagen, the principal collagenous component of articular cartilage. Other cartilage collagen genes studied included the type IX and type XI collagen genes and genes coding for noncollagenous components of the ECM, such as the cartilage oligomeric matrix protein gene (COMP) and the aggrecan gene *AGC1*. On the whole, these studies did not yield convincing data to support a role for common, nonsynonymous mutations in cartilage ECM structural protein genes as risk factors for primary OA.[1,2] It must be concluded, therefore, that these genes have never undergone a mutational event within their amino acid coding sequence that predisposes to primary OA or that if such mutations have occurred, these mutations do not have a sufficiently high frequency to confer a significant population risk.[3]

127

Concurrent with the analysis of ECM structural protein genes, a number of investigators focused on genes coding for proteins influencing bone density. This was driven by the observation that subchondral sclerosis is an early observation in some OA joints and the subsequent suggestion that this sclerosis might damage the cartilage by adversely affecting the transmittance of mechanical load. The vitamin D receptor gene VDR and the estrogen receptor gene (ESR1) have both been investigated by a number of groups. Early studies demonstrated association of both genes with OA. However, these associations were not replicated in all subsequent investigations.[1,2] This is to be expected for a common complex disease such as OA and highlights the fact that any single locus will have at most only a moderate effect on disease occurrence in the population under investigation. A reasonable number of positive reports are now being published, particularly for ESR1.[4] Common variants within this gene are therefore likely to be OA risk factors.

Conclusions

As with other complex disease investigations, OA association studies often suffer from a number of shortcomings. These include the analysis of cohorts of relatively small size and the genotyping of only a few of the known DNA variants within the gene under investigation. The former should be unnecessary for a common disease like OA and makes many studies underpowered and liable to false positives. The latter is becoming avoidable as the cost of genotyping falls and as databases of common variants become more comprehensive in their coverage. Future OA association studies should be designed with these two considerations in mind.

Candidate gene studies have shed some light on OA genetic susceptibility. However, they are constrained by our incomplete knowledge of the biology of OA, which makes candidate selection a fallible act. Investigators have therefore taken a more systematic approach, including genome-wide linkage scans.

GENOME-WIDE LINKAGE SCANS

Four OA genome-wide scans have so far been published, based on small families of affected relatives collected in the U.K.,[5,6] Finland,[7] Iceland,[8] and the USA.[9,10] The U.K. scan was performed on patients ascertained by hip or knee OA, the other scans on patients with hand OA. The hand OA scans were performed using either a global hand OA score or by focusing on particular joints of the hand.

The United Kingdom Study

The first OA genome-wide linkage scan was published by an Oxford group in 1999 and was performed on 481 pedigrees that each contained at least one OA-affected sibling pair (ASP) ascertained by total joint replacement of the hip or the knee.[5,6] With this ascertainment, the investigators were

treating the disease as a discreet trait, since subjects either had or had not undergone joint replacement. The investigators were also focussing on pedigrees that had severe, end-stage OA. Linkages were initially reported to chromosomes 2 and 11, and these were found to be particularly relevant to ASPs concordant for hip OA (chromosome 2) and to female ASPs concordant for hip OA (chromosome 11). A subsequent stratification of the genome scan by sex and by joint replaced (hip or knee) uncovered additional linkages, on chromosome 4 in female ASPs, chromosome 6 in hip ASPs, and chromosome 16 in female ASPs.[6] These were important findings not only because they pointed toward areas of the genome that may encode for OA susceptibility but because they also suggested differences in the nature of the susceptibility between males and females and between different skeletal sites, something that had been suggested by previous epidemiological studies.[1,2]

This original genome scan employed an average of just one microsatellite marker every 15 centiMorgan (cM). This medium density meant that the linkage intervals were relatively large. The Oxford investigators therefore subjected each locus to finer linkage mapping in an expanded cohort of 571 OA pedigrees. This analysis, which employed an average marker density of one marker every 5 cM, succeeded in narrowing each of the linkages and also confirmed or refined their restriction to particular strata. For example, the chromosome 6 linkage was narrowed from a 50-cM interval in hip ASPs to a 12-cM interval in female-hip ASPs. The results of the finer linkage mapping have been published[11–15] and are summarized in Table 6–1. The most significant evidence for linkage from the Oxford study is a logarithm of the odds (LOD) score of 4.8 on chromosome 6.

The Finnish Study

The Finnish scan was performed on 27 pedigrees that each contained at least two affected siblings with radiographic distal interphalangeal (DIP) OA.[7] Nine genomic regions supported linkage and the genotyping of these in additional pedigree members confirmed linkage to chromosomes 2q, 4q, 7p, and the Xcen (Table 6–1). The 2q and 4q linkages do not show overlap with the finer linkage mapped 2q and 4q intervals from the Oxford study and therefore probably represent different loci. The Finnish 2q linkage encompasses the interleukin-1 (IL-1) receptor and ligand gene cluster at 2q12-q13. This cluster has now been associated with OA (discussed later).

The Iceland Study

A genome-wide linkage scan utilizing 1000 microsatellites was performed on 329 Icelandic families containing 1143 individuals with primary hand OA and 939 of their relatives.[8] Each family contained at least two affected individuals related to each other at or within five meioses. Individuals were classed as having hand OA if they exhibited at least two nodes at the DIP joints of each hand or if they demonstrated squaring or dislocation of the first carpometacarpal (CMC1) thumb joint. The highest LOD

TABLE 6–1
LOCI IDENTIFIED FROM THE FOUR OA GENOME-WIDE LINKAGE SCANS

Country	Locus	Strata	LOD	Ref
UK	2q24.3–q31.1	Hip	1.6	11
	4q13.1–q13.2	Female hip	3.1	14
	6p12.3–q13	Female hip	4.8	13,15
	11q13.4–q14.3	Female hip	2.4	12
	16p12.3–p12.1	Female hip	1.7	14
	16q22.1–q23.1	Females	1.9	14
Finland	2q12–q21	Hand (DIP[a]), knee, and hip	2.3	7
	4q26–q27	Hand (DIP[a])	1.9	7
	7p15–p21	Hand (DIP[a])	1.4	7
	Xcen	Hand (DIP[a])	1.0	7
Iceland	19q12–q13.33	Hand	1.83	8
	2p23.2	Hand	1.48	8
	3p13	Hand	1.79	8
	4q32.2	Hand	2.61	8
	2p24.1	CMC1[b] and DIP[a]	4.97	8
	3p13	DIP[a]	1.84	8
	4q32.1	DIP[a]	3.29	8
USA	1p31.1	Hand	2.96	9
	2p23.2	Hand	2.23	9
	7p14.3	Hand	2.32	9
	9q21.2	Hand	2.29	9
	11q13.4	Hand	1.60	9
	12q24.33	Hand	1.66	9
	13q14.11–q14.3	Hand	1.61	9
	19q12–q13.33	Hand	1.83	9
	7q35–q36.1	DIP[a]	3.06	10
	15q22.31–q26.1	CMC1[b]	6.25	10

[a]DIP, distal interphalangeal joint; [b]CMC1, first carpometacarpal joint.

score observed was on chromosome 4 (LOD = 2.61), followed by chromosomes 3 (LOD = 1.79) and 2 (LOD = 1.48) (Table 6–1). The scan was subsequently stratified by site into a DIP cohort (274 families), a CMC1 cohort (204 families), and a DIP and CMC1 cohort (142 families). Linkage in the stratified analysis highlighted the same linkages as those observed in the unstratified scan. However, the evidence for linkage increased at chromosomes 2 and 4, with a LOD score of 4.97 for the CMC1 stratum on chromosome 2, and a LOD score of 3.29 for chromosome 4 in the DIP stratum (Table 6–1). The Icelandic group have gone on to identify an associated variant within the matrilin 3 gene *MATN3* located within their 2p linkage.

The USA Study

The USA study involved 296 small, two-generational families composed of 684 parents and 793 of their offspring from the Framingham cohort.[9,10] Hand OA was characterized radiographically and was assessed in the late 1960s and again in the early 1990s for the parents, and in the 1990s for the offspring. The investigators performed a quantitative linkage analysis that separately tested the degree of joint space narrowing (JSN) and the frequency of osteophytes. They also investigated an overall radiographic score based on the Kellgren and Lawrence (K/L) grading scheme. Linkage was reported to eight chromosomal regions, with the highest LOD score being 2.96 for chromosome 1 in the JSN criteria (Table 6–1). For the overall radiographic score, no LOD exceeded 1.9, and so phenotypic definition was reconsidered by stratifying the linkage scan according to OA disease status in particular joints of the hand that are most susceptible to OA, namely, the DIP joints, the thumb interphalangeal (IP) joint, the proximal interphalangeal (PIP) joint, the metacarpophalangeal (MCP) joints, the wrist joints, and the CMC1 joint at the base of each thumb.[10] This revealed two new loci, one on chromosome 7q in the DIP stratum with a LOD score of 3.06, and one on chromosome 15q in the CMC1 stratum with a LOD score of 6.25 (Table 6–1). Stratification by joint and by sex revealed two further loci in females, one on chromosome 1q in the DIP stratum with a LOD score of 3.03, and one on chromosome 20p in the CMC1 stratum with a LOD score of 3.74. Overall, the USA study had identified at least 12 loci, several of which are restricted to particular joints of the hand.

Intriguingly, the chromosome 2p locus identified in the USA study directly overlapped with the 2p locus identified in the Iceland scan. This might therefore represent an independent confirmation, although a skeptic could argue that so many loci were detected in the USA study, many with relatively low LOD scores, that an overlap is likely to happen by chance alone. Nevertheless, the fact that the Icelandic group has gone on to identify an associated variant within *MATN3* at the 2p locus means that an analysis of this gene in the USA cohort is merited.

Other Osteoarthritis Linkage Studies

As well as the four genome-wide linkage scans reported above, a number of investigators have targeted specific chromosomal regions based on the data from the genome scans. Two groups have investigated the chromosome 6 locus reported by the Oxford study. A Netherlands group investigated 100 small pedigrees composed of probands and their siblings whose OA disease status was assessed radiographically using the K/L scale.[16] Linkage to chromosome 6 was reported in sibling pairs concordant for hip OA but not in sibling pairs concordant for knee, hand, or spinal OA. An Irish group investigated 109 small pedigrees composed of sibling pairs ascertained by hip replacement.[17] No evidence for linkage to chromosome 6 was obtained. The Oxford study had reported that their chromosome 6 linkage was restricted to female sibling pairs concordant for hip OA. Of the 109 pedigrees in the Irish study, only 32 were female-hip sibling pairs. The Irish study therefore had little power to confirm the Oxford report and is likely to represent a false negative result. A group from Israel has investigated linkage to the chromosome 11 locus reported by the Oxford group.[18] This study was conducted on a panel of 295 pedigrees derived from a relatively isolated population of Chuvashians from southern Russia whose hand-OA status had been previously determined using the K/L scale. Moderate evidence of linkage was obtained to the same chromosome 11 locus as that reported by the Oxford group.

Conclusions

The OA genome-wide linkage scans so far reported have revealed some compelling loci based on reasonably high LOD scores for a complex disease (Table 6–1). Several loci also show overlap between the different scans. An important observation from the Iceland and USA scans is that stratification of the hand into its component joints provides more significant evidence for linkage. This highlights the subtle and highly complex way in which OA genetic susceptibility is acting. The U.K. and USA studies stratified their scans by sex and subsequently identified novel loci that were particularly relevant to OA occurrence in women. This supports several epidemiological studies that have suggested that the role of genes in OA may vary between the two sexes.[1,2] More targeted linkage studies have provided some confirmatory evidence for some of the loci detected through the genome scans; however, not all follow-up studies have been positive. This is to be expected for a complex trait where susceptibility loci will have varying frequencies between different cohorts and may be interacting with other loci, or nongenetic factors, in a population-specific manner. Complex traits are, as the name suggests, complex and our understanding of the innumerable factors that interact in their etiology is still at a very basic level.

OSTEOARTHRITIS SUSCEPTIBILITY GENES DETECTED VIA THE GENOME-WIDE LINKAGE SCANS

The genome-wide scans reviewed above have identified a number of relatively broad genomic intervals that may harbor OA susceptibility loci. Several of these intervals have now been subjected to association analyses—principally candidate gene–based studies—and have yielded a number of associated genes.

IL1 Gene Cluster: Chromosome 2q11.2-q13

Although OA is not an inflammatory arthritis, there are instances in which an inflamed synovium can exacerbate the disease. Furthermore, inflammatory mediators such as interleukins are synthesised by articular cartilage chondrocytes and can act in a paracrine and autocrine manner to influence cartilage tissue homeostasis.[19,20] Genes encoding interleukins are therefore plausible OA-susceptibility loci. This notion was supported by the Finnish genome-wide scan discussed above, which reported evidence for linkage to an interval on chromosome 2q that encompassed the interleukin 1 gene cluster. This cluster, which resides at 2q11.2-q13 and covers approximately 12 Mb, contains at least 11 family members. The archetypal members, and those that have been subjected to considerable investigation, are *IL1A* (encoding IL-1α), *IL1B* (encoding IL-1β), *IL1RN* (encoding IL-1 receptor antagonist), and *IL1R1* (encoding the signalling receptor for the above proteins).

The early OA association studies of the IL-1 gene cluster that were reported in the late 1990s and early 2000s were, on the whole, ambiguous, with only marginal evidence for association to OA reported.[1,2] These studies had several weaknesses, including small sample sizes and the analysis of only a small proportion of the known gene variants. In 2004, two new studies were reported that alleviated some of these weaknesses.

The first study, by a group from the Netherlands,[21] was a prospective, population-based analysis of Caucasians from the Rotterdam Elderly Study. A radiographic assessment of the OA status of the hip, knee, hand, and spine was conducted on 886 individuals (347 women, 520 men, and 19 subjects of unrecorded sex) aged between 55 and 65 years. The frequencies of OA were 8% for the hip, 16% for the knee, 4% for the hand, and 62% for the spine, with 17% having no radiographic OA at any of these sites. The patients were genotyped for a single-nucleotide polymorphism (SNP) located within exon 5 of *IL1B* (3953), for a SNP located upstream of *IL1B* (511), and for a variable number of tandem repeat (VNTR) polymorphism located within intron 2 of *IL1RN*. None of the variants was associated with OA when the cohort was analyzed unstratified. However, following stratification by site, the three variants each demonstrated association with hip OA, with *P*-values ranging from 0.004 to 0.001. A haplotype analysis identified a risk and a protective haplotype. Further analyses implied that the three variants themselves were not directly responsible for the associations but were instead in linkage disequilibrium with as yet unidentified functional variants.

The second study, conducted by a group from the U.K. was a case–control association analysis.[22] The cases had radiographically diagnosed knee OA and were collected from two U.K. centers: 141 patients from Bristol (76 females and 65 males, mean age of 62 years) and 163 patients from London (125 females and 38 males, mean age of 71 years). All cases had OA as defined by the American College of Rheumatology (ACR) criteria with at least grade 2 radiological changes. The controls were 195 unrelated healthy blood donors (98 females and 97 males with an unspecified mean age). All individuals were U.K. Caucasians. The cases and controls were genotyped for nine *IL1R1* promoter variants (seven SNPs, one insertion/deletion [indel], and one microsatellite), for two *IL1A* variants (a promoter SNP and a microsatellite located in intron 4), for three *IL1B* variants (the 3953 and 511 SNPs genotyped in the Netherlands study, and a promoter SNP), and for three *IL1RN* variants (the VNTR genotyped in the Netherlands study, a SNP located in intron 3, and a SNP located in exon 4). A linkage disequilibrium analysis revealed that the nine *IL1R1* variants were in strong linkage disequilibrium with each other, as were the eight variants within *IL1A*, *IL1B*, and *IL1RN*. However, *IL1R1* showed only weak linkage disequilibrium with the *IL1A-IL1B-IL1RN* complex, and so these were investigated separately. A haplotype analysis of the nine *IL1R1* variants provided no evidence for association ($P > 0.05$) in either the Bristol or the London cases. However, an analysis of the eight variants within the *IL1A–IL1B–IL1RN* complex provided evidence for an associated risk haplotype in both the Bristol ($P = 0.00043$) and the London ($P = 0.02$) cases. In addition, a protective haplotype was also identified in this complex in the Bristol ($P = 0.0036$) and the London ($P = 0.0000008$) cohorts. These associations were not restricted by sex.

Following the original publications, the U.K. and the Netherlands groups both expanded their studies using each other's findings.[23] The U.K. group investigated hip OA, ascertained by joint replacement. Although the case cohort was small, with only 22 individuals, the use of the eight variants within the *IL1A–IL1B–IL1RN* complex provided very strong evidence for association ($P = 0.0000003$). The Netherlands group increased the number of variants genotyped, thus enabling them to do a comprehensive haplotype analysis akin to the U.K. group. This enabled the Netherlands group to increase the evidence for their hip association. The use of complex haplotypes therefore enabled both groups to identify alleles within the *IL1* gene cluster that increase the risk of hip OA.

MATN3: Chromosome 2p24.1

As noted earlier, a linkage to chromosome 2p has been reported in an Icelandic hand OA cohort.[8] This linkage encompassed *MATN3*, which encodes matrilin 3, an oligomeric protein present in cartilage ECM. The Icelandic group screened the exons and promoter of this candidate gene for common variants in 76 patients and 18 control individuals. Seven SNPs and one indel were identified. The six variants with frequencies greater than 0.05 were genotyped in a larger cohort of 745 patients and 368 controls.

Only one variant showed a significantly greater frequency ($P < 0.05$) in patients versus controls: a nonsynonymous SNP within exon 3 that is predicted to encode the substitution of a threonine by a methionine in the first epidermal growth factor domain of matrilin 3. A subsequent genotyping of a total of 2162 patients and 873 controls reaffirmed the association. However, when the original linkage analysis for chromosome 2p was performed following removal of the mutation carriers, the LOD score remained relatively high, at 3.8. This suggests that other variants, either within the regulatory elements or noncoding regions of *MATN3* or within other nearby genes, must be coding for a significant proportion of the chromosome 2p OA susceptibility. This story is, therefore, still a work in progress.

IL4R: Chromosome 16p12.1

As noted above, an Oxford group has reported a linkage to chromosome 16p in affected sibling-pair families containing females with hip OA. A search of public databases within the linkage interval highlighted the IL-4 receptor α-chain gene *IL4R* (16p12.1) as a strong candidate.[14] IL-4 is a pleiotropic cytokine that is expressed, along with its receptor, in many cell types including adult articular cartilage. Cartilage integrity is partly regulated by mechanotransduction, and IL-4 and its receptor have a pivotal role in the cartilage chondrocyte response to mechanical signals.[24] Molecular genetic analyses of *IL4R* have identified several common coding polymorphisms. As a first stage in the analysis of *IL4R*, the Oxford group genotyped nine common *IL4R* SNPs in the 146 female-hip probands from the families that had provided the 16p linkage and in 399 age-matched female controls.[25] Two of the nine SNPs were located in the *IL4R* promoter, with the remaining seven located in the coding sequence (six nonsynonymous and one synonymous). Two nonsynonymous SNPs were associated in the 146 probands at $P < 0.05$. These two SNPs were also associated in an independent cohort of 310 females with hip OA, as were two other SNPs, while a third approached significance ($P = 0.07$). Five of the nine variants therefore showed some evidence for association to hip OA in female Caucasians. These five positive SNPs defined two distinct groups, with members of each group being in relatively strong linkage disequilibrium with each other. Possessing a copy of an associated allele from both SNP groups was a particular risk factor, with an odds ratio (OR) of 2.4 (95% confidence interval [CI] 1.5-4.1) and a P-value of 0.0008.

FRZB: Chromosome 2q32.1

The chromosome 2q locus identified by the Oxford genome-wide linkage scan mapped to 2q24.3-q31.1.[11] This linkage was restricted to affected sibling-pair families concordant for hip OA and encompassed eight plausible candidate genes: the TNF-α-induced protein 6 gene *TNFAIP6*, the activin A receptor gene *ACVR1*, the fibroblast activation protein α gene *FAP*, the integrin alpha 6 gene *ITGA6*, the activating transcription factor 2 gene *ATF2*, the integrin alpha 4 gene *ITGA4*, the secreted frizzled-related protein 3 gene *SFRP3* (more commonly termed *FRZB*), and the integrin alpha V gene *ITGAV*. Microsatellites within or near to the eight candidates were genotyped in the 378 probands (220 females and 158 males) from the hip families that had provided the linkage and in 760 age-matched controls (399 females and 361 males). Microsatellites targeting *TNFAIP6*, *ITGA6*, and *FRZB* were associated at *P* <0.05.[26] The *TNFAIP6* association was present in all cases whereas the *ITGA6* and *FRZB* associations were restricted to females. Subsequent SNP searches identified a nonsynonymous SNP in *TNFAIP6*, two nonsynonymous SNPs in *FRZB*, but no nonsynonymous SNPs in *ITGA6*. Genotyping of the *TNFAIP6* and *FRZB* SNPs revealed association only to one of the two *FRZB* SNPs, with a *P*-value of 0.04 in the female-hip cases. An additional cohort of 338 female hip cases also showed association to this SNP (*P* = 0.04). The two *FRZB* SNPs are both predicted to encode for the substitution of highly conserved arginine residues—the first in exon 4 (Arg200Trp) and the second in exon 6 (Arg324Gly). It was the exon 6 SNP that was associated. Individuals who possessed a copy of both substituted arginines were at an increased risk of developing OA, with an OR of 3.6 (95% CI 1.6-8.3) and *P*-value of 0.003. This risk was increased in those who had both arginines substituted in the same protein molecule, with an OR of 4.1 (95% CI 1.6-10.7).

The *FRZB* gene product acts as an antagonist of extracellular Wnt ligands.[27] The Wnt signaling pathway has a crucial role in chondrogenesis and secreted frizzled-related protein 3, which is synthesised by adult articular chondrocytes, has been shown to control chondrocyte maturation.[28] Wnt signaling regulates the accumulation of cytoplasmic β-catenin. In the absence of Wnt, the β-catenin is rapidly degraded, whereas in the presence of Wnt, the β-catenin accumulates, is translocated to the nucleus, and instigates gene transcription. The ability of wild-type secreted frizzled-related protein 3 and of the Arg200Trp and Arg324Gly substituted proteins to antagonise Wnt-signalling was therefore investigated by transient transfection of HEK293 cells. Whereas the wild-type protein efficiently inhibited Wnt activity, the Arg324Gly substitution and the Arg200Trp/Arg324Gly double substitution had diminished activity. Similarly, HEK293 cells transfected with the plasmid containing the Arg324Gly substitution required higher levels of expressing plasmid to modestly decrease free cytosolic and nuclear levels of β-catenin. These results clearly demonstrated that the conserved arginines are functionally important, with their substitution reducing the ability of secreted frizzled-related protein 3 to antagonize Wnt signaling.

A Netherlands group very recently genotyped the two FRZB SNPs in a random sample of 1,369 subjects from a population-based cohort scored for radiographic OA in the hip, hand, spine, and knee and in a patient population of 191 ASPs with symptomatic OA at multiple sites.[29] Neither SNP demonstrated association in subjects with hip OA. However, the G-allele of the Arg324Gly SNP was associated (*P* <0.05) in individuals with a generalized OA phenotype. This phenotype constituted OA in at least two of four joint sites (hand, knee, hip, and spine). This is potentially a very important report as it may represent an independent replication, albeit in generalized OA rather than in hip OA, of the original FRZB association. Replicating associations for

complex traits is extremely important in that it not only helps to distinguish true positives from false positives but also provides information regarding the global relevance of a reported find.

LRP5: Chromosome 11q13.2

The chromosome 11 linkage reported by the Oxford and Israel groups encompasses another member of the Wnt-signaling pathway: the low-density lipoprotein receptor-related protein 5 gene *LRP5*. The musculoskeletal community has subjected this gene to considerable investigation since its identification as the susceptibility locus for the osteoporosis-pseudoglioma syndrome[30] and for a high bone mass phenotype.[31] A U.K. group genotyped five LRP5 SNPs in a cohort of 268 cases with knee OA defined using ACR criteria and in 187 controls.[32] No SNP showed evidence of association. However, a haplotype analysis revealed significant differences in haplotype frequencies between the cases and the controls. Since the samples sizes used in this study are relatively small, the results are best considered at this stage as a preliminary indication of an *LRP5* association with OA.

BMP5: Chromosome 6p12.1

The Oxford chromosome 6 linkage was centered at 6p12.3-q13 and was restricted to affected sibling-pair families containing females with hip OA.[13] The linkage encompassed two strong candidate genes: *BMP5* (6p12.1), which encodes bone morphogenetic protein 5, and *COL9A1* (6q13), which encodes the α1 polypeptide chain of type IX collagen. Bone morphogenetic protein 5 is a regulator of articular chondrocyte development,[33] whereas type IX collagen is a quantitatively minor cartilage collagen required for maintaining cartilage integrity.[34] The Oxford group detected all common coding polymorphisms within the two genes but none was associated with OA.[13,35] They subsequently genotyped a relatively high density of microsatellite markers within the linked interval, at an average marker interval of 0.36 cM.[36] Linkage was confirmed, with a LOD score of 4.8. When each marker was tested for association, a marker within intron 1 of *BMP5* was associated (*P* <0.05), as were two markers located immediately downstream of the gene. Mouse studies have revealed that the regulation of the expression of *BMP5* is complex and involves a number of *cis* elements, some of which can reside at some distance from the gene.[37] The Oxford group therefore concluded that variation in *cis* regulatory elements of *BMP5* that influence expression of the gene, as opposed to variants that result in nonsynonymous changes, which they had previously examined and excluded, could account for the linkage result. Any such *cis* variants have not yet been identified, so this conclusion must be considered speculative at this stage.

Conclusions

Candidate gene studies within regions highlighted by genome-wide linkage scans are beginning to yield OA-associated genes. However, several outstanding issues need to be considered regarding the latest results. For example, why do certain associations appear particularly relevant to certain joint sites or to one sex? This implies that there are fundamental differences in the nature of OA genetic susceptibility between different sites and between the two sexes: is this likely or are the studies underpowered to detect associations in all strata? Clarity will come once much larger cohort sizes are investigated. Another important question is do the associations have a broad ethnic relevance or are they restricted to particular populations? To answer this, those in possession of OA cohorts should make it a priority to genotype at least the associated SNPs in their cohorts. Subsequent meta-analyses should enable an accurate determination of how robust and how widespread the associations are.

OSTEOARTHRITIS SUSCEPTIBILITY GENES DETECTED VIA GENOME-WIDE ASSOCIATION STUDIES

Genome-wide linkage scans have been the bedrock for the genetic analysis of common diseases. They provide broad but manageable genomic intervals that can then be interrogated in detail. Their time, however, is drawing to an end, with genome-wide association studies offering a more comprehensive and powerful alternative. This has been driven by major advances in bioinformatics, in the categorization of all common DNA variants within the human genome, in the development of relatively cheap and reliable genotyping platforms, and in the development of robust statistical tools for analyzing the enormous amount of data generated by large association studies. For OA, there has so far been one report of a genome-wide association scan, from a large collaborative group based in Japan. Two exciting finds have emerged from this scan, namely, associations to the asporin gene ASPN[38] and to the calmodulin 1 gene CALM1.[39]

ASPN

Asporin is an ECM macromolecule belonging to the small leucine-rich proteoglycan (SLRP) protein family, other members of which include decorin, biglycan, fibromodulin, and chondroadherin.[40,41] SLRP family members are able to bind other structural components of the ECM, such as collagen, as well as growth factors that temporarily reside in the ECM, such as transforming growth factor β (TGF-β). Asporin is expressed in a number of tissues, including adult articular cartilage. The ASPN gene comprises eight exons and resides on chromosome 9q22.31, a location that had not previously been reported to harbor OA susceptibility in any of the genome-wide linkage scans conducted on European and U.S. families. The Japanese group initially demonstrated that ASPN was expressed in OA articular cartilage. They then sequenced the ASPN exons and flanking regions and identified 21 DNA variants. Eight variants had frequencies greater than 5% and were subsequently genotyped in a population-based cohort of 371 Japanese, comprising 137 individuals (mean age of 75.3, 72% female)

diagnosed as having radiographic knee OA and 234 individuals (mean age of 73.6, 61% female) diagnosed radiographically as unaffected. Only one of the eight variants demonstrated association: a triplet repeat within exon 2, coding for a polymorphic stretch of aspartic acid residues in the N-terminal region of asporin. This repeat polymorphism (given the moniker D-repeat after the one-letter code for aspartic acid) had ten alleles encoding 10–19D residues. The D14 allele was more common in the knee OA individuals than the unaffected individuals ($P = 0.0013$). The D-repeat was then genotyped in a Japanese case–control cohort of 393 cases with knee OA (mean age of 72.5, 84% female) and 374 controls (mean age of 28.8, 56% female). The D14 allele was also associated in this cohort ($P = 0.018$). Combining the two cohorts generated a P-value of 0.00024 and an OR for the D14 allele of 1.87 (95% CI 1.3-2.6). The investigators subsequently genotyped the D-repeat in 593 Japanese individuals with hip OA (mean age of 58.3, 93% female). Again, the D14 allele was associated ($P = 0.0078$). As well as the association to D14, the investigators also noticed that one allele, D13 (i.e., encoding one aspartic acid residue fewer than D14), was consistently underrepresented in the affected individuals. It appeared therefore that an OA-susceptibility allele (D14) and an OA-protective allele (D13) had been detected.

The investigators finally conducted a number of functional studies. These revealed that asporin inhibited the expression of the AGC1 and COL2A1 genes, which code for aggrecan and type II collagen—the principal structural components of cartilage ECM. They also demonstrated that TGF-β induces transcription of AGC1 and COL2A1 and that asporin interacts with TGF-β and inhibits its signaling effect. This inhibitory effect was particularly strong for asporin encoded by the D14 allele and significantly less so for D13-encoded protein. These functional studies therefore provide a plausible model of how the D-repeat polymorphism of ASPN influences susceptibility to OA: firstly, asporin inhibits TGF-β signaling and therefore indirectly regulates the synthesis of aggrecan and type II collagen, critical components of articular cartilage ECM; secondly, this inhibition is strongest for the D14 allele, leading to insufficient quantities of these proteins and therefore a cartilage that is structurally compromised; and finally, D13-encoded asporin has the weakest TGF-β inhibitory effect, resulting in a more structurally resilient cartilage. What still needs determining is exactly how the size of the D-repeat influences protein activity: is the effect via influences on the conformational structure of the protein or does the repeat itself bind directly to TGF-β? Another important question is whether asporin modulates the signalling of other members of the TGF-β superfamily such as the bone morphogenetic proteins, which are also regulators of cartilage development and maintenance.

CALM1

Calmodulin is an intracellular protein that binds to Ca^{2+} and interacts with a number of cellular proteins.[42,43] The Japanese group initially identified an association in patients with hip OA to a SNP within intron 3 of the calmodulin 1 gene *CALM1* (chromosome 14q24-q31). The association was particularly significant in those hip cases that had inherited two copies of the associated allele (i.e., a recessive effect), with a *P*-value of 0.00065 and an OR of 2.40 (95% CI 1.43-4.02). The association was present in both male and female cases, although the majority of the cases were female. The investigators subsequently analyzed all other common variants within *CALM1* to assess whether the intron 3 SNP was in linkage disequilibrium with other polymorphisms. This revealed that the intron 3 SNP was in strong linkage disequilibrium with four other SNPs: a SNP in the core promoter region of *CALM1*, two SNPs in intron 1, and a SNP in the 3'UTR. All these SNPs demonstrated strong association (*P* ≤0.00065) to hip OA.

Of the five associated SNPs that were in linkage disequilibrium, the core promoter SNP was considered the most likely to have a functional effect on calmodulin 1. The investigators demonstrated that *CALM1* was expressed in human articular chondrocytes and also showed higher levels of *CALM1* expression in OA cartilage compared to normal cartilage. They subsequently assessed the effect that the two alleles of the core promoter SNP had on the expression of *CALM1*. This revealed that the associated allele (the T-allele) resulted in reduced transcriptional activity relative to the unassociated allele (the C-allele). The investigators then demonstrated that calmodulin 1 increases the expression of the aggrecan gene *AGC1* and of the type II collagen gene *COL2A1*. These functional studies provide a model of how the core promoter SNP of CALM1 could influence OA susceptibility: firstly, calmodulin 1 naturally increases the synthesis of aggrecan and type II collagen in articular cartilage; and secondly, this synthesis is reduced for the T-allele, particularly in those individuals who are TT homozygotes, leading to insufficient quantities of aggrecan and type II collagen and therefore a structurally compromised cartilage.

Since calmodulin 1 and asporin both regulate the expression of *AGC1* and *COL2A1*, the investigators finally assessed whether the associated allele at *CALM1* (the T-allele of the core promoter SNP) and the risk allele at *ASPN* (the D14-allele of the D-repeat) interacted with each other in an epistatic manner to further increase the risk of developing OA. This revealed that individuals who had inherited two copies of the T-allele and at least one copy of the D14-allele were at a particularly high risk of hip OA, with an OR of 13.16 (95% CI 1.66-104.06). This makes sense, since both the T-allele of *CALM1* and the D14-allele of *ASPN* lead to a reduction in expression of *AGC1* and *COL2A1*. It should be noted however that the broad confidence interval of the OR means that this result is of low statistical certainty.

Conclusions

The Japanese association study has so far identified two very interesting genes associated with the development of large joint OA. Other OA susceptibility loci are likely to follow from this study, since of the 71,880 SNPs genotyped by the Japanese group, 2,219 demonstrated associations at *P* <0.01.[39] The majority of these will be false positives, but as the Japanese group works through these SNPs by genotyping additional cohorts, the genuine positives will emerge. It will be intriguing to see what pathways and mechanisms these highlight, and to note whether the associations to the IL1 gene cluster, *MATN3*, *IL4R*, *FRZB*, *LRP5*, and *BMP5*, reported by European groups are observed in the Japanese study. It will also be interesting to determine whether the *ASPN* and *CALM1* associations detected in Japan have a role in OA development outside of Asia.

OSTEOARTHRITIS SUSCEPTIBILITY GENES DETECTED VIA GENE EXPRESSION ANALYSIS

An alternative strategy to genome-wide linkage or association studies for detecting functional candidates is the identification of those genes that are significantly up- or downregulated in disease versus normal tissue; a difference in expression would imply a role in either disease development or disease progression. Identified genes can then be tested for association. A group based at St. Thomas' Hospital in London recently carried out such an analysis for OA.[44] Using four cDNA libraries constructed from normal cartilage, OA cartilage, normal synovium, and OA synovium, the investigators initially identified 54 genes that showed differential expression between normal and diseased tissue. The investigators next tested the genes for association to OA. They focused on 12 of the 54 genes, with the selection criteria being those that code for proteins whose actions could be therapeutically modified, such as receptors, enzymes, and secreted molecules. They also investigated 12 additional genes that other groups had previously suggested could have a role in OA aetiology. The cohort for the association analysis comprised 749 females (age range of 43–67) who were participating in the U.K. Chingford Study, a population-based investigation of joint diseases. The individuals had undergone a radiographic assessment, including measures of JSN and the occurrence of osteophytes, of knee OA in 1988–1989 and then a decade later. Of the 749 females, 469 were classified as normal (they did not have OA in either knee at both examinations) and 280 were classified as affected. Twenty-six SNPs from the 24 genes were genotyped in the cohort and were tested for association to both OA prevalence and OA progression. SNPs from four genes were associated with OA prevalence: *BMP2* (chromosome 20p12.3), which encodes bone morphogenetic protein 2; *CD36* (7q21.11), which encodes a thrombospondin and collagen receptor; *COX2* (1q25), which encodes a cyclooxygenase; and *NCOR2* (12q24.31), which encodes a nuclear receptor corepressor. Four genes were associated with OA progression: *CILP* (15q22.31), which encodes a cartilage intermediate-layer protein; *OPG* (8q24.12), which encodes osteoprotegerin; *TNA* (3p21.31), which encodes tetranectin; and *ESR1* (6q25.1), which encodes estrogen receptor α. One gene was associated with prevalence and progression: *ADAM12* (chromosome 10q26.2), which encodes a metalloproteinase. When the association data were corrected for the large number of tests performed, only *ADAM12* was still associated, with a corrected *P* of 0.014.

TABLE 6–2
GENES REPORTED TO SHOW EVIDENCE OF ASSOCIATION TO OA

Gene	Protein	Chromosome	Country	Ref
IL1	Interleukin 1 family	2q11.2–q13	Netherlands & UK	21–23
MATN3	Matrilin 3	2p24.1	Iceland	8
IL4R	Interleukin 4 receptor α	16p12.1	UK	25
FRZB	Secreted frizzled-related protein 3	2q32.1	UK	26
LRP5	Low-density lipoprotein receptor-related protein 5	11q13.2	UK	32
BMP5	Bone morphogenetic protein 5	6p12.1	UK	36
ASPN	Asporin	9q22.31	Japan	38
CALM1	Calmodulin 1	14q24–q31	Japan	39
ADAM12	Metalloprotease	10q26.2	UK	44
ESR1	Estrogen receptor α	6q25.1	Several countries	4,44

[a]DIP, distal interphalangeal joint; [b]CMC1, first carpometacarpal joint.

Conclusions

This study has demonstrated an alternative strategy for identifying potential OA susceptibility genes. It has some weaknesses, including the small number of variants tested per gene and the fact that the cDNA libraries used did not provide a complete coverage of all genes. Despite this, a novel locus in *ADAM12* has been identified that merits more comprehensive investigation.

CONCLUDING REMARKS

Considerable progress has been made in recent years in our understanding of the molecular genetic basis of primary OA. Using a variety of techniques and strategies, a number of genes have been identified that are likely to harbor risk alleles for this common arthritis (Table 6–2).

Many of the linkage and association studies do, however, have weaknesses, principally the use of relatively small cohorts and the study of only a small proportion of the genetic variants within the gene of interest. These are potentially major deficiencies. The use of small sample sizes limits the power of the study to detect subtle effects and can increase the likelihood of detecting a false positive. The genotyping of only a proportion of the common gene variants provides only a limited view of the gene and may well lead to loci being disregarded when in fact they do harbor susceptibility. The OA research community needs to be more comprehensive in its approach to mapping OA susceptibility loci. The Japanese reports of associations to *ASPN* and *CALM1* provide a model for others to follow: large sample sizes, all common variants interrogated, and subsequent functional studies to investigate the effect of associated variants on gene activity or protein function.

Of the genes that have so far been implicated as OA susceptibility loci, only two code for structural components of articular cartilage: *MATN3*, which encodes matrilin 3, and *ASPN*, which encodes asporin. The majority of the associated genes code for proteins that regulate joint tissue biology, either as signaling molecules, receptors, or enzymes. This is an important observation as it implies that effects on joint tissue development, maintenance, and homeostasis are the likely paths through which OA genetic susceptibility is acting. Such paths are likely to be more accessible to modification and treatment than are structural defects. One of the major challenges now is how this genetic insight can be used to enhance the care and treatment of patients at risk of developing the disease.

ACKNOWLEDGMENTS

We are grateful to Research into Ageing and the Arthritis Research Campaign who fund our research.

REFERENCES

1. Loughlin J. Genetic epidemiology of primary osteoarthritis. Curr Opin Rheum.13:111–116, 2001.
2. Loughlin J. Genome studies and linkage in primary osteoarthritis. Rheum Dis Clin North Am 28:95–109, 2002.
3. Jakkula E, Melkoniemi M, Kiviranta I, et al. The role of sequence variations within the genes encoding collagen II, IX and XI in nonsyndromic, early-onset osteoarthritis. Osteoarthritis Cartilage 13:497–507, 2005.
4. Bergink AP, van Meurs JB, Loughlin J, et al. Estrogen receptor α gene haplotype is associated with radiographic osteoarthritis of the knee in elderly men and women. Arthritis Rheum 48:1913–1922, 2003.
5. Chapman K, Mustafa Z, Irven CM, et al. Osteoarthritis-susceptibility locus on chromosome 11q, detected by linkage. Am J Hum Genet 65:167–174, 1999.
6. Loughlin J, Mustafa Z, Irven C, et al. Stratification analysis of an osteoarthritis genome screen—suggestive linkage to chromosomes 4, 6 and 16. Am J Hum Genet 65:1795–1798, 1999.
7. Leppävuori J, Kujala U, Kinnunen J, et al. Genome scan for predisposing loci for distal interphalangeal joint osteoarthritis: evidence for a locus on 2q. Am J Hum Genet 65:1060–1067, 1999.
8. Stefánsson SE, Jónsson H, Ingvarsson T, et al. Genomewide scan for hand osteoarthritis: a novel mutation in Matrilin-3. Am J Hum Genet 72:1448–1459, 2003.
9. Demissie S, Cupples LA, Myers R, et al. Genome scan for quantity of hand osteoarthritis. Arthritis Rheum 46:946–952, 2002.

10. Hunter DJ, Demissie S, Cupples LA, et al. A genome scan for joint-specific hand OA susceptibility. Arthritis Rheum 50:2489–2496, 2004.

11. Loughlin J, Dowling B, Mustafa Z, et al. Refined linkage mapping of a hip osteoarthritis susceptibility locus on chromosome 2q. Rheumatology 41:955–956, 2002.

12. Chapman K, Mustafa Z, Dowling B, et al. Finer linkage mapping of primary hip osteoarthritis susceptibility on chromosome 11q in a cohort of affected female sibling pairs. Arthritis Rheum 46:1780–1783, 2002.

13. Loughlin J, Mustafa Z, Dowling B, et al. Finer linkage mapping of a primary hip osteoarthritis susceptibility locus on chromosome 6. Eur J Hum Genet 10:562–568, 2002.

14. Forster T, Chapman K, Marcelline L, et al. Finer linkage mapping of primary osteoarthritis susceptibility loci on chromosomes 4 and 16 in families with affected women. Arthritis Rheum 50:98–102, 2004.

15. Southam L, Dowling B, Ferreira A, et al. Microsatellite association mapping of a primary osteoarthritis susceptibility locus on chromosome 6p12.3-q13. Arthritis Rheum 50:3910–3914, 2004.

16. Alizadeh BZ, Njajou OT, Bijkerk C, et al. Evidence for a role of the genomic region of the gene encoding for the α1 chain of type IX collagen (COL9A1) in hip osteoarthritis. Arthritis Rheum 52:1437–1442, 2005.

17. Meenagh GK, McGibbon D, Nixon J, et al. Lack of support for the presence of an osteoarthritis susceptibility locus on chromosome 6p. Arthritis Rheum 52:2040–2043, 2005.

18. Kalichman L, Kobyliansky E, Malkin I, et al. Search for linkage between hand osteoarthritis and 11q12-13 chromosomal segment. Osteoarthritis Cartilage 11:561–568, 2003.

19. Pelletier J-P, Martel-Pelletier J, Abramson SB. Osteoarthritis, an inflammatory disease. Arthritis Rheum 44:1237–1247, 2001.

20. Goldring MB. The role of the chondrocyte in osteoarthritis. Arthritis Rheum 43:1916–1926, 2000.

21. Meulenbelt I, Seymour AB, Nieuwland M, et al. Association of the interleukin-1 gene cluster with radiographic signs of osteoarthritis of the hip. Arthritis Rheum 50:1179–1186, 2004.

22. Smith AJP, Keen LJ, Billingham MJ, et al. Extended haplotypes and linkage disequilibrium in the IL1R1-IL1A-IL1B-IL1RN gene cluster: association with knee osteoarthritis. Genes Immun 5:451–460, 2004.

23. Smith AJP, Elson CJ, Perry MJ, et al. Accuracy of haplotype association studies is enhanced by increasing number of polymorphic loci examined: comment on the article by Meulenbelt et al. Arthritis Rheum 52:675, 2005.

24. Salter DM, Millward-Sadler SJ, Nuki G, et al. Integrin-interleukin-4 mechanotransduction pathways in human chondrocytes. Clin Orthop 391:S49–S60, 2001.

25. Forster T, Chapman K, Loughlin J. Common variants within the interleukin 4 receptor α gene (IL4R) are associated with susceptibility to osteoarthritis. Hum Genet 114:391–395, 2004.

26. Loughlin J, Dowling B, Chapman K, et al. Functional variants within the secreted frizzled-related protein 3 gene are associated with hip osteoarthritis in females. Proc Natl Acad Sci USA 101:9757–9762, 2004.

27. Jones SE, Jomary C. Secreted frizzled-related proteins: searching for relationships and patterns. Bioessays 24:811–820, 2002.

28. Enomoto-Iwamoto M, Kitagaki J, Koyama E, et al. The wnt antagonist frzb-1 regulates chondrocyte maturation and long bone development during limb skeletogenesis. Dev Biol 251:142–156, 2002.

29. Min JL, Meulenbelt I, Riyazi N, et al. Association of the frizzled-related protein gene with symptomatic osteoarthritis at multiple sites. Arthritis Rheum 52:1077–1080, 2005.

30. Gong Y, Slee RB, Fukai N, et al. LDL receptor-related protein 5 (LRP5) affects bone accrual and eye development. Cell 107:513–523, 2001.

31. Little RD, Carulli JP, Del Mastro RG, et al. A mutation in the LDL receptor-related protein 5 gene results in the autosomal dominant high-bone-mass trait. Am J Hum Genet 70:11–19, 2002.

32. Smith AJP, Gidley J, Sandy JR, et al. Haplotypes of the low-density lipoprotein receptor-related protein 5 (LRP5) gene: are they a risk factor in osteoarthritis? Osteoarthritis Cartilage 13:608–613, 2005.

33. Bailón-Plaza A, Lee AO, Veson EC, et al. BMP-5 deficiency alters chondrocytic activity in the mouse proximal tibial growth plate. Bone 24:211–216, 1999.

34. Eyre D. Collagen of articular cartilage. Arthritis Res 4:30–35, 2002.

35. Southam L, Chapman K, Loughlin J. Genetic association analysis of BMP5 as a potential osteoarthritis susceptibility gene. Rheumatology 42:911–912, 2003.

36. Southam L, Dowling B, Ferreira A, et al. Microsatellite association mapping of a primary osteoarthritis susceptibility locus on chromosome 6p12.3-q13. Arthritis Rheum 50:3910–3914, 2004.

37. DiLeone RJ, Marcus GA, Johnson MD, et al. Efficient studies of long-distance Bmp5 gene regulation using bacterial artificial chromosomes. Proc Natl Acad Sci USA 97:1612–1617, 2000.

38. Kizawa H, Kou I, Iida A, et al. An aspartic acid repeat polymorphism in asporin inhibits chondrogenesis and increases susceptibility to osteoarthritis. Nat Genet 37:138–144, 2005.

39. Mototani H, Mabuchi A, Saito S, et al. A functional single nucleotide polymorphism in the core promoter region of CALM1 is associated with hip osteoarthritis in Japanese. Hum Mol Genet 14:1009–1017, 2005.

40. Lorenzo P, Aspberg A, Önnerfjord P, et al. Identification and characterization of asporin. J Biol Chem 276:12201–12211, 2001.

41. Henry SP, Takanosu M, Boyd TC, et al. Expression pattern and gene characterization of asporin. J Biol Chem 276:12212–12221, 2001.

42. Chin D, Means AR. Calmodulin: a prototypical calcium sensor. Trends Cell Biol 10:322–328, 2000.

43. Haeseleer F, Imanishi Y, Sokal I, et al. Calcium-binding proteins: intracellular sensors from the calmodulin superfamily. Biochem Biophys Res Commun 290:615–623, 2002.

44. Valdes AM, Hart DJ, Jones KA, et al. Association of candidate genes for the prevalence and progression of knee osteoarthritis. Arthritis Rheum 50:2497–2507, 2004.

General Aspects
of Diagnosis

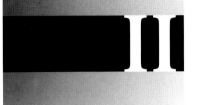

Osteoarthritis: Clinical Presentations

7

Michele M. Hooper   *Roland W. Moskowitz*

The symptomatic osteoarthritic joint presents with pain, limited range of motion, and stiffness; but symptoms are highly variable, depending on which joint is affected, how severely it is affected, and the number of joints involved. Bony enlargement is common and malalignment may occur. Crepitus may be present with or without pain. Effusions may be present, usually without heat or erythema. Certain osteoarthritic joints, such as the spine and hip, can be associated with symptoms related to adjacent nerve compression. Symptoms range in intensity from mild to severe and may lead to altered function and disability. End-stage osteoarthritic joints, especially weight-bearing joints, are extremely painful.

Osteoarthritis (OA) occurring as a result of early trauma, congenital, or genetic abnormalities such as knee OA following anterior cruciate ligament tear, hips with congenital hip disease, or spines in patients with spondyloepiphysial dysplasia may become symptomatic as early as adolescence. Typically, though, osteoarthritic symptoms begin in the fifth decade and increase with aging. Symptomatic hand OA typically begins in women in their 40s. By the age of 60 years, 80% of the population will have radiographic evidence of OA, 40% will be symptomatic, and 10% limited by their arthritis.[1]

Symptomatic OA may be associated with depression, disability, and sleep disturbance; depression in association with hip or knee OA is more predictive of disability than radiographic grade.[2,3] People over the age of 50 years with knee pain also typically have pain at other sites, which compounds the overall pain experience and increases disability.[4] Treatment of the depressed individual with OA with antidepressants can improve pain, function, and quality of life scores.[5]

The differential diagnosis is based on the distribution, number of joints affected, absence of signs of inflammation such as heat, erythema, synovial swelling, and systemic complaints. The presence of bony enlargement (Heberden nodes) of the distal interphalangeal (DIP) joints or arthritis of the first carpometacarpal (CMC) joint is so characteristic of OA that other testing is often not indicated (Table 7–1).

Some OA, particularly of the knee, could be prevented through injury avoidance (athletic or vocational), weight reduction, and exercise. Loss of 11.2 pounds has been associated with a 50% reduction in the risk of developing symptomatic knee OA over a 10-year period.[6] Once established, OA is a chronic disorder. Education in joint sparing, pain control, and coping skills may help to maintain normal function and a good quality of life.[7]

CLINICAL MANIFESTATIONS

Symptoms

Pain

Pain is usually the first and predominant complaint in patients with symptomatic OA. Typical OA pain is exacerbated by use of the joint and relieved with rest. Some patients experience an exacerbation of their pain with changes in barometric pressure. The symptoms may be present at first just with extremes of joint use such as high joint loads or prolonged use, but then may be precipitated with minimal to moderate use, eventually occurring at rest.

As cartilage is aneural, joint pain arises from adjacent structures. Possibilities include a joint capsule stretched by bony enlargement, periosteal reaction, subchondral bone microfractures, increased intra-osseous venous pressure, and synovitis. There is often poor correlation between the amount of pain experienced and the degree of

TABLE 7–1

SIGNS AND SYMPTOMS CHARACTERISTIC OF OSTEOARTHRITIS IN THE MOST FREQUENTLY AFFECTED JOINTS

General: Pain, stiffness, gelling, crepitus, bony enlargement, limited range of motion, malalignment

Hands: DIPs (Heberden nodes), PIPs (Bouchard nodes), CMC; squaring of the base of the hand; medial and lateral deviation at the DIPs and PIPs

Knees: Patellofemoral joint symptoms worse on the stairs than on the flat; varus changes with medial compartment disease, valgus with lateral; Baker's (popliteal) cysts and tenderness of the pes anserine bursa are common

Hips: Typically groin pain, but may present in buttocks; less so in knee or below knee; flexion contractures and Trendelenberg sign may be present

Cervical spine: Local spine pain, muscle spasm, and limited motion (lateral flexion and extension); radicular pain with pain, sensory loss or muscle weakness/atrophy in nerve root distribution; cervical myelopathy with long tract signs, bladder dysfunction

Lumbar spine: Local pain and muscle spasm, limited extension, buttock pain, worse in PM, but not nocturnal; radicular pattern with pain, sensory and motor changes in nerve root distribution; spinal stenosis pattern pain with back/leg pain with standing, walking relieved by sitting

radiographic OA present.[8] Bone marrow edema as demonstrated by magnetic resonance imaging (MRI) correlates well with knee OA pain,[9] and the association is stronger when large bone marrow edema lesions are seen in association with cartilage defects that penetrate to the subchondral bone.[10] Low grade synovitis has been demonstrated in osteoarthritic joints[11] and, on occasion, a very inflammatory reaction may occur, often in the setting of a crystal-related disease such as seen in patients with calcium pyrophosphate dihydrate (CPPD) or hydroxyapatite deposition.

The Joint Commission on the Accreditation of Hospitals has mandated that pain be recorded as the fifth vital sign, with the patient asked to describe their current pain on a visual analog scale.[12] The pain scale rating reveals pain at that particular moment, but it is important to get a sense of the intensity and ranges of joint pain during the previous days, weeks, or months, what actions exacerbate the pain, and what activities have had to be modified or discontinued. OA pain can usually be relieved with resting the joint, but in end-stage OA, pain at rest can occur and is debilitating. Patients can generally describe the source of their pain but there are exceptions: cervical spondylosis symptoms may present with arm pain; some patients perceive first CMC joint pain as wrist pain; buttock pain coming from the lumbar spine is often referred to as hip pain, while the pain from hip OA usually presents in the groin.[13] OA pain may be amplified if there is pain at other sites. In a large survey study, subjects who had knee pain and pain at two or more other sites had more severe knee pain than those who reported the knee as their sole site of pain.[4]

Many individuals feel that their OA pain is exacerbated by cold, damp weather or changes in barometric pressure. Studies of this are contradictory,[14,15] but someone with OA may function better in a warm, dry climate where heavy clothing is not required and walking surfaces are not slippery.

Stiffness

Morning stiffness may occur with OA. It is a sensation that the joints and periarticular musculature are tight and slow to move and usually lasts less than 30 minutes. The stiffness is localized to the region around the affected joint(s) and is not the diffuse morning stiffness characteristic of rheumatoid arthritis. When it occurs during the day following periods of immobilization, it is referred to as gelling. Some individuals perceive stiffness as a painful condition while for others it is a nonpainful resistance to motion.

Limited Joint Function

Individuals with OA may experience decreased function for recreational, vocational, and even self-care activities. They may be limited by their pain; have lost range of motion in the joint because of loss of joint space; have associated muscle weakness due to atrophy of the adjacent muscles; have to work harder to move the joint as the coefficient of friction increases as the cartilage surface fissures and loses integrity; or have joint instability. Joint proprioception is decreased in knee OA, which could impact on function[16] but appears to have minimal clinical impact.[17]

The involvement of more than one joint in a limb or region may greatly limit the individual. Instability of the first metacarpophalangeal (MCP) joint compounds the pain and weakness associated with first CMC disease. A fused osteoarthritic ankle will increase the joint load on the ipsilateral osteoarthritic knee and impair compensatory limping which serves to protect the knee joint. Malalignment and instability of osteoarthritic joints may increase pain and disability.[18]

In addition to the extent and severity of the OA, age, weight, general muscle strength and conditioning, mental health, and alertness may all be factors in determining who becomes disabled and who does not by their OA. As the population ages, and as pain is recognized as an unacceptable symptom and that a sedentary lifestyle is undesirable, more aggressive intervention, particularly for OA of weight-bearing joints, may be appropriate.

Signs

The physical examination serves to verify that the patient's symptoms are coming from a joint and not a periarticular process such as a bursitis. The examination also documents which joints are involved, the number of joints, their range of motion, joint effusion or bony enlargement, malalignment, instability, crepitus, and whether signs such as symmetry or inflammation are present suggesting a more systemic process. Observation includes the gross appearance of the joints and observation for splinting because of pain or muscle spasm, overtly decreased range of motion, and gait assessment for limp.

Each joint is palpated for tenderness, effusion, and crepitus. Passive and active range of motion can be measured. It should be noted if there is pain with motion. A goniometer may be used to obtain precise range of motion measurements. Depending on the site involved, additional findings should be sought, such as pes anserine bursal tenderness with knee OA or a neurological examination with cervical spondylosis and potential myelopathy or radiculopathy.

Tenderness

Tenderness or pain with pressure on the joint or along the joint margin is typical, except for the hip, which is too deep to produce tenderness to palpation. Periarticular structures may be tender secondary to muscle spasm or adjacent bursitis or tendonitis.

Joint Enlargement

Joint enlargement may consist of bony enlargement and/or joint effusions. The bony enlargement is due to osteophytes. These are very characteristic in the DIPs and proximal interphalangeal (PIP) joints of the hand. Effusions are generally noninflammatory. If heat or erythema are present, consideration should be given to the possibility of a crystal arthropathy, joint trauma, or infection.

Crepitus

Crepitus is an audible or palpable sensation of roughness, crunching, or crackling over a joint during active or passive movement. The detection of crepitus in the patellofemoral, tibial, or femoral condyles around the knee correlates well with degenerative findings seen at arthroscopy.[19] However, many people have audible sounds from their joints in the absence of any joint pain. Crepitus is presumably caused by irregularity of joint surfaces or intra-articular debris.

Limitation of Motion

Loss of range of motion in joints may occur with age, such as decreased lateral flexion of the cervical spine and internal rotation of the hip. Subtle losses of motion due to OA may not be noticed by the patient; they may compensate by sparing it or using the joint differently. Range of motion is limited by pain, effusions, flexion contractures, muscle spasm, mechanical inhibition such as loss of cartilage, malalignment, or intra-articular loose bodies. Observing the patient moving during the interview, from fine hand manipulation to walking, can give a good indication about where the source of the pain is and how severe it is. There are characteristic gaits associated with hip and knee OA.

Malalignment

Medial compartment knee OA is frequently associated with a varus malalignment, and lateral compartment degeneration with a valgus angulation. Malalignment is a risk factor for the progression of OA of the knee. The degree of malalignment may be measured with a goniometer or with a full limb length radiograph. Marked angular deviations of the fingers may occur with Heberden's OA. Hallux valgus, or bunion of the first metatarsalphalangeal joint, is a characteristic presentation of OA.

Musculature

The muscles related to the peripheral joints should be assessed for atrophy and for fasiculations in patients with OA of the spine. Motor strength should be assessed. Intrinsic muscle wasting in the hands may reflect cervical spondylosis, and quadriceps femoris atrophy may exist in the presence of knee OA. The latter can be detected by measuring thigh circumference. Muscle mass decreases with age, and rebuilding muscle strength is helpful in restoring function and limiting pain.

CLINICAL PRESENTATIONS

Acuity

The typical pattern for OA is that of a chronic process. An acute inflammatory presentation would suggest a systemic inflammatory arthritis, crystal arthropathy, or infection.

Joint Distribution

OA may be mono- or polyarticular and there are certain joints and patterns that are typical. Multiple joints may be involved with generalized OA or erosive OA. The hands, knees, hips, and spine are the most frequently affected sites. Involvement of the PIP, DIP, and CMC joints is very characteristic of OA. Involvement of unusual sites, such as the MCP joints, the wrists, elbows, and shoulders, should raise suspicion of an underlying process, such as a congenital abnormality, trauma (including direct injury resulting in an intra-articular or subchondral fracture or an injury of an important support structure such as the rotator cuff of the shoulder), or a systemic disease process, including crystal-related and metabolic diseases. Unilateral disease of the hips and knees frequently becomes bilateral in time, and individuals who have had a total hip arthroplasty are at increased risk for developing contralateral knee OA.[20]

Hands

The most typical pattern of hand involvement is the presence of OA in the DIP and the PIP joints. The bony enlargements associated with these joints are referred to as Heberden's nodes and Bouchard's nodes, respectively, and the disorder is referred to as nodal OA. Sisters of women with nodal OA are three times more likely to have it themselves and a strong genetic association has been established.[21]

The clinical picture is typically one of subacute onset of nonpainful firm enlargements on the DIPs and PIPs over several years. Sometimes there is a transient inflammation of the joint, which is usually self-limited and associated with increased pain, swelling, and even erythema. Mucinous cysts, which are soft subcutaneous swellings occurring at the DIPs, may appear. They contain a gelatinous mucoid material, may drain spontaneously, and are usually self-limited. As the osteoarthritic process progresses, significant medial and lateral deviation may occur at the DIPs and PIPs. Pain and loss of function is generally not as severe as the clinical or radiographic picture would suggest.

Osteoarthritic changes involving the first CMC joint are common, especially in association with nodal OA. The base of the thumb is often quite tender and, as osteophytes form, the radial base of the hand becomes squared. Flexor tenosynovitis may develop, presumably as a result of abnormal hand biomechanics, and the thumb may adduct across the palm, sometimes resulting in a fixed adduction. The trapezioscaphoid joint may also become involved and pain may be perceived at the base of the thumb or in the wrist. Individuals who have laxity at the first MCP joint or the IP joint may experience increased instability at these joints as abnormal forces are applied across them to compensate for the involvement of the CMC joint. However, hypermobility at the PIP joints is protective against the development of radiographic PIP OA.[22] Involvement of the first CMC joint is frequently very painful and limits hand function more than DIP and PIP involvement.

The American College of Rheumatology (ACR) criteria for the diagnosis of OA of the hands call for nodal enlargement in at least two of ten joints (DIPs, PIPS, and first CMC), swelling of fewer than three MCP joints, nodal enlargement of at least two DIP joints, and bilateral hand involvement.[23]

Symptomatic OA of the MCP joints is uncommon. Although its presence raises the question of an underlying disorder (hemochromatosis or CPPD disease), it is not that uncommon radiographically, particularly in people who do heavy physical work with their hands.

Knees

There are three compartments of the knee that can be affected by OA: the medial tibiofemoral, the lateral tibiofemoral, and the patellofemoral joint. The medial compartment is more commonly involved (75%) than the lateral compartment (25%). They are rarely both involved and the presence of bicompartmental tibiofemoral knee OA would suggest a previous knee trauma, infection, or other systemic process such as end-stage rheumatoid arthritis. Isolated patellofemoral OA may occur, but it is usually present in association with medial or lateral compartment disease. Aggressive patellofemoral disease with large osteophytes may be a manifestation of primary hyperparathyroidism.

The pain of knee OA typically occurs during weight bearing. Patellofemoral disease is particularly aggravated by walking up and down stairs and arising from chairs. In early disease, the pain should be relieved by rest, but as the disease progresses, pain at rest may also occur. The medial joint line is the most common site of pain, followed by the lateral joint line and then the inferior aspect of the knee.

Stiffness is a frequent complaint with knee OA. This may be present in the morning and usually lasts less than 30 minutes, but frequent gelling following periods of activity may occur throughout the day. Many patients find the stiffness and gelling uncomfortable and as disabling as their pain.

On examination, there may be obvious bony enlargement, tenderness to palpation of the joint, and crepitus which may be heard or palpated over the patellofemoral joint or the femoral or tibial condyles with passive joint motion. Joint effusions may be present, generally without heat or erythema. There may be malalignment of the knee (varus or bow-legged for medial compartment disease and valgus or knock-kneed for lateral compartment disease). Range of motion may be normal. In early knee OA, there is often loss of a few degrees of full flexion and extension and this may progress to the point of contracture. Patellofemoral disease can be detected by compressing the patella of the fully extended knee and asking the patient to raise the leg against resistance which should reproduce the pain. Crepitus is frequently palpable. Popliteal (Baker's) cysts are bursae that communicate with the knee joint space. As synovial fluid accumulates, they become quite large and tense and may cause posterior knee pain. If they become entrapped under the gastrocnemius muscle, they may cause pain and vascular compression mimicking a deep vein thrombosis including pitting edema and a positive Homans sign.[24]

Effusions may be absent or quite large, with visible distention of the suprapatellar pouch. Bony enlargement, usually of the medial femoral condyle, may be detected by inspection or palpation. There is frequent nontender enlargement of the inferior patellar bursa. Quadriceps muscle atrophy may be determined by measuring thigh circumference bilaterally.

People with knee OA may limp. The characteristic gait is slow and associated with less extension of the knee in both the swing phase and stance phases and serves to unload some of the forces generated across it by muscle contraction and gravity. The ACR classification criteria for OA of the knee require knee pain and radiographic osteophytes with at least one of the following: 1) age older than 50 years, 2) morning stiffness less than 30 minutes in duration, or 3) crepitus on motion.[25]

Hips

Classically, hip OA presents with groin pain with weight bearing. Although hip pain may present as buttock pain, more typically patients refer to their buttocks as their hips. As it progresses, patients may note pain during sexual intercourse, difficulty reaching their foot to tie a shoelace, or pain getting in and out of their car. The examination should reproduce the groin pain, typically with limitation of internal rotation and flexion, although all ranges may be limited. A Trendelenburg sign may be present. When the patient stands on the unaffected side, the pelvis as viewed from the back remains level. If the gluteus medius is weak on the painful side as a result of hip OA, when the subject stands on the affected side the unsupported side of the pelvis will droop, producing the characteristic limp of the arthritic hip.[13] Patients with advanced hip OA may develop flexion contractures of the affected hip. This can be demonstrated in the supine patient by flexing the contralateral hip. The upward motion of the pelvis will cause the osteoarthritic hip also to flex and the knee will be lifted off the examination table. Patients with advanced hip OA may also have anterior thigh, knee, and below knee pain because of irritation of the obturator nerve by the osteoarthritic joint.[26] In rare cases, these patients present with just knee pain, but the markedly abnormal hip examination will reveal this inconsistency. Functional shortening of the lower extremity may occur. The ACR classification criteria for OA of the hip require the presence of hip pain with at least two of the following: 1) erythrocyte sedimentation rate below 20 mm/hr, 2) radiographic femoral or acetabular osteophytes, or 3) radiographic joint space narrowing.[27]

Trochanteric bursitis results in lateral hip pain that patients often do not distinguish from an intra-articular process. It presents with lateral upper thigh pain, variable pain with weight bearing, and classically awakening the patient at night when they lie on it. On examination they are tender to touch over the greater trochanter and the pain can be provoked by external rotation of the leg.

Spine

Degenerative changes in the cervical and lumbar intervertebral disks and posterior facet articulations are common, particularly in people older than 60 years. The facet joints are true diarthrodial joints and develop classical OA changes. The osteophyte formation and degeneration of intervertebral disks are often referred to as spondylosis. The intervertebral disk narrowing, hypertrophic spur formation, and disk slippages or spondylolisthesis may lead to impingement of nerves exiting the neural foramina or the spinal cord. Severe radiographic changes may be found in asymptomatic individuals. The spondylosis and osteoarthritic facet joints may create pain and stiffness in the neck and back, respectively. The thoracic spine is relatively spared, presumably because of the stability provided to it by the rib cage.

Cervical Spine. The more common sites of osteoarthritic involvement of the cervical spine are C5 through C7. Neck motion, particularly extension or lateral flexion, may provoke localized neck pain or pain and/or paresthesias in the related nerve root distribution. Compression of the head in the sitting position may provoke similar symptoms. There may be tenderness to palpation over a given segment or at the lateral aspect over a facet joint. Paraspinal and trapezius muscle spasms are common. Sensory changes, weakness, atrophy, and deep tendon reflex abnormalities may also be present in the nerve root distribution. As the cervical neural foramina are relatively small, neurological findings related to facet hypertrophy are common. The relatively large cervical portion of the spinal cord and relatively narrow space for the cord may lead to cervical myelopathy, characterized by leg weakness, bladder dysfunction, and hyperactive lower extremity reflexes. Advanced degenerative changes at the lateral atlantoaxial joints can cause suboccipital neck pain, particularly in older patients. Rarely, compression of the anterior spinal artery may produce vascular occlusion or vertebral insufficiency of the vertebral basilar artery system. Sporadic visual symptoms precipitated by cervical spine motion include vertigo, blurring, diplopia, and field defects. Large anterior cervical vertebral osteophytes may cause dysphagia.

Lumbar Spine. The most common site of involvement is L3 to L5, although vertebral osteophytes may occur at any level. Loss of the lumbar lordosis, pain with extension, and paraspinal muscle spasm are typical findings. Focal tenderness of a lumbar vertebra should lead to consideration of compression fracture or malignancy rather than spondylosis. There may be radicular symptoms of pain, sensory loss, motor weakness, and loss of reflexes.

Stenosis of the lumbar spine results when disk degeneration and facet joint hypertrophy are severe enough to cause compression of the nerve root in the neural foramina or the spinal cord. This may be compounded by the presence of congenital narrowing of the spinal canal or foramina. The classical pain that occurs in the back or buttocks with standing, less so with walking, and that is relieved by flexing at the waist or sitting[28] may mimic arterial claudication. The physical examination may only demonstrate the spasm of the lumbar spine and absent ankle and/or knee reflexes, or the neurological examination may be normal.

Feet and Ankles

The first metatarsophalangeal (MTP) joint sustains the highest loads of any joint in the body and is a frequent site of OA. This may present as hallux valgus or bunion, or as hallux rigidus, where alignment is maintained but range of motion is severely restricted and the joint is unable to be dorsiflexed appropriately for toe-off in gait. With hallux valgus, there is lateral deviation of the first digit at the first MTP joint, which frequently leads to difficulty finding well-fitting shoes and development of calluses or skin breakdown. Extreme valgus changes of the great toe may also cause hammer toe deformities of the second toe and it may overlap the first digit. The inflexible toe of hallux rigidus may respond to a "toe up" shoe which propels the foot forward and minimizes impact on the toe.

The tarsal joints are also subject to osteoarthritic changes, especially in the setting of pes planus. The midfoot may be rigid, and bony enlargement on the dorsum of the foot may cause footwear problems. The tibiotalar and subtalar joints may develop OA, generally secondary to trauma, neuropathy, or foot malalignment. Pain and limited range of motion occur, often with hindfoot valgus and pronation which may cause posterior tibial tendonitis or tarsal tunnel syndrome.

Shoulder Area

OA of the glenohumeral joints is not uncommon in patients with chronic painful shoulders. It usually occurs in association with rotator cuff or glenoid labral injury. Nocturnal pain is frequent as is pain and loss of range of motion. Hydroxyapatite deposition may cause accelerated degeneration of the glenohumeral joint in the elderly, a condition referred to as Milwaukee shoulder.[29] OA of the acromioclavicular joint is common. The joint may be tender or have bony enlargement. Range of motion is usually preserved but its associated osteophytes may impinge upon the supraspinatus tendon causing symptoms of impingement. Sternoclavicular joint OA may present as shoulder pain when the arm is fully abducted.

Temporomandibular Joint

Temporomandibular joint (TMJ) OA accounts for 8% to 12% of patients treated for TMJ pain;[30] the incidence increases with age, presence of malocclusion, tooth loss, disc internal derangement, bruxism, and trauma.[31] Clinically, TMJ OA is associated with limited mandibular motion, including decrease in oral opening and lateral movement and mandibular protrusion. Crepitus, as opposed to the clicking of disc displacement, is present in the majority of osteoarthritic TMJs, as is tenderness of the medial and lateral pterygoid muscles.[32] Facial pain, headache, impaired hearing, tinnitus, and dizziness attributed to OA of the TMJ are likely related to irritation of the facial or auriculotemporal nerve.

Wrists and Elbows

The wrists and elbows are very infrequently affected by OA. The typical scenario would be following an intra-articular fracture with suboptimal anatomic healing or secondary to an underlying disease such as CPPD deposition disease.

SPECIFIC SYNDROMES

Generalized Osteoarthritis

OA occurring in multiple joints, usually in the hands with nodal disease, and some combination of the knees, lumbar spine, and hips is called generalized OA. This is particularly well defined in women between the ages of 45 and 64 years, where the occurrence of OA in multiple joints together exceeds that which would be expected by chance alone. The clinical picture is otherwise similar to isolated OA. There is an increased frequency of symmetrical involvement of the joints and there may be genetic causes.

Radiographic findings are typical. The prognosis for outcome in each joint involved in generalized OA is not worse than that seen in isolated disease.

Erosive Inflammatory Osteoarthritis

Erosive OA is considered a subtype of generalized OA primarily affecting the small joints of the hands. There is a strong familial predisposition and women between the ages of 45 and 55 years are most typically affected. The hand distribution is typical of Heberden and Bouchard nodes, but there is prominent pain, synovial swelling, and erythema. Radiographs demonstrate irregular joint space loss, osteophytes, and bony erosions; bony ankylosis may occur.

Diffuse Idiopathic Skeletal Hyperostosis Syndrome

Diffuse idiopathic skeletal hyperostosis (DISH) syndrome, principally affecting the spine, is not an osteoarthritic condition. While the radiographs demonstrate large hypertrophic spurs, they are not osteophytes, but represent the calcification of the anterior longitudinal ligament. The cartilaginous structures of the facet joints and the disks do not degenerate as a manifestation of the DISH syndrome itself. At peripheral joints, "whiskering" of the periosteum may be seen, mimicking the enthesopathy of a seronegative spondyloarthropathy. However, the sacroiliac joints are spared. DISH is infrequently the cause of significant spine or peripheral joint pain, although stiffness and decreased range of motion of the spine may occur.[33]

CLINICAL DIFFERENTIAL DIAGNOSIS

The differential diagnosis depends on the presenting complaints and physical findings. An acute monoarticular presence warrants consideration of crystal or infectious arthropathy or a seronegative spondyloarthropathy. Polyarticular disease may need to be distinguished from systemic inflammatory arthritis. DIP involvement is typical of psoriatic arthritis and may be seen infrequently in rheumatoid arthritis. Symptomatic MCP involvement is uncommon in OA and typical of rheumatoid arthritis. The presence of warmth and erythema would bode against OA. Evaluation of synovial fluid for total white blood cell count, to detect inflammation, and crystal analysis may be required. Blood tests are indicated if there is a concern about a systemic or inflammatory process; these should be normal in OA. Radiographs will usually distinguish OA from an inflammatory process, but erosive hand OA may be very destructive and difficult to discern from psoriatic arthritis. Pain in a given region and the finding of radiographic OA in a nearby joint does not necessarily confirm OA as the cause of the pain; the differential diagnosis includes tendonopathy, bursitis, an osseous lesion, or pain referred in a radicular or peripheral neuropathic pattern. Unusual patterns (shoulder, wrists, elbows) warrant a further evaluation for an underlying cause (see Chapter 13).

SUMMARY

Symptoms related to clinically active OA range from mildly annoying discomfort to severe and disabling pain. The diagnosis is generally easy to establish for peripheral joints, although consideration of an underlying disorder should be made. The cervical and lumbar spine are more challenging in terms of their diagnosis as imaging studies may be very abnormal in asymptomatic people. OA in many may be an inevitable result of aging, but preventing it where possible (weight loss), early intervention to maintain healthy habits (routine exercise), and respect for the pain and disability of people of all ages is essential as the number of elderly increases yearly.

REFERENCES

1. Lawrence RC, Helmick CG, Arnett FC, et al. Estimates of the prevalence of arthritis and selected musculoskeletal disorders in the United States. Arthritis Rheum 41:778–799, 1998.
2. Van Baar ME, Dekker J, Lemmers JA, et al. Pain and disability in patients with osteoarthritis of hip or knee. J Rheumatol 25:125–133, 1998.
3. Creamer P, Lethbridge-Cejku M, Hochberg MC. Factors associated with functional impairment in symptomatic knee osteoarthritis. Rheumatology 39: 490–496, 2000.
4. Croft P, Jordan K, Jinks C. "Pain elsewhere" and the impact of knee pain in older people. Arthritis Rheum 52:2350–2354, 2005.
5. Lin EHB, Katon W, Von Korff M, et al. Effect of improving depression care on pain and functional outcomes among older adults with arthritis. A randomized controlled trial. JAMA 290: 2428–2434, 2003.
6. Felson DT, Zhang Y, Anthony JM, et al. Weight loss reduces the risk for symptomatic knee osteoarthritis in women: The Framingham Study. Ann Intern Med 116:535–539, 1992.
7. Altman RD, Hochberg MC, Moskowitz RW, et al. Recommendation for the medical management of osteoarthritis of the hip and knee. 2000 update. Arthritis Rheum 43:1905–1915, 2000.
8. Hannan MT, Felson DT, Pincus T. Analysis of the discordance between radiographic changes and knee pain in osteoarthritis of the knee. J Rheumatol 27:1513, 2000.
9. Felson DT, Chaisson CE, Hill CL, et al. The association of bone marrow lesions with pain in knee osteoarthritis. Ann Intern Med 134:541–549, 2001.
10. Sowers MF, Jamadar D, Capul D, et al. Magnetic resonance-detected subchondral bone marrow and cartilage defect characteristics associated with pain and X-ray defined knee osteoarthritis. Osteoarthritis Cart 11:387–393, 2003.
11. Kennedy TD, Plater-Zyberk C, Partridge TA, et al. Morphometric comparison of synovium from patients with osteoarthritis and rheumatoid arthritis. J Clin Pathol 41:847–852, 1988.
12. Phillips DM. JCAHO pain management standards unveiled. JAMA 284:726–733, 2004.
13. Brown MD, Gomez-Martin O, Brookfield KFW, et al. Differential of hip disease versus spine disease. Clin Orthop 419:280–284, 2004.
14. Verges J, Montell E, Tomas E, et al. Weather conditions can influence rheumatic diseases. Proc West Pharmacol Soc 47:134–136, 2004.
15. Wilder FV, Hall BJ, Barret JP. Osteoarthritis pain and weather. Rheumatology; 42:955–968, 2003.
16. Pai YC, Rymer WZ, Change RW, et al. Effect of age and osteoarthritis on knee proprioception. J Rheumatol 40:2260–2265, 1997.
17. Bennell KL, Hinman RS, Metcalf BR, et al. Relationship of knee joint proprioception to pain and disability in individuals with knee osteoarthritis. J Orthop Res 21:792–797, 2003.
18. Cerejo R, Dunlop DD, Cahue S, et al. The influence of alignment on risk of knee osteoarthritis progression according to baseline stage of disease. Arthritis Rheum 46: 2632–2636, 2002.
19. Ike RW, O'Rourke KS. Compartment-directed physical examination of the knee can predict articular cartilage abnormalities disclosed by needle arthroscopy. Arthritis Rheum 38:917–925, 1995.
20. Shakoor N, Block JA, Shott S, et al. Nonrandom evolution of end-stage osteoarthritis of the lower limbs. Arthritis Rheum 46:3185–3189, 2002.
21. Spector TD, Cicutinni F, Baker J, et al. Genetic influences on osteoarthritis in women: a twin study. BMJ 312:940–943, 1996.
22. Kraus VB, Li YJ, Martin ER, et al. Articular hypermobility is a protective factor for hand osteoarthritis. Arthritis Rheum 50: 2178–2183, 2004.
23. Altman R, Alarcon C, Appelroth D, et al. The American College of Rheumatology criteria for the classification and reporting of osteoarthritis of the hand. Arthritis Rheum 33:1601–1610, 1990.
24. Curl WW. Popliteal cysts. Historical background and current knowledge. J Am Acad Orthop Surg 4:129–133, 1996.
25. Altman R, Asch E, Bloch D, et al. Development of criteria for the classification and reporting of osteoarthritis of the knee. Arthritis Rheum 29:1039–1049, 1986.
26. Khan AM, McLoughlin E, Giannakas K, et al. Hip osteoarthritis: where is the pain? Ann R Coll Surg Engl 86:119–121, 2004.
27. Altman RD, Alarcon G, Appelrouth D, et al. The American College of Rheumatology criteria for the classification and reporting of osteoarthritis of the hip. Arthritis Rheum 34:505–514, 1991.
28. Katz JN, Dalgas M, Stucki G, et al. Degenerative lumbar spinal stenosis: diagnostic value of the history and physical examination. Arthritis Rheum 38:1236–1241, 1995.
29. Halverson PB, McCarty DJ, Cheung HS, et al. Milwaukee shoulder syndrome: eleven additional cases with involvement of the knee in seven (basic calcium phosphate crystal deposition disease). Semin Arthritis Rheum 14:36–44, 1984.
30. Crooks MC, Ferguson JW, Edwards JL. Clinical presentation and final diagnosis of patients referred to a temporomandibular joint clinic. NZ Dent J 87:113–118, 1991.
31. Zarb GA, Carlsson GE. Temporomandibular disorders. Osteoarthritis. J Orofac Pain ; 13:295–306, 1999.
32. Martinez-Blanco M, Bagan JV, Fons A, et al. Osteoarthrosis of the temporomandibular joint. A Clinical and radiological survey of 16 patients. Med Oral 9:106–115, 2004.
33. Mata S, Fortin PR, Fitzcharles PA. A controlled study of diffuse idiopathic skeletal hyperostosis. Clinical features and functional status. Medicine (Baltimore) 76:104–117, 1997.

Radiologic Diagnosis

8

Garry Gold   Vijay Chandnani   Donald Resnick

The term osteoarthritis (OA), previously called degenerative joint disease, is applied to a variety of distinct processes affecting joints in extraspinal and spinal locations. There are basic differences in the anatomy of the various types of joints at these sites, and they change in unique fashions. Each type of articular degeneration is associated with characteristic clinical, pathologic, and radiologic features. This chapter discusses the radiologic manifestations of OA at extraspinal joints as well as in the various types of spinal articulations. Methods of quantitation of radiologic changes are also discussed.

OSTEOARTHRITIS OF EXTRASPINAL LOCATIONS

General Considerations

OA, the most frequent articular affliction, was not regarded as a distinct entity until the early twentieth century, when it was clearly differentiated from rheumatoid arthritis.[1,2] OA is the best general phrase to describe degenerative alterations in any type of joint. These alterations may appear in fibrous, cartilaginous, or synovial articulations. The pathologic and radiographic appearances vary from one location to another, but at any site, the abnormalities appear to be related to degeneration of specific articular structures. The terms osteoarthrosis and OA are reserved for OA of synovial joints. Although inflammatory changes are not pronounced in most of these joints, OA is the term used in this chapter because this designation is widely accepted in the United States. Furthermore, in those joints in which significant synovial inflammatory abnormalities do accompany OA, such as in the interphalangeal articulations of middle-aged and elderly women, OA is the more accurate description of the disorder.

Primary and Secondary Osteoarthritis

OA has traditionally been classified into primary (idiopathic) and secondary types. Primary OA has been regarded as a process in which articular degeneration occurs in the absence of any obvious underlying abnormality, whereas secondary OA has been regarded as articular degeneration that is produced by alterations from a preexisting condition. This classification is misleading, because careful evaluation of many examples of "primary" OA will reveal some mechanical deviation in the involved articulation that has led to secondary degeneration of the joint. Examples include infantile and childhood disorders such as congenital dysplasia and a slipped capital femoral epiphysis; when mild, these are easily overlooked, yet later they can lead to OA in the hip. Thus, it appears likely that primary OA does not truly exist, and the use of such a designation seems only to underscore current diagnostic limitations.

Articular degeneration may result from either an abnormal concentration of force across an articulation with normal articular cartilage matrix or a normal concentration of force across an abnormal joint.[3] Eventually, abnormalities of force and articular structure appear together (Table 8–1). This classification emphasizes that there are many potential causes of secondary OA and that these causes may lead to articular degeneration by increasing the amount of stress on cartilaginous and osseous structures or by directly affecting the cartilage or subchondral bone itself. These considerations have relevance to radiologic interpretation of degenerative changes in joints.

Radiographic-Pathologic Correlation

Degenerative changes are found not only in the stressed (pressure) areas of a joint but also in the nonstressed (nonpressure) segments.[4] Therefore, either excessive or

TABLE 8–1
CLASSIFICATION OF OA

ABNORMAL CONCENTRATION OF FORCE ON NORMAL ARTICULATION

Intra-articular malalignment
  Epiphyseal injuries
  Epiphyseal dysplasia
  Neuromuscular imbalance
Extra-articular malalignment
  Inequality of leg length
  Congenital and acquired varus or valgus deformities
  Malunited fractures
  Ligamentous abnormalities
Loss of protective sensory feedback
  Neuroarthropathy
  Intra-articular injection of steroids
Miscellaneous
  Obesity
  Occupational

NORMAL CONCENTRATION OF FORCE ON ABNORMAL ARTICULATION

Normal concentration of force on abnormal cartilage
  Transchondral fractures
  Meniscal tears and diskoid menisci
  Loose bodies
  Preexisting arthritis
  Metabolic abnormalities (gout, calcium pyrophosphate
    dihydrate crystal deposition disease, acromegaly,
    alkaptonuria, mucopolysaccharidoses)
Normal concentration of force on normal cartilage supported by
    weakened subchondral bone
  Osteonecrosis
  Osteoporosis
  Osteomalacia
  Osteitis fibrosa cystica (hyperparathyroidism)
  Neoplasm
Normal concentration of force on normal cartilage supported by
    stiffened subchondral bone
  Osteopetrosis
  Paget disease

From Resnick D. Diagnosis of Bone and Joint Disorders. 4th ed. Philadelphia, WB Saunders, 2002, p 1272.

diminished pressure appears to be deleterious to cartilage. Normally, cartilage derives its nutrition from intermittent intrusion and extrusion of synovial fluid during alternating periods of pressure and rest as well as from vessels in the subchondral bone, which allow material to pass into the basal layer of cartilage.[5-8] Both sources of nutrition become defective in the presence of excessive or diminished stress, leading to degenerative changes.

In the stressed segment, pathologically evident thinning and denudation of the cartilaginous surface and vascular invasion, in addition to infarction and necrosis of the subchondral trabeculae, account for joint space loss, bone sclerosis, and cyst formation that are apparent on the radiographs (Table 8–2). In the nonstressed segment, pathologically evident hypervascularity of marrow and cartilage leads to radiographically detectable osteophytosis.[4]

Cartilage in degenerating joints at first appears discolored, thinned, and roughened; later, crevices, ulcerations, and larger areas of erosion become evident.[9-11] This progressive cartilage loss accounts for one of the fundamental radiographic signs of OA, loss of joint space. This diminution is characteristically located mainly in the area that has been subjected to the greatest pressure, such as the superolateral aspect of an osteoarthritic hip and the medial femorotibial space of an osteoarthritic knee. This focal cartilaginous destruction and resulting loss of the interosseous space allow differentiation from processes such as rheumatoid arthritis that lead to diffuse chondral alterations. Certain sites of involvement are exceptions to this rule; in OA of the interphalangeal or metacarpophalangeal joints of the hands as well as of the sacroiliac joint, diffuse joint space involvement may be noted.

After cartilage loss, bone eburnation becomes evident in the closely applied osseous surfaces, apparently related to deposition of new bone on preexisting trabeculae and to trabecular compression and fracture with callus formation.[12-18] In general, radiographic evidence of joint space loss is present before eburnation becomes apparent. After progressive loss of joint space, sclerosis becomes more apparent, extending vertically into deeper regions of the subchondral bone and horizontally into adjacent osseous segments. The radiodense area may initially appear uniform, but radiolucent areas of varying size eventually appear, reflecting subchondral cyst formation.

Cyst formation is an important finding in OA[19-21] (Fig. 8–1); these lesions have been variously termed synovial cysts,[22] subchondral cysts,[8] subarticular pseudocysts,[23] necrotic pseudocysts,[24] and geodes.[25] Within the stressed segment of the subchondral bone in OA, cystic spaces appear between thickened trabeculae. These cysts are commonly multiple, of varying size (approximately 2 to 20 mm in diameter), and piriform. Communication with the articular space may or may not be identifiable.[26] The cysts seen radiographically in OA characteristically have a sclerotic margin.

Osteophytes (Table 8–3) develop in areas of a degenerating joint that are subjected to low stress; they may be marginal (peripheral), although they may become apparent at other articular locations as well. Osteophytes typically arise as a revitalization or reparative response by remaining cartilage, but they may also develop from periosteal or synovial tissue.[27] The features of conversion of cartilage to bone in OA resemble those accompanying normal endochondral (enchondral) ossification. Marginal osteophytes appear radiographically as lips of new bone around the edges of the joint and are of variable size. The excrescences frequently predominate in one side of the joint, develop initially in areas of relatively normal joint space, and are usually unassociated with significant adjacent sclerosis or cyst formation (Fig. 8–2). Osteophytes may also appear in the central portions of a joint in which remnants of articular cartilage still exist.[27] The hypervascularity of the subchondral bone stimulates endochondral ossification, and the resulting excrescences are often demarcated at their bases by remnants of the original calcified cartilage. Central osteophytes frequently lead to a bumpy articular contour on the radiograph. In certain joints, bone may develop

TABLE 8-2

OA OF SYNOVIAL ARTICULATIONS (OSTEOARTHRITIS): RADIOGRAPHIC-PATHOLOGIC CORRELATION

Pathologic Abnormalities	Radiographic Abnormalities
Cartilaginous fibrillation and erosion	Localized loss of joint space
Increased cellularity and hypervascularity of subchondral bone	Bone eburnation
Synovial fluid intrusion or bone contusion	Subchondral cysts
Revascularization of remaining cartilage and capsular traction	Osteophytes
Periosteal and synovial membrane stimulation	Osteophytes and buttressing
Compression of weakened and deformed trabeculae	Bone collapse
Fragmentation of osteochondral surface	Intra-articular osseous bodies
Disruption and distortion of capsular and ligamentous structures	Deformity and malalignment

From Resnick D. Diagnosis of Bone and Joint Disorders. 4th ed. Philadelphia, WB Saunders, 2002, p 1278.

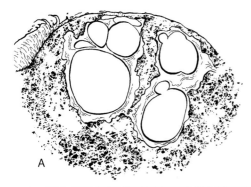

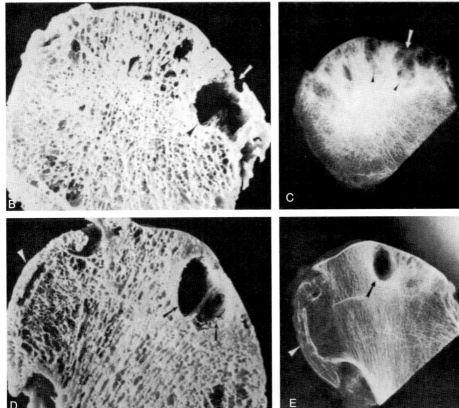

Figure 8–1 Subchondral bone cysts, pathologic and radiographic findings. *A,* A drawing reveals the typical appearance of multiple subchondral cysts of varying size in areas of cartilaginous degeneration or disappearance. They are surrounded by sclerotic bone. *B* and *C,* A photograph and radiograph of a macerated coronal section of a femoral head in a patient with osteoarthritis reveal multiple cystic lesions (arrowheads), which, in places, communicate with the articular cavity (arrows). *D* and *E,* In a different patient with a similar problem, a photograph and radiograph of a coronal section of the femoral head outline subchondral cysts (arrows), which in this instance do not obviously communicate with the articular cavity. They are located on the pressure segment (superolateral aspect) of the femoral head, whereas the osteophytes (arrowheads) are evident on the nonpressure segment. (*A, D,* and *E* from Resnick D. Diagnosis of Bone Joint Disorders. 4th ed. Philadelphia, WB Saunders, 2002, p 1282. *B* and *C* from Resnick D, Niwayama G, Coutts RD. Subchondral cysts [geodes] in arthritic disorders. Pathologic and radiographic appearance of the hip joint. AJR Am J Roentgenol 128: 799–806, 1977. Copyright 1977, American Roentgen Ray Society.)

TABLE 8–3
TYPES OF OSTEOPHYTES

Type	Mechanism	Radiographic Appearance
Marginal osteophyte	Endochondral ossification resulting from vascularization of subchondral bone marrow	Outgrowth at the margins (nonpressure segments) of the joint, producing lips of bone
Central osteophyte	Endochondral ossification resulting from vascularization of subchondral bone marrow	Outgrowth at the central areas of the joint, producing bumpy contour
Periosteal (synovial) osteophyte	Intramembranous ossification resulting from stimulation of periosteal (synovial) membrane with appositional bone formation	Thickening of intra-articular "cortices," producing buttressing
Capsular osteophyte	Capsular traction	Lips of bone extending along the direction of capsular pull

From Resnick D. Diagnosis of Bone Joint Disorders. 4th ed. Philadelphia, WB Saunders, 2002, p 1288.

from cartilaginous stimulation by the periosteum or synovial membrane. This phenomenon, termed buttressing,[28,29] is most characteristic in the medial portion of the femoral neck. On radiographs, a radiodense line of variable thickness extends along part or all of the femoral neck.

OA may be associated with degeneration of other articular structures, such as the fibrocartilage labrum, disks, and menisci.[30–32] Degeneration of tendons, intraosseous ligaments, and membranes is also common, especially near the sites of attachment of these structures to bone (Fig. 8–3).

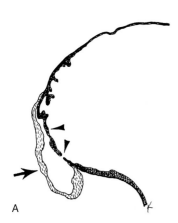

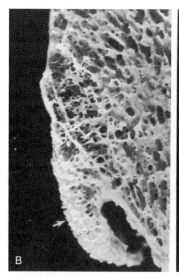

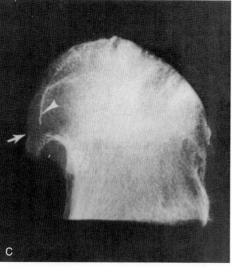

Figure 8–2 Marginal osteophytes, pathologic and radiographic findings. *A,* A diagram indicates the nature of the marginal osteophyte. It develops as a lip of bone (arrow) as a result of vascularization of the subchondral marrow with the inception of endochondral ossification. As it grows, it leaves behind a remnant of the original calcified cartilage (arrowheads). *B* and *C,* A photograph and radiograph of a small to moderate-sized marginal osteophyte (arrows) in these macerated coronal sections of the femoral head reveal the original calcified cartilaginous zone (arrowheads). (From Resnick D. Diagnosis of Bone Joint Disorders. 4th ed. Philadelphia, WB Saunders, 2002, p 1289)

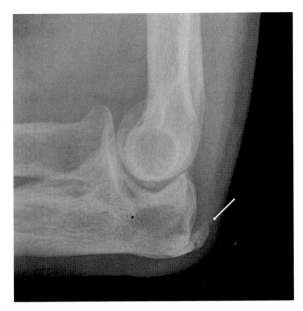

Figure 8–3 Enthesopathy in osteoarthritis. Lateral radiograph of an elbow reveals irregular osseous proliferation at the site of triceps attachment to bone (arrow).

These may manifest radiographically as excrescences that are termed enthesophytes. Tendon and ligament calcification may also be noted.

Osteoarthritis in Specific Locations

Hand and Wrist

OA of the proximal and distal interphalangeal joints of the hand (including the interphalangeal joint of the thumb) is extremely common, especially in middle-aged, postmenopausal women. Involvement of multiple digits of both hands is characteristic. Clinically, the altered digits may reveal malalignment, such as flexion deformity and radial or ulnar deviation at the interphalangeal joints. Bone outgrowths at the distal interphalangeal joints are termed Heberden nodes.[33] Similar outgrowths at the proximal interphalangeal joints are termed Bouchard nodes.

Distal interphalangeal and proximal interphalangeal joints are frequently affected simultaneously and symmetrically; however, extensive alterations at distal interphalangeal joints may occur in the absence of proximal interphalangeal joint abnormalities, and less commonly, isolated abnormalities of proximal interphalangeal joints may be evident.

Radiographs reveal prominent osteophytes and joint space narrowing, providing close apposition of adjacent enlarged osseous surfaces. It is the closely applied, undulating articular surfaces that produce the diagnostic radiographic appearance of the disease, allowing it to be distinguished from erosive disorders, which produce separation of the involved bones. In OA, the wavy contour of the base of the distal phalanx resembles the wings of a bird (i.e., the "seagull" sign) (Fig. 8–4). The involved digits frequently reveal mild to moderate radial and ulnar subluxation at distal interphalangeal or proximal interphalangeal

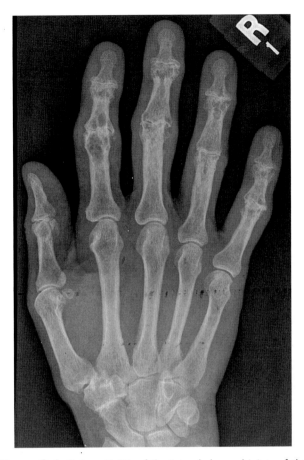

Figure 8–4 Osteoarthritis of the interphalangeal joints of the hand. A typical example of osteoarthritis of both distal interphalangeal and proximal interphalangeal articulations. Note the closely applied interdigitating osseous surfaces, capsular osteophytes, subchondral sclerosis, and wavy contour of the fingers as a result of medial and lateral phalangeal subluxations. On occasion, changes predominate at proximal interphalangeal articulations, resulting in clinically detectable Bouchard nodes. At the interphalangeal articulation of the thumb, prominent osteophytes, ossicles, joint space narrowing, and sclerosis are apparent. Note again the apposition of one bone with its neighbor. The typical distribution of osteoarthritis is illustrated here. Findings are apparent in distal interphalangeal, proximal interphalangeal, and, to a lesser extent, metacarpophalangeal articulations.

joints, producing a zigzag contour. At the margins of the affected joint, focal radiodense lesions (ossicles) are apparent overlying the joint capsule; they resemble intra-articular osseous bodies or fractured osteophytes.

Metacarpophalangeal joint involvement in OA is almost invariably associated with more prominent abnormalities at the proximal and distal interphalangeal joints. Uniform narrowing of one or more metacarpophalangeal interosseous spaces is most characteristic,[34] and cystic lesions and osteophytes may also be apparent. Erosions are absent. One exception to these findings occurs in the first digit, in which isolated alterations at the first metacarpophalangeal joint can be a prominent manifestation of OA.

The radial distribution of OA of the wrist is well known. In the absence of significant accidental or occupational trauma, changes are usually confined to the trapeziometacarpal joint and trapezioscaphoid space of the midcarpal joint. At the

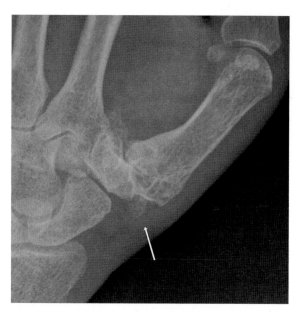

Figure 8–5 Osteoarthritis of the trapeziometacarpal joint. Joint space loss, subchondral sclerosis and cysts, and osteophytes are present at the trapeziometacarpal joint (arrow).

trapeziometacarpal joint, radiographic features of OA are characteristic. Radial subluxation of the metacarpal base, narrowing of the interosseous space, sclerosis, cystic changes in the subchondral bone, osteophytosis, and bone fragmentation become apparent (Fig. 8–5). OA of the trapezioscaphoid space is usually combined with degenerative changes at the trapeziometacarpal joint,[35] although isolated abnormalities have also been reported.[36-38] Typical radiographic features at this location are apparent in a unilateral or bilateral distribution; these include joint space narrowing and sclerosis of apposing surfaces of the trapezium, trapezoid, and scaphoid.

OA localized to other compartments of the wrist is distinctly unusual in the absence of a history of trauma. However, fracture, subluxation, dislocation, or osteonecrosis about the wrist can lead to altered joint motion and can result in secondary OA. Typical examples include OA of the radiocarpal and midcarpal compartments after scaphoid injuries,[39,40] OA of the radiocarpal and inferior radioulnar compartment after osteonecrosis of the lunate (Kienböck disease), and OA of the inferior radioulnar compartment after subluxation of the distal part of the ulna. Arthrosis of the lunate-capitate space, leading to interosseous narrowing, sclerosis, and cyst formation, has been emphasized as an additional post-traumatic degenerative condition.[41] This abnormality is usually combined with scapholunate separation, or dissociation, and narrowing of the radioscaphoid space.[42] The resulting radiographic changes are termed the scapholunate advanced collapse pattern, or SLAC, wrist.[42,43]

Shoulder, Elbow, and Acromioclavicular Joints

OA of the glenohumeral joint has been considered unusual in the absence of trauma. Nontraumatic degenerative changes at this location are usually secondary to other disorders, such as alkaptonuria, acromegaly,

epiphyseal dysplasia, calcium pyrophosphate dihydrate (CPPD), crystal deposition disease, apatite deposition disease (Milwaukee shoulder)[44], and hemophilia.[45-47] The most frequent abnormality in OA at this site is osteophyte formation along the articular margin of the humeral head and the line of attachment of the labrum to the glenoid fossa. These osteophytes predominate along the anteroinferior portions of the joint. Another abnormality seen in OA of the glenohumeral joint is eburnation, manifested as subchondral sclerosis, along the superior and middle portion of the articular surface of the humeral head (Fig. 8–6). Other alterations seen at this location include osseous excrescences with occasional areas of cystic change in the anatomic neck of the humerus. Osteophytes are commonly evident in and around the bicipital groove as well.[48]

OA of the elbow is uncommon and usually follows accidental or occupational trauma, as seen in miners and drillers. Typical radiographic findings include joint space narrowing, sclerosis, cysts, and osteophytes. Olecranon enthesophytes at the ulnar attachment of the triceps tendon may accompany these alterations (Fig. 8–3).

Degenerative changes of the acromioclavicular joint are nearly universal in the elderly. Radiographic examination reveals joint space loss, sclerosis of apposing osseous surfaces, marginal osteophytes, hypertrophy and inferior subluxation of the acromial end of the clavicle, and osseous proliferation on either the superior or inferior surface of the acromion[49,50] (Fig. 8–7).

Hip

OA of the hip is invariably associated with progressive and focal joint space narrowing. With the onset of this narrowing, the femoral head moves toward the acetabulum.

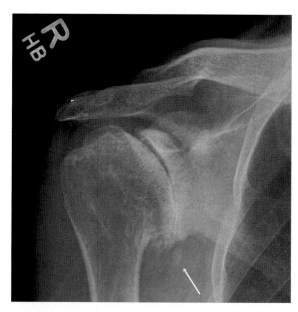

Figure 8–6 Osteoarthritis of the glenohumeral joint. Joint space narrowing, sclerosis, and formation of intra-articular bodies (arrow) are seen.

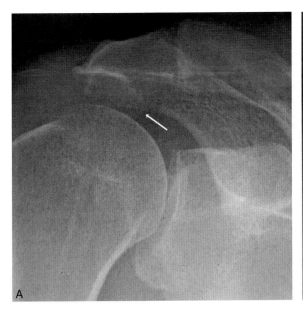
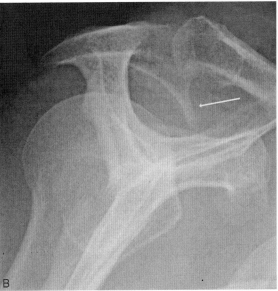

Figure 8–7 Subacromial enthesophytes. *A,* An anteroposterior radiograph of the shoulder in external rotation reveals marked enthesophytic proliferation about the inferior surface of the acromion (arrow). There is also joint space narrowing and subchondral sclerosis at the acromioclavicular joint. *B,* Scapular Y projection also shows the enthesophyte (arrow).

Three basic patterns of migration can be observed: superior migration, medial migration, and axial migration. With superior migration, the femoral head moves in an upward or superior direction with respect to the acetabulum. A medial migration pattern is evident when joint space loss is confined to the inner third of the joint. With axial migration, the femoral head migrates axially along the axis of the femoral neck, and there is diffuse loss of articular space. This classification system relies on changes seen on the frontal radiograph. Anterior or posterior migrations of the femoral head, as seen on lateral radiographs or with computed tomography or magnetic resonance imaging (MRI), may accompany these changes.

Although the pattern of movement of the femoral head with respect to the acetabulum may be variable in OA, thereby influencing the distribution of morphologic changes, the basic radiographic and pathologic changes are similar. These include joint space narrowing, osteophytosis, buttressing, sclerosis, and cyst formation[21,51–67] (Fig. 8–8). The cysts can be single or multiple and are of varying size; they are located on either the femoral or the acetabular side of the joint, or both. Large cystic lesions in the acetabulum are occasionally seen.

Synovial membrane alterations in OA are generally mild, although considerable osseous and cartilaginous debris may become embedded in the synovium of osteoarthritic hips, particularly in the recesses associated with the capsular reflection on the femoral neck.[28] Hypertrophied synovium containing detritus may become prominent in these areas.[65]

Arthrography is occasionally used to outline the location and extent of cartilage loss in OA of the hip,[68] although similar abnormalities may be detected on routine radiography. Arteriography has been used to elucidate the vascular abnormalities of OA of the hip,[69,70] which are manifested as increased number, length, and width of periarticular and intraosseous vessels. Venography may be used to identify a deviation in the normal pattern of venous drainage from the femoral head and neck.[71–74] In OA, increased flow

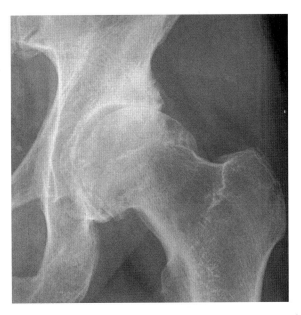

Figure 8–8 Osteoarthritis of the hip. Anteroposterior radiograph of the left hip demonstrates superior migration of the left femoral head, apposition of the femoral head and acetabulum, subchondral sclerosis and cyst formation on both the femoral and acetabular sides of the joint, buttressing of the femoral neck, and large osteophyte formation. These radiographic findings are diagnostic of osteoarthritis of the left hip.

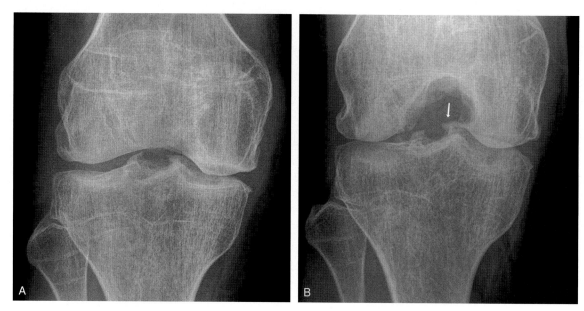

Figure 8–9 Osteoarthritis of the knee, usefulness of "tunnel" view. *A,* The anteroposterior radiograph reveals sclerosis of the lateral and medial tibial articular surfaces and the lateral femoral articular surface. The joint space does not appear diminished. *B,* On a tunnel view, the severity of joint space loss in both lateral and medial femorotibial compartments is evident. In addition, the intra-articular radiodense areas adjacent to the tibial spine are more apparent in this projection (arrow).

initially occurs by way of the femoral shaft; subsequently, pooling of injected contrast material with decreased or absent venous outflow is seen. Radionuclide examination demonstrates increased uptake in periarticular osseous tissue.[75,76] The scintigraphic pattern may be more sensitive, although relatively nonspecific, in detecting the presence and extent of OA. Computed tomography in conjunction with arthrography may be useful in detecting osteocartilaginous debris and in delineating the extent of anteversion of the femoral neck.[77-79] MR imaging or MR arthrography may demonstrate areas of cartilage thinning, tears of the acetabular labrum, increased bone marrow signal on long TE pulse sequences indicative of reactive edema, and presence of intra-articular osteochondral loose bodies.[80-83]

Knee

Many factors contribute to the development of OA in the knee, including prior surgery or trauma, angular deformity, osteonecrosis, osteochondritis dissecans, obesity, and meniscal abnormality. All of these factors lead to an increased stress or force per unit area in the knee.

It is useful to regard the knee joint as consisting of three compartments: the medial femorotibial, the lateral femorotibial, and the patellofemoral. Radiographic changes usually predominate in one or two of these compartments, although pathologic changes are evident in all three areas. Routine radiography is somewhat limited in its sensitivity in detecting early changes.[84,85] Weight-bearing or stress radiographic views better delineate joint space narrowing, sclerosis, cysts, and osteophytes.[84-90] "Tunnel" projections obtained with the knee in flexion may occasionally demonstrate cartilage loss or

osteochondral lesions not well seen on routine views[91] (Fig. 8–9).

Bilateral or unilateral changes may be seen in the femorotibial compartments. Unicompartmental (medial femorotibial compartment)[84,85] or bicompartmental (medial femorotibial and patellofemoral compartments) involvement is typically present in OA (Fig. 8–10). Less commonly, bicompartmental involvement of the lateral femorotibial and patellofemoral compartments is present. Joint space

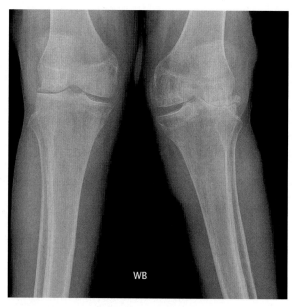

Figure 8–10 Valgus angulation of both the right and left knees with severe bilateral lateral compartment osteoarthritis.

narrowing varies from mild to severe. Subchondral bone sclerosis is more frequent in the proximal portion of the tibia than in the femur. Subchondral cysts are less common in the knee than in the hip and, when present, are usually small and seen in the proximal portion of the tibia. Subchondral cysts are associated with joint space narrowing and eburnation. On occasion, intra-articular surface irregularity and sharpening of the tibial spines are identified. Other radiographic abnormalities in OA of the knee include vacuum phenomenon within the articular space or within a diseased meniscus and meniscal calcification.

In OA, the patellofemoral compartment is commonly involved, although this involvement is usually combined with abnormalities in the femorotibial compartments. Rarely, abnormalities confined to the patellofemoral compartment are present. Radiographic manifestations of patellofemoral OA include joint space narrowing, sclerosis, and osteophytes, particularly on the patellar side of the space. Loss of articular space may be difficult to detect on lateral radiographs but is readily demonstrated on axial views.

Osteophytes at the superior and inferior surface of the patella may, when present, become extremely large. Associated scalloped defects of the anterior cortex of the femur may become prominent.[92,93] This finding appears to arise from pressure erosion of the femoral cortex by the patella and is located at the level the patella assumes on full extension of the knee.

Another degenerative process occurs on the anterior surface of the patella and consists of bone proliferation at the site of osseous attachment of the quadriceps tendon. This is an enthesopathic alteration probably related to abnormal stress on the ligamentous connection to the bone. It produces hyperostosis of the anterior patellar surface and has been termed the "tooth" sign.[94]

Angulation and subluxation at the knee joint are best demonstrated on weight-bearing or stress views of the knee. Varus angulation is more frequent than valgus angulation. The contralateral femorotibial compartment widens as the ipsilateral compartment narrows. Translation or subluxation of the tibia on the femur laterally with varus angulation and medially with valgus angulation is typical (Fig. 8–11).

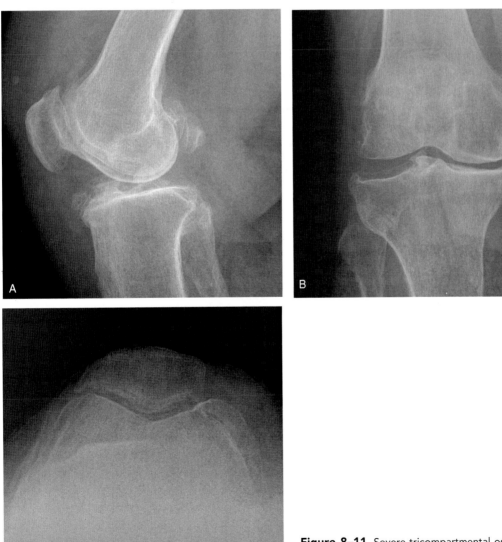

Figure 8–11 Severe tricompartmental osteoarthritis. *A*, Lateral, *B*, Frontal, and *C*, Merchant view radiographs of the left knee reveal joint space obliteration in the medial femoral tibial, lateral femoral tibial, and patellofemoral compartments; varus angulation and lateral subluxation of the tibia; and osteophyte formation.

Cartilaginous and osseous debris arises from the disintegrating surfaces of the bones surrounding the knee joint. Such debris may exist as loose bodies or "joint mice" before being incorporated in the synovial membrane. Specialized techniques such as arthrography, computed tomography, or MR imaging may be useful in the detection and characterization of intra-articular osteochondral bodies.

In OA of the knee, cartilaginous fibrillation and erosion and osseous proliferation can also be observed in the sesamoid fabella. The anterior surface of the fabella may reveal flattening and sclerosis on radiography, and the peroneal nerve may be injured by an enlarged fabella.[95]

Patellofemoral pain syndrome is a term applied to a syndrome of pain and crepitus over the anterior aspect of the knee. It is most commonly seen in young adults.[96–97] The cause of this syndrome is unclear, although it may be related to increased cartilage stress.[98] The patella consists of three facets: the lateral, the medial, and a more medially located odd facet. The medial facet, particularly at the junction of the medial and odd facets, is a classic site of cartilage damage.

Ankle and Foot

OA of the ankle is uncommon in the absence of significant trauma. It may occur after fracture of the neighboring bones, especially when the ankle mortise is disrupted. Degeneration of the ankle may also develop whenever the talocalcaneal joints are altered, as may occur after congenital or surgical fusion. Joint space loss, sclerosis, and osteophytes may appear about the degenerating ankle joint (Fig. 8–12). Capsular traction can produce a talar beak on the dorsal aspect of the bone.[99]

Degenerative changes may develop at the first tarsometatarsal joint and may be manifested as joint space narrowing and sclerosis. Post-traumatic or, rarely, spontaneous changes may develop at other locations, such as the talonavicular portion of the anterior talocalcaneonavicular joint. Small osteophytes arise along the dorsal aspect of the apposing surfaces of the talus and navicular bones.[100]

Persistent hindfoot pain after a calcaneal fracture may result from development of OA in one or both subtalar joints. Plain films are usually inadequate in delineating the degenerative abnormalities; computed tomography provides much more information. Findings include joint space narrowing, irregularity and depression of the articular surfaces, bone sclerosis and cyst formation, and osteophytes.

Plantar and posterior enthesophytes are frequent radiographic findings that can be unassociated with clinical abnormalities. These excrescences develop at the osseous site of attachment of the Achilles tendon, plantar aponeurosis, and long plantar ligament. When they are well defined and sharply marginated, they usually represent no more than an incidental degenerative abnormality related to ligamentous or tendinous traction on bone. Alternatively, a poorly defined or fluffy plantar calcaneal bone outgrowth can be an important radiographic finding of ankylosing spondylitis, psoriasis, and reactive arthritis.[101]

OA of the first metatarsophalangeal joint (hallux rigidus and hallux valgus) is extremely common[102–104] (Fig. 8–13). On radiographs, valgus angulation is frequently associated with pronation of the great toe and bone hypertrophy or osteophytosis, particularly on the medial aspect of the metatarsal head. The enlarged and irregular medial portion

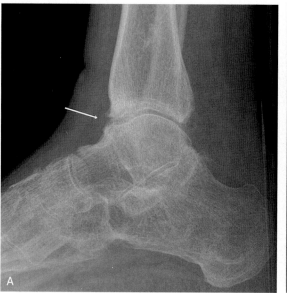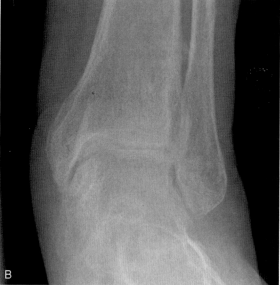

Figure 8–12 Osteoarthritis of the ankle. This middle-aged man developed progressive pain and swelling of the ankle after an injury many years before. Neurologic examination findings were normal. *A,* Lateral view demonstrates anterior osteophyte formation (arrow) and tibiotalar joint space narrowing. *B,* An anteroposterior radiograph of the ankle delineates joint space narrowing, sclerosis, fragmentation, and osteophytosis.

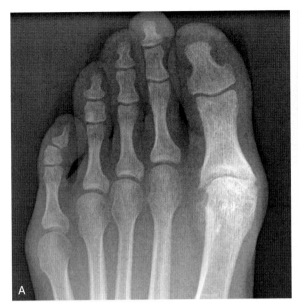
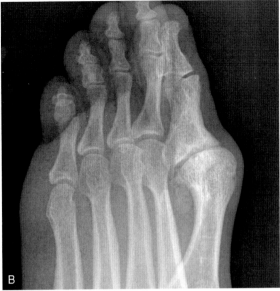

Figure 8–13 Osteoarthritis of the first metatarsophalangeal joint, hallux rigidus. *A,* Frontal and *B,* Oblique radiographs reveal considerable joint space narrowing, sclerosis, and osteophytosis about the first metatarsophalangeal articulation.

of the metatarsal bone may contain cystic lesions and thickened trabeculae. The first tarsometatarsal joint may be obliquely oriented (metatarsus varus) in patients with hallux valgus.[105,106] Changes in the other metatarsophalangeal joints may also become apparent, including subluxation or dislocation. OA of interphalangeal joints of the toes may be detected as an incidental finding on routine radiographs.

Special Types of Osteoarthritis

Generalized Osteoarthritis

The concept of a generalized or polyarticular form of OA is not universally accepted, despite many descriptions of patients with OA in multiple locations, including the joints of the hands, wrists, spine, knees, and hips.[107] When radiographs reveal evidence of degenerative changes in multiple sites, however, diagnoses other than generalized OA must be entertained. Multiple epiphyseal dysplasia, spondyloepiphyseal dysplasia, osteonecrosis, alkaptonuria, Paget disease, acromegaly, occupationally induced articular disorders, CPPD crystal deposition disease, gout, hemophilia, and inflammatory arthritides may lead to similar changes at multiple articular locations.

Inflammatory Osteoarthritis

A peculiar form of interphalangeal OA, characterized by acute inflammatory episodes with eventual ankylosis of some joints, has been described in middle-aged and elderly women.[108] Although some reports have used the term erosive OA, the term inflammatory OA is preferable because the patients with typical clinical findings may not reveal erosive changes on the radiographs.[109-111]

The radiographic changes in inflammatory OA are characterized by a combination of bone proliferation and erosion. Proliferative changes, however, may occur in the absence of any erosive abnormalities. Osteophytosis is present, resembling that seen in noninflammatory OA and predominating in the proximal and distal interphalangeal joints. Joint space narrowing, with associated subchondral sclerosis, is common. Erosions, which commonly begin at the central portion of the joint in the form of sharply marginated, etched defects, are seen frequently in the interphalangeal articulations. Intra-articular bone ankylosis, virtually confined to the interphalangeal joints, is also seen in patients with inflammatory OA[112,113] (Fig. 8–14). In the wrist, joint space narrowing and sclerosis occur on the radial aspect, between the trapezium and the base of the first metacarpal bone and also between the trapezium and the scaphoid; rarely, erosions are seen in these locations. These findings are identical to those in noninflammatory OA.

Complications of Osteoarthritis

In some degenerating joints, malalignment and subluxation of bone may become prominent. Asymmetric loss of joint space is characteristic and may produce varus or valgus angulation. Progressive subluxation may ensue, as evidenced by lateral displacement of the tibia on the femur, lateral displacement of the femoral head with respect to the acetabulum, and radial and proximal displacement of the first metacarpal base in relation to the trapezium.

Bone ankylosis is generally unusual in OA, with notable exceptions, including the ankylosis seen in inflammatory OA and that seen in the sacroiliac joints in noninflammatory OA. Bone bridging may also accompany degenerative changes in the symphyses.

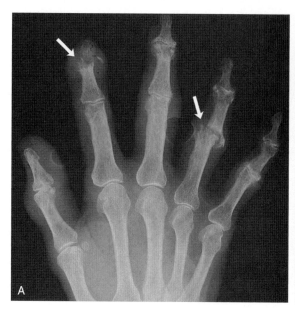
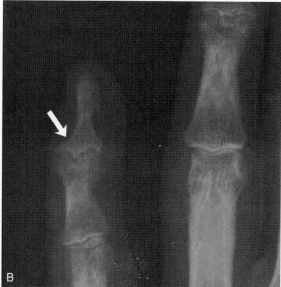

Figure 8–14 Inflammatory (erosive) osteoarthritis, interphalangeal joint abnormalities. *A,* Joint destruction (arrows) in the typical distribution of osteoarthritis is seen. *B,* In a more advanced case, disruption of the entire central aspect of the joint (arrow) is typical. Note the changes in the proximal interphalangeal articulation, which are identical to those of noninflammatory osteoarthritis. The eventual result may be intra-articular osseous fusion, as seen in the distal interphalangeal joint.

Osteocartilaginous bodies may result from several sources: transchondral fractures, disintegration of the articular surfaces, and synovial metaplasia.[114, 115] In OA, fragmentation of the joint surface may occur, and this debris may remain on the joint surface or become dislodged in the joint cavity (Fig. 8–15). This debris may subsequently become embedded at a distal synovial site, eliciting a local inflammatory response. Radiographically dense areas may be present, which can increase or decrease in size. These osteochondral bodies may pass from the joint cavity into a neighboring communicating synovial cyst. The osteochondral bodies seen in OA are generally fewer than ten in number and vary in size, in contrast to idiopathic synovial osteochondromatosis, in which a larger number of uniformly sized osteochondral bodies are present.

OSTEOARTHRITIS OF THE SPINE

General Considerations

The term OA is applied to a variety of distinct processes of spinal joints. Because there are fundamental anatomic differences among the joints of the spine, however, each degenerates in a distinctive fashion. Characteristic clinical, pathologic, and radiologic changes accompany these degenerative processes.

Cartilaginous Joints

The major cartilaginous joint of the spine is the intervertebral disk, consisting of the nucleus pulposus, annulus fibrosus, and adjacent vertebral end plates. These components are intimately associated both anatomically and physiologically. The metabolism of the intervertebral disk in adults is primarily anaerobic[116] and is dependent on diffusion of fluid either from the marrow of the vertebral bodies across the subchondral bone and cartilaginous end plate or through the annulus fibrosus from the surrounding blood vessels.

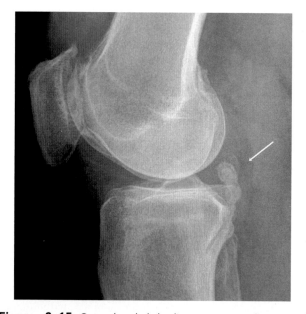

Figure 8–15 Osteochondral bodies as a complication of osteoarthritis. Lateral radiograph of the knee demonstrates osteochondral bodies (arrow) posterior to the joint. These osteochondral bodies typically migrate to the area of lowest pressure within the joint and may eventually become incorporated into the synovium.

Intervertebral Osteochondrosis (Disk Degeneration)

Aging results in dehydration and loss of tissue resiliency in the intervertebral disk, especially in the nucleus pulposus.[117-121] The nucleus pulposus appears desiccated and friable, which is a result of loss of water and proteoglycans. Clefts or crevices appear in the nucleus pulposus that extend to the annulus fibrosus.[122,123]

These earliest changes of osteochondrosis are identified on MR images, which also show dehydration of the nucleus pulposus. Although routine radiography is less sensitive than MR imaging, radiographic changes of intervertebral osteochondrosis include the appearance of characteristic linear or circular radiolucent areas (termed vacuum phenomena).[124-125] These lucent areas are produced by gas, mainly nitrogen, accumulating in the clefts and are accentuated on radiography obtained during extension of the spine. Vacuum phenomena are a reliable indicator of disk degeneration, and their visualization virtually excludes the presence of tumor or infection (Fig. 8–16).

With more advanced intervertebral osteochondrosis, there is diminution of intervertebral disk height, with concomitant degeneration of the cartilaginous end plates and thickening of the adjacent trabeculae. This is manifested on the radiographs as disk space loss and bone eburnation. The sclerosis is generally well defined and linear or triangular; it extends to deeper portions of the vertebral body.[126] Condensation of bone in both vertebral bodies surrounding an involved intervertebral disk is typical. These sclerotic areas are usually homogeneous, although they may contain radiolucent regions representing displaced disk material termed cartilaginous (Schmorl) nodes.

The pathologic and radiographic changes of intervertebral osteochondrosis may be present at any level in the spine, although changes are most prominent in the lower lumbar and cervical regions. Men are affected more commonly than are women.

Spondylosis Deformans

The most obvious pathologic and radiographic OA of the spine is spondylosis deformans, which leads to vertebral outgrowths known as osteophytes (Fig. 8–17). Spinal osteophy-

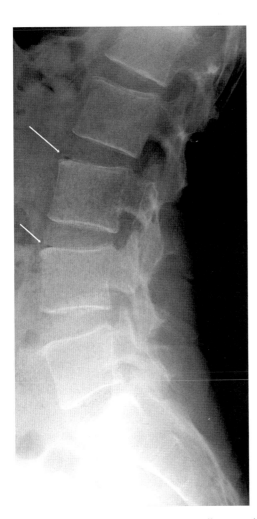

Figure 8–16 Vacuum phenomena. As gas collects in the disk clefts, enlarging radiolucent areas (arrows) appear. The lucent areas are initially circular, but as they progress, linear shadows become evident.

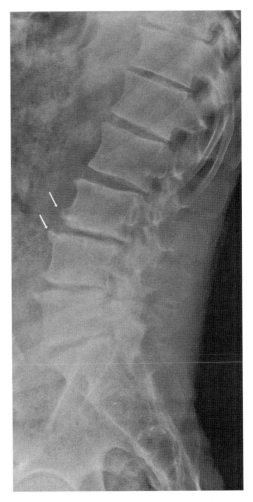

Figure 8–17 Spondylosis deformans. Lateral radiograph of the lumbar spine reveals osteophyte formation (arrows). These initially extend in a horizontal direction and then in a vertical one. Severe apophyseal joint osteoarthritis is also present.

tosis is extremely common.[127,128] By the age of 50 years, approximately 60% of women and 80% of men demonstrate such excrescences. Bone outgrowths are more frequent in the older population and occur more often in men than in women. Any segment of the vertebral column may be affected; in the thoracic spine, right-sided outgrowths predominate and are presumably related to pulsations of the aorta on the left side, which inhibit bone production.

Disruption of the peripheral fibers of the annulus fibrosus is generally accepted to be the initiating event in this disorder. Once disruption occurs, minor degrees of anterior and anterolateral disk displacement is possible. This leads to traction at the site of osseous attachment of the outermost fibers of the annulus fibrosus, known as Sharpey fibers, to the vertebral body. Osteophytes develop at this location, several millimeters from the disk–vertebral body junction. The outgrowths initially extend in a horizontal direction and then turn vertically.

Uncovertebral Joint Arthrosis

Uncovertebral joints (joints of Luschka) are present in the lower five cervical vertebrae (C3 to C7). These vertebral bodies contain bone ridges on each side of their superior surfaces, the uncinate or lunate processes. The uncovertebral joints exist between the superior process of the lower vertebra and the inferior portion of the adjacent vertebral body. The joints have anatomic features of both cartilaginous and synovial articulations.[129,130]

With increasing degeneration of intervertebral disk tissue, there is progressive loss of disk integrity, and the uncinate process of the lower vertebra and the inferior body of the upper vertebra approach each other. Eventually, the articular processes are pressed firmly together and the articulation degenerates.[131] Osteophytes may develop that may impinge on nerve roots or the vertebra at the costotransverse foramen. Radiography in the frontal projection reveals enlarged uncinate processes and joint space narrowing. Similar changes are seen on the oblique and lateral views.

Synovial Joints

Apophyseal Joint Osteoarthritis

The apophyseal joints of the vertebral column are a frequent site of OA. Although any spinal level may be affected, changes commonly predominate in the middle and lower cervical spine, the upper and midthoracic spine, and the lower lumbar spine.[132-134] The degenerative changes are induced by abnormal stress across a joint.[135]

The pathologic and radiographic changes of OA of the apophyseal joints are similar to those occurring in other synovial joints[136,137] and include cartilaginous erosion and denudation manifested radiographically as joint space narrowing. Bone eburnation and osteophytosis are common and may be accompanied by intra-articular osteocartilaginous bodies. Capsular laxity allows subluxation of one vertebral body on another. Bone ankylosis of the joint may ensue.

Fibrous Joints and Entheses

Ligamentous Degeneration

Degenerative abnormalities may become evident in the anterior longitudinal ligament, posterior longitudinal ligament, ligamenta flava, interspinous ligaments, supraspinous ligament, intertransverse ligaments, ligamentum nuchae, and iliolumbar ligaments.

Supraspinous and interspinous ligament abnormalities frequently coexist. Extensive lordosis, or disk space loss, leads to close approximation and contact of spinous processes and to degeneration of intervening ligaments. The "kissing" spinous processes develop reactive eburnation (Baastrup disease)[138,139] and may be associated with considerable pain.[140,141] The characteristic radiographic abnormality in Baastrup disease is the abnormal contact of apposing spinous processes, combined with sclerosis in the superior and inferior portions of adjacent processes. These changes are best demonstrated on lateral radiographs of the flexed and extended spine[142,143] (Fig. 8–18).

Ossification to various degrees in the ligamentum nuchae can be seen and is of no clinical significance.

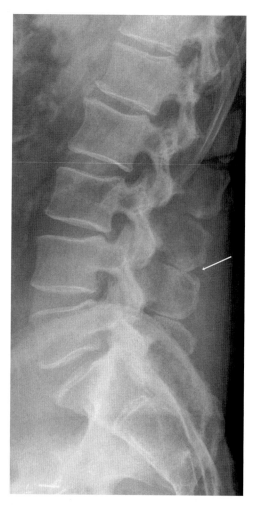

Figure 8–18 Baastrup disease. Lateral radiograph of the lumbar spine shows enlarged spinous processes that are flattened and sclerotic in their inferior and superior portions (arrow).

Ossification may also be present in the iliolumbar ligament and is of unknown pathogenesis and significance. Such ligamentous ossification, however, is more frequent in patients with diffuse idiopathic skeletal hyperostosis.

Complications of Osteoarthritis of the Spine

Alignment Abnormalities

Segmental Instability. Lateral radiographs in the neutral position and with the spine in flexion and extension can be used to evaluate the degree and pattern of motion in the lumbar spine. Radiographic findings suggestive of instability include the presence of gas within the intervertebral disk, osteophytes on adjacent vertebral bodies below the rims of the end plate (i.e., traction spurs), and evidence of a radial spur in the intervertebral disk during diskography. Radiographs should be considered to demonstrate instability when they reveal forward or backward displacement of one vertebra on another, an abrupt change in the length of the pedicles, narrowing of the intervertebral foramina, and loss of height of an intervertebral disk.[144] On frontal radiographs obtained with the patient bending first in one direction and then another, additional abnormalities include asymmetry in the person's ability to bend in both directions, loss of normal vertebral rotation and tilt, abnormal degree of disk closure or opening, malalignment of spinous processes and pedicles, and lateral translation of one vertebra on another as a result of an abnormal degree of rotation.[145]

Degenerative Spondylolisthesis. The term spondylolysis refers to an interruption of the pars interarticularis of the vertebra. Spondylolysis is generally considered to represent an acquired abnormality characterized by a mechanical failure of bone related to abnormal vertebral stress. The term spondylolisthesis refers to displacement of one vertebral body on another, which may be secondary to defects in the neural arch of the vertebra or to OAs of the spine. Radiographic findings of degenerative spondylolisthesis include OA of apophyseal joints (joint space narrowing, sclerosis, and osteophytes), with forward slipping of the superior vertebra on the inferior one.

Another pattern of degenerative spondylolisthesis is associated with intervertebral osteochondrosis (disk degeneration). Intervertebral osteochondrosis results in a decrease in height of the involved disk space, closer approximation of adjacent vertebral bodies, and gliding or telescoping of the corresponding articular processes. Because of the normal oblique inclination of the superior articular processes, there is posterior displacement of the superior vertebra relative to the inferior one.[146–148] Radiographic findings include the typical changes of intervertebral osteochondrosis and apophyseal joint instability and subluxation. In the posterior joints, the initial radiographic appearance is characterized by asymmetry of joint space and tilting of one articular process on another; subsequently, joint displacement is observed, and the inferior articular processes of the superior vertebra extend below the articular surfaces of the superior process.

Senile Kyphosis. Exaggerated thoracic kyphosis is common among the elderly. This may be secondary to osteoporosis (osteoporotic kyphosis) or, less commonly, to degeneration of the annulus fibrosus (senile kyphosis). The radiographic features of senile kyphosis resemble those of intervertebral osteochondrosis, although the disk space narrowing and reactive sclerosis are in a more anterior position in senile kyphosis. Before osseous fusion of vertebral bodies, osteophytosis on the anterior surface of the vertebrae is common; after osseous fusion, the osteophytes may be resorbed.

Degenerative Scoliosis. OAs of the spine do not typically lead to scoliosis, although they may appear during the course of scoliosis and aggravate the condition. Intervertebral osteochondrosis, spondylosis deformans, and OA predominate along the concave portion of the curve.

Intervertebral Disk Displacement

The intervertebral disk is normally a load-bearing structure with hydrostatic properties related to its high water content.[149] As the nucleus pulposus is subjected to increased pressure, it attempts to prolapse from its confined space. The intervertebral disk may be prolapsed anteriorly (spondylosis deformans), posteriorly (intraspinal herniation), or superiorly and inferiorly (cartilaginous nodes).

Posterior displacement of disk material is of great clinical significance because of the intimate relationship between the intervertebral disk and important neurologic structures. Factors that predispose to posterior disk displacement include a somewhat posterior position of the nucleus pulposus, the existence of fewer and weaker annular fibers in this region, and a posterior longitudinal ligament[150] that is not as strong as the anterior longitudinal ligament. The following terms are used to indicate the extent of displacement of the intervertebral disk:

Annular bulge: the annular fibers remain intact but protrude in a localized or diffuse manner into the spinal canal.
Disk prolapse: the displaced nucleus pulposus extends through some of the fibers of the annulus fibrosus but is still confined by the intact outermost fibers.
Disk extrusion: the displaced nucleus pulposus penetrates all of the fibers of the annulus fibrosus and lies beneath the posterior longitudinal ligament.
Disk sequestration: the displaced nucleus pulposus penetrates or extends around the posterior longitudinal ligament and lies within the epidural space, or the displaced nucleus pulposus, although not extending through this ligament, migrates for a considerable distance in a cephalic or caudal direction as a fragment that is separate from the remaining portion of the intervertebral disk.

Although diagnosis of posterior displacement of portions of the intervertebral disk may occasionally be established with routine radiography because of the presence of calcification, other methods are generally required. These include MR imaging, computed tomography with or without intrathecal administration of a contrast agent, and myelography.

Intervertebral Disk Calcification

Many systemic disorders are associated with intervertebral disk calcification. However, in most of these conditions, multiple intervertebral disks are involved. In adults, degenerative calcific deposits may occur in the annulus fibrosus, nucleus pulposus, and cartilaginous end plates; these are usually confined to one or two levels. These changes are generally seen in elderly men and are most apparent at the midthoracic and upper lumbar levels.

Spinal Stenosis

Degenerative disorders of the vertebral column lead to hypertrophic alterations about the involved joints that may compromise spinal contents. Such changes are most common in the lumbar and cervical regions and can be further subdivided on the basis of anatomic location of the stenosis.

Central stenosis occurs in the region of the central canal. Its causes may be developmental or acquired as a result of hypertrophic changes in the joints or ligaments surrounding the central canal. Computed tomography or MR findings in the transaxial plane include distortion of the normal configuration of the canal, compression of the thecal sac, and obliteration of the epidural fat.[151]

Stenosis of the intervertebral foramen may result from disk herniation, osteophytosis of the vertebral bodies or articular process, or various inflammatory and neoplastic diseases. MR imaging and computed tomography are superior to myelography in demonstrating foraminal encroachment and displacement or distortion of the exiting nerve and surrounding epidural fat.[152] These imaging methods are also superior to myelography in demonstrating soft tissue or bone masses.[153]

The subarticular or lateral recess may be compromised by hypertrophy about the apophyseal joint, which may lead to displacement or distortion of adjacent neural elements. These changes are best demonstrated in the transaxial plane with MR imaging or computed tomography.

DIFFUSE IDIOPATHIC SKELETAL HYPEROSTOSIS

Diagnostic Criteria

Diffuse idiopathic skeletal hyperostosis (DISH) is a skeletal disorder producing characteristic alterations in both spinal and extraspinal structures.[154, 155] There are three radiographic criteria for the diagnosis of spinal involvement in DISH:[154]

1. the presence of flowing calcification and ossification along the anterolateral aspect of at least four contiguous vertebral bodies, with or without associated localized pointed excrescences at the intervening vertebral body–intervertebral disk junction (Fig. 8–19);
2. the presence of relative preservation of intervertebral disk height in the involved vertebral segment and the

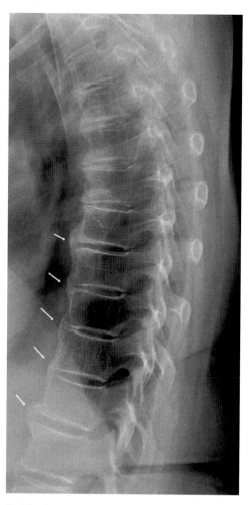

Figure 8–19 Thoracic spine alterations in DISH. Ossification of the anterior longitudinal ligament over five contiguous vertebral bodies. The anterior longitudinal ligament attaches to the midportion of the vertebral bodies (arrows), and ossification within it may be separated from the vertebral bodies at other portions by a lucent area that may measure 1 to 3 mm.

absence of extensive radiographic changes of degenerative disk disease, including vacuum phenomenon and vertebral body marginal sclerosis; and
3. the absence of apophyseal joint bone ankylosis and sacroiliac joint erosion, sclerosis, or intra-articular osseous fusion.

All three radiographic criteria must be fulfilled for a definitive diagnosis of DISH to be established. Each is used to eliminate other spinal disorders that potentially could be confused with DISH, including spondylosis deformans, intervertebral osteochondrosis, and ankylosing spondylitis.

QUANTITATION OF RADIOLOGIC CHANGES

The use of radiography to detect and stage the articular changes of OA is widespread. Conventional radiography, however, is neither sensitive nor specific to the earliest changes of OA. With use of this technique, up to 40% of the population may be diagnosed as having OA while still asymptomatic, and others who have the clinical signs and symptoms of OA have normal findings on radiography. Furthermore, there are differences in interpretation of diagnostic radiographic signs.

A variety of radiographic grading systems have been proposed. No single global staging system may be suitable for the assessment of OA at all sites, however. In the hip joint, the most common radiographic sign seen in OA is joint space narrowing, associated with superior medial or axial migration of the femoral head. With greater severity of the disease, there may be flattening of the femoral head as well as osteophytes seen in the acetabulum and femoral head and neck. Joint space narrowing has been more strongly associated with pain than the presence of osteophytes has, suggesting to some that joint space narrowing may be of more importance than the presence of osteophytes in defining hip OA.[156–165]

In the knee, a grading system has been developed to include joint space narrowing, graded on a scale of 0 to 3; individual features of an osteophyte, graded on a scale of 0 to 3; and sclerosis, graded as being present or absent. Preliminary studies suggest that the best variables in assessing progression of OA of the knee are joint space narrowing followed by the presence of osteophytes.[165]

Buckland-Wright[166,167] proposed a method of quantitation of radiographic changes using magnification radiography. In this technique, a micron-sized x-ray focal spot is used. The joint to be examined is placed close to the x-ray tube and separated by a distance of 1 to 2 meters from the film. This results in a magnified image with high spatial resolution. A standardized protocol for radiographic imaging of different joints has been proposed. Furthermore, methods of standardization and quantification of measurements to ensure accurate interpretation have also been proposed. The most sensitive radiographic signs for detecting the presence of OA are osteophytes, subchondral sclerosis, and juxta-articular lucencies. It is suggested that the only reliable and sensitive parameters for assessing the progression of disease are changes in the number and size of osteophytes and joint space narrowing.

SUMMARY

OA is a common and widespread affliction in extraspinal locations. Abnormalities predominate in the cartilaginous and osseous structures. Typical findings include joint space loss, eburnation, cyst formation, and osteophytosis. Subluxation, malalignment, fibrous ankylosis, and intra-articular osseous and cartilaginous bodies may complicate OA.

The most common extraspinal sites of OA are the interphalangeal and metacarpophalangeal joints of the hand, the first carpometacarpal and trapezioscaphoid areas of the wrist, the acromioclavicular and sternoclavicular joints, the hip, the knee, and the tarsometatarsal and metatarsophalangeal joints of the great toe. At each of these sites, characteristic radiographic findings are present.

Two special forms of OA have been described. Generalized OA may affect multiple articulations. Inflammatory OA is associated with clinical, pathologic, and radiographic manifestations of joint inflammation, including erosions and bone ankylosis, although its distribution is virtually identical to that of noninflammatory digital OA.

OAs of the spine include a variety of processes, each with characteristic radiographic manifestations. Although any one process may predominate, they frequently occur together. These disorders include intervertebral osteochondrosis, which is characterized by vacuum phenomena, disk space narrowing, and reactive sclerosis; spondylosis deformans, which is characterized by osteophytosis; OA, which is characterized by joint space narrowing, bone sclerosis, and hypertrophy; and ligamentous degeneration, which is associated with calcification and ossification. Several complications may occur in the course of such degenerative spine disease, including disorders of alignment, intervertebral disk displacements, disk calcification and ossification, and spinal stenosis.

DISH is a skeletal disorder producing characteristic radiographic findings at both spinal and extraspinal sites. This disorder shares many features with spondylosis deformans, although a qualitative difference between these two conditions is present; the degree of disk displacement and the amount of bone proliferation are greater in DISH than in spondylosis deformans. Spinal ligament calcification and ossification occur in DISH and are not prominent features of spondylosis deformans.

A variety of schemes using conventional and magnification radiography and MR imaging have been proposed to quantitate the changes of OA and to detect and stage progression of the disease. Plain radiography is not as sensitive as magnetic resonance imaging to early changes of OA. However, radiographs remain a valuable clinical and research tool for following the progression of OA.

REFERENCES

1. Garrod AE. Rheumatoid arthritis, osteoarthritis and arthritis deformans. In: Allbutt TC, Rolleston HD, eds. A System of Medicine. Rev ed. Vol 3. London, Macmillan, 1907.
2. Nichols EH, Richardson FL. Arthritis deformans. J Med Res 21:149, 1909.
3. Mitchell NS, Curess RL. Classification of degenerative arthritis. Can Med Assoc J 117:763–765, 1977.
4. Trueta J. Studies of the Development and Decay of the Human Frame. Philadelphia, WB Saunders, 1968.
5. Trueta J, Harrison MHM. The normal vascular anatomy of the femoral head in the adult man. J Bone Joint Surg Br 35:442–461, 1953.
6. Ingelmark BE. The nutritive supply and nutritional value of synovial fluid. Acta Orthop Scand 20:144–155, 1950.
7. Eckholm R, Norback B. On the relationship between articular changes and function. Acta Orthop Scand 21:81–98, 1951.
8. Harrison MHM, Schajowicz F, Trueta J. Osteoarthritis of the hip: a study of the nature and evolution of the disease. J Bone Joint Surg Br 35:598–626, 1953.
9. Redler I. A scanning electron microscopic study of human normal and osteoarthritic articular cartilage. Clin Orthop 103:262–268, 1974.

10. Nimni M, Deshmukh K. Differences in collagen metabolism between normal and osteoarthritic human articular cartilage. Science 181:751–752, 1973.

11. Weiss C, Mirow S. An ultrastructural study of osteoarthritic changes in articular cartilage of human knees. J Bone Joint Surg Am 54:954–972, 1972.

12. Phemister DB. Bone growth and repair. Ann Surg 102:261–285, 1935.

13. Cameron HU, Fornasier VL. Trabecular stress fractures. Clin Orthop 111:266–268, 1975.

14. Todd RC, Freeman MAR, Ririe CJ. Isolated trabecular fatigue fractures in the femoral head. J Bone Joint Surg Br 54:723–728, 1972.

15. Urovitz EPM, Fornasier VL, Risen MI, et al. Etiological factors in the pathogenesis of femoral trabecular fatigue fractures. Clin Orthop 127:275–280, 1977.

16. Havdrup T, Hulth A, Telhag H. The subchondral bone in osteoarthritis and rheumatoid arthritis of the knee. A historical and microradiographical study. Acta Orthop Scand 47:345–350, 1976.

17. Kusakabe A. Subchondral cancellous bone in osteoarthrosis and rheumatoid arthritis of the femoral head. A quantitative histological study of trabecular remodelling. Arch Orthop Unfallchir 88:185–197, 1977.

18. Jeffery AK. Osteogenesis in the osteoarthritic femoral head. A study using radioactive ^{32}P and tetracycline bone markers. J Bone Joint Surg Br 55:262–272, 1973.

19. Landells JW. The bone cysts of osteoarthritis. J Bone Joint Surg Br 35:643–649, 1953.

20. Rhaney K, Lamb DW. The cysts of osteoarthritis of the hip. A radiological and pathological study. J Bone Joint Surg Br 37:663–675, 1955.

21. Ondrouch AS. Cyst formation in osteoarthritis. J Bone Joint Surg Br 45:755–760, 1963.

22. Crane AR, Scarano JJ. Synovial cysts (ganglia) of bone. J Bone Joint Surg Am 49:355–361, 1967.

23. Cruickshank B, Macleod JG, Shearer WS. Subarticular pseudocysts in rheumatoid arthritis. J Fac Radiol Lond 5:218–226, 1954.

24. Bugnion JP. Lesions nouvelles du poignet: pseudokystes necrobiotiques, kystes par herniations capsulaires, arthrite chronique degenerative par osteochondrose marginale. Acta Radiol (Stockh) 90:5, 1951.

25. Resnick D, Niwayama G, Coutts RD. Subchondral cysts (geodes) in arthritic disorders. Pathologic and radiographic appearance of the hip joint. AJR 128:799–806, 1977.

26. Morrissy RT. Acetabular cyst in a child. A case report. J Bone Joint Surg Am 61:609–612, 1979.

27. Jaffe HL. Metabolic, Degenerative and Inflammatory Diseases of Bones and Joints. Philadelphia, Lea & Febiger, 1972.

28. Lloyd-Roberts GC. The role of capsular changes in osteoarthritis of the hip joint. J Bone Joint Surg Br 35:627–642, 1953.

29. Martel W, Braunstein EM. The diagnostic value of buttressing of the femoral neck. Arthritis Rheum 21:161–164, 1978.

30. Hansson T, Oberg T. Arthrosis and deviation in form in the temporomandibular joint. A macroscopic study on a human autopsy material. Acta Odont Scand 35:167–174, 1977.

31. Noble J, Hambien DL. The pathology of the degenerate meniscus lesion. J Bone Joint Surg Br 57:180–186, 1975.

32. Chad K. Horizontal (cleavage) tears of the knee joint menisci in the elderly. J Am Geriatr Soc 20:430, 1972.

33. Heberden W. Commentaries on the History and Cure of Diseases. London, Payne, 1802.

34. Martel W, Snarr JW, Horn JR. The metacarpophalangeal joints in interphalangeal osteoarthritis. Radiology 108:1–7, 1973.

35. North ER, Eaton RG. Degenerative joint disease of the trapezium: a comparative radiographic and anatomic study. J Hand Surg 8:160–166, 1983.

36. Carstam N, Eiken O, Andren L. Osteoarthritis of the trapezio-scaphoid joint. Acta Orthop Scand 39:354–358, 1968.

37. Patterson AC. Osteoarthritis of the trapezioscaphoid joint. Arthritis Rheum 18:375–379, 1975.

38. Dryer RF, Buckwalter JA. Isolated scaphotrapezial trapezoidal arthrosis. Orthopedics 3:213, 1980.

39. Mack GR, Bosse MJ, Gelberman RH, et al. The natural history of scaphoid nonunion. J Bone Joint Surg Am 66:504–509, 1984.

40. Ruby LK, Stinson J, Belsky MR. The natural history of scaphoid nonunion. A review of fifty-five cases. J Bone Joint Surg Am 67:428–432, 1985.

41. Jonsson K, Sigfusson BF. Arthrosis of the lunatecapitate joint. Acta Radiol 24:415–418, 1983.

42. Watson HK, Ballet FL. The SLAC wrist: scapholunate advanced collapse pattern of degenerative arthritis. J Hand Surg 9:358–365, 1984.

43. Watson HK, Ryu J. Degenerative disorders of the carpus. Orthop Clin North Am 15:337–353, 1984.

44. McCarty DJ, Halverson PB, Carrera GF, et al. "Milwaukee shoulder"—association of microspheroids containing hydroxyapatite crystals, active collagenase, and neutral protease with rotator cuff defects. Arthritis Rheum 24:464–473, 1981.

45. Barton NJ. Arthrodesis of the shoulder for degenerative conditions. J Bone Joint Surg Am 54:1759–1764, 1972.

46. Neer CS II. Degenerative lesions of the proximal humeral articular surface. Clin Orthop 20:116–125, 1961.

47. Neer CS II. Replacement arthroplasty for glenohumeral osteoarthritis. J Bone Joint Surg Am 56:1–13, 1974.

48. Cone RO, Danzig L, Resnick D, et al. The bicipital groove: radiographic, anatomic, and pathologic study. AJR 141:781–788, 1983.

49. Zanca P. Shoulder pain: involvement of the acromioclavicular joint (analysis of 1,000 cases). AJR 171:493–506, 1971.

50. Olah J. Das Röntgenbild des akromioklavikularen Gelenkes im Alter. Rofo 127:334–337, 1977.

51. Hermodsson I. Roentgen appearance of coxarthrosis. Relation between the anatomy, pathologic changes, and roentgen appearance. Acta Orthop Scand 41:169–187, 1970.

52. Murray RO. The etiology of primary osteoarthritis of the hip. Br J Radiol 38:810–824, 1965.

53. Gofton J. Studies in osteoarthritis of the hip. Part I. Classification. Can Med Assoc J 104:679–683, 1971.

54. Solomon L. Patterns of osteoarthritis of the hip. J Bone Joint Surg Am 58:176–183, 1976.

55. Hermodsson I. Roentgen appearance of arthritis of the hip. Acta Radiol 12:865–868, 1972.

56. Resnick D. Patterns of migration of the femoral head in osteoarthritis of the hip. Roentgenographic-pathologic correlation and comparison with rheumatoid arthritis. AJR 124:62–74, 1975.

57. Lloyd-Roberts GC. Osteoarthritis of the hip. A study of the clinical pathology. J Bone Joint Surg Br 37:8–47, 1955.

58. Dihlmann W, Hopf A. Das Wiberg-Zeichen, ein Hinweis auf Gestorte Huftgelenksmechanik (Spezielle, weniger beachtete Röntgenbefunde am Stutz- und Gleitgewebe 3). Fortschr Geb Roentgenstr Nuklearmed Erganzungsband 115:572–581, 1971.

59. Ferguson AB Jr. The pathology of degenerative arthritis of the hip and the use of osteotomy in its treatment. Clin Orthop 77:84–97, 1971.

60. Kusakabe A. Subchondral cancellous bone in osteoarthritis and rheumatoid arthritis of the femoral head. A quantitative histological study of trabecular remodelling. Arch Orthop Unfallchir 88:185–197, 1977.

61. Byers PD, Contepomi CA, Farkas TA. Postmortem study of the hip joint. II. Histological basis for limited and progressive cartilage alterations. Ann Rheum Dis 35:114–121, 1976.

62. Byers PD, Contepomi CA, Farkas TA. Postmortem study of the hip joint including the prevalence of the features of the right side. Ann Rheum Dis 19:15–31, 1970.

63. Mankin HJ, Doftman H, Lippiello L, et al. Biochemical and metabolic abnormalities in articular cartilage from osteoarthritic human hips. II. Correlation of morphology with biochemical and metabolic data. J Bone Joint Surg Am 53:523–537, 1971.

64. Vignon E, Arlot M, Meunier P, et al. Quantitative histological changes in osteoarthritic hip cartilage. Morphometric analysis of 29 osteoarthritic and 26 normal human femoral heads. Clin Orthop 103:269–278, 1974.

65. Jeffery AK. Osteophytes and the osteoarthritic femoral head. J Bone Joint Surg Br 57:314–324, 1975.

66. Meachim G, Hardinge K, Williams DR. Methods for correlating pathological and radiological findings in osteoarthritis of the hip. Br J Radiol 45:670–676, 1972.

67. Kashimoto T, Friedenberg ZB. A study of radiographic variations of the hip joint. Acta Orthop Scand 48:487–493, 1977.
68. Tanaka S, Ito T, Yamamoto K. Arthrography in osteoarthritis of the hip. AJR 124:91–95, 1975.
69. Hipp E. Die Gefasse des Hüftkopfes: Anatomie, Angiographie und Klinik. Z Orthop Suppl 96, 1962.
70. Mussbichler H. Arteriographic findings in patients with degenerative osteoarthritis of the human hip. Radiology 107:21–27, 1973.
71. Arnoldi CC, Linderholm H, Mussbichler H. Venous engorgement and intraosseous hypertension in osteoarthritis of the hip. J Bone Joint Surg Br 54:409–421, 1972.
72. Phillips RS, Bulmar JH, Hoyle G, et al. Venous drainage in osteoarthritis of the hip. A study after osteotomy. J Bone Joint Surg Br 49:301–309, 1967.
73. Phillips RS. Phlebography in osteoarthritis of the hip. J Bone Joint Surg Br 48:280–288, 1966.
74. Arnold CC, Djurhuus JC, Heerfordt J, et al. Intraosseous phlebography, intraosseous measurements and ^{99m}Tc-polyphosphate scintigraphy in patients with various painful conditions in the hip and knee. Acta Orthop Scand 51:19–28, 1980.
75. Danielsson LG, Dymling JF, Heripret G. Coxarthrosis in man studied with external counting of Sr^{85} and Ca^{47}. Clin Orthop 31:184–199, 1963.
76. Kolar J, Vyhnanek L, Drapelova D, et al. Degenerativni chorbykloubni pri osteologicke diagnostice se ^{85}Sr. Fysiatr Revmatol Vestn 45:65–72, 1967.
77. Reikeras O, Bjerkreim I, Kolbenstevedt A. Anteversion of the acetabulum and femoral neck in normals and in patients with osteoarthritis of the hip. Acta Orthop Scand 54:18–23, 1983.
78. Reikeras O, Hoiseth A. Femoral neck angles in osteoarthritis of the hip. Acta Orthop Scand 53:781–784, 1982.
79. Terjesen T, Benum P, Anda S, et al. Increased femoral anteversion and osteoarthritis of the hip joint. Acta Orthop Scand 53:571–575, 1982.
80. Hodler J, Trudell D, Pathria MN, et al. Width of the articular cartilage of the hip: quantification by using fat suppression spin-echo MR imaging in cadavers. AJR 159:351–355, 1992.
81. Lecovet FE, Vande Berg BC, Malghem J, et al. MR imaging of the acetabular labrum: variations in 200 asymptomatic hips. AJR 167:1025–1028, 1996.
82. Czerny C, Hofmann S, Neuhold A, et al. Lesions of the acetabular labrum: accuracy of MR imaging and MR arthrography in detection and staging. Radiology 200:225–230, 1996.
83. Petersilge CA, Haque MA, Petersilge WJ, et al. Acetabular labral tears: evaluation with MR arthrography. Radiology 200:231–235, 1996.
84. Thomas RH, Resnick D, Alazraki NP, et al. Compartmental evaluation of osteoarthritis of the knee. A comparative study of available diagnostic modalities. Radiology 116:585–594, 1975.
85. Ahlback S. Osteoarthrosis of the knee. A radiographic investigation. Acta Radiol Diagn (Stockh) Suppl 277:7–72, 1968.
86. Gibson PH, Goodfellow JW. Stress radiography in degenerative arthritis of the knee. J Bone Joint Surg Br 68:608–609, 1986.
87. Harris WR, Kostuik JP. High tibial osteotomy for osteoarthritis of the knee. J Bone Joint Surg Am 52:330–336, 1970.
88. Leach RE, Gregg T, Siber FJ. Weightbearing radiography in osteoarthritis of the knee. Radiology 97:265–268, 1970.
89. Leonard LM. The importance of weight-bearing x-rays in knee problems. J Maine Med Assoc 62:101–106, 1971.
90. Marklund T, Mynerts R. Radiographic determination of cartilage height in the knee joint. Acta Orthop Scand 45:752–755, 1974.
91. Resnick D, Vint V. The "tunnel" view in assessment of cartilage loss in osteoarthritis of the knee. Radiology 137:547–548, 1980.
92. Doppman JL. The association of patellofemoral erosion and synovial hypertrophy. A diagnostic entity. Radiology 82:240–245, 1964.
93. Alexander C. Erosion of the femoral shaft due to patellofemoral osteoarthritis. Clin Radiol 11:110–113, 1960.
94. Greenspan A, Normal A, Tchang FK. "Tooth" sign in patellar degenerative disease. J Bone Joint Surg Am 59:483–485, 1977.
95. Mangieri JV. Peroneal nerve injury from an enlarged fabella. A case report. J Bone Joint Surg Am 55:395–397, 1973.
96. Fredericson, M., Yoon, K. Physical examination and patellofemoral pain syndrome. Am J Phys Med Rehab 59:234–243, 2006.
97. Post, WR. Patellofemoral pain: results of non-operative treatment. Clin Ortho Relat Res. 436:55–59, 2005.
98. Besier TF, Gold GE, Beaupre GS, et al. A modeling framework to estimate patellofemoral cartilage stress in vivo. Med Sci Sports Exerc 37:1924–1930, 2005.
99. Keats TE, Harrison RB. Hypertrophy of the talar beak. Skeletal Radiol 4:37–39, 1979.
100. Resnick D. Talar ridges, osteophytes, and beaks: a radiologic commentary. Radiology 151:329–332, 1984.
101. Resnick D, Feingold ML, Curd J, et al. Calcaneal abnormalities in articular disorders. Rheumatoid arthritis, ankylosing spondylitis, psoriatic arthritis and Reiter's syndrome. Radiology 125:355–366, 1977.
102. Mann RA, Coughlin MJ, DuVries HL. Hallux rigidus. A review of the literature and a method of treatment. Clin Orthop 142:57–63, 1979.
103. Mann RA, Coughlin MJ. Hallux valgus: etiology, anatomy, treatment and surgical considerations. Clin Orthop 157:31–41, 1981.
104. Kato T, Wanatabe S. The etiology of hallux valgus in Japan. Clin Orthop 157:78–81, 1981.
105. Haines RW, McDougall A. The anatomy of hallux valgus. J Bone Joint Surg Br 36:272–293, 1954.
106. Ewald P. Die Atiologie des Hallux valgus. Dtsch Z Chir 114:90, 1912.
107. Kellgren JH, Moore R. Generalized osteoarthritis and Heberden's nodes. Br Med J 1:181–187, 1952.
108. Crain DC. Interphalangeal osteoarthritis characterized by painful inflammatory episodes resulting in deformity of the proximal and distal articulations. JAMA 175:1049–1053, 1961.
109. Ehrlich GE. Inflammatory osteoarthritis. I. The clinical syndrome. J Chronic Dis 25:317–328, 1972.
110. Ehrlich GE. Inflammatory osteoarthritis. II. The superimposition of rheumatoid arthritis. J Chronic Dis 25:635–643, 1972.
111. Ehrlich GE. Osteoarthritis beginning with inflammation. Definitions and correlations. JAMA 232:157–159, 1975.
112. McEwen C. Osteoarthritis of the fingers with ankylosis. Arthritis Rheum 11:734–744, 1968.
113. Smukler NM, Edeiken J, Giuliano VJ. Ankylosis in osteoarthritis of the finger joints. Radiology 100:525–530, 1971.
114. Milgram JW. The classification of loose bodies in human joints. Clin Orthop 124:282–292, 1977.
115. Milgram JW. The development of loose bodies in human joints. Clin Orthop 124:292–303, 1977.
116. King AG. Functional anatomy of the lumbar spine. Orthopedics 12:1588, 1983.
117. Ritchie JH, Fahrni WH. Age changes in lumbar intervertebral discs. Can J Surg 13:65–71, 1970.
118. Joplin RT. Intervertebral disc: embryology, anatomy, physiology, and pathology. Surg Gynecol Obstet 61:591–599, 1935.
119. Coventry MB, Ghormley RK, Kernohan JW. The intervertebral disc: its microscopic anatomy and pathology. II. Changes in the intervertebral disc concomitant with age. J Bone Joint Surg Br 27:233–247, 1945.
120. Coventry MB. Anatomy of the intervertebral disc. Clin Orthop 67:9–15, 1969.
121. Gershon-Cohen J, Schraer H, Sklaroff D, et al. Dissolution of the intervertebral disk in the aged normal. The phantom nucleus pulposus. Radiology 62:383–387, 1954.
122. Fuiks DM, Grayson CE. Vacuum pneumoarthrography and the spontaneous occurrence of gas in the joint spaces. J Bone Joint Surg Am 32:933–938, 1950.
123. Thomas SF, Williams OL. High-altitude joint pains (bends): their roentgenographic aspects. Radiology 44:259–261, 1945.
124. Knutsson F. The vacuum phenomenon in the intervertebral discs. Acta Radiol 23:173–179, 1942.
125. Ford LT, Gilula LA, Murphy WA, et al. Analysis of gas in vacuum lumbar disc. AJR 128:1056–1057, 1977.
126. Battikha JG, Garcia JF, Wettstein P. Aspects of atypical degenerative lesions of vertebrae. Skeletal Radiol 6:103–107, 1981.
127. Bick EM. Vertebral osteophytosis. Pathologic basis of its roentgenology. AJR 73:979–983, 1955.

128. Goldberg RP, Carter BL. Absence of thoracic osteophytosis in the area adjacent to the aorta: computed tomography demonstration. J Comput Assist Tomogr 2:173–175, 1978.

129. Payne EE, Spillane JD. Cervical spine: anatomico-pathologic study of 70 specimens (using special technique) with particular reference to the problem of cervical spondylosis. Brain 80: 571–596, 1957.

130. Bradshaw P. Some aspects of cervical spondylosis. Q J Med 26:177–208, 1957.

131. MacNab I. Cervical spondylosis. Clin Orthop 109:69–77, 1975.

132. Ghormley RK. Low back pain with special reference to the articular facets with presentation of an operative procedure. JAMA 101:1773–1777, 1933.

133. Epstein JA, Epstein BS, Lavine LS, et al. Lumbar nerve root compression at the intervertebral foramina caused by arthritis of the posterior facets. J Neurosurg 39:362–369, 1973.

134. Kirkaldy-Willis WH, Wedge JH, Yong-Hing K, et al. Pathology and pathogenesis of lumbar spondylosis and stenosis. Spine 3:319–328, 1978.

135. Taylor JR, Twomey LT. Age changes in lumbar zygoapophyseal joints. Observations on structure and function. Spine 11: 739–745, 1986.

136. Mannheim H. Freier Korper in einem Zwischenwirbelgelenk nach Trauma. Monatsschr Unfallheilkd 37:67–72, 1930.

137. Hadley LA. Anatomicoroentgenographic studies of the posterior spinal articulations. AJR 86:270–276, 1961.

138. Yamada K, Nishiwaki I, Yasukawa H. Supplemental study upon the pathogenesis of low back pain in Baastrup's disease. Arch Jpn Chir 23:384, 1954.

139. Jacobson HG, Tausend ME, Shapiro JH, et al. The "swayback" syndrome. AJR 79:677–683, 1958.

140. Goobar JE, Clark GM. Sclerosis of the spinousprocesses and low back pain ("cock spur" disease). Arch Interam Rheumatol 5:587–593, 1962.

141. Kattan KR, Pais MJ. The spinous process: the forgotten appendage. Skeletal Radiol 6:199–204, 1981.

142. Resnick D. Degenerative diseases of the vertebral column. Radiology 156:3–14, 1985.

143. Kursunoglu S, Resnick D. Imaging of degenerative disorders of the aging spine. Arch Clin Imaging 1:115–121, 1985.

144. Kirkaldy-Willis WH, Farfan HF. Instability of the lumbar spine. Clin Orthop 165:110–123, 1982.

145. Gillespie HW. Vertebral retroposition (reversed spondylolisthesis). Br J Radiol 25:193, 1951.

146. Johnson R. Posterior luxations of the lumbosacral joint. J Bone Joint Surg 16:867, 1934.

147. Vilaseca Sabater JM, Casademont M. Espondilolistesis y pseudospondilolistesis. Contribucion a su estudio radiologico. Rev Espan Reum 4:293, 1952.

148. Willis TA. Lumbosacral retrodisplacement. AJR 90:1263–1266, 1963.

149. Lipson SJ, Musir H. Proteoglycans in experimental intervertebral disc degeneration. Spine 6:194–210, 1981.

150. Postacchini F, Bellocci M, Massobrio M. Morphologic changes in annulus fibrosus during aging. An ultrastructural study in rats. Spine 9:596–603, 1984.

151. Bolender NF, Schonstrom NSR, Spengler DM. Role of computed tomography and myelography in the diagnosis of central spinal stenosis. J Bone Joint Surg Am 67:240–246, 1985.

152. Osborne DR, Heinz ER, Bullard D, et al. Role of computed tomography in the radiological evaluation of painful radiculopathy after negative myelography: foraminal neural entrapment. Neurosurgery 14:147–153, 1984.

153. Risius B, Modic MT, Hardy RW Jr, et al. Sector computed tomographic spine scanning in the diagnosis of lumbar nerve root entrapment. Radiology 143:109–114, 1982.

154. Resnick D, Shaul SR, Robins JM. Diffuse idiopathic skeletal hyperostosis (DISH): Forestier's disease with extraspinal manifestations. Radiology 115:513–524, 1975.

155. Resnick D, Niwayama G. Radiographic and pathologic features of spinal involvement in diffuse idiopathic skeletal hyperostosis (DISH). Radiology 119:559–568, 1976.

156. Spector RD, Hard DJ, Byrne J, et al. Defining the presence of osteoarthritis of the knee in epidemiologic studies. Ann Rheum Dis 52:790–794, 1993.

157. Croft P, Cooper C, Wickham C, et al. Defining osteoarthritis of the hip for epidemiological studies. Am J Epidemiol 132: 514–522, 1990.

158. Lawrence JS, Bremner JM, Bier F. Osteoarthritis: prevalence in the population and relationship between symptoms and x-ray changes. Ann Rheum Dis 25:1–23, 1966.

159. Kellgren JH, Lawrence JS. Radiological assessment of osteoarthritis. Ann Rheum Dis 16:494–501, 1957.

160. Spector TD, Cooper C. Radiological assessment of osteoarthritis in population studies: wither Kellgren and Lawrence? Osteoarthritis Cartilage 1:203–206, 1994.

161. Kellgren JH, Jeffrey MR, Ball J. The Epidemiology of Chronic Rheumatism. Atlas of Standard Radiographs. Vol 2. Oxford, Blackwell Scientific, 1963.

162. Lawrence JS. Rheumatism in Populations. London, Heinemann, 1977, pp 99–100.

163. Wood PHN. Osteoarthritis in the community. Clin Rheum Dis 2:495–507, 1976.

164. Spector TD, Hochberg MC. Methodological problems in the epidemiological study of osteoarthritis. Ann Rheum Dis 53: 143–146, 1994.

165. Altman RD, Fries JF, Bloch D, et al. Radiographic assessment of progression in osteoarthritis. Arthritis Rheum 30:1214–1225, 1987.

166. Buckland-Wright JC. Quantitative radiography of osteoarthritis. Ann Rheum Dis 53:268–275, 1994.

167. Buckland-Wright JC, Macfarlane DG, Williams SA, et al. Accuracy and precision of joint space width measurements in standard and macroradiographs of osteoarthritic knees. Ann Rheum Dis 54:872–880, 1995.

Magnetic Resonance Imaging

9

Charles G. Peterfy   Julie C. DiCarlo   Manish Kothari

IMAGING OSTEOARTHRITIS WITH MAGNETIC RESONANCE IMAGING

For more than two decades, magnetic resonance imaging (MRI) has been the imaging method of choice for evaluating internal derangements of the knee and other joints. Despite this, however, MRI has thus far played only a minor role in the study or management of osteoarthritis (OA). The main reason for this discrepancy has been the lack of effective structure-modifying therapies for OA. In the absence of therapy, clinicians have little need for methods of identifying patients who are most appropriate for the therapy or for determining how well the therapy worked. However, new insights into the pathophysiology of OA, coupled with advances in molecular engineering and drug discovery, have generated a number of new treatment strategies and raised the possibility of long-term control of this disorder. With this development has come a new demand for better ways of monitoring disease progression and treatment response in patients with OA. Noninvasive imaging techniques, particularly MRI, have drawn considerable attention in this regard. This interest has been intensified by the growing acceptance of structure modification and repair as an independent therapeutic objective in arthritis. Underlying this treatment strategy is the classic disease-illness debate: must therapies that effectively slow or prevent structural abnormalities in arthritis necessarily show an immediate parallel improvement in clinical symptoms and function, as long as they ultimately yield clinical benefits for the patient. Elucidating the structural determinants of the clinical features in arthritis has, accordingly, become a key objective for academia as well as the pharmaceutical industry.

MRI is ideally suited for imaging arthritic joints. Not only is it superior to most other modalities in delineating the anatomy, but also it is capable of quantifying a variety of compositional and functional parameters of articular tissues relevant to the degenerative process and OA.

Moreover, because MRI is nondestructive and free of ionizing radiation, multiple parameters can be analyzed in the same region of tissue, and frequent serial examinations can be performed on even asymptomatic patients.

Accordingly, it is anticipated that MRI will play an increasingly important role in the study of OA and its treatment and that the demand for expertise and experience in evaluating the disease with this technology will increase commensurately. This chapter reviews the current state-of-the-art for MRI of OA and points to areas from where future advances are most likely to come.

MAGNETIC RESONANCE IMAGING TECHNIQUE

The clarity and detail with which MRI depicts cross-sectional anatomy makes interpretation of the images appear deceptively simple. In reality, MRI is a highly sophisticated technology, and some background knowledge is essential to understand the findings, as well as to critically assess conclusions drawn from investigations that employ this technology. The following brief review of basic MRI principles and terminology will aid in understanding the remainder of the chapter and help investigators outside the discipline of Radiology to take better advantage of the growing number of published studies that use MRI. For the interested reader, there are several excellent books and articles that delve deeper into MRI physics and its applications in medicine.[1-5]

Basic Principles of Magnetic Resonance Imaging

MR imaging is based on the response of certain atomic nuclei to the presence of a magnetic field (Fig. 9–1). A number of different nuclei (for example, ^{23}Na, ^{13}C, ^{19}F, and ^{1}H) can be used to generate MR images. Hydrogen nuclei (or protons)

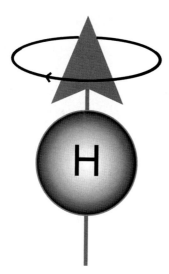

Figure 9–1 The nuclear magnetic moment. Spinning (precessing) anatomic nuclei ("spins") generate small local magnetic fields analogous to the spinning planets. The magnitude of the magnetic moment depends on the rate of precession, or frequency, of the nucleus. The vector sum of individual magnetic moments for a pool of hydrogen nuclei ("protons") in fat or water is the essential parameter measured in clinical MRI. (Courtesy of Synarc, Inc.)

are the most abundant within biological tissue and are therefore the most feasible for clinical imaging. When the tissue is placed within a strong magnetic field in the bore of an MR imaging magnet, these nuclei show a net tendency to align their nuclear magnetic moments along the direction of the static magnetic field. This alignment creates what is referred to as longitudinal magnetization (Fig. 9–2). Exposure of these protons to a second dynamic magnetic field (a radio frequency, or RF field, usually called B_1) that is rotating and perpendicular to the original static field of the magnet torques the protons 90 degrees away from the stronger static field (Fig. 9–3A). This process is known as excitation. The protons that now point in this direction make up what is referred to as transverse magnetization. The spins have a resonant frequency intrinsically tied to the strength of the main magnetic field, by the gyromagnetic ratio:

$$\omega = \gamma B_0$$

Where γ is the spin's gyromagnetic ratio, B_0 is the strength of the main static magnetic field (for example, 1.5 T), and ω is

the proton, or spin resonant frequency in that field. This resonant frequency relationship means that after the spins are tipped into the transverse plane by the B_1 pulse, they precess about the longitudinal axis along B_0. When the RF (B_1) tip-down pulse is turned off, the spins continue to precess. They act as tiny bar magnets, creating their own rotating magnetic field. This changing magnetic field induces a signal across the terminals of the same coil that was used to create the field, because the resonant frequency is the same (Fig. 9–3b). This signal is then used to generate the MR images by computerized Fourier transformation.

MR imaging uses three types of coils. The main magnetic field, B_0, is created by a superconducting magnet enclosed in a cylindrical cryostat. These magnets must be both strong (field strengths range between 0.2 T and 11 T) and very uniform (within 1 part per million in the imaging volume) in order to precisely set spin frequency. Whole-body scanners are currently limited to a maximum strength of 3 T to 4 T, with most clinical systems ranging from 0.5 T to 3 T. The second coil that creates the RF B_1 field is a birdcage-shaped coil that sits permanently within the main B_0 coil. Smaller birdcage coils that fit certain volumes, such as the head or extremities, can be placed in the bore as a substitute. Even smaller ring-shaped coils of 10 mm to 100 mm in diameter can be placed directly on the region to be imaged. There is a great advantage in using the smallest possible receive coil, because these coils are not as sensitive to tissues outside the volume of interest, which contribute significantly to image noise. The greatest gain in image Signal-to-noise ratio (SNR) is then achieved by starting with the most appropriate RF coil. The third type of coil used in MR is the gradient coil, of which there is one for each of the three axes. These coils create much smaller magnetic fields that point in the same direction of B_0, but vary as a function of distance to the coil. The strength of the linearly varying magnetic fields created by these coils is changed rapidly during an MR exam so that only spins in certain locations have frequencies in the range of those to which the receive coil is sensitive. The gradients force spins to move away from each other in frequency and then return to the same frequency to be in phase. This process is referred to as *gradient echo formation*. Both higher gradient amplitudes and faster gradient switching rates achieve echoes more quickly and result in shorter scan times.

The two main types of echoes in MR imaging are the gradient echoes (GREs) previously mentioned and spin

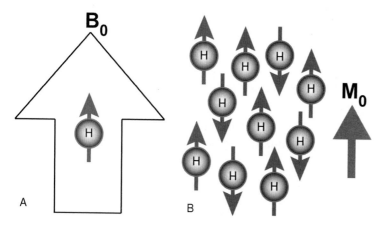

Figure 9–2 Longitudinal magnetization. *A,* Protons placed within the strong magnetic field B_0 (*Large open arrow*) in the bore of a MRI magnet tend to align their magnetic moments (*small arrow*) parallel or anti-parallel with this large magnetic field. *B,* Protons have a slight affinity for parallel alignment, creating a net magnetic moment M_0. The magnitude of this net longitudinal magnetic moment and therefore the maximal signal that could be generated during imaging varies directly with the field strength B_0 of the MRI magnet. (Courtesy of Synarc, Inc.)

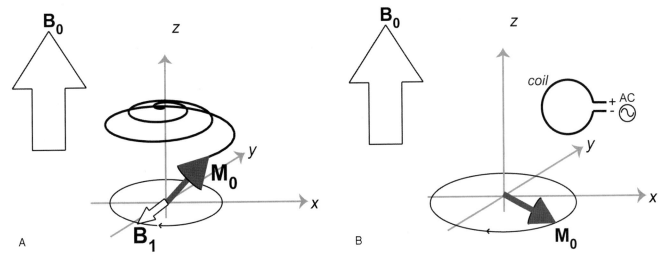

Figure 9–3 RF excitation of transverse magnetization. *A,* The net proton magnetization M_0 that is longitudinally aligned with the high magnetic field B_0 (*large open arrow*) in the MRI magnet bore will realign (resonate) with a second relatively smaller magnetic field B_1 (*small open arrow*) if this new field is tuned to the proton precessional frequency. Since this resonant frequency is in the same range as radio waves, this second field is called a radio-frequency (RF) pulse. *B,* The RF pulse can be played for a specific duration given the pulse amplitude to produce a full 90° rotation of the net magnetization M_0, called the flip angle. This realigned (flipped) magnetic moment (*gray vector arrow*) will continue to rotate transversely once the RF pulse is turned off to induce an alternating current (by Faraday's Law) in the wire of the receiver coil placed near the patient. This induced current is the basis for the MR image. (Courtesy of Synarc, Inc.)

echoes (SEs). SEs rephase protons with a 180 degree RF refocusing pulse. This pulse reverses phase position of the spins, flipping the fastest precessing spins behind the slowest precessing ones. After the phase reversal provided by the refocusing pulse, the fastest-moving spins continue at the same precession speeds and catch up so that all spins refocus to a coherent signal. A useful analogy to this process is a track race, halfway through which, the race is reversed so that all runners finish together at the starting line, assuming they maintain constant running speed.

The time it takes for echo formation is called the echo time, or TE. The total time it takes for both an RF excitation and a gradient echo formation/signal acquisition is the repetition time, or TR. TR can be as short as a few milliseconds or as long as a few seconds. The number of repetition times to form an image depends on the imaging method and whether 2D or 3D images are reconstructed. The length of the TR depends on the way the gradients refocus spins after allowing or forcing them to dephase.

Echoes create the signal for MR images, and TE/TR selection is the mechanism by which contrast is generated between different tissues. As soon as the RF pulse is turned off after excitation, the protons slowly return to their original alignment with the static main field of the magnet (Fig. 9–4). This process of recovering longitudinal magnetization and decaying transverse magnetization is called relaxation. T_1 and T_2 are the time constants with which this occurs. T_1 is the time necessary for the longitudinal magnetization to recover, and T_2 is the time for the transverse magnetization to decay. Both of these vary from tissue to tissue, depending

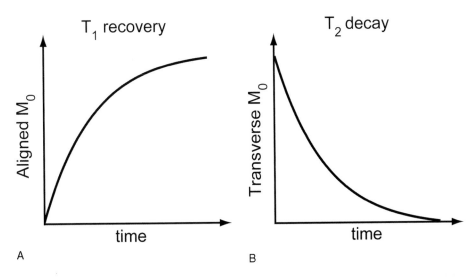

Figure 9–4 T_1/T_2 relaxation. When the rotating 90° RF pulse is turned off, the transversely oriented magnetic moment re-aligns with the static field of the magnet B_0. *A,* This recovery of longitudinal magnetization is called T_1 relaxation, and the parameter, T_1, is a measure of the rate of this recovery. If the 90° RF pulse is repeated before longitudinal magnetization has fully recovered, only this smaller longitudinal component is flipped into the transverse plane and the image signal is correspondingly lower—these protons are said to be partially saturated. *B,* As the longitudinal magnetization re-grows, the transverse component decays. This is called T_2 relaxation. (Courtesy of Synarc, Inc.)

TABLE 9–1

APPROXIMATE T_1 AND T_2 RELAXATION TIMES OF TISSUES IN THE KNEE AT 1.5 T

Tissue	T_1 (ms)	T_2 (ms)	T_1/T_2
Cartilage*	800	30	26.7
Fat	260	80	3.25
Synovial fluid**	2500	200	12.5
Muscle	870	50	17.4

*Measured values for cartilage range between 700 and 1100 ms for T_1 and 20 and 60 ms for T_2.
**Measured values for synovial fluid range between 1400 and 3000 ms for T_1 and 200 and 900 ms for T_2.

on the microenvironments of the different proton populations. T_1 and T_2 are therefore tissue characteristics that allow varying MR acquisition timing to generate contrast between tissues. Table 9–1 gives approximate values of different tissues in the knee at a main field strength of 1.5 T.

T_1 relaxation, for example, occurs rapidly in fat, while water (abundant in muscle) shows slow T_1 relaxation (Fig. 9–5A). T_1 also varies slightly with the magnetic field strength so that relaxation of the longitudinal magnetization back to equilibrium is somewhat shorter at lower main field strengths. Under conditions of rapid RF pulsing, slow T_1 substances such as water are not given sufficient time to recover between the pulses. Thus, there is little longitudinal magnetization available to be tipped again to

create signal, and these substances therefore exhibit low signal intensity. Shorter T_1 substances such as fat need less time for longitudinal regrowth and show higher signal intensity (Fig. 9–5A). Short TR sequences therefore generate contrast (relative signal intensity difference) among tissues on the basis of differences in T_1 and are accordingly referred to as T_1-weighted (Fig. 9–6).

Image contrast is also influenced by T_2 relaxation. While the longitudinal magnetization is regrowing after the RF pulse is turned off, the transverse magnetization is slowly decaying. Although not intuitive, the rate of T_2 relaxation is not necessarily coupled to the rate of T_1 relaxation, other than that the time for T_2 relaxation is always shorter than that for T_1. Although T_1 depends partly on the strength of the main static field, T_2 remains constant across all field strengths. As T_2 relaxation occurs, the transverse magnetization, and therefore signal, decrease. So, although shorter T_1 species are brighter on T_1-weighted images, the longer T_2 species tissue is brightest on T_2-weighted images (Fig. 9–5B). Freely mobile water protons (such as in synovial fluid) show slow T_2 relaxation and therefore retain signal over time, whereas constrained or "bound" water protons (such as by collagen or proteoglycan) show rapid T_2 relaxation and signal decay (Fig. 9–5B, Fig. 9–6).

In addition to the effects of neighboring protons on each other (T_2 relaxation), heterogeneities in the static magnetic field or off-resonance caused by a chemical shift (as with the 220 Hz difference in fat) cause protons to dephase and lose additional transverse magnetization strength. This is noted as T_2' relaxation. The combined effects of proton

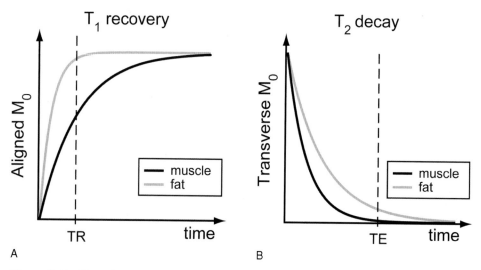

Figure 9–5 Effect of TR/TE on signal intensity. Repetition time (TR) is the time between successive RF pulses in an imaging sequence. Typically, 192 to 256 repetitions are necessary to generate an MR image. If the TR is less than five times the T_1 of a substance, there is insufficient time for complete recovery of longitudinal, or aligned magnetization and signal intensity after subsequent excitations is decreased. A, As TR is shortened, tissues with longer T_1 relaxation times (e.g., muscle) begin to lose signal first, while tissues with shorter T_1 relaxation times (e.g., fat) retain signal until the TR is very short. Short-TR sequences thus generate T_1 contrast among tissues and are called T_1-weighted. Echo time (TE) is the time between the initiating RF pulse and the point at which spins are refocused either by a 180° rephasing RF pulse (spin-echo) or gradient reversal waveform (gradient-echo). Substances with longer T_2 relaxation times (e.g., fat) retain more signal intensity on long-TE (T_2-weighted) sequences. B, As TE is lengthened, signal from tissues with shorter and longer T_2 relaxation times undergo more decay, changing the contrast. Note that for each value of TE and TR, the contrast between any two tissues is proportional to the difference in signal level, or transverse M_0, between the two. In the case of T_1-weighted sequences, reductions in the aligned M_0 translate into reductions in the transverse M_0 after subsequent RF excitations.) (Courtesy of Synarc, Inc.)

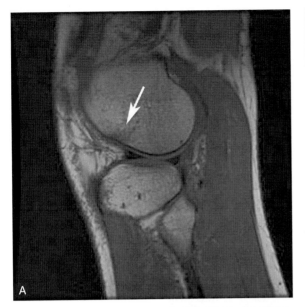
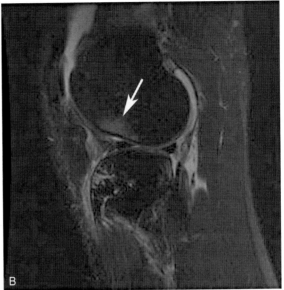
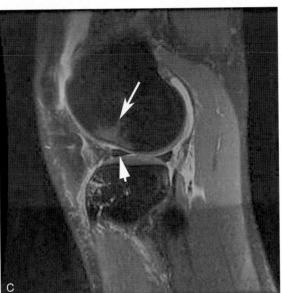

Figure 9–6 T_1, T_2, and PD-weighted MRI. *A*, Sagittal T_1-weighted spin-echo image of a knee depicts structures that contain fat (short T_1) with high signal intensity, and structures that contain water (long T_1) with low signal intensity. The small differences in T_1 relaxation time among synovial fluid, articular cartilage, and muscle do not generate substantial contrast among these structures on this image. It is difficult, therefore, to delineate the entire articular cartilage surface in this slice. *B*, T2-weighted fast spin-echo image of the same knee depicts synovial fluid (long T_2) with higher signal intensity. Water in articular cartilage and muscle is relatively bound (short T_2); these structures therefore show low signal intensity. The dynamic range is much improved with the use of fat suppression, hence the dark marrow in bone. High intrinsic contrast between cartilage and synovial fluid makes this technique useful for delineating the articular surface. *C*, Proton-density weighted, fat-suppressed fast spin-echo image of the same knee uses a shorter echo time, making cartilage signal brighter. Bone marrow edema is visible in all three images (long arrow) and a small meniscal tear is best visualized in the PD-FSE image (short arrowhead). (Courtesy of Synarc, Inc.)

dephasing and T_2 signal loss result in an overall faster decay in transverse magnetization called $T_2{}^*$, which is defined as:

$$\frac{1}{T_2^*} = \frac{1}{T_2} + \frac{1}{T_2'}$$

Signal lost to fixed magnetic heterogeneity, but not that lost to T_2 relaxation, can be recovered using the spin echoes already mentioned.

Local perturbations of the magnetic field typically arise at interfaces between substances that differ considerably in magnetic susceptibility (the degree to which a substance magnetizes in the presence of a magnetic field), such as between soft tissue and gas, metal, or heavy calcification. Severe $T_2{}^*$ at these sites is referred to as magnetic susceptibility effect. Spin-echo refocusing RF pulses correct for fixed magnetic heterogeneities and therefore can provide images with true T_2 contrast. The gradient-echo technique, which relies solely on pre-winding and rewinding gradient waveforms before and after signal acquisition, is faster than spin-echo. However, it does not correct for off-resonance effects and therefore provides only T_2^*-weighted images. These images are highly vulnerable to magnetic susceptibility effects, such as those caused by metallic prostheses, and can result in large signal voids in the vicinities of metal implants. Note that while SNR increases with higher field strength, artifacts from magnetic susceptibility differences become more severe.

Finally, diffusion of protons (for example, water) within a specimen during the acquisition of an MR image results in loss of phase coherence among the protons and therefore a loss in signal. This effect is usually insignificant in conventional MRI but can be augmented with the use of strong magnetic field gradients such as those employed in MR microimaging. Water diffusivity is thus an additional tissue parameter measurable with MRI.[6,7]

Both T_1-weighting (short TR) and T_2-weighting (long TE) involve discarding MR signal. If these effects are eliminated, signal intensity reflects only the proton density. Accordingly, long-TR/ short-TE images are often referred to as proton density-weighted. However, even the shortest finite TE attainable is too long to completely escape T_2 relaxation, and extremely long TRs (>2500 ms) are not practical for imaging in vivo. Therefore, even so-called proton density–weighted images contain some T_1 and T_2 contrast (Fig. 9–6, Fig. 9–14).

Another consequence of the relaxation that occurs from TR to TR is that during the first few repetitions, the signal will be different strengths. Because the magnetization has not fully recovered after the first TR, the second signal acquisition has less available signal to be tipped into the transverse plane. The third acquisition will differ from the second, and so forth. Eventually, however, these differences from TR to TR become smaller and smaller, and the signal is said to be in the steady state. The effort to shorten this transient time to maximize useful imaging time, as well as methods of manipulating spins at the end of each TR to reach this condition more quickly, has been an active area of imaging research.[8-10]

Subtle T_1 contrast (for example, between articular cartilage and synovial fluid) is usually overshadowed on T_1-weighted images by the far greater difference in signal intensity that exists between fat and most other tissues, because the presence of fat increases the dynamic range of the resulting images. However, by selectively suppressing the signal intensity of fat, it is possible to expand the scale of image intensities across smaller differences in T_1 and thus to augment residual T_1 contrast (Fig. 9–7). Another application of fat suppression is to increase contrast between fat and other substances, such as methemoglobin and gadolinium (Gd)-containing contrast material, which also show rapid T_1 relaxation. The most widely used technique for fat suppression is based on the chemical shift phenomenon: Because the frequency of protons in fat differs from that of protons in water, the magnetization of fat

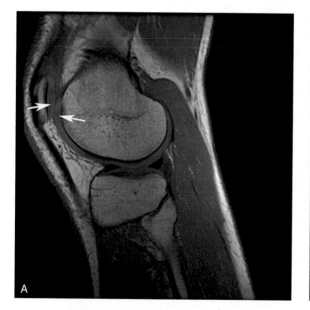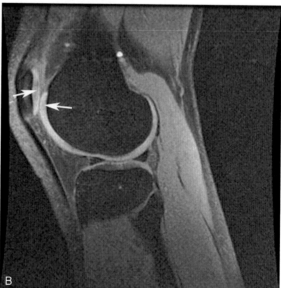

Figure 9–7 Augmenting T1 contrast with fat suppression. *A*, Sagittal, T_1-weighted spin-echo image of a knee acquired with a TR of 500 ms, at the short end of the usual range (500 ms to 700 ms) depicts the articular cartilage (*arrows*) with a slightly higher signal intensity than the adjacent synovial fluid. Contrast between cartilage and water is greater on this shorter-TR image than on the conventional T_1-weighted image shown in Fig. 9–6A (TR = 600 ms), but is still overshadowed by the greater T_1 contrast between fat and other tissues in the image. *B*, The same sequence repeated with fat suppression generates greater contrast between articular cartilage (*arrows*) and synovial fluid as their pixel intensities are rescaled across a broader range of gray scale values. The same effect can be achieved with water-selective excitation. (Courtesy of Synarc, Inc.)

(or water) can be selectively suppressed by a specifically tuned RF pulse at the beginning of the sequence (Fig. 9–8). This RF pulse, which is centered on the fat frequency instead of the water frequency, prematurely tips down the fat spins so that when the sequence RF tip-down pulse is played out, there is no longitudinal magnetization in fat available to produce a signal.

A similar technique can also be used to suppress the signal of water indirectly, through a mechanism called magnetization transfer. In this case, direct suppression of tightly constrained protons in macromolecules such as collagen, which are thermodynamically coupled to freely mobile protons in bulk water, evokes a transfer of magnetization from the water proton pool to the macromolecular pool to maintain equilibrium. This manifests as a loss of longitudinal magnetization and therefore signal intensity from water—in proportion to the relative concentrations of the two proton pools in the tissue and the specific rate constant for the equilibrium reaction. Because collagen (unlike fat) is strongly coupled to water in this way, cartilage and muscle exhibit pronounced magnetization-transfer effects.[11-14]

Magnetization-transfer techniques are therefore useful for imaging the articular cartilage and could potentially be used to quantify the collagen content of this tissue.

The two most important parameters for describing the extent of tissue coverage are image resolution and field of view (FOV). Both of these parameters depend on the strength of the gradients, on gradient switching speed, and on how the gradient waveforms are played out during the acquisition. Finer resolution requires an increase in the number of frequencies that must be sampled and therefore longer gradient waveforms. Images that have larger FOV (that is, are zoomed out to show more anatomy) require frequencies to be more precisely resolved, which means that gradient waveforms must be lower in amplitude and of longer time duration. So, both resolution and FOV are also

dependent on the amount of time available within a single TR to keep scan times reasonable, patient motion reduced, and contrast/signal available despite relaxation effects.

In 2D imaging, a slice is selected during excitation, and the other two spatial axes are localized down and across the image plane during acquisition. Alternatively, 3D data sets can be acquired by exciting all spins and playing localizer gradients on all three axes during acquisition. In either of these cases, dimensions of the individual volume elements, or voxels, comprising it define the spatial resolution of an MR image. Voxel size is determined by multiplying the slice thickness by the size of the in-plane subdivisions of the image, the pixels (picture elements). Pixel size, in turn, is determined by dividing the FOV by the image matrix, which most commonly ranges between 256 × 128 and 256 × 256 for knee imaging. The key point of pixel size is the smaller the pixel, the finer the spatial resolution. Typical sizes for FOV in knee imaging are around 14 cm.

All signals within a single voxel are averaged. Therefore, if an interface with high signal intensity on one side and low signal intensity on the other side passes through the middle of a voxel, then the interface is depicted as an intermediate signal intensity band the width of the voxel (Fig. 9–9). This effect is known as partial-volume signal averaging. However, as voxel size decreases, so does SNR. Accordingly, high-resolution imaging requires sufficient SNR to support the spatial resolution. SNR can be increased by shortening TE (less T_2 decay), increasing TR (more T_1 recovery), imaging at higher field strength (greater longitudinal magnetization), or utilizing specialized coils that reduce noise (small surface coils, quadrature coils, or phased arrays of small coils).[15,16] Specialized sequences, such as those that fully refocus spin dephasing from T_2^* effects, also provide greater SNR.

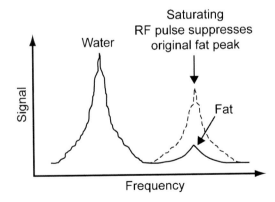

Figure 9–8 Frequency-selective fat suppression. The chemical-shift phenomenon separates the resonant frequencies of water and fat (by 220 Hz at a magnetic field strength of 1.5 T). This allows the longitudinal magnetization of either of these proton pools to be selectively suppressed by an RF pulse tuned to the correct resonant frequency. Since the resonant frequency and the magnitude of the chemical shift both depend on magnetic field strength, this method of fat suppression is dependent on the homogeneity of the static magnetic field and is not feasible at very low field strengths.

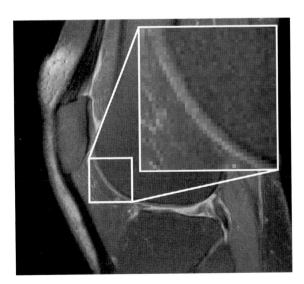

Figure 9–9 Partial volume averaging. The smallest element of an MR image is the individual voxel (pixel size • slice thickness). Different signal intensities within a single voxel are averaged. This effect is most noticeable at high contrast interfaces as shown in the magnified view of the femoral cartilage on this sagittal, fat-suppressed, T_1-weighted gradient-echo image of a knee. (Courtesy of Synarc, Inc.)

IMAGING ARTICULAR CARTILAGE

Magnetic Resonance Imaging Appearance of Articular Cartilage: Contrast Mechanisms

The signal behavior of articular cartilage on MRI reflects the complex biochemistry and histology of this tissue. The high water content (proton density) of articular cartilage forms the basis for MR signal. Water content in this tissue depends on the delicate balance between the swelling pressure of the aggregated proteoglycans and the counter resistance of the fibrous collagen matrix. But, in general terms, changes in cartilage proton density tend to be relatively small (typically <20%). Because the water constitutes approximately 70% of the weight of normal articular cartilage, proton density itself offers little scope for generating image contrast between cartilage and adjacent synovial fluid. However, this fundamental MRI signal in cartilage is modulated by a number of processes, including T_1 relaxation, T_2 relaxation, magnetization transfer, water diffusion, magnetic susceptibility, and interactions with contrast agents. These processes provide many different mechanisms for delineating cartilage morphology and probing its composition.

For comparison, Table 9–1 gives the T_1 and T_2 values of tissues in the knee. The T_1 of articular cartilage at 1.5 T is approximately 800 ms. This time is much shorter than the T_1 of adjacent synovial fluid, (2500 ms) but still longer than the T_1 of subarticular marrow fat (260 ms). The gray scale on a conventional T_1-weighted SE image is then so dominated by fat that the contrast between articular cartilage and adjacent synovial fluid is normally difficult to appreciate (Fig. 9–6). Intrinsic T_1-contrast can be augmented slightly by shortening TR, but a more powerful approach is to suppress the fat signal or selectively excite protons in water, and rescale the smaller residual T_1 contrast across the image. This generates images in which articular cartilage is depicted as an isolated high signal intensity band in sharp contrast with adjacent low signal intensity joint fluid, and nulled fat in adipose tissue (for example, Hoffa's fat pad) and bone.[12,17] Fat suppression also eliminates chemical-shift artifacts that distort the cartilage—bone interface and complicate dimensional measurements.

T_2 relaxation is another tissue characteristic that can be harnessed to image the articular cartilage. Fibrillar collagen in the articular cartilage immobilizes tissue water protons and promotes dipole-dipole interactions among them, increasing T_2 relaxation and therefore signal decay. The T_2 of normal articular cartilage increases from approximately 30 ms in the deep radial zone to 70 ms in the transitional zone[18] (Fig. 9–10). Above the transitional zone, the superficial tangential zone shows extremely rapid T_2 relaxation because of its densely matted collagen fibers. This radial heterogeneity of T_2 gives articular cartilage a laminar appearance on all but extremely short-TE images.[19] The pattern of T_2 variation can be explained, to some extent, by the heterogeneous distribution of collagen in this tissue, but is also affected by the orientation of collagen fibrils relative to the static magnetic field (B_0). T_2 anisotropy in cartilage manifests as decreased signal decay in regions where

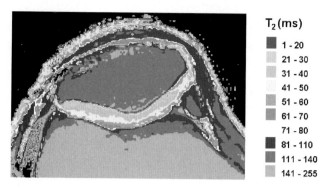

Figure 9–10 T_2 Relaxation of normal adult articular cartilage. T_2 map generated from multislice, multi-echo (11 echoes: TE = 9, 18, . . . 99 ms) spin-echo images acquired at 3 T shows increasing T_2 toward the articular surface. (Courtesy of B. J. Dardzinski, Ph.D. University of Cincinnati College of Medicine.)

the collagen fibrils are oriented at 55° to B_0.[19–22] This so-called "magic-angle" phenomenon is responsible for areas of mildly elevated signal intensity in the radial zone of appropriately oriented cartilage segments on intermediate-TE images (Fig. 9–11). It is also one explanation for the slower T_2 seen in the transitional zone. Collagen fibrils in this zone are slightly sparser than in the radial zone, but more importantly they are also highly disorganized. Accordingly, a significant proportion of the fibrils in the transitional zone are angled at 55° to B_0 regardless of the orientation of the knee in the magnet. With sufficiently long TE (<80 ms), normal articular cartilage appears diffusely low in signal intensity even in regions normally affected by this magic-angle phenomenon.

Superimposed upon these histological and biochemical causes of laminar appearance in articular cartilage are patterns created by truncation artifacts.[23,24] This manifests as one or several thin horizontal bands of low signal intensity midway through the cartilage on short-TE images. Truncation artifacts are less common on high-resolution images, but usually present on fat-suppressed 3D spoiled gradient-recalled (SPGR) images generated with most clinical protocols.

Long-TE images provide high contrast between articular cartilage and adjacent synovial fluid, but poor contrast between cartilage and bone. Shorter-TE images improve

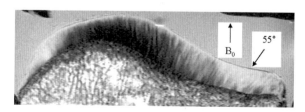

Figure 9–11 Magic-angle phenomenon in articular cartilage. High-resolution spin-echo image of the patellar cartilage shows low signal intensity due to T_2 relaxation in the radial zone of the central portion of the cartilage, where collagen is aligned with the static magnetic field (B_0.) Increased signal intensity (arrow) indicative of prolonged T_2 can be seen in areas where the collagen is oriented at approximately 55° relative to B_0. (Courtesy of D. Goodwin, and J. Dunn, Dartmouth Medical School.)

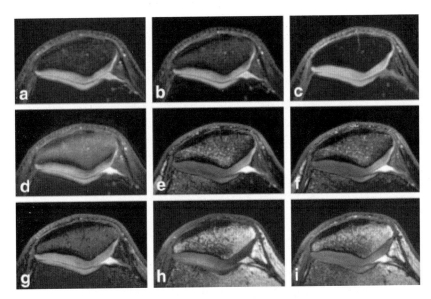

Figure 9–12 Comparison of FSE and SPGR to DEFT and three variants of SSFP. Axial patellofemoral water images from a normal volunteer using *A*, FSE (TR = 1800 ms), *B*, FSE (TR = 3200 ms), *C*, SPGR, *D*, DEFT, *E*, LC-SSFP, *F*, FEMR, and *G*, FS-SSFP. Fat images using LC-SSFP *H*, and FEMR *I*, require no additional scan time. Water images from DEFT *D*, and the SSFP-based techniques (e.g., FS-SSFP, LC-SSFP, and FEMR) all demonstrate both bright cartilage and excellent contrast with synovial fluid. (Hargreaves, B.A., Gold, G.E., Beaulieu, C.F., et al. Comparison of new sequences for high-resolution cartilage imaging. Magn Reson Med 49:700–709, 2003.)

cartilage bone contrast, but are vulnerable to magic-angle effects. Fast SE (FSE) combines T_2 effects with magnetization transfer to decrease signal intensity in articular cartilage.[25,26] Signal loss due to magnetization transfer results from equilibration of longitudinal magnetization between nonsaturated freely mobile protons in water and saturated restricted protons in macromolecules, such as collagen, that have been excited off the resonant frequency of free water during multi-slice imaging.[11,12,14,25–27] The effect is exaggerated with FSE imaging because of the multiple 180° RF pulses used with this technique. Accordingly, intermediate TE (~40 ms) FSE images show relatively low signal intensity in articular cartilage while preserving high signal intensity in synovial fluid and subjacent bone marrow to delineate the articular cartilage with high contrast (Fig. 9–13). Both intermediate and long TE FSE images offer relatively good morphological delineation of articular cartilage in less time than is required for high-resolution fat-suppressed 3D-GRE images. The choice of which TE to use depends on the objectives of the imaging and how they relate to the range of normal and pathological T_2 heterogeneity found in articular cartilage.

Magnetic Resonance Pulse Sequences for Imaging Articular Cartilage Morphology

Two pulse sequences are the clinical workhorses of knee imaging: T_1-weighted spoiled GRE, referred to as SPGR or FLASH (fast low-angle shot) and T_2-weighted fast spin-echo (FSE), or turbo spin-echo (TSE). SPGR provides 3D acquisition in reasonable scan times and is currently the most available clinical option for quantitative measurements of cartilage volume.[28] However, it does not provide strong cartilage-synovial fluid contrast and is susceptible to T_2^* dephasing. FSE is much more robust to off-resonance, and its contrast is not weighted by T_2^*. However, the method requires a longer repetition interval, and therefore scan times for 3D acquisition would be prohibitively long.

Fat-suppressed, T_1-weighted 3D SPGR is easy to use and widely available, and has become a popular MRI technique

for delineating articular cartilage morphology.[12,17,29–32] However, the sequence provides poor cartilage-synovial fluid contrast, making depiction of cartilage surface defects difficult. Driven equilibrium (DE, DEFT, or FR [Fast Recovery] as in FR-SE) produces higher cartilage-synovial fluid contrast than either FSE or SPGR (Fig. 9–12), making it a good choice for imaging cartilage surface defects. The contrast is based on tissue T_2/T_1, which makes synovial fluid brighter. Although DEFT provides shorter scan times and allows for 3D imaging, other sequences with higher SNR efficiency are better choices for cartilage volume measurement.

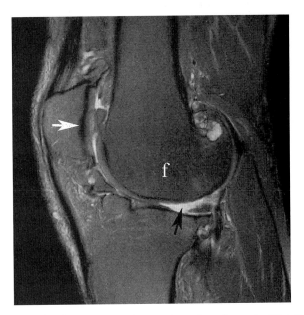

Figure 9–13 Fast spin echo imaging of cartilage. Sagittal T_2-weighted fast spin echo image of the knee shows high contrast between the low signal intensity articular cartilage (*white arrow*) and adjacent high signal intensity synovial fluid (*black arrow*) and intermediate signal intensity subchondral marrow fat (*f*). (Courtesy of Synarc, Inc.)

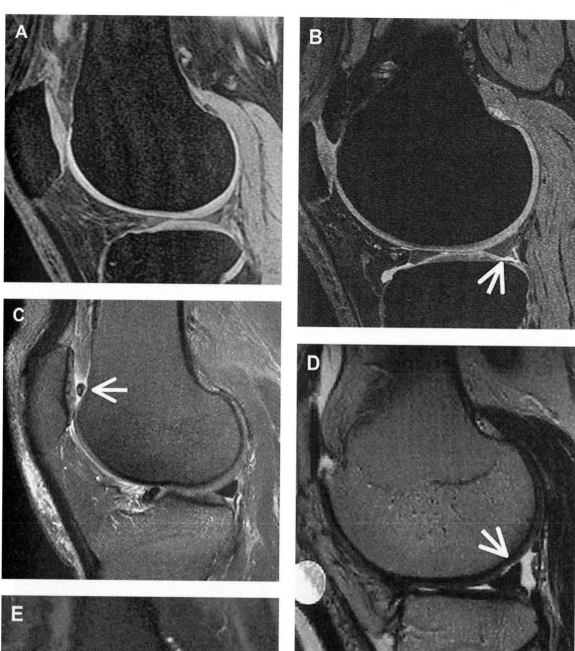

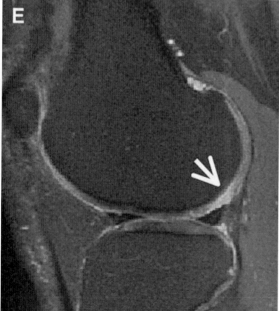

Figure 9–14 Cartilage contrast with various pulse sequences. *A,* Sagittal fat-suppressed T_1-weighted 3D GRE image depicting articular cartilage as a high-signal structure in sharp contrast against adjacent low-signal bone, marrow fat, intra-articular adipose, fluid, ligaments, and menisci. *B,* Sagittal 3D DESS image showing partial-thickness cartilage defect (arrow) over posterior lateral tibia. Note the similarities in contrast properties of fat-suppressed DESS with those of fat-suppressed FSE. *C,* Sagittal fat-suppressed IW 2D FSE shows a loose body (arrow) in the patellofemoral compartment. *D,* Sagittal T_2-weighted 2D FSE image without FS shows a partial-thickness defect (arrow) of the lateral femoral cartilage adjacent to the posterior horn of the meniscus. *E,* Sagittal fat-suppressed T_2-weighted 2D FSE image of a different knee shows a partial-thickness cartilage defect (arrow) in a similar location. (From Peterfy CG, Gold G, Eckstein F, et al. MRI protocols for whole-organ assessment of the knee in osteoarthritis. Osteoarthritis Cartilage, 14 Suppl A:A95–111, 2006)

SPGR sequences are susceptible to T_2^* signal decay because the signal is the average of spins that are dephasing, or falling out of step with the main-field resonant frequency. Balanced steady-state free-precession (bSSFP, SSFP, also FIESTA) or true fast imaging with steady-state free precession (True-FISP) pulse sequences are able to fully refocus spins each acquisition, using symmetric gradient waveforms. This results in a stronger signal and higher SNR images. The number of off-resonant frequencies that can be refocused at high signal strength is inversely proportional to the sequence TR, so imaging times are also inherently shorter. The concept behind SSFP is not new,[33–35] but recent hardware advances resulting in faster gradient switching times has made implementation of SSFP at short TR lengths possible. Figure 9–12 shows a comparison of FSE and SPGR to three variants of SSFP, each with different implementations of fat suppression. As faster hardware becomes more ubiquitous in the clinical setting, 3D fat-suppressed SSFP (FS-SSFP) is a frontrunner to replace 3D FS-SPGR with higher-SNR images.[36] Alternatively, the higher SNR available could be used to improve resolution, which could further improve cartilage segmentation and surface rendering,

adding both sensitivity and specificity to volume and thickness measurements. For imaging cartilage lesions, the frontrunner is another variant, called dual-echo steady-state (DESS) imaging. DESS uses a second gradient echo separated by a refocusing pulse. This lengthens the acquisition window, but results in an image with higher T_2^* weighting, and has been shown to be superior for detecting superficial cartilage lesions.[37] Figure 9–14 shows a comparison of DESS to other GRE and SE sequences.

More recently, projection-reconstruction (PR) based techniques have been developed to image the articular cartilage with ultra-short TE (<0.2 ms) and even greater contrast, fewer chemical shift effects, and lower vulnerability to magnetic susceptibility artifacts (Fig. 9–15).[38] Geometric artifacts that arise from the non-grid sampling inherent to this method should be considered, but some other advantages of this technique include the potential for spectroscopic determination of water content and T_2. Vastly undersampled isotropic projection (VIPR) is one variation of these techniques that has been shown to provide high cartilage-synovial fluid contrast and clear demarcation of cartilage defects.[39] Kijowski et al. have

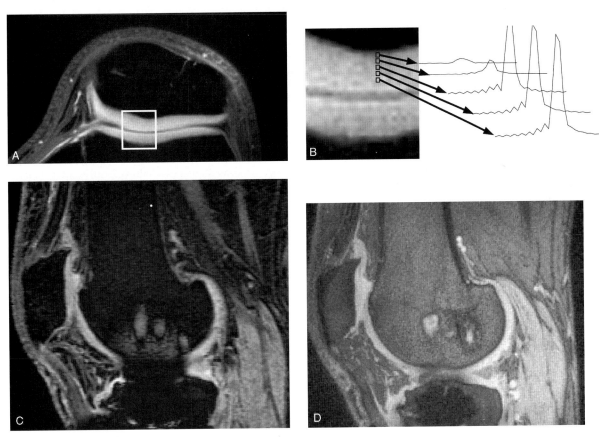

Figure 9–15 Projection-Reconstruction Spiral Imaging of Cartilage. *A* Water frequency image (TE = 200 microseconds, 0.2-mm in-plane resolution, 8-min scan time). *B* Spectra from the voxels indicated in *A*, showing increasing peak area and decreasing width towards articular surface. This indicates increasing water density and T2-relaxation times (Reprinted with permission from the American Journal of Roentgenology: G. Gold, D. Thedens, J. Pauly, K. Fechner, G. Bergman, C. Beaulieu, and A. Macovski. MR Imaging of Articular Cartilage of the Knee: New Methods Using Ultra-Short TE's, AJR Am J Roentgenol 170(5):1223–1226, 1998.) *C* Gradient-recalled echo image from a patient with osteochondral allografts. Metal artifact obscures the articular cartilage. *D* Spectral maximum intensity image (SMIP) of projection-reconstruction spiral imaging of the same slice shows reduced artifacts.(From Gold GE, Bergman AG, Pauly JM, et al. Magnetic resonance imaging of knee cartilage repair. Top Magn Reson Imaging 9(6):377–392, 1998.)

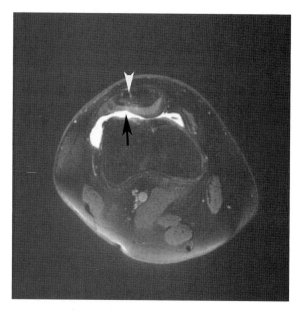

Figure 9–16 Axial VIPR-SSFP image of the knee shows a large defect within the articular cartilage of the lateral facet of the patella (*black arrow*) with adjacent subchondral bone marrow edema (*white arrowhead*). (Courtesy of Richard Kijowski, M.D., University of Wisconsin-Madison.)

demonstrated a variant of VIPR using radial SSFP imaging. The image in Figure 9–16 depicts a large patellar cartilage defect along with adjacent subchondral bone marrow edema using this technique.

There are several new methods of suppressing or separating out fat signal that have been developed for SSFP sequences. In addition to the use of traditional fat saturation pulses (FS-SSFP) or the use of spectrally selective RF pulses that only excite protons at the water frequency, the newer steady-state methods can be broken into two categories. These are: 1) those that create steady-state signals with low or suppressed fat signal, and 2) fat-water separation methods, which provide simultaneous water and fat images with some additional post-imaging reconstruction. The first category includes techniques such as fluctuating equilibrium magnetic resonance (FEMR)[40] and oscillating SSFP.[41,42] These techniques have lower SNR efficiency than FS-SSFP, and are generally less robust than FS-SSFP, so they may be better suited to other applications. The second category includes steady-state fat/water separation methods such as linear combination SSFP (LC-SSFP)[43] and phase-sensitive SSFP (PS-SSFP).[44,45] LC-SSFP requires two acquisitions and is more sensitive to patient motion. PS-SSFP is less sensitive to patient motion, because it images the water-fat difference and requires only one acquisition.[44] It is faster than FS-SSFP and provides excellent cartilage delineation, which makes it a good choice for 3D imaging for volume and thickness assessment.[46] With this method, each voxel is categorized as water or fat based on the majority of voxel tissue content. This method works well in cartilage, but would have difficulty in imaging bone edema, because the marrow fat would contribute partial volume errors to the water-fat separation. Figure 9–17 shows a comparison of PS-SSFP with Proton-density fast

spin-echo (PD-FSE) and fat- suppressed, T_2-weighted FSE in articular cartilage.

In addition to the methods specific to SSFP, there have been recent improvements to Dixon fat-water separation, which uses multiple acquisitions with different echo times to reconstruct water and fat images. *I*terative *Decom*position of water and fat with *E*cho *A*symmetry and *L*east-squares estimation (IDEAL) is a variation of the Dixon technique and can be used with FSE, SPGR, and SSFP.[47,48] IDEAL is very promising for cartilage imaging because it has higher SNR efficiency in both cartilage and synovial fluid, with both SPGR and SSFP.[49,50] Figure 9–18 shows a comparison of the IDEAL and fat saturation pulse methods with SPGR cartilage imaging.

Magnetic Resonance Pulse Sequences for Articular Cartilage Functional Imaging

In addition to delineating cartilage morphology, T_2 relaxation can be used to probe the status of the collagen matrix in articular cartilage. This is because as the collagen network breaks down, tissue water in articular cartilage becomes more fluid and correspondingly less affected by T_2 relaxation. Consistent with this, foci of high signal intensity are often seen within the cartilage of knees of patients with OA on T_2-weighted images (Fig. 9–19). These signal abnormalities have been reported to correspond to arthroscopically demonstrable abnormalities.[51,52] However, they have also been observed in cartilage that appeared normal by arthroscopy.[52-54] This raises questions about the sensitivity of arthroscopy for assessing articular cartilage integrity, at least in very early disease.

A careful assessment of the sensitivity and specificity of subjective evaluations of T_2 abnormalities in articular cartilage using images attainable with conventional MRI hardware and software and histological assessment as the gold standard has yet to be reported. Moreover, most studies that have looked at T_2 abnormalities in cartilage have provided only cross-sectional information. Longitudinal data describing the natural history of this potential marker of cartilage matrix integrity and its association with subsequent cartilage loss and joint failure are scant. In one study,[55] however, 5 (33%) of 15 meniscal surgery patients followed over 3 years postsurgery developed a total of six T_2 lesions in otherwise normal-appearing articular cartilage. Two of these lesions progressed to focal cartilage defects during the study (Fig. 9–20), while three persisted and one regressed. Interestingly, the four lesions that did not progress were in patients who had undergone meniscal repair, while the lesions that progressed were in patients who had meniscal resection. Accordingly, abnormal T_2 may identify cartilage at risk of future loss.

Water diffusion in cartilage also contributes to signal loss on T_2-weighted MR images. This is because water molecules that have changed positions during a portion of the MRI acquisition can no longer be rephased properly and so do not contribute maximally to the net signal. This loss of phase coherence is proportional to the distance traveled by the diffusing water protons and is therefore worse on long TE images. The presence of proteoglycans, particularly

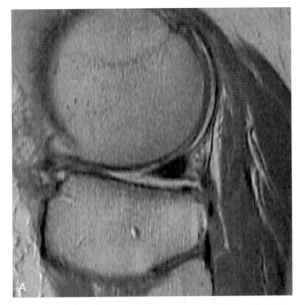

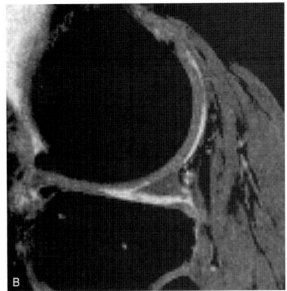

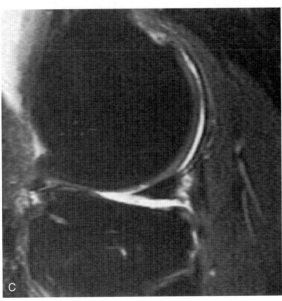

Figure 9–17 Phase-sensitive fat/water separation. *A*, PD-FSE, *B*, PS-SSFP (water), and *C*, T2 FS-FSE sagittal images of the knee, comparing phase-sensitive fat/water imaging with fat-suppressed FSE. (Courtesy of Shreyas S. Vasanawala, M.D., Ph.D., Stanford University.)

chondroitin sulfate, in normal cartilage inhibits water diffusion and keeps this effect relatively small, although with very strong gradients and specialized phase-sensitive pulse sequences, water diffusion can be demonstrated and even quantified in normal articular cartilage.[7] With cartilage degeneration and proteoglycan loss, however, water diffusion has been shown to increase considerably. Accordingly, diffusion may play a more significant role in cartilage signal modulation in osteoarthritic joints.

Burstein et al.[7] showed that treatment of a bovine cartilage sample with trypsin (for proteoglycan removal) resulted in a 20% increase in the measured rate of diffusion. They also showed that a 35% compression of a bovine cartilage sample corresponded with a 19% reduction in the rate of diffusion. Diffusion-weighted imaging of cartilage has also recently been demonstrated in vivo. Gold et al.[56] were able to measure diffusion rates for water in

cartilage using an in-plane resolution of 1.3 × 1.7 mm that were consistent with values determined in vitro at high resolution by Xia et al.[6] Increases in the available gradient strength on clinical systems will be required to fully evaluate the clinical utility of diffusion-weighted imaging for OA. Using a local extremity gradient coil designed to improve the sensitivity and spatial resolution of imaging the knee with MRI, Frank et al.[57] were able to achieve a spatial resolution of the 350 μm × 350 μm in-plane with a slice-thickness of 5 mm. Further advances in local gradient coils and improvements in system gradients will greatly aid the study of cartilage diffusion.

Proteoglycan loss also reduces cartilage hydration and therefore proton density. Since proteoglycan loss usually accompanies collagen loss, prolonged T_2 associated with the collagen loss can be offset by T_2 shortening due to increased diffusion and decreased tissue hydration of cartilage.

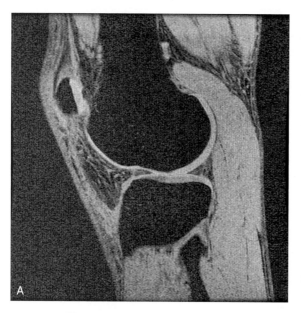
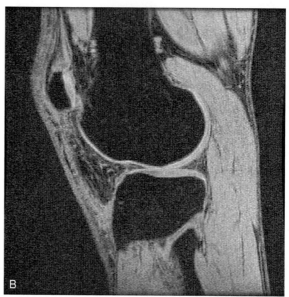

Figure 9–18 Iterative decomposition of water and fat with echo asymmetry and least-squares estimation (IDEAL) fat/water separation. Sagittal images of the knee, comparing IDEAL fat/water separation with fat suppression. Images are 16-cm FOV, acquired using *A*, FS-SPGR, and *B*, IDEAL-SPGR (water image). (Courtesy of Garry E. Gold, M.D., Stanford University.)

In addition to effects on water diffusion and tissue hydration, loss of proteoglycan from cartilage matrix results in decreased ^{23}Na-ion concentration through the associated decrease in fixed negative charge density. Estimation of in vivo ^{23}Na concentration of cartilage by ^{23}Na Nuclear magnetic resonance (NMR) has been proposed as a means to provide an early marker for proteoglycan loss.[58–62]

Despite a high natural abundance in biological systems, the signal from ^{23}Na is approximately 10% of the ^{1}H signal due to a lower NMR sensitivity than protons. NMR

sensitivity is defined as $\gamma^3 I(I+1)$, where γ is the gyromagnetic ratio and I is the spin.[63] The NMR signal is directly proportional to the sensitivity of the nuclei. ^{23}Na imaging is at an initial disadvantage because of these basic differences in the NMR properties of the two nuclei.

The transverse relaxation time (T_2) of ^{23}Na for cartilage exhibits a bi-exponential behavior, with a fast T_2 component between 0.7 and 2.3 ms and a slow T_2 component between 8 and 12 ms.[64] The in vivo longitudinal relaxation time (T_1) of ^{23}Na ranges between 14 and 20 ms.[64] Rapid

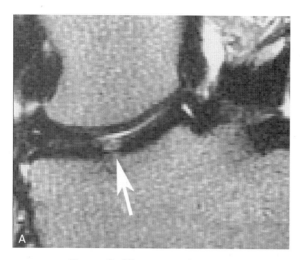
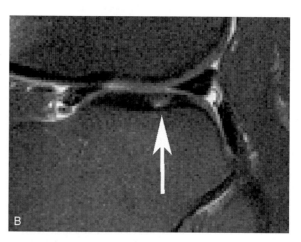

Figure 9–19 Patterns of abnormal cartilage signal. *A*, Coronal FSE image shows focal high signal in the cartilage over the lateral tibial plateau (*arrow*). *B*, In a different knee, a sagittal T_2-weighted FS-FSE image shows a focus of increased signal (*arrow*) in cartilage over the lateral tibial plateau. Note the subchondral bone changes immediately beneath this region. (Courtesy of Synarc, Inc.)

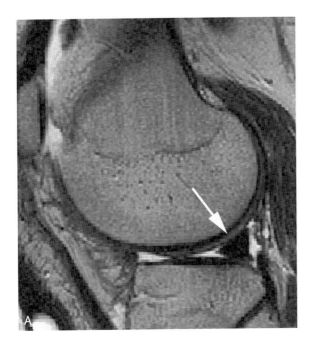 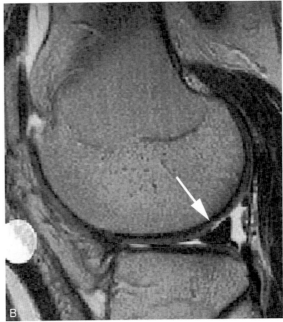

Figure 9–20 Progression of T_2 lesions in articular cartilage. Serial sagittal T_2-weighted fast spin-echo images show a focal T_2 lesion (*arrow*) in the femoral cartilage adjacent to the posterior horn of the lateral meniscus at baseline *A,* Follow-up imaging nine months later *B,* shows a partial-thickness (Grade 2.0) defect at that exact location. (Peterfy, CG. Scratching the surface: articular cartilage disorders in the knee. MRI Clin N Am. 8(2):409–430, 2000.)

transverse relaxation times make imaging more difficult due to the rapid loss of signal during the echo time. [23]Na imaging is aided by a relatively short T_1, which allows rapid signal averaging to partially overcome the poor sensitivity and short transverse relaxation times. Spatial resolution is generally the major concern in [23]Na imaging due to the reduced signal strength. Clinical feasibility of [23]Na imaging was first demonstrated in 1988.[65,66] Granot[65] acquired in vivo sodium images from various tissue structures (including knees) by employing a 3D sequence with short repetition (45 ms) and gradient-echo times (6 ms), concluding that sodium imaging of body organs is clinically feasible.

Several groups have shown in vitro studies that enzymatic degradation of proteoglycans leads to changes in [23]Na relaxation rates.[58,59,61,67] Reddy et al.[64] demonstrated that [23]Na MRI can differentiate between regions of proteoglycan depletion from healthy cartilage when imaging in vitro bovine patella. In addition, they also obtained [23]Na images from a healthy volunteer with a 4T MRI scanner at an in-plane resolution of 1.25 × 2.5 mm and a slice thickness of 4 mm. [23]Na imaging has also been shown to be sensitive to the mechanical deformation of cartilage. Shapiro et al.[68] found that during recovery after exercise (50 deep knee bends), a 15% decrease in the thickness of the lateral facet of the subject's patella cartilage resulted in a 20% reduction in [23]Na signal intensity. A possible cause for the loss in signal was attributed to the expulsion of saline from the cartilage during compression. An in vitro comparison of normal versus PG-depleted cartilage showed both specimens exhibited a decrease in T_1 and T_2 during compression.[69]

[23]Na imaging has been shown to have great potential in characterizing the physiological and mechanical state of cartilage. The major limiting factor to wide clinical usage of these techniques is the available signal strength on the standard 1.5 T system. All of the studies described earlier were performed on systems ranging from 1.5 to 4 T. Improvements in RF coil sensitivity,[70] stronger gradients for shorter echo times, and greater clinical access to high field systems are prerequisites for [23]Na imaging of cartilage to move from the research environment to the clinical setting.

Another interesting marker of cartilage matrix integrity is Gd-DTPA^{2-} uptake.[71–73] Under normal circumstances, anionic Gd-DTPA^{2-} introduced into the synovial fluid (either by i.v. or direct intra-articular injection) is repelled by the negatively charged proteoglycans in normal cartilage. However, in areas of decreased glycosaminoglycan (GAG) content where the fixed negative charge density of cartilage is reduced, Gd-DTPA^{2-} can diffuse into the cartilage and enhance T_1 relaxation. These areas are depicted as conspicuous foci of high signal intensity in the otherwise low signal intensity cartilage on inversion recovery images. Cartilage T_1 values correlate almost linearly with proteoglycan content in the range normally found in cartilage. However, quantifying T_1 can be time consuming and impractical for clinical studies. Further work is necessary to establish the optimal method for acquiring this imaging data. Additional studies are also needed to define the relationship between this marker of proteoglycan matrix damage and elevated T_2 as a marker of collagen matrix damage (Fig. 9–21). Whether one precedes the other and exactly how predictive each of these are—alone or in combination—for subsequent cartilage loss, the development of other structural features of OA, and ultimately for clinical manifestations of OA, have yet to be established. In addition to the use of Gd-DTPA^{2-}, proteoglycan content of

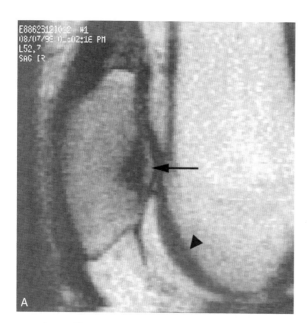
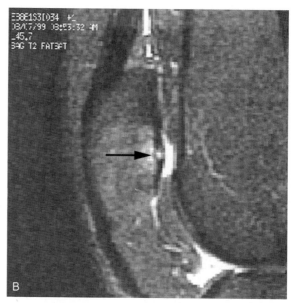

Figure 9–21 Imaging cartilage matrix damage. *A*, Sagittal inversion-recovery image of a knee following i.v. administration of Gd-DTPA shows a region of high signal intensity (*arrow*) in the patellar cartilage indicative of abnormal uptake of anionic Gd-DTPA^{2-}, and therefore, local proteoglycan depletion. Cartilage in the trochlear groove (*arrowhead*) shows low signal intensity indicative of repulsion of Gd-DTPA^{2-} by negatively charged proteoglycans. *B*, Fat-suppressed, T_2-weighted image of the same knee prior to Gd-DTPA^{2-} injection shows a smaller focus of increased signal intensity (*arrow*) in the same location indicative of local collagen matrix loss. This is associated with subarticular marrow edema in the patella. (Courtesy of Synarc, Inc.)

cartilage can be probed with cationic contrast agents such as manganese[74,75] or, as discussed earlier, by imaging sodium instead of hydrogen.[76] Finally, there is currently investigation to determine if $T_{1\rho}$ imaging provides information that correlates with proteoglycan depletion. This method tips protons to the transverse plane, applies a longer, low-power "spin-lock" RF pulse, then tips the spins back to the B_0 axis to prepare them for imaging.[77] This technique has been shown to produce a unique contrast, referred to as $T_{1\rho}$ relaxation contrast,[78] although finding a method that separates this from T_2 effect is difficult due to the nature of T_2 decay.[79]

Monitoring Changes in Articular Cartilage with Magnetic Resonance Imaging

Morphological markers of articular cartilage include both quantitative measures, such as thickness and volume, and semiquantitative measures, that grade cartilage integrity by a variety of scoring methods. Intermediate-TE and long-TE FSE images are usually adequate for most current clinical applications and in circumstances when lengthier high-resolution techniques are not justified (Fig. 9–12, Fig. 9–13). However, thinly partitioned, 3D SPGR images with selective fat suppression or water excitation are preferable for delineating cartilage morphology. Advantages of this latter technique include greater contrast, higher resolution, wide availability, ease of use, stable performance, no chemical shift artifact, and reasonable acquisition time (7 to 10 min). Disadvantages include longer acquisition times than

those required for FSE imaging and vulnerability to magnetic susceptibility and metallic artifacts. These artifacts range from mild distortions arising near small postoperative metallic fragments or gas bubbles introduced into the joint by vacuum phenomenon, to severe distortions caused by metallic implants or other orthopedic hardware following tibial plateau fracture or cruciate ligament repair. Failure of fat suppression due to regional field heterogeneities is generally not a problem because of the cylindrical shape of the knee, but can arise if the knee is bent or if the patella protrudes excessively. Typically, however, failed fat suppression in the region of the patella usually involves the marrow and superficial soft tissues, but does not reach the articular cartilage.

Several studies have evaluated the diagnostic accuracy of fat-suppressed 3D SPGR for identifying areas of cartilage loss in the knee. In a comparison of 3D SPGR with and without fat suppression T_2*-weighted GRE, and conventional T_1-weighted, proton density-weighted and T_2-weighted SE sequences in ten elderly cadaver knees, Recht et al.[29] found fat-suppressed, 3D SPGR (flip angle = 60 degree, TE = 10 ms, voxel size = 469 μm × 938 μm × 1500 μm) to have the greatest sensitivity (96%) and specificity (95%) for demonstrating patellofemoral cartilage lesions visible on pathological sections. Disler et al.[32] similarly showed the same technique in vivo to have 93% sensitivity and 94% specificity for arthroscopically visible cartilage lesions.

Most scoring methods reported thus far simply count articular cartilage defects and grade them according to the depth of the cartilage loss (for example, 0 = normal-thickness, 1 = superficial fraying or isolated signal abnormality, 2 = partial-thickness loss, 3 = full-thickness loss) (Fig. 9–20). Various more complex schemes, which take into account different patterns of cartilage involvement and the distribution of these changes in the knee, have been developed recently.[80] However, the full validity of any of these schemes has not yet been thoroughly established. There is considerable face validity to the link between cartilage loss and clinical outcomes in OA, but the amount of cartilage loss that is clinically relevant has not yet been determined. The issue is complicated by the multifactorial nature of joint failure and the oversimplification that monostructural models suffer. Nevertheless, cartilage loss is currently the most broadly accepted metric of structural progression in OA. Unresolved issues of surrogate validity not withstanding, semiquantitative scoring of cartilage loss can be relatively precise and resolve progression in one year. In a recent study of 29 patients with OA in whom the articular cartilage was scored in 15 locations in the knee using a seven-point scale, the intraclass correlation coefficient between two specially trained radiologists was 0.99.[80] A subsequent examination of 30 subjects from an ongoing cohort study of 3,075 elderly men and women imaged with a 15-min MRI protocol (T_2-weighted FSE) found similar inter-reader precision for femorotibial cartilage using the same scoring method (ICC = 0.91).[81]

Aside from semiquantitative scoring, a number of quantitative markers of cartilage morphology have been developed, including cartilage volume. This measurement can be derived from segmented images of the articular cartilage on fat-suppressed 3D SPGR or SSFP images using any of a variety of image analysis tools currently available (Fig. 9–22). A number of studies have validated the technical accuracy of these methods and established the precision error to range from 2% to 4% coefficient of variation (SD/mean volume)[14,82,83] (Fig. 9–23). In one investigation, 16 elderly women with OA of the knee were imaged with

MRI at yearly intervals for 2 years. The mean annual rate of cartilage loss was determined to be −6.7% ± 5.2% for the femur, −6.33% ± 4.3% for the tibia, and −3.4% ± 2.9% for the patella based on linear regression of the three time points.[84] Eckstein et al.[85] summarized the results of many different evaluations, concluding that annual changes of cartilage volume in most knee compartments in patients with OA are on the order of −4% to −6%. This range is greater than the expected precision error, providing strong evidence that the results are clinically significant.

Limitations of cartilage volume quantification include assumptions used to model cartilage volume change over time. For practical reasons, a linear model is usually the only feasible assumption for most clinical trials and epidemiological studies involving four or fewer time points. More complicated models (quadratic, and so on) may turn out to be more accurate, but until careful natural history studies have refined these models, curve-fitting challenges limit their use in most studies. Regardless, measurement precision for cartilage volume change combines errors related both to the measurement technique and the cartilage loss model used.

Other limitations of cartilage volume as a marker of disease severity and structural progression include insensitivity to small focal defects. These are more easily identified by semiquantitative scoring, or by regional cartilage volume mapping.[86] Measurement precision and therefore statistical power decreases as the subdivisions get smaller. Accordingly, the tradeoff between sensitivity and measurement precision must be carefully balanced. One highly refined method of depicting regional variations in cartilage quantity is thickness mapping.[87,88] As intuitive as cartilage

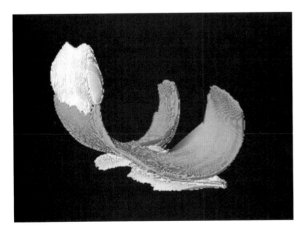

Figure 9–22 Example of cartilage segmentation performed by using fluctuating equilibrium MR imaging in a healthy 32-year-old male volunteer. Cartilage surfaces on the femur (red), patella (yellow), and tibia (blue) are all well seen. (Gold GE, Hargreaves, BA, Vasanawala, SS, Webb, JD, Shimakawa, AS, Brittain, JH, Beaulieu CF: Articular cartilage of the knee: evaluation with fluctuating equilibrium MR imaging—initial experience in healthy volunteers. Radiology 238:712–718, 2006.)

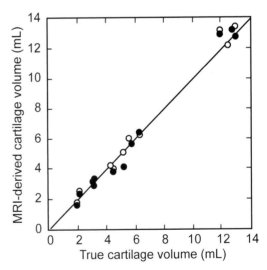

Figure 9–23 Technical accuracy of volumetric quantification of cartilage with MRI. The graph depicts cartilage volumes determined from fat-suppressed, T_1-weighted 3D gradient-echo images (*open circles*) and magnetization transfer subtraction images (*closed circles*) plotted against volumes measured directly by water displacement. A total of 12 cartilage plates (six patellar, three tibial, three femoral) from six knees were included. Line represents theoretical 100% accuracy. (Modified from Peterfy C, van Dijke, CF, Janzen, DL, et al. Quantification of articular cartilage in the knee with pulsed saturation transfer and fat-suppressed MR imaging. Radiology 192:485–491, 1994.)

thickness may seem, however, questions remain as to whether the minimum, maximum, or average thickness is the most relevant, how to deal with multiple lesions, and to what extent the location of a lesion (weight bearing, non-weight bearing) is important.

Perhaps the greatest limitation of all markers of cartilage morphology, however, is their fundamentally irreversible nature and relatively slow responsiveness. Regardless of how precisely change in cartilage morphology can be measured, its rate of change cannot be driven any faster than the disease process itself. For a solution to this problem, one must look upstream to earlier stages in the disease process of cartilage degeneration. Accordingly, there has been a great deal of interest in developing MRI markers of cartilage composition.

MRI in markers of cartilage composition relate principally to the collagen matrix or constituent proteoglycans. The most promising markers of collagen matrix integrity include T_2 relaxation and magnetization transfer coefficient. Markers of proteoglycan integrity include water diffusion, Gd-DTPA^{2-} uptake, $T_{1\rho}$, and ^{23}Na concentration.

As discussed above, disruption of the fibrillar organization of collagen or actual decrease in collagen content reduces T_2 relaxation and increases signal intensity on T_2-weighted images. Areas of elevated signal in otherwise low signal-intensity cartilage on long-TE MR images therefore represent foci of chondromalacia. While several studies have verified this relationship between T_2 relaxation and fibrillar collagen in cartilage, none have meticulously established the diagnostic accuracy (e.g., area under ROC curve, with histological verification) of subjective readings using MRI acquisition techniques that are applicable to multicenter studies or generalizable to clinical use. More importantly, the validity of cartilage T_2 as a biomarker of matrix integrity depends on its predictive power for subsequent cartilage loss. Although there is considerable face validity to this model and some anecdotal longitudinal evidence to support it, further prospective validation is needed. If this hypothesis is indeed true, then abnormal cartilage T_2 may identify cartilage at risk of future loss and thereby identify patients in need of aggressive therapy, hopefully before the point of no return. In addition to subjective evaluations of focal signal abnormalities in articular cartilage, regional changes in T_2 relaxation can be quantified and monitored over time with multi-echo SE imaging.[16,18] Limitations of this approach include technical tradeoffs between image acquisition time and the number of echoes, spatial resolution, and the attainable SNR. Further validation and performance characterization of cartilage T_2 are clearly needed.

Significantly less work has been done with magnetization transfer as a marker of collagen integrity in articular cartilage. Theoretically, this marker could be used almost exactly the same way that cartilage T_2 is used. However, even less is known about its diagnostic accuracy, responsiveness to disease and therapy, dynamic range, and measurement precision. Accordingly, further characterization is needed.

As mentioned above, methods for evaluating the integrity of the proteoglycan matrix by probing regional variations in fixed negative charged density in articular cartilage have recently been developed. The histological and biochemical validity of this approach has been well demonstrated by a number of groups.[71-73] Using cartilage-nulling inversion recovery sequences at high spatial resolutions and high field strength, Bashir et al.[71] demonstrated high histological correlation of the distribution of anionic Gd-DTPA^{2-} with perichondrocytic GAG depletion following incubation of cartilage explants with IL-1 (interleukin-1). Subsequent studies have shown a linear correlation between T_1 associated with Gd-DTPA^{2-} and cartilage GAG ranging from 10 mg/mL to 70 mg/mL as measured directly biochemically.[89] In a study by Trattnig et al.,[73] areas of abnormal Gd-DTPA^{2-} uptake in cartilage specimens harvested at total knee replacement surgery all corresponded to sites of collagen loss based on azan staining at histology. Unfortunately, this study did not report the correlation with areas of abnormal T_2, if any were present. The study also reported marked interindividual variation in the pattern of Gd-DTPA^{2-} uptake in eight normal volunteers that were examined, as well as marked differences in the diffusion times observed for cartilages of different thickness. Accordingly, while Gd-DTPA^{2-} uptake appears to be a valid method for quantifying GAG concentration and its distribution in articular cartilage, with good dynamic range properties relative to GAG concentration, the relationship of this marker to cartilage T_2 has yet to be examined. Does abnormal Gd-DTPA^{2-} uptake precede abnormal T_2 temporally? What is the relative performance of these two markers in terms of sensitivity, specificity, responsiveness to disease and therapy, dynamic range, predictive power for subsequent cartilage loss, other structural changes associated with OA, and clinical outcomes of OA? Finally, what is the optimal in vivo acquisition technique for cartilage Gd-DTPA^{2-} uptake as a marker?

IMAGING OTHER ARTICULAR COMPONENTS IN OSTEOARTHRITIS

In addition to evaluating the articular cartilage, MRI is uniquely capable of imaging all of the other structures that make up the joint, including the synovium and joint fluid, articular bones, intra-articular menisci, labra and discs, cruciate ligaments, collateral and other capsular ligaments, and periarticular tendons and muscles. Moreover, using the same voxel-counting technique employed for quantifying articular cartilage in 3D reconstructed images,[14,90] it is possible to determine the volume of each of these components within the same joint.

Some degree of synovial thickening can be found in a majority of osteoarthritic joints.[91] Whether this synovitis contributes directly to articular cartilage loss in OA, or simply arises in reaction to the breakdown of cartilage by other causes remains a controversy.[92] However, synovitis may be important to the symptoms and disability of OA, and may pose different treatment requirements than those directed only toward "chondroprotection". MRI is capable of imaging thickened or inflamed synovium, but usually this requires the use of special techniques, such as magnetization-transfer subtraction,[12] fat-suppressed, T^1-weighted imaging,[12]

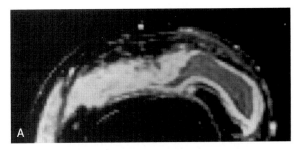
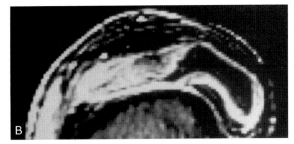

Figure 9–24 Synovial imaging with MRI. Transverse images of the suprapatellar recess of the knee of a patient with rheumatoid arthritis using magnetization-transfer subtraction *A* and fat-suppressed T_1-weighted gradient-echo *B* both delineate the thickened synovial tissue with high contrast. (From Peterfy C, Majumdar S, Lang P, van Dijke CF, Sack K, Genant HK: MR imaging of the arthritic knee: improved discrimination of cartilage, synovium and effusion with pulsed saturation transfer and fat-suppressed, T_1-weighted sequences. Radiology 191:413–419, 1994.)

or intravenous injection of Gd-containing contrast material[12,93–95] (Fig. 9–24). By monitoring the rate of synovial enhancement with Gd-containing contrast over time using rapid, sequential MRI, it is furthermore possible to grade the severity of the synovitis in these patients. The majority of work in this area has, however, focused on rheumatoid arthritis.

Osseous changes in OA are superbly depicted by MRI. Both cortical and trabecular bone can be visualized with MRI, and because of the tomographic nature of this modality, MRI is better at delineating structures, such as osteophytes (Fig. 9–25) and subchondral cysts, that are

often obscured by overlying structures on conventional radiographs. Using high-resolution MRI techniques,[96,97] it may be possible to monitor trabecular changes in the subchondral bone (Fig. 9–26) in order to determine their importance in the development and progression of OA.

In addition to delineating the calcified components of a bone, MRI is uniquely capable of imaging the marrow. Subchondral marrow edema is occasionally associated not only with acute trauma but with progressive OA.[98,99] Focal bone marrow edema in OA may be due to subchondral injuries caused by shifting articular contact points at sites of biomechanically failing cartilage (Fig. 9–27), or pulsion

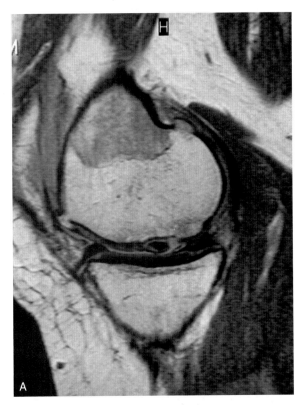
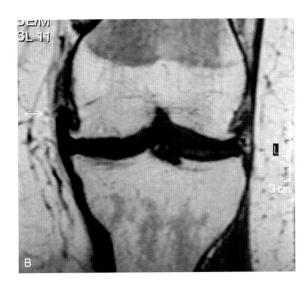

Figure 9–25 Delineating osteophytes with MRI. Sagittal *A*, and coronal *B*, images of a knee of a patient with OA clearly delineate marginal and central osteophytes. (Courtesy of Synarc, Inc.)

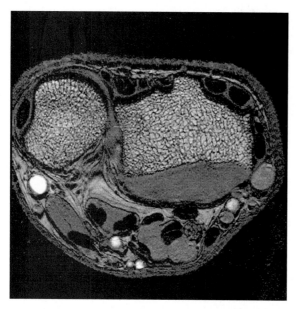

Figure 9–26 High resolution MRI of cortical and trabecular bone. Axial high-resolution (~150 μm in-plane, 500-μm slice thickness) fast 3D GRE image of the distal ulna and radius delineates both cortical and trabecular bone with high detail. (Courtesy of Synarc, Inc.)

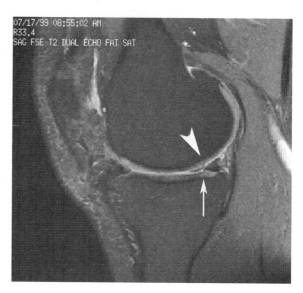

Figure 9–28 MRI of the meniscus. Sagittal, fat-suppressed proton-density image shows a minimally displaced tear (*arrow*) of the posterior horn of the medial meniscus. This is associated with partial-thickness thinning (*arrowhead*) of the femoral articular cartilage immediately adjacent to the torn meniscus. (Courtesy Synarc, Inc.)

of synovial fluid into uncovered subchondral bone. However, osteonecrosis, infection, and infiltrating neoplasms could theoretically produce a similar MRI appearance. Conventional radiographs are usually unremarkable in areas of bone marrow edema; however, bone scintigraphy may show increased uptake in these areas.

The menisci in the knee (Fig. 9–28) and glenoid labrum in the shoulder are important to the stability and functional integrity of these joints. Equally important are the cruciate (Fig. 9–29) and collateral ligaments and the glenohumeral ligaments. The utility of MRI for evaluating these articular structures is already well established.[100]

A whole-organ MRI scoring method (WORMS), has been developed for clinical research in the knee.[101] This scoring method examines 5 articular surface features (articular cartilage, subarticular marrow edema, subarticular cysts, subarticular bone attrition, and marginal osteophytes) in 15 regions of the knee, along with 8 other features (medial and lateral menisci, medial and lateral collateral ligaments, anterior and posterior cruciate ligaments, synovium and synovial effusion, and periarticular bursae and cysts). The test-retest reproducibility of these scores are high when done by trained, experienced radiologists. WORMS is currently being used in numerous longitudinal clinical trials and epidemiological studies.

CHALLENGES IN IMAGING SPECIFIC JOINTS

The Knee

Each joint poses different challenges to proper imaging with MRI. Most work thus far has focused on the knee, because not only is the knee frequently affected by OA and because loss of knee function can be severely disabling, but because the knee is a comparatively easy joint to image. Reasons for this include the large size of this joint, which lowers demands on spatial resolution, and the relatively cylindrical shape of the knee, which minimizes perturbation of the static magnetic field; field homogeneity is critical to the performance of frequency-selective fat suppression or

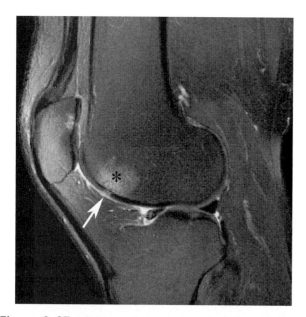

Figure 9–27 Subchondral bone edema in OA. Sagittal fat-suppressed intermediate-weighted FSE image of an osteoarthritic knee showing local bone marrow edema in the antero-lateral femur (*asterisk*). Note the focus of increased signal (arrow) in the articular cartilage overlying this region. Similar findings are also present in the patella of this image. (Courtesy Synarc, Inc.)

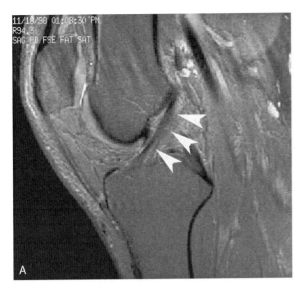 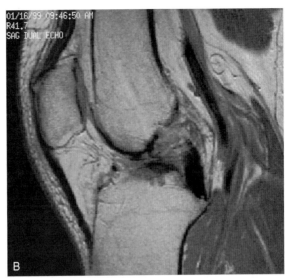

Figure 9–29 MRI of the anterior cruciate ligament. *A,* Sagittal, fat-suppressed proton density–weighted image shows an intact anterior cruciate ligament (*arrowheads*). *B,* Similar image of a different knee shows a torn anterior cruciate ligament. (Courtesy of Synarc, Inc.)

water excitation techniques, and important in quantitative studies based on signal intensity measurements. The cylindrical shape also allows the use of circumferential imaging coils, which show greater homogeneity than surface coils.[15] Additionally, because the knee is a relatively incongruent joint, contact areas between the hyaline cartilage plates in all but the most severely degenerated joints are small. Articular surfaces are therefore easy to separate from each other on MR images. Delineating the articular surfaces is facilitated by the relative abundance of synovial fluid in the knee, which provides high contrast at this interface on T_2-weighted images and fat-suppressed, T_1-weighted images. Because the articular surfaces are only gently curved, partial-volume averaging is not a major problem. Because of these forgiving imaging features and the availability of surgical and arthroscopic therapies for many internal derangements of the knee, MRI experience with the knee is greater than for any other joint in the body.

These advantages, however, are offset to some extent by a number of disadvantages. The knee is a highly complex joint composed of three articular compartments, one of which involves a sesamoid bone—the patella. The hyaline cartilage covering each of the articular surfaces accordingly shows somewhat different biomechanical properties and vulnerabilities. The joint contains two intra-articular ligaments, an intra-articular tendon, two menisci, intracapsular-extrasynovial fat pads, complex capsular ligaments (particularly laterally), and variable ontological remnants (plicas). Joint failure in the knee involves an equally complex interplay among these numerous articular constituents. Because the knee is a large joint, full coverage of the synovial cavity, including the suprapatellar recess, requires a relatively large FOV (12 cm to 18 cm). Because loose bodies tend to collect in the eddy pools within synovial recesses, incomplete coverage can result in important oversights. This can be particularly problematic in cases with large popliteal cysts dissecting down the calf. Larger

fields of view, however, necessitate proportionately larger imaging matrices in order to maintain spatial resolution, and thereby increase the imaging time.[1] A more thorough description of MRI techniques for whole-organ evaluation of the knee joint is provided in a review by Peterfy et al.[102]

The Hip

Next to the knee, the hip is the most important joint affected by OA from a disability standpoint. Despite this, however, the hip has received only scant attention in MRI evaluation for OA. This is at least in part because the hip poses significant challenges to proper imaging with MRI. It is a highly congruent joint, which makes separating the articular surfaces difficult. Delineation of the surfaces is further hampered by the relative lack of joint fluid in the tight synovial cavity of the hip. Moreover, the articular surfaces are highly curved, giving rise to severe partial-volume effects in all planes unless extremely high spatial resolution is employed. Accordingly, cartilage thickness measurements in the hip using MRI have been somewhat disappointing.[103] Achieving high spatial resolution in the hip is, itself, not an entirely straightforward matter. Since the hip is a relatively deep joint, signal drop off with small (<5 cm) surface coils is usually prohibitive. Larger surface coils could be employed, but these offer lower resolution and do not provide homogeneous signal for quantitative measurements. The anatomy of the hip prevents the use of small circumferential coils, which could provide homogeneous images with high resolution. A large circumferential coil, such as the body coil, could be used in this way, but does not provide sufficient SNR to support the high spatial resolution needed. Multiple coils configured in a phased array about the hip offer high SNR along with high spatial resolution (Fig. 9–30) and are probably the best alternative for this purpose.

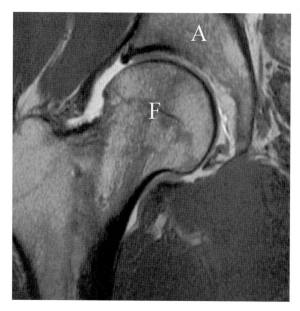

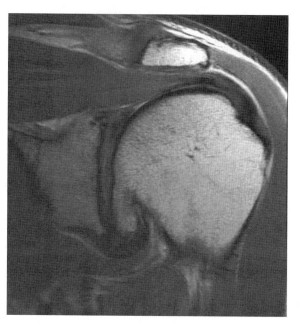

Figure 9–30 MRI of the hip using phased array technique. Coronal T_2-weighted FSE image of a normal hip acquired using multiple coils arranged in a flexible phased array shows high S/N despite the relatively high-resolution employed. F = femoral head, A = superior acetabulum. (Courtesy of Synarc, Inc.)

Figure 9–31 MRI of OA shoulder. Oblique coronal (in plane with the long axis of the supraspinatus tendon), T_1-weighted spin-echo image of an osteoarthritic shoulder shows exuberant osteophyte formation along the inferior margin of the humeral head. (Courtesy of Synarc, Inc.).

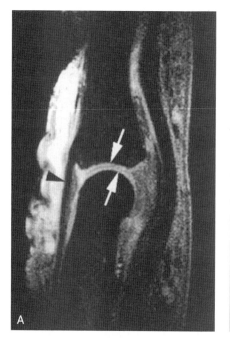

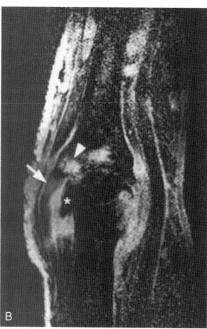

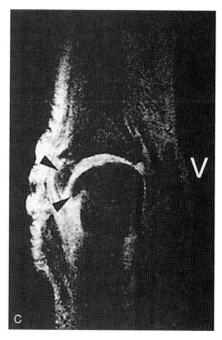

Figure 9–32 MRI of the proximal interphalangeal (PIP) joints using sagittal GRE water-selective excitation imaging. *A,* The articular cartilage (*arrows*) in the proximal interphalangeal (PIP) joint and the normal extensor tendon (*arrowhead*) of a normal subject. *B,* The PIP joint of a patient with severe chronic osteoarthritis, demonstrating complete loss of the articular cartilage. Note the thickening and high signal change in the extensor tendon close to its insertion (*arrow*). Note also the high signal in the bone marrow representing edema at the tendon enthesis site (*arrowhead*) and the large dorsal osteophyte (*). *C,* A commonly seen pattern of cartilage loss predominantly affecting the volar aspect articular surfaces, with more dorsal cartilage preservation. Severe soft tissue swelling around the dorsum of the joint is also present along with prominent dorsal osteophytes (*arrowheads*). V = volar aspect of joint. (From Tan AL, Grainger AJ, Tanner SF, Shelley DM, Pease C, Emery P, McGonagle D. High-resolution magnetic resonance imaging for the assessment of hand osteoarthritis. Arthritis Rheum. 52:2355–2365, 2005.)

The Shoulder

Like the hip, the shoulder is a congruent, ball-in-socket joint with closely opposing articular surfaces[104] (Fig. 9–31). Because of the angular shape of the shoulder, magnetic field heterogeneities tend to develop laterally near the greater tuberosity.[105] Although the field appears relatively undisturbed at the glenohumeral joint, lateral heterogeneities can limit the performance of fat suppression and complicate evaluation of the rotator cuff. Accurate assessment of the tendons of the rotator cuff is important because the shoulder relies heavily on these structures for stability, and rotator cuff tear is an important risk factor for the development of OA in this joint.[106] Shoulder stability is also dependent on the integrity of the glenoid labrum and the glenohumeral ligaments. However, reliable imaging of these labrocapsular structures can be extremely difficult, particularly in the absence of joint distention by significant synovial effusion. This can be improved by intra-articular injection of saline[107] or Gd-containing MRI contrast material (MR arthrography).[108,109]

Hand and Finger Joints

The joint most commonly affected by OA is the distal interphalangeal joint of the finger. The major challenge to imaging this small joint is the demand on spatial resolution. For this reason, small-bore, high-field magnets and small circumferential imaging coils are usually necessary[13,110] (Fig. 9–32). The metacarpophalangeal joints are less frequently affected by OA, but are larger joints, and have been successfully imaged using conventional clinical MRI systems.[90]

ADVANCES IN MRI TECHNOLOGY AND THE IMPACT ON MAGNETIC RESONANCE IMAGING OF OSTEOARTHRITIS

Over the last few years, MRI technology has undergone a significant upgrade, with both higher field scanners (for example 3.0T) and dedicated lower field extremity scanners (0.2T to 1.0T) becoming available. This is a result of scientific advances in the field of superconductivity, digital signal processing, amplifier and networking electronics, and image visualization. The advances in technology make it possible to image joints with higher spatial resolution, lower time, and improved patient comfort.

First generation 3T scanners had a number of limitations that minimized their utility for joint imaging in OA. First of all, the image resolution and characteristics at 1.5T are generally considered satisfactory for clinical imaging of joints and the increased field strength considered unnecessary. Second, the need for additional space and shielding, combined with the poor magnet homogeneity and shortage of FDA approved coils, as well as the increased cost, limited the use of 3T scanners, notwithstanding the ability to visualize various tissue compartments with higher spatial resolution.

Second generation 3T scanners, however, have overcome many of these limitations. Field homogeneity, and thereby fat saturation, is no longer a problem, and a number of coils are available. Enhancements in superconductivity have allowed the bore to become shorter, and the space requirements are now quite similar to 1.5T scanners. Workhorse sequences commonly used on 1.5T such as T_2 FSE and 3D-GRE are also available on the 3T scanner, at a higher SNR. One can take advantage of this improved SNR to either improve the spatial resolution, or to decrease the exam time. In particular, the exam time can be significantly shortened with the use of phased array coils and parallel imaging. Phased array coil technology was originally developed to improve the intensity uniformity of MR images obtained using surface coils, while preserving their inherent gain of SNR. Recently, new methods for encoding the MRI signal are being adopted that fall under the generic name of parallel imaging. Parallel imaging methods use the unique spatial perspective of the signal that comes from individual coils, along with the known sensitivity profiles of the surface coil elements within the array. This strategy allows overall improvement in coverage, which can be traded off for a reduction in the amount of time required to obtain the MR image up to a factor related to the number of independent coil channels within the array. Multiple RF channels are required to process these data independently, and in principle, an eight-channel coil would be able to image eight times as fast. However, practical considerations limit image acceleration to values well below the maximum allowed by theory. The driver for these high field scanners has been neuroimaging and cardiovascular imaging, and OA imaging stands to benefit from the increased presence of 3T scanners. Improved spatial resolution allows for more sensitive assessment of change in slowly progressing markers such as cartilage volume. Alternatively, parallel imaging allows for reductions of 20% to 40% in imaging time, thereby improving patient comfort.

Low-Field Imaging

Another way to improve patient comfort and reduce overall cost burden to the health care system is to use low-field MRI units.[111] Conventional whole-body MRI is still relatively expensive and inconvenient, and although it is free of ionizing radiation, it is contraindicated in patients with pacemakers, aneurism clips, and other metal objects. Additionally, some patients find the experience unpleasant, and about 5% are unable to complete the examination because of claustrophobia. Low field-strength extremity MRI systems were introduced a decade ago as lower-cost alternatives in such circumstances. Because these systems operate at lower magnetic field strength, typically 0.2T to 1.0T, they can be made much smaller and operated less expensively. Also, whereas conventional 1.5T magnets require placing the entire body into the bore, imaging with extremity MRI systems requires patients to insert only their limb into the magnet while sitting or lying next to the unit. This eliminates claustrophobia, and reduces risks associated with metal in the body or in the examination room. Because of the small fringe-field, low weight, and small footprint of these systems, they can operate in environments that were previously inaccessible to MRI, such as medical offices. The smallest extremity MRI system currently available commercially is described by Shellock et al.[112] This system can operate in as little as 4 square meters of space, and is actually portable. Recent work has shown additional utility in one of these scanners[111] in providing a range of magnetic field strengths, which can be used to obtain T_1-dispersion contrast for protein imaging.[113] The main disadvantage of extremity MRI systems is that their low magnetic field strength cannot support as much image resolution or as many image contrast mechanisms as conventional whole-body 1.5T systems.[24] Additionally, the small size of these systems precludes imaging other body parts, such as the shoulders, hips, spine, chest, abdomen, and pelvis, which is a capability that most radiology services require. Because of these limitations, extremity MRI systems were not initially felt by mainstream radiologists to provide sufficient performance for their needs. Higher field strength (1.0T) extremity systems that can support higher spatial resolution and broader contrast mechanisms, as well as larger low-field systems that can accommodate additional anatomical sites, such as the shoulders, have become available, but at the expense of larger space requirements and greater cost, and even these systems still offer some performance deficit in the eyes of many radiologists. It is important to keep in mind, however, that the needs of radiology are not the same as those of orthopedists and rheumatologists. The circumstances and therefore the technical performance requirements for MRI in these disciplines are very different. Orthopedists and rheumatologists do not have as much need to image multiple body parts—at least not in patients with OA. Imaging the knees, and perhaps the hands, is usually sufficient. Fueled by increasing utilization in both OA and rheumatoid arthritis, extremity MRI systems can in turn be expected to continuously improve their technical performance in order to keep pace.

CONCLUSION

MRI is clearly a tool of unprecedented capabilities for evaluating joint disease and its potential treatments. MRI's unparalleled tissue contrast allows it to directly examine all components of a joint simultaneously and thus evaluate the joint as a whole organ and OA as a disorder of organ failure, in which dysfunction may result from any one of a number of different causes. Especially intriguing is the unique potential of this technology for identifying very early changes associated with cartilage degeneration, and its ability to quantify subtle morphological and compositional variations in different articular tissues over time. Employing these techniques, MRI may provide more objective measures of disease progression and treatment response than are currently attainable by other methods. This will facilitate both the assessment of new therapies for OA and investigations of the pathophysiology in this disorder. However, with this growing armamentarium comes a greater need for technical sophistication on the part of the clinician and growing pressures to contain costs. These demands necessitate a deeper understanding of the tradeoffs associated with choosing different diagnostic approaches. There is a partic-

ular need for clinicians to become sophisticated in applications of MRI in this disease, not only to better understand the growing number of studies that utilize this modality, but to assist in directing its development to better serve the needs of clinicians and their patients.

REFERENCES

1. Abragam A. The Principles of Nuclear Magnetism. 1983, London: Oxford University Press.
2. Budinger T, Lauterbur P. Nuclear magnetic resonance technology for medical studies. Science 226:288–298, 1984.
3. Haacke E, Tkach J. Fast MR imaging: techniques and clinical applications. AJR 155:951–964, 1990.
4. Pykett I. NMR imaging in medicine. Sci Am 246:78–88, 1982.
5. Young S. Magnetic Resonance Imaging: Basic Principles. 1988, New York: Raven Press.
6. Xia Y, Farquhar T, Burton-Wurster N, et al. Dffiusion and relaxation mapping of cartilage-bone plugs and excised disks using microscopic magnetic resonance imaging. Magn Reson Med 31:273–282, 1994.
7. Burstein D, Gray ML, Hartman AL, et al. Diffusion of small solutes in cartilage as measured by nuclear magnetic resonance (NMR) spectroscopy and imaging. J Orthop Res 11:465–478, 1993.
8. Hargreaves BA, Vasanawala SS, Pauly JM, et al. Characterization and reduction of the transient response in steady-state MR imaging. Magn Reson Med. 46(1):149–58, 2001.
9. Scheffler K, Heid O, Hennig J. Magnetization preparation during the steady state: fat-saturated 3D TrueFISP. Magn Reson Med 45(6):1075–80, 2001.
10. Hennig J, Speck O, Scheffler K. Optimization of signal behavior in the transition to driven equilibrium in steady-state free precession sequences. Magn Reson Med 48(5):801–9, 2002.
11. Woolf SD, Chesnick S, Frank JA, et al. Magnetization transfer contrast: MR imaging of the knee. Radiology 179: 623–628, 1991.
12. Peterfy CG, Majumdar S, Lang P, et al. MR imaging of the arthritic knee: improved discrimination of cartilage, synovium and effusion with pulsed saturation transfer and fat-suppressed T1-weighted sequences. Radiology 191:413–419, 1994.
13. Hall LD, Tyler JA. Can quantitative magnetic resonance imaging detect and monitor the progression of early osteoarthritis?, in Osteoarthritic Disorders, K.E. Kuetner and V.M. Goldberg, Editors. 1995, American Accadamy of Orthopaedic Surgeons: Rosemont, IL. pp 67–84.
14. Peterfy CG, van Dijke CF, Janzen DL, et al. Quantification of articular cartilage in the knee by pulsed saturation transfer and fat-suppressed MRI: optimization and validation. Radiology 192:485–491, 1994.
15. Kneeland JB, Hyde JS. High-resolution MR imaging with local coils. Radiology 171:1–7, 1989.
16. Mosher T, Dardzinski B, Smith M. Human articular cartilage: influence of aging and early symptomatic degeneration on the spatial variation of T2—preliminary findings at 3 T. Radiology 241(1):259–266, 2000.
17. Chandnani VP, Ho C, Chu P, et al. Knee hyaline cartilage evaluated with MR imaging: a cadaveric study involving multiple imaging sequences and intraarticular injection of gadolinium and saline solution. Radiology 178:557–561, 1991.
18. Dardizinski B, Mosher T, Li S, et al. Spatial variation of T2 in human articular cartilage. Radiology 205:546–550, 1997.
19. Kim DJ, Suh JS, Jeong EK, et al. Correlation of laminated MR appearance of articular cartilage with histology, ascertained by artificial landmarks on the cartilage. J Magn Reson Imaging 10(1):57–64, 1999.
20. Xia Y, Farquhar T, Burton-Wurster N, et al. Origin of cartilage laminae in MRI. JMRI 7:887–894, 1997.
21. Rubenstein JD, Kim JK, Morava-Protzner I, et al. Effects of collagen orientation on MR imaging characteristics of bovine cartilage. Radiology 188:219–226, 1993.

22. Erickson SJ, Prost RW, Timins ME. The "magic angle" effect: background physics and clinical relevance. Radiology 188:23–25, 1993.
23. Erickson SJ, Waldschmidt JG, Caervionke LF, et al. Hyaline cartilage: truncation artifact as a cause of trilaminar appearance with fat suppressed three dimensional spoiled gradient recalled sequences. Radiology 201:260–264, 1996.
24. Frank LR, Brossmann J, Buxton RB, et al. MR imaging truncation artifacts can create a false laminar appearance in cartilage. AJR Am J Roentgenol 168(2): 547–54, 1997.
25. Yao L, Gentili A, Thomas A. Incidental magnetization transfer contrast in fast spin-echo imaging of cartilage. JMRI 6:180–184, 1996.
26. Miyazaki M, Takai H, Kojima F, et al. Control of magnetization transfer effects in fast SE imaging. in Radiological Society of North America. 1994. Chicago, IL.
27. Santyr GE. Magnetization transfer effects in multislice MR imaging. Magn Reson Imaging 11:521–522, 1993.
28. Gold GE, Hargreaves BA, Reeder SB, et al. Controversies in protocol selection in the imaging of articular cartilage. Semin Musculoskelet Radiol 9(2):161–72, 2005.
29. Recht MP, Kramer J, Marcelis S, et al. Abnormalities of articular cartilage in the knee: analysis of available MR techniques. Radiology 187:473–478, 1993.
30. Recht MP, Pirraino DW, Paletta GA, et al. Accuracy of fat-suppressed three-dimensionl spoiled gradient-echo FLASH MR imaging in the detection of patellofemoral articular cartilage abnormalities. Radiology 198:209–212, 1996.
31. Disler DG, McCauley TR, Kelman CG, et al. Fat-suppressed three-dimensional spoiled gradient-echo MR imaging of hyaline cartilage defects in the knee: comparison with standard MR imaging and arthroscopy. AJR 167:127–132, 1996.
32. Disler DG, McCauley TR, Wirth CR, et al. Detection of knee hyaline articular cartilage defects using fat-suppressed three-dimensional spoiled gradient-echo MR imaging: comparison with standard MR imaging and correlation with arthroscopy. AJR 165:377–382, 1995.
33. Carr H.Y. Steady-state free precession in nuclear magnetic resonance. Phys. Rev 112:1693–1701, 1958.
34. Heid O. True FISP cardiac fluoroscopy. In: Proceedings of the 5th International Society for Magnetic Resonance in Medicine, Vancouver, 1997.
35. Duerk JL, Lewin JS, Wendt M, et al. Remember true FISP? A high SNR, near 1-second imaging method for T2-like contrast in interventional MRI at .2 T. J Magn Reson Imaging 8(1):203–8, 1998.
36. Hargreaves BA, Gold GE, Beaulieu CF, et al. Comparison of new sequences for high-resolution cartilage imaging. Magn Reson Med 49(4):700–9, 2003.
37. Mosher TJ, Pruett SW. Magnetic resonance imaging of superficial cartilage lesions: role of contrast in lesion detection. J Magn Reson Imaging 10(2):178–82, 1999.
38. Gold G, Thedens D, Pauly J, et al. MR imaging of articular cartilage of the knee: new methods using ultrashort TEs. AJR 170:1223–1226, 1998.
39. Kijowski R, Lu A, Block WF, et al. Evaluation of the articular cartilage of the knee joint with vastly undersampledisotropic projection reconstruction steady-state free precession imaging. J Magn Reson Imaging. 24(1):168–175, 2006.
40. Vasanawala SS, Pauly JM, Nishimura DG. Fluctuating equilibrium MRI. Magn Reson Med 42(5):876–883, 1999.
41. Absil J, Denolin V, Metens T. Fat attenuation using a dual steady-state balanced-SSFP sequence with periodically variable flip angles. Magn Reson Med 55(2):343–351, 2006.
42. Leupold J, Hennig J, Scheffler K. Alternating repetition time balanced steady state free precession. Magn Reson Med 55(3): 557–565, 2006.
43. Vasanawala SS, Pauly JM, Nishimura DG. Linear combination steady-state free precession MRI. Magn Reson Med 43(1):82–90, 2000.
44. Hargreaves BA, Vasanawala SS, Nayak KS, et al. Fat-suppressed steady-state free precession imaging using phase detection. Magn Reson Med 50(1): 210–213, 2003.
45. Hargreaves BA, Bangerter NK, Shimakawa A, et al. Dual-acquisition phase-sensitive fat-water separation using balanced steady-state free precession. Magn Reson Imaging 24(2):113–122, 2006.
46. Vasanawala SS, Hargreaves BA, Pauly JM, et al. Rapid musculoskeletal MRI with phase-sensitive steady-state free precession: comparison with routine knee MRI. AJR Am J Roentgenol 184(5):1450–1455, 2005.
47. Reeder SB, Pelc NJ, Alley MT, et al. Rapid MR imaging of articular cartilage with steady-state free precession and multipoint fat-water separation. AJR Am J Roentgenol 180(2):357–362, 2003.
48. Reeder SB, Pineda AR, Wen Z, et al. Iterative decomposition of water and fat with echo asymmetry and least-squares estimation (IDEAL): application with fast spin-echo imaging. Magn Reson Med 54(3): 636–644, 2005.
49. Gold G, Reeder S, Yu H, et al. Cartilage Morphology at 1.5T: Comparison of 3D FS-SPGR and IDEAL SPGR Imaging. International Society for Magnetic Resonance in Medicine, Miami, 2005.
50. Kornaat PR, Reeder SB, Koo S, et al. MR imaging of articular cartilage at 1.5T and 3.0T: comparison of SPGR and SSFP sequences. Osteoarthritis Cartilage 13(4):338–344, 2005.
51. Broderick L, Turner D, Renfrew D, et al. Severity of articular cartilage abnormality in patients with osteoarthritis: evaluation with fast spin-echo MR vs arthroscopy. Am J Roentgenol 162:99–103, 1994.
52. Rose PM, Demlow TA, Szumowski J, et al. Chondromalacia patellae: fat-suppressed MR imaging. Radiology 193:437–440, 1994.
53. Yulish BS, Montanez J, Goodfellow DB, et al. Chondromalacia patellae: assessment with MR imaging. Radiology 164:763–766, 1987.
54. Quinn SF, Rose PM, Brown TR, et al. MR imaging of the patellofemoral compartment. MRI Clin N Am 2:425–439, 1994.
55. Zaim S, Lynch JA, Li J, et al. MRI of early cartilage degeneration following meniscal surgery: a three-year longitudinal study. International Society for Magnetic Resonance in Medicine, Glasgow, Scotland, 2001. In proceedings.
56. Gold GE, Butts K, Fechner KP, et al. In vivo diffusion-weighted imaging of cartilage. 6th Annual Meeting of the International Society of Magnetic Resonance in Medicine, Sydney, Australia, 1998.
57. Frank LR, Wong EC, Luh W, et al. Articular cartilage in the knee: mapping of the physiologic parameters at MR imaging with a local gradient coil - preliminary results. Radiology 210:241–246, 1999.
58. Foy BD, LLM, Gray ML, et al. NMR parameters of intersitial sodium in cartilage [abstract]. in Society of Magnetic Resonance in Medicine, Amsterdam, 1989.
59. Jelicks LA, PPK, O'Byrne EM, et al. Hydrogen-1, sodium-23, and ccarbon-13 MR spectroscopy of cartilage degradation in vitro. J Magn Reson Imaging 3:565–568, 1993.
60. Paul PK, O'Byrne EM, Gupta RK, et al. Detection of cartilage degradation with sodium NMR [letter]. Br J Rheumatol 30(4):318, 1991.
61. Bashir A, Gray M, Burstein D. Sodium T1 and T2 in control and defraded cartilage: implications for determination of tissue proteoglycan content. In: Proceedings of the 14th annual meeting of the Society of Magnetic Resonance in Medicine, Nice, 1995.
62. Insko E, Reddy R, Kaufman J, et al. Sodium spectroscopic evaluation of early articular cartilage degradation. In: Proceedings of the 4th annual International Society of Magnetic Resonance in Medicine, New York, 1996.
63. Callaghan P. Principles of Nuclear Magnetic Resonance Microscopy. 1991, New York, Oxford University Press.
64. Reddy R, Insko EK, Noyszewski EA, et al. Sodium MRI of human articular cartilage in vivo. Magn Reson Med 39(5):697–701, 1998.
65. Granot J. Sodium imaging of human body organs and extremities in vivo. Radiology 167(2):547–550, 1988.
66. Ra JB, Hilal SK, Oh CH, et al. In vivo magnetic resonance imaging of sodium in the human body. Magn Reson Med 7(1):11–22, 1988.
67. Insko EK, Kaufman JH, Leigh JS, et al. Sodium NMR evaluation of articular cartilage degradation. Magn Reson Med 41(1):30–34, 1999.
68. Shapiro E, Saha P, Kaufman J, et al. In vivo evaluation of human cartilage compression and recovery using 1H and 23Na MRI. In: Proceedings of the 7th Annual Meeting of the International Society of Magnetic Resonance in Medicine, Philadelphia, 1999.

69. Regatte RR, Kaufman JH, Noyszewski EA, et al. Sodium and proton MR properties of cartilage during compression. J Magn Reson Imaging 10(6):961–967, 1999.

70. Wu E, Gao E, Cham E, et al. Application of HTS RF Coil for sodium imaging on a high field system. In: Proceedings of the 7th Annual Meeting of the International Society of Magnetic Resonance in Medicine. Philadelphia, 1999.

71. Bashir A, Gray ML, Burstein D. Gd-DTPA as a measure of cartilage degradation. Magn Reson Med 36:665–673, 1996.

72. Bashir A, Gray ML, Hartke J, et al. Nondistructive imaging of human cartilage glycosaminoglycan concentration by MRI. Magn Reson Med 41:857–865, 1999.

73. Trattnig S, Mlynarckk V, Breilenseher M, et al. MR visualization of proteoglycan depletion in articular cartilage via intravenous injection of Gd-DTPA. Magn Reson Imaging 17:577–583, 1999.

74. Kusaka Y, Grunder W, Rumpel H, et al. MR microimaging of articular cartilage and contrast enhancement by manganese ions. Magn Reson Med 24:137–148, 1992.

75. Fujioka M, Kusaka Y, Morita Y, et al. Contrast-enhanced MR imaging of articular cartilage: a new sensitive method for diagnosis of cartilage degeneration. In: 40th Annual Meeting, Orthopaedic Research Society, New Orleans, 1994.

76. Lesperance LM, Gray ML, Burstein D. Determination of fixed charge density in cartilage using nuclear magnetic resonance. J Orthop Res 10:1–13, 1992.

77. Borthakur A, Hulvershorn J, Gualtieri E, et al. A pulse sequence for rapid in vivo spin-locked MRI. J Magn Reson Imaging 23(4):591–596, 2006.

78. Li X, Han ET, Ma CB, et al. In vivo 3T spiral imaging based multi-slice T(1rho) mapping of knee cartilage in osteoarthritis. Magn Reson Med 54(4):929–936, 2005.

79. Menezes NM, Gray ML, Hartke JR, et al. T2 and T1rho MRI in articular cartilage systems. Magn Reson Med 51(3):503–509, 2004.

80. Peterfy CG, Guermazi A, Zaim S, et al. Whole-organ evaluation of the knee in osteoarthritis using MRI. in XIV European League Against Rheumatism Congress. Glasgow, Scotland, 1999.

81. Wildy K, Zaim S, Peterfy C, et al. Reliability of the Whole-Organ review MRI scorring (WORMS) method for knee osteoarthritis (OA) in a multicenter study. In: 65th Annual Scientific Meeting of the American College of Rheumatology, San Francisco, Nov. 11–15, 2001.

82. Eckstein F, Sitteck H, Gavazzenia A, et al. Assessment of articular cartilage volume and thickness with magnetic resonance imaging (MRI). Trans Orthop Res Soc 20:194, 1995.

83. Burgkart R, Glaser C, Hyhlik-Dürr A, et al. Magnetic resonance imaging-based assessment of cartilage loss in severe osteoarthritis: Accuracy, precision and diagnostic value. Arthritis Rheum 44(9):2072–2077, 2001.

84. Peterfy C, White D, Zhao J, et al. Longitudinal measurement of knee articular cartilage volume in osteoarthritis. Annual Meeting of Am Coll Rheum. American College of Rheumatology, San Diego, 1998.

85. Eckstein F, Cicuttini F, Raynauld JP, et al. Magnetic resonance imaging (MRI) of articular cartilage in knee osteoarthritis (OA): morphological assessment. Osteoarthritis Cartilage 2006.

86. Pilch L, Stewart C, Gordon D, et al. Assessment of cartilage volume in the femorotibial joint with magnetic resonance imaging and 3D computer reconstruction. J Rheum 21:2307–2321, 1994.

87. Cohen ZA, McCarthy DM, Ateshian GA, et al. In vivo and in vitro knee joint cartilage topography, thickness, and contact areas from MRI. Annual Meeting of Orthopaedic Research Society, San Francisco, February 1997.

88. Eckstein F, Gavazzeni A, Sittek H, et al. Determination of knee joint cartilage thickness using three-dimensional magnetic resonance chondro-Crassometry (3D MR-CCM). Magn Reson Med 36:256–265, 1996.

89. Bashir A, Gray ML, Hartke J, et al. Validation of gadolinium-enhanced MRI for GAG measurement in human cartilage. International Society of Magnetic Resonance in Medicine, Philadelphia, 1998.

90. Peterfy CG, van Dijke CF, Lu Y, et al. Quantification of articular cartilage in the metacarpophalangeal joints of the hand: accuracy and precision of 3D MR imaging. AJR 165:371–375, 1995.

91. Fernandez-Madrid F, Karvonen RL, Teitge RA, et al. Synovial thickening detected by MR imaging in osteoarthritis of the knee confirmed by biopsy as synovitis. Magn Reson Imaging 13:177–183, 1995.

92. Brandt KD. Insights into the natural history of osteoarthritis and the potential for pharmacologic modification of the disease afforded by study of the cruciate-deficient dog, in Osteoarthritic Disorders, K.E. Keutner and V.M. Goldberg, Editors. American Acadamy of Orthopaedic Surgeons: Rosemont, IL 1995, pp 419–426.

93. Palmer WE, Rosenthal DI, Shoenberg OI, et al. Quantification of inflammation in the wrist with gadolinium-enhanced MR imaging and PET with 2-[F-18]-fluoro-2-deoxy-D-glucose. Radiology 196:645–655, 1995.

94. König H, Sieper J, Sorensen M, et al. Contrast-enhanced dynamic MR imaging in rheumatoid arthritis of the knee joint: follow-up study after cortisol drug therapy. In: 77th Scientific Assembly and Annual Meeting of the Radiological Society of North America, Chicago, IL, 1991.

95. Yamato M, Tamai K, Yamaguchi T, et al. MRI of the knee in rheumatoid arthritis: Gd-DTPA perfusion dynamics. J Comput Assist Tomogr 17: 781–785, 1993.

96. Weinstein RS, Majumdar S. Fractal geometry and vertebral compression fractures. J Bone Min Res 9:1797–1802, 1994.

97. Majumdar S, Genant HK, Grampp S, et al. Analysis of trabecular structure in the distal radius using high resolution magnetic resonance images. Euro Radiol 4:517–524, 1994.

98. Vellet AD, Marks P, Fowler P, et al. Occult posttraumatic lesions of the knee, prevalence, classification, and short-term sequelae evaluated with MR imaging. Radiology 178:271–276, 1991.

99. Felson DT, Chaisson CE, Hill CL, et al. The association of bone marrow lesions with pain in knee osteoarthritis. Ann Intern Med 134(7):541–549, 2001.

100. Resnick D. Internal derangements of joints, in Diagnosis of Bone and Joint Disorders, D. Resnick, Ed. W.B. Saunders, Philadelphia, 1995, pp 3063–3069.

101. Peterfy CG, Guermazi A, Zaim S, et al. Whole-Organ Magnetic Resonance Imaging Score (WORMS) of the knee in osteoarthritis. Osteoarthritis Cartilage 12(3):177–190, 2004.

102. Peterfy CG, Gold G, Eckstein F, et al. MRI protocols for whole-organ assessment of the knee in osteoarthritis. Osteoarthritis Cartilage, 14 Suppl A:A95–111, 2006.

103. Hodler J, Trudell D, Pathria MN, et al. Width of the articular cartilage of the hip: quantification by using fat-suppression spin-echo MR imaging in cadavers. AJR 159:351–355, 1992.

104. Hodler J, Loredo R, Longo C, et al. Assessment of articular cartilage thickness of the humeral head: MR-anatomic correlation in cadavers. AJR 165:615–620, 1995.

105. Peterfy C. Technical considerations, in Shoulder Magnetic Resonance Imaging, L. Steinbach, et al. Eds. Lippincott-Raven, Philadelphia, 1998, pp 37–63.

106. Peterfy C, Genant H, Mow V, et al. Evaluating arthritic changes in the shoulder with MRI, in Shoulder Magnetic Resonance Imaging, L. Steinbach, et al., Eds. Lippincott-Raven, Philadelphia, 1998, pp 221–237.

107. Tirman PFJ, Stauffer AE, Crues JV, et al. Saline magnetic resonance arthrography in the evaluation of glenohumeral instability. Arthroscopy 9:550–559, 1993.

108. Palmer WE, Brown JH, Rosenthal DN. Labral-ligamentous complex of the shoulder: evaluation with MR arthrography. Radiology 190:645–651, 1994.

109. Tirman PFJ, Bost FW, Garvin GJ, et al. Posterosuperior glenoid impingement: MRI and MR arthrographic findings with arthroscopic correlation. Radiology 193:431–436, 1994.

110. Tan AL, Grainger AJ, Tanner SF, et al. High-resolution magnetic resonance imaging for the assessment of hand osteoarthritis. Arthritis Rheum 52(8): 2355–2365, 2005.

111. Macovski A, Conolly S. Novel approaches to low-cost MRI. Magn Reson Med 30(2):221–230, 1993.

112. Shellock FG, Stone KR, Crues JV. Development and clinical application of kinematic MRI of the patellofemoral joint using an extremity MR system. Med Sci Sports Exerc 31(6):788–791, 1999.

113. Ungersma SE, Matter NI, Hardy JW, et al. Magnetic resonance imaging with T(1) dispersion contrast. Magn Reson Med 55(6):1362–1371, 2006.

Ultrasound and Alternative Imaging Outcomes

10

Helen I. Keen   Paul Emery   Philip G. Conaghan

Osteoarthritis (OA) is increasingly common in our aging society. Cartilage is not the only anatomic structure involved in the disease: the capsule, ligaments, synovial membrane, and subchondral bone can all be affected in this disease. Consequently it is likely that specific imaging modalities will have benefits for imaging components of the OA process.

Recent years have seen an exciting increase in clinical trials investigating the role of potential disease modifying OA drugs. While the current body of evidence remains inconclusive about the disease modifying properties of these drugs, there is a suggestion that structure modification is potentially measurable.[1] Conventional radiography (CR) has largely been the imaging technique utilized to assess and monitor temporal changes in these and previous OA trials, utilizing joint space narrowing as the outcome. CR is, however, far from an ideal assessment of disease status and outcome measure. It is well documented that clinical symptoms do not correlate with CR changes in OA,[2,3,4] which is explained by multiple factors. Firstly, joint space narrowing which is characteristic of OA on CR is a surrogate measure of cartilage thickness, and really reveals little about cartilage integrity. In addition, CR produces a two-dimensional image of a three-dimensional structure and provides limited information about soft tissue and composite joint structures, including synovial membrane, synovial fluid, the capsule, and ligaments. A further disadvantage of CR is that exposure to ionizing radiation is undesirable in trials that require serial imaging to monitor temporal changes. In addition, the validity of CR in monitoring changes in joint space narrowing over time has also been questioned, particularly in these recent drugs (DMOAD) studies. It is hypothesized

that pain modification in OA may affect the positioning of joints when radiographs are taken, hence altering the apparent joint space narrowing.[1] In addition, radiographs provide no information about the metabolic activity of the joint, or presence or absence of inflammation, which might be vital to understanding the process of OA and the effects of DMOAD drugs. No doubt that future studies are planned to build on this foundation of structure modification in OA, and it is likely alternative imaging techniques will be utilized in order to further understand the disease and the effects of drugs, and monitor disease progression. Recent decades have seen much progress in validating and investigating the role of novel imaging techniques, such as ultrasonography, magnetic resonance imaging (MRI), computer tomography (CT), optical coherence tomography, and scintigraphy in OA. This chapter will focus on the use of novel imaging techniques (with the exception of MRI which, has been covered elsewhere) in understanding, diagnosing, and managing OA.

ULTRASONOGRAPHY

How it Works

Ultrasound (US) utilizes the principle of sound waves reflecting off matter to the source of origin in order to produce an image. Sound waves travel at varying speeds through different matter and are reflected (as echoes) from the interface of materials with differing densities. The reflectivity of an interface is greatest when the two opposing tissues consist of very different properties; for example,

193

the interface between fat and bone will be highly reflective, allowing good visualization of the surface by US imaging.

The development of "B mode" ultrasonography allowed this technique to be applied to medicine. "B mode" ultrasonography produces two-dimensional images in shades of gray: echoes returning to the source are displayed as pixels in varying shades of brightness to produce a picture in gray scale. The pixel brightness is in proportion to the intensity of the echo. Doppler technique can be added to gray scale to provide information about the vascularity of the tissue being imaged. Doppler ultrasonography utilizes the principle that the echo frequency is altered when reflected off moving objects. This principle can be applied to musculoskeletal US as color Doppler or power Doppler (PD). PD displays the amplitude of the Doppler signal as a color spectrum, providing information only about the power of the signal, but is sensitive to low flow. Color Doppler displays the range of frequencies reflected as color, encoding both velocity and directional information. In musculoskeletal imaging, the direction and velocity of vascular flow is often less important than the amplitude of the flow, so PD is the more commonly applied technique in this field.

US Detectable Abnormalities in Osteoarthritis

Utilizing gray scale and PD techniques, US can provide information about the integrity of several structures within the osteoarthritic joint including cartilage, integrity of cortical bone, presence of joint effusions, and synovial hypertrophy. The vascularity of structures can also be assessed, which generally reflects the degree of inflammation.

Cartilage

Animal and in vitro models have been used to demonstrate that US is reliable in measuring cartilage thickness and identifying focal chondral defects.[5,6] US has also been shown to provide qualitative information on cartilage morphology and document real-time change in cartilage in animal models of arthritis.[7]

Imaging of articular cartilage in vivo with noninvasive US techniques is more challenging than in animal and cadaveric models, due to problems of getting adequate visualization of chondral surfaces. When articular cartilage is able to be visualized, general sonography features of osteoarthritic cartilage include loss of normal sharpness of synovial-cartilage interface, loss of clarity of the cartilaginous layer, thinning of joint cartilage, and increased intensity of the posterior bone cartilage interface.[8] While Grassi has demonstrated that articular cartilage can be visualised at the knee, hip, shoulder, elbow, and metacarpal phalangeal joints, with characteristic changes identifiable, the extent on information gathered is dependent on the size of the acoustic window.[8] For example, while a portion of articular cartilage can be visualized at the hip joint, this is usually not the weight-bearing portion, which is most likely to be affected in OA.

However, the reproducibility and precision of using US to determine cartilage thickness compared to MRI and CR has been shown to be good in OA knees,[9-11] and correlate with diagnosis in OA and controls.[10] The correlation

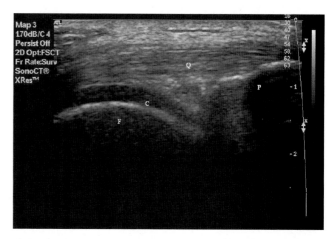

Figure 10–1A Longitudinal US of the distal femur showing articular cartilage. *F* = distal femur; *P* = patella; *Q* = quadriceps tendon; *C* = articular cartilage.

between US and MRI cartilage thickness was not good in normal controls in one study, but this only looked at small numbers.[9] The sharpness and clarity of cartilage on US has correlated with OA or no OA[9] and good correlation with MRI. The clinical significance of imaging articular cartilage at the knee (Figures 10–1A and 10–1B) is uncertain given that weight-bearing portions are unable to be demonstrated reliably.

Bone Changes

Bone is highly echogenic, and the cortical surface is able to be visualized easily with US, as long as an acoustic window is present. General changes detectable with US in OA include bone irregularity and erosions, osteophytes, subchondral bone cysts, decreased joint space, and subluxation of joint surfaces.[12-16]

US has validated against MRI and CT at the acromioclavicular joint and temporomandibular joint, and is found to be as specific but not as sensitive as MRI or CT to cortical irregularities, joint margins, erosions, or osteophytes.[12,15]

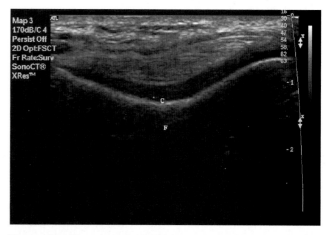

Figure 10–1B Longitudinal US of the distal femur showing articular cartilage. *F* = distal femur; *C* = articular cartilage.

Synovial Inflammation

Many studies have demonstrated the ability of US to detect synovial hypertrophy and joint effusions, common features of OA.[17] The European league against rheumatism (EULAR) study of 600 OA knees demonstrated that knee synovitis or effusions are common; 47% of patients with painful knee OA had either synovitis, effusion, or both on US, with the presence of joint effusion alone being most common (30%). It also demonstrated that in OA of the knee, US is more sensitive to their presence than clinical examination.[17] The study findings are consistent with other studies, whereby US is more sensitive to the presence of synovial effusion than clinical examination.[18-20] Further analysis of the EULAR study found that a formula to allow clinical recognition of inflammation in OA could not be derived, demonstrating that imaging is a more useful method of detecting joint inflammation than clinical pathways.[21]

The reliability of US in detecting effusions and synovial hypertrophy has been validated against CT, MRI, and histopathology at the knee joint[9,10,22,23] and AC joint.[15] US has been shown to demonstrate the presence of effusions in OA at the carpometacarpal joint and shoulder joint.[14,24]

PD technique has been utilized in rheumatology in addition to gray scale to document soft tissue vascularity, which has been demonstrated to reflect inflammatory activity in inflammatory arthritis.[25-27] The use of PD in OA has been validated against histopathology in the knee and hip,[25,28] and has been shown to demonstrate improved differentiation of intra-articular structures compared to gray scale in OA of the knee.[23]

US Contribution to Improved Understanding of Osteoarthritis

As mentioned previously, symptoms of OA do not correlate with CR changes.[2-4] The use of US to image OA has increased our understanding of the structural changes in this disease and their relationship with symptoms. In a study of knee OA, the degree of MRI and US detected cartilage changes, synovial hypertrophy and popliteal cysts increased as radiographic grade increased. In addition, cartilage abnormalities were more common in those with osteophytes.[9] This is in keeping with a study in which the presence of popliteal cysts correlates with grade of OA,[29] suggesting that radiographic grade does reflect the severity of the disease in OA knee.

In a study of 73 patients with symptomatic OA of the knee, pain scores on the woman on the move against cancer (WOMAC) subscale correlated with the osteophyte size and degree of capsular distension on US.[30]

The EULAR study demonstrated that inflammation seen on US correlated with more severe radiological grade, sudden aggravation of pain in the preceding 2 weeks, or the presence of clinically detectable effusion. No correlation existed between pain during recent physical activity and US inflammation. Clinical features such as night pain and early morning stiffness did not correlate well with the presence of inflammation on US. Use of drugs was not associated with US inflammation.[17] Conversely, in a large study of the AC joint, clinical tenderness did not correlate with US changes of inflammation.[15]

The correlation between US changes and more severe radiographic grade found in the EULAR study is interesting, as it adds weight to the theory that inflammation is secondary to chondrolysis, and the inflammation then further accelerates cartilage breakdown.

Outcome Assessment in Osteoarthritis

In animal studies, cartilage changes were demonstrated in a temporal fashion, allowing this to be utilized over time.[7] No human in vivo studies have used US as an outcome measure, although studies demonstrating longitudinal validity assessments of synovitis are stable over time in patients who had dummy steroid (saline) injection.[31] The main disadvantage of utilizing US as an outcome in DMOAD studies is limited visualization of weight-bearing articular cartilage of most joints; cartilage integrity is thought to be integral to the process and progression of OA. The likely role of US in outcome assessment of future OA studies is in those examining the role of inflammation and drugs targeted at inflammation in OA.

COMPUTER TOMOGRAPHY

How it Works

This technology utilizes x-ray images and then digitally creates two- or three-dimensional cross-sectional images of structures. CT revolutionized medical imaging by allowing noninvasive cross-sectional imaging. The use of CT in OA has been phasic; prior to the development of MRI, CT was the only noninvasive technique able to give information about three-dimensional soft tissue structures. Many of the studies investigating the role of CT in rheumatology and OA are several decades old. MRI and US have gained favor as technology improved, accessibility increased, and time and financial costs decreased. Currently, the main use of CT in rheumatology imaging is to define calcified tissues not well visualized with MRI, such as trabecular bone and osteophytes, particularly axial joints such as the spine where CR is also of limited value.[32]

CT Detectable Abnormalities in Osteoarthritis

There is a paucity of published studies examining CT detectable abnormalities in OA, and much of the work was done prior to the widespread availability of MRI. It has been demonstrated that CT reveals knee joint anatomical structures with high accuracy without contrast medium[33] and reliability in detecting pathology at the knee including fluid, meniscal changes, ligamentous injury, or intra-articular bodies using surgery as the Gold standard.[34]

Much of the work utilizing CT in OA has focused on the lumbar facet joints, where CT is superior to radiographs at defining facet joint OA.[35] However, a recent study comparing MRI to CT, where CT was the gold standard, showed good agreement between CT and MRI, with the predominant difference being minor grade differences.[36] The prevailing message of the study, however, was that when an MRI of the lumbar spine had been performed, proceeding to a CT added little clinical benefit.

Outcome Assessment in Osteoarthritis

A study examining facet joint arthritis at the lumbar spine demonstrated response to intra-articular injections in those with CT.[37] There are no studies utilizing CT as an outcome measure in OA; this may be due to a lack of structure modifying OA drugs in the past. It is unlikely that CT is going to be frequently utilized in OA outcome trials in the future, as it has largely been superseded by more novel imaging techniques.

OPTICAL COHERENCE TOMOGRAPHY

How it Works

Optical coherence tomography (OCT) is analogous to B mode US, except it utilizes infrared light (rather than sound) reflected off tissue interfaces. The advantage of OCT over other current imaging techniques is the extremely high resolution, between 2 μm and 20 μm[38] which is up to 20 times that of US MRI or CT[39] and approaches that of histopathology.[40]

Polarization-sensitive OCT (PS-OCT) potentially will be of even greater value. PS-OCT relies on the principle of a change in the polarization status of reflected light. Highly organized tissue such as organized collagen has different refractive indices associated with two polarization states that results in rotation of the axes as light passes through it. Organized collagen is birefringent by light microscopy; it is this same mechanism by which PS-OCT works. This principle allows identification of disorganization in structures that are known to be organized, such as cartilage in the early stages of OA, allowing identification of early disease prior to cartilage thinning or the development of fibrillations.[41]

While the primary advantage of OCT is its resolution, it has other positive features making it a promising tool. Systems are small and portable, and hence suitable for the outpatient clinic. OCT is fiber based and does not require transducers, so OCT arthroscopes are inexpensive and disposable. It is high speed, with imaging acquisition approaching real-time. The addition of PS-OCT can provide information about the biochemical and structural nature of imaged tissue.

Optical Coherence Tomography Detectable Abnormalities in Osteoarthritis

OCT is still a research tool, not utilized widely in clinical practice. Most studies have focused on the appearance of cartilage rather than synovium or synovial fluid. Animal studies have shown that OCT can differentiate between normal cartilage and cartilage of induced arthritis, depicting loss of collagen organization, fibrillations, loss of bone-cartilage interface, and thinning of cartilage.[39,42] Cartilage changes imaged by OCT in an animal model of tissue repair have been validated against histological findings and found to be superior to arthroscopic surface visualization.[40]

In vitro human studies comparing osteoarthritic and normal cartilage have validated OCT findings against histopathology and demonstrated reliability in identifying cartilage fibrillation, fibrosis, and new bone growth.[43] However, discordance in measuring cartilage thickness compared to histopathology was seen, with OCT consistently documenting thinner cartilage. It is unclear whether this was an artefact of histological process or a problem with the technique used in that study, in what remains a relatively new field of imaging.

PS-OCT has been validated in a human in vitro study. The presence of PS-OCT changes correlated with changes by polarization light microscopy, even when routine histopathology was grossly normal.[41] Addition of PS to OTC is a powerful combination utilizing high resolution structural imaging and birefringence detection.

Future studies are underway to refine the technique and determine utility in vivo, and to investigate the role of this imaging technique in soft tissue structures (as synovium and synovial fluid) and other diseases such as inflammatory arthritis.

Outcome assessment in Osteoarthritis

The animal studies published have demonstrated the ability of this technique to monitor temporal changes in response to damage and repair.[39,40,42] While this technique is currently invasive, the ability to detect subtle changes in cartilage prior to macroscopic or histological changes make it attractive for monitoring cartilage-based outcomes in DMOAD studies.

SCINTIGRAPHY

How it Works

Scintigraphy involves the injection of a radioisotope tracer into the vascular system (in bone scans the radioisotope is usually technetium-99m labeled biphosphonate). The tracer is subsequently taken up into the bone, and delayed imaging of the body can detect regional localization of the tracer in skeletal tissue. Areas of greater uptake indicate increased osteoblastic activity at the affected site, and decreased tracer localization is seen in areas of reduced or absent blood flow, as in bone infarction. Scintigraphy uses reduced amounts of radiation compared to CR and is very sensitive to metabolic changes, but can be nonspecific, although technological refinements and recognition of characteristic patterns have increased diagnostic utility. However, limited anatomical information is derived from conventional bone scanning using technetium, particularly about cartilage and surrounding soft tissue structures.

Scintigraphically Detectable Abnormalities in Osteoarthritis

Human in vivo studies have largely concentrated on the knee and the hand in OA. Scintigraphy has been demonstrated as a sensitive way of detecting knee OA.[44] In OA of the knee, scintigraphy has repeatedly shown a generalized increased uptake in the medial compartment consistent with knowledge that radiographic knee OA is predominantly a medial compartment disease.[45,46] Scintigraphy has been shown to be more specific at depicting compartmental disease than CR or arthrography[44] and demonstrates more extensive disease. In small joint OA of the hands, scintography strongly predicts current radiographic OA in symptomatic patients[47,48] and is less predictive in asymptomatic joints.[47] Scintigraphy can detect abnormalities in radiographically normal joints.[47,49]

Scintigraphy Contribution to Improved Understanding of Osteoarthritis

Scintigraphy has driven hypothesis generation regarding the disease process in OA progression. Scintigraphy can detect early structural and biochemical changes of OA, and animal models have shown that in early OA tracer uptake is by endochondreal ossification centers that later develop into osteophytes. Later these lose activity and the uptake is then primarily in subchondral bone under denuded or eburnated surfaces.[50] In human studies of femoral heads removed operatively, uptake first occurs in endochondral ossification zones then in weight-bearing areas, and in the walls of cysts.[51] These studies suggest that OA is a dynamic and phasic process.

Human studies have complemented these animal studies. An MRI and scintographic OA knee study demonstrated a good correlation between technetium uptake and MRI detected subchondral lesions in the knee with chronic knee pain,[46,52] but poor correlation between technetium uptake and MR-detected osteophytes or cartilage defects in OA knee.[52] The authors feel that this is consistent with the theory that increased tracer uptake into subchondral bone may represent an early but growing osteophyte, and that once formed this lesion becomes metabolically less active. This is in keeping with an earlier study in which ostyeophytes that were high signal on MRI correlated with scintigraphy, and that some but not all osteophytes may appear as high signal on MRI because they may be in varying stages of evolution or be a result of heterogeneous pathophysiological processes.[45]

McAlindon demonstrated that OA may be a heterogeneous process with various stages of activity.[45] Several distinct but different patterns of scintigraphic changes were identified in OA of the knee that may reflect various aspects of the disease. A generalized pattern of tracer uptake correlated with pain and radiographic osteophytes, while joint line uptake correlated with subchondral sclerosis on CR, and subchondral uptake correlated with more severe radiographic grade.

Correlation with clinical parameters has also been investigated in OA with varying results. A relationship between pain, raised interosseous pressure, and scintigraphy at the hip has been demonstrated.[53] Poorer correlations between scintography and pain on visual analog scales have been demonstrated in hand OA.[54–56] In contrast, one study demonstrated no correlation between scintigraphy and clinical features (pain, tenderness, or deformity)[48] at baseline, but scintigraphy did predict progression of joint tenderness.[48]

Outcome Assessment in Osteoarthritis

Scintigraphy has been demonstrated to be predictive of progression in OA. Negative scintographic scans have been shown to be strong negative predictors of progression of radiographic OA.[57,58] Positive scans have been demonstrated to predict radiographic progression of OA at the knee and hand. Joints with abnormal scans are more likely to show radiographic progression at follow-up and to a greater degree in most studies.[47,48,54,57,59] In a contrast to these trends, one study of 15 patients with hand OA followed over 5 years found that while positive scans at baseline were predictive of radiographic progression, in those joints that were normal at baseline on scintigraphy 38.5% of joints progressed radiographically.[47] In addition, the magnitude of radiographic progression was higher in joints normal on scintigraphy at baseline than those with abnormal baseline scans, which is again in contrast to other studies. The authors explain the different findings as being a result of using quantitative rather than qualitative definitions of radiographic OA and that radiographs were read in a blinded fashion. They go on to suggest that scintigraphic uptake may be a predictor of what has happened rather than what will happen, which is contrary to other studies where scintigraphy has been shown to be predictive of progression and the hypothesis that isotope retention most likely is related to increased bone remodeling of either osteophytes or subchondral bone. Despite the contrasting findings, it seems clear that OA is a phasic process with periods of scan positivity alternating with scan negativity but a general trend to decreased tracer uptake over time.[57]

Scintigraphy is likely to be a useful tool in assessing outcomes in OA, and while much of this work was done many years ago, it is likely that the utility of scintigraphy in OA will be revisited with the advent of potential disease modifying therapies.

POSITRON EMISSION TOMOGRAPHY

Positron emission tomography (PET) has recently been applied to OA. The principle behind this from of scintigraphy has been known for many decades, but it is only since the development of better instrumentation, hardware, and software that its utility in OA has been examined. The novel feature of PET imaging is that it allows a "functional" image of blood flow or metabolic processes occurring at a cellular level. Neutron poor radionucleotides (such as ^{18}F-fluoride) emit positrons (positively charged beta particles) that interact with electrons to produce energy in the form of two gamma rays simultaneously emitted in opposite directions. The emissions can be detected by receivers placed on either side of the object being imaged. In order for the energy to be recognized as having positron origin, both gamma rays must be recognized simultaneously. The principle allows for high resolution and improved sensitivity over conventional scintigraphy, because in other imaging systems much of the emitted rays need to be discarded to absorb or scatter unwanted background noise.

Traditional bone scan techniques have not allowed good definition or identification of focal lesions and hence had a limited role in OA. Recent use of ^{18}F-Fluoride High Resolution (HR)-PET has allowed high resolution imaging of focal bony metabolic changes and will permit further investigation of OA using this novel technique.

There is little published work validating PET scanning in OA. However, a preliminary report has demonstrated the relationship between regional bone metabolic activity and clinical bony enlargement and pain in OA of the small joints of the hand.[60,61] No relationship was found between clinical soft tissue swelling and HR PET activity. To date there are no published studies utilising PET as an outcome tool in OA.

CONCLUSIONS

Recent years have seen an increase in published trials of purported DMOADs such as glucosamine, chondroitin, doxycyline, and diancerin. Structure modification is now an aim in clinical trials of drug therapy in OA. CR is currently accepted as the usual way of demonstrating OA and monitoring joint space narrowing as a surrogate for cartilage thickness. However, CR is not ideal as an imaging modality in OA trials as it involves ionizing radiation, and provides limited information about cartilage integrity, soft tissue structures, and metabolic status of bones. Novel imaging techniques will have a role in future trials. US is able to reliably and reproducibly demonstrate bony changes and synovial hypertrophy or effusions in OA. OCT remains invasive but can detect early and minor cartilage changes with higher resolution than some histopathology. CT potentially has a role in axial disease where other imaging techniques are of limited use. Scintigraphy provides metabolic information about bone and soft tissue structures, and PET scanning has allowed this to be high resolution. The imaging techniques described have been demonstrated to be largely reliable in determining osteoarthritic damage to joints and sensitivity to temporal changes. In view of this, there is no doubt the future will see further investigation into the disease-modifying effects of these drugs in OA utilizing the imaging techniques described as outcome measures to investigate the structure-modifying effects of drugs and to help us understand more about the common and disabling condition of OA.

REFERENCES

1. Brandt KD, Mazzuca SA. Lessons learned from nine clinical trials of disease-modifying osteoarthritis drugs. Arthritis Rheum 52(11):3349–3359, 2005.
2. Felson DT. An update on the pathogenesis and epidemiology of osteoarthritis. Radiol Clin North Am 42(1):1–9, 2004.
3. Felson DT, Lawrence RC, Dieppe PA, et al. Osteoarthritis: new insights. Part 1: the disease and its risk factors. Ann Internal Med 133(8):635–646, 2000.
4. Hannan MT, Felson DT, Pincus T. Analysis of the discordance between radiographic changes and knee pain in osteoarthritis of the knee. J Rheumatol 27(6):1513–1517, 2000.
5. Myers SL, Dines K, Brandt DA, et al. Experimental assessment by high frequency ultrasound of articular cartilage thickness and osteoarthritic changes. J Rheumatol 22(1):109–116, 1995.
6. Jurvelin JS, Rasanen T, Kolmonen P, et al. Comparison of optical, needle probe and ultrasonic techniques for the measurement of articular cartilage thickness. J Biomech 28(2):231–235, 1995.
7. Nieminen HJ, Saarakkala S, Laasanen MS, et al. Ultrasound attenuation in normal and spontaneously degenerated articular cartilage. Ultrasound Med Biol 30(4):493–500, 2004.
8. Grassi W, Lamanna G, Farina A, et al. Sonographic imaging of normal and osteoarthritic cartilage. Sem Arthritis Rheum 28(6):398–403, 1999.
9. Tarhan S, Unlu Z. Magnetic resonance imaging and ultrasonographic evaluation of the patients with knee osteoarthritis: a comparative study. Clin Rheumatol 22(3):181–188, 2003.
10. Ostergaard M, Court-Payen M, Gideon P, et al. Ultrasonography in arthritis of the knee. A comparison with MR imaging. Acta Radiol 36(1):19–26, 1995.
11. Jonsson K, Buckwalter K, Helvie M, et al. Precision of hyaline cartilage thickness measurements. Acta Radiol 33(3):234–239, 1992.
12. Brandlmaier I, Bertram S, Rudisch A, et al. Temporomandibular joint osteoarthrosis diagnosed with high resolution ultrasonography versus magnetic resonance imaging: how reliable is high resolution ultrasonography? J Oral Rehabil 30(8):812–817, 2003.
13. Iagnocco A, Palombi G, Valesini G. Role of ultrasound in osteoarthritis. Rev Esp Reumatol 28:301–306, 2001.
14. Iagnocco A, Coari G. Usefulness of high resolution US in the evaluation of effusion in osteoarthritic first carpometacarpal joint. Scand J Rheumatol 29(3):170–173, 2000.
15. Alasaarela E, Tervonen O, Takalo R, et al. Ultrasound evaluation of the acromioclavicular joint. J Rheumatol 24(10):1959–1963, 1997.
16. Grassi W, Filippucci E, Farina A, et al. Sonographic imaging of the distal phalanx. Sem Arthritis Rheum 29(6):379–384, 2000.
17. D'Agostino MA, Conaghan P, Le Bars M, et al. EULAR report on the use of ultrasonography in painful knee osteoarthritis. Part 1: Prevalence of inflammation in osteoarthritis. Ann Rheum Dis 64:1703–1709, 2005.
18. van Holsbeeck M, van Holsbeeck K, Gevers G, et al. Staging and follow-up of rheumatoid arthritis of the knee. Comparison of sonography, thermography, and clinical assessment. J Ultrasound Med 7(10):561–566, 1988.
19. Kane D, Balint P, Sturrock R. Ultrasonography is superior to clinical examination in the detection and localization of knee joint effusion in rheumatoid arthritis. J Rheumatol 30:966–971, 2003.
20. Karim Z, Wakefield R, Quinn M, et al. Validation and reproducibility of ultrasonography in the detection of synovitis in the knee: a comparison with arthroscopy and clinical examination. Arthritis Rheum. 50(2):387–394, 2004.
21. Conaghan P, D'Agostino MA, Ravaud P, et al. EULAR report on the use of ultrasonography in painful knee osteoarthritis. Part 2: Exploring decision rules for clinical utility. Ann Rheum Dis 64:1710–1714, 2005.
22. Leeb BF, Stenzel I, Czembirek H, et al. Diagnostic use of office-based ultrasound. Baker's cyst of the right knee joint. Arthritis Rheum 38(6):859–861, 1995.
23. Schmidt WA, Volker L, Zacher J, et al. Color Doppler ultrasonography to detect pannus in knee joint synovitis. Clin Exp Rheumatol 18(4):439–444, 2000.
24. Peetrons P, Rasmussen OS, Creteur V, et al. Ultrasound of the shoulder joint: non "rotator cuff" lesions. Eur J Ultrasound 14(1):11–19, 2001.
25. Walther M, Harms H, Krenn V, et al. Correlation of power Doppler sonography with vascularity of the synovial tissue of the knee joint in patients with osteoarthritis and rheumatoid arthritis. Arthritis Rheum 44(2):331–338, 2001.
26. Terslev L, Torp-Pedersen S, Qvistgaard E, et al. Effects of treatment with etanercept (Enbrel, TNRF:Fc) on rheumatoid arthritis evaluated by Doppler ultrasonography. Ann Rheum Dis 62(2):178–181, 2003.
27. Newman J, Laing T, McCarthy C, et al. Power Doppler sonography of synovitis: assessment of therapeutic response—preliminary observations. Radiology 198(2):582–584, 1996.

28. Walther M, Harms H, Krenn V, et al. Synovial tissue of the hip at power Doppler US: correlation between vascularity and power Doppler US signal. Radiology 225(1):225–231, 2002.

29. Fam AG, Wilson SR, Holmberg S. Ultrasound evaluation of popliteal cysts on osteoarthritis of the knee. J Rheumatol 9(3):428–434, 1982.

30. Do JH, Kang HJ, Kim CH, et al. Correlation of knee joint pain with capsular distension and length of osteophtytes on ultrasonography in patients with osteoarthritis. Arthritis Rheum 46(suppl):S151, 2002.

31. Wu C, Quan A, Hose K, et al. The Response to Intra-articular steroids in knee osteoarthritis as defined by ultrasonographic outcomes: an analysis of the reliability of the sequential ultrasound measurements. Arthritis Rheum 2005,

32. Blackburn WD. Management of osteoarthritis and rheumatoid arthritis: prospects and possibilities. Am J Med 100(2A):24S–30S, 1996.

33. Passariello R, Trecco F, De Paulis F, et al. Computed tomography of the knee joint: technique of study and normal anatomy. J Comput Assist Tomogr 7(6):1035–1042, 1983.

34. Passariello R, Trecco F, De Paulis F, et al. Computed tomography of the knee joint: clinical results. J Comput Assist Tomogr 7(6):1043–1049, 1983.

35. Carrera GF, Haughton VM, Syvertsen A, et al. Computed tomography of the lumbar facet joints. Radiology 134(1):145–148, 1980.

36. Weishaupt D, Zanetti M, Boos N, et al. MR imaging and CT in osteoarthritis of the lumbar facet joints. Skeletal Radiol 28(4):215–219, 1999.

37. Lewinnek GE, Warfield CA. Facet joint degeneration as a cause of low back pain. Clin Orthop Relat Res 213:216–222, 1986.

38. Rogowska J, Brezinski ME. Image processing techniques for noise removal, enhancement and segmentation of cartilage OCT images. Phys Med Biol 47(4):641–655, 2002.

39. Roberts MJ, Adams SB, Jr., Patel NA, et al. A new approach for assessing early osteoarthritis in the rat. Analyt Bioanalyt Chem 377(6):1003–1006, 2003.

40. Han CW, Chu CR, Adachi N, et al. Analysis of rabbit articular cartilage repair after chondrocyte implantation using optical coherence tomography. Osteoarthritis Cartilage 11(2):111–121, 2003.

41. Drexler W, Stamper D, Jesser C, et al. Correlation of collagen organization with polarization sensitive imaging of in vitro cartilage: implications for osteoarthritis. J Rheumatol 28(6):1311–1318, 2001.

42. Patel NA, Zoeller J, Stamper DL, et al. Monitoring osteoarthritis in the rat model using optical coherence tomography. IEEE Trans Med Imaging 24(2):155–159, 2005.

43. Herrmann JM, Pitris C, Bouma BE, et al. High resolution imaging of normal and osteoarthritic cartilage with optical coherence tomography. J Rheumatol 26(3):627–635, 1999.

44. Thomas RH, Resnick D, Alazraki NP, et al. Compartmental evaluation of osteoarthritis of the knee. A comparative study of available diagnostic modalities. Radiology 116(3):585–594, 1975.

45. McAlindon TE, Watt I, McCrae F, et al. Magnetic resonance imaging in osteoarthritis of the knee: correlation with radiographic and scintigraphic findings. Ann Rheum Dis 50(1):14–19, 1991.

46. Boegard T, Rudling O, Dahlstrom J, et al. Bone scintigraphy in chronic knee pain: comparison with magnetic resonance imaging. Ann Rheum Dis 58(1):20–26, 1999.

47. Balblanc JC, Mathieu P, Mathieu L, et al. Progression of digital osteoarthritis: a sequential scintigraphic and radiographic study. Osteoarthritis Cartilage 3(3):181–186, 1995.

48. Olejarova M, Kupka K, Pavelka K, et al. Comparison of clinical, laboratory, radiographic, and scintigraphic findings in erosive and nonerosive hand osteoarthritis. Results of a two-year study. Joint, Bone, Spine 67(2):107–112, 2000.

49. Hutton CW, Higgs ER, Jackson PC, et al. 99mTc HMDP bone scanning in generalised nodal osteoarthritis. I. Comparison of the standard radiograph and four hour bone scan image of the hand. Ann Rheum Dis 45(8):617–621, 1986.

50. Christensen SB. Localization of bone-seeking agents in developing, experimentally induced osteoarthritis in the knee joint of the rabbit. Scand J Rheumatol 12(4):343–349, 1983.

51. Christensen SB, Arnold CC. Distribution of 99mTc-phosphate compounds in osteoarthritic femoral heads. J Bone Joint Surg Am 62(1):90–96, 1980.

52. Boegard T. Radiography and bone scintigraphy in osteoarthritis of the knee—comparison with MR imaging. Acta Radiol Suppl 418:7–37, 1998.

53. Arnoldi CC, Djurhuus JC, Heerfordt J, et al. Intraosseous phlebography, intraosseous pressure measurements and 99mTC-polyphosphate scintigraphy in patients with various painful conditions in the hip and knee. Acta Orthop Scand 51(1):19–28, 1980.

54. Buckland-Wright JC, Macfarlane DG, Fogelman I, et al. Technetium 99m methylene diphosphonate bone scanning in osteoarthritic hands. Eur J Nucl Med 18(1):12–16, 1991.

55. Macfarlane DG, Buckland-Wright JC, Lynch J, et al. A study of the early and late 99technetium scintigraphic images and their relationship to symptoms in osteoarthritis of the hands. Br J Rheumatol 32(11):977–981, 1993.

56. O'Sullivan MM, Powell N, French AP, et al. Inflammatory joint disease: a comparison of liposome scanning, bone scanning, and radiography. Ann Rheum Dis 47(6):485–491, 1988.

57. Dieppe P, Cushnaghan J, Young P, et al. Prediction of the progression of joint space narrowing in osteoarthritis of the knee by bone scintigraphy. Ann Rheum Dis 52(8):557–563, 1993.

58. Hutton CW, Higgs ER, Jackson PC, et al. 99mTc HMDP bone scanning in generalised nodal osteoarthritis. II. The four hour bone scan image predicts radiographic change. Ann Rheum Dis 45(8):622–626, 1986.

59. Macfarlane DG, Buckland-Wright JC, Emery P, et al. Comparison of clinical, radionuclide, and radiographic features of osteoarthritis of the hands. Ann Rheum Dis 50(9): 623–626, 1991.

60. Tan A, Waller M, Bury R, et al. High resolution positron emission tomography study using ^{18}F- fluoride to explore bone metabolism in hand osteoarthritis. Arthritis Rheum (suppl 1844), 2005.

61. Tan A, Waller M, Jeavons A, et al. Heberden's nodes: What Heberden didn't see—a high resolution positron emission tomography with ^{18}F fluoride study of osteoarthritic and normal hands. Rheumatology (suppl OP23), 2005.

Laboratory Findings in Osteoarthritis

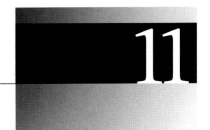

11

Roy D. Altman

As a clinical entity, osteoarthritis (OA) is a constellation of clinical, radiographic, and synovial fluid findings. To date there are no pathognomonic laboratory abnormalities. Blood and urine test results are usually normal, and synovial fluid analysis often yields abnormal but nonspecific results. Nevertheless, tests of body fluids (i.e., blood, urine, and synovial fluid) may serve to exclude other forms of arthritis and identify metabolic disorders that may be associated with secondary OA. This chapter addresses clinically applicable studies and some laboratory studies that may aid in the diagnosis of different subsets of OA.

BLOOD

Cellular Constituents

The cellular components of blood are quantitatively and morphologically normal in uncomplicated primary OA. The platelet count may rise slightly as an acute-phase reactant during certain flares but remains within the normal range.

Acute-Phase Reactants

Although the erythrocyte sedimentation rate (ESR) is most often normal, modest elevations in the ESR may be observed transiently during clinical exacerbations of OA. More persistent elevations may be related to generalized polyarticular OA.[1] To a lesser extent, other acute-phase reactants[2] may be elevated transiently. There is a nonspecific modest increase in ESR with increasing age. Because the prevalence of OA also increases with age, any modest increase in ESR in OA should be addressed with caution.

Hence, marked ESR elevations (above 50 mm/hr) should alert the physician to an unrelated, coexistent disease.

Studies have linked C-reactive protein (CRP) elevations but not ESR with clinical severity of OA of the hip and knee.[3] CRP was significantly associated with disability (as measured by the Health Assessment Questionnaire scale), joint tenderness, pain, fatigue, global severity, and depression. Median CRP was 5.9 µg/mL. ESR was associated with only functional disability. CRP levels were higher in those with erosive (mean 4.7 mg/l), in contrast with nonerosive (mean 2.1 mg/l; $P = 0.001$), interphalangeal OA.[4] Elevated CRP was associated with generalized versus nongeneralized OA.[5] Increased CRP has been correlated with hip pain.[6]

In a longitudinal population-based study of knee OA, levels of CRP were higher in 105 women with radiographic OA compared with 740 women without OA. In the 4-year follow-up, median levels of CRP were higher in the 31 women whose disease progressed at least one Kellgren-Lawrence grade (median, 2.6 µg/mL) than in the ones whose disease did not progress (median, 1.3 µg/mL).[7]

No increase in CRP or relation to activity was noted in 274 patients with knee OA, where high levels of soluble receptors of tumor necrosis factor (TNF)-1 were associated with lower physical function, increased knee symptoms, and higher radiographic scores.[8]

In conclusion, it appears that there is a modest increase in ESR with age that is not related to OA. Sensitive techniques of determining CRP most often demonstrate a modest increase in OA. No studies of CRP elevation in OA have corrected for the presence of cardiovascular disease as another reason for an increase in CRP. The significance in the CRP for diagnostic purposes or in monitoring activity of OA is yet to be determined.

Serum Chemistry

Glucose

OA does not impair glucose tolerance. Conversely, however, diabetes mellitus may accelerate the OA process.[9] In an epidemiologic survey of 1026 patients, the mean fasting plasma glucose level was significantly higher in patients with OA than in normal control subjects.[10] Thus, screening tests for hyperglycemia are indicated in OA patients with early onset or inordinately severe joint disease. Hyperglycemia may suggest hemochromatosis or acromegaly.

Insulin-Like Growth Factor 1

Insulin-like growth factor 1 (IGF-1) serum concentration correlates with the presence and the growth of osteophytes in knee OA and the overall progression of the disease.[11] Serum IGF-1 concentration was linked with the development of distal interphalangeal joint OA and more severe and bilateral knee OA in women.[12]

Insulin

Hyperinsulinemia may be a separate risk factor in the development or progression of OA.[13] In a study of 48 overweight patients, those with OA of the knee had statistically higher serum insulin levels than did those without OA of the knee.

Calcium, Phosphorus, and Alkaline Phosphatase

Results of routine biochemical assessment of bone metabolism are normal in primary OA. Secondary OA from calcium pyrophosphate dihydrate (CPPD) crystal deposition disease ("pseudo-osteoarthritis," McCarty types C and D[14]) (Table 11–1) may raise suspicion of underlying primary hyperparathyroidism.

Plasma growth hormone levels are normal in primary OA. However, in one study,[15] radioimmunoassay growth hormone levels were elevated in menopausal women with OA compared with a control group. Elevation of serum phosphorus concentration in a patient with an OA-like arthropathy may suggest acromegaly.

A minor or marked increase in serum alkaline phosphatase (bone specific) and an increase in urinary levels of markers of type I and II collagen breakdown suggest Paget disease of bone.

Cholesterol

Serum cholesterol may be an independent risk factor for OA.[16] Hypercholesterolemia and high serum cholesterol levels (3rd versus 1st tertile) were independently associated with generalized OA, mostly knee OA. There was no association between cholesterol levels and bilateral OA.

TABLE 11–1

LABORATORY ASSESSMENT OF DISORDERS ASSOCIATED WITH OR CAUSING AN OSTEOARTHRITIS-LIKE ARTHROPATHY

Disorder	Laboratory Studies
CPPD crystal deposition disease	Synovial fluid: positively birefringent, rhomboid crystals Radiography: chondrocalcinosis
CPPD deposition disease induced by hyperparathyroidism	Suggestive: Increased serum calcium, alkaline phosphatase; decreased serum phosphorus Definitive: Increased serum parathyroid hormone
Acromegaly	Suggestive: Increased serum phosphorus and blood glucose Definitive: Increased fasting plasma growth hormone
Hemochromatosis	Suggestive: Increased blood glucose; serum iron >150 µg/dL and >75% saturation of iron-binding capacity Definitive: Tissue (liver, synovium) iron deposition
Ochronosis	Suggestive: Darkening of urine on standing; pigmented shards in synovial fluid ("ground pepper" sign) Definitive: Increased serum and urine homogentisic acid
Wilson disease	One or more of the following: serum nonceruloplasmin copper >25 µg/dL; serum ceruloplasmin <20 mg/dL; urine copper >100 µg/24 hr; liver copper >250 µg/g dry weight

---

Cartilage Matrix Components

Sensitive and specific assays for cartilage proteoglycan components and degradation products[17] have been developed. Although of interest, serum sampling appears of limited value because of several metabolic factors, including dilution in serum from a single joint dysfunction and unknown influences of renal or liver function.[18,19]

Keratan sulfate in humans is a distinct and unique sugar derived primarily (95%) from articular and intervertebral disk cartilage. Elevations of serum keratan sulfate levels have been found in patients with OA, but there is a considerable variation in values in both cross-sectional and longitudinal studies.

Plasma levels of hyaluronate in OA were twice that in rheumatoid arthritis (RA) and seven times that in control subjects.[20] Elevated hyaluronate was found to correlate with the patients' functional capacity. Another study of 94 patients with tibiofemoral OA showed that serum hyaluronate values at entry correlated with disease duration, minimum joint space, and previous surgery.[21] In this retrospective review, radiographic progression or knee surgery correlated with higher baseline hyaluronate levels.

Levels of serum hyaluronate failed to show a correlation with the Lequesne algofunctional index, duration of symptoms, CRP, or severity of radiographic changes. In a cross-sectional study, serum hyaluronan levels correlated with radiographic OA, ethnicity, sex, and age even after adjustment for multiple variables (P <0.0045).[22] In a 2-year follow-up, those with knee OA and higher hyaluronan levels at baseline had faster radiographic progression (P <0.005).[23] Serum hyaluronan was followed in a 3-year study of knee OA.[23] Baseline hyaluronan levels did not correlate with progression. However, reduction in hyaluronan found at the first year correlated with radiographic progression at 3 years ($r = 0.27$, $P = 0.02$) (similar findings were present for an increase in serum osteocalcin).

In knee OA, elevation of cartilage oligomeric matrix protein (COMP) related to progression.[24] COMP increases may directly relate to physical exercise, even walking.[25,26] Pain of hip OA has been correlated with increased COMP.[27] Of 81 patients observed for 5 years, progression was defined as those having a decrease of 2 mm or more in joint space on radiographic examination or those requiring knee surgery during the 5-year follow-up.[28] Serum COMP levels increased by a mean of 6.42 µg/mL in patients whose OA progressed compared with a mean of 0.07 µg/mL in those whose OA did not progress. In another study of 48 with hip OA and observed prospectively with radiographs and serum samples, levels of COMP correlated with rapidly progressing OA of the hip.[29] In the same study, serum levels of bone sialoprotein (BSP) correlated inversely with osteophyte grade and sclerosis grade in OA of the hip.

COMP related to progression of knee OA in a 5-year follow-up and patterns of progression suggested that knee OA progression is episodic or phasic.[30] The authors suggested that large individual variation precludes the use of COMP for predicting progression, but that sequential COMP measurements may help identify OA progression.

Metalloproteinases

Stromelysin (matrix metalloproteinase 3 [MMP-3]) has been found to be elevated in the serum of patients with OA and correlated strongly with the articular index.[31] Levels of collagenase (MMP-1) or of tissue inhibitor of matrix metalloproteinases (TIMP-1) were within normal limits. In a study of 36 patients, MMP-3 and MMP-9 were significantly increased in patients with rapidly destructive hip OA versus OA in patients awaiting total hip prosthesis.[32]

Sex Hormones

Serum sex hormones have been measured in patients with OA. An association has not been found between endogenous estrogen levels and OA or its severity.[33]

Miscellaneous Components

Nonspecific elevation of plasma substance P levels was seen in patients with OA compared with normal individuals, but it did not occur to the degree of elevation in patients with reactive arthritis.[34]

When there is a reduction of serum iron levels in patients with OA, it is secondary to another illness, such as gastrointestinal blood loss (increased iron-binding capacity) or "chronic disease" (reduced iron-binding capacity). Increased serum iron concentration in OA may be secondary to another illness (e.g., hemochromatosis).

Serum copper and ceruloplasmin levels are normal in patients with primary OA. Increased serum copper concentrations with secondary OA of the large joints may be the result of Wilson disease (Table 11–1). Wilson disease of small joints may be related to chondrocalcinosis.

Immunologic Studies

Studies of the immune system to date have failed to identify aberrant cellular or humoral immunity in the pathogenesis of OA.

Cellular Studies

Sensitization to proteoglycan antigens was demonstrated in 9 of 22 patients with OA by the lymphocytotoxin production test[35] but in only 1 of 14 patients by the lymphocyte transformation test.[36] It remains unclear whether this cellular immune response contributes to joint damage or reflects the incidental unmasking of proteoglycan antigenic sites during cartilage breakdown.

Humoral Studies

The prevalence of serum rheumatoid factor in OA parallels that observed in the general population. Because the frequency of rheumatoid factor increases with advancing age, low-titer serum rheumatoid factor is anticipated in 5% to 20% or more of patients with OA.[37,38] Otherwise, circulating immune complexes have not been observed.[39]

Low-titer antinuclear antibodies may infrequently be encountered in patients with OA, with a prevalence equivalent to that of a similarly aged healthy population without OA.[40,41]

Antiproteoglycan antibodies have been noted in the serum of patients with severe OA.[42] This finding appears to be an epiphenomenon of joint destruction and is not of etiologic or diagnostic significance.

Complement Studies

Levels of serum total hemolytic complement or specific complement components are normal. In one study,[43] the ninth component of complement was elevated twofold in patients with OA compared with control subjects, similar to values observed in RA and nonrenal systemic lupus erythematosus.

URINE

Results of urine studies are normal in patients with primary OA. Urinary calcium and phosphorus levels vary widely, depending on dietary intake. Urinary estrogen and gonadotropin excretion is similar in postmenopausal women with and without OA.[44]

Urinary abnormalities may be noted in patients with some forms of secondary OA. In ochronosis, alkaline urine may darken on standing. Ochronotic urine reduces alkaline copper solutions, producing a false-positive result in the Benedict test for glycosuria. Confirmation requires enzymatic assay of urine (or serum) for homogentisic acid. Renal tubular acidosis associated with the OA of Wilson disease may produce hyposthenuria, glycosuria, aminoaciduria, proteinuria, and hyperuricosuria.

Any increase in urinary pyridinium collagen cross-links (pyridinoline and deoxypyridinoline) have failed to correlate with grades of severity of OA[45] except in a study of women with OA of the knee.[46] In one study, the elevation was more notable in patients with OA of the knee than in those with OA of the hip or hand. Treatment with intra-articular depocorticosteroids led to a decrease in levels of the urinary cross-links.[47] In contrast, in another study, no elevation of urinary hydroxypyridinium cross-links was found in patients with OA compared with control subjects.[48]

SYNOVIAL FLUID

Synovial fluid in primary OA is generally considered "non-inflammatory" (Ropes and Bauer classification type I[49]). However, increased volume of joint fluid, frequent decrease in viscosity, mild but significant pleocytosis, and modest elevation of synovial fluid protein indicate inflammatory synovitis (Table 11–2).

TABLE 11–2
SYNOVIAL FLUID FINDINGS IN NORMAL AND PRIMARY OSTEOARTHRITIC JOINTS

	Normal (17 patients)	OA (17 patients)
Number of fluid specimens	29	27
Appearance	Yellow, clear	Yellow, clear
Mucin clot	Good	Good
Mean total white blood cell count (cells/mm³)	63	720
Range	13–180	20–3600
Percentage polymorphonuclear	<25%	<25%
Mean total protein (g/dL)	1.7*	3.1†
Range	1.1–2.1*	1.3–4.9†
Viscosity	Normal	Normal–decreased

*Ten synovial fluid specimens.
†Sixteen synovial fluid specimens.

Volume

The volume of synovial fluid in the knee may vary from normal (0.5 to 1.5 mL)[50] to greater than 100 mL in OA. In general, smaller increases in synovial fluid may be evident in other joints with OA. Indeed, the mechanisms that control the volume of synovial fluid are poorly understood and can be explained only partially by vascular hydrostatic pressure. Inexplicably, minimal radiographic evidence of OA may be associated with large synovial effusions; conversely, severe radiographic evidence of OA may elicit only minimal or no synovial effusion.

Intra-articular volumes of synovial fluid as determined by radiolabeling were high (109 ± 35 mL) and were higher than the volume that could be aspirated (59 ± 28 mL).[50] Mean clearance rate for the synovial fluid was 0.039 ± 0.030 mL (SD) per minute, somewhat slower than fluids from patients with RA.

Appearance

The normal synovial fluid usually appears pale yellow, dark yellow, or clear. Along with an increased viscosity, it is reminiscent of the derivation of the term synovial (syn, like; ovum, egg "white"). It may infrequently be blood tinged or frankly bloody. Joint bleeding most often occurs in affected glenohumeral and unstable knee joints and is often associated with an acutely painful exacerbation, trivial trauma, or increased activity. Hemarthrosis may reflect "pinching" of synovium between contiguous osteophytes or irregular joint surfaces or, less frequently, a microfracture of subchondral or osteophytic bone or a tear of the rotator cuff (shoulder) or anterior cruciate ligament (knee). In these cases, the bloody fluid is evident throughout the arthrocentesis procedure, and the fluid often fails to clot. In contrast, bloody fluid resulting from traumatic aspiration technique clears during the course of withdrawal, or, alternatively, blood is seen to enter the syringe and mix with initially yellow fluid during joint aspiration. Repeated aspiration of bloody fluid from a single joint should suggest pigmented villonodular synovitis, particularly if the synovial effusion has a "port wine" color.

In primary OA, shed cartilage "shard" fragments are visible as floating white specks and particles. In OA associated with ochronosis, pigmented shards of cartilage may assume the appearance of ground pepper in joint fluid.[51]

Clarity

Synovial fluid in OA is clear and occasionally faintly turbid.

Viscosity

Synovial fluid viscosity is dependent on a protein–hyaluronic acid complex. The hyaluronate complex consists of an unbranched glycosaminoglycan macromolecule of approximately 2000 kDa composed in turn of polymerized disaccharide dimers of glucuronic acid–glucosamine coiled into a spherical or ellipsoid

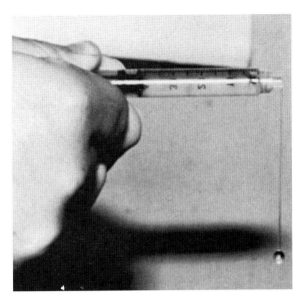

Figure 11–1 High viscosity allows the synovial fluid to "string" when it is dropped from a syringe.

conformation. This conformation allows the structure to occupy a solvent domain considerably larger than the volume of the polymer chain. Hyaluronate depolymerization or synovial membrane secretion of a poorly polymerized hyaluronate or a hyaluronate complex with altered conformation results in diminished viscosity.

In OA, viscosity is inversely related to clinical evidence of inflammation; fluid from palpably "cool" joints usually has a normal viscosity and produces a "string" sign (Fig. 11–1). Markedly poor viscosity, in which the fluid drops like water from the syringe, is uncommon and may reflect coexistent pseudogout or another inflammatory arthritis. Conversely, extremely thick, viscous fluid should suggest osteochondromatosis or hypothyroidism.[52] Pseudomucinous synovial cysts, found over the dorsum of osteoarthritic distal interphalangeal joints, contain pale, gelatinous fluid similar to that observed in ganglia.

Mucin

The precipitation of the protein salt of hyaluronic acid after acidification of joint fluid is the basis of the mucin clot or "Ropes" test.[49] An aliquot of synovial fluid is added to a beaker containing a four times greater volume of 2% acetic acid and mixed with a glass rod. The resulting mucin clot (hyaluronate protein) reflects the degree of polymerization of hyaluronic acid. In OA, a tight, ropy mass is formed (graded good); whereas in RA and other inflammatory arthritides, the mass shows friable edges (graded poor). The mucin clot is almost invariably good in OA, even when viscosity is significantly diminished.

If it is uncertain whether synovial fluid has been aspirated, mucin clot formation and metachromatic staining are capable of detecting as little as 0.5 μL of synovial fluid.[53]

Synovial Fluid Microscopy

Leukocytes

Synovial fluid in OA may be relatively acellular, but a mild increase in the white blood cell count (1000 to 3500 cells/mm^3) often indicates inflammatory synovitis. Synovial pleocytosis in excess of 5000 cells/mm^3 is uncommon (Table 11–2). The majority of leukocytes are lymphocytes (Table 11–2), predominantly T cells.[54] Synovial fluid total and differential white blood cell counts can now be counted by an automated hematology analyzer by pretreatment with hyaluronidase at 37°C for 10 minutes.[55]

Cytoplasmic Inclusions

Leukocytes containing refractile intracytoplasmic inclusions by phase contrast microscopy are sparse in comparison with the numerous "ragocytes"[56] of RA and other arthritides. In OA, these spherical inclusions, measuring 0.5 to 2.0 μm in diameter, appear to be composed largely of triglycerides[57] (Fig. 11–2). In interphalangeal osteoarthritis, synovial cysts may contain large polymorphonuclear leukocytes containing multiple fat staining inclusions similar to those seen in ganglia.

Fragments of type II collagen can be detected in synovial fluid phagocytes by immunohistologic staining and immunoelectron microscopy.[58] This technique may be a sensitive indicator of cartilage erosion but does not separate OA from RA.

Synovial Lining Cells

Large exfoliated mononuclear synovial lining cells, measuring 20 to 40 μm in length, may be seen singly (Fig. 11–3) or in sheets;[59,60] they can be identified on wet mount microscopy but are best identified with Wright stain. The nucleus, which often has prominent nucleoli, is eccentric and encompasses less than half the cell volume. These cells may be distinguished from macrophages by their smaller nuclei and lack of stain by Sudan black.[61]

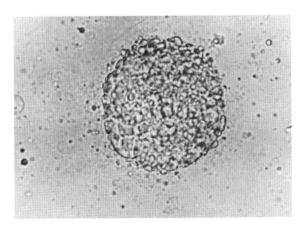

Figure 11–2 Wet mount microscopic preparation of synovial fluid in OA may demonstrate cells containing many inclusions, composed mostly of triglycerides.

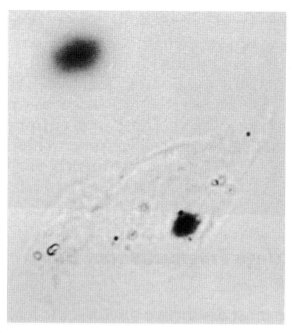

Figure 11–3 Wet mount microscopic preparation of synovial fluid in OA may reveal synovial lining cells. Better cellular definition would necessitate fixation and Wright staining.

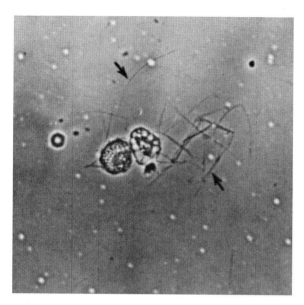

Figure 11–4 Wet mount microscopic preparation of synovial fluid in OA may demonstrate occasional polymorphonuclear leukocytes and fibrils of fibrin or collagen fibers (arrows). These are thin and should not be confused with crystals. (Phase contrast microscopy.)

Cartilage Fragments and Bone Cells

The most distinctive microscopic feature of OA synovial fluid is the occasional presence of multinucleated cells, probably osteoclasts. These cells appear singly or, more often, in sheets or clusters. Cartilage fragments may contain mononuclear chondrocytes. These chondrocytes may be normal in appearance but often display varying degrees of degeneration and stain inconsistently for proteoglycans (e.g., with safranin O or dimethylene blue). In OA of ochronotic origin, sloughed cartilage fragments exhibit a golden (ocher) hue.

Fibrils

Faintly positively birefringent "fibrin" strands that are morphologically indistinguishable from sloughed collagen fibers may be visualized on wet mount microscopy[62] (Fig. 11–4). The collagen fiber of osteoarthritic synovial fluid appears to be type II, derived from articular hyaline cartilage.[63] Fibril presence correlated with progression of OA.[64]

These fibrils may have the appearance of pseudogout "rod-like" crystals. However, in contrast to CPPD crystals, they are resistant to addition of acid (e.g., acetic acid), whereas crystals would dissolve.

Crystals

Calcium hydroxyapatite crystals detected by electron microscopy have been implicated in flares of OA.[65,66] Occasional clumps of hydroxyapatite crystals appear as nonbirefringent amorphous globular matter on routine wet mount microscopy. A semiquantitative technique employing ^{14}C-labeled etidronate disodium binding has detected crystals in OA joint fluid that seem to be hydroxyapatite.[67] There was a correlation between the presence of hydroxyapatite crystals and evidence of cartilage loss by radiography. Synovial fluid microspherules containing hydroxyapatite crystals, active collagenase, and neutral protease have been identified in patients with glenohumeral OA and rotator cuff defects ("Milwaukee shoulder" syndrome).[68]

Cholesterol crystals are most typical in the joint fluid of patients with chronic rheumatoid synovitis. However, cholesterol crystals have been identified by light microscopy in synovial fluids of patients with recurrent OA knee effusions.[69] In the presence of cholesterol crystals, synovial fluid white blood cell counts varied from 125 to 3100 cells/mm³. The cholesterol crystals showed a large (10 to 80 μm) "notched plate" configuration with occasional irregular rod- and needle-shaped (1 to 5 μm) structures. Previous experiments have established that cholesterol crystals may exert a mild phlogistic effect,[70,71] and thus these crystals appear to contribute to the synovitis of OA.

Weakly positively birefringent, rhomboid CPPD crystals may be noted in the fluid of joints affected with the pseudo-OA or pseudogout syndrome associated with calcium pyrophosphate crystal deposition disease.[72] In one study, CPPD and basic calcium crystals too small or few to be detected by light microscopy were found in 11 of 12 patients with OA but in only 1 of 5 with RA by use of analytic electron microscopy and x-ray powder diffraction.[73] Crystals were present in 52% or 330 patients with OA and synovial effusions (CPPD 21%, hydroxyapatite 47%).[64] In those in whom sequential synovial fluids were available, crystals appeared with progression of OA (CPPD 19% first and 34% last aspiration; hydroxyapatite 23% first and 58% last aspiration).

Electrolytes

The synovial fluid is largely an ultrafiltrate of plasma. Concentrations of sodium, potassium, chloride, and bicarbonate in OA synovial fluid approximate those in the serum.

Cartilage Markers

Various markers have been measured in an attempt to find a reliable measure of cartilage matrix turnover. In one study, the relative content of aggrecan and COMP was measured in synovial fluid. The aggrecan/COMP ratio was significantly higher in those with radiographic knee OA than in control subjects.[74]

Sugars and Proteoglycans

The glucose levels of OA synovial fluid parallel serum values. In the fasting state, synovial fluid glucose concentration is usually within 5 to 10 mg/dL of serum levels. Marked depression of glucose to less than half of serum values is most often associated with septic arthritis but can occur in rheumatoid and crystal-induced arthritides; it is not observed in OA.

Synovial fluid levels of sulfated sugars such as chondroitin sulfate and glucosamine sulfate are elevated in OA.[75,76] However, the levels have failed to correlate with radiologic grade or to differentiate radiographically progressive OA in patients observed for up to 2 years.[77]

Sensitive and specific assays of cartilage proteoglycan components and degradation products[17] are potentially useful in analysis of synovial fluids. Proteoglycan analysis has limited value in OA because diseases with more inflammatory synovitis reflect higher synovial fluid proteoglycans,[78-80] with an inverse relationship to the radiographic stage of disease.[81] A prospective study of patients with anterior cruciate ligament rupture or meniscus tear of the knee suggests that proteoglycan epitope is elevated at the time of trauma.[82] The majority of patients have a gradual decrease of the antigen with time, although some have persistent elevation. Other cartilage matrix fractions are under investigation.[83] Aggrecan fragments are released from joint cartilage and into the joint fluid after trauma and in OA.[84]

YKL-40 is a human glycoprotein of the Chitinase protein family. Its levels in synovial fluid have correlated with the degree of synovitis in patients with OA.[85] Fibronectin is a glycoprotein found in the extracellular matrix of most types of cells. Its presence has been associated with enhanced metalloproteinase expression by synovial fibroblasts. Fibronectin has been detected in OA synovial fluid.[86]

Lipids

Normal synovial joint fluid contains small quantities of cholesterol and phospholipids but lacks triglycerides.[87] Cholesterol, phospholipids, and triglycerides were detected in OA synovial fluid.[88]

Synovial fluid contains lower concentrations of lipids and apoproteins than plasma does, particularly those associated with very low-density and low-density lipoproteins (triglycerides, apoprotein B, and apoprotein C-III), so that high-density lipoproteins are the dominant synovial fluid lipoproteins.[89]

In addition, there is a shift of synovial fluid high-density lipoprotein-cholesterol and its major apoproteins (apoproteins A-I and A-II) to lower density, implying cholesterol enrichment of high-density lipoprotein. The apoprotein E–rich fraction of high-density lipoprotein, thought to play an important role in high-density lipoprotein-cholesterol transport, contained larger particles in synovial fluid than in plasma. The plasma and synovial fluid lipid/apoprotein ratios are higher in OA than in RA patients, suggesting that the filtration barrier to plasma lipoproteins is greater in OA. Thus, like lymph, synovial fluid from patients with OA and RA contains a preponderance of large cholesterol- and apoprotein-rich high-density lipoproteins. This suggests that filtered lipoproteins interact with synovial tissue and therefore play a role in the metabolism of inflamed synovial tissue.

The fatty acid composition of synovial fluid is similar to that of serum.[90] Total fatty acids in synovial fluid are approximately a third of those in sera. Palmitic, oleic, and linoleic acids represent nearly 80% of the total fatty acids; myristic, palmitoleic, stearic, and arachidonic acids constitute minor components. Synovial fluid findings in OA and RA are similar. Joint fluid fatty acid concentration and leukocyte count did not correlate, and fatty acid analysis failed to differentiate between inflammatory and noninflammatory effusions.

Succinic acid, a short-chain fatty acid, is not present in synovial fluid. Its presence, as detected by gas-liquid chromatography, suggests septic arthritis and can be used in that differential diagnosis.[91]

Oxygen Tension and pH

Lund-Olesen[92] noted that the mean oxygen tension in 13 OA knee joint cavities was 43 mm Hg (range, 20 to 71 mm Hg), lower than the mean oxygen tension in traumatic effusions (63 mm Hg; range, 42 to 87 mm Hg) ($P <.01$) and higher than that in RA effusions (27 mm Hg; range, 0 to 91 mm Hg) ($P <.01$). PCO_2 values correlated with those for PO_2. Effusions greater than 50 mL were associated with synovial fluid PO_2 levels below 50 mm Hg. Richman and colleagues[93] postulated that high intra-articular pressure resulting from sizable effusions may shunt blood from the synovium by collapse of subsynovial capillaries. Synovial fluid pH paralleled that in the serum until joint fluid PO_2 decreased below 45 mm Hg; at that point, further reductions in PO_2 were associated with proportional reductions in pH.

Enzymes

Lactate Dehydrogenase

Lactate dehydrogenase is slightly increased in synovial fluid of patients with OA, especially fractions 3 and 4. This correlates with the synovial fluid leukocytosis. Synovial fluid levels are lower than those in patients with RA.[94]

Lysosomal Enzymes

The concentrations of a variety of lysosomal enzymes, including acid phosphatase, glycosidase, β-glucuronidase, and N-acetylglucosaminidase, are elevated in the synovial fluid[60,95] in OA. Enzyme activity is directly related to synovial fluid pleocytosis and is less than that in joint fluid in RA. It is uncertain whether these enzymes play a role in the degradation of articular glycosaminoglycans.

Lysozyme

Synovial fluid lysozyme, derived from leukocytic lysosomes and nonlysosomal cartilage matrix, is elevated in OA.[94] Lysozyme activity reflects both synovial inflammation and cartilage degradation.

Collagenase

Free and latent collagenase (MMP-1) has been detected in osteoarthritic synovial fluid[95,96] but is particularly elevated in idiopathic destructive arthropathy of the shoulder.[97] Increase in MMP-1 was also present in injury and pseudogout.[98]

Stromelysin

Stromelysin (MMP-3) levels in synovial fluid increase with inflammation and are significantly higher in RA than in OA.[99] Increase in MMP-3 was also present in injury and pseudogout.

Aggrecanase

Aggrecanase was determined in 40 synovial fluids from OA temporomandibular joints with 15 controls.[100] Aggrecanase was present in OA and in higher values in severe OA and anterior disc displacement.

Tissue Inhibitor of Metalloproteinases

TIMP is elevated in primary OA, post-traumatic OA, and pyrophosphate-related arthritis. The ratio of the matrix metalloproteinases to TIMP seems to be increased in these patients.[101]

Insulin-Like Growth Factor

In a study of 41 patients, levels of both IGF-1 and IGF-binding proteins were found to be elevated in both OA and RA patients compared with normal control subjects.[102]

Neuroregulatory Enzymes

Dopamine β-hydroxylase mediates the conversion of dopamine to norepinephrine and is released from sympathetic neuron synaptic vesicles. The enzyme was detected in normal synovial fluid and, in significantly higher concentrations, in OA joint fluid.[103] Conceivably, dopamine hydroxylase may influence the secretory function of articular cells. Elevated levels of synovial fluid substance P in OA exceeded serum levels.[34]

Hyaluronidase

The synovial fluid in OA contains small amounts of plasma-filtrated hyaluronidase with a molecular mass of 60 kDa.[104] The concentration of the enzyme correlates with synovial fluid white blood cell counts and the presence of synovial debris.[105]

Mast Cell Products

Mast cell counts and histamine concentration have been reported to be increased in OA synovial fluid compared with RA fluid.[106]

Hormones

Corticotropin-releasing hormone levels are elevated in OA synovial fluid although to a lesser extent than in RA.[107]

Proteins

The total protein concentration of synovial fluid in patients with OA is slightly elevated compared with normal (Table 11-2). The relative concentrations of various protein moieties (immunoglobulins G, M, and A; transferrin; and β$_2$-macroglobulin) parallel normal serum values.[108,109] A higher ratio of synovial fluid/serum concentration for non-immunoglobulin proteins, haptoglobin, β$_2$-macroglobulin, orosomucoid, transferrin, and ceruloplasmin is seen in OA joints compared with normal joints.[110-112] The enhanced concentrations correlated with the molecular weight of the particular protein. Synovial inflammation by biopsy did not correlate with increased protein concentration. However, the greatest protein concentration was observed when histologic changes suggested a "proliferative" phase with synovial edema and large numbers of dilated venules and capillaries.

Type II collagen, characteristic of hyaline articular cartilage, was observed in two of six OA effusions. The presence of collagen in sufficient amounts to be detected correlated with decreased radiographic joint space and synovial fluid pH.[42] Synovial fluid concentrations of the C-propeptide of type II collagen have been observed to correlate independently with OA stage in the knee and with body mass index.[113] C-telopeptide fragments of type II collagen (CTX-II) were elevated in knee synovial fluid from OA, pseudogout, and trauma.[114]

Elevated synovial fluid tenascin-C, an extracellular matrix glycoprotein, was found in severe knee OA and correlated with progression of disease.[115] CD44 isoforms v5 and v6, another glycoprotein, were elevated in synovial fluid in 46 patients with OA of the knee, v6 upregulated in the presence of inflammation.[116] Knee synovial fluid cartilage–derived retinoic acid-sensitive protein (CD-RAP) was higher in moderately severe OA than in RA.[117]

Clotting Factors

Normal synovial fluid lacks fibrinogen and contains only trace amounts of plasminogen. Both fibrinogen and plasminogen are detectable in osteoarthritic joint fluid but in lower concentrations than those observed in traumatic and inflammatory arthritides.[118]

Immunologic Studies

Cellular

Lymphokines have been noted occasionally in synovial fluid from patients with OA.[119] The presence of this soluble mediator of cellular immunity possibly reflects an autoimmune response to OA joint debris.

Humoral

Significant titers of synovial fluid antinuclear antibody are absent.[120] Other autoantibodies may be detectable in joint fluid when they are simultaneously present in the serum.[121] Serum antibodies to types I, II, III, IV, and V native or denatured collagens were present in 5% to 25% of patients with OA. This frequency is far less than that found in other rheumatic diseases such as RA.[122]

Immune complexes (immunoglobulins and complement) have been detected in the synovial membranes and hyaline articular cartilage of OA joints but have not been reported as yet in synovial fluid.[123]

Cryoprecipitates may be detected in OA synovial fluid.[124] In contrast to RA, they do not contain immunoglobulin M, infrequently contain immunoglobulin G, and seem largely composed of nonspecific cold-insoluble proteins.

Complement

Synovial fluid complement levels are not depressed in OA, in contrast to those in RA.[125,126] None of 12 OA synovial fluid specimens showed joint fluid total hemolytic complement less than 10% of mean normal serum values.[127] No relationship was found among synovial fluid complement activity, clinical activity, protein concentration, and leukocyte count.

Inflammatory Mediators

Levels of interleukin-1β, TNF-α, and interleukin-6 can be found in the synovial fluid of most patients with OA. The concentrations are lower than in synovial fluid from patients with RA.[128] In the same study, phospholipase A_2 activity was increased in OA and was not statistically different from that in RA. In another study, phospholipase A_2 activity was elevated in OA synovial fluid compared with synovial fluids from RA[129] and did not seem to correlate with degree of joint inflammation. In contrast, synovial fluid prostaglandin E levels were normal in OA (<1.5ng/mL).[130] Patients in this group were refractory to nonsteroidal anti-inflammatory agents. Superoxide radical is detectable in OA synovial fluid[131] and is capable of reducing hyaluronate viscosity[132] and degrading cartilage proteoglycans and collagen in vitro.[133] Other studies have detected an increase in the concentration of kinins in the synovial fluid of OA.[134]

Nitric Oxide

Nitric oxide has been detected in higher concentrations in the OA joint fluid compared with controls.[135]

Bone and Cartilage

Hydroxyproline

Small-fragment, dialyzable hydroxyproline is increased in OA synovial fluid, presumably reflecting accelerated collagen metabolism. Nondialyzable hydroxyproline is normal.[136]

Inorganic Pyrophosphate

Synovial fluid inorganic pyrophosphate is increased in OA,[137,138] as well as in CPPD, compared with normal fluids (or serum). Inorganic pyrophosphate is the major product of adenosine triphosphate catabolism in synovial fluid.[139] The degree of elevation seems to correlate with the radiographic severity of the joint disease. However, in a study of 135 consecutive patients with knee OA observed prospectively for a mean of 2.5 years, high levels of extracellular inorganic pyrophosphate in synovial fluid were associated with slower radiographic progression as judged by Kellgren-Lawrence grade.[140]

SYNOVIAL HISTOLOGIC EXAMINATION

Synovial histologic examination in primary OA reveals nonspecific changes of chronic, mild inflammation.[141-143] Closed needle or open biopsy of the synovium is seldom necessary. However, in selected cases, synovial biopsy may serve to exclude other arthritides or to confirm the presence of OA associated with ochronosis or hemochromatosis.

Primary Osteoarthritis

In early cases, the synovium may appear normal. Focal hyperemia and edema are often evident. Not infrequently, villous hypertrophy is noted, but usually not to the degree observed in RA. Light microscopy reveals proliferation of synovial lining cells with scattered collections of lymphocytes and plasma cells. Venules and arterioles may be dilated with extravasation of red blood cells. Iron may be noted within occasional macrophages of the synovial intima and in both macrophages and the stroma of subintimal and deeper synovial layers.[144]

Inflammatory synovial changes in OA are anatomically restricted to areas near the cartilage and are of varied intensity.[145] The synovial inflammation of OA may be

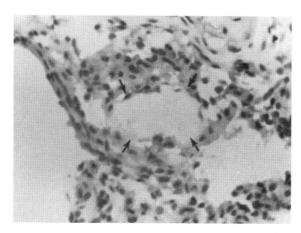

Figure 11–5 Synovial biopsy specimen demonstrates mild synovial proliferation with a degenerating cartilage fragment engulfed by the synovium (arrows).

indistinguishable from synovitis of RA. Fragments of calcified and uncalcified cartilage are sometimes embedded in the synovium, and synovial lining cells may ingest cartilage debris (Fig. 11–5). In more advanced cases, synovial fibrosis may be evident.

Although nonspecific, immunoreactive P component without amyloid can be identified with synovial fibrosis.[146] Fibronectin was more widely distributed and, when accompanied by CRP and laminin, was associated with inflammatory synovitis.

Electron microscopic studies have demonstrated ultrastructural abnormalities in synovial lining cells, including 1) increased rough endoplasmic reticulum with dilated cisternae, 2) decreased number and size of Golgi apparatus and smooth-walled cytoplasmic vesicles, and 3) increased number of lysosomes.

REFERENCES

1. Kellgren JH, Moore R. Generalized osteoarthritis and Heberden's nodes. Br Med 1:181–187, 1952.
2. Denko CW, Gabriel P. Serum proteins—transferrin, ceruloplasmin, albumin, α_1-acid glycoprotein, α_1-antitrypsin—in rheumatic disorders. J Rheumatol 6:664–672, 1974.
3. Wolfe F. The C-reactive protein but not erythrocyte sedimentation rate is associated with clinical severity in patients with osteoarthritis of the knee or hip. J Rheumatol 24:1486–1488, 1997.
4. Punzi L, Ramonda R, Oliviero F, et al. Value of C reactive protein in the assessment of erosive osteoarthritis of the hand. Ann Rheum Dis 64:955–957, 2005.
5. Takahashi M, Naito K, Abe M, et al. Relationship between radiographic grading of osteoarthritis and the biochemical markers for arthritis in knee osteoarthritis. Arthritis Res Ther 6:R208–212, 2004.
6. Garnero P, Mazieres B, Gueguen A, et al. Cross-sectional association of 10 molecular markers of bone, cartilage and synovium with disease activity and radiological joint damage in patients with hip osteoarthritis: the ECHODIAH cohort. J Rheumatol 32:578–579, 2005.
7. Spector TD, Hart DJ, Nandra D, et al. Low-level increases in serum C-reactive protein are present in early osteoarthritis of the knee and predict progressive disease. Arthritis Rheum 40:723–727, 1997.
8. Penninx BW, Abbas H, Ambrosius W, et al. Inflammatory markers and physical function among older adults with knee osteoarthritis. J Rheumatol 31:2027–2031, 2004.
9. Waine H, Nivinny D, Rosenthal J, et al. Association of osteoarthritis and diabetes mellitus. Tufts Folia Med 7:13–17, 1961.
10. Cimmino MA, Cutolo M. Plasma glucose concentration in symptomatic osteoarthritis: a clinical and epidemiological survey. Clin Exp Rheumatol 8:251–257, 1990.
11. Schouten JS, Van den Ouweland FA, Valkenburg HA, et al. Insulin-like growth factor-1: a prognostic factor of knee osteoarthritis. Br J Rheumatol 32:274–280, 1993.
12. Lloyd ME, Hart DJ, Nandra D, et al. Relation between insulin-like growth factor-1 concentrations, osteoarthritis, bone density, and fractures in the general population: the Chingford study. Ann Rheum Dis 55:870–874, 1996.
13. Silveri F, Brecciaroli D, Argentati F, et al. Serum levels of insulin in overweight patients with osteoarthritis of the knee. J Rheumatol 21:1899–1902, 1994.
14. McCarty D. Calcium pyrophosphate deposition disease: pseudogout, articular chondrocalcinosis. In: McCarty DJ, ed. Arthritis and Allied Conditions. Philadelphia, Lea & Febiger, 1979, p 1285.
15. Franchimont P, Denis F. Détermination du taux de la somatotrophine et des gonadotrophines dans des cas d'arthrose apparaissant lors de la ménopause. J Belge Rhum Med Phys 23:59–64, 1968.
16. Sturmer T, Sun Y, Sauerland S, et al. Serum cholesterol and osteoarthritis. The baseline examination of the Ulm Osteoarthritis Study. J Rheumatol 25:1827–1832, 1998.
17. Ristch L, Risteli J. Analysis of extracellular matrix proteins in biological fluids. Methods Enzymol 145:391–411, 1987.
18. Sweet MBE, Coelho A, Schnitzler CM, et al. Serum keratan sulfate levels in osteoarthritis patients. Arthritis Rheum 31:648–652, 1988.
19. Wood KM, Curtis CG, Powell GM, et al. The metabolic fate of intravenously injected peptide-bound chondroitin sulfate in the rat. Biochem J 158:39–46, 1976.
20. Goldberg RL, Huff JP, Lenz ME, et al. Elevated plasma levels of hyaluronate in patients with osteoarthritis and rheumatoid arthritis. Arthritis Rheum 34:799–807, 1991.
21. Sharif M, George E, Shepstone L, et al. Serum hyaluronic acid level as a predictor of disease progression in osteoarthritis of the knee. Arthritis Rheum 38:760–767, 1995.
22. Elliott AL, Kraus VB, Luta G, et al. Serum hyaluronan levels and radiographic knee and hip osteoarthritis in African Americans and Caucasians in the Johnston County Osteoarthritis Project. Arthritis Rheum 52:105–111, 2005.
23. Pavelka K, Forejtova S, Olejarova M, et al. Hyaluronic acid levels may have predictive value for the progression of knee osteoarthritis. Osteoarthritis Cartilage 12:277–283, 2004.
24. Bruyere O, Collette JH, Ethgen O, et al. Biochemical markers of bone and cartilage remodelingin prediction of longterm progression of knee osteoarthritis. J Rheumatol 30:910–912, 2003.
25. Mundermann A, Dyrby CO, Andriacchi TP, et al. Serum concentration of cartilage oligomeric protein (COMP) is sensitive to physiological cyclic loading in healthy adults. Osteoarthritis Cartilage 13:34–38, 2005.
26. Kersting UG, Stubendorff JJ, Schmidt MC, et al. Changes in knee cartilage volume and serum COMP concentration after running exercise. Osteoarthritis Cartilage 13:925–934, 2005.
27. Balblanc JC, Hartmann D, Noyer D, et al. L'acide hyaluronique serique dans l'arthrose. Rev Rhum Ed Fr 60:194–202, 1993.
28. Sharif M, Saxne T, Shepstone L, et al. Relationship between serum cartilage oligomeric matrix protein levels and disease progression in osteoarthritis of the knee joint. Br J Rheumatol 34:306–310, 1995.
29. Conrozier T, Saxne T, Fan CS, et al. Serum concentration of cartilage oligomeric matrix protein and bone sialoprotein in hip osteoarthritis: a one year prospective study. Ann Rheum Dis 57:527–532, 1998.
30. Sharif M, Kirwan JR, Elson CJ, et al. Suggestion of nonlinear or phasic progression of knee osteoarthritis based on measurements of serum cartilage oligomeric matrix protein levels over five years. Arthritis Rheum 50:2479–2488, 2004.

31. Manicourt DH, Fujimoto N, Obata K, et al. Serum levels of collagenase, stromelysin-1, and TIMP-1. Age- and sex-related differences in normal subjects and relationship to the extent of joint involvement and serum levels of antigenic keratan sulfate in patients with osteoarthritis. Arthritis Rheum 37:1774–1783, 1994.
32. Masubara K, Nakai T, Yamaguchi K, et al. Significant increases in serum and plasma concentrations of matrix metalloproteinas 3 and 9 in patients with rapidly destructive osteoarthritis of the hip. Arthritis Rheum 46:2625–2631, 2002.
33. Cauley JA, Kwoh CK, Egeland G, et al. Serum sex hormones and severity of osteoarthritis of the hand. J Rheumatol 20:1170–1175, 1993.
34. Marshall KW, Chiu B, Inman RD. Substance P and arthritis: analysis of plasma and synovial fluid levels. Arthritis Rheum 33:87–90, 1990.
35. Herman JH, Houk JL, Dennis MV. Cartilage antigen dependent lymphotoxin release: immunopathological significance in articular destructive disorders. Ann Rheum Dis 33:446–452, 1974.
36. Herman JH, Wiltse DW, Dennis MV. Immunopathologic significance of cartilage antigenic components in rheumatoid arthritis. Arthritis Rheum 16:287–297, 1973.
37. Mikkelson WM, Dodge HJ, Duff IF, et al. Estimates of the prevalence of rheumatic disease in the population of Tecumseh, Michigan, 1950-60. J Chronic Dis 20:351–369, 1967.
38. Bennett PH, Wood PHN, eds. Population Studies of the Rheumatic Diseases. Amsterdam, Excerpta Medica, 1968.
39. Lambert PH, Casali P. Immune complexes and the rheumatic diseases. Clin Rheum Dis 4:617–642, 1978.
40. Cammarata RJ, Rodnan GP, Fennell RH Jr, et al. Serologic reactions and serum protein concentrations in the aged [abstract]. Arthritis Rheum 7:297, 1964.
41. Robitaille P, Zvaifler J, Tan EM. Antinuclear antibodies and nuclear antigens in rheumatoid synovial fluids. Clin Immunol Immunopathol 1:385–397, 1973.
42. Herman JH, Carpenter BA. Immunobiology of cartilage. Semin Arthritis Rheum 5:1–40, 1975.
43. Ruddy S, Everson LK, Schur PH, et al. Hemolytic assay of the ninth complement component: elevation and depletion in rheumatic diseases. J Exp Med 134:2595–2755, 1974.
44. Rogers FB, Lansbury J. Urinary gonadotrophin excretion in osteoarthritis. Am J Med Sci 232:419–420, 1956.
45. Astbury C, Bird HA, McLaren AM, et al. Urinary excretion of pyridinium crosslinks of collagen correlated with joint damage in arthritis. Br J Rheumatol 33:11–15, 1994.
46. Thompson PW, Spector TD, James IT, et al. Urinary collagen crosslinks reflect the radiographic severity of knee osteoarthritis. Br J Rheumatol 31:759–761, 1992.
47. MacDonald AG, McHenry P, Robins SP, et al. Relationship of urinary pyridinium crosslinks to disease extent and activity in osteoarthritis. Br J Rheumatol 33:16–19, 1994.
48. Graverand MP, Tron AM, Ichou M, et al. Assessment of urinary hydroxypyridinium cross-links measurement in osteoarthritis. Br J Rheumatol 35:1091–1095, 1996.
49. Ropes MW, Bauer W. Synovial Fluid Changes in Joint Disease. Cambridge, MA, Harvard University Press, 1953.
50. Wallis WJ, Simkin PA, Nelp WB, et al. Intraarticular volume and clearance in human synovial effusions. Arthritis Rheum 28:441–449, 1985.
51. Hunter T, Gordon DA, Ogryzlo MA. The ground pepper sign of synovial fluid: a new diagnostic feature of ochronosis. J Rheumatol 1:45–53, 1974.
52. Dorwart BB, Schumacher HR. Joint effusions, chondrocalcinosis, and other rheumatic manifestations in hypothyroidism. A clinicopathologic study. Am J Med 59:780–789, 1975.
53. Goldenberg DL, Brandt KD, Cohen AS. Rapid, simple detection of trace amounts of synovial fluid. Arthritis Rheum 16:487–490, 1973.
54. van de Putte LBA, Meijer CJLM, Lafeber GJM, et al. Lymphocytes in rheumatoid and nonrheumatoid synovial fluids. Ann Rheum Dis 35:451–455, 1976.
55. Sugiuchi H, Ando Y, Manabe M, et al. Measurement of total and differential white blood counts in synovial fluid by means of an automated hematology analyzer. J Lab Clin Med 146:36–42, 2005.
56. Hollander JL, McCarty DJ, Rawson AJ. The "RA cell," "ragocyte," or "inclusion body cell." Bull Rheum Dis 16:382–385, 1965.
57. Hersko C, Michaeli D, Shibolet S, et al. The nature of refractile inclusions in leukocytes of synovial effusions. Isr J Med Sci 6:838–846, 1967.
58. Moreland LW, Stewart T, Gay RE, et al. Immunohistologic demonstration of type II collagen in synovial fluid phagocytes of osteoarthritis and rheumatoid arthritis patients. Arthritis Rheum 32:1458–1464, 1989.
59. Naib ZM. Cytology of synovial fluids. Acta Cytol 17:299–309, 1973.
60. Broderick PA, Corvese N, Pierik MG, et al. Exfoliative cytology interpretation of synovial fluid in joint disease. J Bone Joint Surg Am 58:396–399, 1976.
61. Shehan HL, Storey GW. Improved method of staining leukocyte granules with Sudan black. Br J Pathol Bacteriol 59:336–337, 1947.
62. Kitridou R, McCarty DJ, Prockop DJ, et al. Identification of collagen in synovial fluid. Arthritis Rheum 12:580–588, 1969.
63. Cheung HS, Ryan LM, Kozin F, et al. Identification of collagen subtypes in synovial fluid sediments from arthritic patients. Am J Med 68:73–79, 1980.
64. Nalbant S, Martinez JA, Kitumnuaypong T, et al. Synovial fluid features and their relations to osteoarthritis severity: new findings from sequential studies. Osteoarthritis Cartilage 11:50–54, 2003.
65. Dieppe PA, Huskisson EC, Crocker P, et al. Apatite deposition disease. A new arthropathy. Lancet 1:266–270, 1976.
66. Schumacher HR Jr. Pathogenesis of crystal-induced synovitis. Clin Rheum Dis 3:105–131, 1977.
67. Halverson PB, McCarty DJ. Identification of hydroxyapatite crystals in synovial fluid. Arthritis Rheum 22:389–395, 1979.
68. McCarty DJ, Halverson PB, Carrera GF, et al. "Milwaukee shoulder"—association of microspheroids containing hydroxyapatite crystals, active collagenase, and neutral protease with rotator cuff defects. II. Synovial fluid studies. Arthritis Rheum 24:474–483, 1981.
69. Fam AG, Pritzker KPH, Cheng PT, et al. Cholesterol crystals in osteoarthritic joint effusions. J Rheumatol 8:273–280, 1981.
70. Bland JH, Gierthy JF, Suhre ED. Cholesterol in connective tissue of joints. Scand J Rheumatol 3:199–203, 1974.
71. Pritzker KPH, Fam AG, Omar SA, et al. Experimental cholesterol crystal arthropathy. J Rheumatol 8:281–290, 1981.
72. McCarty DJ. Calcium pyrophosphate dihydrate crystal deposition disease—1975. Arthritis Rheum 19:275–285, 1976.
73. Swan A, Chapman B, Heap P, et al. Submicroscopic crystals in osteoarthritic synovial fluids. Ann Rheum Dis 53:467–470, 1994.
74. Petersson IF, Sandqvist L, Svensson B, et al. Cartilage markers in synovial fluid in symptomatic knee osteoarthritis. Ann Rheum Dis 56:64–67, 1997.
75. Sweet MBE. An ultracentrifugal analysis of synovial fluid. S Afr Med J 45:1205–1206, 1971.
76. Belcher C, Yaqub R, Fawthrop F, et al. Synovial fluid chondroitin and keratan sulfate epitopes, glycosaminoglycans, and hyaluronan in arthritic and normal knees. Ann Rheum Dis 56:299–307, 1997.
77. Fawthrop F, Yaqub R, Belcher C, et al. Chondroitin and keratan sulfate epitopes, glycosaminoglycans, and hyaluronan in progressive versus non-progressive osteoarthritis. Ann Rheum Dis 56:119–122, 1997.
78. Saxne T, Heinegard D, Wollheim FA. Therapeutic effects on cartilage metabolism in arthritis asmeasured by release of proteoglycan structures into the synovial fluid. Ann Rheum Dis 45:491–497, 1986.
79. Saxne T, Heinebard D, Wollheim FA. Cartilage proteoglycans in synovial fluid and blood in inflammatory joint disease: relation to systemic treatment. Arthritis Rheum 30:972–980, 1987.
80. Witter J, Roughley PJ, Webber C, et al. The immunological detection and characterization of cartilage proteoglycan degradation products in synovial fluids of patients with arthritis. Arthritis Rheum 30:519–529, 1987.
81. Saxne T, Heinegard D, Wollheim FA, et al. Difference in cartilage proteoglycan level in synovial fluid in early rheumatoid arthritis and reactive arthritis. Lancet 2:127–128, 1985.

82. Lohmander LS, Dahlberg L, Ryd L, et al. Increased levels of pro-teoglycan fragments in knee joint fluid after injury. Arthritis Rheum 32:1434–1442, 1989.

83. Fife RS, Brandt KD. Cartilage matrix glycoprotein is present in serum in experimental canine osteoarthritis. J Clin Invest 84:1432–1439, 1989.

84. Lohmander LS. The release of aggrecan fragments into synovial fluid after joint injury and in osteoarthritis. J Rheumatol Suppl 43:75–77, 1995.

85. Johansen JS, Hvolris J, Hansen M, et al. Serum YKL-40 levels in healthy children and adults. Comparison with serum and syn-ovial fluid levels of YKL-40 in patients with osteoarthritis or trauma of the knee joint. Br J Rheumatol 35:553–559, 1996.

86. Xie DL, Meyers R, Homandberg GA. Fibronectin fragments in osteoarthritic synovial fluid. J Rheumatol 19:1448–1452, 1992.

87. Bole GG. Synovial fluid lipids in normal individuals and patients with rheumatoid arthritis. Arthritis Rheum 5:589–601, 1962.

88. Chung AC, Shanahan JR, Brown EM Jr. Synovial fluid lipids in rheumatoid and osteoarthritis. Arthritis Rheum 5:176–183, 1962.

89. Altman RD, Goldberg RB, Gibson JC, et al. Synovial fluid (SF) contains large, cholesterol rich high density lipoproteins. Arthritis Rheum 29(suppl):S39(A), 1986.

90. Kim IC, Cohen AS. Synovial fluid fatty acid composition in patients with rheumatoid arthritis, gout and degenerative joint disease. Proc Soc Exp Biol Med 123:77–80, 1966.

91. Borenstein DG, Gibbs C, Jacobs RP. Synovial fluid (SF) analysis by gas-liquid chromatography (GLC): succinic acid (SA) and lac-tic acid (LA) as markers for septic arthritis [abstract]. Arthritis Rheum 24:590, 1981.

92. Lund-Olesen K. Oxygen tension in synovial fluids. Arthritis Rheum 13:769–776, 1970.

93. Richman AI, Su EY, Ho G Jr. Reciprocal relationship of synovial fluid volume and oxygen tension. Arthritis Rheum 24:701–705, 1981.

94. Veys EM, Wieme RJ. Lactate dehydrogenase in synovial fluid diagnostic evaluation of total activity and isoenzyme patterns. Ann Rheum Dis 27:569–576, 1968.

95. Abe S, Shinmel M, Nagai Y. Synovial collagenase and joint dis-eases: the significance of latent collagenase with special reference to rheumatoid arthritis. J Biochem 73:1007–1011, 1973.

96. Peltonen L. Collagenase in synovial fluid. Scand J Rheumatol 7:49–54, 1978.

97. Dieppe PA, Cawston T, Mercer E, et al. Synovial fluid collagenase in patients with destructive arthritis of the shoulder joint. Arthritis Rheum 30:882–890, 1988.

98. Tchetverikov I, Lihmander LA, Verzijl N, et al. MMP protein and activity levels in synovial fluid from patients with joint injury, inflammatory arthritis, and osteoarthritis. Ann Rheum Dis 64:694–698, 2005.

99. Sasaki S, Iwata H, Ishiguro N, et al. Detection of stromelysin in synovial fluid and serum from patients with rheumatoid arthritis and osteoarthritis. Clin Rheumatol 13:228–233, 1994.

100. Yoshida K, Takatsuka S, Tanaka E, et al. Aggrecanase analysis of synovial fluid of temporomandibular joint disorders. Oral Dis 11:299–302, 2005.

101. Lohmander LS, Hoerrner LA, Lark MW. Metalloproteinases, tis-sue inhibitor, and proteoglycan fragments in knee synovial fluid in human osteoarthritis. Arthritis Rheum 36:181–189, 1993.

102. Fernihough JK, Billingham ME, Cwyfan-Hughes S, et al. Local disruption of the insulin-like growth factor system in the arthritic joint. Arthritis Rheum 39:1556–1565, 1996.

103. Sanchez-Martin M, Garcia AG. Dopamine betahydroxylase in human synovial fluid. Experientia 33:650–652, 1977.

104. Stephens RW, Ghosh P, Taylor TKF. The characterization and function of the polysaccharidases of human synovial fluid in rheumatoid and osteoarthritis. Biochim Biophys Acta 399:101–112, 1975.

105. Palmer DG. Total leukocyte enumeration in pathologic synovial fluids. Am J Clin Pathol 49:813–814, 1968.

106. Renoux M, Hilliquin P, Galoppin L, et al. Release of mast cell mediators and nitrites into knee joint fluid in osteoarthritis—comparison with articular chondrocalcinosis and rheumatoid arthritis. Osteoarthritis Cartilage 4:175–179, 1996.

107. Crofford LJ, Sano H, Karalis K, et al. Corticotropin-releasing hor-mone in synovial fluids and tissues of patients with rheumatoid arthritis and osteoarthritis. J Immunol 151:1587–1596, 1993.

108. Panush RS, Bianco NE, Schur PH. Serum and synovial fluid IgG, IgA and IgM antigammaglobulins in rheumatoid arthritis. Arthritis Rheum 14:737–747, 1971.

109. Veys EM. Comparative investigation of protein concentration in serum and synovial fluid. Scand J Rheumatol 3:1–12, 1974.

110. Nettelbladt E, Sundblad L, Jonsson E. Permeability of the synovial membrane to proteins. Acta Rheum Scand 9:28–32, 1963.

111. Reinmann I, Arnoldi CC, Nielsen OS. Permeability of synovial membrane to plasma proteins in human coxarthrosis: relation to molecular size and histologic changes. Clin Orthop 147:296–300, 1980.

112. Scudder PR, McMurray W, White AG, et al. Synovial fluid copper and related variables in rheumatoid and degenerative arthritis. Ann Rheum Dis 37:71–72, 1978.

113. Kobayashi T, Yoshihara Y, Samura A, et al. Synovial fluid concen-trations of the C-propeptide of type II collagen correlate with body mass index in primary knee osteoarthritis. Ann Rheum Dis 56:500–503, 1997.

114. Lohmander LS, Atley LM, Pietka TA, et al. The release of crosslinked peptides from type II collagen into human synovial fluid is increased soon after joint injury and in osteoarthritis. Arthritis Rheum 48:3130–3039, 2003.

115. Hasegawa M, Hirata H, Sudo A, et al. Tenascin-C concentration in synovial fluid correlates with radiographic progression of knee osteoarthritis. J Rheumatol 31:2021–2026, 2004.

116. Fuchs S, Rolauffs B, Arndt S, et al. CD44H and the isoforms CD44v6 and CD 44v6 in the synovial fluid of osteoarthritic human knee joint. Osteoarthritis Cartilage 11:839–844, 2003.

117. Saito S, Kondo S, Mishima S, et al. Analysis of cartilage-derived retinoic-acid-sensitive protein (CD-RAP) in synovial fluid from patients with osteoarthritis and rheumatoid arthritis. J Bone Joint Surg Br 84:1066–1069, 2002.

118. Anderson RB, Gormsen J. Fibrin dissolution in synovial fluid. Acta Rheum Scand 16:319–333, 1970.

119. Stastny P, Rosenthal M, Andreis M, et al. Lymphokines in the rheumatoid joint. Arthritis Rheum 18:237–243, 1975.

120. MacSween RNM, Dalakos TK, Jasani MK, et al. Antinuclear fac-tors in synovial fluids. Lancet 1:313–314, 1967.

121. Wordsworth P, Ebringer R, Jones D, et al. Thyroid antibodies in synovial effusions [letter]. Lancet 1:660, 1980.

122. Stuart JM, Huffstutter EH, Townes AS, et al. Incidence and specificity of antibodies to types I, II, III, IV, and V collagen in rheumatoid arthritis and other rheumatic diseases as meas-ured by ^{125}I radioimmunoassay. Arthritis Rheum 26:832–840, 1983.

123. Cooke TDV, Bennett EL, Ohno O. Identification of immunoglob-ulin and complement components in articular collagenous tis-sues of patients with idiopathic osteoarthritis. In: Nuki G, ed. The Aetiopathogenesis of Osteoarthritis. Tunbridge Wells, England, Pitman Medical, 1980, pp 144–154.

124. Ludivido CL, Myers AR. Survey of synovial fluid cryoprecipitates. Ann Rheum Dis 39:253–259, 1979.

125. Ruddy S, Fearon DT, Austin KF. Depressed synovial fluid levels of properdin and properdin factor B in patients with rheumatoid arthritis. Arthritis Rheum 18:289–295, 1975.

126. Perrin LH, Nydegger UE, Zublev RH, et al. Correlation between levels of breakdown products of C3, C4 and properdin factor B in synovial fluid from patients with rheumatoid arthritis. Arthritis Rheum 20:647–656, 1977.

127. Sheppeard H, Lea DJ, Ward DJ. Synovial fluid total hemolytic complement activity in rheumatic diseases: a reappraisal. J Rheumatol 8:390–397, 1981.

128. Vignon E, Balblanc JC, Mathieu P, et al. Metalloproteinase activ-ity, phospholipase A_2 activity and cytokine concentration in osteoarthritis synovial fluids. Osteoarthritis Cartilage 1:115–120, 1993.

129. Pruzanski W, Vadas P, Stefanski E, et al. Phospholipase A_2 activity in sera and synovial fluids in rheumatoid arthritis and osteoarthritis. Its possible role as a proinflammatory enzyme. J Rheumatol 12:211–216, 1985.

130. Tokunaga M, Ohuchi K, Yoshozawa S, et al. Change of prostaglandin E level in joint fluids after treatment with flurbiprofen in patients with rheumatoid arthritis and osteoarthritis. Ann Rheum Dis 40:462–465, 1981.
131. Lunec J, Halloran P, White AG, et al. Free radical oxidation (peroxidation) products in serum and synovial fluid in rheumatoid arthritis. J Rheumatol 8:233–245, 1981.
132. Greenwald RA, Moy WW. Effect of oxygen-derived free radicals on hyaluronic acid. Arthritis Rheum 23:448–454, 1980.
133. Greenwald RA, Moy WW, Lazarus D. Degradation of cartilage proteoglycans and collagen by superoxide radical [abstract]. Arthritis Rheum 19:799, 1976.
134. Bond AP, Lemon M, Dieppe PA, et al. Generation of kinins in synovial fluid from patients with arthropathy. Immunopharmacology 36:209–216, 1997.
135. Ni J, Ding R, Wang W, et al. Change in nitric oxide contents of knee joint fluid from patients with degenerative osteoarthritis. Hunan I Ko Ta Hsueh Pao 22:333–334, 1997.
136. Manicourt D, Rao VH, Orloff S. Serum and synovial fluid hydroxyproline fractions in microcrystalline arthritis and osteoarthritis. Scand J Rheumatol 8:193–198, 1979.
137. Altman RD, Muniz OE, Pita JC, et al. Articular chondrocalcinosis: microanalysis of pyrophosphate (PPi) in synovial fluid and plasma. Arthritis Rheum 16:171–178, 1973.
138. Camerlain M, McCarty DJ, Silcox DC, et al. Inorganic pyrophosphate pool size and turnover rate in arthritic joints. J Clin Invest 55:1373–1381, 1975.
139. Park W, Masuda I, Cardenal-Escarcena A, et al. Inorganic pyrophosphate generation from adenosine triphosphate by cell-free human synovial fluid. J Rheumatol 23:665–671, 1996.
140. Doherty M, Belcher C, Regan M, et al. Association between synovial fluid levels of inorganic pyrophosphate and short term radiographic outcome of knee osteoarthritis. Ann Rheum Dis 55:432–436, 1996.
141. Lloyd-Roberts GC. Osteoarthritis of the hip; study of clinical pathology. J Bone Joint Surg Br 37:8–47, 1955.
142. Roy S. Ultrastructure of synovial membrane in osteoarthritis. Ann Rheum Dis 26:517–527, 1967.
143. Arnoldi CC, Reimann I, Bretlau P. The synovial membrane in human coxarthrosis: light and electron microscopic studies. Clin Orthop 148:213–220, 1980.
144. Darrell JOH, Fornaiser VL. Synovial iron deposition in osteoarthritis and rheumatoid arthritis. J Rheumatol 7:30–36, 1980.
145. Lindblad S, Hedfors E. Arthroscopic and immunohistologic characterization of knee joint synovitis in osteoarthritis. Arthritis Rheum 30:1081–1088, 1987.
146. Butler MG, D'Ardenne AJ, Scott DL. P component in the synovium in rheumatoid and osteoarthritis. Ann Rheum Dis 47:463–467, 1988.

Noninvasive Biochemical Markers in Osteoarthritis

12

Patrick Garnero

INTRODUCTION

Osteoarthritis (OA) is a highly prevalent age-related disease characterized by an abnormal and degraded cartilage, associated with synovitis and variable subchondral bone reaction, resulting in pain and severe mobility impairment. Synovitis can be evaluated using systemic inflammation. Parameters of inflammation such as highly sensitive assay for C-reactive protein (CRP) or cytokine levels. However, because these biological markers are not specific of alteration of joint tissues, they are poorly correlated with cartilage damage at the individual level. Thus, the most established method for assessing the extent of joint destruction in OA remains plain radiography. This technique provides direct information on bone, but only indirect estimation of cartilage loss via the measurement of the distance between opposing articular cortices (described as joint-space width, JSW). Radiography is rather insensitive and does not allow an early detection of joint tissue damage nor an efficient monitoring of the efficacy of treatment aimed at preventing joint destruction. Magnetic resonance imaging (MRI) is more sensitive than radiography and provides direct, accurate, and precise evaluation of the key joint structures including articular cartilage, osteophytes, bone marrow, synovium, ligaments, and menisci, although most of these studies focused on cartilage assessment.[1] Complementary to these imaging modalities, there has recently been a considerable interest in identifying specific biological markers which could reflect quantitative and dynamic variations in joint tissue remodeling. In this chapter we will review the recent development in biochemical markers for bone, cartilage, and synovium tissue turnover

and then review their potential clinical role for the management of OA.

ASSAYS FOR BIOCHEMICAL MARKERS OF JOINT TISSUE TURNOVER

Joints are enclosed in a strong fibrous capsule. The inner surfaces of the joint capsule are lined with a metabolically active tissue, the synovium, which secretes the synovial fluid that provides the nutrients required by the tissues within the joint. Each articular bone end within the joint is lined by a thin layer of hydrated soft tissue, i.e., the articular cartilage. In joint diseases, there is a loss of the normal balance between the synthesis and the degradation of the macromolecules that provide articular cartilage with its biomechanical and functional properties. Concomitantly, changes occur in the metabolism of the synovium and in the microarchiture and turnover of the subchondral bone. Consequently, for a comprehensive assessment of the physiopathological processes that lead to joint failure in OA, it is important to gain access to highly specific biochemical markers of cartilage, bone, and synovium tissue turnover (Table 12–1).

Biochemical Markers of Cartilage Turnover

Articular cartilage is a multiphasic material with two major phases: a fluid phase composed of water and electrolytes, and a solid phase composed of collagen, proteoglycans, glycoproteins, other proteins, and the chondrocytes. Each of

215

TABLE 12–1
BIOCHEMICAL MARKERS OF BONE, CARTILAGE, AND SYNOVIUM TURNOVER

	Synthesis	Degradation
Cartilage Type II collagen	• N- and C-propeptides (PIICP, PIIANP, and PIIBNP)	• PYD • Type II collagen C-telopeptide (CTX-II) • Type II collagen collagenase neoepitope (C2C, C12C, TIINE) • Type II collagen helical fragments (Helix-II, Coll 2-1)
Aggrecan	• Chondroïtin sulfate (epitopes 846, 3B3, 7D4)	• Core protein MMPs and aggrecanase neoepitopes • Keratan sulfate (epitopes 5D4, ANP9)
Nonaggrecan and noncollagen proteins	• Chitinase 3-like proteins 1 and 2 (YKL-40 and YKL-39)	• Cartilage oligomeric matrix protein (COMP)
Bone Type I collagen	• N- and C-propeptides (PICP, PINP)	• Pyridinoline (PYD) • Deoxypyridinoline (DPD) • C- and N-telopeptide (CTX-I, NTX-I, ICTP) • Helical peptide
Noncollagen proteins	• Osteocalcin • Bone alkaline phosphatase	• Bone sialoprotein (BSP) • Tartrate resistant acid phosphatase (TRACP, 5b isoenzyme) • Cathepsin K • Urinary osteocalcin fragments
Synovium/synovitis Type I/III collagen	• Type I/Type III N propeptide (PINP/PIIINP)	• PYD • CTX-I, NTX-I • Glucosyl-galactosyl-pyridinoline (Glc-Gal-PYD)
Noncollagen proteins Proteases	• Hyaluronic acid • YKL-40 • COMP	
Systemic inflammation	• MMP-1, 2, 3, 9 Ultrasensitive C-reactive protein (CRP)	

the phases contributes to its mechanical and physiological properties. Of the organic components, the collagens—mostly collagen type II—provide the quantitatively major component, followed by proteoglycans, especially aggrecan[2] (Fig. 12–1). Although the other proteins are not major components in terms of the absolute solid phase, they may approach the molar concentration of collagen and aggrecan. The maintenance of cartilage integrity is dependent on a tight balance between the synthesis and degradation activities of chondrocytes, which is altered in OA.

Markers of Type II Collagen Turnover

The predominant type of collagen is type II, which is cartilage specific and forms the basic fibrillar structure of the extracellular matrix. Types IX and XI are also cartilage specific and are present together with type II collagen. There is evidence that many collagens, including types II, IX, and XI in cartilage, exist as hybrid molecules. In contrast, type VI collagen forms distinct microfibrils that appear concentrated in the capsular matrix surrounding individual chondrocytes or groups of chondrocytes.

Markers of Type II Collagen Synthesis. Type II collagen is synthesized and secreted by the chondrocytes as a precursor, the procollagen. Type II procollagen is constituted by the type II collagen molecule—comprising the major triple helix ($[\alpha 1 \ (II)]_3$) and the linear N- and C-telopeptides—and the N and C-terminal propeptides at the two extremities. The propeptides are removed by specific proteinases before the mature molecules are incorporated into fibrils in matrix following which they are released into biological fluids, and their levels are believed to reflect type II collagen synthesis. Type II procollagen is synthesized in two splice forms, type IIA and type IIB. Type IIA contains an additional 207 base pair exon (exon 2) encoding the 69 amino acid cysteine-rich domain of the N-propeptide; it is expressed mainly by fetal tissues but can be re-expressed in osteoarthritic cartilage,[3] whereas the IIB variant is the major form of adult cartilage. The two forms of aminoterminal propeptide of type III procollagen (PIINP) (PIIANP and PIIBNP) and procollagen type II carboxy-terminal propeptide (PIICP) may thus serve as markers of type II collagen synthesis. An enzyme-Linked immunosorbent assay (ELISA) for PIIANP was recently developed using a specific polyclonal

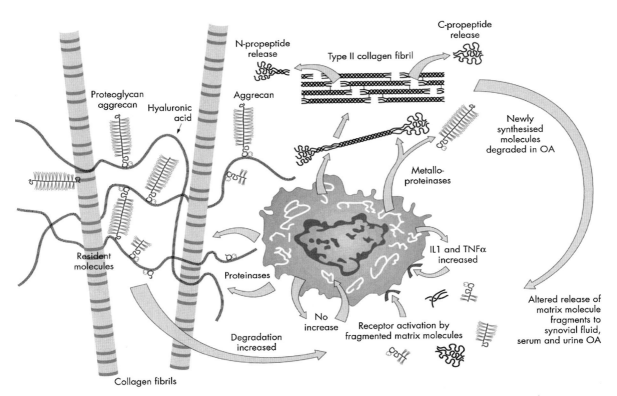

Figure 12–1 Schematic representation of the main constituents of articular cartilage matrix and their turnover: Type II collagen fibrils form an endoskeleton and associated with them in interfibrillar sites resides the proteoglycan aggrecan aggregated with hyaluronic acid. There is physiological active pericellular turnover of extracellular matrix involving proteolysis mediated by matrix metalloproteinases (MMPs). In OA there is increased damage to resident matrix molecules more remote from chondrocytes with upregulation of synthesis of collagen and proteoglycan in early disease. These new molecules are also subject to degradation. Biochemical markers of synthesis and degradation of collagen and aggrecan are released to body fluids where they can be detected. (From Poole AR, Kobayashi M, Yasuda T, et al. Type II collagen degradation and its regulation in articular cartilage in osteoarthritis. Ann Rheum Dis 61 [Suppl 2]:ii;78–81, 2002.)

antibody raised against recombinant exon-2 protein. Compared to healthy sex- and age-matched controls, increased serum levels of PIIANP were reported in early knee OA,[4] whereas decreased values[5] were found in patients with advanced disease. These results obtained from analysis of systemic levels of PIIANP are in agreement with direct measurements of type II collagen in human OA cartilage using proline incorporation which show that type II collagen synthesis is increased in early stages of cartilage degeneration, but progressively decreased in late stages.[6] These data indicate that in early OA, chondrocytes upregulate their biosynthetic activities to compensate for increased damage, but this anabolic response may become deficient in advanced OA. Because type IIB collagen is the major form of adult cartilage, the development of an assay for PIIBNP would be very useful as it may provide different information compared to PIIANP in OA.

Markers of Type II Collagen Degradation. Type II collagen is degraded by proteolytic enzymes secreted by the chondrocytes and the synoviocytes of the synovium tissue, including the matrix metalloproteinases (MMP) and the cysteine proteases.[7,8] Among the MMPs, the collagenases cleave the triple helical region of type II collagen at a single site between residues 778 and 776 generating two

fragments representing three fourths and one fourth, respectively, of the intact collagen molecule. Other MMPs, including the gelatinases and stromelysins, especially stromelysin 1 (also named MMP-3), can cleave denaturated collagen within the triple helical domain and the telopeptides. Stomelysin 1, which attacks type II collagen within the telopeptides, may not have a major role in this process[9] but could contribute indirectly to collagen breakdown by activating the other MMPs. MMP-13, whose expression is increased in OA, could be one of the major enzymes involved in the increased type II collagen degradation.[7,10] Although MMPs are likely to play a major role in degradation of type II collagen in OA, several cysteine proteases have also been suggested to contribute to cartilage destruction. Among them, numerous reports have shown increased expression of cathepsins B, L, K, and S.[8] Cathepsins B and L have been shown to cleave type II collagen within the nonhelical telopeptide of collagens, whereas cathepsin K is capable of cleaving collagen at multiple sites within the triple helix of type I and type II collagen[11,12] and has recently been suggested to be the major cysteine protease expressed in OA cartilage.[13,14] Cathepsin S is unique in that it is the only cysteine protease to be active at neutral and slightly alkaline pH and thus can participate in extracellular matrix degradation of articular cartilage. Although cathepsin S has a weak collagenolytic activity, it is very efficient in hydrolyzing aggrecan[15] and thus may play a deleterious role in the integrity of the aggrecan-type II collagen network.

The development of assays specific for type II collagen breakdown represents a breakthrough in the field of biological markers for OA, given that degradation of collagen fibers is associated with irreversible cartilage destruction. Antibodies recognizing different type II collagen fragments have been developed (Fig. 12–2). Those directed against the neoepitopes generated by the collagenases include the so-called COL2-3/4 long mono or C2C which is specific of type II collagen and the COL2-3/4C Short or C1,2C which detects cleavages of both type II and type I collagen[10] and the type II collagen neoepitope (TIINE). These collagenase neoepitopes have mainly been used to demonstrate increased type II collagen cleavage in OA cartilage explants, although more recently they have been applied in synovial fluid and serum immunoassays both in animal models of OA[16] and in patients with knee OA.[17] More recently, other type II collagen markers have been identified including fragments of the triple helical domain (Helix-II, Coll 2-1)[18,19] and a fragment of the C-telopeptide (CTX-II)[20] (Fig. 12–2). Helix-II, Coll 2-1, and CTX-II have been shown to be increased in patients with knee and hip OA and rheumatoid arthritis (RA). The different type II collagen degradation fragments are likely to be released from articular cartilage by different biological pathways. Indeed, in vitro studies showed that Helix-II and CTX-II are released

from human cartilage by different cathepsins and MMPs, and immunohistochemistry experiments also indicate that Helix-II and CTX-II have distinct distributions in tissue sections of human articular OA cartilage.[21,22] Thus, their combination may better characterize the complex mechanisms of cartilage damage in arthritis than the use of one of these two biochemical markers alone. This also provides a biological basis for the independent and additive information given by Helix-II and CTX-II on disease progression in patients with hip OA[23] and in early RA.[18]

Cartilage matrix molecules including type II collagen can undergo post-translational modifications which can either be mediated by an enzymatic process or be spontaneous and age related. Measuring post-translational–modified cartilage matrix proteins may lead to the development of biochemical markers which can give valuable information on altered biological processes related to OA. Chondrocytes can express high levels of inducible and neuronal forms of nitric oxide synthetase which generate nitric oxide. Nitric oxide can then react with superoxide radical to form peroxynitite, a potent oxidizing radical that can in turn react with tyrosine residues of proteins to form nitrotyrosine. Two different assays recognizing a sequence—which can be either un-nitrosylated (Coll 2-1) or nitrosylated (Coll 2-1 NO_2) of the triple helix of type II collagen—have recently been developed.[19] Increased serum levels of Coll 2-1 and Coll 2-1 NO_2 have been reported in patients with knee OA. One-year changes of their urinary levels—but not baseline values—were modestly related to more rapid disease

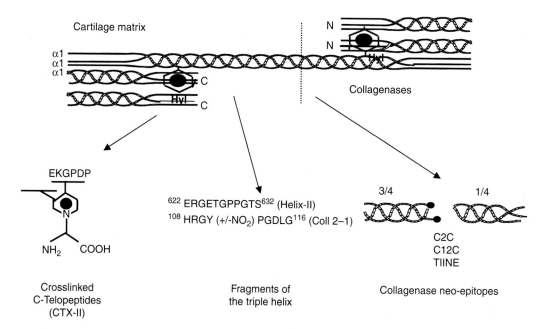

Figure 12–2 Type II collagen fragments as specific biological markers of cartilage degradation. Type II collagen is formed by the association of three identical α1 chains in triple helix except at the ends (telopeptides). In the extracellular matrix of cartilage, collagen molecules are cross-linked by pyridinoline (PYD) involving the telopeptide regions. During cartilage degradation, different molecules are released in synovial fluid, serum, and urine. These include neoepitopes generated by the collagenases (e.g., C2C, C12C, and TIINE), fragments of the triple helix (Helix-II and Col 2-1), and C terminal cross-linking telopeptides (CTX-II). See text for details.

progression of knee OA over 3 years.[24] It remains unclear, however, from these studies whether there is an additive value of investigating the nitrosylated form of type II collagen fragments in OA.

Markers of Aggrecan Turnover

Aggrecans are proteoglycans composed of a protein (core protein) and glycosaminoglycan (GAGs) chains that are covalently attached to the core protein (Fig. 12–1). The core protein of aggrecan has a molecular mass of approximately 230 kDa and consists of three globular domains, G1, G2, and G3, and two GAGs attachment domains, the keratan sulfate (KS) and the chondroitin sulfate (CS) domains. The total molecular mass can reach approximately 2.200 kDa.[25] The *G1 domain* has a structure consisting of three disulfide-bonded loops and interacts with hyaluronan in the formation of proteoaglycan aggregates. *The interglobular domain (IGD)* between the G1 and G2 domains is 90 amino-acid residues long, has a rod-shape, and contains proteolytic cleavage sites susceptible to a variety of proteinases including MMPs, aggrecanases including members of the *A Disintegrin And Metalloproteinase with ThromboSpondin* motifs family (ADAMTS) such as ADAMTS-5,[26] serine proteases such as plasmin and leukocyte elastase, and cysteine proteases such as cathepsin B and K.[7,8] After synthesis of the core protein by the chondrocytes, up to 50 *KS* chains [Gal β(14) GlucNAc β(1-3)] and 100 *CS* chains [GlcA β(1-3) GalNAc β](1-4)] are added during post-transcriptional processing, and together these carbohydrates make up more than 90% of the molecular mass. The *G3 domain* located at the C-terminus consists of three modules: epidermal growth factor (EGF)-like module, C-type lectin module, and complement regulatory proteins module. With aging, the population of aggrecan without the G3 domain increases in cartilage because of its proteolytic cleavage.

Putative markers of aggrecan synthesis include epitopes located on the CS chains of the aggrecan such as the 3-B-3, 7-D-4, and 846 epitope. The 3-B-3 (–) antibody recognizes atypical structures at the nonreducing terminal of the CS glycaminonoglycan side chains of the proteoglycans. The 7-D-4 antibody is directed against another atypical structure (sulfation pattern) in native CS GAGs of proteoglycans.[27,28] Epitopes 3-B-3 (–) and 846[29] are present in high concentration in fetal cartilage and almost absent in mature normal cartilage.[30–32] In contrast, epitope 7-D-4 is frequently found in normal adult cartilage.

The development of a specific biochemical marker of aggrecan degradation would be very interesting as aggrecan is more easily degraded than type II collagen and may thus be a sensitive indicator of early cartilage damage. However, increased levels of aggrecan fragments in synovial fluid and serum should be interpreted with caution. Indeed, although newly synthesized aggrecan molecules are particularly susceptible to degradation, the concentration of aggrecan fragments can actually increase as a result of an upregulation of aggrecan synthesis. Keeping this limitation in mind, it has been shown that the majority of aggrecan fragments found in the joint fluid from injured or OA

joints are large, but have lost the G1 domain.[33] These degradation fragments can be measured by immunoassays using antibodies against KS or the core protein. The ELISA using the antibody 5D4 (also called AgKS) remains the most used assay for quantifying smaller aggrecan-related molecules in serum.[34] Although several research groups have recently developed assays for the various neoepitopes in the protein portion of aggrecan, it is still unclear which of these epitopes is the most relevant to be measured in biological fluids, and clinical data are still limited.

Nonaggrecan and Noncollagen Proteins

Cartilage Oligomeric Matrix Protein (COMP). Among noncollagenous proteins, the most investigated cartilage marker is the protein so-called COMP. COMP is a 524 kDa homopentameric extracellular matrix glycoprotein (5 identical units of 755 amino acid), which belongs to the thrombospondin family. Each monomer is composed of an amino-terminal cysteine-rich domain, four epithelial growth factor (EGF)-like domains, eight calmodulin-like repeats, and a C-terminal globular domain.[35–37] The biological function of COMP is still unclear. Bovine and human proteins—but not rat protein—contain an Arg-Gly-Asp (RGD) sequence, suggesting that COMP may mediate cell binding through integrin. The carboxy-terminal globular domain binds to collagen I, II, and IX, suggesting that COMP may be involved in regulating fibril formation and maintaining integrity of collagen network. The fact that COMP may have important functions is also illustrated by the data showing that two human dominant skeletal dysplasias, pseudoachondroplasia and multiple epiphyseal dysplasia,[38–40] are associated with a mutation in the potentially Ca-binding domain of COMP gene. However, COMP-deficient mice do not have cartilage abnormalities,[41] suggesting that these human diseases are probably not caused by a reduced amount of COMP but by other mechanisms such as folding defects or extracellular assembly alterations due to potentially dysfunctional mutated COMP.

Originally felt to be cartilage specific, over the last years COMP has been identified in all structures of the joints including ligaments, meniscus, tendons, and synovium.[42] COMP was also found to be secreted by osteoblasts and vascular smooth muscle. In cartilage, synovial fluid, and serum of patients with OA, COMP has been shown to be present as the intact molecule and several fragments.[43] These fragments are likely to result from the activity of MMPs such as MMP-1, MMP-13, MMP-9, and ADAMTS4,[44] although it remains unknown which of these enzymes play the major role of COMP degradation in vivo. A careful epitope mapping is required and monoclonal antibodies specific for intact molecules and fragments would be very useful, especially for assessing the efficacy of MMP inhibitors in preventing cartilage destruction in patients with OA. Currently, however, available immunoassays based on polyclonal[45] or monoclonal antibodies[46] appear to detect both the intact molecule and fragments in body fluids.

Chitinase 3-like Protein 1 (YKL-40) and Chitinase 3-like Protein 2 (YKL-39). Chitinase 3-like protein 1 (YKL-40, also named human cartilage glycoprotein 39) and Chitinase 3-like protein 2 (YKL-39) are two different mammalian glycoproteins related in sequence to family 18 of bacterial and fungal Chitinases.[47] YKL-40 does not exhibit glycosidase activity against Chitinase substrates, as the glutamate in the active site Trp-Glu-Tyr-Pro is replaced by another amino acid. It was originally described as a major gene product of chondrocytes and synovial cells.[48] Subsequently however, mRNA for YKL-40 has also been detected in high amounts in the liver, which may be the main source of circulating YKL-40-, weakly in brain, kidney, and placenta, and undetectable in heart, lung, skeletal muscle, mononuclear cells, and skin fibroblasts.[48,49] The function of YKL-40 is unknown. One hypothesis is that increased expression of this protein by human articular chondrocytes and/or synovial cells in patients with OA/RA could increase the degradative capacity of these cells, although no proteolytic activity has been yet demonstrated including against hyaluronan.[48] Although serum YKL-40 has been reported to be increased in patients with knee OA or hip OA in some,[50,51] but not in all[52] studies, its clinical utility in OA remains unclear as it does not correlate with radiological damage[52] and progression.[53] YKL-40 may be a more interesting marker of disease progression in patients with RA[54] or cancer.[55-57]

It has been shown that YKL-39, but not YKL-40, was overexpressed in cartilage from patients with OA compared to healthy cartilage.[58,59] Autoantibodies to YKL-39 have also been reported in a proportion of patients with OA similar to patient with RA, suggesting that humoral response to this molecule may be involved in the pathophysiology of these arthritic diseases.[60,61] All together these preliminary data suggest that YKL-39 may be more specific for cartilage that YKL-40 and may prove to be a more sensitive biochemical marker of joint damage in OA, although data for synovial fluid and serum YKL-39 are still lacking.

Biochemical Markers of Bone Turnover

Bone turnover is characterized by two opposite activities, the formation of new bone by osteoblasts and the resorption of old bone by osteoclasts. The rate of formation or degradation of bone matrix can be assessed either by measuring an enzymatic activity of the bone-forming or bone-resorbing cells—such as alkaline and tartrate resistant acid phosphatase (TRACP)—or by measuring bone matrix components released into the circulation during formation or resorption (Table 12–1). Current bone turnover markers cannot discriminate between turnover changes in a specific skeletal envelope, i.e., trabecular versus cortical, or compartment, i.e., skeletal versus subchondral, but mainly reflect whole body net changes. These markers are usually separated into markers of formation and resorption, but it should be kept in mind that in disease states or following certain treatment where both events are coupled and change in the same direction, any marker will reflect the overall rate of bone turnover. Increasingly, specific

biochemical markers for bone remodelling have been identified in recent years and used mainly in osteoporosis (reviewed in Garnero and Delmas[62]).

At present, the most sensitive markers for bone formation are serum total osteocalcin—an hydroxyapatite-binding noncollagenous protein exclusively synthesized by osteoblasts, odontoblasts, and hypertrophic chondrocytes—bone alkaline phosphatase, and the procollagen type I N-terminal propeptide (PINP). Procollagen propeptides are cleaved by specific propeptidases and are partly released into the circulation from where they are cleared by liver endothelial cells. Most of the circulating propeptide pool originates from bone formation.

The majority of bone resorption markers are degradation products of collagen type I, which is the most abundant protein of bone tissue, except for TRACP isoenzyme 5b which reflects mainly the number of osteoclasts, some specific fragments of osteocalcin, and bone sialoprotein (BSP). During bone resorption, osteoclasts secrete different factors such as acid, matrix MMPs, and cathepsin K. These enzymes degrade type I collagen into several products including the hydroxypyridinium crosslinks of collagen pyridinoline (PYD) and deoxypyridinoline (DPD), the MMP product carboxyterminal telopeptide of type I collagen (ICTP), and the combined MMP and cathepsin K products type I cross-linked N- and C-telopeptide (NTX and CTX).[62] Partly degraded type I collagen is taken up by the osteoclast into vesicles. To these vesicles the enzyme TRACP 5b is added intracellularly which can further degrade the type I collagen breakdown products. The content of this vesicle is excreted from the cell at the apical side.[63] Immunological assays are now available for PYD and DPD in urine, for ICTP in serum, and for CTX, NTX both in serum or urine. Most of these biochemical marker assays are now available on automatic platforms with increased precision over manual assays and high throughput which allow convenient accurate measurements in large number of individuals.

The different type I collagen-related markers can respond differently in the presence of diseases and treatments, although there is limited data in OA. For example, serum and urine CTX and NTX levels are markedly increased in postmenopausal women with osteoporosis and their values decrease markedly and rapidly with antiresorptive therapy, contrasting with the slight and nonsignificant modifications of ICTP in these two conditions.[64] In contrast, serum ICTP is a sensitive marker in other pathological conditions including malignant bone diseases and RA.[65,66] These different responses are likely to result form differences in the enzymatic pathways leading to the release of CTX/NTX and ICTP from bone type I collagen (Fig. 12–3). Indeed, it has been shown that the peptide ICTP recognized by the antibody used in the immunoassay can be cleaved by cathepsin K, an osteoclastic- specific cysteine protease which is the key enzyme responsible for bone collagen degradation in normal physiological conditions. Thus, when cathepsin K is active, ICTP will be destroyed and not anymore recognized by the immunoassay resulting in low serum levels. Conversely, the peptide ICTP can be released from type I collagen by some MMPs including MMP-2.[67,68] Because of the important role played by MMPs in pathological bone degradation including bone

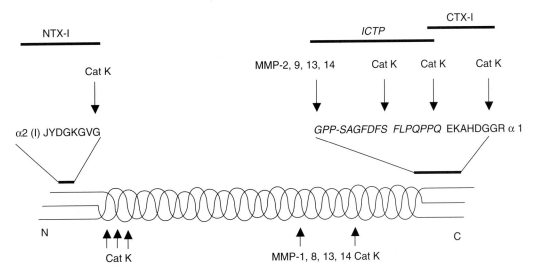

Figure 12–3 Schematic representation of the different type I collagen peptides used as markers of bone resorption and sites of cleavage by cathepsin K (Cat K) and matrix metalloproteases (MMPs). The NTX-I epitope and CTX-I epitopes in the N- and C-telopeptide regions, respectively, are efficiently generated by Cat K—the main enzyme responsible for type I collagen degradation in physiological conditions—but not directly by MMP which have been proposed to participate in bone resorption in physiological conditions, but also in arthritis. In contrast, ICTP epitope is destroyed by the action of Cat K and is generated by MMPs, especially MMP-2, and MMP-13.

metastases and arthritis, ICTP may be a sensitive marker in these conditions, although no data have yet been published in OA. In contrast, the CTX and NTX peptides are directly generated by the action of cathepsin K on collagen and their immunoreactivity can be further increased by subsequent degradation by MMPs.[68] The understanding of these enzymatic pathways is of crucial importance for the clinical interpretation of data under treatments especially with anti proteases.

More recently, new biochemical markers and assays for bone turnover have emerged. These include immunoassays for serum TRACP which preferentially detect the isoenzyme 5b, an enzyme predominantly expressed by the osteoclast.[69] TRACP 5b isoenzyme is likely to represent mainly the number and activity of osteoclasts and not directly the rate of bone matrix degradation in contrast to the type I collagen–related markers.

Although most of the newly synthesized osteocalcin is captured by bone matrix, a small fraction is released into the blood where it can be detected by immunoassays and is currently considered as a specific bone formation marker. Circulating osteocalcin is constituted of different immunoreactive forms including the intact molecule, but also various fragments.[70] It has been shown that the majority of circulating fragments arises from the in vivo degradation of the intact molecule and thus also reflects bone formation.[70] However, some of these fragments could also be released from the degradation of bone matrix, resistant to glomeral filtration and accumulated in urine.[71] Using urine samples from patients with Paget disease, a peptide has recently been isolated corresponding to the mid 14-28 molecule sequence of human osteocalcin, and elevated levels were reported in osteoporotic postmenopausal women.[72] From a theoretical point of view, urinary osteocalcin

fragments may be more specific for bone resorption than type I collagen-related markers, although their clinical value in OA remains to be evaluated.

BSP, a 60- to 70-kDa phosphorylated glycoprotein, could be involved in the mineralization process. Interestingly, and in contrast to the other bone proteins, BSP has a relatively restricted distribution to the osteocartilagenous interfaces that are involved early in OA.[73] The early involvement of this area in OA has led to the suggestion that serum BSP may be a sensitive indicator for alterations of subcondral bone turnover. Various assays for BSP have been developed including that of the group of Heinegard which has been used in several studies.[74] In serum, BSP was shown to be increased in knee OA, with highest levels in those patients with bone scan abnormalities.[75] Although baseline levels were not different between progressors and nonprogressors in patients with early stage OA[76] and in hip OA,[77] an increase of BSP over 3 years was reported to be associated with progressive OA. However, available immunoassays require technical improvements especially in the characterization of the different circulating immunoreactive forms and few studies using this marker in OA have been published in the last few years. Finally, an emerging bone resorption marker is serum cathepsin K. An immunoassay for serum cathepsin K has recently been developed, and increased levels were reported in patients with RA, levels correlating with radiological damage.[78] Whether measurement of serum cathepsin K will prove to be useful in OA remains to be investigated. In summary, although bone turnover markers may reflect the focal abnormalities of bone metabolism in OA, circulating and urinary levels are more likely to reflect the overall skeletal turnover, which may be influenced by a variety of conditions including age, menopausal status, osteoporosis, and other bone diseases. This may explain the discordant results observed with bone markers across the different studies in patients with OA (for a review, see Garnero[79]). Consequently, most studies have concentrated on the development of specific biochemical markers of cartilage and synovium turnover.

Biochemical Markers of Synovium Turnover and Systemic Inflammation

Investigation of synovial tissue metabolism in OA has received little attention. However, there is increasing evidence indicating alterations in synovial tissue metabolism in a significant proportion of patients with OA[80] as well as a correlation between the severity of synovitis and the progression of joint destruction.[81] Thus, the development of biological markers specific to the synovial membrane is of particular interest. Several markers have been proposed to assess synovitis and inflammation in OA. Increased systemic inflammation in OA can be detected by ultrasensitive assays for CRP; discrepant findings have been generated. Although most studies found an association between serum CRP levels with the degree of joint damage and/or progression of the disease in OA,[82,83] this relationship may be confounded by obesity as recently shown in American populations.[84] In addition, CRP is not joint specific and can be affected by other chronic medical conditions, suggesting that it is unlikely to be a useful marker in OA. Consequently, developing biochemical markers more specifically reflecting the activity of the synoviocytes or the turnover of the synovial tissue may be an attractive approach to investigate the importance of synovitis in OA initiation or progression.

Synovium Tissue Structure

The essential elements of synovium are a surface layer of cells (or intima or synovial lining), a superficial microvasculature net, and a connective tissue substratum (or subintima, or subsynovium).[85] The synovial lining (or intima) is only a few cell layers deep, typically around 3. It averages about 50 μm in normal human knee. Most of the cells are macrophages or specialized fibroblasts. Immediately beneath the synovial lining, there is a net of capillaries which promote rapid transfer of water and lipid soluble solutes like electrolytes, glucose, amino acids, and nonprotein-bound drugs. The passive ultrafiltrate of plasma and exit of leucocytes across the walls of the synovial capilarities forms the synovial fluid.[86] All proteins of plasma are also found in the synovial fluid but at decreased concentration due to molecular sieving by the capillary wall. Albumin is the predominant protein of the synovial fluid and dominates the colloid osmotic pressure. The components that make the synovial fluid unusual are *hyaluronan* (HA) and *lubricin*, two biopoymers that are actively secreted by the synovial lining cells. HA is a high molecular weight glycosaminoglycan consisting of alternating units of β(1-4) linked N-acetyl-β-D-glucosamine and β(1-3) linked β-D-glucuronic acid. Its molecular weight in synovial fluid from healthy adults is approximately 3 to 5.10^6 MW and its concentration range is 3 to 5.10^6 Da mg/mL. Lubricin, a product of the gene proteoglycan 4 (*PRG4*), is a major component of synovial fluid and participates in the boundary lubrication of synovial fluids.[87,88] The synovial lining has no distinct outer border. However, at a depth of about 20 to 50 μm, the lining gives way to the *subsynovium*. Subsynovium contains a plexus of fine *lymphatic vessels* which are important for synovial fluid regulation because they drain excess fluid from the joint cavity, maintaining a subatmospheric pressure in the joint. These lymphatics are also the unique route by which macromolecules like plasma protein, hyaluronan, and partly degraded cartilage macromolecules are removed from the joint.[89] The only other means of removal of intra-articular macromolecules is by local degradation. *Subsynovium extracellular* matrix is mainly composed of type I and type III collagens, which differ in structure from type I and type III collagens of other connective tissues by posttranslational modifications including glycosylations of hydroxylysine residues. In addition to collagens, the extracellular matrix of subsynovium is composed of GAG (sulfates GAGs and hyaluronan) and structural glycoproteins including fibronectin, laminin, entactin (a sulfated glycoprotein with high affinity for laminin), and tenascin. Both chondroitine 4 sulfate (S) and 6S are secreted by synovial cells.

Biochemical Markers of Synovial Tissue Activity

Based on the above structure, the activity of the synovial membrane can be more specifically evaluated by the measurement of serum levels of N-propeptide of type I and type III procollagen, reflecting the synthesis of the most abundant collagens of subsynovium, noncollagenous proteins such HA, and the various enzymes secreted by the synoviocytes including MMP-3.

HA can be measured by employing the specific binding of the G1 domain of aggrecan to HA.[90] HA is carried from the joint to the blood by lymph and it is rapidly taken up by the liver, although a minor part may be removed by the kidney and thus its levels are markedly increased in patients with liver diseases.[91] Increased HA serum levels have been reported in patients with knee and hip OA, levels correlating with the number of joints involved[92] and independently with sex, age, body mass index and comorbidities (Fig. 12–4), and radiological progression.[93,94] Thus, serum HA appears as a potential prognostic marker of joint destruction in OA provided that hepatic function is not altered.

As discussed before, proteases such as the collagenases MMP-1 and MMP-13 and stromelysin-1 (MMP-3) are considered to play an important role in joint damage associated with OA. When synovitis is present, these enzymes are secreted by synovial cells in increased amounts. In patients with OA, increased levels of MMP-3 in the synovial fluid have been observed.[95] More recently, higher serum levels of MMP-3 have been reported to be associated with greater risk of radiological progression in women with knee OA.[96]

All biochemical markers discussed above are not specific to synovial tissue. We have characterized a glycosylated

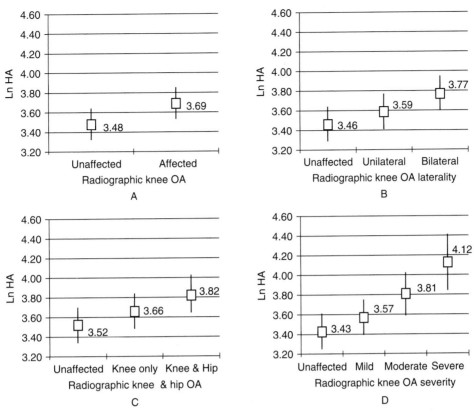

Figure 12–4 Serum levels of hyaluronic acid (HA) according to radiographic knee osteoarthritis (OA), radiographic knee OA laterality, radiographic knee and hip OA, and radiographic knee severity in 753 individuals from the Johnston County Osteoarthritic Project cohort. The figures show the mean levels of log-transformed HA values in each subgroup adjusted for ethnicity, sex, age, body mass index, gout, and circulation problems. Differences in HA levels were statistically significant for all comparisons ($P < 0.005$). (From Elliot AL, Kraus VB, Luta G, et al. Serum hyaluronan levels and radiographic knee and hip osteoarthritis in African Americans and Caucasians in the Johnston County Osteoarthritis Project. Arthritis Rheum 52:105–111, 2005.)

pyridinoline derivative, glucosyl-galactosyl-pyridinoline (Glc-Gal-PYD), which is found in large amounts in human synovium and in very low levels in the cartilage and other soft tissues.[97] The specificity of Glc-Gal-PYD for synovial tissue has also been demonstrated in ex vivo models of human joint tissue degradation, indicating that this marker was released in the supernatant of synovium tissue but not of cartilage and bone. Urinary Glc-Gal-PYD has been found to be significantly increased in patients with knee OA,[52,98,99] especially in those presenting with knee swelling[98] (Fig. 12–5). Increased levels were also found to be associated with decreased joint space width[98,99] and worse clinical symptoms.[52]

New Marker Methodologies

Current OA biochemical markers are individually measured by immuno- or chromatographic assays. Because OA is an organ disease with different tissues and biological processes involved, a combination of a panel of biochemical markers will probably be more powerful to investigate joint damage than single biomarker assessment. This strategy has been recently supported by an analysis of ten different biochemical markers each measured by single immunoassay in the Evaluation of the

CHOndromodulating effect of DIAcerein in osteoarthritis of the Hip (ECHODIAH) cohort of patients with hip OA. Using principal component analysis we could segregate the ten markers into five independent clusters which were believed to be representative of different pathophysiological processes such as cartilage and bone turnover, synovitis, systemic inflammation, and MMP-1 and MMP-9 activities.[100] Interestingly, new approaches have recently been applied for identifying and assaying OA biochemical markers including genomics, proteomics, and metabolomics. These new methodologies coupled with sophisticated data analysis methods should allow the simultaneous analyses of multiple markers.

Marshall et al.[101] used a genomic approach based on isolation of mRNA from circulating blood to identify six genes which were significantly downregulated in patients with mild OA—according to arthroscopy assessment—compared to healthy controls. A combination of these six genes in a multiple variable model was able to correctly identify 85% with mild OA and controls. Proteomic generally involves separation of proteins by two-dimensional (2D) electrophoresis followed by their identification using mass spectroscopy. Proteomic analysis has recently been successfully used to identify biochemical markers related to disease development and progression but also

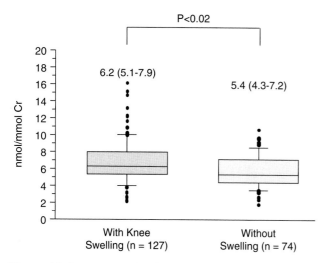

Figure 12–5 Urinary levels of glucosyl-galactosyl pyridinoline, a biochemical marker of synovial tissue activity, in patients with knee osteoarthritis presenting with or without knee swelling. (From Gineyts E, Mo JA, Ko A, et al. Effects of ibuprofen on molecular markers of cartilage and synovium turnover in patients with knee osteoarthritis. Ann Rheum Dis 63:857–861, 2004.)

autoimmunity in OA. Applying 2D electrophoresis to human chondrocyte extracts followed by reaction with serum samples from 20 patients with OA, 20 patients with RA, and 20 healthy controls, Xiang et al.[102] identified 19 auto-antigens specific to OA, 11 specific to RA, and 22 which were common to the two diseases. Triosephosphate isomerase (TPI) was subsequently identified by mass-spectroscopy as one of the unique OA autoantigens. Indeed, immunoglobulin anti-TPI auto-antibodies were detected in about 25% of OA serum and synovial fluid samples but in fewer than 6% of patients with RA or lupus. Presence of anti-TPI autoantibodies in patients with OA was associated with lower radiographic grade. This study underscores the importance of autoimmunity, which is a well-recognized etiologic factor in RA, in the physiopathology of OA, and in the potential of using autoantibodies as diagnostic biochemical markers of OA. Another new approach is metabolomics which consists in the determination of a profile of metabolites specific to patients with OA. Using nuclear MR spectroscopy followed by principal component analysis, it has been reported that urinary hydroxybutyrate, pyruvate, creatine/creatinine, and glycerol were increased in 45 patients with knee or hip OA compared to healthy controls, suggesting altered energy utilization in OA.[103]

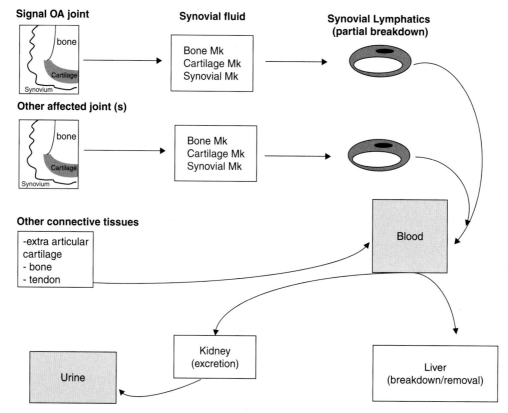

Figure 12–6 Sources and metabolism of biochemical markers of joint tissue turnover. Biochemical markers generated by synthesis or degradation of cartilage matrix, bone, or synovial tissue are released into the joint fluid compartment. They are then cleared through the synovial membrane into lymphatic vessels and then released in the circulation. Some fragments found in blood can also originate from turnover of the matrix of extra-articular connective tissues. Most of the markers are taken up and degraded in the liver and some specific fragments are further excreted by the kidney and found in urine. (Adapted from Young-Min SA, Cawston TE, Griffiths ID. Markers of joint destruction: principles, problems, and potential. Ann Rheum Dis 60:545–549, 2001.)

These technical developments will ultimately allow identifying a panel of biochemical markers which could then be assessed simultaneously by microarray platforms. This strategy was recently used in a case control study of the Baltimore Longitudinal Study of Aging to analyze 160 candidate blood proteins implicated in tissue matrix degradation, cellular activation, and inflammation. It was shown that a combination of a few of these proteins were already differently expressed in the 21 patients with no OA at the time of investigation who developed OA in the following 10 years compared to the 66 individuals who remained free of radiological disease.[104] Because the outcome of the studies using these novel technologies is highly dependent on sample collection and data processing—for which standardization is still lacking—these findings obtained on a small number of patients will have to be independently replicated in larger samples.

Factors that Influence Interpretation of Osteoarthritis Biochemical Markers

Levels of biochemical markers measured in blood or urine (because assessment of synovial fluid is often impracticable) provide information on systemic skeletal tissue turnover and are not necessarily specific of the alterations occurring in the signal joint (Fig. 12–6). For example, it has been shown that degenerative disease of the knees, hips, hands, and lumbar discs contributed independently and additively to urinary CTX-II levels, clearly illustrating the total body contribution to systemic levels.[105,106] The potential contribution of intervertebral discs is of particular relevance because disc degeneration is common with aging. Accordingly, adjusting systemic levels by a total body OA score based on radiographic damage and cartilage volume estimated by quantitative MRI would be an attractive approach to analyze and clinically interpret data of OA biochemical markers.[107] The normal extra-articular turnover of connective tissue matrix may also contribute to the pool of circulating biochemical markers. Thus any contribution from affected joints is small and may not always significantly alter the overall level (Fig. 12–6). The clearance of the markers from the joint compartment to body fluids is complex and can involve changes in structure or metabolism of the markers. The processing of the markers in the liver and kidney which occur before levels reach a steady state in blood and urine varies across individuals and can increase with inflammation, after joint mobilization and exercise.[108-110] Serum and urinary levels of most biochemical markers also vary with sex, age, menopausal status, and ethnicity, and OA risk factors such as body mass index. In a 6-week randomized controlled trial of patients with painful knee OA, it has been reported that ibuprofen (and also the COX-2 specific inhibitor rofecoxib) prevented the significant elevation of CTX-II and Glc-Gal-PYD observed in patients receiving placebo.[98] Although it remains to be determined whether nonsteroidal anti-inflammatory drugs have disease-modifying effects, these data underscore that commonly prescribed therapy in OA may be a confounding factor in biochemical marker clinical studies.

CLINICAL USES OF BIOLOGICAL MARKERS FOR OSTEOARTHRITIS

Early Diagnosis

Several cross-sectional studies have found elevated or decreased levels of biological markers in knee and hip OA, as compared to healthy sex- and age-matched controls. Because the levels of most of these markers in unaffected subjects are influenced by sex, age, body mass index (BMI), and hormone replacement therapy, it is important to adjust for these factors to judge the diagnostic value of markers. Most of these cross-sectional studies also showed an association between serum and urinary levels of the markers with the extent of radiological joint damage and/or clinical indices of disease activity (for a review, see Garnero[79]). These studies however clearly demonstrated that there is a large overlap in marker levels between OA patients and healthy age- and sex-matched controls, indicating that the measurement of a single one of the currently available markers are probably insufficiently sensitive to be useful for the diagnosis of OA. Important limitations to these cross-sectional studies need, however, to be considered. Indeed, most of the studies did not perform radiological assessment in apparently healthy individuals. Thus, it is likely that a significant proportion of controls have asymptomatic OA in one or a few joints which would then lead to an underestimation of the true diagnostic accuracy of the markers. Another issue is that these studies included mainly patients with advanced disease as the selection was based on a radiological Kelgreen and Lawrence (K/L) score at or above 2. Because biochemical markers reflect dynamic changes in tissue turnover, their levels are likely to be altered well before radiological damage. Consequently, for assessing the diagnostic utility of biochemical markers, it may be more appropriate to include patients with early OA which may be identified using sensitive imaging modalities such as MRI. We recently reported an association between urinary CTX-II and and MRI findings related to the severity of bone marrow abnormalities suggested to be an early feature of OA[111] (Fig. 12–7). In the near future, many more studies relating biochemical markers with the various MRI features of the joint will be undertaken and should bring valuable information for the biological interpretation of both of these two diagnostic modalities.

Prediction of Progression

Progression in OA shows considerable variation across individuals and the predictive capacity of clinical indices is poor. Because of the current inability to differentiate patients who will progress from nonprogressors, both groups of patients are included in clinical trials of disease modifying OA (DMOAD). This usually results in a limited sensitivity in measurement of disease progression and consequently adds to duration, number of patients, and ultimately to the cost of the study. Having the possibility of recruiting a more homogeneous population of OA progressors in clinical trails would thus be highly

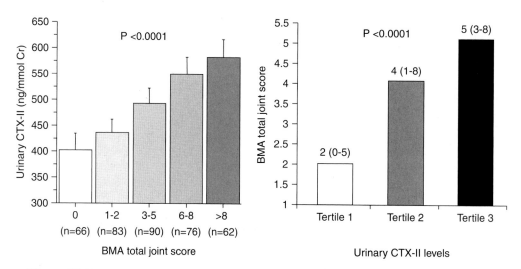

Figure 12–7 Association between the extent of knee bone marrow abnormalities (BMA) and urinary CTX-II levels in 377 patients with painful knee osteoarthritis (OA). Femoral and tibial condyles and patella were divided into eight sites for scoring of BMA. A BMA was defined as an area of increased signal on T_2-weighted images by magnetic resonance imaging of the subchondral bone. *Left panel*: Patients were categorized according to the extent of total joint BMA. The bars show the mean + SE of urinary CTX-II levels. *Right panel*: Patients were categorized in tertile of urinary CTX-II. The bars represent the median (25; 75 percentile) of total joint BMA score in each tertile of urinary CTX-II levels. *P* values for differences between groups after adjustment for age, gender, and body mass index. (From Garnero P, Peterfy C, Zaim S, et al. Bone marrow abnormality on magnetic resonance imaging is associated with type II collagen degradation in knee osteoarthritis: a three-month longitudinal study. Arthritis Rheum 52:2822–2829, 2005.)

advantageous to faster drug development. Recent longitudinal studies are in this respect encouraging as they suggest that a combination of some new biochemical markers may have a role in predicting disease progression. In a large population-based cohort of 1235 men and women, it was found that baseline levels of urinary CTX-II in the highest quartile was associated with a six- to eightfold higher risk of radiological progression of knee and hip OA in the subsequent 6.6 years compared to individuals with levels in the lowest quartile. Importantly, this association was independent of other risk factors of disease progression such as age, sex, body mass index, lower limb disability index, and baseline radiographic OA.[112] Increased baseline COMP levels were also shown to be associated with loss of JSW over 3 years in a small population of patients with established knee OA.[113] Sharif et al.[114] followed a group of patients with early knee OA (37% with a K/L score <2) prospectively for 5 years (Fig. 12–8). They showed that progression was not linear over this period and that serum COMP, which was measured every 6 months, was associated with this phasic pattern of progression.[114] One could argue that assessment of progression in these studies is unreliable because they were based on the measurement of joint space narrowing (JSN) using standard standing anterior-posterior radiographs. This concern is especially relevant for short-term studies in knee OA but of less critical importance for the hip and long-term evaluation. Interestingly, higher levels of serum MMP-3 have recently been reported to be associated with greater JSN measured over 30 months using state-of-the-art radiography positioning in women with knee OA participating in a randomized trail of doxycycline.[96]

Progression of joint destruction in OA is complex as it involves interaction of several tissues and different pathophysiologic pathways that are likely to not be adequately represented by the measurement of a single biochemical marker. In a prospective study of 52 patients with established knee OA, we found that low serum levels of PIIANP (in late OA type II collagen synthesis decreases) or high urinary CTX-II excretion were associated with faster joint destruction as evaluated over a 1-year period, either by plain radiographs or by arthroscopy.[115] Combining these two biological markers to obtain an index of uncoupling of type II collagen synthesis and breakdown was more effective in predicting cartilage destruction than measurements of a single marker (Fig. 12–9). Similar findings were reported in a longitudinal 5-year study of 84 patients with early knee OA, where the combination of increased serum PIIANP (in early OA type II collagen synthesis increases) with increased urinary CTX-II allowed identification of 92% of patients who showed radiological progression whereas one of these two markers when used alone could identify 40% to 70% of patients who progressed.[4] In the evaluation of the chondromodulating effect of diacerein in. OA of the hip (ECHODIAH) cohort of patients with hip OA followed over 3 years, we found that among ten different molecular markers, increased serum levels of hyaluronic acid and urinary CTX-II were significantly associated with increased risk of progression independently of other risk factors (Table 12–2).[53] Interestingly, the combination of urinary CTX-II with HA was more predictive than one of these markers alone. Indeed, the third of patients with the highest levels of CTX-II *or* HA had a risk of progression which was

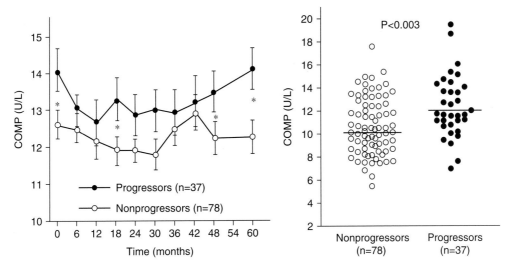

Figure 12–8 Longitudinal changes of serum cartilage oligomeric matrix protein (COMP) in patients with early knee osteoarthritis (OA) with and without progression. Serum COMP was measured every 6 months for 5 years in 115 patients with early knee OA (37% of patients with Kellgren-Lawrence score <2). Over 5 years, 37 patients progressed (joint space narrowing ≥2 mm or total knee replacement), whereas the other 78 did not show progression. *Left panel*: shows the mean and SE values in progressor and nonprogressor patients at each time point (*P <0.05 vs. nonprogressors). *Right panel*: shows individual 5-year average COMP values in progressor and nonprogressor patients. (From Sharif M, Kirwan JR, Elson CJ, et al. Suggestion of nonlinear or phasic progression of knee osteoarthritis based on measurements of serum cartilage oligomeric matrix protein levels over 5 years. Arthritis Rheum 50:2479–2488, 2004.)

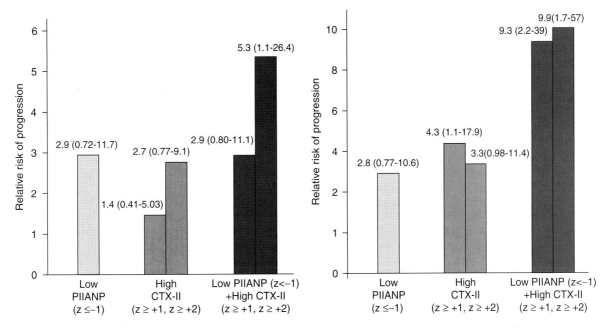

Figure 12–9 Relative risk (95% confidence interval) of disease progression over 1 year in patients with low and high levels of biochemical markers of type II collagen synthesis and degradation at baseline in 52 patients with established knee osteoarthritis. Low levels of serum N-propeptide of type IIA procollagen (PIIANP, marker of type II collagen synthesis) were those below the mean − 1 SD of healthy controls (Z ≤–1). High levels of urinary C-terminal cross-linking telopeptide of type II collagen (CTX-II, type II collagen degradation) were those which exceeded the mean + 1SD (z ≥+1) or 2SD (z ≥+2) of healthy controls. *Left panel*: Progression was assessed by changes in joint space width (JSW) on radiography (decrease of JSW 0.5 mm). *Right panel*: Progression was assessed by changes of a visual analogue scale (VAS) score of artroscopic chondropathy (VAS increase >8 units). (From Garnero P, Ayral X, Rousseau J-C, et al. Uncoupling of type II collagen synthesis and degradation predicts progression of joint damage in patients with knee osteoarthritis. Arthritis Rheum 46:2613–2624, 2002.)

TABLE 12–2

BIOCHEMICAL MARKERS OF CARTILAGE DEGRADATION (URINARY CTX-II) AND SYNOVITIS (SERUM HYALURONIC ACID, HA) AS INDEPENDENT PREDICTOR OF DISEASE PROGRESSION IN HIP OSTEOARTHRITIS (OA): THE ECHODIAH COHORT*

Parameters at Baseline	Cut-offs		Percent of Patients with Progression at 3 years		Relative Risk (95% CI)	P
Sex	Male	Female	57%	62%	1.20 (0.88–1.63)	0.2504
Age	<66 (yr)	≥66 (yr)	56%	67%	1.21 (0.90–1.63)	0.2099
Functional impairment (Lesquenes index)	<2	≥2	50%	65%	1.52 (1.10–2.07)	0.0101
Joint space width	≥2 mm	<2 mm	54%	70%	1.36 (1.02–1.82)	0.0373
Femoral head migration	Superomedial/ concentric	Lateral	45%	67%	2.34 (1.66–3.30)	<0.0001
Treatment modalities	Placebo	Diacerein	64%	55%	0.72(0.54–0.96)	0.0274
CTX-II (ng/mmol crea	≤346 (low and medium tertile)	>346 (highest tertile)	51%	77%	2.00 (1.49–2.70)	<0.0001
sHA (mg/mL)	≤137 (low and medium tertile)	>137 (highest tertile)	54%	73%	1.69 (1.25-2–27)	0.0006

*Three hundred and three patients with painful hip OA were randomized to diacerein or placebo in a multicenter, prospective, double-blind, 3-year follow-up trial. Structural progression was defined as a joint space decrease ≥0.5 or greater) 0.5 mm or requirement for total hip replacement. The table shows the relative risks of structural progression associated with clinical and radiographic parameters and biochemical marker levels at baseline. From Mazières B, Garnero P, Guéguen A, et al. Molecular markers of cartilage breakdown and synovitis at baseline as predictors of structural progression of hip osteoarthritis. The Echodiah cohort. Ann Rheum Dis, 65:354–359, 2006.

increased by 1.8- to 2-fold compared to the rest of the patients, whereas this risk was multiplied by 3.7 in the 13% of patients that had *both* markers elevated.

Monitoring Efficacy of Disease Modifying Osteoarthritis Treatment

One of the main issues which currently impair efficient development of structure OA modifying therapies is the low sensitivity of plain radiographs requiring long-term studies involving large number of patients to show a significant difference between placebo and active-drug treated patients. Biological markers may prove capable of providing earlier information compared to demonstration of slowing of JSN by x-ray (Fig. 12–10). The paucity of data on the potential role of biological markers for monitoring the treatment of OA is chiefly ascribed to the absence of medications with established chondroprotective activity. In a randomized clinical trial of 137 subjects with knee pain, no significant effect of glucosamine sulfate could be demonstrated on the serum and urinary levels of the type II collagen neopitopes C2C and C12C after 6 months of treatment.[17] Similar findings were reported in another 3-year placebo controlled trial of glucosamine sulfate using CTX-II as a marker of cartilage breakdown.[116] These negative findings can be explained either by the lack of sensitivity of the particular markers utilized in these studies to this particular treatment or the lack of efficacy of glucosamine sulfate to decrease cartilage damage as the disease-modifying activity of this compound is still debated. However, in the second trial a significant effect of glucosamine sulfate on

urinary CTX-II was observed in the subgroup of patients that had high pretreatment CTX-II levels,[116] suggesting that patients with high cartilage turnover may have a greater therapeutic response to DMOADs.

Antiresorptive bone agents currently used for the treatment of postmenopausal osteoporosis have been suggested to play a role as DMOADs mainly because of the importance of subchondral bone remodeling in OA initiation and/or progression. Animal models of OA have

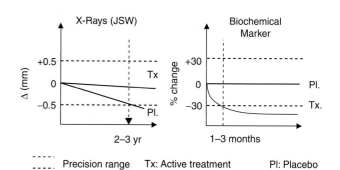

Figure 12–10 Radiography and biochemical markers to monitor efficacy of disease modifying osteoarthritis treatment. *Left panel:* Based on the reproducibility and sensitivity to change of measurement of joint space width by plain radiography, duration of 2 to 3 years is usually required to demonstrate differences of progression between active treated patients (Tx) and those receiving a placebo (Pl). *Right panel:* Although the variability of biochemical measurements is larger than that of radiography, the change under treatment is larger and faster. Consequently, a significant difference between Tx. and Pl. groups is likely to be observed within 1 to 3 months.

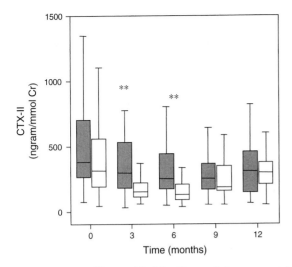

Combined discriminative capacity of urinary CTX-II (absolute values), measured at baseline and 3 months after the start of therapy, for detecting patients with no long-term radiographic progression		
CTX-II levels* (baseline/3months)	No progression (<2 Sharp-units/year)	Odds ratio of no progression (95% CI)
Increased/increased (n=71)	18**	1.0 (reference)
Increased/normal (n=20)	50**	4.5 (1.5 to 13)***
Normal/normal (n=13)	69**	10 (2.7 to 38)***

*The cut-off value between normal and increased levels is 150 ng/mmol creatinine
**Figures are percentages of patients with no progression at 5 years per group of CTX-levels
***Odds ratios relative to the reference category

Figure 12–11 Effects of disease modyfing antirheumatic therapy (DMARD) on urinary CTX-II and relationships with long-term radiological progression in rheumatoid arthritis (RA): The COBRA study. One hundred and ten patients with early RA (<2 years, median 4 months, no previous DMARD) were randomized to either an aggressive step-down combination therapy (COBRA, including temporary high-dose prednisolone, temporary low-dose methotrexate, and sulfasalazine) or mild monotherapy (sulfasalazine). Urinary CTX-II was measured at baseline and 3, 6, 9, and 12 months after treatment initiation. Radiographs of the hands, wrists, and feet were obtained at baseline, week 28, and week 56 and approximately every year thereafter for 5 years. Radiographs were read according to van der Heijde's modification of the Sharp-score, using the mean of two independent readers. *Left panel:* Changes of urinary CTX-II in patients treated with COBRA (empty boxes) or sulfasalazine (filled boxes). * *P* <0.001 for differences in changes between the two groups. From the bottom up, the box indicates the 25th, 50th (median), and 75th percentiles, while the bars indicate the 10th and 90th per-centiles, respectively. *Right panel:* Relative risk of no radiological progression at 5 years according to baseline and 3-month levels of urinary CTX-II in combined COBRA and sulfasalazine treated patients. (From Landewé R, Geusens P, Maarten B, et al. Markers for type II collagen breakdown predict the effect of disease modifying treatment on long-term radiographic progression in patients with RA: The Cobra study. Arthritis Rheum 50:1390–1399, 2004.)

indeed shown that agents such as the bisphosphonates risedronate, alendronate, and zoledronate, calcitonin, estrogens, and selective estrogen-receptor modulators (SERM) could partially prevent progression of joint damage. A series of recent studies has investigated the effects of these treatments on urinary CTX-II using stored samples from randomized placebo-controlled clinical trials in post-menopausal women. They showed that bone-effective doses of oral and transdermal 17β estradiol[117] the SERM levormeloxifene,[118] and the bisphosphonates alendronate and ibandronate[119] significantly decreased urinary CTX-II within 3 to 6 months. The decrease of CTX-II was dose dependent for the bisphosphonates and calcitonin, but not for estradiol and levormeloxifene. The magnitude of reduction of CTX-II was about 50% lower than that observed for the type I collagen biochemical markers of bone resorption urinary NTX-I or CTX-I, with the exception of levormeloxifene. More recently, a dose-dependent effect of the bisphosphonate risedronate on urinary CTX-II was also found in patients with knee OA.[120,121] The biological and clinical interpretation of these findings requires further investigation. Indeed, the decrease of CTX-II could result from indirect effects of these drugs on subchondral bone turnover or a direct action on cartilage metabolism which has been suggested, for example, for calcitonin. Because it remains to be shown that these therapies indeed have disease-modifying activity in humans with OA, the clinical relevance of these changes to predict efficacy on

joint damage also remains to be investigated. RA may serve as a model to validate biochemical markers as surrogate markers of efficacy because efficient disease-modifying antirheumatic drugs (DMARDs) are available. In a ran-domized study of the combined sulphasalazine-methotrexate-prednisone therapy in early RA, we showed that the magnitude of CTX-II decrease at 3 months was associated with changes in radiological scores after 5 years independently of the changes in disease activity and inflammation[122] (Fig. 12–11). These data suggest that early changes of biochemical markers of cartilage turnover may predict long-term structural efficacy of treatment in RA and potentially in OA, a hypothesis that will be possible to val-idate once effective DMOADs are available.

CONCLUSION

Biochemical markers of OA are increasingly tissue and process specific. The influences of the various factors that could obscure their clinical interpretation need to be better characterized. The panel of new markers is likely to expand with the optimization of genomic/proteomic-based tech-nologies. An optimal combination of biochemical markers is likely to be useful for identifying OA patients at increased risk for disease progression and to speed the development of DMOADs.

REFERENCES

1. Gray ML, Eckstein F, Peterfy C, et al. Toward imaging biomarkers for osteoarthritis. Clin Orthop Relat Res 427(Suppl):S175–181, 2004.
2. Heinegard D, Bayliss M, Lorenzo P. Biochemistry and metabolism of normal and osteoarthritic cartilage. In Brandt KD, Doherty M, Lohmander LS, eds. Osteoarthritis, Oxford, UK, Oxford Medical Publications, 1998.
3. Aigner T, Zhu Y, Chansky HH, et al. Re-expression of type II A procollagen by adult articular chondrocytes in osteoarthritic cartilage. Arthritis Rheum 42:1443–1450, 1999.
4. Garnero P, Sharif M, Charni1 N, et al. A 5 year longitudinal study of type II collagen synthesis and degradation and their association with disease progression in early knee osteoarthritis. Arthritis Rheum 52(Suppl):S74, 2005.
5. Rousseau JC, Sandell LJ, Delmas PD, et al. Development and clinical application in arthritis of a new immunoassay for serum type IIA procollagen NH2 propeptide. Human Reproduction. Methods Mol Med 101:25–38, 2004.
6. Lippielllo L, Hall D, Mankin HJ. Collagen synthesis in normal and osteoarthritic human cartilage. J Clin Invest 59:593–600, 1997.
7. Burrage PS, Mix KS, Brinckerhoff CE. Matrix metalloproteinases: role in arthritis. Front Biosci. 11:529–543, 2006.
8. Yasuda Y, Kaleta J, Brömme D. The role of cathepsins in osteoporosis and arthritis: rational for the design of new therapies. Adv Drug Delivery Rev 57:973–993, 2005.
9. Mudget JS, Hutchinson NI, Chatrain NA, et al. Susceptibility of stromelysin 1-deficient mice to collagen-induced arthritis and cartilage destruction. Arthritis Rheum 41:110–121, 1998.
10. Billinghurst RC, Dahlberg L, Ionescu M, et al. Enhanced cleavage of type II collagen by collagenase in osteoarthritic articular cartilage. J Clin Invest 99:1534–1545, 1997.
11. Garnero P, Borel O, Byrjalsen I, et al. The collagenolytic activity of cathepsin K is unique among mammalian proteinases. J Biol Chem 273:32347–32352, 1998.
12. Kafienah W, Bromme D, Buttle DJ, et al. Human cathepsin K cleaves native type I and II collagens at the N-terminal end of the triple helix. Biochem J 331:727–732, 1998.
13. Konttinen YT, Mandelin J, Li TF, et al. Acidic cysteine endoproteinase cathepsin K in the degeneration of the superficial articular hyaline cartilage in osteoarthritis. Arthritis Rheum 46:953–960, 2002.
14. Morko JP, Soderstrom M, Saamanen AM, et al. Up regulaton of cathepsin K expression in articular chondrocytes in a transgenic mouse model for osteoarthritis. Ann Rheum Dis 63:649–655, 2004.
15. Hou WS, Li Z, Buttner FH, et al. Cleavage site specificity of cathepsin K toward cartilage proteoglycans and protease complex formation Biol Chem 384(6):891–897, 2003.
16. Chu Q, Lopez M, Hayashi K, et al. Elevation of collagenase generated type II collagen neoepitope and proteoglycan epitopes in synovial fluid following induction of joint instability in the dog. Osteoarthritis Cartilage 10:662–669, 2002.
17. Cibere J, Thorne A, Kopec JA, et al. Glucosamine sulfate and cartilage type II collagen degradation in patients with knee osteoarthritis: randomized discontinuation trial employing biomarkers. J Rheumatol 32:896–902, 2005.
18. Charni N, Juillet F, Garnero P. Urinary type II collagen helical peptide (Helix II) as a new biochemical marker of cartilage degradation in patients with osteoarthritis and rheumatoid arthritis. Arthritis Rheum 52:1081–1090, 2005.
19. Deberg M, Labasse A, Christgau S, et al. New serum biochemical markers (Coll 2-1 and Coll 2-1 NO2) for studying oxidative-related type II collagen network degradation in patients with osteoarthrtitis and rheumatoid arthritis. Osteoarthritis Cartilage 13:1059–1062, 2005.
20. Christgau S, Garnero P, Fledelius C, et al. Collagen type II C-Telopeptide fragments as an index of cartilage degradation. Bone 29:209–215, 2001.
21. Garnero P, Desmarais S, Charni N, et al. The type II collagen fragments HELIX-II and CTX-II reveal distinct enzymatic pathways of cartilage collagen degradation: Diagnostic and therapeutic implications in rheumatoid arthritis and osteoarthritis. Arthritis Rheum 44(suppl):S56, 2005.·
22. Bay Jensen AC, Charni N, Andersen TL, et al. The type II collagen degradation markers, Helix-II and CTX-II, have distinct distributions in tissue sections of human articular cartilage, and are affected differently by menopause. Osteoarthritis Cartilage 13(Suppl A5): S41, 2005.
23. Garnero P, Conrozier T, Juillet F, et al. Urinary type II collagen helical peptide (HELIX-II) levels are increased in patients with a rapidly destructive hip osteoarthritis. Ann Rheum Dis 64(suppl. 3): OP0117, 2005.
24. Deberg M, Labasse AH, Collette J, et al. One year increase of Coll 2-1, a new marker of type II collagen is highly predictive of radiological OA progression. Osteoarthritis Cartilage 13:258–265, 2005.
25. Watanabe H, Yamada Y, Kimata K. Roles of aggrecan, a large chondroitin sulfate proteoglycan, in cartilage structure and function. J Biochem 124:667–683, 1998.
26. Glasson S, Askew R, Sheppard N, et al. Deletion of active ADMATS5 prevents cartilage degradation in a murine model of osteoarthritis. Nature 644–648, 2005.
27. Caterson B, Christner JE, Baker JR, et al. Production and characterization of monoclonal antibodies directed against connective tissue proteoglycans. Fed Proc 44:386–393, 1985.
28. Visco DM, Johnstone B, Jolly Ga, et al. Immunohistochemical analysis of 3B3 (−) and 7D4 epitope expression in canine osteoarthritis. Arthritis Rheum 36:1718–1725, 1993.
29. Rizkalla G, Reiner A, Bogoch E, et al. Studies of the articular cartilage proteoglycan aggrecan in health and osteoarthritis. Evidence for molecular heterogeneity and extensive molecular changes in disease. J Clin Invest 30:2268–2277, 1992.
30. Glant TT, Mikecz K, Roughley PJ, et al. Age-related changes in protein-related epitopes of human articular cartilage proteoglycans. Biochem J 236:71–75, 1986.
31. Slater RR, Bayliss MT, Lachiewicz PF, et al. Monoclonal antibodies that detect biochemical markers of arthritis in humans. Arthritis Rheum 5:665–659, 1995.
32. Antoniou J, Steffen T, Nelson F, et al. The human intervertebral disc: evidence for changes in the biosynthesis and denaturation of the extracellular matrix with growth maturation, aging and degeneration. J Clin Invest 98:996–1003, 1996.
33. Lohmander LS, Neame PJ, Sandy ID. The structure of aggrecan fragments in human synovial fluid. Evidence that aggrecanase mediates cartilage degradation in inflammatory joint disease, joint injury, and osteoarthritis. Arthritis Rheum 36:1214–1222, 1993.
34. Thonar EJ-MA, Lenz ME, Klintworth GK, et al. Quantification of keratn sulfate in blood as a marker of cartilage catabolism. Arthritis Rheum 28:1367–1376, 1985.
35. Hedhom E, Antonsson P, Hjerpe A, et al. Cartilage matrix proteins: an acidic oligomeric protein (COMP) detected only in cartilage. J Biol Chem 267:6132–6136, 1992.
36. Morgelin M, Heinegard D, Engel J, et al. Electron microscopy of native cartilage oligomeric matrix protein purified from the Swarm rat chondrosarcoma revealed a five-armed structure. J Biol Chem 267:6137–6141, 1992.
37. Oldberg A, Antonsson P, Lindblom K, et al. COMP (Cartilage Oligomeric Matrix Protein) is structurally related to the thrombospondins. J Biol Chem 267,22346–22350, 1992.
38. Briggs MD, Hoffman SM, King LM, et al. Pseudoachondroplasia and multiple epiphyseal dysplasia due to mutations in the cartilage oligomeric matrix protein gene. Nat Genet 10:330–336, 1995.
39. Hecht JT, Nelsaon LD, Crowder E, et al. Mutations in exon 17B of cartilage oligomeric matrix protein (COMP) cause pseudoachondroplasia. Nat Genet 10:325–329, 1995.
40. Posey KL, Hayes E, Haynes R, et al. Role of TSP-5/COMP in pseudoachondroplasia. Int J Cell Biol 36:1005–1012, 2004.
41. Svensson L, Aszodi A, Heinegard D, et al. Cartilage oligomeric matrix protein-deficient mice have normal skeletal development. Mol Cell Biol 22:4366–4371, 2002.
42. Muller G, Michel A, Altenburg E. COMP (Cartilage Oligomeric Matrix Protein) is synthesized in ligament, tendon, meniscus, and articular cartilage. Connect Tissue Res 39:233–244, 1998.
43. Di Cesare PE, Carlson CS Stolerman ES, Hauser N, et al. Increased degradation and altered tissue distribution of cartilage oligomeric matrix protein in human rheumatoid and osteoarthritic cartilage. J Orthop Res 14:946–955, 1996.

44. Dickinson SSC, Vankemmelbeke MN, Buttle DJ, et al. Cleavage of cartilage oligomeric matrix protein (thrombospondin-5) by matrix-metalloproteinases and a disintegrin and metalloproteinase with thrombospondin motifs. Matrix Biol 22:267–278, 2003.

45. Saxne T, Heinegard D. Cartilage oligomeric matrix protein: a novel marker turnover detectable in synovial fluid and blood. Brit J Rheumatol 31:583–591, 1992.

46. Vilim V, Voburka Z, Vytasek R, et al. Monoclonal antibodies to human cartilage oligomeric matrix protein: epitope mappling and characterization of sandwich ELISA. Clin Chim Acta 328: 59–69, 2003.

47. Henrissat B, Bairoch A. New families in the classification of glycosyl hydrolases based on amino-acid sequences similarities. Biochem J 293:781–788, 1993.

48. Hakala BE, White C, Recklies AD. Human cartilage gp-39, a major secretory product of articular chondrocytes and synovial cells, is a mammalian member of a Chitinase protein family. J Biol Chem 293:781–788, 1993.

49. Hu B, Trinh K, Figueira WF, et al. Isolation and sequence of a novel human chondrocytes protein related to mammalian members of the Chitinase protein family. J Biol Chem 271:19415–19420, 1996.

50. Johansen JS Hvolris J, Hansen M, Backer V, et al. Serum YKL-40 levels in healthy children and adults. Comparison with serum and synovial fluid levels of YKL-40 in patients with osteoarthritis or trauma of the knee joint. Brit J Rheumatol 35:553–559, 1996.

51. Conrozier T, Carlier MC, Mathieu P, et al. Serum levels of YKL-40 and C reactive protein in patients with hip osteoarthritis and healthy subjects: a cross sectional study. Ann Rheum Dis 59(10): 828–831, 2000.

52. Garnero P, Piperno M, Gineyts E, et al: Cross sectional evaluation of biochemical markers of bone, cartilage and synovial tissue metabolism in patients with knee osteoarthritis: Relations with disease sctivity and joint damage. Ann Rheum Dis 60:619–626, 2001.

53. Mazieres B, Garnero P, Gueguen A, et al. Molecular markers of cartilage breakdown and synovitis are strong independent predictors of structural progression of hip osteoarthritis. The ECHODIAH cohort. Ann Rheum Dis (in press).

54. Johansen JS, Stoltenberg M, Hansen M, et al. Serum YKL-40 concentrations in patients with rheumatoid arthritis: relation to disease activity. Rheumatology (Oxford) 38:618–626, 1999.

55. Johansen JS, Cintin C, Jorgensen M, et al: Serum YKL-40: a new potential marker of prognosis and location of metastases of patients with recurrent breast cancer. Eur J Cancer 31A: 1437–1442, 1995.

56. Johansen JS, Drivsholm L, Price PA, et al. High serum YKL-40 level in patients with small cell lung cancer is related to early death. Lung Cancer 46(3):333–340, 2004.

57. Brasso K, Christensen IJ, Johansen JS, et al. Prognostic value of PINP, bone alkaline phosphatase, CTX-I, and YKL-40 in patients with metastatic prostate carcinoma. Prostate, 66:503–513, 2006.

58. Steck E, Breit SD, Breusch SJ, et al. Enhanced expression of the human Chitinase 3-like 2 gene (YKL-39) but not chitrinase 3-like 1 gene (YKL-40) in osteoarthritic cartilage. Biochem Biophys Res Commun 299:109–115, 2002.

59. Knorr T, Obermayr F, Bartnick E, et al. YKL-39 (Chitinase 3-like protein 2), but not YKL-40 (Chitinase 3-like protein 1) is up regulated in osteoarthritic chondrocytes. Ann Rheum Dis 62:995–998, 2003.

60. Tsuruha J, Masuko-hongo K, Kato T, et al. Autoimmunity against YKL-39, a human cartilage derived protein, in patients with osteoarthritis. J Rheumatol 29:1459–1466, 2002.

61. Du H, Masuko-Hongo K, Nakamura H, et al. The prevalence of autoantibodies against cartilage intermediate layer protein, YKL-39, osteopontin and cyclic citrullinated pin patients with early-stage knee osteoarthritis: evidence of a variety of autoimmune processes. Rheumtol Int 26:35–41, 2005.

62. Garnero P, Delmas PD. Investigation of Bone: Bone Turnover in Rheumatology, 4rd edition, Hochberg MC, Silman AJ, Smolen JS, et al. eds, Harcourt Health Sciences Ltd, London, UK, (in press),

63. Halleen JM, Alatalo SL, Suominen H, et al. Tartrate-resistant acid phosphatase 5b: a novel serum marker of bone resorption. J Bone Miner Res 15(7):1337–1345, 2000.

64. Garnero P, Shih WJ, Gineyts E, et al. Comparison of new biochemical markers of bone turnover in late postmenopausal osteoporotic women in response to alendronate. J Clin Endocrinol Metab 79:1693–1700, 1994.

65. Blomqvist C, Risteli L, Risteli J, et al. Markers of type I collagen degradation and synthesis in the monitoring of treatment responses in bone metastases from breast cancer. Br J Cancer 73: 1074–1079, 1996.

66. Sassi ML, Aman S, Hakala M, et al. Assay for crosslinked carboxyterminal telopeptide of type I collagen (ICTP) unlike Crosslaps assay reflects increased pathological degradation of type I collagen in rheumatoid arthritis. Clin Chem Lab 41:1038–1044, 2003.

67. Sassi ML, Eriksen H, Risteli L, et al. Immunochemical characterization of assay for carboxyterminal telopeptide of human type I collagen: Loss of antigenicity by treatment with cathepsin K. Bone 26:367–373, 2000.

68. Garnero P, Ferreras M, Karsdal MA, et al. The type I collagen fragments ICTP and CTX reveal distinct enzymatic pathways of bone collagen degradation. J Bone Miner Res 18:859–867, 2003.

69. Oddie GW, Schenk G, Angel N, et al. Structure, function and regulation of tartrate-resistant acid phosphatase. Bone 27:575–584, 2000.

70. Garnero P, Grimaux M, Seguin P, et al. Characterization of immunoreactive forms of human osteocalcin generated in vivo and in vitro. J Bone Miner Res 255–264, 1994.

71. Taylor AK, Linkhart S, Mohan RA, et al. Multiple osteocalcin fragments in human urine and serum detected by a midmolecule osteocalcin radioimmunoassay. J Clin Endocrinol Metab 70: 467–472, 1990.

72. Srivastava AK, Mohan FR, Singer FR, et al. A urine midmolecule osteocalcin assay shows higher discriminatory power than a serum midmolecule osteocalcin assay during short-term alendronate treatment of osteoporotic patients. Bone 31:62–69, 2002.

73. Debri E, Reinholt FP, Heinegard D, et al. Bone sialoprotein and osteopontin distribution at the osteocartilagineous interface. Clin Orthop 330:251–260, 1996.

74. Saxne T, Zunino L, Heinegard D. Increased release of bone sialoprotein into synovial fluid reflects tissue destruction in rheumatoid arthritis. Arthritis Rheum 1:82–90, 1995.

75. Petersson IF, Boegard T, Dahlstrom J, et al. Bone scan and serum markers of bone and cartilage in patients with knee pain and osteoarthritis. Osteoarthritis Cartilage 6:33–39, 1998.

76. Peterson IF, Boegard T, Svensson B, et al. Changes in cartilage and bone metabolism identified by serum markers in early osteoarthritis of the knee joint. Brit J Rheumatol 37:46–50, 1998.

77. Conrozier T, Saxne T, Fan CS, et al. Serum concentrations of cartilage oligomeric matrix protein and bone sialoprotein in hip osteoarthritis: A one year prospective study. Ann Rheum Dis 9: 527–532, 1998.

78. Skoumal M, Haberhauer G, Kolarz G, et al. Serum cathepsin K levels of patients with lonstanding rheumatoid arthritis: correlation with radiological destruction. Arthritis Res Ther 7:565–570, 2005.

79. Garnero P, Rousseau JC, Delmas PD. Molecular basis and clinical use of biochemical markers of bone, cartilage, and synovium in joint diseases. Arthritis Rheum 43:953–968, 2000.

80. Pelletier J-P, Martel-Pelletier J, Abramson SB. Osteoarthritis, an inflammatory disease. Arthritis Rheum 44:1237–1247, 2001.

81. Ayral X, Pickering EH, Woodworth TG, et al. Synovitis: a potential predictive factor of structural progression of medial tibiofemoral knee osteoarthritis—results of a 1 year longitudinal arthroscopic study in 422 patients. Osteoarthritis Cartilage 13(5):361–367, 2005.

82. Spector TD, Hart DJ, Nandra D, et al. Low-levels increases in serum C-reactive protein are present in early osteoarthritis of the knee and predict progressive disease. Arthritis Rheum 40:723–727, 1997.

83. Sharif M, Shepstone L, Elson CJ, et al. Increased serum C reactive protein may reflect events that precede radiographic progression in osteoarthritis of the knee. Ann Rheum Dis 59(1):71–74, 2000.

84. Sowers M, Jannausch M, Stein E, et al. C-reactive protein as a biomarker of emergent osteoarthrtitis. Osteoarthritis Cartilage 10:595–601, 2002.

85. Edwards JC. The nature and origin of synovium: experimental approaches to the study of synoviocyte differentiation. J Anat 184:493–501, 1994.

86. Stevens CR, Blacke DR, Merry P, et al. A comparative study by morphometry of the microvasculature in normal and rheumatoid synovium. Arthrirtis Rheum 34:150–1513, 1991.

87. Swann DA, Radin EL. The molecular basis of articular lubrication. I. Purification and properties of a lubricating fraction from bovine synovial fluid. J Biol Chem 40:414–418, 1972.

88. Jay GD, Britt DE, Cha CJ. Lubricin is a gen product of megakaryocyte stimulating factor gene expression by human synovial fibroblasts. J Rheumatol 27:594–600, 2000.

89. Brown TJ, Laurent UBG, Fraser JRE. Turnover of hyaluronan in synovial joints. Exp Physiol 76:125–134, 1991.

90. Golderg R. Enzyme-linked immunosorbent assay for hyaluronate using cartilage proteoglycan and an antibody for keratan sulfate. Anal Biochem 174:448–458, 1988.

91. Laurent TC, Larent UBG, Fraser RE. Serum hyaluronan as a disease marker. Ann Med 28:241–253, 1996.

92. Elliot AL, Kraus VB, Luta G, et al. Serum hyaluronan levels and radiographic knee and hip osteoarthritis in African Americans and Caucasians in the Johnston County Osteoarthritis Project. Arthritis Rheum 52:105–111, 2005.

93. Sharif M, George L, Shepstone J, et al. Serum hyaluronic acid level as a predictor of disease progression in osteoarthritis of the knee. Arthritis Rheum 38:760–767, 1995.

94. Pavelka K, Forejtova S, Olejarova M, et al. Hyaluronic acid levels may have predictive value for the progresson of knee osteoarthrtitis. Osteoarthrtitis Cartilage 12:277–283, 2004.

95. Lohmander LS, Hoerrner LA, Lark MW. Metalloproteinases-tissue-inhibitor and proteoglycan fragments in knee synovial fluid in human osteoarthritis. Arthrtitis Rheum 191–189, 1993.

96. Lohmander LS, Brandt KD, Mazzuca SA, et al. Use of plasma stromelysin (matrix metalloproteinase 3) concentration to predict joint space narrowing in knee osteoarthritis. Arthritis Rheum 52:3160–3167, 2005.

97. Gineyts E, Garnero P, Delmas PD. Urinary excretion of glucosyl-galactosyl pyridinoline: a specific biochemical marker of synovium degradation. Rheumatology 40:315–323, 2001.

98. Gineyts E, Mo JA, Ko A, et al. Effects of ibuprofen on molecular markers of cartilage and synovium turnover in patients with knee osteoarthritis. Ann Rheum Dis 63:857–861, 2004.

99. Jordan KM, Syddall HE, Garnero P, et al. Urinary CTX-II and glucosyl-galactosyl-pyridinoline are associated with presence and severity of radiographic knee osteoarthritis in men. Ann Rheum Dis, 65:871–877, 2006.

100. Garnero P, Mazières B, Guéguen A, et al. Cross sectional association of ten molecular markers of bone, cartilage and synovium with disease activity and radiological joint damage in hip osteoarthritis patients: the ECHODIAH Cohort. J Rheumatol 32:697–703, 2005.

101. Marshall KW, Zhang H, Yager TD, et al. Blood-based biomarkers for detecting mild osteoarthritis. Osteoarthritis Cartilage 13:861–871, 2005.

102. Xiang Y, Sekine T, Nakamura H, et al. Proteomic surveillance of autoimmunity in osteoarthritis: identification of triosephosphate isomerase as an autoantigen in patients with osteoarthritis. Arthritis Rheum 50:1511–1521, 2004.

103. Lamers RJAN, van Nessselrooij JHJ, Kraus VB et al. Identification of a urinary profile associated with osteoarthritis. Osteoarthritis Cartilage, 2005.

104. Ling QM, Patel D, Zhan M, et al. Changes in selected proteins associated with osteoarthritis development in the Baltimore Longitudinal study of aging (BSLA). Arthritis Rheum 52 (suppl): S256, 2005.

105. Garnero P, Sornay-Rendu E, Arlot M, et al. Association between spine disc degeneration and type II collagen degradation in postmenopausal women: the OFELY study. Arthritis Rheum 50:3137–3144, 2004.

106. Meulenbelt I, Kloppenburg M, Kroon HM, et al. Urinary CTX-II levels are associated with radiographic subtypes of osteoarthritis (OA) in hip, knee, and facet joints in subject with familial OA at multiple sites: the GARP study. Ann Rheum Dis Aug 3, 2005.

107. Moskowitz RW, Holderbaum D, Hooper MM. Total quantitative osteoarthritis load (TQOL) assessment tool: a proposed methodology for biomarker correlations. Arthritis Rheum 52 (supp.): S71, 2005.

108. Crisione LG, Elliot AL, Stabler T, et al. Variation of serum hyaluronan with activity in individual with knee osteoarthritis. Osteoarthritis Cartilage 13:837–840, 2005.

109. Kerstin UG, Studbendorff JJ, Schmidt MC, et al. Changes in knee cartilage volume and serum COMP concentration after running exercise. Osteoarthritis Cartilage 13:925–934, 2005.

110. Mundermann A, Dyrby CO, Andriacchi TP, et al. Serum concentration of oligomeric matrix protein (COMP) is sensitive to physiological cyclic loading in healthy adults. Osteoarthritis Cartilage 13:34–38, 2005.

111. Garnero P, Peterfy C, Zaim S, et al. Bone marrow abnormality on magnetic resonance imaging is associated with type II collagen degradation in knee osteoarthritis: a three-month longitudinal study. Arthritis Rheum, 52:2822–2829, 2005.

112. Reijman M, Hazes JM, Bierna-Zeinstra SM, et al. A new marker for osteoarthritis: cross-sectional and longitudinal approach. Arthritis Rheum 50:2471–2476, 2004.

113. Vilim V, Olejarova M, Machacek S, et al. Serum levels of cartilage oligomeric matrix protein (COMP) correlate with radiographic progression of knee osteoarthritis. Osteoarthritis Cartilage 10:707–713, 2002.

114. Sharif M, Kirwan JR, Elson CJ, et al. Suggestion of nonlinear or phasic progression of knee osteoarthritis based on measurements of serum cartilage oligomeric matrix protein levels over five years. Arthritis Rheum 50:2479–2488, 2004.

115. Garnero P, Ayral X, Rousseau JC, et al. Uncoupling of type II collagen synthesis and degradation predicts progression of joint damage in patients with knee osteoarthritis. Arthritis Rheum 46:2613–2624, 2002.

116. Christgau S, Henrotin Y, Tanko LB, et al. Osteoarthritis patients with high cartilage turnover show increased responsiveness to the cartilage protecting effect of glucosamine sulfate. Clin Exp Rheumatol 22:36–42, 2004.

117. Ravn P, Warning L, Christgau S, et al. The effect on cartilage of different forms of application of postmenopausal estrogen therapy: comparison of oral and transdermal therapy. Bone 35:1216–1221, 2004.

118. Christgau S, Tanko LB, Cloos PAC, et al. Suppression of elevated cartilage turnover in postmenopausal women and in ovariectomized rats by estrogen and a selective estrogen-receptor modular (SERM). Menopause 11:508–518, 2004.

119. Lehmann HJ, Mouritzen U, Christgau S, et al. Effect of bisphosphonates on cartilage turnover assessed with a newly developed assay for collagen type II degradation products. Ann Rheum Dis 61:530–533, 2002.

120. Spector TD, Conaghan PG, Buckland-Wright JC, et al. Effect of risedronate on joint structure and symptoms of knee osteoarthritis: results of the brisk: randomized, controlled trial [ISRCTN01928173]. Arthritis Res Ther 7:R625–R633, 2005.

121. Garnero P, Bingham CO III, Aronstein W, et al. Treatment with risedronate reduced urinary CTX-II, a specific biochemical marker of cartilage type II collagen degradation in a 24-month study of knee OA. Arthritis Rheum 50(suppl): 5636, 2004.

122. Landewé R, Geusens P, Maarten B, et al. Markers for type II collagen breakdown predict the effect of disease modifying treatment on long-term radiographic progression in patients with rheumatoid arthritis: The Cobra study. Arthritis Rheum 50:1390–1399, 2004.

Secondary Osteoarthritis

13

H. Ralph Schumacher, Jr.   *Lan X. Chen*   *Joseph Buckwalter*

In increasing percentages of patients, osteoarthritis (OA) can now be classified as secondary on the basis of an identifiable congenital, developmental, traumatic, or systemic disease that appears to explain the degenerative changes in the articular cartilage. All diseases considered in this chapter have clinical, radiologic, and pathologic features in common with "idiopathic" OA to varying degrees. However, there are also unique features that suggest each underlying cause. These distinguishing features are emphasized, along with brief descriptions of each disease process. Although osteoarthritic changes associated with these underlying diseases are emphasized, other musculoskeletal symptoms produced by these diseases that may be confused with osteoarthritic manifestations are also described. The systemic diseases causing arthritis deserve major emphasis because 1) in some patients, the OA may be an early or, even initial, clue to a potentially dangerous and treatable systemic disease; 2) these secondary osteoarthritides may have specific therapies, in contrast to the largely symptomatic treatment used in most osteoarthritides; and 3) the mechanisms identified in these examples of secondary OA may provide helpful clues to mechanisms in idiopathic disease.

Specific treatments of underlying diseases or diseases related to them are also discussed in this chapter. Unless otherwise noted, symptomatic and general therapy is as described in Section III for general management of OA.

SYSTEMIC METABOLIC DISEASES

Hemochromatosis

Hemochromatosis is a chronic disease characterized by excess iron deposition and fibrosis in a variety of tissues. Most hemochromatosis is idiopathic. Ninety percent of idiopathic cases are associated with homozygosity for a tyrosine substitution at position 282 on the HFE gene.[1] There are a variety of other less common mutations.[2] This is not a rare disease. Estimated incidences of clinically detectable disease have varied; homozygosity for the gene in white populations is about 1 in 500. Mutations and disease are much less common in Blacks and Asians.[3] Frequent manifestations are hepatomegaly and cirrhosis, increased skin pigmentation (in large part because of increased melanin), diabetes, other endocrine deficiency, and cardiomyopathy. Iron overload usually requires many years to develop, so that most patients have onset of symptoms between the ages of 40 and 60 years. Hemochromatosis is uncommon in premenopausal women, presumably because of menstrual blood loss. The largest iron deposits are in the liver, and biopsy is frequently performed for diagnosis. Elevation of fasting serum iron levels with saturation of iron-binding capacity greater than 62% or elevated serum ferritin levels can help suggest the diagnosis. Genetic testing can be supportive. Liver function abnormalities are often minimal, even with advanced hepatic deposition of iron.

OA-like changes in hemochromatosis were first described in 1964[4] but have since been recognized to occur in 20% to 50% of patients; one study showed radiographic changes in 81%.[5] Age at onset of the arthritis has varied from 26 to 70 years but is most common in the fifth decade. Arthritis generally coincides closely with the onset of other manifestations of hemochromatosis but may antedate other findings and be the first clue to the disease.[6,7]

The hands, knees, and hips are most commonly involved, although virtually any joint, including those in the ankles and feet,[8,9] can be affected. Helpful in diagnosis is the characteristic involvement of metacarpophalangeal (MCP) joints as well as proximal interphalangeal (PIP)

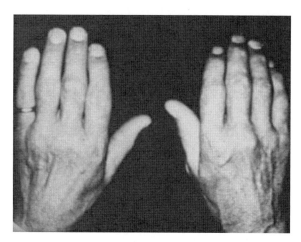

Figure 13–1 Bony osteoarthritis–like enlargement of some of the distal interphalangeal, proximal interphalangeal, and metacarpophalangeal joints in hemochromatosis.

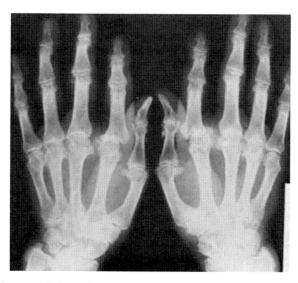

Figure 13–2 Radiograph of the hands in hemochromatosis showing joint space narrowing, subluxations, subchondral cysts, periarticular sclerosis, spurs, and soft tissue calcifications, all most prominent at the second to fourth metacarpophalangeal joints.

and distal interphalangeal (DIP) joints with a firm, bony, and often only mildly tender enlargement that is different from that seen in rheumatoid arthritis (Fig. 13–1). Involvement of the second and third MCP joints is particularly characteristic, although it can also occasionally be seen in patients with generalized OA, in manual laborers, and in association with calcium pyrophosphate deposition disease. Joints are stiff and become limited in motion, but morning stiffness is not prominent.

Joint effusions have been noninflammatory, with leukocyte counts less than 2000/mm², except during the infrequent attacks of associated pseudogout. Cells are predominantly mononuclear and occasionally contain iron on staining with Prussian blue.[10] Measurements of iron levels in synovial fluid are comparable to those in serum.

Synovial tissue shows a striking deposition of iron that is most prominent in the synovial lining cells and, as seen by electron microscopy, is actually greatest in the type B or synthetic cells.[11] By light microscopy, the iron is golden and may be missed unless it is specifically looked for. Other synovial changes are only mild lining cell proliferation, fibrosis, and scattered chronic inflammatory cells. Although few cases have been studied, iron is also demonstrable in the chondrocytes of articular cartilage and at the line of ossification. There are degenerative changes in cartilage.[12] All cartilages studied to date by electron microscopy have also shown either apatite or calcium pyrophosphate dihydrate (CPPD) crystals, which may be important in pathogenesis.[12]

Radiographic studies show the characteristic joint distribution that often includes MCP joints. There is joint space narrowing and irregularity; subchondral sclerosis; and often large cystic erosions, hook-like bone proliferation, and even subluxation (Fig. 13–2). In up to 60% of patients, chondrocalcinosis and periarticular soft tissue calcification are seen. Aside from the distribution and frequency of calcifications, the involvement at the hips and other sites seems indistinguishable from idiopathic OA. Three cases have been reported with aseptic necrosis at the

hip.[13] Whether this underlies some hip OA in these patients needs further study.

Musculoskeletal manifestations other than OA are also seen. As noted earlier, pseudogout attacks can occur from CPPD crystals. Apatite may also be involved in some crystal-induced arthritis. Osteopenia is seen and may be related to the cirrhosis or to androgen or other endocrine deficiency.

Mechanisms involved in the arthritis are not established, although there are intriguing possibilities.[14] Iron deposition in the chondrocytes could alter the proteoglycans, collagen, or enzymes released by these cells, leading to the degenerative change in the matrix. Iron could promote the formation of toxic free radicals or could bind directly to some proteoglycans and alter their function, as it has been shown to do in vitro. In vitro iron can downregulate prostaglandin E_2 production by synovial fibroblasts. The balance of this effect on these cells could have deleterious or beneficial results.[15] Iron, in vitro, also inhibits the enzyme pyrophosphatase and could thus contribute to the deposition of CPPD crystals. Because the iron and calcium crystal depositions are not spatially related, iron would appear to promote calcification in some indirect way, or alternatively, the calcifications may be a result of unrelated mechanisms or related inherited factors. Although cartilage appears to be primarily involved in the OA, the synovium also has heavy deposits of iron, and stimulation of release of cytokines or enzymes from the synovium might contribute to the process. Synovial siderosis might alter the clearance of factors involved in calcification.[16] The possibility has been raised that the HFE mutation may predispose to hand or other OA even without iron overload.[17] This has not been confirmed to date for hip and knee OA.[18]

Hemochromatosis can be treated and many systemic features reversed or prevented by removal of excess iron with intensive and continued phlebotomies or with the chelating agent deferoxamine. Alcohol, which increases the risk of liver damage, and vitamin C ingestion, which increases iron absorption, should be avoided. Once established, joint disease has not been reversed, and in fact, some patients have had their first joint symptoms or exacerbations of arthritis after phlebotomy. In vitro studies suggest that iron could even inhibit CPPD deposition so that depletion of iron might possibly exacerbate chondrocalcinosis.[19] Episodes of acute crystal-induced arthritis should be watched for and can be treated with nonsteroidal antiinflammatory agents. Prosthetic hip and knee replacements have been successfully performed for chronic changes. Family members of all patients with hemochromatosis should be screened for iron overload as early treatment may prevent arthritis and other manifestations.

Wilson Disease (Hepatolenticular Degeneration)

Wilson disease is an uncommon familial disease associated with a variety of mutations in a gene (ATPTB) on chromosome 13 q14.3.[20] The most frequent mutation is a substitution of glutamine for histidine at amino acid 1069.[20] The disease is characterized by the Kayser-Fleischer ring, consisting of brown pigment at the corneal margin; cirrhosis; and basal ganglion degeneration leading to tremor, rigidity, or other neurologic problems. Many patients also develop renal tubular acidosis. The onset of symptoms occurs between the ages of 4 and 50 years. A disorder of copper metabolism can be demonstrated by an increase in urinary excretion of copper and a general decrease in the serum copper-binding protein ceruloplasmin. Copper concentration is increased in liver, brain, and other tissues. A rapid polymerase chain reaction (PCR) test can be used to document the most common mutation in ATPTB.[20]

Arthropathy is rare in children but occurs in up to 50% of adults.[21,22] The OA may be asymptomatic despite radiographic findings or may be markedly symptomatic with worsening on activity. More commonly involved joints have been the wrists, elbows, shoulders, hips, and knees and, occasionally, the fingers. The early age at onset and the prominent involvement of the wrists in many patients suggest a difference from primary OA.[14,21,22]

Joint effusions are usually small and consist of clear, viscous fluid. Leukocyte counts have been approximately 200 to 300/mm^3 with predominantly mononuclear cells. Synovial biopsy specimens have shown mild lining cell hyperplasia and few chronic inflammatory cells.[14,22,23] Cartilage has been examined in four patients and was shown to contain copper by energy-dispersive elemental analysis in two.[23] Copper has also been found in synovium, where it might alter cytokine and protease production.[24,25] CPPD crystals were not noted in our patients but have been reported in an intervertebral disk.[26] Joint hypermobility occurred in 9 of 32 patients in one series.[27]

Radiographic joint findings have included subchondral bone fragmentation and sclerosis, subchondral cysts, cortical irregularity, cartilage space narrowing, periarticular cysts, vertebral wedging,[14,21,22,25] osteochondritis dissecans,[27] and severe chondromalacia patellae.[22] Periarticular calcifications are common. Some calcifications have been thought to represent bone fragments, and chondrocalcinosis has been described.[23]

No correlation has been found between total disease severity, spasticity or tremor, osteopenia, or liver or renal disease and the arthritis. Experimental studies of only short-term copper loading have not produced an arthropathy. Although the nature of most joint calcifications is not yet known, McCarty and Pepe[28] showed that cupric (as well as ferrous) ions could inhibit pyrophosphatase in vitro, suggesting a possible cause for deposition of CPPD crystals. In vitro copper loading of articular chondrocytes has altered matrix synthesis and caused increased collagen production.[29]

Wilson disease is associated with osteopenia in 25% to 50% of patients in different series. It is usually asymptomatic but can be painful in the presence of pathologic fractures. Some of the bone demineralization results from definite rickets or osteomalacia attributed to the renal tubular disease.

This is a treatable disease; penicillamine appears to be the most effective chelating agent for mobilizing copper from the tissues, although zinc may also be used. Treatment is continued for life. Although neurologic improvement is often reported, there is no evidence that the established arthropathy has been helped; in fact, some penicillamine-treated patients have subsequently developed the OA. Whether early diagnosis and treatment can prevent the arthritis is not yet known. Family members should always be checked to try to establish an early diagnosis. Penicillamine seems occasionally to produce polymyositis, lupus, inflammatory polyarthritis,[27] and other immunologic syndromes.

Ochronosis

Ochronosis is the result of a hereditary deficiency of a liver enzyme, homogentisic acid oxidase; the defect is now mapped to chromosome 3q with a wide variety of mutations reported.[14,30,31,32] Lack of this enzyme allows accumulation of homogentisic acid, which, when excreted in large amounts, imparts a dark brown or black color to the urine. This is termed alkaptonuria. Freshly passed urine usually appears normal but darkens with standing or with alkalinization. This inherited defect is thought to be transmitted as a simple autosomal recessive.

Ochronosis occurs when polymers of homogentisic acid become deposited in connective tissue. The exact mechanisms of affinity of homogentisic acid for connective tissue are not known. Deposition is reversible until the homogentisic acid is polymerized. Mechanisms of tissue injury may include a demonstrated inhibitory effect of homogentisic acid on in vitro chondrocyte growth.[33] Ochronotic pigment is black when it is viewed grossly in masses in tissues; when it is seen in thin histologic sections under the light microscope, it is ocher or golden yellow.

Infants may have black staining of diapers. By the fourth decade, ochronotic pigment becomes detectable as a blue-black hue in the external ear cartilage or tympanic membrane, as scleral pigmentation, or as malar and other cutaneous darkening. Pigment deposits in the mitral and aortic valves can deform the leaflets and cusps, producing murmurs in 15% to 20% of patients. Calcified prostatic calculi containing ochronotic pigment occur in a large percentage of men with ochronosis.

Deposition of the pigment in intervertebral disks and in articular cartilages leads to degenerative disk disease and peripheral arthropathy. The majority of patients older than 30 years develop spondylosis, which may present with low back stiffness and aching or, in about 15% of patients, herniation of a lumbar nucleus pulposus. Involvement of the dorsal and cervical spine occurs only later. Symptoms may be minimal despite prominent radiographic changes.

Peripheral arthropathy generally occurs later and is milder than the spondylosis. The knees, shoulders, and hips are most commonly involved.[35] In peripheral joints, symptoms may antedate detected radiographic changes. As with other forms of OA, symptoms are predominantly pain, crepitation, limited motion, and stiffness.

Joint effusions occur in about 50% of involved knees. Synovial fluid is clear, viscous, and yellow. On occasion, dark specks of ochronotic cartilage can be seen floating in the fluid.[36,37] Cartilage fragments seen microscopically in joint fluid are golden yellow. Leukocyte counts are generally in the noninflammatory range, with counts from 112 to 700/mm³; mononuclear cells predominate. Joint fluids have been described with CPPD crystals without inflammatory reaction or with acute attacks of pseudogout superimposed on the degenerative arthropathy.[38] Although small amounts of homogentisic acid occur in joint fluid, the amount is insufficient to cause darkening with alkalinization.[35]

The earliest radiographic changes suggestive of ochronosis are calcification and even ossification in the lumbar intervertebral disks. Hydroxyapatite has been identified as the calcium salt in the disks. Although typical of ochronosis, disk calcification (Fig. 13–3) is not diagnostic

because it has also been seen with CPPD deposition disease, hemochromatosis, chronic respiratory paralytic poliomyelitis, ankylosing spondylitis, acromegaly, amyloidosis, tuberculosis, and trauma or without any identifiable systemic disease. The calcification in ochronosis is followed later by disk space narrowing; osteophytes tend to be small but may bridge occasional vertebrae. The sacroiliac joints can show narrowing but do not fuse; typical syndesmophytes like those found in ankylosing spondylitis are not seen.

On radiographic examination, peripheral joints do not differ in appearance from those in other forms of OA except in the distribution of ochronosis. Ochronosis tends to involve the larger joints and spare or only mildly involve the hands and feet. Protrusio acetabuli has been reported in one case.[35] Loose bodies occur in some peripheral joints.[35] Chondrocalcinosis may be seen. As in the spine, the osteophytes tend to be small.

Ochronotic pigment deposition is initially in the deeper and midzone cartilage but eventually produces grossly visible diffuse blackening of cartilage (Fig. 13–4). This cartilage is so friable that it progressively erodes, with fragments breaking loose into synovial fluid. Pigmented shards become embedded in synovial membrane (Fig. 13–5). Cartilage collagen and associated substances appear to be primary sites of the pigment deposition.[35,39] Ochronotic pigment is probably secondarily phagocytosed by chondrocytes and synovial cells. Because chondrocytes show some degenerative changes in virtually all cases studied by electron microscopy, they may also be affected in some way early in the disease.[35] The matrix ochronotic pigment and the cellular changes result in a dramatically friable cartilage that predictably degenerates in early middle age. Joint loose bodies appear to arise from osteochondrometaplasia around the ochronotic shards embedded in synovium.[35]

No satisfactory therapy for the enzymatic defect has yet been developed. Unfortunately, a diet low in phenylalanine and tyrosine precursors has been too unpalatable to demonstrate whether it might have any long-term clinical benefit, although urinary homogentisic acid levels can be

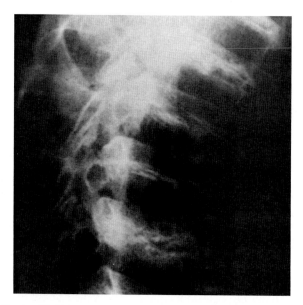

Figure 13–3 Intervertebral disk ossification in ochronosis.

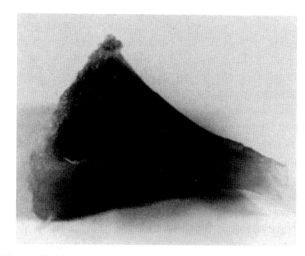

Figure 13–4 Blackening of the knee meniscus in ochronosis.

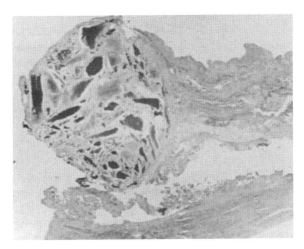

Figure 13–5 Golden brown pigmented shards from the friable cartilage embedded in synovium in ochronosis.

decreased with it.[14,35] High doses of ascorbic acid, although they do not decrease total urinary homogentisic acid, have been reported to inhibit binding to connective tissue in experimental alkaptonuria of rats.[40] High levels of ascorbic acid in vitro can prevent the inhibitory effect of homogentisic acid on chondrocyte growth.[33] Nitisinone is an experimental agent that has had initial clinical studies and has been shown to decrease homogentisic acid levels.[40a] Corrective orthopedic measures have been effective and without any special problems.[41,42]

Gaucher Disease

Gaucher disease is an inherited metabolic disease characterized by the accumulation of glucocerebroside in distinctive Gaucher cells, most prominently in the liver, spleen, and bone. The glucocerebroside deposits occur because of a deficiency of the enzyme glucocerebrosidase.[43] The disease is more common in, but not restricted to, people of Ashkenazi Jewish background. Clinical severity can vary widely. Different clinical types with different prognoses have been defined. Some individuals are disabled by the age of 30 years, whereas others lead relatively symptom-free lives to old age.[44,45] Common findings in adults are splenomegaly, hepatomegaly, anemia and thrombocytopenia (caused by hypersplenism and, occasionally, marrow replacement), pingueculae, and bone marrow expansion causing such findings as the Erlenmeyer flask appearance of the distal femur. Neurologic problems are more common in children. The age at onset and severity tends to correlate with the degree of glucocerebrosidase deficiency.[43]

Definitive diagnosis can be made by bone marrow biopsy or by biochemical study of leukocytes detecting low levels of beta glucosidase. Gaucher cells are large reticuloendothelial cells with profuse, "wrinkled," pale pink cytoplasm on hematoxylin-eosin staining and with one or more small nuclei. Electron microscopy shows that the cytoplasm of these cells is occupied by membrane-bound inclusions filled with tubular structures typical of glucocerebroside. Acid phosphatase is demonstrable within the

tubules in some vacuoles. Chemical analysis also shows iron and other components in the vacuoles.[43] Gaucher-like cells are not diagnostic of Gaucher disease; they have also been seen in thalassemia[46] and chronic myelogenous leukemia.[47]

Elevated serum levels of acid phosphatase are observed and may be helpful in suggesting a diagnosis of Gaucher disease. Increased angiotensin-converting enzyme[48] and relative factor IX deficiency have been reported.

The degenerative arthritis in Gaucher disease follows marrow infiltration, aseptic necrosis, or pathologic fracture,[49] with resulting joint distortion. It is most common in the hip but has also been seen in the shoulders and knees. Joint space narrowing is secondary.

Synovial fluid has rarely been examined. In one patient with pathologic fractures of tibial plateaus, joint fluid was clear yellow and contained 600 white blood cells, 7050 red blood cells, and no crystals under polarized light.[49] Actual infiltration of Gaucher cells into cartilage has not been noted.

In addition to aseptic necrosis, radiographic changes of the skeleton include demineralization and cortical thinning as a result of the medullary expansion, foci of sclerosis, and pathologic fractures. Epiphyseal and diaphyseal areas of long bones are prominently involved. Shafts of long bones may be widened with the infiltrative process, as is most typically described in the distal femur.

Not all musculoskeletal symptoms are caused by the OA; they also appear to result from pathologic fractures, episodic periostitis or painful bone crises possibly due to ischemia (often with fever) that may be difficult to distinguish from osteomyelitis[50] and deep aching bone pain.[51] Many bone lesions detected radiographically are asymptomatic. Amyloidosis[52] has been noted in two reports in association with Gaucher disease and might offer a secondary cause for musculoskeletal problems.

Reconstructive joint surgery,[50] including total hip replacement, has been successful, but hemorrhage has been an important complication. Increased postoperative infections have been reported.

Replacement of the deficient enzyme has been performed, but how effective it will be for bone disease is not known.[53] Other theoretical treatments such as gene therapy, extracorporeal degradation of the glucocerebroside, stimulation of residual endogenous enzyme, and alteration of other normal related enzymes have been considered and may be clinically possible in the future.[43,54]

Hemoglobinopathies

Sickle Cell Disease

Sickle cell disease is by far the most common hemoglobinopathy associated with musculoskeletal manifestations.[55] Homozygous sickle cell disease is an inherited disease most common in Blacks and caused by a substitution of valine for glutamic acid as the sixth amino acid in the β-chain of hemoglobin. This results in sickling of erythrocytes, which presumably occludes small vessels, causing painful crises and bone lesions.[56] Other manifestations described include hemolytic anemia, renal involvement with hyposthenuria, leg ulcers, hyporegenerative crises, increased infections (especially with salmonellae), and a variety of rheumatic or bone and joint problems.

Diagnosis is generally made by hemoglobin electrophoresis or with allele specific oligonucleotide probes. Hemoglobin S comprises 76% to 100% of hemoglobin in homozygous sickle cell disease.

Aseptic necrosis appears to be the basis for any OA in these patients.[55] As with other causes of aseptic necrosis, homozygous sickle cell disease, sickle cell–hemoglobin C disease, sickle cell–thalassemia, and possibly sickle cell trait[57,58] can lead to OA as a result of the incongruity of the joint space and loss of normal bony support for the articular cartilage. This is most common at the hip but can also involve the spine, knee,[59] shoulder[60] (Fig. 13–6), and occasionally other joints.

In addition to aseptic necrosis, radiographic changes in sickle cell disease can include coarse trabeculae with hair-on-end appearance in the skull, osteopenia, vertebral indentations, medullary infarctions, and periosteal elevation.

Other bone and joint problems in sickle cell disease that are clearly more typical than OA for this disease include infarction of bone away from joints, hyperuricemia and occasional gout,[58] the "hand-foot syndrome" in young children, osteomyelitis and rare septic arthritis, muscle necrosis, and acute joint effusions, usually but not always with low leukocyte counts.[55,61] An element of synovitis for which there is no clear explanation[62] and a diffuse chondrolysis[63] can damage cartilage and contribute to the later development of OA.

Total hip and knee arthroplasties[55,64,65] have been performed for the secondary OA after avascular necrosis and have been highly successful. Preoperative transfusions have been used to decrease the chances of sickling during surgery. Tourniquets should be avoided to reduce anoxia and stasis, which contribute to thrombosis. Good hydration and efforts during anesthesia to avoid any hypoxia and acidosis are also warranted.[64]

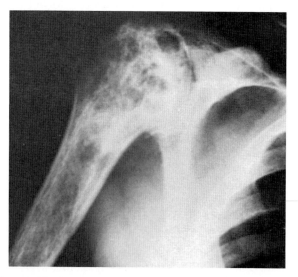

Figure 13–6 Severe marrow infarctions at the shoulder with associated OA in sickle cell disease.

Thalassemia

β-Thalassemia describes a group of inherited disorders of hemoglobin synthesis resulting in a relative decrease in β-chains. Hemoglobin α-chains accumulate, producing unstable hemoglobin, Heinz bodies, and hypochromic microcytic erythrocytes. Early erythrocyte death results in marrow expansion and splenomegaly. Levels of hemoglobin F or A_2 are elevated.

Frequent transfusions are required and often lead to secondary iron overload. Thalassemia major with severe anemia often leads to death in the second or third decade. Milder thalassemia minor may be asymptomatic and may not require therapy.

OA has been described as developing prematurely in thalassemia major and minor. Weight-bearing joints (including the ankles) were predominantly involved in one series, but shoulders, wrists, and elbows have been equally affected in other studies.[66-70] The speculation is that marrow hyperplasia may weaken the subchondral bone and allow microfractures that then alter the normal support required by the articular cartilage.[69,70] Osteomalacia has been confirmed in the areas of microfractures.[70] Multiple transfusions and iron overload might contribute to osteoarthropathy in some patients, as is described in hemochromatosis,[71] but early OA has also been described without iron overload.[69] Juxta-articular osteopenia and bone cysts[67] may be seen on radiographs. Osteonecrosis has been reported, but whether it is increased in incidence has not been established.[68,72] Widened medullary spaces with thin cortices, coarse trabeculations, and microfractures are seen in bone with marrow expansion. Synovial fluid, when studied, has been noninflammatory. Tophaceous gout has been described.[73]

Dull, aching pain, especially at the ankles, has been described after strenuous exercise.[70] Because the cartilage space was normal on radiography, the pain was attributed to the periarticular bone involvement.[70]

No specific treatment is available for the established OA caused by thalassemia. Transfusions may decrease excessive erythropoiesis with its associated marrow expansion and bone loss. Bone marrow or stem cell transplantation has been used for some patients for the thalassemia.[74] Total hip replacements have been performed.[75]

Ehlers–Danlos Syndrome and Other Joint Hypermobility

The Ehlers–Danlos syndrome consists of a group of heritable disorders of connective tissue[76] with features that include hypermobility of joints (Fig. 13–7), hyperextensible skin, poor wound healing, bruising, and cigarette paper scars. At least seven different types of Ehlers–Danlos syndrome have been identified, with clinical differences, different inheritance, and, in some cases, identified biochemical defects.

The most serious type of Ehlers–Danlos syndrome is the type IV vascular or ecchymotic type; patients with this form of the syndrome rarely survive past 20 years of age.

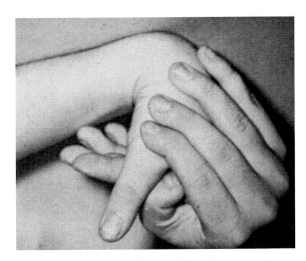

Figure 13–7 Joint hypermobility in Ehlers–Danlos syndrome.

Restriction fragment length polymorphisms for the type III collagen gene have been described.[77] Such diagnostic testing has allowed identification of milder variants of this type. Type III Ehlers–Danlos syndrome with benign hypermobility is inherited as an autosomal dominant trait and is one of the types in which secondary OA can become prominent. The biochemical defect is not known. Type I has large, irregular collagen fibers by electron microscopy. It is also inherited as an autosomal dominant trait and has been associated with premature OA.[78]

Quantification of the degree of hypermobility has been described.[79] A typical collapsing skeletal structure on the initial handshake may be a clue.

The development of OA seems to be directly related to the severity of hypermobility and the frequency and degree of trauma to which any given joint is exposed.[80] OA associated with Ehlers–Danlos syndrome or other hypermobility has been reported in the hands, knees, ankles, and shoulders. It often appears before the age of 40 years, but not all reviews can confirm an association with OA.[81] Beighton[80] reported finding no cases of OA of the hip associated with the Ehlers–Danlos syndrome.

Synovial effusions studied have had few cells. Synovial biopsy specimens have shown no distinctive changes by light microscopy.[82] Pathologic studies of articular cartilage have not been reported. Abnormal bone morphology has been suggested.[83] Radiographs of joints have no unique features, and subluxations, when correctable, may not be appreciated on films.

Mechanisms of production of the OA are suspected to include abnormal cartilage structure or wear caused by excessive motion and inadequate protection from trauma. Whether structural abnormalities related to abnormal collagen occur in capsule and cartilage is not yet known. Studies based on pressure-volume relationships in the knee during distention showed no definite evidence of altered collagen functional properties.[84]

In addition to OA, joints may be involved by dislocations, instability, noninflammatory effusions, and spinal deformities (kyphoscoliosis).[82,85] Other potentially con-fusing and complicating problems include fibromyalgia,[81] increased muscle cramps, and spasm; peripheral circulatory disease, especially in type IV Ehlers–Danlos syndrome; congenital abnormalities of bones; and periarticular hemorrhage.

Treatment in symptomatic patients should include educational efforts to help avoid activities that hyperextend joints. Swimming can be used to strengthen muscles to try to aid joint support. Surgery may be made difficult by unpredictable increased bleeding and poor wound healing, but total knee arthroplasties have been performed successfully.[86]

Isolated joint hypermobility without Ehlers–Danlos syndrome also seems to be associated with an increased incidence of OA in some reports and, in one study,[87] with chondrocalcinosis. These were not prospective studies, so the exact reasons for such relationships are not clear.[88] Scott and associates[88] found more OA in patients with mild idiopathic joint hypermobility than in age-matched control subjects. The neck, thumb, and knee are involved with OA in patients before the age of 30 years.[79] In other studies, no correlation could be found between "benign hypermobility" and OA, other arthritis, or arthralgias.[89,90] Kraus et al.[91] actually found a protective effect of hypermobility on hand OA. It has been proposed that occupational stresses and hypermobility have an additive effect in causing cases of intercarpal OA.[92] Recurrent subluxation of the patella can lead to patellofemoral OA, but Crosby and Insall[93] actually found that OA was more common in patients in their series after attempted surgical realignment to prevent dislocation.

Other causes of hypermobility that have been described include Larsen syndrome[85] (a congenital condition characterized by depressed bridge of the nose and other altered facial features); Desbuquois syndrome, with prominent eyes and a variety of hand problems; spondyloepimetaphyseal dysplasia; the occipital horn syndrome caused by copper deficiency (formerly type IX Ehlers–Danlos syndrome) or the similar Menkes syndrome; acromegaly; Marfan syndrome; Jaccoud arthropathy after rheumatic fever, in systemic lupus erythematosus, or in KID (keratitis, ichthyosis, and deafness) syndrome[72]; hyperparathyroidism; hereditary osteochondrodysplasia; progressive arthroophthalmopathy[97]; Wilson disease; and Noonan syndrome.[95] Interestingly, OA does not develop in all of these patients, despite the hypermobility.

ENDOCRINE DISEASES

Acromegaly

A growth hormone–secreting tumor of the anterior pituitary in adults leads to slowly progressive overgrowth of soft tissue, bone, and cartilage. Because linear growth is not possible at this time, enlargement is prominent in the acral parts, with gradually increasing size of the hands and feet as well as of the nose and mandible. There is typical coarsening of features. Patients with acromegaly often have increased sweating and moist, thick skin. Mild glucose intolerance occurs in 50% of patients, because hyperexcretion of growth hormone causes insulin resistance. Diagnosis is based on clinical findings together with laboratory confirmation by demonstration of elevated levels of insulin-like growth factor 1 (somatomedin C) or serum growth hormone levels and failure of suppression of growth hormone with glucose. The severity of acromegaly does not correlate directly with growth hormone levels, probably at least partly because growth hormone effects are mediated indirectly through somatomedins produced in the liver.[96]

Peripheral and spinal OA is common in acromegaly. Peripheral joint symptoms occur in about 60% of acromegalic individuals.[97–99] The joints most commonly involved have been the knees, hips, shoulders, elbows, and occasionally ankles. Although soft tissue swelling, widened distal phalanx bone tufts, and carpal tunnel syndrome are present in the hands, there is little OA. Hip and knee involvement has been disabling in severe acromegaly. Crepitus is very common. There may be small or, rarely, large effusions and apparent synovial thickening, but acute inflammation has not been reported.

Backache occurs frequently, but back motion (as well as peripheral joint motion) is often normal or increased. This is tentatively attributed to the thickened disks and cartilages plus laxity of acromegalic ligaments.[100] A kyphotic posture is common. There can be spinal demineralization.[101]

Synovial effusions have been noninflammatory, as in other osteoarthritides. Fluids with high leukocyte counts have been seen in our series only in patients who also have rheumatoid arthritis or gout.[102] Synovial biopsy specimens have shown only mild villous proliferation, focal increased lining cells, and increased vascularity.[98,102]

The early increased cartilage thickness producing wide "joint spaces" on radiographs can be seen at various joints. Later, joint space narrowing, osteophytes, and subchondral sclerosis occur. Chondrocalcinosis, capsular calcification, and osteochondromas have occasionally been seen. Remodeling of phalanges can produce thickening of the shaft at the tendon and capsular attachments, but thin metacarpal shafts have also been seen, possibly caused by remodeling. In the spine, large anterior osteophytes and ossification in widened disks and in ligaments can be seen. Increased new bone formation can be similar to that seen in diffuse idiopathic skeletal hyperostosis and may be related to increased somatomedins.[103,104] Vertebral bodies often develop anteroposterior elongation.[100]

Mechanisms involved in the secondary OA appear to include dramatic cartilage overgrowth that produces joint incongruity and abnormal wear. Whether abnormal cartilage composition also contributes to degeneration is not known. Hypermobility might also contribute to cartilage abuse. Hypermobility was severe in seven patients studied by Kellgren and coworkers,[100] with actual subluxations in two. Chondrocalcinosis seen on radiographs[105] and apatite crystals seen so far mainly in synovial biopsy specimens[102] might also contribute to OA by either local mechanical effects in the cartilage or low-grade inflammation. Histologic studies of articular cartilage show hyperplasia

and hypertrophy of the columnar and basal zones of chondrocytes. Superficial fibrillation and erosion of cartilage at weight-bearing sites occur with time. Marginal osteophyte formation is often excessive.

As noted previously, musculoskeletal symptoms in acromegaly are caused not only by OA but also by carpal tunnel syndrome, hypermobility, and possibly other related endocrine deficiencies.

Acromegaly can be treated by medical therapy with octreotide or bromocriptine, surgical resection of small adenomas, or occasional adjunct pituitary irradiation. There is no suggestion that this alters established OA, although associated arthralgias and conditions resulting from overgrowth of soft tissue, such as the carpal tunnel syndrome, are dramatically relieved.[97,98]

When needed, surgery such as total hip arthroplasty has been successful; the firm trabecular bone of acromegaly appears to tolerate the prosthesis well. Careful evaluation of other endocrine values is essential before surgery. Adrenal insufficiency secondary to hypopituitarism, for example, may require steroid supplementation.

Hypothyroidism

Only fairly severe hypothyroidism with detectable clinical features such as cold intolerance, weight gain, lethargy, and constipation has been definitely associated with arthropathy. In addition to low serum triiodothyronine and thyroxine levels, reported cases have highly elevated levels of thyrotropin (also known as thyroid-stimulating hormone), suggesting that they are caused by primary thyroid disease rather than pituitary insufficiency.

OA has been described in association with hypothyroidism,[106] but whether it is definitely increased above the expected frequency in the population is not known. Hip OA changes in a young man led to a review of possible epiphyseal dysgenesis as a factor.[107] Chondrocalcinosis and CPPD deposition do occur and could explain some cases of OA.[108] Kashin-Beck disease has been reported to be more severe in areas with iodine deficiency and hypothyroidism.

Radiographic examination may or may not show chondrocalcinosis, even if CPPD crystals are found in the synovial fluid. Some patients have a destructive OA.[106]

Other manifestations of hypothyroidism cause musculoskeletal symptoms that can be confused with OA. These include carpal tunnel syndrome, viscous joint effusions, myalgias, myopathy, secondary gout, flexor tenosynovitis, and fibrositis. Serum creatine kinase may be elevated and may cause confusion with polymyositis.

There is no evidence that treating hypothyroidism alters any associated OA, but thyroid hormone replacement may relieve some of the associated symptoms. The clinician should be aware that patients with CPPD crystals but no inflammatory reaction can and do develop acute pseudogout with thyroid hormone therapy.[108] Thyroxine has actually been shown to stimulate transglutaminase and a hypertrophic phenotype that favors mineralization of articular chondrocytes.[109] How this fits with thyroid disease and OA remains to be seen.

Hyperparathyroidism

Increased levels of parathyroid hormone, whether primary or secondary, can produce a wide variety of rheumatic problems in addition to the classic features of osteitis fibrosa cystica. Other systemic manifestations include peptic ulcer disease, nephrolithiasis, symptoms caused by hypercalcemia, pancreatitis, and a variety of other less common problems. Serum calcium levels are usually elevated at some time; hyperparathyroidism can be confirmed by elevated parathyroid hormone levels. Serum uric acid levels may be increased.

OA has been described as complicating hyperparathyroidism,[110] and two major mechanisms have been postulated. These are

1) cartilage damage from the mechanical or inflammatory effects of the frequently associated CPPD crystal deposition (chondrocalcinosis, which has been reported in up to 25% of patients with primary hyperparathyroidism[111])
2) subchondral bone erosion caused by the resorptive effects of parathyroid hormone, leading to subchondral bone change and secondary collapse of articular cartilage.

This has been seen most often at the DIP, PIP, MCP, and wrist joints.[110] Parathyroid hormone increases collagenase activity, which also contributes to tendon ruptures and avulsions.[112] The resulting instability might be a factor in some cases of OA.

Radiographs classically show subperiosteal bone resorption along the middle phalanges or elsewhere and osteolytic, cystic, or sclerotic changes in bone, and may show typical chondrocalcinosis.[113,114]

Synovial effusions may contain CPPD crystals, and these are sometimes accompanied by elevated leukocyte counts. Because of the impaired urate clearance, urate crystals can also be present. Concomitant occurrence of synovial fluid urates and CPPD should suggest a search for hyperparathyroidism.[115]

Other musculoskeletal problems[116] seen in hyperparathyroidism include gout related to impaired renal clearance of urate, proximal neuromyopathy, fatigue that is probably partially caused by hypercalcemia, and ischemic problems resulting from intravascular calcification in secondary hyperparathyroidism. Parathyroidectomy does not consistently alter the chondrocalcinosis, and in fact, attacks of pseudogout can occur postoperatively coincident with the fall in serum calcium.[113,117,118] Bone resorption can be reversed, and systemic features such as the neuromyopathy and fatigue should resolve, although established OA will not.

Diabetes Mellitus

Although diabetes has been mentioned as a possible cause of OA,[119] known mechanisms through which OA may develop seem to be limited so far to the neuropathic joints complicating diabetes. These are discussed separately with Charcot joints. In experimental diabetes in rats, cartilage collagen and other protein production was diminished. This was reversible with insulin therapy.[120]

Diabetes does have other effects on the musculoskeletal system that can confuse or complicate the management of OA.[121] These include distal neuropathy, a proximal muscle weakness probably caused by neuropathy and termed diabetic amyotrophy, diabetic muscle infarction,[122] gout, adhesive capsulitis at the shoulders, phalangeal flexion contractures[123] with or without Dupuytren contracture, septic joints, and osteolysis. Diffuse idiopathic skeletal hyperostosis is more common in diabetics (and acromegalics) but should not be confused with OA.

Aspirin has a mild hypoglycemic effect that occasionally must be considered in management of patients. Intra-articular steroids for treatment of OA should be used cautiously in light of their known systemic absorption and ability to cause temporary control problems in severe diabetes.

CALCIUM CRYSTAL DEPOSITION DISEASES

Calcium Pyrophosphate Deposition Disease

Deposition of CPPD crystals, which is virtually confined to joints and bursae, can have various overlapping or separate presentations. The crystals can be phagocytosed by synovial fluid cells,[124-127] and can be associated with acute or chronic gout-like arthritis with clearly inflammatory joint effusions. Chronic forms may closely mimic joint involvement in rheumatoid arthritis. CPPD can be present in asymptomatic form in articular cartilage and can then be detected only by radiographic or histologic examination. Such "chondrocalcinosis" was described in 1957 by Zitnan and Sitaj,[128] and the synovial fluid crystals and their apparent role in inflammation were discovered by McCarty and Hollander[129] in 1961. CPPD crystals are also commonly found in many osteoarthritic joint fluids, where they are sometimes but not invariably associated with appreciable inflammation.[130,131]

Calcium pyrophosphate deposition is most often idiopathic, although it clearly increases with age and has been identified in familial clusters in Czechoslovakia,[132] Chile,[133] and elsewhere. The mode of inheritance is not clear. CPPD crystals have been identified in 3.2% to 6.8% of cadavers and have been suspected radiographically in 2.2% to 4.6% of subjects in their sixth decade and in as many as 27% of a group of elderly people with a mean age of 83 years.[124,134] CPPD deposition has also been described to be increased in association with a number of important, largely metabolic diseases, including hyperparathyroidism, hemochromatosis, myxedematous hypothyroidism, hypophosphatasia, hypomagnesemia, and possibly amyloidosis, ochronosis, acromegaly, and Wilson disease. Possible molecular factors involved in CPPD deposition have been reviewed.[135]

CPPD crystals are identified in tissue or synovial fluid as rod-shaped or rhomboid crystals that are usually 3 to 15 μm in length. With compensated polarized light, they have weakly positive or absent birefringence. Light microscopic morphologic and birefringence characteristics are highly suggestive of CPPD crystals but are not pathognomonic, because other rod-like, positively birefringent crystals, including depot steroids, some calcium oxalate,[136] and calcium hydrogen phosphate dihydrate,[137,138] can also occasionally be seen in joint effusions. Lithium heparin used in test tubes as an anticoagulant may also yield crystals that resemble CPPD.[139]

Crystals can be concentrated and prepared for x-ray diffraction study as described by Kohn and coworkers.[140] If specimens have adequate numbers of crystals, this is definitive.

Electron microscopic examination for crystals can be done with standard glutaraldehyde or other fixation, as is done for routine transmission electron microscopy, because the CPPD crystals are minimally soluble in the water-based solutions used. CPPD crystals are electron dense and foamy after exposure to the electron beam (Fig. 13–8). CPPD crystals are hard and can be dislodged from sections, causing them to be missed. A rapid technique allowing transmission electron microscopic processing for examination in less than 4 hours[141] may prove useful in prompt diagnosis of problem cases. Small CPPD crystals can be missed by light microscopy and found by electron microscopy.

Drops of crystal-containing synovial fluid can also be dried on Formvar-coated grids or processed for scanning electron microscopy for rapid identification of the presence of crystals. With all these electron microscopic techniques, crystals can then be further characterized by either electron diffraction[137] or electron probe elemental analysis, which can confirm a calcium to phosphorus ratio of approximately 1:1, as is seen with CPPD.[137,142]

CPPD crystals can be identified in the midzone of involved articular cartilage (Fig. 13–9) and in tophus-like deposits in synovial biopsy specimens.[138,143] The only

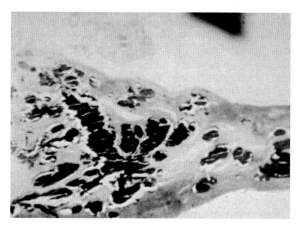

Figure 13–9 von Kossa staining of CPPD crystals is most profuse in the midzone of a knee meniscus.

required precaution is to avoid decalcification, which might be done by error if the specimen is submitted with fragments of bone. Serum calcium and phosphorus levels are usually normal, except in hyperparathyroidism.

There is clearly an increased association of CPPD with OA that appears to be more consistent at the knee than at the hip.[144,145] The basis for this association can be related to at least two patterns:

1. Obvious CPPD deposition antedates significant OA. As cartilage degenerates, OA with joint distribution typical of that of CPPD deposition disease develops (i.e., prominent involvement of the knees, wrists, and second and third MCP joints). Not all patients with CPPD deposition progress to significant OA, so further studies are needed.

2. The second pattern is OA, either idiopathic or related to some other primary cause, in which CPPD crystal deposition develops late in the disease. This is presumably a result of cartilage and other damage, as is also seen in chronic rheumatoid arthritis, gout, and other joint diseases. It is speculated that a cartilage matrix change in these various situations favors CPPD precipitation. Adequate sequential studies have not been done to fully establish this suggested sequence. In our laboratory about 52% of osteoarthritic synovial fluids have contained either CPPD or apatite crystals. In sequential studies only 19% had CPPD on the initial aspiration while 34% had developed CPPD on the final fluid.[146]

Synovial fluids in chronic OA with CPPD crystals are typically still noninflammatory, with predominantly mononuclear cells. Only during attacks of crystal-induced arthritis do leukocyte counts rise.

Radiographic findings include the typical linear calcification in articular cartilages and menisci. Visible calcification, however, may disappear with loss of cartilage or may rarely be seen only as punctuate deposits spread throughout the joint. Other CPPD deposits may be too small to be detected by radiography. Joint space narrowing, subchondral sclerosis, and cysts in joints typically involved in CPPD deposition disease should also suggest

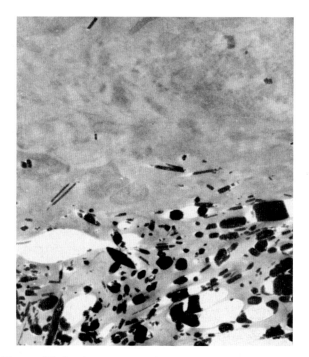

Figure 13–8 Electron-dense foamy CPPD crystals in articular cartilage (approximately ×18,000).

this diagnosis. Osteophyte formation is variable and inconstant. Occasional joints show severe destruction mimicking Charcot joints even without neurologic disease. Rarely, bone fusion may occur.

Mechanisms of the production of OA with CPPD deposition[147] may include mechanical effects of the crystals[148] in the cartilage and acute or chronic inflammation induced by the crystals with release of enzymes destructive to cartilage. An element of low-grade inflammation has been documented in naturally occurring[130,131] and experimental OA.[149] Crystals are one possible factor contributing to this, although studies in our laboratory do not show any clear correlation between the severity of synovial fluid inflammatory cell response and the presence of crystals. Injection of CPPD crystals into joints in a lapine model of OA accelerated the OA.[150,151]

Many joint fluids, including those of idiopathic OA, have been reported to have higher than normal concentrations of pyrophosphate,[150] but whether this is followed by increased precipitation of CPPD crystals is not known.

Treatment of inflammatory episodes with nonsteroidal anti-inflammatory drugs usually controls bouts of acute pseudogout. Colchicine may also be effective, especially if it is administered intravenously. In patients with repeated episodes of inflammation, daily low-dose prophylactic administration of nonsteroidal agents or colchicine can help control symptoms. There is no evidence that this has any beneficial effect on the cartilage degeneration. Hydroxychloroquine has been used by some patients with erosive OA with CPPD crystals with anecdotal benefit. Magnesium and probenecid have also been suggested.[135] Hyaluronate use has been controversial but there are apparently no increased risks of pseudoseptic flares in patients with CPPD.[152]

Massive numbers of crystals can be aspirated with at least theoretical advantage to the joint involved, but no method to deplete CPPD crystals, comparable to the use of allopurinol or probenecid in gout, is available. Associated metabolic disease should be sought and treated when possible.

Apatite Crystal Deposition Disease

Hydroxyapatite, $Ca_3OH(PO_4)_3H_2O_2$, and related basic calcium phosphates have been recognized to be involved in the acute soft tissue syndromes of calcific tendinitis, bursitis, and periarthritis[153,154] and the subcutaneous calcifications in scleroderma and dermatomyositis. Although suspected[155] and shown[156] to be present in some articular cartilages, a role for apatite in joint disease was not strongly considered until reports in the 1970s by Dieppe and colleagues[157] and Schumacher and coworkers.[142,158] Clumps of apatite crystals can be phagocytosed in vivo or in vitro[159] and can induce inflammation when they are injected into the knee joints of dogs.[142] Like CPPD or urate crystals, they can be present without appearing to cause symptoms or can be associated with acute transient or chronic erosive arthritis.[160] Intra-articular apatite crystals have been seen in collagen-vascular disease,[161] in rheumatoid and other patients with rice bodies,[162] renal failure being treated with dialysis, hypothyroidism,

hemochromatosis, CPPD deposition disease, and OA,[142] as discussed later. Crystals have also been seen without any evident underlying cause,[142] suggesting still incompletely explained systemic factors in their deposition. Trauma is clearly an inadequate explanation for the multifocal deposits. Knee effusions have been studied most often, but there are no good data as to the frequency of involvement of various joints, the ages of individuals affected, and the epidemiologic patterns.

Clumps of apatite crystals are not birefringent and thus are not more readily detected with compensated polarized light. Clumps appear as glossy, homogeneous, and round or angular chunks measuring 1 to 15 µm in diameter. Clumps stain strongly with alizarin red or von Kossa stains. X-ray diffraction can be diagnostic if sufficient numbers of crystals are present. Smaller numbers of crystals can be identified by electron microscopy as tiny needles measuring 75 to 25 nm in diameter (Fig. 13–10). Electron probe elemental analysis shows a calcium to phosphorus ratio of approximately 1.6:1.[142,172] This can be done with either transmission or scanning electron microscopy.

OA with identifiable apatite crystals has to date shown no features different from any other OA except that the presence of apatite correlates with radiographic evidence of more severe OA.[163] Whether this is a result or a cause of the OA is not known. Patients with severe destructive OA as in the Milwaukee shoulder or comparable rapidly progressive OA of other joints virtually always have apatite or CPPD crystals in joint fluids.[164] Nine of 34 osteoarthritic joint fluid specimens studied by Huskisson and associates[131] had apparent apatite by scanning electron microscopy, whereas we have found apatite by alizarin red staining and transmission electron microscopy in approximately 50% of 100 osteoarthritic joint fluid samples we have studied.[130] Virtually every fluid specimen with CPPD crystals also contains apatite.

Synovial effusions in most OA associated with apatite have had leukocyte counts of less than 600/mm², although occasional elevated leukocyte counts and inflammatory

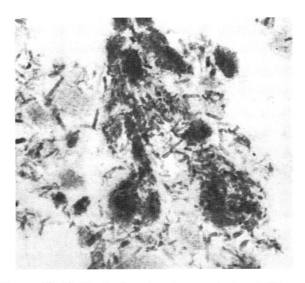

Figure 13–10 Needle-shaped apatite crystals at ×90,000 magnification by electron microscopy.

infiltrates or proliferative changes in synovium can be seen. These seem to correlate with the severity of OA as well as with the presence of crystals,[130] so that the role of the crystals versus other factors in the development of inflammation has not been established.

Apatite clumps can be demonstrated in synovium in OA[130,131] and, most intriguingly, can be found in articular cartilage by electron microscopy[130,165] much more often than had been appreciated by light microscopy or radiography (Fig. 13–11). Quantitation of crystal frequency and amount in different joints, ages, and patterns of OA is still needed. Basophilia and von Kossa staining in calcified areas can be an important clue to the presence of crystals.[165] Ali[165] has emphasized that the initial apatite deposition is in matrix vesicles, although this is not clearly true in all studies.

Radiographs in OA commonly show small periarticular calcifications that have previously been little appreciated but can now be shown to correlate with both the severity of OA and the presence of apatite.[130,131,166]

Severe degenerative changes of shoulders and other large joints in association with apatite-containing particles have been described.[167,168] Synovial fluid samples show apatite crystals and, in the initial studies, collagenase and neutral protease activity. It was suggested that enzymatic release of hydroxyapatite crystals from the synovium and endocytosis by synovial macrophage-like cells, with subsequent crystal-stimulated release of collagenase and neutral protease into the joint fluid, were components of the pathogenic cycle of this entity. The origin of apatite in such severely destroyed joints is not established; much of it may be from bone debris. In a recent study of 30 patients with rotator cuff tears, those with apatite crystals identified by alizarin red stains had more glenohumeral OA but not higher leukocyte counts, PGE2, or proteinase levels.[169]

As noted previously, mechanisms relating apatite to low-grade inflammation and OA are still under study. One possibility is that other materials in the fluid or coating the apatite clumps may influence their inflammatory potential. Apatite may also be contributing to OA by its physical presence in the cartilage, as was also suggested with CPPD. Naturally occurring[170] and experimental[171] apatite deposition in rabbit articular cartilage has been documented and should allow study of any of its effects on cartilage with further aging. A series of elegant studies have shown that apatite and other basic calcium phosphates can induce metalloproteinase synthesis by fibroblasts,[172] can induce TNF expression,[173] PGE2 production[174] and can induce mitogenesis that might cause synovial proliferation[175] but also preserve cells. It is not known whether apatites are always deleterious or might have some physiologic protective role. Different basic calcium phosphate composition of deposits might alter effects in the joint. Inflammatory properties vary among octacalcium phosphate, hydroxyapatite, and carbonated apatite.[176]

As yet, there are no recommended alterations in the routine treatment of OA that can be predicated on the presence of apatite crystals in synovial fluid.

OTHER SYSTEMIC DISEASES

Neuropathic Arthropathy (Charcot Joints)

Neuropathy resulting from various causes can be complicated by an arthropathy that has elements of unusually severe OA. The neuropathy may vary from mild loss of sensation of pain or proprioception to a severe neurologic problem, including anesthesia.[177] Since the early description by Charcot in 1868, diseases that have been associated with neuropathic joints include diabetes mellitus,[178] syringomyelia, meningomyelocele, syphilis with tabes dorsalis, leprosy, congenital insensitivity to pain,[179] amyloidosis,[180] and hereditary sensory neuropathies.[181] Other less common causes of neurologic dysfunction have also been described with Charcot joints.[177,182,183] Sites of involvement tend to vary among diseases and are discussed later.

The arthropathy clinically presents with swelling that may be massive, crepitus from the typically severe destruction of cartilage and bone, instability, palpable loose bodies, and, later, large osteophytes. Some pain may be present and is worse on use. When it is present, pain tends to be much less than would be expected from the appearance of the joint. Effusions are often intermittent and may be associated with erythema.

Synovial effusions are generally noninflammatory or hemorrhagic. Cells in the fluid have been mostly mononuclear. In occasional patients with associated calcium pyrophosphate deposition, higher leukocyte counts and more neutrophils are seen.

Synovial biopsy specimens show cartilage and bone debris ground deeply into the membrane, along with

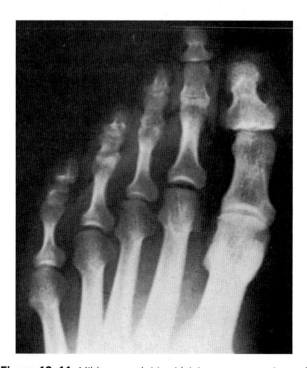

Figure 13–11 Mild osteoarthritis with joint space narrowing and sclerosis at the first metatarsophalangeal joint. Acute inflammation that was proved to be caused by apatite crystals developed at this joint.

hemosiderin and metaplastic bone formation.[184,185] Pannus-like synovial proliferation has been described.[186] Mild to moderate infiltration of chronic inflammatory cells has been noted without specific relationship to calcified areas.[187] Histologic examination of cartilage has shown the sequence of changes seen in other OA.[188] Bone has been described as histologically normal except for the fractures.[189]

In tabes dorsalis, the knees are most prominently involved; hip, ankle, foot, and spine disease is also seen in some patients. About 10% of patients with tabes develop arthropathy. In syringomyelia, about 25% of afflicted individuals develop Charcot joints, which in this disease occur most often in the shoulder (Fig. 13–12). Other sites of involvement, in order of frequency, are the elbow, wrist, and cervical spine.

In diabetes mellitus, about 5% of patients with chronic disease and neuropathy develop neuropathic arthropathy in the feet. The tarsal and tarsometatarsal joints are commonly involved (Fig. 13–13). Osteomyelitis can be difficult to exclude especially in patients with local cutaneous ulcers and may require biopsy.[190] Osteolysis in the phalanges may accompany disease there. Other sites are affected much less often.

Radiographs initially show only soft tissue swelling, but this is soon followed by subluxation and changes seen with any OA. Differentiating features may include enormous and bizarre osteophytes, transverse fractures, osteolysis, prominent osseous fragments, or calcifications. The diagnosis should often be suspected on clinical grounds before the more advanced distinctive changes appear. Chondrocalcinosis has been seen, but it is not clear whether this is merely a result of the cartilage

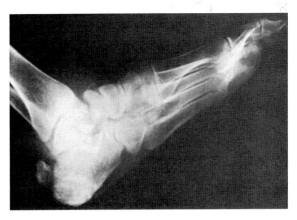

Figure 13–13 Charcot foot in diabetes mellitus. Note fracturing, calcifications, and intertarsal narrowing.

degeneration or if a more destructive arthritis results when the neurologic deficit is added to a preexisting calcium pyrophosphate deposition.[191,192]

Mechanisms involved almost certainly include repeated joint abuse because of loss of normal pain and proprioceptive protection. Experimental studies have supported this; protection of denervated animal limbs from trauma has been reported to prevent fractures and other changes.[189] Microvascular disease has been thought to be a possible contributing factor in diabetic patients.

Treatment should include any effort possible to slow or halt the various associated neurologic diseases. Protection from trauma is more critically important than in most primary osteoarthritides. Splinting, braces, special shoes, and canes are often helpful. Aspiration of large joint effusions can help prevent the stretching of supporting structures. Successful surgical fusions of unstable joints have been performed, but some difficulties have been encountered in obtaining a fusion, especially if complete, long-duration immobilization is not achieved. Complete removal of the proliferated synovium and detritus, excision of an adequate amount of the damaged bone, and internal fixation seem to improve the chances for success of the fusion.[188]

Charcot joints may become secondarily infected, and this needs to be watched for and treated. Joint replacements have rarely been used and are generally contraindicated. In one instance, limited success at one hip was complicated by poor healing and by recurrent dislocations.[193] Fractures of fragments, other than small ones, require internal fixation. Osteotomy may provide some help by aligning severely subluxated knees.

Paget Disease (Osteitis Deformans)

Paget disease is a skeletal disorder of unknown cause characterized by thickened trabeculae with disorganized osteoid seams. Both new bone formation and absorption are increased, leading to softening and enlargement of bones and bowing of the long bones. Other well-demarcated areas of bone are normal. Commonly involved sites include the tibiae, clavicles, femora, pelvis, sternum, skull, and spine.

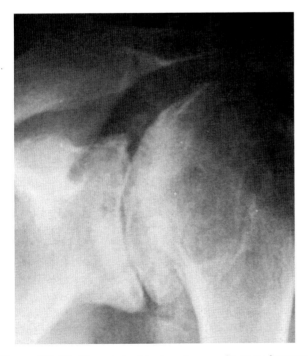

Figure 13–12 Charcot shoulder in syringomyelia. Note fragmentation, sclerosis, osteophytes, and joint space narrowing.

Blood flow is increased in the lesions, occasionally leading to bruits and even high-output heart failure. Serum alkaline phosphatase levels are increased. Hydroxyproline released from sites of bone resorption is excreted, giving elevated urinary levels. Bone biopsy is needed only occasionally when the diagnosis is unclear. The disease is frequently asymptomatic.

Disease of the hip joint with features of OA (i.e., pain on use and limited motion) can result from distortion of the femoral heads or acetabulum as a result of the underlying bone disease. Altman[194] found OA of the hips in 30% of patients with Paget disease. The knee was involved in 11% of the patients. OA can develop in other joints, including even the first metatarsophalangeal joint (Fig. 13–14), because of distortion of the joint by adjacent pagetic bone involvement. Asymptomatic Paget disease in one leg may lead to painful OA on the opposite side as a result of leg length discrepancy. Juxta-articular bone enlargement is sometimes evident.

Lumbar spine pain is common[194] and in many patients is associated with straightening of the low back and some hip and knee flexion. Back pain has complex factors related to posture, some pagetic involvement, and secondary or unrelated OA. Results of synovial fluid examinations or synovial biopsies have not been reported in the studies reviewed.

Radiographs of areas involved with Paget disease show mottled increase in bone density, coarse trabeculae, and incomplete fractures as well as a variety of deformities caused by the bone softening. Protrusio acetabuli with adjacent osteophytes can develop from the pressure of the femoral head into the soft acetabulum.[195] Joint space narrowing occurs. It has been suggested[196] that this is at least

partially caused by accelerated endochondral ossification and replacement of the deeper layers of cartilage by pagetic bone. Pagetic changes have been seen in the spinal ossifications of ankylosing hyperostosis.[194]

Mechanisms for the OA include distortion of joint configuration by the abnormal bone, leading to abnormal wear, alteration in the properties of subchondral bone, accelerated endochondral ossification, and altered biomechanics from bowing and leg length discrepancies.[194,197]

Pain obviously also arises from bone itself more often than from the joint disease, and this must be differentiated. Any dramatic increase in pain or swelling should suggest fracture or osteogenic sarcoma, which has an increased incidence in pagetic bone. Some patients have had overproduction of uric acid and gouty arthritis has been associated.[198] CPPD deposition disease has also been reported,[199] but the frequency of this is not convincingly increased compared with that in the nonpagetic population.[194]

Treatment of Paget disease can include the use of aspirin or other nonsteroidal anti-inflammatory agents that seem to help both bone pain and the pain of the secondary OA. Oral bisphosphonates given in courses of 2 to 4 months may decrease pain and lower alkaline phosphatase levels. Mithramycin has also been used in refractory disease but is now rarely needed.

Total joint replacements have been performed successfully in joints with pagetic bone involvement,[200] and osteotomies can be used to correct bowing deformities. Vascular pagetic bone may bleed at surgery. Treatment with a bisphosphonate before any surgery may decrease the hypervascularity and limit the risk of bleeding at operation.

Osteopetrosis

Osteopetrosis is a rare disease[201–206] that is characterized by generalized skeletal osteosclerosis, hard but fragile bone leading to easy fracture, and obliteration of the marrow cavity.

Patients with the severe "congenital" autosomal recessive form have not survived past 20 years of age; a milder Type II autosomal dominant form (Albers-Schonberg disease) also occurs and can cause secondary OA. The disease mechanism involves defective absorption of calcified cartilage, with the persistence of primitive bone. Bone biopsies show increased trabecular bone that blends with the cortex and cartilage cores within trabeculae. Varying appearances of osteoclasts have been described. Serum calcium and phosphorus levels are usually normal, but the alkaline phosphatase level is often increased. Renal tubular acidosis has been associated with osteopetrosis in several cases and may actually have ameliorated the osteosclerosis.

Bone marrow encroachment can cause anemia, thrombocytopenia, leukopenia, and extramedullary hematopoiesis. Cranial nerve compression at foramina can occur. Infections may be increased and include osteomyelitis in the abnormal bone.

OA has been noted especially at the hips.[201–204] Hip OA developed in 27% of one large series and required total joint arthroplasty in 9 of the 16 affected hips.[204] Factors that may

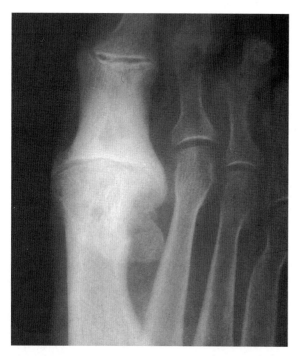

Figure 13–14 Paget disease of the first toe metatarsal and phalanx causing OA of the MT-P joint.

be involved include loss of the normal shock-absorbing qualities for cartilage with this hard bone, subchondral fractures weakening support for the initially normal cartilage, and, in a few of the reported cases, malalignment problems from deformities or aseptic necrosis resulting from femoral neck fractures.[201]

Radiographs of bones[206] show diffuse, extreme laminar cortical thickening with a chalky appearance, loss of normal trabeculations, and varying degrees of obliteration of the marrow cavity. Margins of the cortex usually remain sharp, not fuzzy as in metastatic tumor. A "shaft-within-a-shaft" appearance can be seen in long bones. Other causes of relatively diffuse, dense sclerotic bone that should be differentiated include fluorosis,[207] sickle cell disease, Paget disease, hyperparathyroidism, lymphoma, multiple myeloma,[208] mastocytosis, polyvinylpyrrolidone toxicity,[209] heavy metal poisoning, sarcoidosis, renal osteodystrophy,[210] and myelofibrosis. At least some of these conditions have also been associated with bone necrosis, fractures, and secondary OA.

Although there have been some difficulties and complications with surgery on this brittle bone, successful total hip and knee replacement surgery has been performed.[201, 202,204] The absence of a medullary canal and the hard bone can lead to fractures during insertion of prostheses.[204,205] The basic defect in osteopetrosis may include defective osteoclast activity. Osteoclast replacement by marrow transplantation and transplantation of hematopoietic stem and progenitor cells from placental blood have been used.[211]

OSTEOARTHRITIS FOLLOWING JOINT INJURY (POST-TRAUMATIC OSTEOARTHRITIS)

The end-stage of post-traumatic OA, the OA that follows joint injury, is identical to that of primary OA, but patients with post-traumatic OA are often young or middle age adults, and have a well-defined precipitating insult.[212,213] Clinical experience and epidemiologic studies show that meniscal, ligament, and joint capsule tears; joint dislocations; and intra-articular fractures increase the risk of the progressive joint degeneration that causes post-traumatic OA.[213-216] Participation in sports that expose joints to high levels of impact or torsional loading also increases the risk of joint degeneration.[217-220]

The risk of OA following joint injury varies with the type of injury: meniscal and ligamentous injuries have a lower risk than intra-articular fractures. A study of 1321 former medical students[213] found that 13.9% of those who had a knee injury (including meniscal, ligamentous, or bone injuries) during adolescence and young adulthood developed knee OA, as compared with 6.0% of those who did not have a knee injury. A study of patients who suffered ligamentous and meniscal injuries of the knee reported that they had a tenfold increased risk of osteoarthritis as compared with patients who do not have joint injury.[221] Intra-articular fractures have the greatest risk of OA. About one in four patients develop OA after fractures of the acetabulum,[222-224] between 23% and 44%

of patients develop knee OA after intra-articular fractures of the knee,[225-227] and more than 50% of patients with fractures of the distal tibial articular surface develop OA.[214,228-231]

The time interval between joint injury and the development of OA varies from a less than a year in patients with severe intra-articular fractures to a decade or more in some patients with ligamentous or meniscal injuries.[212,214,221,224,227] Because many joint injuries occur in young adults, the population of patients with post-traumatic OA includes many individuals under 50 years of age, but older individuals may have an increased risk of OA after joint injuries. Studies of patients with intra-articular fractures of the knee show that patients older than 50 years of age have a twofold to fourfold greater risk of developing OA than younger patients.[225,226,232] Patients over 40 years who have acetabular fractures[223,233,234] and patients over 50 years who have displaced ankle fractures may also have a greater risk of OA than younger patients who have similar injuries,[235] and age increases the risk of knee joint degeneration after anterior cruciate ligament injury.[236]

The causes of OA following joint injury are poorly understood.[212,237] The relationships between severity of acute articular surface injury and risk of joint degeneration have not been well defined, and the mechanisms responsible for progressive loss of grossly normal articular surfaces after joint injuries have received little attention. Furthermore, the risk of post-traumatic osteoarthritis varies among joints and among individuals.[214,238] The available evidence indicates that the acute joint injury kills chondrocytes[239] and that post-traumatic joint incongruity, instability, and malalignment compromise repair of the articular surface and increase the risk of progressive degeneration of residual grossly normal articular cartilage.[212,214] Current approaches to minimizing the risk of post-traumatic OA include accurate assessment of the type and severity of acute joint injuries including use of CT and MRI, restoring joint alignment, stability, and joint surface congruency following injury, and promoting articular surface repair.[212,214,237]

JOINT DYSPLASIA

The abnormal shapes of dysplastic joints apparently increases the risk of joint degeneration.[240-243] In some forms of joint dysplasia, abnormalities of the articular cartilage may contribute to the degeneration of the joint, but in others the articular surface structure and composition appear to be normal. In these latter instances, the abnormal shape presumably leads to joint degeneration by causing increased stress on parts of the articular surface and joint instability.

Although any joint presumably can develop an abnormal shape,[240,244-248] the most extensively studied form of joint dysplasia occurs in the hip, a condition referred to as developmental dysplasia of the hip.[241,249,250] Patients with developmental dysplasia of the hip have a shallow acetabulum that does not provide complete coverage of the femoral head. The risk of OA associated with hip dysplasia appears to vary with the degree to which the shallow acetabulum increases articular surface contact stress between the femoral head and the acetabulum. Evaluation of 83 patients with unilateral hip dysplasia at an average of 29.2 years from the time of diagnosis showed a strong relationship between the calculated articular surface contact pressure and the development of joint degeneration.[251,252] These observations have led surgeons to recommend osteotomies to deepen the acetabulum in patients with hip dysplasia and symptoms or signs of OA.[253-256] Although these procedures decrease symptoms in many patients, their role in delaying or preventing the progression of OA is uncertain.

OSTEOARTHRITIS AFTER MISCELLANEOUS SYSTEMIC DISEASES WITH OTHER INITIAL MECHANISMS OF JOINT DAMAGE

Inflammatory or proliferative joint diseases of many kinds involving synovium can produce cartilage damage that leads to progressively severe OA that can persist with or without continued activity of the inflammatory disease. Some examples are rheumatoid arthritis, septic arthritis, gout, seronegative spondyloarthropathies, and hemophilia. Release of destructive enzymes from inflammatory and proliferative cells is a major factor in the cartilage degeneration. In gout, crystals can also become deposited in cartilage and adjacent bone, and can destroy cartilage.

Treatment directed effectively at early control of the synovial involvement and systemic features of these diseases can prevent the later OA.

Frostbite

Severe cold injury, generally with actual frostbite recalled as occurring before closure of epiphyses, has resulted in premature OA of the hands.[257,258] The soft tissue changes appropriately evoke the greatest concern at the time of frostbite, because there are usually no identifiable joint symptoms at the time of injury. Joint pain begins months to years later, is often worse in the winter, and is initially associated with few objective findings.

Osteoarthritic involvement is usually identified in the DIP and PIP joints. In addition to bone enlargement, stiffness, and crepitus, shortening of the distal phalanges is common and can be a suggestive clue. The age at onset of symptomatic OA has varied from younger than 10 years to older than 40 years. Unilateral involvement (Fig. 13–15) has been seen after unilateral frostbite[257] including one case with severe frostbite in a young marine.[259] Biopsy specimens or joint aspirations have not been studied.

Radiographic studies in children shortly after severe frostbite show destruction of epiphyses. In milder cases and older subjects, the first radiographic changes of periarticular bone cysts in hands (or feet) do not occur until after 5 to 12 months. There may be some periosteal new bone formation. Later radiographs show OA, with shortening of the fingers sometimes the clue differentiating this entity from idiopathic OA.

Possible mechanisms involved include vascular impairment and direct injury to cartilage and subchondral bone

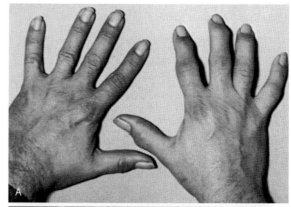
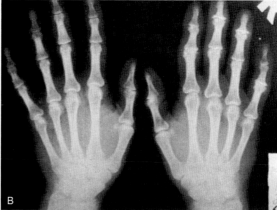

Figure 13–15 *A* and *B*, Unilateral osteoarthritis occurring after frostbite. Radiographic study corroborated the severe osteoarthritic changes seen clinically to involve the distal and proximal interphalangeal joints of the right hand.

in response to cold. Widespread vascular occlusion can be shown after cold injury in rabbits.[260] Freezing of a localized area of articular hyaline cartilage induced minimal degenerative changes at 6 months.[261] When animals were studied at 12 months, however, progressive degenerative changes were observed.[262] Peripheral nerve damage can also occur with cold and can complicate symptoms and care.

No specific treatment is available once destruction of the epiphyseal area has occurred. It is not clear whether sympathectomy or other measures to improve blood flow to the bone at the time of frostbite will prevent the later sequelae,[263] although there is some support for this. Rarely, patients with severe deformity resulting from both the OA and the overlying skin changes may benefit from reconstructive surgery.[264]

CONCLUSION

Searches for underlying causes of OA can identify treatable associated diseases and prevent some systemic disease progression. Less often identification of secondary OA may suggest some unique requirements for the treatment of the OA. Finally some secondary OA is due to familial disease such as hemochromatosis for which screening of families can prevent disease.

REFERENCES

1. Beutler E. Targeted disruption of the HFE gene. Proc Natl Acad Sci USA 95:2033–2034, 1998.
2. Pietrangelo A. Hereditary hemochromatosis–a new look at an old disease. N Engl J Med 350;23:2383–2397, 2004.
3. Adams PC, Reboussin DM, Barton JC, et al. Hemochromatosis and iron-overload screening in a racially diverse population. N Engl J Med 352:1769–1778, 2005.
4. Schumacher HR. Hemochromatosis and arthritis. Arthritis Rheum 7:41–50, 1964.
5. Sinigaglia L, Fargion S, Fracanzani AL, et al. Bone and joint involvement in genetic hemochromatosis: role of cirrhosis and iron overload. J Rheumatol 24:1809–1813, 1997.
6. Schumacher HR, Straka PC, Krikker MA, et al. The arthrospathy of hemochromatosis. Ann NY Acad Sci 526:224–233, 1988.
7. M'seffar A, Fornasier VL, Fox IM. Arthropathy as the major clinical indicator of occult iron storage disease. JAMA 238:1825–1828, 1977.
8. Budiman-Mak E, Weitzner R, Lertratanakul Y. Arthropathy of hemochromatosis. Arthritis Rheum 20:1430–1432, 1977.
9. Schmid H, Struppler C, Braun GS, et al. Ankle and hindfoot arthropathy in hereditary hemochromatosis. J Rheumatol 30:196–199, 2003.
10. Kra SJ, Hollingsworth JW, Finch SC. Arthritis with synovial iron deposition in a patient with hemochromatosis. N Engl J Med 272:1268–1271, 1965.
11. Schumacher HR. Ultrastructural characteristics of the synovial membrane in idiopathic haemochromatosis. Ann Rheum Dis 31:465–473, 1972.
12. Schumacher HR. Articular cartilage in the degenerative arthropathy of hemochromatosis. Arthritis Rheum 25:1460–1468, 1982.
13. Rollot F, Wechsler B, du Boutin LTH, et al. Hemochromatosis and femoral head aseptic osteonecrosis: a nonfortuitous association? J Rheumatol 32:376–378, 2005.
14. Schumacher HR. Ochronosis, hemochromatosis and Wilson's disease. In Koopman WJ and Moreland LW, eds. Arthritis and Allied Conditions. Philadelphia, Lippincott, Williams & Wilkins, 2005, pp 2459–2471.
15. Histakawa N, Nishiya K, Tahara K, et al. Down regulation by iron of prostaglandin E_2 production by human synovial fibroblasts. Ann Rheum Dis 57:742–746, 1998.
16. McCarty DJ, Palmer DW, Garancis JC. Clearance of calcium pyrophosphate dihydrate crystals in vivo. III. Effects of synovial hemosiderosis. Arthritis Rheum 24:706–710, 1981.
17. Ross JM, Kowalchuk RM, Shaulinsky J, et al. Association of heterozygous hemochromatosis C282Y gene mutation with hand osteoarthritis. J Rheumatol 30:121–125, 2003.
18. Loughlin J, Carr A, Chapman K. The common HFE variants C282Y and H63D are not associated with primary Osteoarthritis of the hip or knee. J Rheumatol, 32:391–392, 2005. (letter to editor)
19. Cheng P-K, Pritzker KPH. Ferrous but not ferric ions inhibit de novo formation of calcium pyrophosphate dihydrate crystals: possible relationships to chondrocalcinosis and hemochromatosis. J Rheum 15:321–324, 1988.
20. Maier-Dobersberger T, Ferenci P, Polli C, et al. Detection of the His 1069 Gln muation in Wilson's disease by rapid polymerase chain reaction. Ann Intern Med 127:21–26, 1997.
21. Finby N, Bearn AG. Roentgenographic abnormalities of the skeletal system in Wilson's disease (hepatolenticular degeneration). Am J Roentgenol 79:603–611, 1958.
22. Feller E, Schumacher HR. Osteoarticular changes in Wilson's disease. Arthritis Rheum 15:259–266, 1972.
23. Meherey KA, Eider W, Brewer GJ, et al. The arthropathy of Wilson's disease; clinical and pathologic findings. J Rheum 15:331–337, 1988.
24. Kramer U, Weinberger A, Yarom R, et al. Synovial copper distribution as a possible explanation for arthropathy in Wilson's disease. Bull Hosp J Dis 52:46–49, 1993.
25. Kataoka M, Tsumura H, Itonaga I, et al. Subchondral cyst of the tibia secondary to Wilson disease. Clin Rheumatol 23:460–463, 2004.
26. McClure J, Smith PS. Calcium pyrophosphate dihydrate deposition in the intervertebral discs in a case of Wilson's disease. J Clin Pathol 36:764–768, 1983.
27. Golding DN, Walshe JM. Arthropathy of Wilson's disease. Ann Rheum Dis 36:99–111, 1997.
28. McCarty DJ, Pepe PE. Erythrocyte neutral inorganic pyrophosphatase in pseudogout. J Lab Clin Med 79:277–284, 1972.
29. Heraud F, Sanneau C, Harmand M-F. Copper modulation of extra-cellular matrix synthesis by human articular chondrocytes. Scand J Rheum 31:279–284, 2002.
30. LaDu BN, Zannoni VG, Laster L, et al. The nature of the defect in tyrosine metabolism in alcaptonuria. J Biol Chem 230:251–260, 1968.
31. Janocha S, Wolzw, Soren S, et al. The human gene for alkaptonuria maps to chromosome 3q. Genomics 19:5–8, 1994.
32. Phornphutkul C, Introne WJ, Gahl WA. Alkaptonuria. N Engl J Med, 348:1408, 2003.
33. Angeles AP, Badger R, Gruber HE, et al. Chondrocyte growth inhibition induced by homogentisic acid and its partial prevention with ascorbic acid. J Rheumatol 16:512–517, 1989.
34. Suwannarat P, O'Brien K, Perry MB, et al. Use of nitisinone in patients with alkaptonuria. Metabolism 54:719–728, 2005.
35. Schumacher HR, Holdsworth DE. Ochronotic arthropathy. I. Clinicopathologic studies. Semin Arthritis Rheum 6:207–246, 1977.
36. Hunter T, Gordon DA, Ogryzlo MA. The ground pepper sign of synovial fluid. A new diagnostic feature of ochronosis. J Rheumatol 1:45–53, 1974.
37. Reginato AJ, Schumacher HR, Martinez VA. Ochronotic arthropathy with calcium pyrophosphate crystal deposition. A light and electron microscopic study. Arthritis Rheum 16:705–714, 1973.
38. Rynes RI, Sosman JL, Holdsworth DE. Pseudogout in ochronosis. Report of a case. Arthritis Rheum 18:21–25, 1975.
39. O'Brien WM, LaDu BN, Bunim JJ. Biochemical, pathologic and clinical aspects of alcaptonuria, ochronosis and ochronotic arthropathy. Review of world literature (1584–1962). Am J Med 34:813–838, 1963.
40. Lustberg TD, Schulman JD, Seegmiller JE. Decreased binding of ^{14}C-homogentistic acid induced by ascorbic acid in connective tissues of rats with experimental alcaptonuria. Nature 228:770–771, 1970.
40a. Suwannarat P, O'Brien K, Perry MB, et al. Use of nitisinone in patients with alkaptonuria. Metabolism 54:719–728, 2005.
41. Detenbeck LC, Young HH, Underdahl LO. Ochronotic arthropathy. Arch Surg 100:215–219, 1970.
42. Carrier DA, Harris CM. Bilateral hip and bilateral knee arthroplasties in a patient with ochronotic arthropathy. Orthop Rev 19:1005–1009, 1990.
43. Peters SP, Lee RE, Glew RH. Gaucher's disease. A review. Medicine (Baltimore) 56:425–442, 1977.
44. Beutler E. Gaucher's disease in an asymptomatic 72-year-old. JAMA 237:2529–2530, 1977.
45. Stowens DW, Teitelbaum SL, Kahn AJ, et al. Skeletal complications of Gaucher's disease. Medicine (Baltimore) 64:310–322, 1985.
46. Zaino EC, Rossi MB, Pham TD, et al. Gaucher's cells in thalassemia. Blood 38:457–562, 1971.
47. Kattlove HE, Williams JC, Gaynor E, et al. Gaucher cells in chronic myelocytic leukemia: an acquired abnormality. Blood 33:379–390, 1969.
48. Silverstein E, Pertschuk LP, Friedland J. Immuno-fluorescent detection of angiotensin-converting enzyme (ACE) in Gaucher cells. Am J Med 69:408–410, 1980.
49. Seinsheimer F, Mankin HJ. Acute bilateral symmetrical pathologic fractures of the lateral tibial plateaus in a patient with Gaucher's disease. Arthritis Rheum 20:1550–1555, 1977.
50. Goldblatt J, Jacks S, Beighton P. The orthopedic aspects of Gaucher's disease. Clin Orthop 137:208–214, 1978.
51. Brady RO, Pentchev PG, Gal AE, et al. Replacement therapy for inherited enzyme deficiency. Use of purified glucocerebrosidase in Gaucher's disease. N Engl J Med 291:989–993, 1974.
52. Hanash SM, Rucknagel DL, Heidelberger KP, et al. Primary amyloidosis associated with Gaucher's disease. Ann Intern Med 89:639–641, 1978.

53. NIH Technology Assessment Panel on Gaucher Disease. Gaucher disease: current issues in diagnosis and treatment. JAMA, 275: 548–553, 1996.

54. Robbins PD, Tahara H, Mueller G, et al. Retroviral vectors for use in human gene therapy for cancer, Gaucher disease and arthritis. Ann NY Acad Sci 716:72–88, 1994.

55. Schumacher HR. Rheumatological manifestations of sickle cell disease and other hereditary hemoglobinopathies. Clin Rheum Dis 1:37–52, 1975.

56. Taylor PW, Thorpe WP, Trueblood MC. Osteonecrosis in sickle cell trait. J Rheumatol 13:643–645, 1986.

57. Dorwart BB, Goldberg MA, Schumacher HR, et al. Absence of increased frequency of bone and joint disease with hemoglobin AS and AC [letter]. Ann Intern Med 86:66–67, 1977.

58. Rothschild BM, Sienknecht CW, Kaplan SB, et al. Sickle cell disease associated with uric acid deposition disease. Ann Rheum Dis 39:392–396, 1980.

59. Bahebeck J, Atangana R, Techa A, et al. Relative rates and features of musculoskeletal complications in adult sicklers. Acta Orthop Belg, 70:107–111, 2004.

60. Hernigou P, Allain J, Bachir D, et al. Abnormalities of the adult shoulder due to sickle cell osteonecrosis during childhood. Rev Rhum Engl Ed 65:27–32, 1998.

61. Espinoza LR, Spilberg I, Osterland CK. Joint manifestations of sickle cell disease. Medicine (Baltimore) 53:295–305, 1974.

62. Schumacher HR, Dorwart BB, Bond J, et al. Chronic synovitis with early cartilage destruction in sickle cell disease. Ann Rheum Dis 36:413–419, 1977.

63. Schumacher HR, Van Linthoudt D, Manno CS, et al. Diffuse chondrolytic arthritis in sickle cell disease. J Rheumatol, 20: 385–389, 1993.

64. Habermann ET, Grayzel AI. Bilateral total knee replacement in a patient with sickle cell disease. Clin Orthop 100:211–215, 1974.

65. Alonge TO, Shokunbi WA. The choice of arthroplasty for secondary osteoarthritis of the hip joint following avascular necrosis of the femoral head in sicklers. J Natl Med Assoc, 96:678–681, 2004.

66. Schlumpf U, Gerber N, Bunzli H, et al. Arthritiden bei Thalassemia minor. Schweiz Med Wochenschr 107:1156–1162, 1977.

67. Arman MI, Bektas S. Rheumatologische Befunde bei patienten mit Beta-thalassemia major und intermedia. Z Rheumatol 48: 68–72, 1989.

68. Abourizk NN, Nasr FW, Frayha RA. Aseptic necrosis in thalassemia minor. Arthritis Rheum 20:1141–1142, 1977.

69. Dorwart BB, Schumacher HR. Arthritis in β-thalassemia trait: clinical and pathological features. Ann Rheum Dis 40:185–189, 1981.

70. Gratwick G, Bullough PG, Bohne WHO, et al. Thalassemic arthropathy. Ann Intern Med 88:494–501, 1978.

71. Sella EJ, Goodman AH. Arthropathy secondary to transfusion hemochromatosis. J Bone Joint Surg Am 55:1077–1081, 1973.

72. Schlumpf U. Thalassemia minor and aseptic necrosis. A coincidence. Arthritis Rheum 21:280, 1978.

73. Kumar V, Gruber B. Tophaceous gout in a patient with thalassemia. J Clin Rheumatol 9:380–384, 2003.

74. Boulard F, Gardina P, Gillo A, et al. Bone marrow transplantation for homozygous beta thalassemia: The Memorial Sloan Kettering experience. Ann NY Acad Sci 850:498, 1998.

75. Wayne AS, Zelicof SB, Sledge CB. Total hip arthroplasty in beta thalassemia: case report and review of the literature. Clin Orthop 294:149, 1993.

76. Byers PH. The Ehlers-Danlos syndromes. In: Rimoin DL, Connor JM, Pyeritz RE, eds. Principles and Practice of Medical Genetics. 3rd ed. New York, Churchill Livingstone, 1997, pp 1067–1081.

77. Superti-Fuga A, Gugler E, Gitzelmann R, et al. Ehlers-Danlos syndrome type IV: a multi-exon deletion in one of the two COL3A1 alleles affecting structure, stability and processing of type III procollagen. J Biol Chem 263:6226–6232, 1988.

78. Beighton P, Horan E. Orthopaedic aspects of Ehlers-Danlos syndrome. J Bone Joint Surg Br 51:444–453, 1969.

79. Kirk JA, Ansell BM, Bywaters EGL. Hypermobility syndrome. Musculoskeletal complaints associated with generalized joint hypermobility. Ann Rheum Dis 26:419–425, 1967.

80. Beighton P. Articular manifestations of the Ehlers-Danlos syndrome. Semin Arthritis Rheum 1:246–261, 1971.

81. Hudson N, Starr MR, Esdaile JM, et al. Diagnostic associations with hypermobility in rheumatology. Br J Rheumatol 34: 1157–1161, 1995.

82. Schumacher HR. Musculoskeletal manifestations of the Ehlers-Danlos syndrome. A clinicopathologic study [abstract]. Arthritis Rheum 8:467–468, 1965.

83. Julkenen H, Rokkanen P, Jounela A. Bone changes in Ehlers-Danlos syndrome. Ann Med Int Fenn 56:55–59, 1967.

84. Steer G, Jayson MIV, Dixon ASJ, et al. Joint capsule collagen. Analysis by the study of intraarticular pressure during joint distention. Measurements in the knees of control subjects and patients with rheumatoid arthritis and Ehlers-Danlos syndrome. Ann Rheum Dis 30:481–486, 1971.

85. Robertson FW, Kozlowski K, Middleton RW. Larsen's syndrome. Clin Pediatr 14:53–60, 1975.

86. Rose PA, Johnson CA, Hungerford DS, et al. Total knee arthroplasty in Ehlers-Danlos syndrome. J Arthroplasty, 19:190–196, 2004.

87. Bird HA, Tribe CR, Bacon PA. Joint hypermobility leading to osteoarthritis and chondrocalcinosis. Ann Rheum Dis 37:203–211, 1978.

88. Scott D, Bird HA, Wright V. Joint hypermobility in osteoarthritis [abstract]. Ann Rheum Dis 38:495, 1979.

89. Dolan AL, Hart DJ, Doyle DV, et al. The relationship of joint hypermobility, bone mineral density, and osteoarthritis in the general population: the Chingford Study. J Rheumatol, 30: 799–803, 2003.

90. Jessee EF. The benign hypermobile joint syndrome. Arthritis Rheum 23:1053–1056, 1980.

91. Kraus VB, Li YJ, Martin ER, et al. Articular hypermobility is a protective factor for hand osteoarthritis. Arthritis Rheum, 50:2178–2183, 2004.

92. Martin JR, Ives EJ. Familial articular hypermobility and scaphotrapezial/trapezoid osteoarthritis in two siblings. Rheumatology 41:1203–1206, 2002.

93. Crosby EB, Insall J. Recurrent dislocation of the patella. Relation of treatment to osteoarthritis. J Bone Joint Surg Am 58:9–13, 1976.

94. Leventhal LJ, Straka PC, Schumacher HR. Jaccoud arthropathy and acroosteolysis in KID syndrome. J Rheumatol 16:1274–1277, 1989.

95. Boulton MR, Rugh DM, Mattioli LF, et al. The Noonan syndrome: a family study. Ann Intern Med 80:626–629, 1974.

96. Golde DW, Herschman HR, Lusis AJ, et al. Growth factors. Ann Intern Med 92:650–652, 1980.

97. Layton MW, Fudman EJ, Barkan A, et al. Acromegalic arthropathy: characteristics and response to therapy. Arthritis Rheum 31:1022–1027, 1988.

98. Lacks S, Jacobs RP. Acromegalic arthropathy: a reversible rheumatic disease. J Rheumatol 13:634–636, 1986.

99. Detenbeck LC, Tressler HA, O'Duffy JD, et al. Peripheral joint manifestations of acromegaly. Clin Orthop 91:119–127, 1973.

100. Kellgren JH, Ball J, Tutton GK. The articular and other limb changes of acromegaly. Q J Med 21:405–424, 1952.

101. Diamond T, Nery L, Posen S. Spinal and peripheral bone mineral densities in acromegaly. The effects of excess growth hormone and hypogonadism. Ann Intern Med 111:S67–S73, 1989.

102. Weinberger A, Schumacher HR. Unpublished observations, 1981.

103. Littlejohn GO, Hall S, Brand CA, et al. New bone formation in acromegaly. Clin Exp Rheum 4:99–104, 1986.

104. Bijlsma JWJ, Duursma SA. Serum concentrations of somatomedins and growth hormone in relation to bone metabolism in acromegaly and thyroid dysfunction. Clin Exp Rheum 4:105–110, 1986.

105. Lamotte M, Segresta JM, Krassine G. Arthrite microcristalline calcique (pseudogout) chez un acromègale. Sem Hop Paris 42:2420–2424, 1966.

106. Bland JH, Frymoyer JW. Rheumatic syndromes of myxedema. N Engl J Med 282:1171–1174, 1970.

107. McLean RM, Podell DN. Bone and joint manifestations of hypothyroidism. Semin Arthritis Rheum 24:282–290, 1985.

108. Dorwart BB, Schumacher HR. Joint effusions, chondrocalcinosis and other rheumatic manifestations in hypothyroidism. Am J Med 59:780–790, 1975.

109. Rosenthal AK, Heinkel D, Gohr CM. Thyroxine stimulates transglutaminase activity in articular chondrocytes. Osteoarthritis Cartilage, 11:463–470, 2003.

110. Bywaters EGL, Dixon AStJ, Scott JT. Joint lesions in hyperparathyroidism. Ann Rheum Dis 22:171–185, 1963.

111. Hamilton EBD. Diseases associated with CPPD deposition disease. Arthritis Rheum 19:353–357, 1976.

112. Preston FS, Adicoff A. Hyperparathyroidism with avulsion of 3 major tendons. N Engl J Med 266:968–971, 1962.

113. Pritchard MH, Jessop JD. Chondrocalcinosis in primary hyperparathyroidism. Influence of age, metabolic bone disease and parathyroidectomy. Ann Rheum Dis 36:146–151, 1977.

114. Franco M, Bendini J-C, Blaimont A, et al. Distal phalangeal brachydactyly and osteosclerosis in a case of secondary hyperparathyroidism. Joint Bone Spine, 70:143–145, 2003.

115. Grahame R, Sutor DJ, Mitchener MB. Crystal deposition in hyperparathyroidism. Ann Rheum Dis 30:597–604, 1971.

116. Lipson RL, Williams LE. The "connective tissue disorder" of hyperparathyroidism. Arthritis Rheum 11:198–205, 1971.

117. O'Duffy JD. Pseudogout syndrome in hospital patients. JAMA 225:42–44, 1973.

118. Rynes R, Merzig EG. Calcium pyrophosphate crystal deposition disease and hyperparathyroidism. A controlled, prospective study. J Rheumatol 5:460–468, 1978.

119. Lee P, Rooney PJ, Sturrock RD, et al. The etiology and pathogenesis of osteoarthritis. A review. Semin Arthritis Rheum 3:189–218, 1974.

120. Umpierrez GE, Goldstein S, Phillips LS, et al. Nutritional and hormonal regulation of articular collagen production in diabetic animals. Diabetes 38:758–763, 1989.

121. Cagliero E. Rheumatic manifestations of diabetes mellitus. Curr Rheumatol Rep 5:189–194, 2003.

122. Kapur S. McKendry J. Treatment and outcomes of diabetic muscle infarction. J Clin Rheumatol, 11:8–12, 2005.

123. Rosenbloom AL, Sliverstein JH, Lezotte DC, et al. Limited joint mobility in childhood diabetes mellitus indicates increased risk for microvascular disease. N Engl J Med, 305:191–194, 1981.

124. McCarty DJ. Calcium pyrophosphate deposition disease—a current appraisal of the problem. In: Holt PJL, ed., Current Topics in Connective Tissue Disease. Edinburgh, Churchill Livingstone, 1975, pp 181–197.

125. Schumacher HR. Gout and Pseudogout. Garden City, NY, Medical Examination Publishing, 1978, pp 53–73.

126. Moskowitz RW, Garcia F. Chondrocalcinosis articularis (pseudogout syndrome). Arch Intern Med 132:87–91, 1973.

127. Schumacher HR. Pathogenesis of crystal-induced synovitis. Clin Rheum Dis 3:105–131, 1977.

128. Zitnan D, Sitaj S. Calcifications multiples du cartilage articulaire. 9th International Congress sur les Maladies Rhumatismales 2:291, 1957.

129. McCarty DJ, Hollander JL. Identification of urate crystals in gouty synovial fluid. Ann Intern Med 54:452–460, 1961.

130. Schumacher HR, Gordon G, Paul H, et al. Osteoarthritis, crystal deposition and inflammation. Semin Arthritis Rheum 11:116–119, 1981.

131. Huskisson EC, Dieppe PA, Tucker AK, et al. Another look at osteoarthritis. Ann Rheum Dis 38:423–428, 1979.

132. Zitnan D, Sitaj S. Natural course of articular chondrocalcinosis. Arthritis Rheum 19:363–390, 1976.

133. Reginato AJ, Schiapachasse V, Zmijewski CM, et al. HLA antigens in chondrocalcinosis and ankylosing chondrocalcinosis. Arthritis Rheum 22:928–932, 1979.

134. Ellman MH, Levin B. Chondrocalcinosis in elderly persons. Arthritis Rheum 18:43–47, 1975.

135. Pay S, Terkeltaub R. Calcium pyrophosphate dehydrate and hydroxyapatite crystal deposition in the joint: new developments relevant to the clinician. Curr Rheumatol Rep 5:235–243, 2003.

136. Hoffman GS, Schumacher HR, Paul H, et al. Calcium oxalate crystal associated arthritis in chronic renal failure [abstract]. Arthritis Rheum 24:573, 1981.

137. Moskowitz RW, Harris BK, Schwartz A, et al. Chronic synovitis as a manifestation of calcium crystal deposition disease. Arthritis Rheum 14:109–116, 1971.

138. Gaucher A, Faure G, Netter P, et al. Identification des cristaux observés dans les arthropathies destructices de la chondrocalcinose. Rev Rhum 44:407–414, 1977.

139. Tanphaiachit RK, Spilberg I, Hahn BH. Lithium heparin crystals simulating CPPD crystals. Arthritis Rheum 19:966–968, 1976.

140. Kohn NN, Hughes RE, McCarty DJ, et al. The significance of calcium pyrophosphate crystals in synovial fluid of arthritic patients: the pseudogout syndrome. II. Identification of crystals. Ann Intern Med 56:738–745, 1962.

141. Cherian PV, Schumacher HR. Diagnostic potential of rapid electron microscopic analysis of joint effusions. Arthritis Rheum 25:98–100, 1982.

142. Schumacher HR, Somlyo AP, Tse RL, et al. Arthritis associated with apatite crystals. Ann Intern Med 87:411–416, 1977.

143. Reginato AJ, Schumacher HR, Martinez V. The articular cartilage in familial chondrocalcinosis. Arthritis Rheum 17:977–992, 1974.

144. Sokoloff L, Varma AA. Chondrocalcinosis in surgically respected joints. Arthritis Rheum 31:750–756, 1988.

145. Mitrovic DR, Stankovic A, Iriate-Borda O, et al. The prevalence of chondrocalcinosis in the human knee joint. An autopsy study. J Rheumatol 15:633–641, 1988.

146. Nalbant S, Martinez JAM, Kitumnuaypong, et al. Synovial fluid features and their relations to osteoarthritis severity: new findings from sequential studies. Osteoarthritis Cartilage, 11:50–54, 2003.

147. Schumacher HR. The role of inflammation and crystals in the pain of osteoarthritis. Semin Arthritis Rheum 18(suppl 2):81–85, 1989.

148. Hayes A, Harris B, Dieppe PA, et al. Wear of articular cartilage: the effects of crystals. Proc Inst Mech Eng 207:41–58, 1993.

149. Moskowitz RW, Goldberg VM, Berman L. Synovitis as a manifestation of degenerative joint disease. An experimental study [abstract]. Arthritis Rheum 19:813, 1976.

150. Fam AG, Morava-Protzner EM, Purcell C, et al. Acceleration of experimental lapine osteoarthritis by calcium pyrophosphate microcrystalline synovitis. Arthritis Rheum 58:201–210, 1995.

151. Howell DS, Muniz O, Pita JC, et al. Extrusion of pyrophosphate in extracellular media by osteoarthritis cartilage incubates. J Clin Invest 56:1473–1480, 1975.

152. Pullman-Mooar S, Mooar P, Sieck M, et al. Are there distinctive inflammatory flares after hylan G-F 20 intraarticular injections? J Rheumatol, 29:2611–2614, 2002.

153. Pinals RS, Short CL. Calcified periarthritis involving multiple sites. Arthritis Rheum 7:359–367, 1964.

154. McCarty DJ, Gatter RA. Recurrent acute inflammation associated with focal apatite crystal deposition. Arthritis Rheum 9:804–819, 1966.

155. Bennet GA, Waine H, Bauer W. Changes in the Knee Joint at Various Ages. New York, The Commonwealth Fund, 1942, p 97.

156. McCarty DJ, Hogan JM, Gatter RA, et al. Studies on pathological calcification in human cartilage. I. Prevalence and types of crystal deposits in the menisci of 215 cadavers. J Bone Joint Surg Am 48:209–235, 1966.

157. Dieppe PA, Crocker P, Huskisson EC, et al. Apatite deposition disease. A new arthropathy. Lancet 1:266–269, 1976.

158. Schumacher HR, Tse R, Reginato AJ, et al. Hydroxyapatite-like crystals in the synovial fluid cell vacuoles: a suspected new cause for crystal-induced arthritis [abstract]. Arthritis Rheum 19:821, 1976.

159. Maurer KH, Schumacher HR. Hydroxyapatite phagocytosis by human polymorphonuclear leukocytes. Ann Rheum Dis 38:84–88, 1979.

160. Schumacher HR, Miller JL, Ludivico C, et al. Erosive arthritis associated with apatite crystal deposition. Arthritis Rheum 24:31–37, 1981.

161. Reginato A, Schumacher HR. Synovial calcification in a patient with collagen-vascular disease: light and electron microscopic studies. J Rheumatol 4:261–271, 1977.

162. Li-Yu J, Clayburne GM, Sieck MS, et al. Calcium apatite crystals in synovial fluid rice bodies. Ann Rheum Dis, 61:387–390, 2002.

163. Bardin T, Bucki B, Lequesne M, et al. Synovial fluid crystals and rapidity of osteoarthritis progression [abstract]. Arthritis Rheum 32 (suppl 4):836, 1989.

164. Zakraoui L, Schumacher HR, Rothfuss S, et al. Idiopathic destructive arthropathies. J Clin Rheum 2:9–17, 1996.

165. Ali SY. Matrix vesicles and apatite nodules in arthritic cartilage. In: Willoughby DA, Giroud JP, Velo GP, eds. Perspectives in Inflammation. Baltimore, University Park Press, 1977, pp 211–223.

166. Shitama K. Calcification of aging articular cartilage in man. Acta Orthop Scand 50:613–619, 1979.

167. McCarty DJ, Halverson PB, Carrera GF, et al. "Milwaukee shoulder"—association of microspheroids containing hydroxyapatite crystals, active collagenase, and neutral protease with rotator cuff defects. I. Clinical aspects. Arthritis Rheum 24:464–473, 1981.

168. Campion GV, McCrae F, Alwan W, et al. Idiopathic destructive arthritis of the shoulder. Semin Arthritis Rheum 17:232–245, 1988.

169. Antoniou J, Tsai A, Baker D, et al. Milwaukee shoulder: correlating possible etiologic variables. Clin Orthop Relat Res 407: 79–85, 2003.

170. Yosipovich ZH, Glimcher MJ. Articular chondrocalcinosis, hydroxyapatite deposition disease in adult mature rabbits. J Bone Joint Surg Am 54:841–853, 1972.

171. Reginato AJ, Schumacher HR, Brighton CT. Experimental hydroxyapatite articular calcification [abstract]. Arthritis Rheum 21:585–586, 1978.

172. McCarthy GM, Macius AM, Christopherson PA, et al. Basic calcium phosphate crystals induce synthesis and secretion of 92 kDa gelatinase (gelatinase B/matrix metalloprotease 9) in human fibroblasts. Ann Rheum Dis 57:56–60, 1998.

173. Meng ZH, Hudson AP, Schumacher HR, et al. Monosodium urate, hydroxyapatite and calcium pyrophosphate crystals induce tumor necrosis factor-a expression in a mononuclear cell line. J Rheumatol, 24:2385–2388, 1997.

174. Morgan M, Fitzgerald D, McCarthy C, et al. Basic calcium phosphate crystals cause increased production of prostaglandin E2 by induction of both cyclooxygenase-1 and cyclooxygenase-2 in human fibroblasts. Arthritis Rheum 43:S281, 2000.

175. Hamilton JA, McCarthy GM, Whitty G. Inflammatory micro-crystals induce murine macrophage survival and DNA synthesis. Arthritis Res 3:242–246, 2001.

176. Prudhommeaux F, Schiltz C, Liote F, et al. Variation in the inflammatory properties of basic calcium phosphate crystals according to crystal type. Arthritis Rheum 39:1319–1326, 1996.

177. Bruckner FE, Howell A. Neuropathic joints. Semin Arthritis Rheum 2:47–69, 1972.

178. Sinha S, Munichoodappa CS, Kozak GP. Neuroarthropathy (Charcot joints) in diabetes mellitus. Clinical study of 101 cases. Medicine (Baltimore) 51:191–210, 1972.

179. Abell JM, Hayes JT. Charcot knee due to congenital insensitivity to pain. J Bone Joint Surg Am 46:1287–1291, 1964.

180. Peitzman ST, Miller JL, Ortega L, et al. Charcot arthropathy secondary to amyloid neuropathy. JAMA 235:1345–1347, 1981.

181. Pruzanski W, Baron M, Shupak R. Neuroarthropathy (Charcot's joints) in familial amyloid polyneuropathy. J Rheumatol 8: 477–481, 1981.

182. Brucker FE. Double Charcot's disease. Br Med J 2:603–604, 1968.

183. Wolfgang GL. Neurotrophic arthropathy of the shoulder—a complication of progressive adhesive arachnoiditis. Clin Orthop 87:217–220, 1972.

184. Horwitz T. Bone and cartilage debris in the synovial membrane—its significance in the early diagnosis of neuro-arthropathy. J Bone Joint Surg Am 30:579–588, 1948.

185. Lloyd-Roberts GC. The role of capsular changes in osteoarthritis of the hip joint. J Bone Joint Surg Br 35:627–642, 1953.

186. Floyd W, Lovell W, King RE. The neuropathic joint. South Med J 52:563–569, 1959.

187. Beetham WP, Kaye RL, Polley HF. Charcot's joints. Ann Intern Med 58:1002–1012, 1963.

188. Drennan DB, Fahey JJ, Maylahn DJ. Important factors in achieving arthrodesis of the Charcot knee. J Bone Joint Surg Am 53:1180–1193, 1971.

189. Johnson JTH. Neuropathic fractures and joint injuries. J Bone Joint Surg Am 49:1–30, 1967.

190. Berendt AR, Lipsky B. Is this bone infected or not? Differentiating neuro-osteoarthropathy from osteomyelitis in the diabetic foot. Curr Diab Rep, 4:424–429, 2004.

191. Rondier J, Cayla J, Guiraudon C, et al. Arthropathie tabétique et chondrocalcinose articulaire. Rev Rhum 44:671–674, 1977.

192. Jacobelli S, McCarty DJ. Calcium pyrophosphate dihydrate crystal deposition in neuropathic joints. Ann Intern Med 79: 340–347, 1973.

193. Ritter MA, DeRosa P. Total hip arthroplasty in a Charcot joint. A case report with a 6 year follow-up. Orthop Rev 6:51–53, 1977.

194. Altman RD. Musculoskeletal manifestations of Paget's disease of bone. Arthritis Rheum 23:1121–1127, 1980.

195. Machtey I, Rodnan GP, Benedek TG. Paget's disease of the hip joint. Am J Med Sci 251:524–531, 1966.

196. Steinbach HL. Some roentgen features of Paget's disease. Am J Roentgenol 86:950–964, 1961.

197. Hadjipavlou A, Lander P, Srolovitz H. Pagetic arthritis. Pathophysiology and management. Clin Orthop 208:15–19, 1986.

198. Lluberas-Acosta G, Hansell JR, Schumacher HR. Paget's disease of bone in patients with gout. Arch Intern Med 146:2389–2392, 1986.

199. Doury P, Delahaye RF, Leguay G, et al. Chondrocalcinose articulaire diffuse et maladie de Paget. Rev Rhum 42:551–554, 1975.

200. Detenbeck LC, Sim FH, Johnson EW. Symptomatic Paget disease of the hip. JAMA 224:213–217, 1973.

201. Cameron HU, Dewar FP. Degenerative osteoarthritis associated with osteopetrosis. Clin Orthop 127:148–149, 1977.

202. Casden AM, Jaffe FF, Kastenbaum DM, et al. Osteoarthritis associated with osteopetrosis treated by total knee arthroplasty: report of a case. Clin Orthop 247:202–207, 1989.

203. Jaffe HL. Metabolic, Degenerative, and Inflammatory Diseases of the Bones and Joints. Philadelphia, Lea & Febiger, 1972, p 492.

204. Benichou OD, Laredo JD, de Vernejoul MC. Type II autosomal dominant osteopetrosis (Albers-Schonberg disease): clinical and radiological manifestations in 42 patients. Bone, 26:87–93, 2000.

205. Strickland JP, Berry DJ. Total joint arthroplasty in patients with osteopetrosis: a report of 5 cases and review of the literature. J Arthroplasty, 20:815–820, 2005.

206. Beighton P, Hamersma H, Cremin B. Osteopetrosis in South Africa. S Afr Med J 55:659–665, 1979.

207. Klemmer PJ, Hadler NM. Subacute fluorosis. A consequence of abuse of an organo-fluoride anesthetic. Ann Intern Med 89: 607–611, 1978.

208. Clarisse PDT, Staple TW. Diffuse bone sclerosis in multiple myeloma. Radiology 99:327–328, 1971.

209. Mazieres B, Durroux R, Jambon E. Densification osseuse et nécrose de la tête fémorale par thesaurismose à la polyvinyl-pyrrolidone. Rev Rhum 47:257–265, 1980.

210. Garver P, Resnick D, Niwayama G. Epiphyseal sclerosis in renal osteodystrophy simulating osteonecrosis. Am J Radiol 136: 1239–1241, 1981.

211. Coccia PF, Krivit W, Cervenka J, et al. Successful bone-marrow transplantation for infantile malignant osteopetrosis. N Engl J Med 302:701–708, 1980.

212. Buckwalter JA, Brown TD. Joint injury, repair, and remodeling: roles in post-traumatic osteoarthritis. Clin Orthop Relat Res 7–16, 2004.

213. Gelber AC, Hochberg MC, Mead LA, et al. Joint injury in young adults and risk for subsequent knee and hip osteoarthritis. Ann Intern Med 133:321–328, 2000.

214. Marsh JL, Buckwalter J, Gelberman R, et al. Articular fractures: does an anatomic reduction really change the result? J Bone Joint Surg Am 84–A:1259–1271, 2002.

215. Cooper C, Inskip H, Croft P, et al. Individual risk factors for hip osteoarthritis: obesity, hip injury, and physical activity. Am J Epidemiol 147:516–522, 1998.

216. Nelson F, Billinghurst RC, Pidoux I, et al. Early post-traumatic osteoarthritis-like changes in human articular cartilage following rupture of the anterior cruciate ligament. Osteoarthritis Cartilage 14:114–119, 2006.

217. Buckwalter JA, Lane NE. Athletics and osteoarthritis. Am J Sports Med 25:873–881, 1997.

218. Roach KE, Persky V, Miles T, et al. Biomechanical aspects of occupation and osteoarthritis of the hip: A case-control study. J Rheumatol 21:2334–2340, 1994.

219. Yoshimura N, Sasaki S, Iwasaki K, et al. Occupational lifting is associated with hip osteoarthritis: A Japanese case-control study. J Rheumatol 27:434–440, 2000.

220. Coggon D, Kellingray S, Inskip H, et al. Osteoarthritis of the hip and occupational lifting. Am J Epidemiol 147:523–528, 1998.
221. Gillquist J, Messner K. Anterior cruciate ligament reconstruction and the long-term incidence of gonarthrosis. Sports Med 27:143–156, 1999.
222. Laird A, Keating JF. Acetabular fractures: a 16-year prospective epidemiological study. J Bone Joint Surg Br 87:969–973, 2005.
223. Matta JM. Fractures of the acetabulum: accuracy of reduction and clinical results in patients managed operatively within three weeks after the injury. J Bone Joint Surg 78A:1632–1645, 1996.
224. Saterbak AM, Marsh JL, Nepola JV, et al. Clinical failure after posterior wall acetabular fractures: the influence of initial fracture patterns. J Orthop Trauma 14:230–237, 2000.
225. Honkonen SE. Degenerative arthritis after tibial plateau fractures. J Orthop Trauma 9:272–277, 1995.
226. Volpin G, Dowd GSE, Stein H, et al. Degenerative arthritis after intra-articular fractures of the knee: long-term results. J Bone Joint Surg 72B:634–638, 1990.
227. Weigel DP, Marsh JL. High-energy fractures of the tibial plateau. Knee function after longer follow-up. J Bone Joint Surg Am 84–A:1541–1551, 2002.
228. Bonar SK, Marsh JL. Unilateral external fixation for severe pilon fractures. Foot Ankle 14:57–64, 1993.
229. Bourne RB, Rorabeck CH, Macnab J. Intra-articular fractures of the distal tibia: the pilon fracture. J Trauma 23:591–596, 1983.
230. Etter C, Ganz R. Long-term results of tibial plafond fractures treated with open reduction and internal fixation. Arch Orthop Trauma Surg 110:277–283, 1991.
231. Kellam JF, Waddell JP. Fractures of the distal tibial metaphysis with intra-articular extension—the distal tibial explosion fracture. J Trauma 19:593–601, 1979.
232. Stevens DG, Beharry R, McKee MD, et al. The long-term functional outcome of operatively treated tibial plateau fractures. J Orthop Trauma 15:312–320, 2001.
233. Pennal GF, Davidson J, Garside H, et al. Results of treatment of acetabular fractures. Clin Orthop 151:115–123, 1980.
234. Ivory JP, Rigby M, Foy MA. The hip. In: Foy MA, Fagg PS, eds. Medicolegal Reporting in Orthopaedic Trauma. London, Churchill Livingstone, 2002, pp 235–259.
235. Beauchamp CG, Clay NR, Thexton PW. Displaced ankle fractures in patients over 50 years of age. J Bone Joint Surg 65B:329–332, 1983.
236. Sommerlath K, Lysholm J, Gillquist J. The long-term course after treatment of acute anterior cruciate ligament ruptures: A 9 to 16 year followup. Am J Sports Med 19:156–162, 1991.
237. Martin JA, Brown T, Heiner A, et al. Post-traumatic osteoarthritis: the role of accelerated chondrocyte senescence. Biorheology 41:479–491, 2004.
238. Saltzman CL, Salamon ML, Blanchard GM, et al. Epidemiology of ankle arthritis: report of a consecutive series of 639 patients from a tertiary orthopaedic center. Iowa Orthop J 25:44–46, 2005.
239. Kim HT, Lo MY, Pillarisetty R. Chondrocyte apoptosis following intraarticular fracture in humans. Osteoarthritis Cartilage 10:747–749, 2002.
240. Smith SP, Bunker TD. Primary glenoid dysplasia. A review of 12 patients. J Bone Joint Surg 83B:868–872, 2001.
241. Ponseti IV. Morphology of the acetabulum in congenital dislocation of the hip. Gross, histological and roentgenographic studies. J Bone Joint Surg 60A:586–599, 1978.
242. Christie PT, Curley A, Nesbit MA, et al. Mutational analysis in X-linked spondyloepiphyseal dysplasia tarda. J Clin Endocrinol Metab 86:3233–3236, 2001.
243. Hicks J, De Jong A, Barrish J, et al. Tracheomalacia in a neonate with kniest dysplasia: histopathologic and ultrastructural features. Ultrastruct Pathol 25:79–83, 2001.
244. Bensahel H, Souchet P, Pennecot GF, et al. The unstable patella in children. J Pediatr Orthop B 9:265–270, 2000.
245. Azouz EM, Kozlowski K. Small patella syndrome: A bone dysplasia to recognize and differentiate from the nail-patella syndrome. Pediatr Radiol 27:432–435, 1997.
246. Kocyigit H, Arkun R, Ozkinay F, et al. Spondyloepiphyseal dysplasia tarda with progressive arthropathy. Clin Rheumatol 19:238–241, 2000.
247. Walch G, Badet R, Boulahia A, et al. Morphologic study of the glenoid in primary glenohumeral osteoarthritis. J Arthroplasty 14:756–760, 1999.
248. Ahmad M, Haque MF, Ahmad W, et al. Distinct, autosomal recessive form of spondyloepimetaphyseal dysplasia segregating in an inbred Pakistani kindred. Am J Med Genet 78:468–473, 1998.
249. Lindstrom JR, Ponseti IV, Wenger DR. Acetabular development after reduction in congenital dislocation of the hip. J Bone Joint Surg 61A:112–118, 1979.
250. Ishii Y, Ponseti IV. Long-term results of closed reduction of complete congenital dislocation of the hip in children under one year of age. Clin Orthop:167–174, 1978.
251. Hadley NA, Brown TD, Weinstein SL. The effects of contact pressure elevations and aseptic necrosis on the long-term outcome of congenital hip dislocation. J Orthop Res 8:504–513, 1990.
252. Maxian TA, Brown TD, Weinstein SL. Chronic stress tolerance levels for human articular cartilage: two nonuniform contact models applied to long-term follow-up of CDH. J Biomech 28:159–166, 1995.
253. Ito H, Matsuno T, Minami A. Chiari pelvic osteotomy for advanced osteoarthritis in patients with hip dysplasia. J Bone Joint Surg Am 87 (Suppl 1):213–225, 2005.
254. Clohisy JC, Barrett SE, Gordon JE, et al. Periacetabular osteotomy in the treatment of severe acetabular dysplasia. J Bone Joint Surg Am 88:65–83, 2006.
255. Pogliacomi F, Stark A, Wallensten R. Periacetabular osteotomy. Good pain relief in symptomatic hip dysplasia, 32 patients followed for 4 years. Acta Orthop 76:67–74, 2005.
256. Yasunaga Y, Ochi M, Shimogaki K, et al. Rotational acetabular osteotomy for hip dysplasia: 61 hips followed for 8–15 years. Acta Orthop Scand 75:10–15, 2004.
257. Schumacher HR. Unilateral osteoarthritis of the hand. JAMA 191:180–181, 1965.
258. Pettit TM, Finger DR. Frostbite arthropathy. J Clin Rheum 4:316–318, 1998.
259. Turner M, Smith RW. Unusual and memorable. Ann Rheum Dis, 57:271, 1998.
260. Kulka JP. Cold injury of the skin. The pathogenic role of microcirculatory impairment. Arch Environ Health 11:484–497, 1965.
261. Simon WH, Green WT. Experimental production of cartilage necrosis by cold injury: failure to cause degenerative joint disease. Am J Pathol 64:145–152, 1971.
262. Simon WH, Richardson S, Herman W, et al. Long-term effects of chondrocyte death on rabbit articular cartilage in vivo. J Bone Joint Surg Am 58:517–526, 1976.
263. Golding MR, Dejong P, Saqyer PN, et al. Protection from early and late sequelae of frostbite by regional sympathectomy: mechanism of "cold sensitivity" following frostbite. Surgery 53:303–308, 1963.
264. Bigelow DR, Ritchie GW: The effects of frostbite in childhood. J Bone Joint Surg Br 45:122–131, 1963.
265. Solomon L. Patterns of osteoarthritis of the hip. J Bone Joint Surg Br 58:176–183, 1976.

General Aspects
of Management

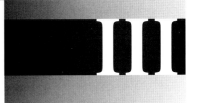

Baseline Program

14

Todd Stitik   Marc C. Hochberg

An estimated 21 million adults, or 12% of the U.S. population aged 25 to 74 years, have signs and symptoms of osteoarthritis (OA), making this group of conditions a major public health concern among the musculoskeletal diseases.[1] OA may affect any of the diarthrodial joints in the body; the most common extremity joints that are involved and cause individuals to come to clinical attention are the knee, hip, and small joints of the hands and feet.

Once the diagnosis of OA is established, the development of a therapeutic program needs to take into consideration the different symptoms, signs, and functional limitations when different joints are affected, which implies different therapeutic options.[2] The correlation of pain severity, functional limitation, and impaired health-related quality of life with the extent of structural changes as measured by the radiograph is only modest; hence, management decisions should not be made solely on the presence and severity of radiographic changes.[3] The basic therapeutic program summarized in this chapter focuses on nonpharmacologic measures of management, stressing a team care approach that touches on the educational, physical, and social needs of the patient with OA.

MANAGEMENT OBJECTIVES

The goals of management of the individual patient with symptomatic OA are to 1) control pain so that the patient reaches an acceptable symptom state, 2) reduce functional limitation and disability, 3) improve health-related quality of life, and 4) avoid over-treatment with potentially harmful pharmacologic agents.

Guidelines have been proposed for management of OA at the knee and the hip[4-9]; the Osteoarthritis Research Society International (OARSI) is presently involved in updating and harmonizing these recommendations with the goal of publication in 2007 (Nuki G, personal communication). Recommendations published by the European League of Associations of Rheumatology (EULAR) include a series of ten propositions with a supporting evidence-based review of randomized clinical trials.[8,9] The first recommendation stresses that "The optimal management of OA requires a combination of nonpharmacological and pharmacological treatment modalities." Furthermore, the non-pharmacological treatment modalities ". . . should include education, exercise, appliances and weight reduction." The evidence supporting the use of these nonpharmacologic modalities will be reviewed in this chapter.

Patient Education

Education is important for all people with OA; for many, it is the most important intervention. Pain and disability, the two greatest concerns of patients with OA, are concerns that should be addressed by educational programs for the patient. The literature suggests that education of the patient with OA can increase the practice of healthy behaviors, improve health status, and decrease health care utilization. Lorig and colleagues carried out a series of studies on the Arthritis Self-Management Program™ that is taught in the community by teams of trained lay leaders who conduct 2-hour weekly group sessions with 10 to 15 people.[10-13] Study participants increased their level of physical activity, increased their use of cognitive pain management techniques, and reported decreased pain. Reinforcement after 1 year did not add to the effect, and subjects who were observed for up to 4 years continued to demonstrate reduced pain; they also had fewer arthritis-related visits to physicians. The Arthritis Self-Management Program™ is now sponsored by the Arthritis Foundation, a national voluntary arthritis organization with chapters throughout the United States, and modifications are used throughout the world.

Despite the widespread recommendation that education be part of the basic program for management of patients with symptomatic OA, the supporting evidence suggests only a weak effect of education on pain and functional limitation.[14,15] Superio-Cabuslay and colleagues performed a meta-analysis of controlled trials of patient education interventions in OA and rheumatoid arthritis and compared the effects on pain and functional disability to effects obtained in a meta-analysis of placebo-controlled trials of nonsteroidal anti-inflammatory drugs (NSAIDs).[14]

They identified 23 patient education trials, 19 of which met their inclusion criteria; 10 of these trials included patients with OA, either exclusively or predominantly. Sample size in these 10 OA trials ranged from 85 to 707 and the median duration of the trials was 16 weeks. The weighted average effect size for reduction in pain in the OA trials was 0.15 (95% confidence interval [CI] –0.43, 0.73) and for reduction in physical disability, –0.02 (95% CI –0.51, 0.47); neither of these changes was statistically significant.

A more recent meta-analysis by Warsi and colleagues produced similar results.[15] These authors identified 35 controlled trials of which 17 met their inclusion criteria; 9 of these trials included patients with OA. Of the 16 trials that reported pain outcomes, the pooled effect size was 0.12 (95% CI 0.00, 0.24); of the 12 trials that reported disability outcomes, the pooled effect size was 0.07 (95% CI 0.00, 0.15) (Fig. 14 –1). The authors noted significant heterogeneity among the trials for effects on pain but not for effects on disability. In a preplanned subgroup analysis of trials that used the Arthritis Self-Help Course™, there was no evidence of statistically significant efficacy for either pain or disability. These authors did not present results for studies of patients with OA separately. Based on the results of these two meta-analyses, the effects of patient education on pain and functional limitation are small at best. Beneficial effects of patient education on helplessness and coping skills may be present, however, without significant measurable effects on pain. Nonetheless, patient education has now become the standard of care and was incorporated as part of the usual care control treatment group in two large randomized trials of other nonpharmacologic interventions.[16,17]

Weight Loss

Being overweight is the single most important potentially modifiable risk factor for the development of lower limb OA.[18] Furthermore, in epidemiological studies, weight loss was associated with a reduced risk of symptomatic knee OA.[19] Unfortunately, until recently, the evidence supporting the recommendation of weight loss for overweight patients with lower limb OA was based on nonrandomized studies that demonstrated improvement in knee pain in overweight patients with knee OA.[20-22] A pilot randomized study of exercise plus diet compared to exercise alone in only 24 patients with symptomatic knee OA showed significantly greater weight loss in the exercise plus diet group but significant improvement in both pain and function in both groups over 24 weeks; however, the study was not powered to demonstrate differences in symptomatic improvement between the groups.[23] Based on these preliminary data, Messier and colleagues subsequently conducted a definitive study of exercise plus diet in overweight patients with symptomatic knee OA.[24]

The Arthritis, Diet and Activity Promotion Trial (ADAPT) was a single-blind, randomized, controlled trial designed to compare the effects of exercise, dietary weight loss, and the combination compared to usual care in sedentary patients with symptomatic knee OA aged 60 and above with body mass index of 28 kg/m² or greater.[24] A total of 316 subjects with a mean age of 69 years and a mean body mass index of 34 kg/m² were enrolled. Patients randomized to the weight loss only group lost an average of 4.9% of body weight during the 18-month intervention and had a significant 18% improvement in physical

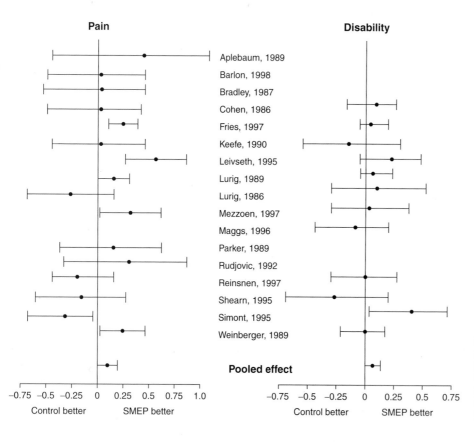

Figure 14–1 Estimated effect size of education on arthritis pain and disability and 95 percent confidence intervals for individual studies included in meta-analysis by Warsi and colleagues.[15] *SMEP* = self management education program.

function and a significant 15% improvement in pain as measured by the Western Ontario and McMaster Universities Osteoarthritis Index (WOMAC) physical function and pain subscales, respectively. These improvements in physical function and pain, however, were not significantly different from those seen in the usual care control group. Indeed, the only group that showed significant improvement compared to the usual care control group was the group randomized to both exercise and diet. These findings led the authors to conclude that the combination of weight loss plus moderate exercise provides better overall improvement in both symptoms and function compared with usual care. This study had several limitations including the enrollment of patients who were not only overweight but obese and very obese, the achieved weight loss was only modest leaving patients still obese on average at the end of the study, and the adherence rate in the groups randomized to either diet alone or diet plus exercise was less than 75%.[25] Nonetheless, these results support the recommendations of weight loss, in the setting of exercise plus dietary counseling, for overweight patients with symptomatic knee OA.

Physical Therapy Interventions

It is generally accepted that a therapeutic exercise program can improve functional capability and provide an analgesic effect in OA patients without exacerbating their symptoms.[26] The general sentiment that therapeutic exercise is beneficial in OA patients is supported by a meta-analysis.[27] Furthermore, a consensus panel agreed that prescription of both general (aerobic fitness training) and local (strengthening) exercises is an essential core aspect of management of every patient with hip or knee OA.[28] The panel also published the statement that there are few contraindications to the prescription of strengthening or aerobic exercise in these patients. With varying degrees of scientific evidence, other consensus recommendations related to therapeutic exercises in hip and knee OA patients include the following: 1) exercise therapy should be individualized and patient-centered so as to take into account factors such as age, comorbidity, and overall mobility; 2) to be effective, exercise programs should include advice and education to promote a positive lifestyle change with an increase in physical activity; 3) group exercise and home exercise are equally effective and patient preference should be considered; 4) adherence is the principle predictor of long-term outcome from exercise; 5) strategies to improve and maintain adherence should be adopted; and 6) improvements in muscle strength and proprioception gained from exercise programs may reduce OA progression. The American College of Rheumatology recommends that patients with symptomatic lower limb OA be enrolled in a physical therapy program including aerobic and strengthening exercises.[4-6] It should be noted, however, that it is still unclear as to whether a therapeutic exercise program is better delivered in a center-based setting or a home-based setting as a meta-analysis on this topic did not find any studies that specifically compared these approaches in OA.[29]

TABLE 14–1
TYPICAL PHYSICAL THERAPY PROGRAM CONTENT

Modalities
Range of motion exercises
Stretching exercises
Muscle strengthening exercises
Mobility training (ambulation, elevations, stairs, assistive device trials)
Aerobic conditioning
Patient education
Home exercise program development

Although an exact physical therapy "formula" for OA patients has not been developed, a general rehabilitation medicine teaching principle is that a physical therapy program should consist of at least several components (Table 14–1).[30-33] Patients are usually enrolled in an initial 4-week course of physical therapy on a two-to-three times a week basis. Ideally, the practitioner should perform an assessment after 1 month at which time the physical therapy summary progress note is available for the physician's review. The physician then can make an informed decision regarding the necessity for additional physical therapy and can make modifications in the physical therapy orders as needed. Depending on how the patient progresses with this initial therapy course and upon insurance coverage eligibility, an additional month or two can then be prescribed prior to the patient being discharged to a home exercise program.

The ideal exercise intensity within the physical therapy program is unclear. For aerobic exercise, one study of 39 knee OA patients found that both high intensity and low intensity aerobic exercise was equally effective in improving a patient's functional status, gait, pain, and aerobic capacity.[34] Another study found that a 6-week high-intensity exercise program had no effect on pain or function in middle-aged patients with moderate to severe radiographic knee OA. However, some benefit resulted in improved quality of life in the exercise group compared to the control group.[35]

Specific Modalities

Typical modalities administered alone or in combination to OA patients by physical therapists include thermotherapy (the therapeutic use of heat), cryotherapy (the therapeutic use of cold), and electrical stimulation. Although it is still unclear as to how to optimally use each of these modalities, some basic principles exist; for example, it has traditionally been taught that cold is more likely than heat to be beneficial in acute arthritic flares characterized by pain and swelling. The basis behind this principle is that cold-induced vasoconstriction helps to limit tissue edema formation and has an anti-inflammatory effect presumably by lowering joint temperature, collagenase activity, and white blood cell counts within arthritic joints.[36] Although a review of the effects of locally applied heat or cold on the deeper tissues of joints and on joint temperature in patients did not find consistent results, locally applied heat generally increases and locally applied cold generally decreases the temperature of the skin, superficial and deeper tissues, and joint cavity.[37]

However, actual studies comparing the clinical effects of these thermal modalities in OA patients have largely been lacking. A Cochrane systematic review examined randomized controlled trials on participants with clinical and/or radiological confirmation of OA of the knee and interventions using heat or cold therapy compared with standard treatment or placebo.[38] Three randomized controlled trials involving 179 patients were identified. Ice massage had a statistically significant beneficial effect on range of motion, function, and knee strength compared to control. While cold packs decreased swelling, hot packs had no beneficial effect on edema compared with placebo or cold application. However, ice packs did not affect pain significantly compared to control. The authors concluded that more well-designed studies with a standardized protocol and adequate numbers of subjects are needed to evaluate the effect of thermotherapy in the treatment of knee OA.

Heat is used in OA patients in order to enhance stretching exercises by increasing tissue elasticity and in order to provide analgesia.[39] The purported heat-induced analgesia is believed to occur via direct suppression of free nerve endings, via vasodilatation-enhanced removal of metabolic byproducts, and by the suppression of skeletal muscle hyperactivity through activation of descending pain-inhibitory systems by unknown mechanisms.[40] Heating modalities can be classified into those that heat superficially, and those that heat deeply. Superficial heat can be further subclassified into conduction (the direct transfer of thermal energy between two objects that are in physical contact with one another, such as occurs with a water bottle), convection (the exchange of heat by movement of the current the molecules in the air or liquid across the body's surface, such as occurs in a heated whirlpool), or radiation (the transfers of heat by the absorption of electromagnetic energy, such as occurs with an infrared lamp).

Perhaps the most common superficial heating modality used within a physical therapy facility is a hydrocollator pack (a canvas bag filled with silicon dioxide absorbs heat and releases it on direct contact with the patient). A typical example of the use of a hydrocollator pack is the application on the cervical paraspinal/trapezius muscles of a patient with cervical spondylosis prior to stretching of these muscle groups. While studies on the use of the hydrocollator pack in OA are lacking, other forms of superficial heat have been studied. A randomized controlled trial using tap water found a significant pain reduction in knee OA patients.[41] Two other studies found reductions in pain with the use of hydrotherapy for OA patients with peripheral joint involvement and spa therapy for patients with OA of the hip, knee, and lumbar spine.[42,43] One final form of superficial heating, infrared light therapy, was found to provide pain relief in knee OA and erosive inflammatory hand OA, respectively.[44,45]

Therapeutic ultrasound (the conversion of high-frequency sound waves into heat at deep tissue interfaces) is the most commonly used deep heating modality and is often administered with the belief that it has analgesic properties. However, a meta-analysis of studies involving ultrasound found only one placebo-controlled study of knee OA and this study showed no difference in pain relief between the ultrasound and placebo groups.[46] The combination of ultrasound and therapeutic exercise did not show a statistically significant improvement in pain over exercise alone in hip or knee OA patients.[47] In contrast, one randomized study involving 120 knee OA patients found that those treated with ultrasound in addition to exercise had significant improvements in range of motion and ambulation speed.[48] This study concluded that ultrasound treatment could increase the effectiveness of isokinetic exercise for functional improvement of knee OA, and pulsed ultrasound had a greater effect than continuous ultrasound. Another use of therapeutic ultrasound in OA patients is to facilitate stretching of deep structures such as hip and shoulder capsules; for example, a patient with OA of the glenohumeral joint and concomitant shoulder capsule tightness might be administered therapeutic ultrasound over the capsule prior to performing stretching exercises.

Cryotherapy is most commonly applied over arthritic joints with effusions. In a physical therapy gym setting, this is generally done using a simple gel ice pack. Patients are often instructed to apply ice at home as part of the self-management of acute inflammation. There have been no published randomized controlled trials on the therapeutic use of cold in OA patients in the non-arthroplasty setting.

Electrical stimulation in the form of direct electrical stimulation strong enough to cause muscle contraction (galvanic stimulation), pulsed electromagnetic field stimulation, and transcutaneous electrical nerve stimulation (TENS) has not been extensively studied in OA. Galvanic stimulation is generally believed to be effective in relieving involuntary skeletal muscle contraction in myofascial pain syndromes. TENS involves stimulation of large-diameter cutaneous nerve fibers, which in turn inhibit the transmission of painful stimuli to the spinal cord via gate control theory.[49] TENS has been used most often for myofascial pain and neuropathic pain. Pulsed electrical stimulation is believed to act at the level of hyaline cartilage by maintaining proteoglycan composition of articular cartilage via the down regulation of its turnover.[50] There are two published galvanic stimulation studies in OA patients;[51,52] neither of the studies, however, has shown efficacy greater than that of placebo. There is one published multicenter, double-blind, randomized-controlled 4-week trial involving 78 knee OA patients who received pulsed electrical stimulation.[53] This study investigated three primary efficacy variables including pain, function, and physician global evaluation of patients' condition. Patients treated with pulsed electrical stimulation showed statistically, significantly greater improvement than the placebo group for all primary efficacy variables in comparisons of mean change from baseline to the end of treatment. A study of knee and cervical spine OA patients who were treated for 4 to 6 weeks reported a significant improvement in pain relief and mobility compared with sham groups.[54] TENS has been studied in knee OA patients and most, but not all, studies have found it to be superior to placebo and useful as an effective adjunct to therapeutic exercise or

NSAIDs with respect to pain relief.[55–61] Specific protocols for TENS are now being studied; however, the optimal one has yet to be identified.[55,62]

Range of Motion Exercises

A general therapeutic exercise principle is that an osteoarthritic joint should be put through a full functional range of motion on a regular basis. Range of motion exercises are generally felt to be important in order to help prevent motion loss that can occur within the osteoarthritic joint. Loss of knee or hip flexion can be particularly disabling as it can interfere with the patient's ability to negotiate elevations, including stairs and curbs. Ideally, the physical therapy program should be tailored according to a patient's ability to independently perform range of motion, for example, if the patient has full and unrestricted range of motion and adequate strength to move the joint themselves. In contrast, if the patient has limitation of motion or inadequate strength to range the joint, the therapist should perform active assisted range of motion exercises. Research evidence for the performance of range of motion exercises in OA patients in the nonarthroplasty setting is limited. One pilot study examined the effects of continuous passive motion (CPM) in 21 patients with hip OA and found that there were significant improvements in patient assessment of pain on visual analog scale, Sickness Impact Profile, self-selected walking speed, and decreased medication usage.[63] While CPM has been employed in the postarthroplasty inpatient rehabilitation and acute care setting, it is not generally used in the manner described above as range of motion exercises are most often performed without the use of any equipment.

Stretching Exercises

Another basic therapeutic exercise principle is that all muscle groups crossing a joint should be stretched so as to prevent abnormal force generation to develop across a joint as might occur if that muscle group is tight. Stretching exercises are felt to be most effective if performed on a daily basis, particularly after tissue has been heated as heating enables collagen to be maximally stretched. Formal evidence that stretching is efficacious in OA is very limited. One study in hip OA did find increased range of hip abduction after a stretching program.[64] Indirect evidence for the beneficial effects of stretching as an intervention to provide pain relief comes from studies in which stretching was incorporated as part of an exercise program.[65]

Muscle Strengthening Exercises

Evidence-based recommendations for the role of strengthening exercises in the management of hip and knee OA are based on the fact that strengthening has been shown to be effective in 16 randomized controlled trials for knee OA and 1 randomized controlled trial for hip OA.[28] Although one observational study suggested that greater baseline quadriceps strength increased the likelihood of OA progression in malaligned or lax knees, this finding cannot be extrapolated to therapeutic exercise-induced strength improvements.[66]

Some controversy exists with respect to the prescription of open chain (terminal limb not in direct contact with a surface [e.g., leg extension exercises]) as opposed to closed chain (terminal limb in direct contact with a surface [e.g., wall slides and leg press exercises]) kinetic strengthening exercises. There is evidence that open chain kinetic exercises may pathologically increase forces within the knee including tibiofemoral compressive forces, patellofemoral compressive forces, and tibiofemoral shear forces;[67–69] for this reason, some physiatrists will specify in the physical therapy orders that open chain exercises are not to be included in the physical therapy program. Simple strengthening exercises such as wall slides and quadriceps sets can be taught to patients either as part of a formal physical therapy program or during physician office visits. These exercises offer the advantage of not requiring any specific equipment. They can then readily be incorporated into a home exercise program.[70]

Mobility Training (Ambulation, Elevations, Stairs, Assistive Device Trials)

Mobility generally encompasses transfers, ambulation, elevations (including ramps and curbs), and stair negotiation (ascending/descending). In order to maximize function, lower limb OA patients should be assessed with respect to mobility and should be given specific training if deficits are found. In order to optimally perform these activities, a patient might benefit from an assistive device for transfers or ambulation. Transferring from low-level surfaces, such as chairs, toilet seats, beds, and car seats, can be difficult, especially if pain is present or range of motion is limited. Assistive devices such as elevated toilet seats, grab bars, and sliding boards may help to facilitate these transfers. With respect to ambulation, it has been generally accepted that assistive devices such as straight canes are capable of partially unloading painful weight-bearing joints.[71] The degree to which canes are capable of reducing hip contact forces has been calculated to be a maximum of no more than 60% of body weight.[72] With respect to the hip, use of the assistive device contralateral to the more symptomatic hip is most effective. Contralateral use shifts the center of gravity away from the painful hip and also generates a ground reaction force with a longer lever arm so as to assist the gluteus medius with hip abduction and therefore limit the amount of compressive forces that this muscle will exert on the hip. Evidence suggests that contralateral use is also preferable for the knee.[73] Unfortunately, compliance with assistive devices for ambulation is less than ideal. One study found that although 44% of 187 OA patients owned a walking aid, 30% did not actually use it.[74] While ownership correlated with advanced age and higher disability, actual usage correlated with older age, pain intensity, disability level, a decrease in morning stiffness by the aid, and a positive evaluation of the aid. Besides straight canes, more supportive mobility devices such as narrow and wide-based quad canes, Loftstrand crutches, standard walkers, rolling walkers, and wheelchairs can also be prescribed depending on the level of assistance needed. The cane length should be determined with the cane held with the patient erect and the elbow flexed to about 20 degrees.

Aerobic Conditioning

Aerobic conditioning exercises are generally believed by expert opinion to be safe and effective in patients with OA of the hips and knees, and their incorporation into patient management is supported by reviews of randomized controlled trials.[75,76] After participation in such a program, a goal is for the patient to be discharged to a long-term home exercise program that incorporates aerobic conditioning.

Incorporation of the aerobic conditioning exercises into a therapeutic exercise program is logical, as OA patients have decreased aerobic capacity that may have an adverse impact on overall morbidity and mortality compared with age-matched controls.[77] The mechanism by which aerobic conditioning exercises yield an analgesic effect is not completely clear. However, there is evidence that aerobic conditioning exercises cause the release of endogenous opioids.[78,79] Other benefits include improvement in symptoms of depression and anxiety.[80] Aerobic conditioning exercises include both land-based exercises and aquatic exercises. Aquatic aerobic exercise has traditionally been offered to OA patients by the Arthritis Foundation. This mode of aerobic exercise has in fact been studied in OA patients and was found to be efficacious in a randomized controlled trial.[81]

Home Exercise Programs

Even if a patient has made good progress with a physical therapy–based exercise program, the patient will eventually be discharged to a home exercise program that will be performed either at home or, less commonly, in a gym-type setting. Long-term compliance with a home exercise program is a major goal as good exercise compliance has been found to be associated with improved physical function in overweight and obese older adults with knee OA.[82,83] However, long-term compliance with a home exercise program is a difficult challenge. The Fitness Arthritis Seniors Trial (FAST) assessed exercise compliance during 18 months (a 3-month center-based phase and a 15-month home-based phase) in 439 knee OA patients.[82] Despite monitoring exercise compliance during the home-based phase with random phone calls and home visits, overall compliance in this group of patients over age 60 was only 50%; post hoc analysis found that exercise adherence was significantly associated with the magnitude of improvement with respect to pain and functional limitation. A literature review of exercise adherence and the factors that influence it among OA patients revealed multiple determinants of exercise adherence. However, these determinants have not been carefully studied in OA patients.[84]

Occupational Therapy Interventions

The major goals of participation in an occupational therapy program include assessment of and training in activities of daily living (ADLs) and instrumental ADLs (more

TABLE 14–2
JOINT PROTECTION TECHNIQUES

Ask for help with tasks
Avoid extreme joint flexion
Avoid maintaining a given joint position for prolonged
    time periods
Avoid overuse
Balance rest and activity
Control your weight
Distribute pressure
Simplify tasks
Respect pain
Unload a joint if it becomes painful
Use biomechanically correct motion patterns
Use your strongest muscles and joints

complex activities needed for independent community living including household management, housework, and transportation), provision of assistive devices designed to increase function, pain reduction and instruction in joint protection techniques, and energy conservation techniques (Table 14–2).[85,86] An example of a joint protection technique is the use of a long-handled shoe horn to help limit the amount of hip and knee flexion required to put on shoes. Whether these interventions actually protect the joint over time has yet to be proven. Energy conservation can be important, because pain and low-level inflammation can cause OA patients to have fatigue.

Although there may be some overlap with physical therapy in terms of program content (e.g., modality use might be taught by both the occupational and physical therapist), some clear differences usually exist. For example, the duration and frequency of a typical course of occupational therapy are usually less than that of a physical therapy program. Although there may be an exercise component to the occupational therapy program, it most typically places more of an emphasis on patient education and functional training, two activities that can usually be accomplished in a shorter amount of time compared to a therapeutic exercise program. An exception is occupational therapy for hand OA patients, as this often includes demonstration of specific therapeutic exercises, including intrinsic hand muscle strengthening and range of motion exercises for fingers and wrists. Various custom splints for the arthritic hand (e.g., thumb base splints to immobilize the trapezioscaphoid joint) are sometimes custom-fabricated by the occupational therapist.[87] Studies on the use of occupational therapy in OA are very limited.

Orthotic Management

Orthotic intervention is recommended for some patients with knee or hip OA; a comprehensive review of footwear alterations and bracing as treatments for knee OA concluded that a biomechanical approach should be included in the treatment plan for patients with knee OA in order to improve patients' function and possibly reduce disease progression.[88] Lateral wedge foot orthoses have been shown in some biomechanical and clinical studies to reduce the load on the medial compartment and/or to improve the symptoms of medial compartment knee OA.[89-91] The addition of a subtalar strap to a lateral-wedge insole may provide added benefit.[92,93] Foot orthoses prescribed to knee OA patients include simple viscoelastic inserts such as the Viscoped S silicone insert, and antisupinator orthotics that are used in the setting of knee OA with varus malalignment.

Orthotic options for knee OA, including braces ranging from simple knee sleeves to hinged-adjustable knee unloader braces that correct varus or valgus malalignment, act by two possible mechanisms including improving proprioception and providing mechanical support. Patellofemoral type orthoses are also sometimes used and range from simple infrapatellar bands and straps, to patellar stabilizing sleeves that redirect patellar motion (e.g., the Palumbo patellar stabilizer). An alternative to patellofemoral orthoses is medial taping of the patella.[94]

The theory that orthoses can slow knee OA disease progression is based in part on studies that correlated knee malalignment with the subsequent development of knee OA. Despite the fact that varus and valgus knee malalignment lead to knee OA and the evidence that foot orthoses and some knee braces alter knee varus moments and lead to symptomatic relief, direct evidence that orthoses can actually slow osteoarthritic disease progression is lacking.

Hip-girdle orthoses are rarely used in nonsurgical management. Orthoses are regularly used in clinical practice for patients with hand OA and for the rare patient with ankle OA. Examples of orthoses used for patients with hand OA mainly include first CMC joint splints. On occasion, other splints such as simple wrist splints can be used depending on the location of the OA and the treatment goals. Orthoses that are available for patients with ankle OA are designed to unload the ankle or provide simple compression to help limit any ankle joint and/or associated soft tissue swelling that may be present. These orthoses include simple elastic ankle sleeves, lace-up ankle braces (e.g., Swede-O ankle lock brace, RocketSoc® brace), and hard plastic ankle stirrup braces with Velcro closures (e.g., Ankle Aircast® brace). There are few studies that support the use of orthoses for patients with ankle OA.[95,96]

REFERENCES

1. Lawrence RC, Helmick CG, Arnett FC, et al. Estimates of the prevalence of arthritis and selected musculoskeletal disorders in the United States. Arthritis Rheum 41:778–799, 1998.
2. Liang MH, Fortin P. Management of osteoarthritis of the hip and knee. N Engl J Med 325:125–127, 1991.
3. Hochberg M, Lawrence RC, Everett DF, et al. Epidemiologic association of pain in osteoarthritis of the knee: data from the National Health and Nutrition Examination Survey and the National Health and Nutrition Examination-I epidemiologic follow-up survey. Semin Arthritis Rheum 18(suppl 2):4–9, 1989.
4. Hochberg MC, Altman RD, Brandt KD, et al. Guidelines for the medical management of osteoarthritis. Part I. Osteoarthritis of the hip. Arthritis Rheum 38:1535–1540, 1995.
5. Hochberg MC, Altman RD, Brandt KD, et al. Guidelines for the medical management of osteoarthritis. Part II. Osteoarthritis of the knee. Arthritis Rheum 38:1541–1546, 1995.
6. American College of Rheumatology Subcommittee on Osteoarthritis Guidelines: Recommendations for the medical management of osteoarthritis of the hip and knee. Arthritis Rheum 43:1905–1915, 2000.
7. Pendleton A, Arden N, Dougados M, et al. EULAR recommendations for the management of knee osteoarthritis: report of a task force of the Standing Committee for International Clinical Studies Including Therapeutic Trials (ESCISIT). Ann Rheum Dis 59:936–944, 2000.
8. Jordan KM, Arden NK, Doherty M, et al. EULAR Recommendations 2003: an evidence based approach to the management of knee osteoarthritis: Report of a Task Force of the Standing Committee for International Clinical Studies Including Therapeutic Trials (ESCISIT). Ann Rheum Dis 62:1145–1155, 2003.
9. Zhang W, Doherty M, Arden N, et al. EULAR evidence based recommendations for the management of hip osteoarthritis: report of a task force of the EULAR Standing Committee for International Clinical Studies Including Therapeutics (ESCISIT). Ann Rheum Dis 64:669–681, 2005.
10. Lorig K, Kraines RG, Holman HR. A randomized prospective study of the effects of health education for people with arthritis. Arthritis Rheum 24(suppl 4):S90, 1981.
11. Lorig K, Holman HR. Long term outcomes of an arthritis self-management study: effects of reinforcement efforts. Soc Sci Med 29:221–224, 1989.
12. Lorig K, Mazonson P, Holman HR. Evidence suggesting that health education for self-management in patients with chronic arthritis has sustained health benefits while reducing health care costs. Arthritis Rheum 36:439–446, 1993.
13. Lorig K, Seleznick M, Lubeck D, et al. The beneficial outcomes of the arthritis self-management course are inadequately explained by behavior change. Arthritis Rheum 32:91–95, 1989.
14. Superio-Cabuslay E, Ward MM, Lorig KR. Patient education interventions in osteoarthritis and rheumatoid arthritis: a meta-analytic comparison with nonsteroidal anti-inflammatory drug treatment. Arthritis Care Res 9:292–301, 1996.
15. Warsi A, LaValley MP, Wang PS, et al. Arthritis self-management education programs: a meta-analysis of the effect on pain and disability. Arthritis Rheum 48:2207–2213, 2003.
16. Ettinger WH, Burns R, Messier SP, et al. A randomized trial comparing aerobic exercise and resistance exercise with a health education program in older adults with knee osteoarthritis. The Fitness Arthritis and Seniors Trial (FAST). JAMA 277:25–31, 1997.
17. Berman BM, Lao L, Langenberg P, et al. Effectiveness of acupuncture as adjunctive therapy in osteoarthritis of the knee: a randomized, controlled trial. Ann Intern Med 141:901–910, 2004.
18. Felson DT, Zhang Y, An update on the epidemiology of knee and hip osteoarthritis with a view to prevention. Arthritis Rheum 41:1343–1355, 1998.
19. Felson DT, Zhang Y, Anthony JM, et al. Weight loss reduces the risk for symptomatic knee osteoarthritis in women: The Framingham study. Ann Intern Med 116:535–539, 1992.
20. Toda Y, Toda T, Takamura S, et al. Change in body fat, but not body weight or metabolic correlates of obesity, is related to symptomatic relief of obese patients with knee osteoarthritis after a weight control program. J Rheumatol 25:2181–2186, 1998.
21. Huang M-H, Chen C-H, Chen T-W, et al. The effects of weight reduction on the rehabilitation of patients with knee osteoarthritis and obesity. Arthritis Care Res 13:398–403, 2000.
22. Martin K, Fontaine K, Goldberg A, Hochberg MC: J Clin Rheumatol 7:219–223, 2001.
23. Messier SP, Loeser RF, Mitchell MN, et al. Exercise and weight loss in obese older adults with knee osteoarthritis: a preliminary study. J Am Geriatr Soc 48:1062–1072, 2000.
24. Messier SP, Loeser RF, Miller GD, et al. Exercise and weight loss in overweight and obese older adults with osteoarthritis: the Arthritis, Diet and Activity Promotion Trial. Arthritis Rheum 50:1501–1510, 2004.
25. Fransen M: Dietary weight loss and exercise for obese adults with knee osteoarthritis: modest weight loss targets, mild exercise, modest effects. Arthritis Rheum 50:1366–1369, 2004.

26. Ytterberg SR, Mahowald ML, Krug HE. Exercise for arthritis. Baillieres Clin Rheumatol. 8(1):161–189, 1994.
27. Roddy E, Zhang W, Doherty M. Aerobic walking or strengthening exercise for osteoarthritis of the knee? A systematic review. Ann Rheum Dis. 64(4):544–548, 2005.
28. Roddy E, Zhang W., Doherty M, et al. Evidence-based recommendations for the role of exercise management of osteoarthritis of the hip or knee-the MOVE consensus. Rheumatology 44:67–73, 2005.
29. Ashworth NL, Chad KE, Harrison EL, et al. Home versus center based physical activity programs in older adults. Cochrane Database Syst Rev. 1:CD004017, 2005.
30. Stitik TP, Foye PM, Stiskal D, et al. Osteoarthritis. In: DeLisa JA, ed. Physical Medicine and Rehabilitation: Principles and Practice. 4th ed. Philadelphia, Lippincott Williams & Wilkins, 2005, 765–778.
31. Shiller AD. Osteoarthritis. In: Frontera WR, Silver K, eds. Essentials of Physical Medicine and Rehabilitation. Philadelphia, Hanley & Belfus, Inc., 2002, 638–644.
32. Lennard TA. Physical Medicine and Rehabilitation Pearls. Philadelphia, Hanley & Belfus, Inc., 2001.
33. Hicks JE, Gerber LH. Rehabilitation of the patient with arthritis and connective tissue disease. In: DeLisa JA, ed. Physical Medicine and Rehabilitation: Principles and Practice. 1st ed. Philadelphia, JB Lippincott, 1988, 765–794.
34. Brosseau L, MacLeay L, Robinson V, et al. Intensity of exercise for the treatment of osteoarthritis. Cochrane Database Syst Rev. 2:CD004259, 2003.
35. Thorstensson CA, Roos EM, Petersson IF, et al. Six-week high-intensity exercise program for middle-aged patients with knee osteoarthritis: a randomized controlled trial. BMC Musculoskelet Disord. 6:27, 2005.
36. Oosterveld FG, Rasker JJ. Effects of local heat and cold treatment on surface and articular temperature of arthritic knees. Arthritis Rheum 37:1578–1582, 1994.
37. Oosterveld FG, Rasker JJ. Treating arthritis with locally applied heat or cold. Semin Arthritis Rheum. 24(2):82–90, 1994.
38. Brosseau L, Yonge KA, Robinson V, et al. Thermotherapy for treatment of osteoarthritis. Cochrane Database Syst Rev 4:CD004522, 2003.
39. Lehman JF, Masock AJ, Warren CG, et al. Effect of therapeutic temperature on tendon extensibility. Arch Phys Med Rahabil 51:481–487, 1970.
40. Cox JS, Andrish JT, Implicito PA, et al. Heat modalities. In: Drez D, ed. Therapeutic Modalities for Sports Injuries. St. Louis, Mosby Year Book, 1989, 1–23.
41. Szucs L, Ratko I, Lesko T, et al. Double-blind trial on the effectiveness of the Puspokladany thermal water on arthrosis of the knee-joints. J R Soc Health. 109(1):7–9, 1989.
42. Ahern M, Nicholls E, Simionato E. Clinical and psychological effects of hydrotherapy rheumatic diseases. Clin Rehabil 9:204–212, 1995.
43. Nguyen M, Revel M, Dougados M. Prolonged effects of 3 week therapy in a spa resort on lumbar spine, knee and hip osteoarthritis: follow-up after 6 months. A randomized controlled trial. Br J Rheumatol. 36(1):77–81, 1997.
44. Stelian J, Gil I, Habot B, et al. Improvement of pain and disability in elderly patients with degenerative osteoarthritis of the knee treated with narrow-band light therapy. J Am Geriatr Soc 40(1):23–26, 1992.
45. Favoro L, Frisoni M, Baffoni L, et al. Successful treatment of hand erosive osteoarthritis by infrared radiation. Europa Medicophysics 30, 1994.
46. Gam AN, Johannsen F. Ultrasound therapy in musculoskeletal disorders: a meta-analysis. Pain 63(1):85–91, 1995.
47. Puett DW, Griffin MR. Published trials of non-medicinal and non-invasive therapies for hip and knee osteoarthritis. Ann Intern Med 121:133–140, 1994.
48. Huang MH, Lin YS, Lee CL, et al. Use of ultrasound to increase effectiveness of isokinetic exercise for knee osteoarthritis. Arch Phys Med Rehabil. 86(8):1545–1551, 2005.
49. Melzack R, Wall PD. Pain mechanisms. A new therapy. Science 150:971–979, 1965.
50. Liu H, Abbott J, Bee JA. Pulsed electromagnetic fields influence hyaline cartilage extracellular matrix composition without affecting molecular structure. Osteoarthritis Cartilage 4(1):63–76, 1996.
51. Oldham JA, Howe TE, Petterson T, et al. Electrotherapeutic rehabilitation of the quadriceps in elderly osteoarthritis patients. A double-blind assessment of patterned neuromuscular stimulation. Clin Rehabil 9:10–20, 1995.
52. Svarcova J, Trnavsky K, Zvarova J. The influence of ultrasound, galvanic currents and shortwave diathermy on pain intensity in patients with osteoarthritis. Scand J Rheumatol Suppl. 67:83–85, 1987.
53. Zizic TM, Hoffman KC, Holt PA, et al. The treatment of osteoarthritis of the knee with pulsed electrical stimulation. J Rheumatol. 22(9):1757–1761, 1995.
54. Trock DH, Bollet AJ, Markoll R. The effect of pulsed electromagnetic fields in the treatment of osteoarthritis of the knee and cervical spine. Report of randomized, double blind, placebo controlled trials. J Rheumatol. 21(10):1903–1911, 1994.
55. Law PP, Cheing GL. Optimal stimulation frequency of transcutaneous electrical nerve stimulation on people with knee osteoarthritis. J Rehabil Med 36(5):220–225, 2004.
56. Cheing GL, Hui-Chan CW. Would the addition of TENS to exercise training produce better physical performance outcomes in people with knee osteoarthritis than either intervention alone? Clin Rehabil 18(5):487–497, 2004.
57. Ng MM, Leung MC, Poon DM. The effects of electro-acupuncture and transcutaneous electrical nerve stimulation on patients with painful osteoarthritic knees: a randomized controlled trial with follow-up evaluation. J Altern Complement Med 9(5):641–649, 2003.
58. Yurtkuran M, Kocagil T. TENS, electroacupuncture and ice massage: comparison of treatment for osteoarthritis of the knee. Am J Acupunct. 27(3–4):133–140, 1999.
59. Lewis B, Lewis D, Cumming G. The comparative analgesic efficacy of transcutaneous electrical nerve stimulation and a non-steroidal anti-inflammatory drug for painful osteoarthritis. Br J Rheumatol 33(5):455–460, 1994.
60. Cheing GL, Hui-Chan CW, Chan KM. Does four weeks of TENS and/or isometric exercise produce cumulative reduction of osteoarthritic knee pain? Clin Rehabil 16(7):749–760, 2002.
61. Lewis D, Lewis B, Sturrock RD. Transcutaneous electrical nerve stimulation in osteoarthrosis: a therapeutic alternative? Ann Rheum Dis 43(1):47–49, 1984.
62. Cheing GL, Tsui AY, Lo SK, et al. Optimal stimulation duration of Tens in the management of osteoarthritic knee pain. J Rehabil Med 35(2):62–68, 2003.
63. Simkin PA, de Lateur BJ, Alquist AD, et al. Continuous passive motion for osteoarthritis of the hip: a pilot study. J Rheumatol 26(9):1987–1991, 1999.
64. Leivseth G, Torstensson J, Reikeras O. Effect of passive muscle stretching in osteoarthritis of the hip. Clin Sci (Lond) 76(1):113–117, 1989.
65. Rogind H, Bibow-Nielsen B, Jensen B, et al. The effects of a physical training program on patients with osteoarthritis of the knees. Arch Phys Med Rehabil 79(11):1421–1427, 1998.
66. Sharma L, Dunlop DD, Cahue S, et al. Quadriceps strength and osteoarthritis progression in malaligned and lax knees. Ann Intern Med 138(8):613–619, 2003.
67. Escamilla RF, Fleisig GS, Zheng N, et al. Biomechanics of the knee during closed kinetic chain and open kinetic chain exercises. Medicine & Science in Sports & Exercise 30(4):556–559, 1998.
68. Lutz GE, Palmitier RA, An KN, et al. Comparison of tibiofemoral joint forces during open-kinetic-chain and closed-kinetic-chain exercises. J Bone Joint Surg Am 75(5):732–739, 1993.
69. Stuart MJ, Meglan DA, Lutz GE, et al. Comparison of intersegmental tibiofemoral joint forces and muscle activity during various closed chain kinetic exercises. Am J of Sports Med 24(6):792–799, 1996.
70. Stitik TP, Foye PM, Blacksin M, et al. Intra-articular hyaluronan therapy and concomitant home exercise strengthening–an additive therapeutic algorithm for osteoarthritis of the knee. Arch Phys Medication Rehabil 85:9, 2004.
71. Blount WP. Don't throw away the cane. J Bone Joint Surg Am 38:695–698, 1956.
72. Brand RA, Crowninshield RD. The effect of cane use on hip contact force. Clin Orthop Relat Res (147):181–184, 1980.
73. Chan GN, Smith AW, Kirtley C, et al. Changes in knee moments with contralateral versus ipsilateral cane usage in females with knee osteoarthritis. Clin Biomech (Bristol, Avon) 20(4): 396–404, 2005.

74. Van der Esch M, Heijmans M, Dekker J. Factors contributing to possession and use of walking aids among persons with rheumatoid arthritis and osteoarthritis. Arthritis Rheum. 49(6):838–842, 2003.

75. Roddy E, Zhang W, Doherty M. Aerobic walking or strengthening exercise for osteoarthritis of the knee? A systematic review. Ann Rheum Dis 64(4):544–548, 2005.

76. van Baar ME, Assendelft WJ, Dekker J, et al. Effectiveness of exercise therapy in patients with osteoarthritis of the hip or knee: a systematic review of randomized clinical trials. Arthritis Rheum 42(7):1361–1369, 1999.

77. Fontaine KR, Heo M, Bathon J. Are U.S. adults with arthritis meeting public health recommendations for physical activity? Arthritis Rheum 50:624–628 , 2004.

78. Goldfarb AH, Jamurtas AZ. Beta-endorphin response to exercise. An update. Sports Med 24(1):8–16, 1997.

79. Schwarz L, Kindermann W. Changes in beta-endorphin levels in response to aerobic and anaerobic exercise. Sports Med. 13(1): 25–36, 1992.

80. Minor MA. Exercises treatment of osteoarthritis. Rheum Dis Clin North Am 25:3907–415, 1999.

81. Cochrane T, Davey RC, Matthes Edwards SM. Randomised controlled trial of the cost-effectiveness of water-based therapy for lower limb osteoarthritis. Health Technol Assess 9(31):iii–iv, ix–xi, 1–114, 2005.

82. Ettinger WH Jr, Burns R, Messier SP, et al. A randomized trial comparing aerobic exercise and resistance exercise with a health education program in older adults with knee osteoarthritis. The Fitness Arthritis and Seniors Trial (FAST). JAMA 277(1):25–31, 1997.

83. van Gool CH, Penninx BW, Kempen GI, et al. Effects of exercise adherence on physical function among overweight older adults with knee osteoarthritis Arthritis Rheum 53(1):24–32, 2005.

84. Marks R, Allegrante JP. Chronic osteoarthritis and adherence to exercise: a review of the literature. J Aging Phys Act 13(4): 434–460, 2005.

85. Moran M. Osteoarthritis and occupational therapy intervention. In: Stitik TP, ed. Osteoarthritis. Physical Medicine and Rehabilitation State of the Art Reviews. Philadelphia, Hanley & Belfus, Inc., 2001, 65–82.

86. Furst G, Gerber L, Smith C. Rehabilitation through learning: energy conservation and joint protection. Bethesda, MD, National Institutes of Health, 1982.

87. Towheed TE. Systematic review of therapies for osteoarthritis of the hand. Osteoarthritis Cartilage 13(6):455–462, 2005.

88. Krohn K. Footwear alterations and bracing as treatments for knee osteoarthritis. Curr Opin Rheumatol 17(5):653–656, 2005.

89. Kerrigan DC, Lelas JL, Goggins J, et al. Effectiveness of a lateral-wedge insole on knee varus torque in patients with knee osteoarthritis. Arch Phys Med Rehabil 83(7):889–893, 2002.

90. Pham T, Maillefert JF, Hudry C, et al. Laterally elevated wedged insoles in the treatment of medial knee osteoarthritis: a two-year prospective randomized controlled study. Osteoarthritis Cartilage 12:46–55, 2004.

91. Maillefert JF, Hudry C, Baron G, et al. Laterally elevated wedged insoles in the treatment of medial knee osteoarthritis: a prospective randomized controlled study. Osteoarthritis Cartilage 9: 738–745, 2001.

92. Toda Y, Tsukimura N. A six-month followup of a randomized trial comparing the efficacy of a lateral-wedge insole with subtalar strapping and an in-shoe lateral-wedge insole in patients with varus deformity osteoarthritis of the knee. Arthritis Rheum 50:3129–3136, 2004.

93. Toda Y, Tsukimura N, Kato A. The effects of different elevations of laterally wedged insoles with subtalar strapping on medial compartment osteoarthritis of the knee. Arch Phys Med Rehabil 85:673–677, 2004.

94. Cushnaghan J, McCarthy C, Dieppe P. Taping the patella medially: a new treatment for osteoarthritis of the knee joint? BMJ 308(6931):753–755, 1994.

95. Pruitt AL. Orthotic and brace use in the athlete with degenerative joint disease with angular deformity. Clin Sports Med 24(1): 93–99, 2005.

96. Bono CM, Berberian WS. Orthotic devices. Degenerative disorders of the foot and ankle. Foot Ankle Clin 6(2):329–340, 2001.

The Pharmacologic Treatment of Osteoarthritis

15

Lee S. Simon   *Vibeke Strand*

Osteoarthritis (OA), a heterogeneous disorder that affects a majority of people older than 60 years, is typically observed as an inflammatory and/or painful process once a patient finally presents to a treating clinician. The precipitating event may not be temporally related to inflammation but instead may be associated with a mechanical process; that initial event may have been remote in time. The patient usually presents with complaints of pain with or without obvious inflammation and occasionally limited range of motion.

Once the patient has pursued nonpharmacologic interventions, it is likely that therapy with a drug will be required. The choice of which specific drug or combination treatment to use remains to be individualized (Table 15–1). Most therapies are targeted to symptomatic response, although therapeutic interventions designed to stimulate new cartilage growth or to change the natural history of cartilage damage appear to be on the horizon. An understanding of the currently available therapies, their effectiveness and limitations, and their safety profile is of obvious import.

SIMPLE ANALGESICS

The initial use of acetaminophen was recommended by Bradley and colleagues,[1–3] who demonstrated that 1000 mg four times a day was equal in its effects to ibuprofen at either 1200 or 2400 mg/day in the treatment of patients with OA of the knee or hip. The one difference in efficacy observed was that anti-inflammatory doses of ibuprofen (2400 mg/24 hr), rather than lower doses (1200 mg, an

"analgesic" dose), or acetaminophen alone improved pain at rest.[2] Acetaminophen was better tolerated than either dose of ibuprofen. It is certainly worthwhile to initiate a trial of acetaminophen, known to be beneficial in OA patients with mild to moderate pain, on the basis of the risk/benefit ratio and cost. However, studies suggest that nonsteroidal anti-inflammatory drugs (NSAIDs) are associated with better efficacy. Pincus and coworkers[4,5] demonstrated that Arthrotec (a combination of diclofenac and misoprostol) at 75 mg twice daily provided greater benefit than acetaminophen, 4000 mg/day, in treating patients with OA of the hip or knee[4] and celecoxib 200 mgs q day was also better in terms of same outcomes.[5] Outcomes were measured by the patient's self-assessed functional scores, including the Western Ontario and McMaster Universities Osteoarthritis Index (WOMAC, a functional assessment that is a disease-specific tool for OA)[6] and the multidimensional Health Assessment Questionnaire (a quality-of-life measure for patients with arthritis).[7] In the celcoxib comparator study the patients also preferred the COX-2 selective inhibitor. Nonetheless, acetaminophen offered better gastrointestinal tolerability.

Although an absolute understanding of the mechanism of action of acetaminophen remains elusive, it has been demonstrated to be an excellent analgesic and antipyretic while not possessing effective anti-inflammatory activity.[8–11] It has been shown at high doses to have effects in vitro on the inhibition of prostaglandin synthesis.[12] It is believed that acetaminophen affects the brain and spinal cord, perhaps through the inhibition of PG (E_2) synthesis, while having no effect on prostaglandin synthesis in peripheral tissues.[13]

267

TABLE 15-1
AGENTS TO TREAT PAIN AND/OR INFLAMMATION

Simple analgesics
    Acetaminophen
    Tramadol
Topical agents
    Capsaicin
Nonsteroidal anti-inflammatory drugs
COX-2 selective inhibitors
Intra-articular glucocorticoid injections
Intra-articular hyaluronic acid injections
Opioid analgesics
Nutraceuticals
    Glucosamine
    Chondroitin sulfate
Experimental therapies
    Metalloproteinase inhibitors
Tetracyclines

Other data have shown that acetaminophen is metabolized uniquely in the brain into an agonist of TRPV1, thus suggesting that its main mode of action of antipyresis and analgesia may be modulated in the brain through the vanilloid receptor and may not have much to do with direct effects on cyclooxygenase activity.[14]

Issues regarding acetaminophen-induced toxicity have reached prominence. This includes hepatotoxicity as well as potential renal damage.[15-20] Acute overdose is associated with liver damage, which at times can be irreversible. If patients are taking more than 2 ounces of alcohol on a daily basis, the dose of acetaminophen should be decreased to a maximum of 2 to 2.5 g/24 hr.[21,22,22a] Perneger and colleagues[17] demonstrated in a case-controlled study that chronic use of acetaminophen may be associated with interstitial kidney damage leading to chronic renal failure. Investigators recruited patients from the End-Stage Renal Disease Program in the United States and an age-matched control population without kidney disease. Telephone interviews queried patients about regular acetaminophen or ASA use during the preceding 10 years. Patients with renal failure had taken significantly more acetaminophen and ASA than the control population did. Unfortunately, there are significant confounders to these observations. Patients in the End-Stage Renal Disease Program in the United States are typically allowed to use acetaminophen only for pain relief; thus, there is intrinsic bias in this study. Nonetheless, it is possible that chronic use of acetaminophen may lead to interstitial nephritis similar to that reported for the parent product, phenacetin. However, given its broad use as a pain reliever worldwide, this is likely to be a rare event.

Data have suggested that acetaminophen, long considered to be safe when it is used with clinically important anticoagulation therapy such as warfarin, has a potential effect on the prothrombin time. In patients requiring a higher international normalized ratio (INR) for control of their clotting tendency, the concomitant use of acetaminophen at high dose is a risk; therefore, more frequent monitoring of the INR should be planned.[23,24]

There is also accumulating evidence of concern regarding the potential cardiovascular (CV) risk of acetaminophen. Chan et al. published a prospective cohort study nested within the nurses health study (NHS) that demonstrated that acetaminophen, when taken more than 15 days of the month chronically, is associated with an increased incidence of CV events which is similar to that seen with both the nonselective NSAIDs and the cyclooxygenase-2 (COX-2) selective inhibitors.[25]

The risk/benefit ratio for use of acetaminophen in patients with little inflammation but mild to moderate pain and who derive benefit argues for its continued broad use. Its ubiquity and low cost means that most patients will already have tried acetaminophen, often at less than maximum doses; although a number of patients will have only a limited therapeutic response, it is important to ascertain whether the patient has given the drug a fair trial before determining this treatment to be a failure. Intermittent use or inadequate daily doses should be followed with a several-week trial of acetaminophen of up to 4 g/24 hr with care toward monitoring for untoward events, particularly the development of worsening hypertension.[26]

TOPICAL ANALGESICS

Topical agents with significant local effects have been used for years as tried and true home remedies, including menthol rubs, alcohol rubs, and substances such as camphor. Few clinical trials demonstrate adequate evidence to support recommendations for their use. The process of application may be the important therapeutic event, and massage is also a source of benefit. If there is benefit, there is also little risk.

In contrast, capsaicin 0.025 or 0.075%, derived from pepper, is a counterirritant. When it is used regularly, substance P and calcitonin gene–related peptide (CGRP), important neurotransmitters for pain, are depleted in the local tissues within a week.[27,28] Clinical trials have shown benefit when the cream or ointment is applied four times daily. Toxicity is minimal, predominantly associated with application of the cream or ointment where it is not indicated. Care needs to be taken, and hands should be washed quickly to prevent accidental application of the drug to mucous membranes or the eyes. The counterirritant effect of the pepper derivative, which may be important for clinical effect, can occasionally be intolerable and may also induce rashes.[22,27,28]

There is increasing evidence to support the use of topical NSAIDs. Although as of this writing there are still none approved in the United States, these drugs have been available around the world for years. These authors await further publications as these products have been studied more extensively in recent years.

NONSTEROIDAL ANTI-INFLAMMATORY DRUGS

NSAIDs are anti-inflammatory, analgesic, and antipyretic agents. They are widely used to reduce pain, to decrease the gelling phenomenon, and to improve function in patients with OA and rheumatoid arthritis, and for treatment of pain, including headache, dysmenorrhea, and postoperative pain.[29–31] Whether their clinical effects are solely due to their anti-inflammatory or analgesic effects or other possible properties is not known.[29] There are at least 20 different NSAIDs currently available in the United States (Table 15–2). In addition, COX-2–selective inhibitors (e.g., celecoxib) with similar efficacy but significantly decreased gastrointestinal and platelet effects are available.[32–35]

Prior to events surrounding the identification of increased cardiovascular risk with chronic use of nonselective and selective NSAIDs, these drugs represented one of the most commonly used classes of drugs in the world. It has been estimated that more than 17,000,000 Americans used these agents on a daily basis. With the aging of the U.S. population, the Centers for Disease Control and Prevention predicts a significant increase in the prevalence of painful rheumatic conditions and thus an increased burden on the need for drugs like NSAIDs.[36,37] Approximately 60 million NSAID prescriptions were written each year in the United States, the number for elderly patients exceeding that for younger patients by approximately 3.6-fold.[36] ASA ibuprofen, naproxen, and ketoprofen are also available over the counter. At equipotent doses, the clinical efficacy and tolerability of the various

TABLE 15–2
THE NONSTEROIDAL ANTI-INFLAMMATORY DRUGS

NSAID	Trade Name	Usual Dose	Approved Use*
CARBOXYLIC ACIDS			
ASA (acetylsalicylic acid)	Multiple	2.4–6 g/24 hr in 4–5 divided doses	RA, OA, AS, JCA, ST
Buffered ASA	Multiple	Same	Same
Enteric-coated salicylates	Multiple	Same	Same
Salsalate	Disalcid	1.5–3.0 g/24 hr bid	Same
Diflunisal	Dolobid	0.5–1.5 g/24 hr bid	Same
Choline magnesium trisalicylate	Trilisate	1.5–3 g/24 hr bid–tid	RA, OA, pain, JCA
PROPRIONIC ACIDS			
Ibuprofen	Motrin, Rufen, OTC	OTC: 200–400 mg qid Rx: 400, 600, 800 mg max 3200 mg/24 hr	RA, OA, JCA
Naproxen	Naprelan, Anaprox, Naprosyn EC	250, 375, 500 mg bid	RA, OA, JCA, ST
Fenoprofen	Nalfon	300–600 mg qid	RA, OA
Ketoprofen	Orudis	75 mg tid	RA, OA
Flurbiprofen	Ansaid	100 mg bid–tid	RA, OA
ACETIC ACID DERIVATIVES			
Indomethacin	Indocin, Indocin SR	25, 50 mg tid or qid SR: 75 mg bid; rarely >150 mg/24 hr	RA, OA, G, AS
Tolmetin	Tolectin	400, 600, 800 mg; 800–2400 mg/24 hr	RA, OA, JCA
Sulindac	Clinoril	150, 200 mg bid (some ↑ to tid)	RA, OA, AS, ST, G
Diclofenac	Voltaren, Arthrotec	50 mg tid, 75 mg bid	RA, OA, AS
Etodolac	Lodine	200, 300 mg bid to qid max: 1200 mg/24 hr	OA, pain
FENAMATES			
Meclofenamate	Meclomen	50–100 mg tid–qid	RA, OA
Mefenamic acid	Ponstel	250 mg qid	RA, OA
ENOLIC ACIDS			
Piroxicam	Feldene	10, 20 mg qd	RA, OA
NAPHTHYLKANONES			
Nabumetone	Relafen	500 mg bid up to 1500 mg/24 hr	RA, OA
COXIBS			
Celecoxib	Celebrex	100 mg bid 200 mg qd–bid	OA, RA acute pain

*FDA approved.
RA, rheumatoid arthritis; OA, osteoarthritis; AS, ankylosing spondylitis; G, gout; JCA, juvenile chronic polyarthritis; ST, soft tissue injury.

NSAIDs are similar; however, individual responses are highly variable.[29,30,36,37] Although it is believed that it is reasonable to try another NSAID from a different class if a patient fails to respond to one NSAID of one class, no one has studied this in a prospective controlled manner.[29,30] As will be discussed, the use of simple analgesics and opioids has increased with the debate continuing regarding the overall risk and benefit of the NSAIDs.

Sodium salicylic acid was discovered in 1763. Impure forms of salicylates had been used as analgesics and antipyretics throughout the previous century. Once it was purified and synthesized, the acetyl derivative of salicylate, acetylsalicylic acid (ASA), was found to provide more anti-inflammatory activity than salicylate alone. Because of the toxicity of ASA, phenylbutazone, an enolic acid derivative, was introduced in the early 1950s. This was the first nonsalicylate NSAID developed for use in patients with painful and inflammatory conditions. This drug, a weak prostaglandin synthase inhibitor, induced uricosuria and was rapidly found to be useful in patients with ankylosing spondylitis and gout. However, owing to concerns related to bone marrow toxicity, particularly in women older than 60 years, this compound is now rarely prescribed. Indomethacin, an indoleacetic acid derivative, was subsequently developed in 1958 to substitute for phenylbutazone. It had significant toxicity as well, and the search for safer (particularly gastrointestinally safer)— and at least equally effective—NSAIDs ensued. Other issues have driven the development of newer agents, such as once- or twice-daily dosing to improve compliance.

The choice of NSAID is typically based on the physician's prescribing behavior. Historically, ASA congeners including enteric-coated ASA were the first choice for treating inflammatory and degenerative arthritic conditions. Although cost is low, gastrointestinal intolerance and the requirement of multiple regular doses throughout the day to maintain adequate anti-inflammatory blood levels pose a problem. Depending on body mass, concomitant drug use, serum albumin levels, and other physiologic factors, 10 to 20 plain ASA tablets daily, taken no more than 8 hours apart, are usually required to achieve anti-inflammatory salicylate blood levels. Doses may need to be increased if enteric-coated ASA is chosen because of variable absorption within the bowel.

Although low dose ASA has been extensively studied and used to inhibit platelet aggregation as a prophylaxis against second myocardial infarction as well as suggestive evidence of decrease in primary events, there are little data that describe higher dose ASA as beneficial except as an anti-inflammatory agent. Recently a small study of prevention of recurrent colon polyps demonstrated an increased risk of stroke which was statistically significant and dose dependent.[38] Furthermore there is experimental evidence that concomitant use of ibuprofen may alter the cardiovascular benefit of prophylactic low doses of ASA.[39]

Mechanism of Action

Some NSAIDs appear to be potent inhibitors of prostaglandin synthesis, whereas others more prominently affect nonprostaglandin-mediated biologic events.[29,30,40-45] Differential clinical effects have also been attributed to variations in the enantiomeric state of the agent as well as its pharmacokinetics, pharmacodynamics, and metabolism.[29,30,40-47] The theoretical and real differences between NSAIDs have been reviewed by Brooks and Day[29] and Furst.[30] Although variability can be explained in part by absorption, distribution, and metabolism, potential differences in mechanism of action must be considered an important explanation for their variable effects.[29,30,47]

NSAIDs are primarily anti-inflammatory and analgesic by decreasing production of prostaglandins of the E series.[48] Prostanoic acids are proinflammatory and increase vascular permeability and sensitivity to the release of bradykinins. NSAIDs have also been shown to inhibit the formation of prostacyclin and thromboxane, resulting in complex effects on vascular permeability and platelet aggregation, undoubtedly contributing to the overall clinical effects of these compounds.

Polyunsaturated fatty acids including arachidonic acid, constituents of all cell membranes, exist in ester linkage in the glycerols of phospholipids and are ultimately converted to prostaglandins or leukotrienes first through the action of phospholipase A_2 or phospholipase C.[48] Free arachidonic acid released by the phospholipase acts as a substrate for the prostaglandin endoperoxide (PGH) synthase complex, which includes both cyclooxygenase and peroxidase. The enzymes catalyze the conversion of arachidonic acid to the unstable cyclic endoperoxide intermediates Prostaglandin G2 (PGG_2) and prostaglandin H2 (PGH_2). These arachidonic acid metabolites are then converted to the more stable PGE_2 and PGF_2 compounds by specific tissue prostaglandin-synthases. NSAIDs specifically inhibit cyclooxygenase and thereby reduce the conversion of arachidonic acid to PGG_2.

There are at least two isoforms of the cyclooxygenase enzymes. Although they share 60% homology in the amino acid sequences considered important for catalysis of arachidonic acid, they are products of two different genes. They differ most importantly in their regulation and expression.[49,50] COX-1 or prostaglandin synthase H_1 is a "house-keeping enzyme" that regulates normal cellular processes and is stimulated by hormones or growth factors. It is constitutively expressed in most tissues and is inhibited by all NSAIDs to varying degrees, depending on the applied experimental model system used to measure drug effects.[51-54] It is important in maintaining the integrity of the gastric and duodenal mucosa, and many of the toxic effects of the NSAIDs on the gastrointestinal tract are attributed to its inhibition.[55-60]

The other isoform, prostaglandin synthase H_2 or COX-2, is an inducible enzyme and is usually undetectable in most tissues. Its expression is increased during states of inflammation or experimentally in response to mitogenic stimuli. For example, in monocyte-macrophage systems, endotoxin stimulates COX-2 expression; in fibroblasts, various growth factors, phorbol esters, and interleukin-1 do so.[61] This isoform is also constitutively expressed in the brain (specifically cortex and hippocampus), in the female reproductive tract, in the male vas deferens, in bone, and at least in some models in human kidney.[49,50] The expression of COX-2 is inhibited by glucocorticoids.[49,50,62] COX-2 is also inhibited by all of the presently available NSAIDs to a greater or lesser degree.[51-54]

The in vitro systems used to define the actions of the available NSAIDs are based on cell-free systems, pure enzyme systems, or whole cell systems.[51] Each drug studied to date has demonstrated different measurable effects within each system. As an example, it appears that nonacetylated salicylates inhibit the activity of COX-1 and COX-2 in whole cell systems but are not active against either COX-1 or COX-2 in recombinant enzyme or cell membrane systems. This suggests that salicylates act early in the arachidonic acid cascade, similar to glucocorticoids, perhaps by inhibition of enzyme expression rather than by direct inhibition of cyclooxygenase.

Evidence has accumulated that several NSAIDs are selective for COX-2 enzyme effects over COX-1. For example, in vitro effects of etodolac demonstrate an approximately tenfold inhibition of COX-2 compared with COX-1 at low doses.[63,64] However, at higher anti-inflammatory doses, this specificity appears to be mitigated, because both enzymes are affected. Celecoxib is the only COX-2 selective inhibitor that is currently available in the U.S.[64] This COX-2–selective inhibitor has been shown to be as effective at inhibiting OA pain, dental pain, and the pain and inflammation associated with rheumatoid arthritis as naproxen (500 mg twice daily), ibuprofen (800 mg three times daily), and diclofenac (75 mg twice daily), without endoscopic evidence of gastroduodenal damage and without affecting platelet aggregation.[32–35,65,66] Unfortunately, owing to the design of the randomized clinical trials, many of the important questions regarding the renal effects of this COX-2 inhibitor remain unanswered.[49,50]

Arachidonic acid can also serve as a substrate for 5- or 12-lipoxygenase. These enzymes catalyze the conversion of arachidonic acid to biologically active leukotriene and hydroxyeicosatetraenoic acids. None of the presently available NSAIDs inhibits 5-lipoxygenase directly, although several compounds presently under development may have inhibitory effects on both cyclooxygenase and lipoxygenase. It remains to be seen whether these will be clinically useful.

NSAIDs are lipophilic and become incorporated in the lipid bilayer of cell membranes and thereby may interrupt protein–protein interactions important for signal transduction.[40,41,56] For example, stimulus-response coupling, which is critical for recruitment of phagocytic cells to sites of inflammation, has been demonstrated in vitro to be inhibited by some NSAIDs.[31,40,41] There are data suggesting that NSAIDs inhibit activation and chemotaxis of neutrophils as well as reduce toxic oxygen radical production in stimulated neutrophils.[12,31,67] There is also evidence that several NSAIDs scavenge superoxide radicals.[68]

Salicylates have been demonstrated to inhibit phospholipase C activity in macrophages. Some NSAIDs have been shown to affect T lymphocyte function experimentally by inhibiting rheumatoid factor production in vitro. Another newly described action not directly related to prostaglandin synthesis inhibition is interference with neutrophil–endothelial cell adherence, which is crucial to migration of granulocytes to sites of inflammation; expression of L-selectins is decreased.[43] NSAIDs have been demonstrated in vitro to inhibit NF-κB (nuclear transcription factor)–dependent transcription, thereby inhibiting inducible

nitric oxide synthase.[42,45] Anti-inflammatory levels of ASA have been shown to inhibit expression of inducible nitric oxide synthase and subsequent production of nitrite in vitro. At pharmacologic doses, sodium salicylate, indomethacin, and acetaminophen were studied and had no effect; but at suprapharmacologic dosages, sodium salicylate inhibited nitrite production.[42]

It has been described that prostaglandins inhibit apoptosis (programmed cell death) and that NSAIDs, by inhibition of prostaglandin synthesis, may reestablish more normal cell cycle responses.[49,50,69] There is also evidence suggesting that some NSAIDs may reduce PGH synthase gene expression, thereby supporting the clinical evidence of differences in activity in NSAIDs in sites of active inflammation.

The importance of these prostaglandin- and non-prostaglandin-mediated processes in reducing clinical inflammation is not entirely clear. Although nonacetylated salicylates have been shown in vitro to inhibit neutrophil function and to have equal efficacy in patients with rheumatoid arthritis,[70] there is no clinical evidence to suggest that biologic effects other than prostaglandin synthase inhibition are more important.

Pharmacology

Bioavailability

All NSAIDs are completely absorbed after oral administration. Absorption rates may vary in patients with altered gastrointestinal blood flow or motility and when certain NSAIDs are taken with food.[29,30] For example, taking naproxen with food may decrease absorption by 16%, although this is not likely to be clinically important. Enteric coating may reduce direct effects of NSAIDs on the gastric mucosa but may also reduce the rate of absorption.

Most NSAIDs are weak organic acids; once absorbed, they are more than 95% bound to serum albumin. This is a saturable process. Clinically significant decreases in serum albumin levels or institution of other highly protein bound medications may lead to an increase in the free component of NSAID in serum. This may be important in patients who are elderly or are chronically ill, especially with associated hypoalbuminemic states. Importantly, because of increased vascular permeability in localized sites of inflammation, this high degree of protein binding may result in delivery of higher levels of NSAIDs.

Metabolism

NSAIDs are metabolized predominantly in the liver by the cytochrome P450 system and the CYP2C9 isoform and excreted in the urine. This must be taken into consideration in prescribing NSAIDs for patients with hepatic or renal dysfunction. Some NSAIDs, such as oxaprozin, have two metabolic pathways whereby some portion is directly secreted into the bile and another part is further metabolized and excreted in the urine. Others (e.g., indomethacin, sulindac, and piroxicam) have prominent enterohepatic circulation resulting in a prolonged half-life and should be used with caution in the elderly. In patients with renal insufficiency, some inactive metabolites may be resynthesized in vivo to the active compound. Two of the traditional NSAIDs, diclofenac and flurbiprofen, and celecoxib are metabolized in the liver and should be used with care and at the lowest possible doses in patients with clinically significant liver disease and patients with significant liver dysfunction, this means patients with significant liver dysfunction, such as patients with cirrhosis with or without ascites, prolonged prothrombin times, falling serum albumin levels, or important elevations in liver transaminases in blood.

Salicylates are the least highly protein bound NSAID, at approximately 68%. Zero-order kinetics are dominant in salicylate metabolism. Thus, increasing the dose of salicylates is effective over a narrow range, but once the metabolic systems are saturated, incremental increases in dose may lead to high serum salicylate levels. Thus, changes in salicylate doses need to be carefully considered at chronic steady-state levels, particularly in patients with altered renal or hepatic function.

Plasma Half-Life

Significant differences in plasma half-lives of the NSAIDs may be important in explaining their diverse clinical effects. Those with long half-lives typically do not attain maximal plasma concentrations quickly, and clinical responses may be delayed. Plasma concentrations can vary widely owing to differences in renal clearance and metabolism. Piroxicam has the longest serum half-life of currently marketed NSAIDs, 57 ± 22 hours. In comparison, diclofenac has one of the shortest, 1.1 ± 0.2 hours (Table 15–3). Although drugs have been developed with long half-lives to improve the compliance of patients, the fact that piroxicam has such a long half-life is not that attractive for the elderly patient at risk for specific NSAID-induced toxic effects. In the older patient, it is sometimes preferable to use drugs of shorter half-life so that the unwanted effects may more rapidly disappear when the drug is discontinued.

Sulindac and nabumetone are "prodrugs" in which the active compound is produced after first-pass metabolism through the liver. Prodrugs were developed to decrease the exposure of the gastrointestinal mucosa to the local effects of the NSAIDs. Unfortunately, as noted before, with adequate inhibition of COX-1, the patient is placed at substantial risk for an NSAID-induced upper gastrointestinal tract event as long as COX-1 activity is inhibited. This is true for drugs such as ketorolac given by injection, indomethacin given rectally, and for these prodrugs when they are given in adequate therapeutic doses.[71, 72]

Once steady state has been achieved, synovial fluid concentrations of NSAIDs do not vary much. Although theoretically important for clinical effect, this has not been shown in vivo.[29, 30] Thus, choices to prescribe specific NSAIDs are largely based on issues of safety, convenience, and compliance.

Miscellaneous

Other pharmacologic properties may be important clinically. NSAIDs that are highly lipid soluble in serum will penetrate the central nervous system more effectively and may occasionally produce striking changes in mentation, perception, and mood.[73,74] Indomethacin has been

TABLE 15–3

PLASMA HALF-LIVES OF THE NSAIDs AND THE COXIBs

Chemical Class	Drug Name	Plasma Half-Life (hr)
Carboxylic acids	Acetylsalicylic acid	4–15
	Choline magnesium trisalicylate	4–15
	Salsalate	4–15
	Diflunisal	7–15
Propionic acids	Ibuprofen	1.5–2
	Naproxen	13
	Fenoprofen	3
	Ketoprofen	2
	Flurbiprofen	3–9
	Oxaprozin	36–40
Acetic acids	Indomethacin	3–11
	Tolmetin	1–1.5
	Sulindac	13–16
	Diclofenac	1–2
	Etodolac	2–4
	Ketorolac	2
Fenamic acids	Mefenamic acid	2
	Meclofenamic acid	2–3
Enolic acids	Piroxicam	30–86
Naphthylkanones	Nabumetone	19–30
Coxibs	Celecoxib	11
	Rofecoxib	17

associated with many of these side effects, even after a single dose, particularly in the elderly.

Adverse Effects

Mechanism-Based Adverse Effects

Risk for Anaphylaxis and Pulmonary Effects. Many adverse reactions attributed to NSAIDs are due to inhibition of prostaglandin synthesis in local tissues (Table 15–4). Patients with allergic rhinitis, nasal polyposis, or a history of asthma are the broadest example; in these patients, all NSAIDs effectively inhibit prostaglandin synthase and increase their risk for anaphylaxis. In high doses, even nonacetylated salicylates may sufficiently decrease prostaglandin synthesis to induce an anaphylactic reaction in sensitive patients.[75] Although the exact mechanism for this effect remains unclear, it is known that E prostaglandins serve as bronchodilators. When cyclooxygenase activity is inhibited in patients at risk, a decrease in synthesis of prostaglandins that contributes to bronchodilation results. Another explanation implicates other enzymatic pathways that use the arachidonate pool after it is converted from phospholipase, whereby shunting of arachidonate into the leukotriene pathway occurs when cyclooxygenase is inhibited. The leukotriene pathway converts arachidonate by 5-lipoxygenase, leading to products such as leukotriene B_4 and others, which are clearly associated with anaphylaxis. This explanation implies that release

TABLE 15–4

ADVERSE REACTIONS OF THE NSAIDs

Gastrointestinal	Nausea, vomiting, dyspepsia, diarrhea, constipation
	Gastric mucosal irritation, superficial erosions, peptic ulceration, increased fecal blood wasting
	Major gastrointestinal hemorrhage, penetrating ulcers
	Small bowel erosions; induce "diaphragm" development in small bowel
	Hepatotoxicity, hepatitis, fulminant hepatic failure
Renal	Glomerulopathy, interstitial nephritis, alterations in renal plasma flow leading to fall in glomerular filtration rates; interfere with natriuresis induced by diuretics; inhibit renin release; induce edema
	Alterations in tubule functions
Central nervous system	Headaches, confusion, hallucinations, depersonalization reactions, depression, tremor
	Aseptic meningitis, tinnitus, vertigo, neuropathy, toxic amblyopia, transient transparent corneal deposits
Hematologic	Anemia, marrow depression, Coombs-positive anemia
	Decrease platelet aggregation
Hypersensitivity	Asthma, asthma/urticaria syndrome, urticaria, rashes, photosensitivity, Stevens-Johnson syndrome
Other	Drug interactions, such as displacement of oral hypoglycemics and warfarin from protein binding sites and from sites of metabolism
	Interference with the actions of β-blockers and some diuretics

of large stores of arachidonate in certain inflammatory situations leads to excess substrate for leukotriene metabolism. This results in release of products that are highly reactive, leading to increased bronchoconstriction and the risk for anaphylaxis in the right patient.[76] Whether the main mechanism of effect is inhibition of prostaglandin synthesis or shunting of arachidonate into conversion by 5-lipoxygenase or a combination of the two, it is clear that patients who are sensitive are at great risk when NSAIDs are used.

The nonacetylated salicylates as a group have been considered a safe choice in these patients because they are known to possess anti-inflammatory activity but are relatively weak cyclooxygenase inhibitors. Stevenson and associates[77] have demonstrated that in general, this continues to be true; however, their study suggests a bit of caution. They studied ten ASA–sensitive patients who had developed asthma previously when treated with ASA. In a double-blinded, placebo-controlled, crossover oral challenge, these patients received either ASA or 2 g of salsalate (a nonacetylated condensation product of two salicylate moieties). All but two patients tolerated the salsalate dose

well; in these two patients, an increase in airway resistance with salsalate therapy was demonstrated. When they were desensitized to ASA, the two patients who were previously intolerant showed improvement in tolerance to the salsalate, which suggests crossover in the mode of action. Thus, not all patients who develop bronchospasm to NSAIDs are safe when they are prescribed a nonacetylated salicylate, and if it is absolutely required, the patient should be monitored carefully, perhaps with an airflow meter after a single dose of the chosen drug to determine whether bronchospasm develops. Alternatively, the patient should be desensitized before the start of therapy.

We know little about the importance of the activities of either of the two cyclooxygenase isoforms in the lung parenchyma.[49]

Platelet Effects. Platelet aggregation and thus the ability to clot are primarily induced through stimulating thromboxane production with activation of platelet COX-1. There is no COX-2 in the platelet. NSAIDs and ASA inhibit the activity of COX-1, but the COX-2–specific inhibitors have no effect on COX-1 at clinically effective therapeutic doses.[49]

The effect of the nonsalicylate NSAIDs on platelet function is reversible and related to the half-life of the drug, whereas the effect of ASA is to acetylate the COX-1 enzyme, thereby permanently inactivating it. Because platelets cannot synthesize new cyclooxygenase enzyme after exposure to ASA, the platelet does not function appropriately for its life span. Therefore, the effect of ASA on the platelet does not wear off as the drug is metabolized, as with the nonsalicylate NSAIDs. Patients awaiting surgery should therefore stop their NSAIDs at a time determined by four to five times the serum half-life; ASA needs to be discontinued 1 to 2 weeks before the planned procedure to allow repopulation of platelets that have been unexposed to ASA.

There is also little information about the use of the COX-2–selective inhibitors in patients at risk for thrombosis.[49] The randomized clinical trials of the COX-2–selective inhibitors were not designed to address this question; thus, we have to await postmarketing surveillance to help resolve this problem. Furthermore, there is little information demonstrating that the traditional NSAIDs are safer or more useful than the COX-2–selective inhibitors in this regard. Only ASA has been studied prospectively, and low-dose ASA should be given concomitantly with either NSAIDs or selective COX-2 inhibitors in patients at risk for thrombosis. Given the additive ulcerogenic potential associated with the use of multiple NSAIDs, it is advisable to use selective COX-2 inhibitors with ASA when combination cardioprotective and anti-inflammatory therapies are considered. It is recommended that frail patients who are at increased risk for gastrointestinal (GI) complications when prescribed a COX-2 selective inhibitor combined with low-dose aspirin should also receive a proton-pump inhibitor as well.

The most clinically significant adverse effects associated with NSAIDs occur either in the gastrointestinal mucosa or are related to the potential risks for thromboembolic events.

Gastrointestinal Tract. The GI effects appear to be due to local or systemic inhibition of prostaglandin synthesis.[55–60,78–87] NSAIDs cause a wide range of gastrointestinal tract problems, including esophagitis, esophageal stricture, gastritis, mucosal erosions, hemorrhage, peptic ulceration or perforation, obstruction, and death.[57] There is increasing evidence that the mucosa of the large and small bowel is affected. These agents may also induce stricture formation,[29,30,40,78] which may manifest as diaphragms that precipitate small or large bowel obstruction and can be difficult to detect on contrast radiographic studies.

In addition, there is evidence to suggest that NSAIDs interfere with permeability of the gastrointestinal tract mucosa. The weakly acidic NSAIDs rapidly penetrate the superficial lining cells of the gastrointestinal tract mucosa, leading to oxidative uncoupling of cellular metabolism, local tissue injury, and ultimately cell death. This can result in local erosions, hemorrhages, and formation of clinically significant ulcers in the patients.[40,78]

Endoscopic studies have clearly demonstrated that NSAID administration results in shallow erosions and submucosal hemorrhage; although these occur at any site in the gastrointestinal tract, they are more commonly observed in the stomach near the prepyloric area and the antrum.[55] These lesions are typically asymptomatic, making prevalence data difficult to determine.[87,88] Nor do we know the number of lesions that spontaneously heal or that progress to ulceration, frank perforation, gastric or duodenal obstruction, serious gastrointestinal hemorrhage, or subsequent death. Risk factors for development of gastrointestinal toxicity in patients receiving NSAIDs include age older than 60 years; prior history of peptic ulcer disease; prior use of antiulcer therapies for any reason; concomitant use of glucocorticoids, particularly in patients with rheumatoid arthritis; comorbidities, such as significant cardiovascular disease; and severe rheumatoid arthritis.[55,60,80,81,85,89,90] Another risk factor is increasing dose of specific and singular NSAIDs.[74]

The magnitude of risk for gastrointestinal adverse events is controversial. The U.S. Food and Drug Administration (FDA) reports an overall risk of 2% to 4% for NSAID-induced gastric ulcer development and its complications.[55,56] In general, on the basis of multiple clinical trials, the relative risk is estimated to be 4.0 to 5.0 for gastric ulcer, 1.1 to 1.6 for duodenal ulcer, and 4.5 to 5.0 for clinically significant gastric ulcers with hemorrhage, perforation, obstruction, or death. Although many epidemiologic studies have been designed to prove causal associations, most have had inherent design flaws that have prevented accurate estimations of true risk.

As noted, other sites in the gastrointestinal tract including the esophagus and small and large bowel may also be affected. Exposure to NSAIDs is probably a major factor in the development of esophagitis and subsequent stricture formation.[91,92] Effects on small and large bowel have been increasingly reported.[84] An autopsy study of 713 patients showed that small bowel ulcerations defined as ulcers more than 3 mm in diameter were observed in 8.4% of patients exposed to NSAIDs compared with 0.6% of nonusers of NSAIDs.[94] Ulcerations of stomach and duodenum were observed in 22% of NSAID users compared with 12% of nonusers.

Knowledge of increased risk for NSAID-induced small and large bowel damage becomes important with evidence accumulated with capsular endoscopy.[93] This technique allows visualization of the lower GI tract. These data have confirmed the previously noted information that NS NSAIDs damage the lower GI tract and proton pump inhibitors (PPIs) do not protect the lower GI tract from these effects as they do in the upper GI tract. Furthermore, the COX-2 selective inhibitors that have been studied do not induce similar lower GI lesions. Although these lower GI tract abnormalities are not observed as frequently as upper GI lesions, they were reported to be the cause of 40% of the complications noted in the Vioxx gastrointestinal outcomes research (VIGOR) trial of rofecoxib compared with naproxen.[94]

Epidemiologic studies suggest that the nonacetylated salicylates are less likely to result in an NSAID-induced adverse gastrointestinal event. Other newer agents, such as nabumetone, are usually listed together with similar effects.[71,72] NSAIDs with prominent enterohepatic circulation and significantly longer half-lives, such as sulindac and piroxicam, have been linked to increased potential for gastrointestinal toxicity attributed to prolonged reexposure of gastric and duodenal mucosa to bile reflux and the active moiety of the drug.[91]

Endoscopic data from large numbers of patients treated with COX-2–selective inhibitors strongly suggest that ulcers occur at the same rate as in patients who received placebo, whereas the traditional NSAID active comparators induced ulcers (as documented by endoscopy) in 15% (diclofenac, 75 mg twice daily; ibuprofen, 800 mg three times daily) to 19% (naproxen, 500 mg twice daily) after 1 week of treatment in healthy volunteers[33] and in 26% (naproxen, 500 mg twice daily) of patients with OA and rheumatoid arthritis after 12 weeks of treatment.[32-34] In addition, the extent of ulcer complications has been shown to be decreased by about two- to threefold with both rofecoxib and celecoxib. Both trials recruited about 8000 patients with either rheumatoid arthritis or OA, treated with two to four times the recommended dose of the COX-2 selective inhibitor and compated the GI complication rate with that produced by either naproxen 500 mg twice daily, ibuprofen 800 mg three times daily or diclofenac 75 mg twice daily[95,96] It is possible that patients with preexisting ulcer may experience delay in healing when they are treated with a COX-2–selective inhibitor, but only long-term outcome clinical trials will clarify whether this is a risk.[97-101]

Cardiovascular Effects. During the VIGOR trial in which rofecoxib 50 mgs was compared with naproxen 500 mg BID, there was a surprising secondary outcome of increased thromboembolic events favoring naproxen with a fivefold increased incidence of nonfatal myocardial infarction (MI) in the rofecoxib-treated patient group.[95] A similar difference was not observed in the celebrex long-term arthritis safety study (CLASS) trial comparing 800 mg celecoxib with ibuprofen 800 mg three times daily or diclofenac at 75 mg twice daily.[102] In this study, the incidence was about 1% for all comparators but no placebo arm was included. It was unclear what this meant as these were secondary outcomes in trials not designed to explore cardiovascular outcomes, and it could be suggested that naproxen actually served to decrease the incidence of these events or rofecoxib could be implicated in inducing these events; however, it is not known why they were not observed in the CLASS trial. There were similar numbers of patients recruited into both trials, but there were far fewer patient-years of exposure in the CLASS trial due to nonuniform dropout of patients from all arms approaching 50%.

With the development of another COX-2 selective inhibitor, lumiricoxib, a larger study was instituted with cardiovascular outcomes a priori defined as secondary outcomes and an adjudication committee established before the study was begun. Although there were 18,000 patients recruited into the study, there were only approximately 7000 patient years of exposure to either naproxen 500 mgs twice daily, lumericoxib 400 mgs once daily, or ibuprofen 800 mgs three times daily. Similar to the CLASS trial results, there were no statistical differences between the three comparators in terms of composite cardiovascular outcomes.[103,104]

Thus when time came to study the potential of these drugs to prevent colonic polyposis, the companies included a priori defined secondary outcomes along with appropriate adjudication committees to ascertain CV risk. These studies were planned to be long term and employ true placebo, but unfortunately not study patients with arthritis or pain.

The Cardiovascular Risk of the NSAIDs

Current data do not support extrapolation of the cardioprotective effects of ASA to other NSAIDs. ASA exerts its antiplatelet effects by irreversibly acetylating a serine residue in platelet COX-1, inhibiting the production of thromboxane A_2 for the lifetime of the platelet, since the platelet lacks the machinery to synthesize new cyclooxygenase.[105,106] In contrast, conventional NSAIDs bind reversibly at the active site of the enzyme, depressing thromboxane A_2 production for only part of the dosing interval[107] except in unusual cases. Case-controlled analyses confirm that the incomplete and reversible inhibition of cyclooxygenase by NSAIDs is unlikely to produce clinically detectable CV protection comparable to that achieved by low-dose ASA.[108–110]

Data from the VIGOR trial also were the first to suggest unusual CV risk among patients receiving rofecoxib. In this study, patients with rheumatoid arthritis (RA) received a mean of 9 months of rofecoxib 50 mg/day, a dose two to four times higher than that usually recommended for long-term treatment of arthritis.[95] Patients enrolled in the VIGOR trial were not permitted to take ASA and other NSAIDs after randomization. Although the overall mortality rate and rate of death from CV causes was similar in the rofecoxib and naproxen arms, the rate of nonfatal MI was significantly lower in the naproxen-treated group (0.1%) than in the rofecoxib group (0.5%). This difference was largely due to a high rate of MI among patients at high risk for coronary events. Among patients who did not have an indication for secondary prophylaxis with ASA , the rates of MI were similar in the two treatment groups.[95] Some have attributed this difference in risk to a cardioprotective effect associated with naproxen; however, this interpretation has been controversial.[111,112] In interpreting results of VIGOR, it is important to remember that this randomized controlled trial was designed to assess GI effects. CV events were not prespecified as outcomes and, therefore, were collected only from spontaneous reports of investigators, without any standardized definitions, and without prospective balancing of treatment arms for cardiovascular risk.

However, a meta-analysis of 18 randomized, controlled trials and 11 observational studies of rofecoxib support the CV results of VIGOR. Overall, patients who received rofecoxib in these studies were at a 2.3-fold increased risk of myocardial infarction compared with those receiving placebo or other NSAIDs.[113] Importantly, the meta-analysis result was largely driven by the VIGOR data and, like VIGOR, none of the other trials included in the meta-analysis had prespecified documentation or definition of CV events.

The results of VIGOR gain more credence because similar results were reported in the Adenomatous Polyp Prevention on Vioxx (APPROVe) trial, a study of patients with a history of colorectal adenomas in which CV events were prospectively defined and collected.[114] The 2586 study subjects were randomly assigned to therapy with rofecoxib 25 mg/day or placebo. Among patients assigned to rofecoxib, 46 patients had a confirmed CV event (acute MI, stroke, or sudden death) during 3059 patient-years of follow-up, compared with 26 patients in the placebo group during 3327 patient-years of follow-up, a 1.92-fold increase in risk of CV events associated with rofecoxib. A divergence in risk of serious CV events was observed after 18 months of therapy, primarily reflecting a greater number of MIs and strokes in the rofecoxib group.[114]

An increase in CV events has also been observed in patients who received valdecoxib and its intravenous prodrug, parecoxib, as treatment for postoperative pain following coronary-artery bypass grafting.[115] After an initial, small study (CABG-1) suggesting increased CV risk with sequential therapy consisting of intravenous parecoxib followed by oral valdecoxib, a second study (CABG-2) was undertaken in 1671 patients randomized to either (a) intravenous parecoxib for at least 3 days, followed by oral valdecoxib through day 10, (b) intravenous placebo followed by oral valdecoxib, or (c) placebo alone for 10 days. Compared with the group receiving placebo, in groups that received parecoxib and valdecoxib or placebo and valdecoxib, a higher proportion of patients suffered at least one confirmed adverse event (4.0% in the placebo group vs. 7.4% in the parecoxib plus valdecoxib and valdecoxib alone groups). Cardiovascular adverse events (e.g., MI, cardiac arrest, stroke, and pulmonary embolism) were significantly more frequent in the group that received parecoxib plus valdecoxib than in those who received placebo (2.0% vs. 0.5%; $P = 0.03$). These data indicate that even short-term COX-2 inhibition, with the drugs and doses employed in this study, is associated with an increase in CV events in some subsets of patients with coronary artery disease.

In contrast to the results observed in the VIGOR and APPROVe trials, no between-group differences were detected in the incidence of CV events among patients enrolled in the CLASS trial, another GI outcome trial that was analyzed post hoc for CV risk regardless of ASA use.[96] Similarly, in a meta-analysis of multiple trials involving more than 31,000 patients with arthritis, there was no significant difference in MI frequency in patients taking celecoxib compared with those receiving placebo, any nonselective NSAID, or, specifically, naproxen, regardless of concomitant ASA use. Celecoxib use was associated with a trend toward a lower risk of MI in all patients (RR = 0.85; 95% CI, 0.23, 3.15) and in those not receiving ASA (RR = 0.60; 95% CI, 0.11, 3.29) compared with placebo.[102] However, like VIGOR and the rofecoxib meta-analysis, CLASS and the celecoxib studies included in the meta-analysis did not prospectively define CV events or their documentation; moreover, like the rofecoxib studies (other than VIGOR and, later, APPROVe), the randomized controlled celecoxib studies were of relatively short duration.

Based on the experience with VIGOR and APPROVe, CV event documentation and adjudication were prospectively mandated prior to trial completion in the several randomized trials of celecoxib for prevention of colonic adenomas and for retardation of progression of Alzheimer's disease. In one of these trials (Adenoma Prevention with Celecoxib [APC]), CV events segregated significantly with celecoxib among 2035 patients with a history of colorectal neoplasia.[116] In this study, patients were randomly assigned to 200 mg or 400 mg celecoxib twice daily or to placebo. During a follow-up period of 2.8 to 3.1 years, the composite endpoint of death from CV causes, myocardial infarction, stroke, or heart failure was reached in 7 of 679 patients in the placebo group (1.0%), 16 of 685 patients in the celecoxib 200 mg twice daily group (2.3% [95% CI, 0.9 to 5.5]), and 23 of 671 patients in the celecoxib 400 mg twice daily group (3.4%, [statistically 95% CI, 1.4 to 7.8]). Approximately half of the events in the celecoxib groups comprised MI.[116] These findings led the trial's data and safety monitoring board to recommend study discontinuation prior to its planned completion.

The results of the other randomized trials have not yet been published, fully adjudicated, or presented in public in their entirety, but a recent presentation to the FDA indicated that, in one of them, the Prevention of Spontaneous Adenomatous Polyps (PreSAP) trial, no difference was seen in the frequency of CV events among patients receiving placebo and those receiving celecoxib (total dose 400 mg per day). In the Alzheimer's Disease Anti-Inflammatory Prevention Trial (ADAPT), stopped prematurely because of the cessation of APC, there also was no evidence that either naproxen 220 mg twice daily or celecoxib (200 mg bid) was associated with an increased risk of CV events.[117]

An additional source of useful data on CV risk is available from large epidemiologic studies that have been enabled in recent years by massive medical insurance databases on drug prescriptions and discharge diagnoses following hospitalizations. These epidemiologic studies suffer from lack of randomization and the resulting potential for unintentional channeling biases, lack of rigorous documentation of drug actually taken and of nonprescription drugs administered concomitantly, and from dependence on diagnoses defined to meet coding requirements for insurance payments, without supporting documentation or detailed event descriptions. However, they have an advantage over randomized clinical trials in that, unlike randomized trials that typically exclude 90% of the population at risk so as to avoid influences that might confound unambiguous data interpretation, the large databases include a highly representative proportion of the populations of interest. As a result, estimates of absolute event risk drawn from these database studies are likely to reflect more realistically the expectations for the population at large than do event rates drawn from randomized clinical trials.

Several epidemiologic studies indicate that the CV risk associated with COX-2 inhibitors generally is similar to that in patients receiving conventional nonselective NSAIDs and that small but potentially important within-group and between-group variability in CV risk may exist. For example, among high-risk patients receiving non-naproxen NSAIDs, Shaya and colleagues collected medical and prescription claims data on 1005 patients using COX-2 inhibitors and 5245 patients using nonselective NSAIDs. Overall, the odds of experiencing a CV event among patients who were using COX-2 inhibitors was 1.09 compared with patients using non-naproxen NSAIDs.[118]

Another retrospective cohort study using a large state Medicaid database illustrates the differences in risk that may be associated with usage of individual NSAIDs and COX-2 inhibitors. In this study, the risk of acute MI and fatal coronary heart disease (CHD) was compared in patients receiving rofecoxib, celecoxib, ibuprofen, and naproxen. Patients between 50 and 84 years of age who did not have life-threatening noncardiovascular illnesses were eligible for inclusion in the analysis. Of the new drug users in the study, patients who received more than 25 mg/day of rofecoxib exhibited a significantly higher incidence of serious CV events compared with those receiving other NSAID treatments, including low-dose rofecoxib (≤25 mg/day) ($P = 0.024$). Compared with celecoxib, the high-dose (>25 mg/day) rofecoxib group exhibited 2.2 times the rate of serious CHD events ($P = 0.014$).[119]

Among the largest epidemiologic studies was a nested case-controlled analysis of information from the Kaiser-Permanente database.[120] This study, involving data from more than 1.3 million patients and 2.3 person-years of follow-up, found that rofecoxib at doses greater than 25 mg/day was associated with a threefold higher incidence of MI and/or cardiac deaths than were recorded among nonusers or remote users of anti-inflammatory drugs. Rofecoxib at ≤25mg/day also was associated with significantly more events than among remote drug users, with an absolute rate comparable to those of several conventional NSAIDs. Interestingly, in this study, celecoxib nominally was associated with a lower event rate than that seen in remote drug users (not a statistically significant finding, though the celecoxib event rate was significantly lower than that associated with naproxen, among other conventional NSAIDs).

Increased Cardiovascular Risk in Patients Receiving NSAIDs and COX-2 Inhibitors: Some Plausible Pathophysiologic Bases

All NSAIDs, conventional and COX-2 selective, have the capacity to increase sodium and water retention and, thereby, to increase blood pressure and to cause or potentiate congestive heart failure. Blood pressure exerts an important influence on CV event rate; hypertension is a primary risk factor for CV events. Epidemiologic data indicate that an average blood pressure increase of even 2 mm Hg to 3 mm Hg, achievable with some NSAIDs and COX-2 inhibitors, can have a measurable impact on CV risk.

Admission rates for heart failure in elderly patients are substantially higher among those who receive rofecoxib or nonselective NSAIDs; however, celecoxib has not been associated with an increase in risk of admission for heart failure. Heart failure risk also may be related to NSAID-associated increases in blood pressure. An early meta-analysis found that when data from all nonselective NSAIDs (including ASA) were pooled, supine mean blood pressure was increased by 5.0 mm Hg compared with non-use.[121]

The Celecoxib Rofecoxib Efficacy and Safety in Comorbidities Evaluation Trial (CRESCENT) investigators reported that patients with hypertension, OA, and type 2 diabetes treated with rofecoxib 25 mg/day but not celecoxib 200 mg/day or naproxen 500 mg/bid had a significant increase in 24-hour systolic BP (130.3 mm Hg to 134.5 mm Hg, $P < 0.001$) after 6 weeks of therapy,[122] suggesting a possible basis for differing rates of CV adverse events associated with these agents.

A more recent meta-analysis of COX-2 inhibitors found that, overall, these agents were associated with a higher relative risk of hypertension than placebo. In comparison with celecoxib, rofecoxib was associated with a 50% greater risk of developing clinically important systolic BP elevation.[123] It appears that all NSAIDs—both conventional and COX-2-selective—have the capacity to increase sodium and water retention and to cause or potentiate hypertension and heart failure, although celecoxib appears to have a lower propensity for causing blood pressure elevations than rofecoxib. These data suggest that a plausible explanation for the apparent association of NSAIDs and COX-2 inhibitors with CV risk is the effect of these drugs on blood pressure. Fortunately, this is a remediable problem, as the blood pressure effects of the drugs usually can be reversed with appropriate therapy.

Another mechanistic hypothesis has been advanced for the adverse cardiac effects of COX-2 inhibitors.[124] Data indicate that COX-2 activity, rather than COX-1, is the dominant source of prostaglandin I_2 in the human epithelium. Prostaglandin I_2 is involved in inhibiting platelet aggregation, in causing vasodilation, and in preventing the proliferation of vascular smooth muscle cells. In contrast, thromboxane A_2, which is largely produced by the COX-1 enzyme, is involved in platelet aggregation, vasoconstriction, and smooth muscle proliferation. While ASA and traditional NSAIDs suppress the activities of both COX-1 and COX-2, and therefore reduce both thromboxane A_2 and prostaglandin I_2, COX-2 inhibitors selectively suppress the production of prostaglandin I_2 without affecting thromboxane A_2 synthesis. As a result, patients in whom COX-2 is selectively suppressed might be expected to have elevated blood pressure, accelerated atherogenesis, and an exaggerated thrombotic response to plaque rupture. This attractive hypothesis does not easily account for the observation from clinical trials, discussed earlier, that ASA use does not appear to have influenced the relation of CV event rates observed between COX-2 inhibitors and comparators among patients in randomized trials. In addition, pharmacoepidemiologic studies show approximately similar event rates with the nonselective NSAIDs and with at least some doses of certain COX-2 selective inhibitors. Thus, any relation between COX-2 inhibition and cardiovascular events is likely to be more complex than can be explained solely by an imbalance between COX-1 and COX-2 inhibition.

An additional hypothesis suggests that at least some anti-inflammatory drugs may *prevent* CV events at some doses because of salutary effects on vascular endothelium or on the inflammatory components of atherosclerosis. One study, conducted by Chenevard and colleagues, found that COX-2 inhibition improved endothelium-dependent vasodilation and reduced low-grade chronic inflammation and oxidative stress in patients with severe coronary artery disease.[125] Indeed, this may be particularly important in systemic inflammatory conditions, such as adult RA, that appear to enhance risk of CV events, presumably by potentiating vascular inflammation.

"CLASS" EFFECTS OF NSAIDs AND COX-2 INHIBITORS

Taken together, data from clinical trials and epidemiologic studies suggest that NSAIDs as a group may potentiate CV risk at some doses whether or not they are selective for COX-2. The data also suggest some interdrug variability in these effects, and a potentially important relation of CV effects and dose with at least some of these drugs. The problem seems most apparent when rofecoxib is employed at doses ≥25 mg/day, but conventional NSAIDs at some commonly used doses may be associated with similar problems. Among the COX-2 agents tested thus far at their labeled doses, CV and GI safety profiles generally have been similar, though studies suggest that celecoxib may have a slightly better safety profile compared with other COX-2 inhibitors or NSAIDs. A possible basis for this is suggested by the study of Whelton and colleagues, in which 810 elderly patients with OA and hypertension were randomly assigned to therapy with once-daily celecoxib 200 mg or to rofecoxib 25 mg.[126] Nearly twice as many patients who received rofecoxib experienced edema compared with those who received celecoxib. Moreover, systolic blood pressure increased significantly in 17% of patients who received rofecoxib, compared with 11% of patients who received celecoxib. Mean blood pressure after 6 weeks of therapy was increased 2.6 mm Hg in patients who received rofecoxib; in contrast, blood pressure was reduced 0.5 mm Hg in the celecoxib group.

Approach to the Patient at Risk for NSAID-Induced Gastrointestinal Tract Adverse Events

The approach to the patient with OA at risk for an NSAID-induced gastrointestinal tract event remains controversial. Many patients with dyspepsia or upper gastrointestinal distress have superficial erosions evident on endoscopy that frequently heal spontaneously without change in therapy. Even more difficult to evaluate is whether cytoprotective agents actually alter NSAID-associated symptoms that may or may not predict significant gastrointestinal tract events. Although one clinical study demonstrated that more than 80% of patients who developed significant NSAID-induced endoscopic abnormalities were asymptomatic,[87,88] several prospective observational trials indicated that patients were more symptomatic with NSAID-induced toxicities than was previously thought.[87]

The patient who develops a gastric or duodenal ulcer while taking NSAIDs should have treatment discontinued and therapy instituted for ulcer disease, either histamine H_2 receptor antagonists or proton pump inhibitors (PPIs).[57-60] If NSAIDs must be continued concomitantly, the patient will be required to receive antiulcer therapy for longer periods. Most patients with uncomplicated gastric or duodenal ulcers will typically heal within 8 weeks of initiating PPIs. If NSAID treatment is continued, perhaps 16 weeks of therapy may be necessary for adequate healing. Diagnostic tests to determine whether *Helicobacter pylori* is present should be performed, and if the patient has measurable antibodies, specific antibiotic therapy to eradicate the infection should be administered.[58]

Prophylaxis to prevent NSAID-induced gastric or duodenal ulcers is more complicated. To date, there has been no evidence that agents other than misoprostol will prevent NSAID-induced gastric ulceration and its complications.[89,90,127] Although H_2 antagonists or proton pump inhibitors have been demonstrated to prevent NSAID-induced duodenal ulcers, prevention of gastric ulcerations and their complications has not been clearly shown.[128,129] Endoscopy trials have shown that famotidine at twice the approved dose (40 mg twice daily) significantly decreased the incidence of both gastric and duodenal ulcers.[130] Similarly, an endoscopy trial demonstrated that treatment with omeprazole (a proton pump inhibitor) decreased gastroduodenal ulcers.[129] Preliminary evidence suggests that the COX-2 inhibitors will also decrease bleeding complications.[131]

Misoprostol is a prostaglandin analogue believed to locally replace prostaglandins whose synthesis in the gastroduodenal mucosa is inhibited by NSAIDs.[89,90] A large prospective trial evaluated 8843 patients with rheumatoid arthritis to determine whether misoprostol would decrease the incidence of ulcers and their complications. Patients were prescribed various NSAIDs and were observed for 6 months receiving either misoprostol cotherapy or placebo. The study was powered on the basis of endoscopic observations of an 80% decrease with concomitant misoprostol therapy in endoscopically proven ulcers more than 0.3 to 0.5 cm in diameter in the gastric and duodenal mucosa.[127] Misoprostol successfully inhibited development of ulcer complications such as bleeding, perforation, and obstruction. There was a 40% reduction in patients treated with misoprostol as opposed to those receiving placebo.[89] Further analysis demonstrated that patients with Health Assessment Questionnaire scores above 1.5 (thus worse disease) had an 87% reduction in risk for an NSAID-induced toxic event if they were concomitantly treated with misoprostol.[90]

These data suggest that high-risk patients may benefit from concomitant misoprostol therapy if NSAID treatment is indicated. Gabriel and colleagues[132] have demonstrated the pharmacoeconomic utility of such therapy in the high-risk patient. Unfortunately, the major adverse event causing withdrawal in approximately 10% of patients was diarrhea, and 30% of patients complained of diarrhea. Therefore, medications such as stool softeners and cathartics should be stopped. There are data suggesting that concomitant treatment with misoprostol once an ulcer develops will allow healing. These data are preliminary, at best.[129]

Renal Adverse Effects. The effects of NSAIDs on renal function include retention of sodium, changes in tubular function, interstitial nephritis, and reversible renal failure due to alterations in filtration rate and renal plasma flow.[133] Prostaglandins and prostacyclins are important for maintenance of intrarenal blood flow and tubular transport. All NSAIDs except nonacetylated salicylates have the potential to induce reversible impairment of glomerular filtration rate. This effect occurs more frequently in patients with congestive heart failure; in established renal disease with altered intrarenal plasma flow, including diabetes, hypertension, and atherosclerosis; and with induced hypovolemia—salt depletion or significant hypoalbuminemia.[133,134] Triamterene-containing diuretics, which increase plasma renin levels, may predispose patients receiving NSAIDs to precipitously develop acute renal failure. NSAIDs have been implicated in the development of acute and chronic renal insufficiency as a result of inhibition of vasodilating prostaglandins, thereby reducing renal blood flow.[133,135]

NSAID-associated interstitial nephritis is typically manifested as nephrotic syndrome, characterized by edema or anasarca, proteinuria, hematuria, and pyuria.[133,136] The usual stigmata of drug-induced allergic nephritis, such as eosinophilia, eosinophiluria, and fever, are not typically present. Interstitial infiltrates of mononuclear cells are seen histologically with relative sparing of the glomeruli. Phenylpropionic acid derivatives such as fenoprofen, and tolmetin along with the indoleacetic acid derivative indomethacin are most commonly associated with the development of interstitial nephritis. Of interest, indomethacin has been suggested as a treatment to decrease proteinuria in patients with nephrotic syndrome from other causes.[137-140]

Inhibition of prostaglandin synthesis intrarenally by NSAIDs decreases renin release and thus produces a state of hyporeninemic hypoaldosteronism with resulting hyperkalemia.[133] This effect may be amplified physiologically in patients taking potassium-sparing diuretics. Salt retention precipitated by some NSAIDs, which may lead to peripheral edema, is probably due to inhibition of intrarenal prostaglandin production, which decreases renal medullary blood flow and increases tubular reabsorption of sodium chloride, as well as to direct tubular effects. NSAIDs have also been reported to increase antidiuretic hormone effect, thereby reducing excretion of free water, resulting in hyponatremia.[133] Thiazide diuretics may produce an added effect on the NSAID-induced hyponatremia. All NSAIDs have been demonstrated to interfere with medical management of hypertension and heart failure.

All NSAIDs with the exception of the nonacetylated salicylates have been associated with increases in mean blood pressure.[141-143] Patients receiving antihypertensive agents including β-blockers, angiotensin-converting enzyme inhibitors, and thiazide and loop diuretics must be checked regularly when therapy is initiated with a new NSAID to ensure that there are no significant continued and sustained rises in blood pressure.

The mechanism of acute renal failure induced in the "at-risk" patient treated with NSAIDs is believed to be prostaglandin mediated.[133] However, the role of COX-2 in maintenance of renal homeostasis in the human remains unclear. COX-2 activity is notably present in the macula densa and tubules in animals and humans, and it is upregulated in salt-depleted animals.[49,144] In humans, COX-1 is an important enzyme for control of intrarenal blood flow. Unfortunately, at this time there is not sufficient evidence to indicate whether the new COX-2–specific inhibitors will be safer than traditional NSAIDs in terms of renal function. Until the appropriate clinical trials are done, any patient at high risk for renal complications should be monitored carefully. No patient with a creatinine clearance of less than 30 mL/min should be treated with either an NSAID or a COX-2–specific inhibitor.

Hepatic Effects. NSAID-induced elevation in hepatic transaminase levels is not uncommon, although it occurs more often in patients with juvenile rheumatoid arthritis or systemic lupus erythematosus. Although there are many reports indicating that elevated serum transaminases are common in patients taking NSAIDs, unless elevations exceed two or three times the upper limit of normal or serum albumin, or prothrombin times are altered, these effects are not usually considered clinically significant.[145,146] Nonetheless, overt liver failure has been reported after use of many NSAIDs, including diclofenac, flurbiprofen, and sulindac.[147] Of all NSAIDs, sulindac has been associated with the highest incidence of cholestasis in certain countries.[145] Therefore it is recommended that patients at risk for liver toxicity be observed carefully. When NSAID treatment is initiated, all patients should be evaluated again within 8 to 12 weeks and serious consideration given to performance of blood analysis for serum transaminase changes.

Idiosyncratic Adverse Effects. Many of the untoward effects of NSAIDs are related to their mechanism of action through prostaglandin inhibition, but they also have important idiosyncratic effects. A typical nonspecific reaction that includes rash and photosensitivity is associated with all currently available NSAIDs and particularly the phenylpropionic acid derivatives.[13] The phenylpropionic acid derivatives may also induce aseptic meningitis, especially in patients with systemic lupus erythematosus.[30] The underlying mechanism of action remains unknown. This class of NSAIDs has been associated with a reversible toxic amblyopia.[13]

Owing to the antiplatelet effects of all NSAIDs except the nonacetylated salicylates, concomitant therapy with warfarin (Coumadin) puts patients at great risk for bleeding. Because concomitant NSAID therapy would displace warfarin from its albumin binding sites, the prothrombin time may be prolonged; in addition, given the increased relative risk for NSAID-induced gastroduodenal ulcers and bleeding, there is an increased risk for bleeding when the NSAIDs are used concomitantly with warfarin. In that the COX-2–specific inhibitors do not cause ulcers of the gastrointestinal tract or alter platelet function, the patient taking warfarin would have less risk for a significant gastrointestinal bleed with these drugs than with traditional NSAIDs. Effects such as these may also be seen with phenytoin (Dilantin) or other

highly protein-bound drugs such as antibiotics. The NSAIDs inhibit the renal excretion of lithium and should be used with caution in patients taking this drug. Cholestyramine, an anion exchange resin, reduces the rate of NSAID absorption and its bioavailability.

The central nervous system side effects of NSAIDs include aseptic meningitis, psychosis, and cognitive dysfunction.[29,30,73,74] These changes are more commonly seen in elderly patients treated with indomethacin, whereas the phenylpropionic acid derivatives are more commonly associated with the development of aseptic meningitis and toxic amblyopia. Tinnitus is a common problem with higher doses of salicylates as well as with the nonsalicylate NSAIDs. The mechanism is unknown. Interestingly, the young and the elderly may not complain of tinnitus but only of hearing loss. Other NSAIDs may also induce tinnitus in specific patients. Decreasing the dose usually alleviates the effect. In all circumstances, tinnitus is reversible with discontinuation of medication.

There is ample evidence that traditional use of NSAIDs does not lead to osteoporosis.[148–150] It is clear that COX-2 is upregulated in the osteoblasts near the periosteum in association with stretching and with the effects of gravity.[148,149] The role of COX-1 remains unclear. Although inflammation in the joint leads to juxta-articular osteopenia, this is the result of increased prostaglandin synthesis in the inflamed joint, which is likely to be directly related to increased COX-2 activity.

Some of the early available NSAIDs have been associated with an increased risk for bone marrow failure. This is particularly true of phenylbutazone and indomethacin. Strom and associates[151] have described the incidence of neutropenia as a toxic effect of the NSAIDs. In a case-controlled study performed with use of Medicaid claims data, these investigators determined that the adjusted odds ratio for neutropenia in patients treated with NSAIDs is 4.2 (CI, 2.0 to 8.7). When patients treated with either phenylbutazone or indomethacin were excluded, the odds ratio for the development of neutropenia remained robust at 3.5 (CI, 1.6 to 7.6). In general, given the common use of NSAIDs, the risk for neutropenia is small.

It has been shown that COX-2 is important for ovulation through the peroxisome proliferator-activated receptor-γ.[49] In addition, COX-2 is upregulated with implantation of a fertilized ovum or in decidualization. Although there are a few case reports of reversible infertility associated with the use of NSAIDs, given the large numbers of patients who regularly use NSAIDs, there does not appear to be a generalized epidemic of infertility. There are few data documenting the effects of the NSAIDs on pregnancy or the fetus.[152] In animal models, the NSAIDs have been shown to increase the incidence of dystocia, postimplantation loss, and delay of parturition.[152] The effect of prostaglandin inhibition may result in premature closure of the ductus arteriosus. ASA has been associated with smaller babies and neonatal bruising; however, it has been used for many years in the treatment of patients who require NSAIDs while they are pregnant. Therapy with ASA is typically stopped about 8 weeks before delivery to decrease the risk of interference with ductus closure. In animals, there is no evidence that ASA is a teratogen. The NSAIDs are excreted in breast milk. It is believed that salicylates in normally recommended doses are not dangerous to nursing infants. Although it is possible to use ASA in pregnancy, the decision to use any drug during pregnancy should be made after careful consideration of the potential consequences, and the drug should be deemed essential for appropriate management. Most of the data demonstrating safety of ASA were obtained either in animal models or after empirical observation. For obvious reasons, randomized clinical trials have not been performed.

Bone and Cartilage Effects

Although NSAIDs are known to decrease pain and inflammation and to be antipyretic, they have not been shown to decrease erosions in rheumatoid arthritis, to retard osteophyte formation in OA, or to protect cartilage from mechanical or inflammatory injury. Interestingly, however, pretreatment with NSAIDs has repeatedly been demonstrated to decrease heterotopic bone formation after joint replacement.[153] Specific NSAIDs have been shown in vitro to inhibit chondrocyte proteoglycan synthesis.[154] A few case reports suggest that the chronic use of some NSAIDs accelerated cartilage damage in OA, and some investigators believe the data to be compelling enough to preclude the use of NSAIDs in standard therapy for OA.[155] Although this effect may have profound implications clinically, the evidence is inferential that chronic use of NSAIDs clearly damages cartilage in humans or worsens the clinical course of OA. There is ample evidence to support the popular use of NSAIDs and now the safer COX-2–specific inhibitors in the treatment of OA.[156-159]

TRAMADOL

If the patient continues to complain of pain despite acetaminophen, NSAIDs, COX-2–selective therapy at full doses, or if little or no inflammation is evident, or if the benefit to risk ratio is unwarranted, tramadol should be considered. It is possible that tramadol may become a more important drug for OA with the conflicting information about the overall benefit to risk of the NSAIDs, and this may be particularly true if improved formulations are developed. This is neither an NSAID nor a classic opiate. Although it binds to the μ opioid receptor, it is also a serotonin and norepinephrine uptake inhibitor, and it is probably this combination that affords pain relief.[160-163] An effective analgesic, it is not antipyretic. Schnitzer and colleagues[164] and others have demonstrated that the drug can spare the use of traditional NSAIDs in that combination therapy with naproxen allowed lower doses of NSAID for control of symptoms. It has been shown to be effective in some patients with fibromyalgia.[165]

It is available as a 50-mg tablet as well as extended release formulas and in tablets with acetaminophen and can be prescribed in doses up to 400 mg/day. However, patients who suffer chronic renal insufficiency or who are older than 60 years should not receive doses higher than 250 to 300 mg/day. The drug cannot be given with monoamine oxidase inhibitors.[162]

Although tramadol is reasonably safe, there are, unfortunately, significant adverse events associated with its use. In particular, some effects, such as nausea and vomiting as well as some dysphoric reactions, appear to be directly related to the initial starting dose.[162] Clinical studies have demonstrated that slow titration decreases the incidence of these effects,[166,167] and it is suggested to start at a dose of 50 mg once per day and slowly increase to a split dose of three or four times a day in the elderly. For some patients who derive benefit, it may be necessary to initiate therapy with only 25 mg (half a tablet).

An uncommon but unacceptable adverse effect that may be dose related is seizure.[168,169] The incidence of seizures appears to be increased in those in whom high doses are rapidly titrated and in patients with systemic lupus erythematosus. Therefore, again, a slow increase in the dose is recommended over several weeks. Addiction has been reported, and most often occurs in those with prior addiction.

OPIOID ANALGESICS

The treatment of pain is important, and there are some patients who will not achieve relief with the interventions already considered. Although various opioid drugs have frequently been used for short periods in patients with severe pain associated with significant flares of OA who obtain minimal relief with simple analgesics or NSAIDs, their chronic use has generally been avoided. More recently, there has been increased acceptance of the benefits of this therapy in selected types of patients. Some patients who might benefit from opioid analgesics are those with advanced symptomatic OA suffering unrelenting pain, and in particular night pain, who are not candidates for surgery. In addition, there are those patients with comorbid conditions that might preclude the use of other therapies.[170,171] Judicious use of these potent analgesics will provide flexibility for the patients who suffer severe disease.

INTRA-ARTICULAR THERAPY

Viscosupplementation or Hyaluronic Acid Replacement Therapy

Since it has been demonstrated that hyaluronic acid is abnormal in the synovial fluid of patients with OA, it has been believed that replacement with either synthetic or biologically derived hyaluronic acid would be benefical.[172] To date, hyaluronic acid (hyaluronan) therapy has been shown to modulate pain in OA of the knee with variable evidence of potential disease-modifying effects on articular cartilage.[173-183] Further detailed discussion of the use of this form of intra-articular therapy is presented in Chapter 16.

INTRA-ARTICULAR GLUCOCORTICOIDS

For those patients with prominent inflammation in one or two joints, an intra-articular glucocorticoid injection may be helpful.[184-187] The typical glucocorticoid used for injection is a crystalline form, allowing prolonged residence in the joint.

Injections should generally not be repeated more than four times per year in any one joint.[188,189] A detailed discussion of this therapeutic modality, including the indications, techniques for injection, risks, and anticipated outcomes, is found in Chapter 16.

DISEASE-MODIFYING OSTEOARTHRITIS DRUGS

Unfortunately, no drug as yet has been reproducibly shown to alter the natural history of this disease. There are reports of patients with atypical forms of OA, such as inflammatory erosive OA, who respond to drugs such as hydroxychloroquine.[190–192] This drug used for rheumatoid arthritis alters cell processes related to inflammation; thus, in such a subset of patients with a disease not dissimilar to rheumatoid arthritis, it might be an effective therapy.[190] Its use in OA is not FDA approved, and its administration for this purpose remains investigational.

Although there has been significant interest in the use of metalloproteinase inhibitors to alter the disease, there are as yet few data in humans that have demonstrated an important effect.

NUTRACEUTICALS AND OTHER INVESTIGATIONAL AGENTS

Although the nutraceuticals glucosamine and chondroitin sulfate continue to be controversial, evidence is accumulating to suggest that, individually or in combination, they yield significant improvement in pain compared with placebo.[188,193–202] Furthermore, there has been evidence of a potential structure-modifying effect in humans with 3 years of treatment with glucosamine sulfate. Reginster and colleagues[189] reported benefit with decreased pain and improved structural outcome as measured by radiography. These data, although preliminary, suggest that long-term use of such a nutraceutical may not only decrease pain but may also affect the natural history of the disease. However, routine standing weight-bearing radiographs of the knee were the applied radiologic techniques in this clinical trial, rather than the semiflexed weight-bearing position; accordingly, radiographic benefit ascribed to active therapy may have been due to increased knee extension after pain relief rather than to true preservation of cartilage structure. In a different approach, McAlindon and coworkers[203] demonstrated in a case-controlled study that patients who consumed antioxidants regularly and at high dose (particularly vitamin C) suffered a less progressive course of OA. There was a suggestion of less damage as measured by radiography as well. Further details about these and other investigational agents, including those targeted to modify disease activity, such as the metalloproteinase inhibitors, are discussed in Chapter 17.

SUMMARY AND GUIDELINES

The treatment of the patient with OA is easy but complex. In a heterogeneous disease with such an unpredictable course, it is important to first remember to do no harm.

Second, it is difficult to apply a hierarchical treatment algorithm to a heterogeneous disease population, much less the individual who is suffering. Therefore, this section outlines a suggested treatment approach that should be tailored to the needs of the patient, taking into consideration the benefit/risk ratio of the therapy and what is currently known about the potential for positive outcomes. The risk of such an approach in a textbook is that it will be rapidly out of date. However, this is unlikely if the suggestions remain based on evidence and the approach is flexible.

One of the first important considerations is whether the patient is suffering pain alone or whether the pain is associated with inflammation. In the past, it had been assumed that a significant number of patients suffer only pain without clinically significant inflammation and thus might benefit from analgesia alone without concomitant anti-inflammatory therapies. This belief combined with the concerns about the risk/benefit ratio of the known NSAIDs initially led to guidelines such as the 1995 American College of Rheumatology guidelines for the treatment of OA of the hip or knee.[21,22] These guidelines suggest that after nonpharmacologic interventions fail, the appropriate treatment is the use of simple analgesics up to a full dose (such as acetaminophen, 1000 mg four times daily) as first-line therapy. If that fails, topical agents such as capsaicin (in combination with acetaminophen or alone) should be considered for everything but OA of the hip. The next escalation considers analgesic doses of nonacetylated salicylates, low-dose nonsalicylate NSAIDs, or other forms of more substantial analgesia such as tramadol. Finally, if there are still problems, full-dose NSAIDs along with local injections of glucocorticoids or hyaluronic acid supplementation should be considered. In those patients prescribed an NSAID and who are at high risk for an NSAID-induced gastrointestinal tract adverse event, prophylactic therapy with misoprostol, or a proton pump inhibitor, should be added to the NSAID regimen.

Although this remains a useful algorithm, there is increasing evidence to warrant the use of anti-inflammatory therapies earlier in the treatment plan.[204] Unfortunately, data are also accumulating that acetaminophen is not as safe as was previously assumed. In addition, clinical data such as those from Pincus and coworkers[5,6] demonstrate that NSAIDs provide more benefit than simple analgesics alone, an opinion shared by a large contingent of practicing rheumatologists.

With the favorable GI benefit/risk ratio afforded by the COX-2–selective inhibitors over the traditional NSAIDs, these "GI" safer anti-inflammatory and analgesic agents may appropriately be considered reasonable first-line prescription therapeutics, particularly in patients with moderate to severe pain with or without inflammatory findings such as joint tenderness and synovial effusion. However, these benefits must be weighed against the rare risk of CV complication.[22a] Patients when treated with an NSAID must be observed for the emergence of important salt and water balance issues, including even small changes in both systolic or diastolic blood pressure or evidence of edema, and if noted, treated appropriately. In patients who achieve an inadequate response or who are intolerant of the COX-2–selective inhibitors, traditional NSAIDs should be considered modified by the same caveats. If traditional NSAIDs are to be used, the clinician should ensure that appropriate prophylactic therapy is considered in those patients who are at risk for an NSAID-induced gastrointestinal tract event. Because almost all patients with OA are older than 60 years, most possess at least one of these important risk factors.

However, with the presently available information that the COX-2 selective inhibitors possess the same increased CV risk as do the nonselective NSAIDs (or at least drugs like ibuprofen and diclofenac), the at-risk GI patient might be best served by treatment with a nonselective NSAID and low-dose ASA if they are at increased CV risk with aggressive control of any incipient blood pressure elevation or peripheral edema and the concomitant use of a PPI.

At any time, the patient may benefit from a glucocorticoid injection into an inflamed joint. Repetitive injections should be limited. Hyaluronic acid injections are an alternative for patients when available nonpharmacologic interventions and full doses of simple analgesics fail. Their safety profile makes them advantageous for consideration in patients with NSAID intolerance or in patients with a relative contraindication to NSAID therapy.

The use of nutraceuticals is attractive to patients because they are able to try these without visiting a physician or accessing their health plan. Unfortunately, as physicians, we do not yet have enough information to categorically recommend any of these products. However, we do not discourage patients from trying them, as long as their safety record remains as substantial as it has been to date.

Most patients will be helped with nonpharmacologic and currently available pharmacologic therapies. Those who are not helped may require referral to an orthopedic surgeon for consideration of surgical approaches, such as arthroscopic surgery or joint replacement.

It is likely that the idea of single-drug interventions will rapidly disappear in the treatment paradigm of patients with OA as it has in the treatment of patients with rheumatoid arthritis. It is hoped that soon we will have therapies that will alter the natural history of the process to complement our current abilities to alleviate pain and improve function.

REFERENCES

1. Bradley JA, Brandt KD, Katz BP, et al. Treatment of knee osteoarthritis: relationship of clinical features of joint inflammation to the response to a nonsteroidal antiinflammatory drug or pure analgesic. J Rheumatol 19:1950–1954, 1992.
2. Bradley J, Brandt K, Katz B, et al. Comparison of an antiinflammatory dose of ibuprofen, an analgesic dose of ibuprofen, and acetaminophen in the treatment of patients with osteoarthritis of the knee. N Engl J Med 325:87–91, 1991.
3. Brandt KD. Toward pharmacologic modification of joint damage in osteoarthritis. Ann Intern Med 122:874–875, 1995.
4. Pincus T, Koch GG, Sokka T, et al. A randomized, double-blind, crossover clinical trial of diclofenac plus misoprostol versus acetaminophen in patients with osteoarthritis of the hip or knee.Arthritis Rheum 44(7):1587–1598, 2001.
5. Pincus T, Koch G, Lei H, et al. Patient preference for Placebo, Acetaminophen (paracetamol) or Celecoxib Efficacy Studies (PACES): two randomised, double blind, placebo controlled, crossover clinical trials in patients with knee or hip osteoarthritis. Ann Rheum Dis 63(8):931–939, 2004. Epub Apr 13, 2004.
6. Bellamy, N, Buchanan WW, Goldsmith CH, et al. Validation study of WOMAC: a health status instrument for measuring clinically important patient relevant outcomes to antirheumatic drug therapy in patients with osteoarthritis of the hip or knee. J Rheumatol 15:1833–1840, 1988.
7. Pincus T, Swearingen C, Wolfe F. Toward a Multidimensional Health Assessment Questionnaire (MDHAQ): assessment of advanced activities of daily living and psychological status in the patient-friendly health assessment questionnaire format. Arthritis Rheum 42:2220–2230, 1999.
8. Watson MC, Brookes ST, Kirwan JR, et al. Osteoarthritis: the comparative efficacy of non-ASA non-steroidal anti-inflammatory drugs for the management of osteoarthritis of the knee (Cochrane Review). In: The Cochrane Library. Oxford, Update Software, 1998, p 3.
9. Williams HJ, Ward JR, Eggar MJ, et al. Comparison of naproxen and acetaminophen in a two year study of treatment of osteoarthritis of the knee. Arthritis Rheum 36:1196–1206, 1993.
10. Towheed TE, Hochberg MC. A systematic review of randomized controlled trials of pharmacological therapy in osteoarthritis of the knee. Semin Arthritis Rheum 27:755–770, 1997.
11. Towheed TE, Hochberg MC. A systematic review of randomized controlled trials of pharmacological therapy in osteoarthritis of the hip. J Rheumatol 24:349–357, 1997.
12. Cryer B, Feldman M. Cyclooxygenase-1 and cyclooxygenase-2 selectivity of widely used nonsteroidal anti-inflammatory drugs. Am J Med 104:413–421, 1998.
13. Simon LS, Mills LS. Drug therapy: nonsteroidal antiinflammatory drugs. N Engl J Med 302:1179–1185, 1237–1243, 1980.
14. Hogestat ED, Jonssan BAG, Ermund A, et al. Conversion of acetaminophen to the bioactive N-acylphenolamine AM404 via fatty acid amide hydrolase-dependent arachidonic acid conjugation in the nervous system. J Biol Chem 280:31406–31412, 2006.
15. Schiodt FV, Rochling FA, Casey DL, et al. Acetaminophen toxicity in an urban country hospital. N Engl J Med 337:1112–1117, 1997.
16. Whitcomb DC, Block GD. Association of acetaminophen hepatotoxicity with fasting and ethanol use. JAMA 274:1845–1850, 1994.
17. Perneger TV, Whelton PK, Klag MJ. Risk of kidney failure associated with the use of acetaminophen, ASA, and nonsteroidal antiinflammatory drugs. N Engl J Med 331:1675–1679, 1994.
18. Barrett BJ. Acetaminophen and adverse chronic renal outcomes: an appraisal of the epidemiologic evidence. Am J Kidney Dis 28(suppl):S14–S19, 1996.
19. Perez Gutthann S, Garcia Rodriguez LA, Raiford DS, et al. Nonsteroidal anti-inflammatory drugs and the risk of hospitalization for acute renal failure. Arch Intern Med 156:2433–2439, 1996.
20. Buckalew VM Jr. Habitual use of acetaminophen as a risk factor for chronic renal failure: a comparison with phenacetin. Am J Kidney Dis 28(suppl):S7–S13, 1996.
21. Hochberg MC, Altman RD, Brandt KD, et al. Guidelines for the medical management of osteoarthritis. I. Osteoarthritis of the hip. Arthritis Rheum 38:1535–1540, 1995.
22. Hochberg MC, Altman RD, Brandt KD, et al. Guidelines for the medical management of osteoarthritis. II. Osteoarthritis of the knee. Arthritis Rheum 38:1541–1546, 1995.
22a. American College of Rheumatology. American college of rheumatology subcommittee on osteoarthritis guidelines recommendations for the medical management of osteoarthritis of the hip and knee. Arthritis Rheum 43:1905–1915
23. Hyiek EM, Heiman H, Skates SJ, et al. Acetaminophen and other risk factors for excessive warfarin anticoagulation. JAMA 279:657–662, 1998.
24. Fitzmaurice DA, Murray JA. Potentiation of anticoagulant effect of warfarin. Postgrad Med J 73:439–440, 1997.
25. Chan AT, Manson JE, Albert CM, et al. Nonsteroidal antiinflammatory drugs, acetaminophen and the risk fo cardiovascular events. Circulation 113:1578–1587, 2006.
26. Curhan GC, Willett WC, Rosner B, Stampfer MJ Frequency of analgesic usse and risk of hypertension in younger women. Arch Int Med 162:2204–2208, 2002.

27. Schnitzer TJ. Non-NSAID pharmacologic treatment options for the management of chronic pain. Am J Med 105:45S–52S, 1998.

28. Rehman Q, Lane NE. Getting control of osteoarthritis pain. An update on treatment options. Postgrad Med 106:127–134, 1999.

29. Brooks PM, Day RO. Nonsteroidal antiinflammatory drugs: differences and similarities. N Engl J Med 324:1716–1725, 1991.

30. Furst DE. Are there differences among nonsteroidal antiinflammatory drugs? Comparing acetylated salicylates, nonacetylated salicylates, and nonacetylated nonsteroidal antiinflammatory drugs. Arthritis Rheum 37:1–9, 1994.

31. Abramson SB, Weissman G. The mechanisms of action of nonsteroidal antiinflammatory drugs. Arthritis Rheum 32:1–9, 1989.

32. Simon LS, Lanza FL, Lipsky PE, et al. Preliminary study of the safety and efficacy of SC-58635, a novel cyclooxygenase 2 inhibitor: efficacy and safety in two placebo-controlled trials in osteoarthritis and rheumatoid arthritis, and studies of gastrointestinal and platelet effects. Arthritis Rheum 41:1591–1602, 1998.

33. Simon LS, Weaver AL, Graham DY, et al. The anti-inflammatory and upper gastrointestinal effects of celecoxib in rheumatoid arthritis: a randomized, controlled trial. JAMA 282:1921–1928, 1999.

34. Laine L, Harper S, Simon T, et al. A randomized trial comparing the effect of rofecoxib, a cyclooxygenase-2 specific inhibitor, with that of ibuprofen on gastroduodenal mucosa of patients with osteoarthritis. Gastroenterology 117:776–783, 1999.

35. Hawkey CJ. COX-2 inhibitors. Lancet 353:307–314, 1999.

36. Baum C, Kennedy DL, Forbes MB. Utilization of nonsteroidal anti-inflammatory drugs. Arthritis Rheum 28:686–691, 1985.

37. Phillips AC, Simon LS. NSAIDs and the elderly: toxicity and the economic implications. Drugs Aging 10:119–130, 1997.

38. Baron JA, Cole BF, Sandler RS, et al. A randomized trial of ASA to prevent colorectal adenomas. N Engl J Med 348(10):891–899. 2003.

39. Catella-Lawson F, Reilly MP, Kapoor SC, et al. Cyclooxygenase inhibitors and the antiplatelet effects of ASA. N Engl J Med 345:1809–1817, 2001.

40. Mahmud T, Rafi SS, Scott DL, et al. Nonsteroidal antiinflammatory drugs and uncoupling of mitochondrial oxidative phosphorylation. Arthritis Rheum 39:1998–2003, 1996.

41. Abramson SB, Leszczynska-Piziak J, Clancy RM, et al. Inhibition of neutrophil function by ASA-like drugs (NSAIDs): requirement for assembly of heterotrimeric G proteins in bilayer phospholipids. Biochem Pharmacol 47:563–572, 1994.

42. Amin AR, Vyas P, Attur M, et al. The mode of action of ASA-like drugs: effect on inducible nitric oxide synthase. Proc Natl Acad Sci USA 92:7926–7930, 1995.

43. González F, González-Alvero I, Companero MR, et al. Prevention of in vitro neutrophil-endothelial attachment through shedding of L-selectin by nonsteroidal antiinflammatory drugs. J Clin Invest 95:1756–1765, 1995.

44. Dingle JT. Cartilage maintenance in osteoarthritis: interaction of cytokines, NSAIDs and prostaglandins in articular cartilage damage and repair. J Rheumatol Suppl 28:30–37, 1991.

45. Pelletier JP. The influence of tissue cross-talking on OA progression: role of nonsteroidal antiinflammatory drugs. Osteoarthritis Cartilage 7:374–376, 1999.

46. Walker JS, Sheather-Reid RB, Carmody JJ, et al. Nonsteroidal antiinflammatory drugs in rheumatoid arthritis and osteoarthritis: support for the concept of "responders" and "nonresponders." Arthritis Rheum 40:1944–1954, 1997.

47. Simon LS, Strand V. Clinical response to nonsteroidal antiinflammatory drugs. Arthritis Rheum 40:1940–1943, 1997.

48. Smith WL. Prostanoid biosynthesis and mechanisms of action. Am J Physiol 263:F181–F191, 1992.

49. Crofford LJ, Lipsky PE, Brooks P, et al. Basic biology and clinical application of cyclooxygenase-2. Arthritis Rheum 43:4–13, 2000.

50. Dubois RN, Abramson SB, Crofford L, et al. Cyclooxygenase in biology and disease. FASEB J 12:1063–1073, 1998.

51. Mitchell JA, Akarasereenont P, Thiemermann C, et al. Selectivity of nonsteroidal antiinflammatory drugs as inhibitors of constitutive and inducible cyclooxygenase. Proc Natl Acad Sci USA 90:11693–11697, 1994.

52. Patrignani P, Panara MR, Greco A, et al. Biochemical and pharmacological characterization of the cyclooxygenase activity of human blood prostaglandin endoperoxide synthases. J Pharmacol Exp Ther 271:1705–1712, 1994.

53. Meade EA, Smith WL, Dewitt DL. Differential inhibition of prostaglandin endoperoxide synthase (cyclooxygenase) isoenzymes by ASA and other non-steroidal anti-inflammatory drugs. J Biol Chem 268:6610–6614, 1993.

54. Laneuville O, Breuer DK, DeWitt DL, et al. Differential inhibition of human prostaglandin endoperoxide H synthases-1 and -2 by nonsteroidal antiinflammatory drugs. J Pharmacol Exp Ther 271:927–939, 1994.

55. Fries JP, Miller SR, Spitz PW. Toward an epidemiology of gastropathy associated with nonsteroidal antiinflammatory drug use. Gastroenterology 96:647–655, 1989.

56. Gabriel SE, Jaakkimainen L, Bombardier C. Risk for serious gastrointestinal complications related to use of nonsteroidal antiinflammatory drugs: a meta-analysis. Ann Intern Med 115: 787–796, 1991.

57. Wolfe MM, Lichtenstein DR, Singh G. Gastrointestinal toxicity of the nonsteroidal antiinflammatory drugs. N Engl J Med 340: 1888–1899, 1999.

58. Scheiman JM. NSAIDs, gastrointestinal injury and cytoprotection. Gastroenterol Clin North Am 25:279–298, 1996.

59. Laine L. Nonsteroidal antiinflammatory drug gastropathy. Gastrointest Endosc Clin North Am 6:489–504, 1996.

60. Hollander D. Gastrointestinal complications of nonsteroidal anti-inflammatory drugs: prophylactic and therapeutic strategies. Am J Med 96:274–281, 1994.

61. Charleson S, Cartwright M, Frank J, et al. Characterization of prostaglandin G/H synthase 1 and 2 in rat, dog, monkey, and human gastrointestinal tracts. Gastroenterology 111:445–454, 1996.

62. DeWitt DL, Meade EA, Smith WL. PGH synthase isoenzyme selectivity: the potential for safer nonsteroidal antiinflammatory drugs. Am J Med 95(suppl 2A):40S–44S, 1993.

63. Glaser K, Sung M-L, O'Neill K, et al. Etodolac selectively inhibits human prostaglandin G/H synthase 2 (PGHS-2) versus human PGHS-1. Eur J Pharmacol 281:107–111, 1995.

64. Lipsky PE, Abramson SB, Crofford L, et al. The classification of cyclooxygenase inhibitors [editorial]. J Rheumatol 25:2298–2303, 1998.

65. Bensen WG, Fiechtner JJ, McMillen JI, et al. Treatment of osteoarthritis with celecoxib, a cyclooxygenase-2 inhibitor: a randomized controlled trial. Mayo Clin Proc 74:1095–1105, 1999.

66. Ehrich EW, Dallob A, De Lepeleire I, et al. Characterization of rofecoxib as a cyclooxygenase-2 isoform inhibitor and demonstration of analgesia in the dental pain model. Clin Pharmacol Ther 65:336–347, 1999.

67. Friman C, Johnston C, Chew C, et al. Effect of diclofenac sodium, tolfenamic acid and indomethacin on the production of superoxide induced by N-formyl-methionyl-leucyl-phenylalanine in normal human polymorphonuclear leukocytes. Scand J Rheumatol 15:41–46, 1986.

68. Gay JC, Lukens JN, English DK. Differential inhibition of neutrophil superoxide generation by nonsteroidal antiinflammatory drugs. Inflammation 8:209–222, 1984.

69. Lu X, Xie W, Reed D. Nonsteroidal antiinflammatory drugs cause apoptosis and induce cyclooxygenases in chicken embryo fibroblasts. Proc Natl Acad Sci USA 92:7961–7965, 1995.

70. Bombardier C, Peloso PM, Goldsmith CH. Salsalate, a nonacetylated salicylate, is as efficacious as diclofenac in patients with rheumatoid arthritis. Salsalate-Diclofenac Study Group. J Rheumatol 22:617–624, 1995.

71. Simon LS, Zhao SZ, Arguelles LM, et al. Economic and gastrointestinal safety comparisons of etodolac, nabumetone and oxaprozin from insurance claims data from patients with arthritis. Clin Ther 20:1218–1235, discussion 1192–1193, 1998.

72. Agrawal NM, Caldwell J, Kivitz AJ, et al. Comparison of the upper gastrointestinal safety of Arthrotec 75 and nabumetone in osteoarthritis patients at high risk for developing nonsteroidal anti-inflammatory drug–induced gastrointestinal ulcers. Clin Ther 21:659–674, 1999.

73. Saag KG, Rubenstein LM, Chrischilles EA, et al. Nonsteroidal antiinflammatory drugs and cognitive decline in the elderly. J Rheumatol 22:2142–2147, 1995.

74. Hoppmann RA, Peden JG, Ober SK. Central nervous system side effects of nonsteroidal antiinflammatory drugs. Aseptic meningitis, psychosis, and cognitive dysfunction. Arch Intern Med 151:1309–1313, 1991.

75. Simon LS. Biology and toxic effects of nonsteroidal antiinflammatory drugs. Curr Opin Rheumatol 10:153–158, 1998.

76. Robinson DR, Skosliewicz M, Bloch KJ, et al. Cyclooxygenase blockade elevates leukotriene E$_4$ production during acute anaphylaxis in sheep. J Exp Med 163:1509–1517, 1986.

77. Stevenson DD, Hougham, Schrank PJ, et al. Salsalate cross-sensitivity in ASA-sensitive patients with asthma. J Allergy Clin Immunol 86:749–758, 1990.

78. Bjarnson I, Hyllar J, MacPherson AJ, et al. Side effects of the nonsteroidal antiinflammatory drugs on small and large intestine. Gastroenterology 104:1832–1847, 1993.

79. Garcia Rodriguez LA, Walker AM, Perez Gutthann S. Nonsteroidal antiinflammatory drugs and gastrointestinal hospitalizations in Saskatchewan: a cohort study. Epidemiology 3:337–342, 1992.

80. Griffin MR, Piper JM, Daugherty JR, et al. Nonsteroidal antiinflammatory drug use and increased risk for peptic ulcer disease in elderly persons. Ann Intern Med 114:257–263, 1991.

81. Garcia Rodriguez LA. Nonsteroidal antiinflammatory drugs, ulcers and risk: a collaborative meta-analysis. Semin Arthritis Rheum 26(suppl):16–20, 1997.

82. Bjarnson I, Thjodleifsson B. Gastrointestinal toxicity of nonsteroidal anti-inflammatory drugs: the effect of numesulide compared with naproxen onthe human gastrointestinal tract. Rheumatology 38(suppl):24–32, 1999.

83. Holt S, Rigoglioso V, Sidhu M, et al. Nonsteroidal antiinflammatory drugs and lower gastrointestinal bleeding. Dig Dis Sci 38:1619–1623, 1993.

84. Wilcox CM, Alexander LN, Cotsonis GA, et al. Nonsteroidal antiinflammatory drugs are associated with both upper and lower gastrointestinal bleeding. Dig Dis Sci 42:990–997, 1997.

85. Traversa G, Walker AM, Ippolito FM, et al. Gastroduodenal toxicity of different nonsteroidal antiinflammatory drugs. Epidemiology 6:49–54, 1995.

86. Wallace JL, Bak A, McKnight W, et al. Cyclooxygenase I contributes to inflammatory responses in rats and mice: implications for gastrointestinal toxicity. Gastroenterology 115:101–109, 1998.

87. Singh G, Ramey DR, Morfeld D, et al. Gastrointestinal tract complications of nonsteroidal antiinflammatory drug treatment in rheumatoid arthritis. A prospective observational study. Arch Intern Med 156:1530–1536, 1996.

88. Larkai EN, Smith JL, Lidsky MD, et al. Gastroduodenal mucosa and dyspeptic symptoms in arthritic patients during chronic nonsteroidal anti-inflammatory drug use. Am J Gastroenterol 82:1153–1158, 1987.

89. Silverstein FE, Graham DY, Senior JR, et al. Misoprostol reduces serious gastrointestinal complications in patients with rheumatoid arthritis receiving nonsteroidal anti-inflammatory drugs. Ann Intern Med 123:241–249, 1995.

90. Simon LS, Hatoum HT, Bittman RM, et al. Risk factors for serious nonsteroidal-induced gastrointestinal complications: regression analysis of the MUCOSA trial. Fam Med 28:202–208, 1996.

91. Minocha A, Greenbaum DS. Pill-esophagitis caused by nonsteroidal antiinflammatory drugs. Am J Gastroenterol 86:1086–1089, 1991.

92. Eng J, Sabanathan S. Drug-induced esophagitis. Am J Gastroenterol 86:1171–1133, 1991.

93. Goldstein JL, Eisen GM, Lewis B, et al. Video capsule endoscopy to prospectively assess small bowel injury with celecoxib, naproxen plus omeprazole, and placebo. Clin Gastroenterol Hepatol.3:133–141, 2005.

94. Laine L, Connors LG, Reicin A, et al. Serious lover gastrointestinal clinical events with non selective NSAID or coxib use. Gastroenterology 124:288–292, 2003.

95. Bombardier C, Laine L, Reicin A, et al. Comparison of upper gastrointestinal toxicity of rofecoxib and naproxen in patients with rheumatoid arthritis. N Engl J Med 343:1520–1528, 2000.

96. Silverstein FE, Faich G, Goldstein JL, et al. Gastrointestinal toxicity with celecoxib vs. nonsteroidal anti-inflammatory drugs for osteoarthritis and rheumatoid arthritis. JAMA 284:1247–1255, 2000.

97. Reuter BK, Asfaha S, Buret A, et al. Exacerbation of inflammation-associated colonic injury in rats through inhibition of cyclooxygenase-2. J Clin Invest 98:2076–2085, 1996.

98. McCarthy CJ, Crofford LJ, Greensom J, et al. Cyclooxygenase-2 expression in gastric antral mucosa before and after eradication of *Helicobacter pylori* infection. Am J Gastroenterol 94:1218–1223, 1999.

99. Eckmann L, Stenson WF, Savidge TC, et al. Role of intestinal epithelial cells in the host secretory response to infection by invasive bacteria. Bacterial entry induces epithelial prostaglandin H synthase-2 expression and prostaglandin E$_2$ and F$_2$ production. J Clin Invest 100:296–309, 1997.

100. Singer I, Kawka DW, Schloemann S, et al. Cyclooxygenase 2 is induced in colonic epithelial cells in inflammatory bowel disease. Gastroenterology 115:297–306, 1998.

101. Mizuno H, Sakamoto C, Matsuda K, et al. Induction of cyclooxygenase 2 in gastric mucosal lesions and its inhibition by the specific antagonist delays healing in mice. Gastroenterology 12:387–397, 1997.

102. White WB, Faich G, Borer JS, et al. Cardiovascular thrombotic events in arthritis trials of the cyclooxygenase-2 inhibitor celecoxib. Am J Cardiol 92:411–418, 2003.

103. Schnitzer TJ, Burmester GR, Mysler E, et al. TARGET Study Group. Comparison of lumiracoxib with naproxen and ibuprofen in the Therapeutic Arthritis Research and Gastrointestinal Event Trial (TARGET), reduction in ulcer complications: randomised controlled trial. Lancet 364:665–674. 2004.

104. Farkouh ME, Kirshner H, Harrington RA, et al. TARGET Study Group.comparison of lumiracoxib with naproxen and ibuprofen in the Therapeutic Arthritis Research and Gastrointestinal Event Trial (TARGET), cardiovascular outcomes: randomised controlled trial. Lancet 364:675–684, 2004.

105. Funk CD, Funk LB, Kennedy ME, et al. Human platelet/erythroleukemia cell prostaglandin G/H synthase: cDNA cloning, expression, and gene chromosomal assignment. FASEB J 5(9):2304–2312, 1991.

106. FitzGerald GA. Mechanisms of platelet adtivation: thromboxane A$_2$ as an amplifying signal for other agonists. Am J Cardiol 68:11B–15B, 1991.

107. Pedersen AK, FitzGerald GA. Cyclooxygenase inhibition, platelet function, and metabolite formation during chronic sulfinpyrazone dosing. Clin Pharmacol Ther 37:36–42, 1985.

108. Garcia Rodriguez LA, Varas C, Patrono C. Differential effects of ASA and non-ASA nonsteroidal antiinflammatory drugs in the primary prevention of myocardial infarction in postmenopausal women. Epidemiology 11:382–387, 2000.

109. Ray WA, Stein CM, Hall K, et al. Non-steroidal anti-inflammatory drugs and risk of serious coronary heart disease: an observational cohort study. Lancet. 359:118–123, 2002.

110. Mamdani M, Rochon P, Juurlink DN, et al. Effect of selective cyclooxygenase 2 inhibitors and naproxen on short-term risk of acute myocardial infarction in the elderly. Arch Intern Med 163(4):481–486, 2003.

111. Rahme E, Pilote L, LeLorier J. Association between naproxen use and protection against acute myocardial infarction. Arch Intern Med 162:1111–1115, 2002.

112. Konstam MA, Weir MR, Reicin A, et al. Cardiovascular thrombotic events in controlled, clinical trials of rofecoxib. Circulation 104:2280–2288, 2001.

113. Juni P, Nartey L, Reichenbach S, et al. Risk of cardiovascuolar events and rofecoxib: cumulative meta-analysis. Lancet 364:2021–2029, 2004.

114. Bresalier RS, Sandler RS, Quan H, et al., and the Adenomatous Polyp Prevention on Vioxx (APPROVe) Trial Investigators. Cardiovascularevents associated with rofecoxib in a colorectal adenoma chemoprevention trial. N Engl J Med 352:1092–1102, 2005.

115. Nussmeier NA, Whelton AA, Brown MT, et al. Complications of the COX-2 Inhibitors parecoxib and valdecoxib after cardiac surgery. N Engl J Med 352:1081–1091, 2005.

116. Solomon SD, McMurray JJV, Pfeffer MA, et al. Adenoma Prevention with Celecoxib (APC) Study Investigators. Cardiovascular risk associated with celecoxib in a clinical trial for colorectal adenoma prevention. N Engl J Med 352:1071–1080, 2005.

117. http://www.fda.gov/ohrms/dockets/ac/05/minutes/2005-4090M1_Final.htm

118. Shaya FT, Blume SW, Blanchette CM, et al. Selective cyclooxygenase-2 inhibition and cardiovascular effects: anj observational study of a Medicaid population. Arch Intern Med 165:181–186, 2005.

119. Ray WA, Stein CM, Daugherty JR, et al. COX-2 selective non-steroidal anti-inflammatory drugs and risk of serious coronary heart disease. Lancet 360:1071–1073, 2002.

120. Graham DJ, Campen D, Hui R, et al. Risk of acute myocardial infarction and sudden cardiac death in patients treated with cyclo-oxygenase 2 selective and non-selective non-steroidal anti-inflammatory drugs: nested case-control study. Lancet. 2005; 365:475–481.

121. Johnson AG, Nguyen TV, Day RO. Do nonsteroidal anti-inflammatory drugs affect blood pressure? A meta-analysis. Ann Intern Med. 1994 Aug 15;121(4):289–300.

122. Sowers, JR, White WB, Pitt B, et al., for the Celecoxib Rofecoxib Efficacy and Safety in Comorbidities Evaluation Trial (CRESCENT) Investigators. The effects of cyclooxygenase-2 inhibitors and nonsteroidal anti-inflammatory therapy on 24-hour blood pressure in patients with hypertension, osteoarthritis and type 2 diabetes. Arch Intern Med. 2005;165:161–168.

123. Aw TJ, Haas SJ, Liew D, et al. Meta-analysis of cyclooxygenase-2 inhibitors and their effects on blood pressure. Arch Intern Med. 2005;165:490–496.

124. FitzGerald GA. Coxibs and cardiovascular disease. N Engl J Med. 2004;351:1709–1711.

125. Chenevard R, Hurlimann D, Bechir M, et al. Selective COX-2 inhibition improves endothelial function in coronary artery disease. Circulation. 2003;107:405–409.

126. Whelton A, Fort JG, Puma JA, et al., for the Success Study Group. Cyclooxygenase-2—specific inhibitors and cardiorenal function: a randomized, controlled trial of celecoxib and rofecoxib in older hypertensive osteoarthritis patients. Am J Ther. 2001; (8):85–95.

127. Graham DY, White RH, Moreland LW, et al. Duodenal and gastric ulcer prevention with misoprostol in arthritis patients taking NSAIDs. Ann Intern Med 119:257–262, 1993.

128. Levine LR, Cloud ML, Enas NH. Nizatidine prevents peptic ulceration in high-risk patients taking nonsteroidal anti-inflammatory drugs. Arch Intern Med 153:2449–2454, 1993.

129. Hawkey CJ, Karrasch JA, Szczepanski L, et al. Omeprazole compared with misoprostol for ulcers associated with nonsteroidal antiinflammatory drugs. N Engl J Med 338:727–734, 1998.

130. Taha AS, Hudson N, Hawkey CJ, et al. Famotidine for the prevention of gastric and duodenal ulcers caused by nonsteroidal anti-inflammatory drugs. N Engl J Med 334:1435–1439, 1996.

131. Hawkey CJ. Omeprazole and bleeding peptic ulcer, or "how case-control studies can tell you what you suspected all along." Epidemiology 10:211–213, 1999.

132. Gabriel SE, Jaakkimainen RL, Bombardier C. The cost-effectiveness of misoprostol for nonsteroidal antiinflammatory drugs–associated adverse gastrointestinal events. Arthritis Rheum 36: 447–459, 1993.

133. Schlondorff D. Renal complications of nonsteroidal anti-inflammatory drugs. Kidney Int 44:643–653, 1993.

134. Clive DM, Stoff JS. Renal syndromes associated with the nonsteroidal anti-inflammatory drugs. N Engl J Med 310:563–572, 1984.

135. Whelton A, Hamilton CW. Nonsteroidal anti-inflammatory drugs: effects on kidney function. J Clin Pharmacol 31:588–598, 1991.

136. Whelton A. Nephrotoxicity of nonsteroidal anti-inflammatory drugs: physiologic foundations and clinical implications. Am J Med 106:13s–24s, 1999.

137. Golbetz H, Black V, Shemesh O, et al. Mechanism of the antiproteinuric effect of indomethacin in nephrotic humans. Am J Physiol 256:F44–F51, 1989.

138. Garini G, Mazzi A, Buzio C, et al. Renal effects of captopril, indomethacin and nifedipine in nephrotic patients after an oral protein load. Nephrol Dial Transplant 11:628–634, 1996.

139. Espinoza LR, Jara LJ, Martinez-Osuna P, et al. Refractory nephrotic syndrome in lupus nephritis: favorable response to indomethacin therapy. Lupus 2:9–14, 1993.

140. Curhan GC, Willett WC, Rosner B, Stampfer MJ Frequency of analgesic usse and risk of hypertension in younger women Arch Int Med 2002; 162: 2204–2208.

141. Pope JE, Anderson JJ, Felson DT. A meta-analysis of the effects of nonsteroidal anti-inflammatory drugs on blood pressure. Arch Intern Med 153:477–484, 1993.

142. Johnson AG, Simons LA, Simons J, et al. Non-steroidal anti-inflammatory drugs and hypertension in the elderly: a community-based cross-sectional study. Br J Clin Pharmacol 35:455–459, 1993.

143. Chrischilles EA, Wallace RB. Nonsteroidal anti-inflammatory drugs and blood pressure in an elderly population. J Gerontol 48:M91–M96, 1993.

144. Harris RC, McKanna JA, Aiai Y, et al. Cyclooxygenase-2 is associated with the macula densa of rat kidney and increases with salt restriction. J Clin Invest 94:2504–2510, 1994.

145. Garcia Rodriguez LA, Williams R, Derby LE, et al. Acute liver injury associated with nonsteroidal antiinflammatory drugs and the role of risk factors. Arch Intern Med 154:311–316, 1994.

146. Walker AM. Quantitative studies of the risk of serious hepatic injury in persons using nonsteroidal antiinflammatory drugs. Arthritis Rheum 40:201–208, 1997.

147. Helfgott SM, Sandberg-Cook J, Zakim D, et al. Diclofenac-associated hepatotoxicity. JAMA 264:2660–2662, 1990.

148. Kawaguchi H, Pilbeam CC, Harrison JR, et al. The role of prostaglandins in the regulation of bone metabolism. Clin Orthop 313:36–46, 1995.

149. Pilbeam CC, Fall PM, Alander CB, et al. Differential effects of nonsteroidal anti-inflammatory drugs on constitutive and inducible prostaglandin G/H synthase in cultured bone cells. J Bone Miner Res 12:1198–1203, 1997.

150. Bauer DC, Orwell ES, Fox KM, et al. Aspirin and NSAID use in older women: effect on bone mineral density and fracture risk. Study of Osteoporotic Fractures Research Group. J Bone Miner Res 11:29–35, 1996.

151. Strom BL, Carson JL, Schinnar R, et al. Nonsteroidal anti-inflammatory drugs and neutropenia. Arch Intern Med 153:2119–2124, 1993.

152. Ostensen M, Ostensen H. Safety of nonsteroidal anti-inflammatory drugs in pregnant patients with rheumatic disease. J Rheumatol 23:1045–1049, 1996.

153. Nilsson OS, Persson PE. Heterotopic bone formation after joint replacement. Curr Opin Rheumatol 11:127–131, 1999.

154. Amin AR, Attur M, Patel RN, et al. Superinduction of cyclooxygenase-2 activity in human osteoarthritis-affected cartilage. Influence of nitric oxide. J Clin Invest 15:1231–1237, 1997.

155. Huskisson EC, Berry H, Gishen P, et al. Effects of anti-inflammatory drugs on the progression of osteoarthritis of the knee. LINK Study Group. Longitudinal investigation of nonsteroidal anti-inflammatory drugs in knee osteoarthritis. J Rheumatol 22:1941–1946, 1995.

156. Dieppe P, Cushnaghan J, Jasani MK, et al. A 2 year placebo controlled trial of non-steroidal anti-inflammatory therapy in osteoarthritis of the knee joint. Br J Rheumatol 32:595–600, 1993.

157. Scholes D, Stergachis A, Penna PM, et al. Nonsteroidal anti-inflammatory drug discontinuation in patients with osteoarthritis. J Rheumatol 22:708–712, 1995.

158. Pincus T, Callahan LF. Clinical use of multiple nonsteroidal anti-inflammatory drug preparations within individual rheumatology private practices. J Rheumatol 16:1253–1258, 1989.

159. Hoyeraal HM, Fagertun H, Ingemann-Hansen T, et al. Characterization of responders and nonresponders to tiaprofenic acid and naproxen in the treatment of patients with osteoarthritis. J Rheumatol 20:1747–1752, 1993.

160. Schnitzer TJ. Non-NSAID pharmacologic treatment options for the management of chronic pain. Am J Med 105:45S–52S, 1998.

161. Roth SH. Efficacy and safety of tramadol HCL in breakthrough musculoskeletal pain attributed to osteoarthritis. J Rheumatol 27:1358–1363, 1998.

162. Katz WA. Pharmacology and clinical experience with tramadol in osteoarthritis. Drugs 52(suppl 3):39–47, 1996.

163. Aronson MD. Nonsteroidal anti-inflammatory drugs, traditional opioids, and tramadol: contrasting therapies for the treatment of chronic pain. Clin Ther 19:420–432, discussion 367–368, 1997.
164. Schnitzer TJ, Kamin M, Olson WH. Tramadol allows reduction of naproxen dose among patients with naproxen-responsive osteoarthritis pain: a randomized, double blind, placebo controlled trial. Arthritis Rheum 42:1370–1377, 1999.
165. Biasi G, Manca S, Manganelli S, et al. Tramadol in the fibromyalgia syndrome: a controlled clinical trial versus placebo. Int J Clin Pharmacol Res 18:13–19, 1998.
166. Petrone D, Kamin M, Olson W. Slowing the titration rate of tramadol HCl reduces the incidence of discontinuation due to nausea and/or vomiting: a double blind randomized trial. J Clin Pharm Ther 24:115–123, 1999.
167. Ruoff GE. Slowing the initial titration rate of tramadol improves tolerability. Pharmacotherapy 19:88–93, 1999.
168. Jick H, Derby LE, Vasilakis C, et al. The risk of seizures associated with tramadol. Pharmacotherapy 18:607–611, 1998.
169. Kahn LH, Alderfer RJ, Graham DJ. Seizures reported with tramadol [letter]. JAMA 278:661, 1997.
170. American Geriatrics Society Panel on Chronic Pain in Older Persons. The management of chronic pain in older persons. J Am Geriatr Soc 46:635–651, 1998.
171. The use of opioids for the treatment of chronic pain. A consensus statement from the American Academy of Pain Medicine and the American Pain Society. Clin J Pain 13:6–8, 1997.
172. Balazs EA, Denlinger JL. Viscosupplementation: a new concept in the treatment of osteoarthritis. J Rheumatol Suppl 39:3–9, 1993.
173. Adams ME, Atkinson MH, Lussier AJ, et al. The role of viscosupplementation with hylan G-F 20 (Synvisc) in the treatment of osteoarthritis of the knee: a Canadian multicenter trial comparing hylan G-F 20 alone, hylan G-F 20 with non-steroidal anti-inflammatory drugs (NSAIDs) and NSAIDs alone. Osteoarthritis Cartilage 3:213–226, 1995.
174. Altman RD, Moskowitz R, and the Hyalgan Study Group. Intraarticular sodium hyaluronate (Hyalgan) in the treatment of patients with osteoarthritis of the knee: a randomized clinical trial. J Rheumatol 25:2203–2212, 1998.
175. Corrado EM, Peluso GF, Gigliotti S, et al. The effects of intra-articular administration of hyaluronic acid on osteoarthritis of the knee: a clinical study with immunological and biochemical evaluations. Eur J Rheumatol Inflamm 15:16–25, 1995.
176. Listrat V, Ayral X, Patarnello F, et al. Arthroscopic evaluation of potential structure modifying activity of hyaluronan (Hyalgan) in osteoarthritis of the knee. Osteoarthritis Cartilage 5:153–160, 1997.
177. Dougados M, Nguyen M, Listrat V, et al. High molecular weight sodium hyaluronate (hyalectin) in osteoarthritis of the knee: a 1 year placebo controlled trial. Osteoarthritis Cartilage 1:97–103, 1993.
178. Jones AC, Pattrick M, Doherty S, et al. Intra-articular hyaluronic acid compared to intra-articular triamcinolone hexacetonide in inflammatory knee osteoarthritis. Osteoarthritis Cartilage 3:269–273, 1995.
179. Lohmander LS, Dalen N, Englund G, et al. Intra-articular hyaluronan injections in the treatment of osteoarthritis of the knee: a randomized double blind placebo controlled multicenter trial. Ann Rheum Dis 55:424–431, 1996.
180. Lussier A, Cividino AA, McFarlane CA, et al. Viscosupplementation with hylan for the treatment of osteoarthritis: findings from clinical practice in Canada. J Rheumatol 23:1579–1585, 1996.
181. Dahlberg L, Lohmander LS, Ryd L. Intraarticular injections of hyaluronan in patients with cartilage abnormalities and knee pain: a one year double blind placebo-controlled study. Arthritis Rheum 37:521–528, 1994.
182. Henderson EB, Smith EC, Pegley F, et al. Intra-articular injection of 750 kD hyaluronan in the treatment of osteoarthritis: a randomised single-center double-blind placebo-controlled trial of 91 patients demonstrating lack of efficacy. Ann Rheum Dis 53:529–534, 1994.
183. Brandt KD, Smith GN Jr, Simon LS. Intraarticular injection of hyaluronan as treatment for knee osteoarthritis: what is the evidence? Arthritis Rheum 2000 Jun;43(6):1192–1203.
184. Kirwan JR, Rankin E. Intra-articular therapy in osteoarthritis. Baillieres Clin Rheumatol 11:769–794, 1997.
185. Grillet B, Dequeker J. Intra-articular steroid injection. A risk benefit assessment. Drug Saf 5:205–211, 1990.
186. Caldwell JR. Intra-articular corticosteroids. Guide to selection and indications for use. Drugs 52:507–514, 1996.
187. Hunter JA, Blyth TH. A risk-benefit assessment of intra-articular corticosteroids in rheumatic disorders. Drug Saf 21:353–365, 1999.
188. Howell DS, Altman RD. Cartilage repair and conservation in osteoarthritis. A brief review of some experimental approaches to chondroprotection. Rheum Dis Clin North Am 19:713–724, 1993.
189. Reginster J-Y, Deroisy R, Rovati LC, et al. Long-term effects of glucosamine sulfate in osteoarthritis progression: a randomised, placebo-controlled clinical trial. Lancet 357:251–256, 2000.
190. Bryant LR, des Rosier KF, Carpenter MT. Hydroxychloroquine in the treatment of erosive osteoarthritis. J Rheumatol 22:1527–1531, 1995.
191. Utsinger PD, Resnick D, Shapiro RF, et al. Roentgenologic, immunologic, and therapeutic study of erosive (inflammatory) osteoarthritis. Arch Intern Med 138:693–697, 1978.
192. Belhorn LR, Hess EV. Erosive osteoarthritis. Semin Arthritis Rheum 22:298–306, 1993.
193. Deal CL, Moskowitz RW. Nutraceuticals as therapeutic agents in osteoarthritis. The role of glucosamine, chondroitin sulfate, and collagen hydrolysate. Rheum Dis Clin North Am 25:379–395, 1999.
194. Hardingham T. Chondroitin sulfate and joint disease. Osteoarthritis Cartilage 6(suppl A):3–5, 1998.
195. Uebelhart D, Thonar EJ, Delmas PD, et al. Effects of oral chondroitin sulfate on the progression of knee osteoarthritis: a pilot study. Osteoarthritis Cartilage 6(suppl A):39–46, 1998.
196. Pipitone VR. Chondroprotection with chondroitin sulfate. Drugs Exp Clin Res 17:3–7, 1991.
197. Verbruggen G, Goemaere S, Veys EM. Chondroitin sulfate: S/DMAOD (structure/disease modifying anti-osteoarthritis drug) in the treatment of finger joint OA. Osteoarthritis Cartilage 6(suppl A):37–38, 1998.
198. Bussci L, Poor G. Efficacy and tolerability of oral chondroitin sulfate as a symptomatic slow-acting drug for osteoarthritis (SYSADOA) in the treatment of knee osteoarthritis. Osteoarthritis Cartilage 6(suppl A):31–36, 1998.
199. Bourgeois P, Chales G, Dehais J, et al. Efficacy and tolerability of chondroitin sulfate 1200 mg/day vs chondroitin sulfate 3 × 400 mg/day vs placebo. Osteoarthritis Cartilage 6(suppl A):25–30, 1998.
200. McCarty MF. Enhanced synovial production of hyaluronic acid may explain rapid clinical response to high-dose glucosamine in osteoarthritis. Med Hypotheses 50:507–510, 1998.
201. Ronca F, Palmieri L, Panicucci P, et al. Anti-inflammatory activity of chondroitin sulfate. Osteoarthritis Cartilage 6(suppl A): 14–21, 1998.
202. Kelly GS. The role of glucosamine sulfate and chondroitin sulfate in the treatment of degenerative joint disease. Altern Med Rev 3:27–39, 1998.
203. McAlindon TE, Jacques P, Zhang Y, et al. Do antioxidant micronutrients protect against the development and progression of knee osteoarthritis? Arthritis Rheum 39:648–656, 1996.
204. Altman RD, Hochberg MC, Moskowitz RW, et al. Recommendations for the medical management of osteoarthritis of the hip and knee: 2000 update. Arthritis Rheum 43:1905–1915, 2000.

Intra-Articular Therapy

16

David H. Neustadt   Roy Altman

INTRA-ARTICULAR STEROIDS IN OSTEOARTHRITIS

In 1951, hydrocortisone was introduced and popularized for local intra-articular administration. Observations and a vast experience accumulated during the intervening years have confirmed the value of this compound and of other corticosteroid suspensions for combating pain and inflammation when they are given at the local tissue level.[1-3]

Although the value of intra-articular steroids in the treatment of rheumatoid arthritis and other inflammatory arthropathies is undoubted, their use in the therapy for osteoarthritis (OA) has been controversial.[4] Early experimental studies suggested the possibility of a neuropathic Charcot-like arthropathy after multiple corticosteroid injections,[5-7] and studies performed on small animals (i.e., mice, rats, and rabbits) indicated evidence of altered cartilage protein synthesis and damage to the cartilage.[3,8-12] These deleterious effects curbed the enthusiasm for intra-articular corticosteroid therapy in OA. However, other investigators reported that clinical observations after repeated administration of intra-articular steroids to knees demonstrated no significant evidence of destruction or accelerated deterioration.[13-14] A detailed study of the effects of steroid injections on monkey joints disclosed no appreciable joint damage, suggesting that primate joints probably respond in a different way from those of mice and rabbits.[15] Most authorities now consider intra-articular corticosteroid therapy in OA of considerable value when administered appropriately and judiciously. Intra-articular steroid therapy is always considered as an adjunctive form of therapy added to a conventional management program.

Rationale

The major objective of intrasynovial therapy in OA is to enter the joint space, aspirate any fluid, and instill the corticosteroid suspension that suppresses inflammation and provides the most effective relief for the longest period of time.

The metabolic pathway and fate of corticosteroids within the joint have not been completely elucidated.[3] Some evidence of the injected steroid can be detected in the synovial fluid cells for 48 hours after injection. Prednisolone trimethylacetate has been identified in synovial fluid 14 days after its injection. The rate of absorption and duration of action are related to the solubility of the compound instilled.[16] Triamcinolone hexacetonide is the most insoluble preparation currently available.[1]

An antilymphocytic action is considered a possible mechanism of steroid benefit on rheumatoid synovial lining. Corticosteroids inhibit prostaglandin synthesis and decrease collagenase and other enzyme activity. The major basis of benefit in OA remains somewhat unclear. Saxne and coworkers[17] measured the release of proteoglycans into synovial fluid to monitor the effects of therapy on cartilage metabolism. Their data strongly suggest that intra-articular corticosteroid injections reduce the production of mediators such as interleukin (IL)-1, TNF-alpha, and other so-called protease enzymes that may induce cartilage degradation.

Systemic "spillover" with absorption may occur, varying with the size of the dose and the solubility of the preparation injected. One study showed that 40 mg of methylprednisolone acetate was sufficient to induce a transient adrenal suppression, as reflected in depressed cortisol levels for up to 7 days.[16] A postinjection rest regimen (Table 16–1) or partial limitation of motion of the injected joint probably delays "escape" of the intra-articular steroid and minimizes systemic overflow effects.[18]

Indications

It is important to emphasize that intra-articular steroid therapy must be considered an adjunct to basic measures. Except in treating a strict regional problem such as

TABLE 16-1

POSTINJECTION REST REGIMEN

- Remain at rest for 3 days, except for meals and bathroom needs.
- After the 3 days of bed rest, use a walking aid (cane, crutches, or walker, as directed) for 3 weeks for any outside distance walking.

traumatic synovitis or olecranon bursitis, it should be thought of as a component modality included in a comprehensive management program.

The indications for the use of intra-articular steroids are summarized in Table 16-2. In addition to the goal of introducing a drug into the joint cavity, arthrocentesis permits the aspiration of synovial fluid, which is useful as a diagnostic aid. Examination of the synovial fluid permits an estimation of the presence and degree of inflammation. An experienced observer can usually distinguish rheumatoid from traumatic or osteoarthritic fluid by its gross appearance and viscosity. Only a few drops of fluid may suffice to establish the diagnosis of an accompanying crystal synovitis (gout or pseudogout).

When usual conventional therapy has failed to control the symptoms adequately or prevent disability, local steroid therapy deserves consideration. A tense or painful effusion is the strongest indication for prompt arthrocentesis, followed by a corticosteroid injection, pending synovial fluid findings to exclude infection.

Relief of pain with preservation or restoration of joint motion is the major objective of therapy. When one or more joints are resistant to systemic therapy, consideration should be given to intrasynovial injections. Local joint injections are often helpful in preventing adhesions and correcting flexion deformities of the knee. In large, tense,

TABLE 16-2

INDICATIONS FOR INTRASYNOVIAL CORTICOSTEROIDS

1. To provide pain relief and suppress the inflammation of synovitis.
2. To provide adjunctive therapy for one or two joints not responsive to other systemic therapy.
3. To facilitate a rehabilitative and physical therapy program or orthopedic corrective procedures.
4. To prevent capsular and ligamentous laxity (large knee effusion).
5. To bring about a "medical synovectomy."
6. To treat patients unresponsive to or intolerant of oral systemic therapy.
7. To treat acute effusions occurring with associated crystal deposition disease.

or boggy effusions, the capsule and ligaments may become stretched, and this can be combated effectively with intra-articular therapy. Finally, in longstanding or recurrent effusions of the knee, a so-called "medical synovectomy" can be performed by instilling a relatively large dose (30 to 50 mg) of an insoluble preparation such as triamcinolone hexacetonide, followed by a strict postinjection rest regimen (Table 16-1).

Clinical Efficacy

Numerous authors reported favorably on the use of intra-articular steroids in the treatment of OA.[3,19-23] Balch and associates[13] reported on repeated intrasynovial injections given over a period varying from 4 to 15 years. The minimum number of injections given was 15 during a period of 4 years, with the interval between injections being not less than 4 weeks. Their results strongly supported the conclusion that this was a "very useful" form of treatment.

Although certain controlled trials[24,25] failed to demonstrate significant efficacy of steroid injections, these studies did not take into consideration such important factors as adequate dosage, the presence or absence of fluid, removal of excess fluid (dilution factor), and the injection technique. Most important, there was no attempt to regulate the postinjection physical activity of the patient.

Dieppe and colleagues[26] reported a beneficial response with significantly greater reduction of pain and tenderness compared with placebo in a controlled trial in which 20 mg of triamcinolone hexacetonide were injected into 48 osteoarthritic knees. These results were obtained even though injections were made into the infrapatellar pouch and only 5 mL of fluid were aspirated from each knee at the time of the procedure. In another report[27] of 42 patients with OA in whom triamcinolone hexacetonide, betamethasone acetate, and betamethasone disodium were compared, the results confirmed that intra-articular steroid treatment of OA was highly effective. In another other study[27,28] including a similar comparative assessment in a group consisting of 19 patients with OA of the knee, favorable results were obtained.[28] The duration of effect varied with different preparations and dosage.

These carefully performed randomized double-blind and single-blind studies support the results of Hollander's[1] 30 years of experience with a large number of injections. He reported that in a 10-year follow-up of the first 100 patients who had been given repeated intra-articular steroids in osteoarthritic knees, 59 patients no longer needed injections, 24 continued to require occasional injections, and only 11 did not obtain a worthwhile response.[23]

My own experience is similar to that of Hollander and the other authors cited previously. Striking relief of pain, frequently coupled with increased motion, occurred in the majority of injected joints. However, the success of short-term beneficial response must be balanced against the all-important duration of effect and any potential iatrogenic deleterious response.

Contraindications and Complications

The role of intra-articular corticosteroids in OA remains somewhat controversial despite extensive use and reported beneficial response because of some reports of the development of steroid induced (Charcot-like) arthropathy after multiple injections.[5,7]

Contraindications are relative and are listed (Table 16–3). Local infection or recent serious injury overlying the structure to be injected or the presence of a generalized infection with possible bacteremia is an obvious contraindication to the local instillation of a corticosteroid or any local injection. In patients with systemic infections, intra-articular therapy might be performed under the "cover" of appropriate antibiotic therapy, if the indication is considered urgent. The risk of provoking serious bleeding in patients receiving anticoagulants must be determined after a review of the patient's general status, including determination of the prothrombin time. Joints of the lower extremities that demonstrate considerable underlying damage (e.g., an unstable knee) should not be injected with corticosteroids unless there is a relatively large inflammatory effusion and the patient will cooperate by adhering to a non-weight-bearing rest schedule for several weeks after the procedure.

Complications of intra-articular therapy are listed in Table 16–4. Despite some systemic "spillover," physical evidence of hypercortisonism or other undesirable steroid effects rarely occur from intermittent intra-articular therapy. If "moon" face appears, injections may have been administered too frequently.[29] Although the possibility of introducing an accidental infection is the most serious potential complication, review of our extensive experience and that of others discloses that infections occurring as an aftermath of joint injections are extremely rare.[1,3,30]

Local adverse reactions are minor and reversible. The so-called postinjection flare is a rare complication that begins shortly after the injection and usually subsides within a few hours, rarely continuing up to 48 to 72 hours. Some

TABLE 16–3

RELATIVE CONTRAINDICATIONS TO INTRA-ARTICULAR THERAPY

1. Infection (local or systemic)
2. Anticoagulant therapy
3. Hemorrhagic effusions
4. Uncontrolled diabetes mellitus
5. Severe joint destruction and/or deformity
6. Extreme overnutrition

TABLE 16–4

COMPLICATIONS OF INTRA-ARTICULAR THERAPY

Infection
Postinjection flare
Crystal-induced synovitis
Cutaneous atrophy (local)
Steroid arthropathy (rare)

investigators consider these reactions to be a true crystal induced synovitis caused by corticosteroid ester crystals.[2,31] The application of ice to the site of injection and oral analgesics usually control after-pain until the reaction abates. In a few instances, the postinjection synovitis has been sufficiently severe to require aspiration of the joint to obtain relief.

Another infrequent complication is localized subcutaneous or *cutaneous atrophy*.[2,3] This cosmetic change can be recognized as a thin or depressed area at the site of the injection, sometimes associated with depigmentation. As a rule, the skin appearance will be restored to normal when the crystals of the corticosteroid have been completely absorbed. Rarely, capsular (periarticular) calcification at the site of the injection has been noted in roentgenograms taken after treatment. The calcifications usually disappear spontaneously and are not of clinical significance.[18] Careful technique to prevent the steroid suspension from leaking along the needle track to the skin surface will avoid or minimize this problem. A small amount of 1% lidocaine (or equivalent) or normal saline solution can be utilized to flush the needle used to administer the crystalline suspension before removing the needle.

An occasional patient may complain of transient warmth and flushing of the skin. There may be central nervous system and cardiovascular reactions to local anesthetics if used in combination with the steroid for injection. It has been suggested that the abolition of pain after the introduction of steroids permits the patient to "overwork" the involved joint, causing additional cartilage and bone deterioration and finally giving rise to a Charcot-like or steroid arthropathy.[32] In addition, experimental evidence in rabbit joints indicates that frequently repeated injections of corticosteroids may interfere with normal cartilage protein synthesis.[3,12] As stated earlier, studies on primate joints failed to confirm evidence of significant cartilage damage caused by repeated administration of intra-articular steroids, suggesting that the steroid effect on primate joints, including human joints, is probably temporary.[15] Indeed, evidence of a "protective effect" of corticosteroids against cartilage damage and osteophyte formation has been shown with triamcinolone hexacetonide in a guinea pig knee model of experimental arthritis.[33]

TABLE 16–5
INJECTABLE CORTICOSTEROIDS

Repository Preparations (mg)*	mg/mL	Range of Usual Dosage
Hydrocortisone tebutate (hydrocortone TBA)	50	25–100
Betamethasone acetate and betamethasone sodium phosphate (Celestone Soluspan)	6[†]	1.5–6
Methylprednisolone acetate (DepoMedrol[‡])	20	4–40
Triamcinolone acetonide (Kenalog 40)	40	5–40
Triamcinolone diacetate (Aristocort Forte)	40	5–40
Triamcinolone hexacetonide (Aristospan)	20	5–40

*Amount will vary depending on the size of the joint to be injected.
[†]Available as 3 mg of acetate and 3 mg of phosphate.
[‡]Supplied in 20 mg/mL, 40 mg/mL, and 80 mg/mL preparations.

Available Compounds and Choice of Drugs

Hydrocortisone and a variety of available repository preparations are listed in Table 16–5. All corticosteroids, with the exception of cortisone and prednisone, can produce a significant and prompt anti-inflammatory effect in an inflamed joint. The most soluble corticosteroid suspension is absorbed rapidly and has a short duration of effect. Tertiary butyl acetate (TBA, tebutate) ester prolongs the duration of action as a result of decreased solubility, which probably causes its dissociation by enzymes to proceed at a lower rate. Although an occasional patient may obtain greater benefit from one steroid derivative than from another, no single steroid agent has demonstrated a convincing margin of superiority, with the exception of triamcinolone hexacetonide.[6,23,34] Prednisolone tebutate has the virtues of price advantage and longtime usage; unfortunately, it is currently relatively unavailable because of "manufacturing" problems. Depomethylprednisolone and triamcinolone hexacetonide may be substituted. Triamcinolone hexacetonide is the least water-soluble preparation currently available. It is 2.5 times less soluble in water than prednisolone tebutate and usually provides the longest duration of effectiveness. There is minimal systemic "spillover" with this agent.

Dosage and Administration

The dose of any microcrystalline suspension employed for intrasynovial injection must be arbitrarily selected. Factors that influence the dosage and the anticipated results are listed in Table 16–6.

TABLE 16–6
FACTORS THAT INFLUENCE RESPONSE TO INTRA-ARTICULAR INJECTIONS

Size of joints
Volume of synovial fluid
Choice of corticosteroid preparation
Dosage and technique
Severity (and extent) of synovitis
Postinjection activity

For estimating dosage, a useful guide is as follows:

For small joints of the hand and foot, 2.5 to 10 mg of methylprednisolone acetate suspension or an equivalent glucocorticoid
For medium-sized joints such as the wrist and elbow, 10 to 25 mg
For the knee, ankle, and shoulder, 20 to 40 mg
For the hip, 25 to 40 mg

It is occasionally necessary to give larger amounts to obtain optimal results. For intrabursal therapy, such as for the hip (trochanteric) or the knee (anserine) bursa, 15 to 40 mg is usually an adequate dose.

The longer the intervals between injections, the better. I usually recommend a 4-week minimum between intra-articular procedures, and in weight-bearing joints, I prefer an interval of at least 6 to 12 weeks between injections. Injections should not be repeated on a "regular" routine basis, and rarely should more than two to three injections into a specific weight-bearing joint be repeated per year. Injections into soft tissue sites of para-articular inflammation may be given on a more frequent basis. After knee injection, I advise the patient to adhere to the following rest regimen (Table 16–1). The patient should remain in bed for 3 days, with the exception of getting up for bathroom privileges and meals; crutches are then prescribed, to be used with "three-point" gait to protect the injected knee during distance walking for 2 to 4 weeks. A cane may be substituted at times when crutches are considered inappropriate or uncomfortable. This postinjection rest regimen facilitates a sustained improvement and avoids the hazard of "overworking" or abusing the injected joint. An additional benefit is that the inactivity reduces any systemic effect by delaying absorption of the steroid from the synovial joint cavity. This program is optimal for achieving maximal therapeutic benefit and reducing possible deleterious effects of joint overuse after injection. However, as with all therapeutic programs, rheumatologists may vary the regimen based on the individualized needs of the given patient. Experimental evidence indicates that during exercise of the inflamed human knee, there is a large increase in intra-articular (hydrostatic) pressure, which causes intra-articular hypoxia.[35] On cessation of exercise, there is oxidative damage to lipids and immunoglobulin G (IgG) within the joint. The lipid peroxidation products in synovial fluid are not found in resting knees. Reperfusion of the synovial membrane occurs when exercise is stopped.

During the past several years, I have hospitalized five patients with OA of the knees who had intractable, recurrent synovitis resistant to frequent arthrocenteses and repeated intra-articular injections. After the administration of a steroid (usually triamcinolone hexacetonide) and the completion of the strict rest period, these patients obtained complete resolution of effusions for up to a year or longer.

Preparation of Injection Site

Preparation of the site for injection of a steroid requires rigid adherence to aseptic technique. Landmarks are outlined with a skin pencil or ball point pen. The point of entry is then cleansed with an antibacterial cleanser (antimicrobial soap or the equivalent) or a povidone-iodine solution, and alcohol is sponged on the area. Sterile drapes and gloves are not ordinarily considered necessary. Sterile 4-inch × 4-inch gauze pads are useful for drying the area.

Injection Techniques

General Considerations

Arthrocentesis is easily and relatively painlessly performed in a joint that is distended with fluid or when boggy synovial proliferation is present. For most joints, the usual point of entry is on the extensor surface, avoiding the large nerves and major vessels that are usually present on the flexor surface. Optimal joint positioning should be accomplished to stretch the capsule and separate the joint "ends" to produce maximal enlargement and distraction of the joint or synovial cavity to be penetrated.

A local anesthetic may be desirable, especially when a relatively "dry" joint is being entered or when only a small amount of fluid is present. A small skin wheal made by infiltration with lidocaine or the equivalent or spraying (frosting) the skin with a vapocoolant such as chloroethane (ethyl chloride) usually provides adequate anesthesia.

Aspiration of as much synovial fluid as possible prior to instillation of the corticosteroid suspension reduces the possible dilution factor. After the therapeutic agent is injected in large joints, it may be advisable to reaspirate and reinject several times within the barrel of the syringe (barbotage) to obtain good "mixing" and dispersion of the therapeutic compound throughout the joint and synovial cavity. I often instill a small amount of air just prior to removing the needle to ensure adequate diffusion. Finally, gentle manipulation, carrying the joint through its full excursions of motion, facilitates maximal dispersion of the injected medication.

Specific Joints and Adjacent Sites

The joints most frequently considered for corticosteroid injection in OA include the knee, the distal and proximal interphalangeal joints, the first carpometacarpal joint, and the first metatarsophalangeal joint. The hip and temporomandibular joints are less commonly injected. Shoulder joints are rarely involved in primary OA but, like the elbow, may develop OA on a secondary, underlying basis.

Technique for Knee Injection

The knee joint contains the largest synovial space in the body and is the most commonly aspirated and injected joint. Demonstrable, visible, or palpable effusions often develop, making it the easiest joint to enter and inject with medication. When a large amount of fluid is present, entry is as simple as puncturing a balloon.

Aspiration of the knee is usually performed with the patient lying on a table with the knee supported and extended as much as possible. The usual site of entry is medial at about the midpoint of the patella or just below the point where a horizontal line tangential to the superior pole of the patella crosses a line paralleling the medial border. The needle (1.5- to 2-inch, 20-gauge) is directed downward or upward, sliding into the joint space beneath the undersurface of the patella (Fig. 16–1). Aspiration of the knee can be facilitated by applying firm pressure with the palms cephalad to the patella over the site of the suprapatellar bursa. If cartilage is touched, the needle is withdrawn slightly and the fluid is aspirated. A similar approach can be used on the lateral side especially if the maximal fluid bulge is present laterally. The lateral approach is especially convenient if there is a large effusion in the suprapatellar bursa. The point of penetration is lateral and superior to the patella. An approach that is used less frequently is the infrapatellar anterior route, which is useful when the knee cannot be fully extended and there is only minimal fluid present. With the knee flexed to approximately 90°, the needle is directed either medially or laterally to the inferior patellar tendon and cephalad to the infrapatellar fat pad. It is difficult to obtain fluid with this approach, and there is a slight possibility of injury to the joint surface.

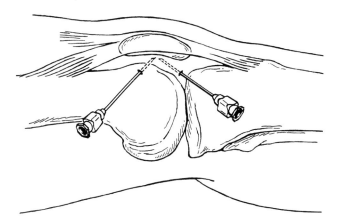

Figure 16–1 Arthrocentesis of the knee joint, medial approach, the usual entry site. (From Steinbrocker O, Neustadt DH. Aspiration and Injection Therapy in Arthritis and Musculoskeletal Disorders: A Handbook on Technique and Management. Hagerstown, MD, Harper & Row, 1972.)

Knee Region

Although radiographic evidence of degenerative changes involving the knee may be present, the "knee" pain and associated disabling symptoms sometimes result from extra-articular causes. Some of these painful conditions in the knee region, often associated with OA, may respond to local injection therapy.

These disorders include bursitides of the knee with involvement of the prepatellar, suprapatellar, and anserine bursae. Other disorders adjacent to the knee that may be responsive to injection therapy include semimembranosus tenosynovitis, Pelegrini-Stieda syndrome, and painful points around the edge of the patella associated with patellofemoral OA. The differential diagnosis between OA of the knee and these disorders is based on a thorough history and the physical findings.

Prepatellar Bursitis. Prepatellar bursitis ("housemaid's knee"), characterized by swelling and effusion of the superficial bursa overlying the patella, is easily recognized. The chronic bursal reaction commonly occurs from repetitive activity or pressure, such as kneeling on a firm surface ("rug cutter's knee" and "nun's knee"). Pain is relatively minimal except on direct pressure, and motion is usually preserved. Aspiration, which may yield a small amount of clear, serous fluid, is performed, and then 1 to 2 mL of lidocaine and 10 to 20 mg of a prednisolone suspension are instilled. This bursa is not usually a single cavity but a multilocular structure in which loose areolar tissue separates the walls of the bursa. Thus, in some cases, the procedure may need to be repeated once or a few times to obtain a lasting result. Whenever possible, the activity provoking the bursitis should be eliminated.

Suprapatellar Bursitis. Suprapatellar bursitis is usually associated with synovitis of the knee cavity. On occasion, the suprapatellar bursa is largely separated developmentally from the synovial cavity. In these cases, effusion is especially prominent in the suprapatellar region.

Anserine Bursitis. Anserine bursitis ("cavalryman's disease") now mainly occurs in obese women with disproportionately heavy thighs in association with OA of the knee. The bursa is located at the anteromedial surface of the tibia just below the joint line of the knee, at the site of the insertion of the conjoined tendon of the sartorius, semitendinosus, and gracilis muscles, and superficial to the medial collateral ligament. The entity may simulate or coexist with OA of the knee. A relatively abrupt increase in knee pain, localized tenderness with a sensation of fullness in the vicinity of the site of the bursa, or the development of an angular knee deformity should strongly suggest consideration of this often overlooked disorder. Injection of a few millimeters of lidocaine and approximately 1 to 1.5 mL of a corticosteroid suspension from an anteromedial approach with a 1.5-inch, 22-gauge needle frequently produces prompt symptomatic relief. The duration of effect is variable and may correlate with the patient's weight-bearing activities.

Semimembranosus Tenosynovitis. Semimembranosus ("popliteal") tenosynovitis is characterized by pain in the posterior or posteromedial aspect of the knee. Localized tenderness over the superoposterior area of the medial condyle of the tibia (the semimembranosus groove) supports the diagnosis. Protective muscle spasm of the medial hamstrings causes a "pseudolocking" of the knee. This condition is usually superimposed on underlying OA, and the onset is relatively sudden. Treatment with local steroid injection to the points of greatest tenderness is frequently beneficial.

Pellegrini-Stieda Syndrome. This syndrome occurs as an aftermath of trauma. Calcification develops in the region of the medial tibial collateral ligament. The major manifestation is progressively impaired knee joint flexion. The diagnosis is made by roentgenographic study disclosing the calcification 3 to 4 weeks after the injury. Early local injections of steroids and/or an anesthetic are the most beneficial form of treatment.

Another area where pain may arise in the "unswollen" knee is around the edge of the patella in association with patellofemoral OA. Occasionally one or two localized tender points are detected. Injection of these "pain spots" with 1 mL of lidocaine and 0.5 to 0.75 mL of a steroid suspension may produce significant relief. The injection has to be made under pressure into the actual fibrous tissue attachments of the capsule to the edge of the patella. The use of a relatively short needle (7/8 to 1 inch) will help prevent advancing the needle too far and entering the knee cavity.

The Shoulder

Scapulohumeral Joint. Of the approaches to the shoulder, the anterior route provides the simplest entry. A needle is directed mediodorsally in the groove between the medial aspect of the humeral head at a point just inferior to the tip of the coracoid process (Fig. 16–2). A 1.5- or 2-inch, 20- or 22-gauge needle is advanced into the scapulohumeral interspace; any fluid if present is aspirated, and 20 to 30 mg of prednisolone suspension is introduced with or without 2 to 3 mL of lidocaine.

The posterior approach is often preferable, because it is done out of the patient's line of vision. Internal rotation of the shoulder with adduction of the patient's arm across the chest wall and with the hand resting on the opposite shoulder tends to open up the joint space. The site of needle entry is just below (1 to 2 cm) the posterolateral angle of the posterior aspect of the acromion. A 1.5- or 2-inch, 20- or 22-gauge needle is introduced through a cutaneous wheal to a point within a free space, visualized as the capsule of the scapulohumeral joint. Aspiration, which rarely yields fluid, is performed, and 20 to 30 mg of a steroid preparation is instilled.

Acromioclavicular Joint. Entry is made through a cutaneous lidocaine wheal over the interosseous groove at the point of maximal tenderness. The joint is relatively superficial, and a 7/8- or 1-inch, 22-gauge needle is adequate. One to 2 mL of lidocaine and 0.75 to 1 mg of a prednisolone suspension are instilled. It is not necessary to advance the needle beyond the proximal margin of the joint surfaces.

Sternoclavicular Joint. OA of the sternoclavicular joint is seldom the cause of much pain. However, in the rare instance that involvement is considered clinically significant, the joint is easily located and injected by sliding a

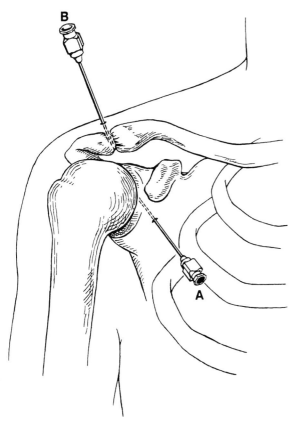

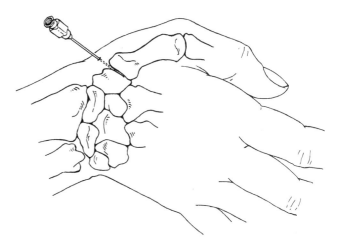

Figure 16–3 Arthrocentesis of the first carpometacarpal joint (thumb base). (From Steinbrocker O, Neustadt DH. Aspiration and Injection Therapy in Arthritis and Musculoskeletal Disorders: A Handbook on Technique and Management. Hagerstown, MD, Harper & Row, 1972.)

Figure 16–2 Arthrocentesis of the scapulohumeral joint, anterior approach (*A*), and injection of the acromioclavicular joint (*B*). (From Steinbrocker O, Neustadt DH. Aspiration and Injection Therapy in Arthritis and Musculoskeletal Disorders: A Handbook on Technique and Management. Hagerstown, MD, Harper & Row, 1972.)

7/8-inch, 25-gauge needle between the articular surfaces, and then 0.25 mL of a steroid suspension is instilled.

The Elbow

The elbow (humeroulnar) joint can usually be readily entered by the posterolateral approach. With the joint incompletely extended and held in a relaxed position, the bulge of any synovial effusion is noted posterolaterally, just outside of the olecranon process and inferior to the humeral lateral epicondyle. The needle is introduced at the outer aspect of the olecranon and just below the lateral epicondyle. It is directed medially, proximal to the radial head. The radial head can be easily identified by pronating and supinating the forearm. Aspiration of any fluid is performed, followed by intra-articular injection of 1 to 1.5 mL of a corticosteroid suspension.

Because the elbow region is subject to frequently occurring extraarticular soft tissue forms of pathology such as epicondylitis, it must be kept in mind that the presence of OA may not be the source of pain.

Finger and Toe Joints

First Carpometacarpal Joint. The carpometacarpal joint of the thumb is commonly affected with OA (thumb base

OA). With the thumb adducted and held in flexion within the palm, steroid injection is performed from the dorsal side, inserting the needle at the point of maximal tenderness. It is not usually necessary to actually slide the needle between the trapezium (greater multiangular) and the base of the thumb metacarpal (Fig. 16–3).

Interphalangeal Joints. Small hand joints are entered on the dorsal surface, utilizing 7/8-inch, 25-gauge needles. The needle is slipped beneath the extensor tendon from either the lateral or the medial side. Aspiration does not usually yield fluid. In small joints, it is necessary to use a gentle teasing technique with the needle in combination with efforts to distract the joint, but frequently, periarticular injection produces an adequate response, indicating that it is not always necessary to instill the therapeutic suspension directly into the joint space. Aspiration and steroid injection of distal joints are performed in a fashion similar to those of the proximal joints. Steroids may be injected into toe joints by utilizing traction to facilitate insertion of the needle between the phalangeal joint surfaces.

Injecting a tender, inflamed Heberden node with a steroid is usually accomplished through a point frozen by spraying chloroethane (ethyl chloride); a fine needle, such as a 7/8-inch, 27-gauge one, is used, and any effort to aspirate fluid is avoided. The needle is gently teased through the point of entry into the capsule, depositing the steroid without attempting to enter the tiny joint space. Ready transport of the corticosteroid occurs through inflamed tissue.

Mucous (synovial) cysts associated with Heberden nodes at the dorsum of the affected joint can be "unroofed," inspissated fluid can be removed, and a small dose of corticosteroid suspension can be instilled. If the result is not satisfactory after one or two injections and the cyst is troublesome, surgical excision should be considered.

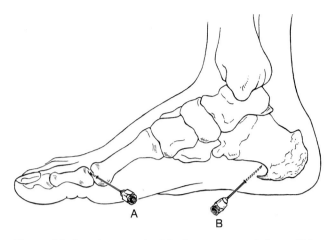

Figure 16–4 Arthrocentesis of the first metatarsophalangeal joint (*A*) and injection of calcaneal bursitis with heel spur (*B*). (From Steinbrocker O, Neustadt DH: Aspiration and Injection Therapy in Arthritis and Musculoskeletal Disorders: A Handbook on Technique and Management. Hagerstown, MD, Harper & Row, 1972.)

Metatarsophalangeal Joints. The metatarsophalangeal joints may be entered through a mediodorsal approach by teasing with 24- or 25-gauge needles. Rarely, a metatarsophalangeal joint is approached from the plantar surface by a subcutaneous entry.

The first metatarsophalangeal joint (bunion joint) may be the site of acute or chronic synovitis. It may be entered through a mediodorsal approach by teasing with a 25-gauge needle. Five to 10 mg of prednisolone suspension may be injected. Subcutaneous entry of the swollen capsule for aspiration and injection or deposit of the dosage over the joint space is usually sufficient.

Freezing the skin with a vapocoolant chloroethane (ethyl chloride) spray before needling small joints is usually preferred to the injection of lidocaine (Fig. 16–4).

Hip Region

Periarticular Pain Points. Localized tender points are found occasionally in the abundant musculature and fibrous tissues in the vicinity of the hip joint and may be associated with OA of the hip. These secondary sites of irritation may produce pain and tenderness adjacent to the joint. Injection of the sore joint may prove helpful at one or more circumscribed sites of tenderness. The injections are given deeply with a 2- or 2.5-inch, 20-gauge needle, administering 3 to 4 mL of 1% lidocaine and 0.5 to 1 mL (10 to 20 mg) of prednisolone suspension (Fig. 16–5).

Trochanteric Bursa. Involvement of the trochanteric bursa may simulate osteoarthritic hip pain. If the bursa is calcified, it is easily located by roentgenogram. Trochanteric bursitis occurs over or below the greater trochanter, and tenderness is localized over the greater trochanter. Active abduction of the hip when lying on the opposite side typically accentuates the discomfort. Intrabursal injection of 3 to 5 mL of lidocaine and 1 to 2 mL (20 to 40 mg) of prednisolone suspension is frequently effective in suppressing the pain (Fig. 16–6).

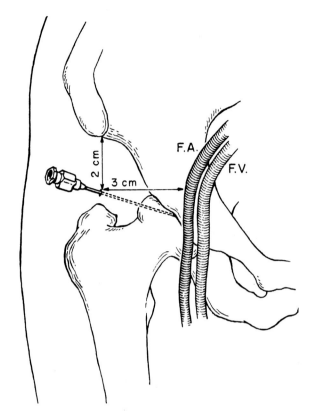

Figure 16–5 Arthrocentesis of the hip joint, anterior approach. (From Steinbrocker O, Neustadt DH: Aspiration and Injection Therapy in Arthritis and Musculoskeletal Disorders: A Handbook on Technique and Management. Hagerstown, MD, Harper & Row, 1972.)

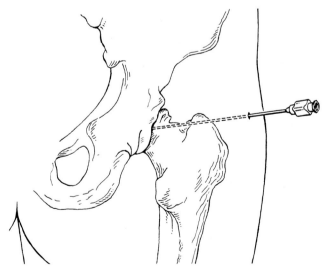

Figure 16–6 Arthrocentesis of the hip joint, lateral approach. (From Steinbrocker O, Neustadt DH. Aspiration and Injection Therapy in Arthritis and Musculoskeletal Disorders: A Handbook on Technique and Management. Hagerstown, MD, Harper & Row, 1972.)

Ankle Joint (Tibiotalar Joint)

OA affecting the ankle joint is relatively rare except as an aftermath of trauma or special activities or occupations such as ballet dancing. Local steroid injections are often ineffective in suppressing osteoarthritic ankle pain.

The ankle joint may be difficult to enter. The usual technique includes holding the foot in slight plantar flexion. The point of entry is just medial to the extensor hallucis longus tendon. The needle is directed somewhat laterally from a point approximately 1 cm above and 1 cm lateral to the medial malleolus (Fig. 16–7). A slight depression can be felt between the medial malleolus and the extensor hallucis longus tendon. Plantar flexion tends to open up the ankle joint, providing a larger area for injection.

Foot

Calcaneal Bursitis with Spur. The major condition of the foot associated with OA for which steroid injection therapy is suitable is calcaneal bursitis (plantar fasciitis) with painful heel spurs. If simple measures including orthopedic shoe corrections and aids are ineffective, steroid injec-

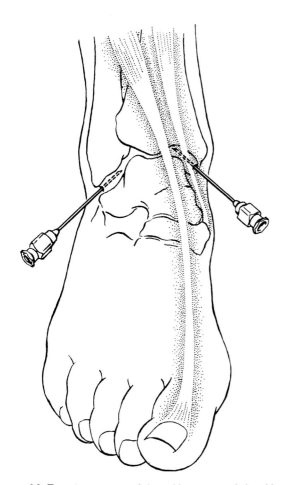

Figure 16–7 Arthrocentesis of the ankle joint, medial and lateral entries. (From Steinbrocker O, Neustadt DH. Aspiration and Injection Therapy in Arthritis and Musculoskeletal Disorders: A Handbook on Technique and Management. Hagerstown, MD, Harper & Row, 1972.)

tion of the painful heel is often beneficial. At the site of maximal tenderness, a 1-inch, 22- to 24-gauge needle is inserted into the plantar surface at a 90° angle, sliding into the space at the midpoint of the calcaneus. The tip of the needle lies in the aponeurosis of the attachment to the os calcis (Fig. 16–4). One milliliter of lidocaine and 10 to 20 mg of prednisolone suspension are instilled.

Crystal Synovitis and Osteoarthritis

Calcium Pyrophosphate Dihydrate Deposition

The link between OA and calcium pyrophosphate dihydrate (CPPD) deposition is extremely strong. The majority (about 70%) of cases of CPPD are associated with a chronic arthritis identical to OA, usually involving the hips, wrists, and knees.[36]

In those patients who develop an acute or subacute attack ("pseudogout"), arthrocentesis permits diagnostic confirmation and thorough aspiration of synovial fluid; introduction of 1 to 2 mL of a corticosteroid suspension generally suppresses the inflammatory process in the knee. Involved joints other than the knee may respond satisfactorily to intrasynovial steroid therapy.

Hydroxyapatite Crystals and Osteoarthritis

The possible relationship of hydroxyapatite crystal deposition and OA was first reported by Dieppe and associates in 1976.[37] The notion that the inflammation may be caused by apatite crystals was based on the finding of the crystals in synovial fluid from osteoarthritic patients. Specific diagnosis is made by electron microscopy or x-ray diffraction of crystals. Although clinical recognition of apatite crystals is difficult, when acute or subacute arthritis with an effusion develops, especially in patients on dialysis, it is reasonable to aspirate the contents of the synovial cavity and instill a corticosteroid suspension.

Corticosteroid Postinjection Crystal Synovitis

The rare postinjection flare that occurs within a few hours after the administration of a local corticosteroid injection usually subsides spontaneously in several to 24 hours. In some cases, a true crystal induced synovitis caused by microcrystalline corticosteroid ester crystals occurs. If the reaction is severe, a thorough aspiration of the joint contents provides prompt relief. Oral administration of analgesics or nonsteroidal anti-inflammatory agents for several days is also beneficial when symptoms are severe.

NONSTEROIDAL INTRA-ARTICULAR THERAPEUTIC AGENTS

Intra-articular injections were performed with a variety of compounds for relief of symptoms long before the advent of corticosteroids. However, none of the preparations available before corticosteroids had dependable or durable effects. Agents that have been injected include lactic acid, phenylbutazone, cytotoxic compounds, sodium salicylate, and aspirin (dissolved in saline solution).[38] Phenylbutazone is beneficial but causes considerable local irritation.[39] In my experience and that of others, nitrogen mustards and thiotepa produced only minimal benefit and occasionally caused toxic effects with high fever.[40–42]

The terms chemical synovectomy and radiation (nonsurgical) synovectomy have been introduced to describe the effects of potent agents such as osmic acid and radioisotopes such as gold 198 ([198]Au) and yttrium 90 (^{90}Y).

Osmic Acid

Failure to produce predictable prolonged local remissions after corticosteroid injections prompted the use of chemical agents such as osmic acid. Osmic acid is an aqueous solution of osmium tetroxide in a 1% or 2% concentration. Intra-articular injection of osmic acid has been used in synovitis of the knee since 1950 in Scandinavia.[45] The drug is relatively widely used in other countries, especially France, and more than 4000 injections have been given at the Rheumatism Foundation Hospital in Finland.[43] To my knowledge, osmic acid therapy has not been used in human joints in the United States.

Radioisotopes

The use of radioactive gold in the treatment of malignant pleural effusions prompted its trial use in cases of persistent synovial effusions.[46] Despite successful results, the concern with minimizing unwanted radiation led to subsequent studies with ^{90}Y, erbium 169 ([169]Er), and other radioactive isotopes.[47,48] Satisfactory results have been reported from Europe, including more than 9000 joints treated with radioisotope injections in France.[44]

The fear of leakage of radioactivity from the joint and the uncertain long-term biologic hazards of radiation has limited this form of therapy in the United States to experimental studies in animals.[49,50] The most recently introduced isotope, dysprosium 165, has the advantage of avoiding extra-articular radioactive leakage because of its short half-life.[51] Unfortunately, its use would be limited by cost and the necessity for a nearby reactor to produce the radioisotope. Some comparative clinical studies indicate that radioisotope therapy is not superior to "long-acting" steroids, including methylprednisolone and triamcinolone hexacetonide.[44,52,53]

In a recent double-blind, placebo-controlled trial comparing radiation synovectomy with intra-articular ^{90}Y plus glucocorticoids with intra-articular steroids for persistent knee arthritis, there was no evidence of additional benefit in the radiosynovectomy group.[54]

INTRA-ARTICULAR HYALURONATE (HYALURONIC ACID, HYALURONAN)

Normal

In the normal joint, synovial fluid is an ultrafiltrate of plasma composed of water and low molecular weight solutes transuded from blood. Hyaluronate (HA) is

---

TABLE 16–7

HYALURONAN FUNCTIONS IN THE NORMAL DIATHRODIAL JOINT

Stabilize joint function
  Lubrication function at low shear
  Increased friction at high shear

Mechanical barrier
  Viscoelastic properties—thin layer of HA acts as a shock absorber between cartilage/cartilage and cartilage/meniscal surfaces

Exclusion properties
  Large molecular weight solutes

Physical barrier to entry of polymorphonuclear leukocytes into the synovial cavity

Anti-inflammatory
  Medium and high molecular weight HA are anti-inflammatory, in part by binding inflammatory mediators
  Reduces IL-1β and some MMP activity of synovium

Analgesic
  Coats pain receptors—prevents binding to peptide agonists

Modulates synovial cell behavior
  Binds CD-44 and Toll 2 and 4 receptors
  Creates a physical meshwork around cells
  Stimulates HA synthesis
  Reduces gaps between synovial cells
  Binds RHAMM receptor

Modulates chondrocyte behavior
  Binds CD-44 and Toll 2 and 4 receptors
  Reduces ICAM-1
  Increases proteoglycan production
  Binds to link glycoprotein
  Increases tissue inhibitor of metalloproteinase (TIMP)-1 release
  Reduces nitric oxide–induced chondrocyte apoptosis

---

secreted by the synovial cells as a long chain polymer of about 5000 repeating disaccharide units of N-acetyl-D-glucosamine and beta-glucoronic acid. Each unit of HA is about 2.5 μm in length and has a high viscosity. Although synovial cavity HA has a turnover of about 12 hours, it is 10 times slower than small solutes and proteins.[55] Within the joint, HA is metabolized by the synovial lining cells. Potential functions of HA in the normal joint are listed in Table 16–7. Normal synovial fluid HA molecular weight is $3.5-5 \times 1,000$ kDa.

Osteoarthritis

In OA, most often HA molecular weight decreases, reversing the actions listed in Table 16–7. In contrast, osteochondromatosis, associated with OA, may present with an increase in synovial fluid HA and related viscosity. However, in OA, the total amount of HA in the synovial cavity is often increased due to the larger volume of synovial fluid.[56]

Hyaluronan Therapy

The principle of replacement therapy with HA for OA stems from the work of Balazs.[57,58] The initial HAs for medical use were extracted from rooster combs. The purification process results in a relatively pure HA with limited cross-allergy of those with allergic reactions to fowl products. Newer HA extracts are derived from biological fermentation of streptococcal origin. These are generally of high molecular weight and contain fewer impurities than the HA of rooster comb origin.

There are differences between the various products available. The differences relate to molecular weight, viscosity, and cross-linking. At present, there is no evidence that one molecular weight, viscosity, or cross-linking has better clinical performance than another. There are differences in the residence times in the joint, also of unknown clinical significance. Because there are no clinical efficacy differences between HAs demonstrated to date, this chapter will discuss the HAs without reference to specific products. There may be differences in adverse reactions to HAs, as discussed later.

The HAs are administered intra-articularly in 1, 3, 4, or 5 injection series, depending on the agent. The HA is injected into the joint, usually following aspiration of excessive effusion. Research into the dosing schedules as well as the volume used in the injection has been empiric. This approach to the application of the HAs in OA will assuredly remain empiric until more is understood on the mechanism of action, and a scientific approach to dosing, volume, and interval can be developed.

Most of the testing for HA has been for OA of the knee. More recent clinical research has explored therapy with HA for OA of other joints. Some of the more common HAs available for OA are listed in Table 16–8.

TABLE 16–8
SOME COMMERCIALLY AVAILABLE HYALURONANS FOR OSTEOARTHRITIS AND THEIR MOLECULAR WEIGHTS

BioHy (Arthrease)	300–600 kDa
Durolane	1000 kDa
Euflexxa	2400–3600 kDa
Hyalgan	500–730 kDa
Hylan G-F 20 (Synvisc)*	5000–6000 kDa
NRD101	1900 kDa
Orthovisc	1000–2900 kDa
Ostenil	1200 kDa
Sinovial	800–1200 kDa
Supartz (Artz, Artzal)	620–1200 kDa
Suplasyn	500–730 kDa

Human synovial fluid HA is 350–500 kDa.
* Cross-linked, contains formaldehyde and vinyl sulfone.

Mechanism of Action

The mechanism of action of HA therapy for OA is unknown. Although often labeled as viscosupplementation, the resident half-life of HA in the joint varies from 24 hours to 2 weeks, with the longest resident time ranging from 5 to 30 days (depending on the product). Beyond the resident time in the joint, the device is no longer present and cannot provide biomechanical properties. Hence, if benefit is achieved beyond the resident time in the joint, the benefit must be from some other action and not by its biomechanical properties.

Beyond their mechanical properties, HA has many other potential roles.[59] These are outlined in Table 16–7. The presence of HA in the synovial cavity restricts the entry of large plasma proteins and cells into the cavity; at the same time HA facilitates solute exchange between the joint tissues such as cartilage and synovial capillaries.[60] HA can form a pericellular coat around cells (e.g., nerve endings), interact with proinflammatory mediators, and bind to cell receptors to modulate cell proliferation, migration, and gene expression. HA reduces the proliferation of human macrophages with an increase in apoptotic macrophages.[61] HA induces an increase in human synovial fluid nitric oxide (NO) levels.[62] In contrast, NO was reduced in human articular chondrocyte culture fluid, with an increase in proteoglycan, in the presence of both IL-1 beta and HA.[63] In a lapine model, there was a reduction in apoptosis and NO in cultured cartilage.[64] HA reduces the NO level in joint fluid, reduces the release and degradation of aggrecan, and/or enhances the synthesis of aggrecan in cartilage.[65] HA decreases synovial fluid IL-6 but not IL-8 or tumor necrosis factor (TNF)-alpha.[66] HA suppressed mRNA expression of matrix metralloproeinase (MMP)-3 in lapine synovium, but not cartilage.[67] There was no change in mRNA for MMP-1 or tissue inhibitor of metalloproteinase (TIMP)-1 in cartilage or synovium. HA may act as a 'sink,' binding inflammatory mediators. In a human cartilage explant culture, HA suppressed fibonectin fragment-mediated cartilage damage by trapping the fibronectin.[68] Although the mechanism is not understood, HA appears to increase synovial cell production of HA.

Cluster determinant (CD) 44 is a membrane glycoprotein and the major cell-surface receptor of hyaluronate. It is present on many cells including synovial cells and chondrocytes. The results of HA binding to CD44 can be contradictory and seem to relate to the size of the HA.[60] HA binding to the CD44 receptor in many tissues participates in leukocyte recruitment while activating various inflammatory cells. This pro-inflammatory activity is not present with HA at molecular weights above 300 kDa. HA also enters cells and inhibits neutrophil adhesion which may involve ICAM-1 and not CD44.[69] CD44 with HA have an important role in the maintenance of cartilage homeostasis.[70]

Efficacy of Hyaluronan for Osteoarthritis of the Knee

HA has been shown to be effective in OA of the tibiofemoral joint of the knee in several studies as summarized in a thorough Cochrane review of the literature.[71]

Indeed, HA in OA of the knee has been demonstrated to be of benefit in other reviews of the literature, including most meta-analyses.[72-75] In the 5- to 13-week postinjection period, there was an 11% to 54% improvement in pain and a 9% to 15% improvement in function compared to baseline.[71] There is not a dramatic effect size for HA therapy that may relate to several problems of the conduct of clinical trials, e.g., instruments that are less sensitive to change than desired, high placebo response to intra-articular therapy (particularly intra-articular saline as the placebo), confounding benefit of escape analgesia, high expectations of subjects, and patient response confounded by lack of benefit to other joints with OA.

There appears to be a subset of patients (perhaps 20% of those treated) who achieve dramatic benefit with minimal or no resultant pain.[76,77] There is also a subset of patients who have no benefit to HA therapy at all. In clinical trial subset analysis, no factors could be identified that would allow one to predict which patients will respond or not respond.

In general, clinical trials included patients with mild to moderate radiographic grade of OA (e.g., Kellgren Lawrence grades 2 and 3). At present, there are insufficient data on severe radiographic OA (e.g., Kellgren Lawrence grade 4). There are also insufficient evidence to state whether or not HA therapy will delay joint replacement surgery.

There was no significant change in the use of rescue medication allowed in most trials (mostly acetaminophen).

HA injections improved knee muscle contraction strength (concentric and eccentric) in 25 patients with knee OA 1 week following a five-injection series of HA,[78] but the dynamics of gait need longer-term follow-up.

In a 20-week study, the younger patients with OA had a lesser benefit than those over age 60,[79] suggesting a better response in the older patients.

Length of Effectiveness of HA Therapy. The benefit of a single course of HA is most often limited and symptoms frequently recur. Although studies vary, perhaps related to the HA used and/or the number of injections, the recurrence time in responders is most often between 6 and 12 months. In a study of 110 patients, 1 year efficacy was appreciated in 77% of those on HA (vs. 54% for placebo).[80] Relief of symptoms was reported in 55% of 59 patients 1 year after HA therapy.[81]

Effectiveness of Retreatment with HA. There are limited numbers of studies that address retreatment.[82] Most indicate that retreatment is effective, but the length of time of the benefit of retreatment is unclear. Reduced effectiveness with retreatment may suggest progression of disease.

Comparison of HA to Intra-articular Depocorticosteroids. *Concomitant use:* In a 47-patient 1-year study of HA with and without triamcinolone acetonide, both groups improved, with the combination-therapy subjects improving sooner using the Western Ontario and McMaster Universities OA Index (WOMAC) pain subscale and pain visual analog scales (VAS).[83] In an open study, dexamthasone injected with HA was more effective than HA alone 1 week after the completion of five HA injections.[84]

Comparative use: HA was compared to a depocorticosteroid (betamethasone) in a 6-month trial that demonstrated improved WOMAC in both groups, with a lesser response by women (this is the only study to point out a sex difference in response).[85] In another 6-month study comparing HA to triamcinolone hexacetonide, there was improvement from baseline in the completer analysis for both groups without a significant difference between treatment groups or placebo.[86] In this study there was a trend in favor of the HA. In general, depocorticosteroid therapy has an earlier onset of benefit that is limited in time, while the HA has a slower onset of benefit and remains effective.[71]

In a study of Hip OA, three HA injections were not better than placebo, whereas the depocorticosteroid was effective up to day 28 after injections.[87] In a study of the first carpometacarpal joint, triamcinolone injections provided more pain relief at 2- to 3-weeks postinjection, but less benefit at 26 weeks follow-up.[88]

Additive Effects of HA with Anti-inflammatory or Analgesic Agents

Although combining therapies that attack different causes of pain seems appropriate, there are few studies that have examined combination therapy. Hence, at this time it is uncertain if there is an additive benefit of combining an anti-inflammatory drug or primary analgesic with an HA. A lack of an additive effect is suggested by a 12-week study with a 26-week telephone interview; HA with and without a nonsteroidal anti-inflammatory drug (NSAID) were equally effective with both superior in pain relief to the NSAID alone.[77]

There was no difference in the effectiveness between a five-injection series of HA versus naproxen 1000 mg daily in a 26-week trial.[76] Indeed, a greater percent of patients had no pain or minimal pain in the HA group. There was equal clinical improvement of HA to diacerein in a 1-year study.[89]

Comparison of Hyaluronans

There are an increasing number of studies that compare different HAs.[90-94] To date, no single HA has been proven clinically superior to the other as to efficacy. The studies compared a variety of products of different molecular weights and viscosities. In one study that examined more than the clinical changes, there was an equal reduction in synovial fluid intercellular adhesion molecule-1 (ICAM-1) and vascular cell adhesion molecule-1 (VCAM-1), suggesting an equal reduction in inflammation.[95]

Efficacy of Hyaluronan for Osteoarthritis of Other Joints

HA therapy for OA has been studied in the patellofemoral joint,[96] hip,[97] shoulder,[98] ankle,[99] and first carpometacarpal joint.[88] All showed improvement with HA over placebo, sometimes only numerically. Many of the trials were uncontrolled or open label, and more information is needed. Ultrasound has been demonstrated to be effective in guiding intra-articular therapy, particularly for the hip.[100] Because intra-articular injections are not always intra-articular, it may be appropriate to use ultrasound for other joints as well.

Hyaluronan for Structure Modification of Osteoarthritis

As stated earlier, support for the potential for structure (disease) modification includes preclinical as well as clinical data.[101] The potential for HA to alter the course of OA of the knee clinically was suggested by an arthroscopic and imaging study of 39 patients reexamined at 1 year.[102] In another arthroscopic study at 6 months, cartilage biopsies demonstrated reconstitution of the superficial layer and improved chondrocyte density and territorial matrix appearance for HA in contrast to those treated with methylprednisolone acetate.[103] Additional evidence stems from a 1-year trial of HA in which patients with an initial mean joint space width of the medial tibiofemoral compartment of greater than 4.6 mm had less progression of joint space narrowing than those with joint space widths of less than 4.6 mm.[104] However, another 1-year study failed to show preservation of the joint space by HA.[89]

Adverse Reactions to Hyaluronans

Intra-articular HA is generally well tolerated, with injection site pain reported in 3% to 8% of patients. In clinical trials, the injection site pain was rarely problematic, where few discontinued the trial because of the pain. It has been suggested that the frequency of injection site pain is related to the skill of the person performing the injection and their ability to place the needle in the joint, in contrast to the periarticular region.

Flares of pseudogout have been reported following intra-articular HA.[105,106] Pseudoseptic reactions have been reported and may be unique to certain HAs.[107–109] These tend to occur with repeat injections of HA and are characterized by an acute flare of synovitis within 24 to 72 hours of injection and require therapy to resolve. Mononuclear cells may dominate the synovial fluid cell count, suggesting the pseudoseptic reaction. The flare responds to aspiration, injection of depocorticosteroids, and oral anti-inflammatory drugs. One should be alert as septic arthritis following HA has been reported.[110] In addition, acute pseudogout needs to be ruled out.

Granulomatous synovitis with histocytic and multinucleated giant cells has also been reported with HA for the knee.[111] Inflammatory reactions in synovial biopsies have been identified around hylan gel particles.[112] This proliferative synovitis may be associated with certain of the HAs and usually follows more than one series of injections. No specific therapy has been described, other than to discontinue the HA therapy. Laboratory support for the immunogenicity of certain HAs has been demonstrated in Guinea pigs and mice.[113]

REFERENCES

1. Hollander JL. Intrasynovial corticosteroid therapy in arthritis. Md Med J 19:62–66, 1972.
2. Steinbrocker O, Neustadt DH. Aspiration and Injection Therapy in Arthritis and Musculoskeletal Disorders: A Handbook on Technique and Management. Hagerstown, MD, Harper & Row, 1972.
3. Gray RG, Tenenbaum J, Gottlieb NL, et al. Local corticosteroid injection treatment in rheumatic disorders. Semin Arthritis Rheum 10:231–254, 1981.
4. Intraarticular steroids. Br Med J 1:600–601, 1978. Editorial.
5. Chandler GN, Jones GT, Wright V, et al. Charcot arthropathy following intraarticular hydrocortisone. Br Med J 1:952–953, 1959.
6. Neustadt DH. Chemistry and Therapy of Collagen Diseases. Springfield, IL, Charles C Thomas, 1963, p. 54.
7. Chandler GN, Wright V. Deleterious effect of intraarticular hydrocortisone. Lancet 2:661–663, 1958.
8. Silberberg M, Silberberg R, Hasler M, et al. Fine structure of articular cartilage in mice receiving cortisone acetate. Arch Pathol 82:569–582, 1966.
9. Meyer WL, Kunin AS. Decreased glycolytic enzyme activity in epiphyseal cartilage of cortisone treated rats. Arch Biochem Biophys 129:431–437, 1969.
10. Mankin HJ, Conger KA. The acute effects of intraarticular hydrocortisone on articular cartilage in rabbits. J Bone Joint Surg 48A:1383–1388, 1966.
11. Moskowitz RW, Davis W, Sammarco J, et al. Experimentally induced corticosteroid arthropathy. Arthritis Rheum 13:236–243, 1970.
12. Behrens F, Shepherd N, Mitchel N. Alterations of rabbit articular cartilage by intraarticular injection of glucocorticoids. J Bone Joint Surg 57A:1157–1160, 1976.
13. Balch HW, Gibson JMC, El Ghobarey AF, et al. Repeated corticosteroid injections into knee joints. Rheumatol Rehabil 16:137–140, 1977.
14. Keagy RD, Keim HA. Intraarticular steroid therapy: Repeated use in patients with chronic arthritis. Am J Med Sci 253:45–51, 1967.
15. Gibson T, Burry HC, Poswillo D, et al. Effect of intraarticular corticosteroid injections in primate cartilage. Ann Rheum Dis 36:74–79, 1976.
16. Armstrong RD, English J, Gibson T, et al. Serum methylprednisolone levels following intraarticular injections of methylprednisolone acetate. Ann Rheum Dis 40:571–574, 1981.
17. Saxne T, Heinegard D, Wollheim FA, et al. Therapeutic effects on cartilage metabolism in arthritis as measured by release of proteoglycan structures into the synovial fluid. Ann Rheum Dis 45:491–497, 1986.
18. McCarty DJ. Treatment of rheumatoid joint inflammation with triamcinolone hexacetonide. Arthritis Rheum 15:157–173, 1972.
19. Bornstein J, Silver M, Neustadt DH, et al. Intraarticular hydrocortisone acetate in rheumatic disorders. Geriatrics 9:205–210, 1954.
20. Zuckner J, Machek O, Caciolo C, et al. Intraarticular injections of hydrocortisone, prednisolone and their tertiarybutylacetate derivatives in patients with rheumatoid arthritis and osteoarthritis. J Chronic Dis 8:637–644, 1958.
21. Hydrocortisone and osteoarthritis. JAMA 170:1451, 1959. Foreign letters.
22. Kehr MJ. Comparison of intraarticular cortisone analogues in osteoarthritis of the knee. Ann Rheum Dis 18:325–328, 1959.
23. Hollander JL. Osteoarthritis: Perspectives on treatment. Postgrad Med 68:161–168, 1980.
24. Miller JH, White J, Norton TH, et al. The value of intraarticular injection in osteoarthritis of the knee. J Bone Joint Surg 40A:636–643, 1958.
25. Friedman DM, Moore ME. The efficacy of intraarticular steroids in osteoarthritis: A doubleblind study. J Rheumatol 7:850–856, 1980.
26. Dieppe PA, Sathapatayavongs B, Jones HE, et al. Intraarticular steroids in osteoarthritis. Rheumatol Rehabil 19:212–217, 1980.
27. Valtonen EJ. Clinical comparison of triamcinolone hexacetonide and betamethasone in the treatment of osteoarthrosis of the knee joint. Scand J Rheumatol 41(suppl):3–7, 1981.
28. Clemmesen S. Triamcinolone hexacetonide in intraarticular and intramuscular therapy. Acta Rheumatol Scand 17:273–278, 1971.
29. Neustadt DH. Complications of local corticosteroid injection. JAMA 246:835–836, 1981. Letter to the Editor.
30. Fitzgerald RH. Intrasynovial injection of steroids: Uses and abuses. Mayo Clin Proc 51:655–659, 1976.
31. Gordon GV, Schumacher HR. Electron microscopic study of depo corticosteroid crystals with clinical studies after intraarticular injection. J Rheumatol 6:7–14, 1979.

32. Sweetnam R. Corticosteroid arthropathy and tendon rupture. J Bone Joint Surg 51B:397–398, 1969. Editorial.

33. Williams JM, Brandt KD. Triamcinolone hexacetonide protects against fibrillation and osteophyte formation following chemically induced articular cartilage damage. Arthritis Rheum 28:1267–1274, 1985.

34. Bain LS, Balch HW, Wetherly JMR, et al. Intraarticular triamcinolone hexacetonide: Doubleblind comparison with methylprednisolone. Br J Clin Pract 26:559–561, 1972.

35. Blake BR, Merry P, Unsworth J, et al. Hypoxic reperfusion injury in the inflamed human joint. Lancet 1(8633):289–293, 1989.

36. McCarty DJ. Calcium pyrophosphate dihydrate crystal deposition diseasea current appraisal of the problem. In Holt PJL, ed.: Current Topics in Connective Tissue Disease. New York, Longman, Inc., 1975, p. 184.

37. Dieppe PA, Crocker P, Huskisson EC, et al. Apatite deposition disease. A new arthropathy. Lancet 1:266–269, 1976.

38. Rylance HJ, Chalmers TM, Elton RA, et al. Clinical trials of intraarticular aspirin in rheumatoid arthritis. Lancet 2:1099–1102, 1980.

39. Neustadt DH, Steinbrocker O. Observations of the effects of intraarticular phenylbutazone. J Lab Clin Med 47:284–288, 1956.

40. Henderson ED, Nathan FF. Experience with injection of nitrogen mustard into joints of patients with rheumatoid arthritis. South Med J 62:1455–1458, 1969.

41. Zuckner J, Uddin J, Ramsey RH, et al. Evaluation of intraarticular thiotepa in rheumatoid arthritis. Ann Rheum Dis 25:178–183, 1966.

42. Gristina AG, Pace NA, Kantor TG, et al. Intraarticular thiotepa compared with depomedrol and procaine in the treatment of arthritis. J Bone Joint Surg 52A:1603–1610, 1970.

43. Nissila M. Absence of increased frequency of degenerative joint changes after osmic acid injections. Scand J Rheumatol 7:81–84, 1978.

44. Menkes CJ. Is there a place for chemical and radiation synovectomy in rheumatic diseases? Rheumatol Rehabil 18:65–77, 1979.

45. Anttinen J, Oka M. Intraarticular triamcinolone hexacetonide and osmic acid in persistent synovitis of the knee. Scand J Rheumatol 4:125–128, 1975.

46. Makin M, Robin GC. Chronic synovial effusions treated with intraarticular radioactive gold. JAMA 188:725–728, 1964.

47. Ingrand J. Characteristics of the radioisotopes for intraarticular therapy. Ann Rheum Dis 32(suppl):3–9, 1973.

48. Yates DB, Scott JT, Ramsay N, et al. Double blind trial of yttrium 90 for chronic inflammatory synovitis of the knee. Ann Rheum Dis 36:481, 1977.

49. Sledge CB, Noble J, Hnatowich S, et al. Experimental radiation synovectomy by dyferric hydroxide macroaggregate. Arthritis Rheum 20:1334–1342, 1977.

50. Lee P. The efficacy and safety of radiosynovectomy. J Rheumatol 9:165–168, 1982. Editorial.

51. Sledge CB, Zuckerman JD, Zalutsky MR, et al. Treatment of rheumatoid synovitis of the knee with intraarticular injection of dysprosium165-ferric oxide macroaggregates. Arthritis Rheum 29:153–159, 1986.

52. Ruotsi A, Hypen M, Rekonen A, et al. Erbium169 versus triamcinolone hexacetonide in the treatment of rheumatoid finger joints. Ann Rheum Dis 38:45–47, 1979.

53. Gumpel JM, Matthews SA, Fisher M, et al. Synoviortheses with erbium169: A double blind controlled comparison of erbium169 with corticosteroids. Ann Rheum Dis 38:341–343, 1979.

54. Jahangier ZN, Jacobs JWG, Lafeber FPJG, et al. Is radiation synovectomy for arthritis of the knee more effective than intraarticular treatment with glucocorticoids? Arthritis Rheum 52(11):3391–3402, 2005.

55. Brown TJ, Laurent UBG, Fraser JRE, et al. Turnover of hyaluronan in synovial joints: elimination of labeled hyaluronan from the knee joint of rabbit. Exp Physiol 76:125–134, 1991.

56. Dahl LB, Dahl IM, Engstrom-Laurent A, et al. Concentration and molecular weight of sodium hyaluronate in synovial fluid from patients with rheumatoid arthritis and other arthropathies. Ann Rheum Dis 44:817–822, 1985.

57. Balazs EA, Wadson D, Duff IF, et al. Hyaluronic acid in synovial fluid I. Molecular parameters of hyaluronic acid in normal and arthritic human fluids. Arthritis Rheum 10:357, 1967.

58. Balazs EA, Denlinger JL. Viscosupplementation: a new concept in the treatment of osteoarthritis. J Rheumatol 20 (Suppl 39):3–9, 1993.

59. Liao YH, Jones SA, Forbes B, et al. Hyaluronan: pharmaceutical characterization and drug delivery. Drug Deliv 12:327–342, 2005.

60. Ghosh P, Guidolin D. Potential mechanism of action of intra-articular hyaluronan therapy in osteoarthritis: are the effects molecular weight dependent? Semin Arthritis Rheum 32:10–37, 2002.

61. Sheehan KM, DeLott LB, Day SM, et al. Hyalgan has a dose-dependent differential effect on macrophage proliferation and cell death. J Orthop Res 21:744–751, 2003.

62. Karatay S, Kiziltunc A, Yildirim K, et al. Effects of different hyaluronic acid products on synovial fluid NO levels in knee osteoarthritis. Clin Rheumatol 24:497–501, 2005.

63. Fiorayanti A, Cantarini L, Chellini F, et al. Effect of hyaluronic acid (MW 500-730 kDa) on proteoglycan and nitric oxide production in human osteoarthritic chondrocyte cultures exposed to hydrostatic pressure. Osteoarthritis Cartilage 13:688–696, 2005.

64. Diaz-Gallego L, Prieto JG, Coronel P, et al. Apoptosis and nitric oxide in an experimental model of osteoarthritis in rabbit after hyaluronic acid treatment. J Orthop Res 23:1370–1376, 2005.

65. Kobayashi K, Matsuzaka S, Yoshida Y, et al. The effects of intraarticularly injected sodium hyaluronate on levels of intact aggrecan and nitric oxide in the joint fluid of patients with knee osteoarthritis. Osteoarthritis Cartilage 12:536–542, 2004.

66. Sezgin M, Demirel AC, Karaca C, et al. Does hyaluronan affect inflammatory cytokines in knee osteoarthritis? Rheumatol Int 25:264–269, 2005.

67. Qui B, Liu SQ, Peng H, et al. The effects of sodium hyaluronate on mRNA expressions of matrix metalloproteinas-1, -3 and tissue inhibitor of metalloproteinas-1 in cartilage and synovium of traumatic osteoarthritis model. Chin J. Traumatol 8:8–12, 2005.

68. Kang Y, Eger W, Koepp H, et al. Hyaluronan suppresses fibronectin fragment-mediated damage to human cartilage explant cultures by enhancing proteoglycan synthesis. J Orthop Res 17:858–869, 1999.

69. Alam CA, Seed MP, Freemantle C, et al. The inhibition of neutrophil-endothelial cell adhesion by hyaluronan independent of CD44. Inflammopharmacology 12:535–550, 2005.

70. Knudaon W, Lowser RF. CD44 and integrin matrix receptors participate in cartilage homeostasis. Cell Mol Life Sci 59:36–44, 2002.

71. Bellamy N, Campbell J, Robinson V, et al. Visco-supplementation for the treatment of osteoarthritis of the knee. Cochrane Database Syst Rev Issue 2, Art No CD005321, Pub 2, 2006.

72. Arrich J, Piribauer F, Mad P, et al. Intra-articular hyaluronic acid for the treatment of osteoarthritis of the knee: systematic review and meta-analysis. CMAJ 172:1039–1043, 2005.

73. Lo GH, LaValley M, McAlindon T, et al. Intra-articular hyaluronic acid in treatment of knee osteoarthritis. A meta-analysis. JAMA 290:3115–3121, 2003.

74. Modawal A, Ferrer M, Choi HK, et al. Hyaluronic acid injections relieve knee pain. J Fam Pract 54:758–767, 2005.

75. Wang D-T, Lin J, Chang C-J, et al. Therapeutic effects of hyaluronic acid on osteoarthritis of the knee. A meta-analysis of randomized controlled trials. J Bone Joint Surg Am 86-A:538–545,2004.

76. Altman RD, Moskowitz RW. Intraarticular sodium hyaluronate (Hyalgan) in the treatment of patients with OA of the knee: a randomized clinical trial. J Rheumatol 25:2203–2212, 1998.

77. Adams ME, Atkinson MH, Lusssier AJ, et al. The role of viscosupplementation with hylan G-F 20 (Synvisc) in the treatment of osteoarthritis of the knee: a Canadian multicenter trial comparing hylan G-F 20 alone, hylan G-F 20 with non-steroidal anti-inflammatory drugs (NSAIDs) and NSAID alone. Osteoarthritis Cartilage 3:213–225, 1995.

78. Tang SF, Chen CP, Chen MJ, et al. Improvement of muscle strength in osteoarthritic knee patients after intraarticular knee injections of hyaluronan. Am J Phys Med Rehabil 84:274–277, 2005.

79. Lohmander LS, Dalen N, Englund G, et al. Intra-articular hyaluronan in the treatment of osteoarthritis of the knee: a randomized, double blind, placebo controlled multicentre trial. Hyaluronan Multicentre Trial Group. Ann Rheum Dis 56:424–431, 1997.

80. Dougados M, Nguyen M, Listrat V, et al. High molecular weight sodium hyaluronate (hyalectin) in osteoarthritis of the knee: a 1 year placebo-controlled trial. Osteoarthritis Cartilage 1:97–103, 1993.

81. Kotz R, Kolarz G. Intra-articular hyaluronic acid: duration of effect and results of repeat treatment cycles. Am J Orthop 28(11 Suppl):5–7, 1999.

82. Pagnano M, Westrich G. Successful nonoperative management of chronic osteoarthritis pain of the knee: safety and efficacy of retreatment with intra-articular hyaluronans. Osteoarthritis Cartilage 13:751–761, 2005.

83. Ozturk C, Atamaz F, Hepguler S, et al. The safety and efficacy of intraarticular hyaluronan with/without corticosteroid in knee osteoarthritis: 1-year, single blind, randomized study. Rheumatol Int 26:314–319, 2006.

84. Grecomoro G, Piccione F, Letizia G, et al. Therapeutic synergism between hyaluronic acid and dexamethasone in the intra-articular treatment of osteoarthritis of the knee: a preliminary open study. Curr Med Res Opinion 13:49–55, 1992.

85. Leopold SS, Redd BB, Warme WJ, et al. Corticosteroid compared with hyaluronic acid injections for the treatment of osteoarthritis of the knee. J Bone Joint Surg Am 85-A:1197–1203, 2003.

86. Jones AC, Pattrick M, Doherty S, et al. Intra-articular hyaluronic acid compared to intra-articular tramcinolone hexacetonide in inflammatory knee osteoarthritis. Osteoarthritis Cartilage 3:269–273, 1995.

87. Ovistgaard E, Christensen R, Torp-Pedersen S, et al. Intra-articular treatment of hip osteoarthritis: a randomized trial of hyaluronic acid, corticosteroid, and isotonic saline. Osteoarthritis Cartilage 14:163–170, 2006.

88. Fuchs S, Monikes R, Wohlmeiner A, et al. Intra-articular hyaluronic acid compared with corticoid injections for the treatment of rhizarthrosis. Osteoarthritis Cartilage 14:82–88, 2006.

89. Pham T, Le Henanff A, Dieppe P, et al. Evaluation of the symptomatic and structural efficacy of a new hyaluronic acid compound, NRD101, in comparison with diacerein and placebo in a 1 year randomized controlled study in symptomatic knee osteoarthritis. Ann Rheum Dis 63:1611–1617, 2004.

90. Karatosun V, Unver B, Gocen Z, et al. Comparison of two hyaluronan drugs in patients with advanced osteoarthritis of the knee. A prospective, randomized, double-blind study with a long term follow-up. Clin Exp Rheumatol 23:213–218, 2005.

91. Atamaz F, Kirazil Y, Akkoc Y, et al. A comparison of two different intra-articular hyaluronan drugs and physical therapy in the management of knee osteoarthritis. Rheumatol Int DOI 10.1007.

92. Tikiz C, Unlu Z, Sener A, et al. Comparison of the efficacy of lower and higher molecular weight viscosupplementation in the treatment of hip osteoarthritis. Clin Rheumatol 24:244–250, 2005.

93. Kirchner M. Marshall D. A double-blind randomized controlled trial comparing alternate forms of high molecular weight hyaluronan for the treatment of osteoarthritis of the knee. Osteoarthritis Cartilage 14:154–162, 2006.

94. Kotevoglu N, Iyibozkurt PC, Hiz O, et al. A prospective randomized controlled clinical trial comparing the efficacy of different molecular weight hyaluran solutions in the treatment of knee osteoarthritis. Rheumatol Int 26:325–330, 2006.

95. Karatay S, Kiziltunc A, Yildirim K, et al. Effects of different hyaluronic acid products on synovial fluid levels of intercellular adhesion molecule-1 and vascular cell adhesion molecule-1 in knee osteoarthritis. Ann Clin Lab Sci 34:330–335, 2004.

96. Clarke S, Lock V, Duddy J, et al. Intra-articular hylan G-F 20 (Synvisc) in the management of patellofemoral osteoarthritis of the knee (POAK). Knee 12:57–62, 2005.

97. Conrozier T, Vignon E. Is there evidence to support the inclusion of viscosupplementation in the treatment paradigm for patients with hip osteoarthritis? Clin Exp Rheumatol 23:711–716, 2005.

98. Altman RD, Moskowitz R, Jacobs S, et al. A double-blind, randomized trial of intra-articular injection of sodium hyaluronate (Hyalgan®) for the treatment of chronic shoulder pain. Arthritis Rheum 52 (Suppl):S461, 2005.

99. Salk RS, Chang TJ, D'Costa WF, et al. Sodium hyaluronate in the treatment of osteoarthritis of the ankle: a controlled, randomized, double-blind pilot study. J Bone Joint Surg Am 88:295–302, 2006.

100. Pourbagher MA, Ozalay M, Pourbagher A. Accuracy and outcome of sonographically guided intra-articular sodium hyaluronate injections in patients with osteoarthritis of the hip. J Ultrasound Med 24:1391–1395, 2005.

101. Goldberg VM, Buckwalter JA. Hyaluronans in the treatment of osteoarthritis of the knee: evidence for disease-modifying activity. Osteoarthritis Cartilage 13:216–224, 2005.

102. Listrat V, Ayral X, Patarnello F, et al. Arthroscopic evaluation of potential structure modifying activity of hyaluronan (Hyalgan) in osteoarthritis of the knee. Osteoarthritis Cartilage 5:153–160, 1997.

103. Guidolin DD, Ronchetti JP, Lini E, et al. Morphological analysis of articular cartilage biopsies from a randomized, clinical study comparing the effects of 500-730 kDa sodium hyaluronate (Hyalgan) and methylprednisolone acetate on primary osteoarthritis of the knee. Osteoarthritis Cartilage 9:371–381, 2001.

104. Jubb RW, Piva S, Beinat L, et al. A one-year, randomized, placebo (saline) controlled clinical trial of 500-730 kDa sodium hyaluronate (Hyalgan) on the radiological change in osteoarthritis of the knee. Int J Clin Pract 57:467–474, 2003.

105. Luzar MJ, Altawil B. Pseudogout following intraarticular injection of sodium hyaluronate. Arthritis Rheum 41:939–941, 1998.

106. Kroesen S, Schmid W, Theiler R. Induction of an acute attack of calcium pyrophosphate dihydrate arthritis by intra-articular injection of hylan G-F 20 (Synvisc). Clin Rheumatol 19(2):147–149, 2000.

107. Goldberg VM, Coutts RD. Pseudoseptic reactions to hylan viscosupplementation: diagnosis and treatment. Clin Orthop Relat Res 419:130–137, 2004.

108. Leopold SS, Warme WJ, Pettis PD, et al. Increased frequency of acute local reaction to intra-articular hylan GF-20 (synvisc) in patients receiving more than one course of treatment. J Bone Joint Surg Am 84-A:1619–1623, 2002.

109. Roos J, Epaulard O, Juvin R. Acute pseudoseptic arthritis after Intraarticular sodium hyaluronan. Joint Bone Spine 71:352–354, 2004.

110. Albert C, Brocq O, Gerard D, et al. Septic knee arthritis after intra-articular hyaluronate injection. Joint Bone Spine DOI 10.1016.

111. Michou L, Job-Deslandre C, de Pinieux G, et al. Granulomatous synovitis after Intraarticular Hylan GF-20. A report of two cases. Joint Bone Spine 71:438–440, 2004.

112. Zardawi IM, Chan I. Synvisc perisynovitis. Pathology 33:519–520, 2001.

113. Sasaki M, Miuazaki T, Nakamura T, et al. Immunogenicity of hylan g-f 20 in guinea pigs and mice. J Rheumatol 31:943–950, 2004.

Complementary and Alternative Medicine

17

Sharon L. Kolasinski

INTRODUCTION

In 1993, the publication of a survey on the use of what was then termed "unconventional medicine"[1] surprised many in the traditional medical community. The report showed that in a nationwide sample of 1539 adults, 34% said they used some form of what has come to be known as complementary and alternative medicine (CAM) in the preceding year. In addition, it was estimated that expenditures on these types of therapies cost close to $14 billion, more than out-of-pocket annual expenditures on hospitalizations in the United States. In the ensuing years, it has become clear that the use of CAM has grown. More recently, the 2002 Centers for Disease Control National Health Interview Survey estimated from a sample of 31,044 U.S. adults that 49.8% have used CAM for health reasons.[2] Furthermore, a number of studies looking specifically at patients with rheumatic diseases, including osteoarthritis (OA), have found that they use CAM more frequently than the general public.[3] A 1997 survey showed that 63% of 232 patients surveyed with either rheumatoid arthritis (RA) or OA used some type of alternative care for their arthritis.[4] A 2001 survey of 480 elderly subjects with arthritis showed that 66% had used CAM for their arthritis.[5] The array of therapies has expanded as well. The Institute of Medicine estimated that in 2004, 29,000 products were on the market with 1,000 new products being developed annually.[6] Sales of dietary supplements alone accounted for $16 billion in annual sales,[6] and others have estimated that total costs for CAM to be comparable to the total out-of-pocket expenditures for physician services in the United States.[7]

The National Center for Complementary and Alternative Medicine (NCCAM) was established by Congress in 1998 to explore CAM therapies in a rigorous scientific context, train researchers, and disseminate authoritative information to the public and to health care professionals. NCCAM has defined CAM as a group of diverse medical and health care systems, practices, and products that are not presently considered to be part of conventional medicine. This definition is subject to change over time as various therapies are adopted into the standard treatment for OA or other diseases. The NCCAM divides these therapies into five categories: biologically based therapies such as dietary supplements and herbal products; alternative medicine systems such as homeopathy, naturopathy, traditional Chinese medicine, and Ayurvedic medicine; manipulative and body-based therapies such as chiropractic, osteopathy, and massage; mind-body interventions such as meditation and prayer; and energy therapies such as qi gong, Reiki, therapeutic touch, and the application of magnetic fields.

The reasons patients give for choosing CAM therapies are varied. Many arthritis patients cite "pain control" as the most important reason.[4] This may reflect the inadequacy of their current analgesia, but might also reflect the sense that patients using CAM are doing so on their own initiative. In addition, patients may view CAM therapies as less toxic than prescription medications.[4] Nonetheless, most CAM users are likely to be taking prescription medications along with their alternative therapies and to be under the care of medical physicians.[5] In fact, CAM users often feel that CAM used in combination with conventional medicine is more likely to help than either alone.[2]

GLUCOSAMINE

OA patients are cited as frequent CAM users in large part because of their high rate of consumption of glucosamine compounds. Glucosamine and chondroitin are used by over 5 million Americans each year[2] and accounted for close to $750 million in annual sales in 2004.[8] Glucosamine is an amino-monosaccharide and one of the basic constituents of the disaccharide units of articular cartilage glycosaminoglycans. Glucosamine is reduced in osteoarthritic cartilage, and, therefore, the notion of replenishing glucosamine by taking dietary supplements is appealing. However, just how useful glucosamine is as a therapy for OA, either for symptom relief or disease modification, remains controversial.

A considerable amount of in vitro and animal data has been amassed regarding potential mechanisms of action by which glucosamine could treat OA. Work from the 1990s suggested that glucosamine could stimulate proteoglycan synthesis by human chondrocytes and become incorporated into glycosaminoglycans.[9]

However, some have questioned whether or not glucosamine is absorbed in amounts large enough to significantly influence macromolecular synthesis in humans and whether glucosamine would be likely to arrive intact within articular cartilage and become available to the chondrocytes there. In vitro experiments in human chondrocytes show that more than 99% of the galactosamine in chondroitin sulfate (CS) is produced from endogenously produced glucose rather than from exogenously available H-glucosamine.[3,10] The circumstances under which proteoglycan production by chondrocytes would preferentially rely on exogenously administered glucosamine are unclear.[11]

Experiments have shown that orally administered glucosamine is detectable in rats given about 17 times the usual human dose (maximum level 100 μmol/L)[12] and in dogs given 8 times the human dose (maximum level 50 μmol/L).[13] Recently, glucosamine has been detected in human serum using high performance liquid chromatography after oral glucosamine ingestion.[14] Glucosamine levels were initially undetectable in all 18 subjects with OA tested. Subjects received 1500 mg of crystalline glucosamine sulfate mixed in water. In one subject, glucosamine levels remained undetectable throughout the subsequent 3 hours of testing. In the others, serum glucosamine levels reached a maximum of 4.8 (range 0-11.5) μmol/L at a mean of 2 hours after ingestion. Interestingly, subjects who had previously taken glucosamine had an earlier onset of a detectable level, delayed time to maximum level, and higher maximum levels. In two subjects, additional measurements showed a considerable reduction in glucosamine levels at 5 hours and a return to baseline undetectable levels at 8 hours. Based on these pharmacokinetic data, the investigators felt it was unlikely that glucosamine contributes to chondroitin synthesis in vivo.

Other work has suggested that glucosamine might have additional effects and some of these might be relevant to a potential beneficial mechanism of action in OA. They include countering enzymatic or inflammatory processes leading to degradation of cartilage. At concentrations of 50 to 400 μmol/L, glucosamine inhibits IL-1β–induced matrix metalloproteinase activity in human OA articular chondrocytes.[15] At concentrations of 5 mmol/L, glucosamine inhibits aggrecanase-mediated degradation of aggrecan in explant cultures of bovine articular cartilage.[16] Glucosamine at concentrations of 1 to 4.5 mg/mL in culture with rat chondrocytes antagonizes IL-1β–induced nitric oxide and prostaglandin E2 production.[17] It was recently shown that glucosamine effects on MMP-13, aggrecanase 1, and IL-1β–induced expression of inducible nitric oxide synthase and cyclooxygenase 2 may occur at the level of gene expression. Reductions in corresponding levels of mRNA were detected in normal equine chondrocyte culture at glucosamine concentrations of only 10 μg/mL.[18] Interestingly, it has recently been shown that orally administered glucosamine sulfate, dosed at 1500 mg/d for 14 days, is detectable in the plasma and synovial fluid of subjects with knee OA at concentrations of 7.9 $\pm$ 3.9 μM and 7.2 $\pm$ 3.2 μM, respectively,[19] 3 hours after the last dose has been given.

Many short term clinical trials were carried out over a number of years to assess the analgesic efficacy of glucosamine in the treatment of osteoarthritis. Each was small and short term and meta-analyses were subsequently carried out on a number of these trials to clarify their conclusions. One meta-analysis of many of the early trials[20] suggested that there was short-term analgesic benefit from the use of glucosamine and that short-term use was safe. The magnitude of the effect was comparable to that seen with nonsteroidal anti-inflammatory drugs (NSAIDs) but delayed in onset by weeks by comparison. Larger trials have since been carried out and further meta-analyses done. The first of the larger and longer term trials involved 212 subjects with osteoarthritis of the knee who received either oral glucosamine at a dose of 1500 mg daily or placebo for 3 years.[21] Subjects were evaluated using the Western Ontario and McMaster Universities Osteoarthritis Index (WOMAC) and with weight-bearing anteroposterior view radiographs of the knees. Fluoroscopy was used to correct lower limb positioning for the radiographs. The trial showed that subjects who received glucosamine had modest pain reduction based on the WOMAC (average of 11.7% reduction in WOMAC score in the intention to treat analysis), while those in the placebo group worsened (average of 9.8% worsening) and the difference between these average scores was statistically significant. Radiographs of those who received placebo showed a mean of 0.31 mm (range: 0.13-0.48 mm loss) of joint space narrowing in the medial joint compartment at the end of 3 years in the intention to treat analysis. Those who received glucosamine had a mean of 0.06 mm of joint space narrowing (range: 0.22-mm loss to 0.09-mm gain). The difference between these two mean figures was statistically significant. Interestingly, there was no correlation between the improvement of symptoms and radiographic findings. The side effects of glucosamine did not differ from those of placebo.

A subsequent study of 202 subjects used a similar trial design and got similar results.[22] Participants were randomized to receive either 1500 mg of crystalline glucosamine sulfate or placebo for 3 years. In the intention to treat analysis at 3 years, the subjects treated with glucosamine had a mean reduction of 8 points in their WOMAC total scores (from a total of 30.48 points at baseline), while those in the placebo group had a mean reduction of 4.9 points (from a total of 30.70 points at baseline). This was a statistically significant difference. Intention to treat analysis of radiographs of those who received placebo showed a mean of 0.19 mm (range: 0.09-0.29 mm loss) of joint space narrowing on anteroposterior weight-bearing radiographs of the knee in full extension with fluoroscopic positioning of the center of the x-ray beam. In the glucosamine treated group, there was a mean gain in joint space of 0.04 mm (range: 0.06 mm loss to 0.14 mm gain). This difference was statistically significant. Again, glucosamine did not differ from placebo in the frequency or type of side effects noted.

Both of these studies have been interpreted to support the contention that glucosamine is a disease-modifying treatment for osteoarthritis. Acceptance of this conclusion hinges on the interpretation of the radiographic outcome measures used. Subsequent studies have suggested that the reliability and reproducibility of the anteroposterior knee radiograph as a measure of OA progression can be influenced by a number of technical[23] and patient specific[24] factors. Unequivocal evidence of the ability of glucosamine to modify structure in OA awaits the development of more precise outcome measures.

Additional studies and meta-analyses have cast doubt on the ability of glucosamine to modify symptoms in a meaningful way in OA. One discontinuation trial has recently been published.[25] This study enrolled 137 current users of glucosamine (whether subjects used the sulfate or hydrochloride formula was not specified) who had experienced subjective improvement in their knee pain when they started using glucosamine. Participants were randomized to receive either 1500 mg of glucosamine sulfate in tablet form or placebo for 6 months. They were assessed throughout the trial for the presence of a disease flare, defined as either the patient's perception of worsening of symptoms with a concomitant increase of at least 20 mm in WOMAC pain on walking (using a visual analog scale) or a worsening of the physician global assessment by at least 1 grade (on a 1 to 5 scale). In the intention to treat analysis, 28 (42%) of the 66 subjects in the placebo group and 32 (45%) of the 71 subjects in the glucosamine group experienced a disease flare. These were statistically indistinguishable.

Many had hoped that the National Institutes of Health-sponsored Glucosamine/Chondroitin Arthritis Intervention Trial (GAIT) would clarify whether or not glucosamine was a significant agent for symptom or structure modification. Radiographic data have yet to be published, but the data on symptom relief recently reported failed to end the controversy about the utility of glucosamine.[26] The GAIT trial was innovative in its use of a five-arm intervention of either glucosamine 1500 mg daily; chondroitin 1200 mg daily; the combination of glucosamine and chondroitin; a cyclooxygenase inhibitor; and placebo. Overall, glucosamine, chondroitin, and the combination of the two were no better at relieving OA symptoms than placebo

measured by WOMAC, health assessment questionnaire, or patient or physician global assessments. Use of chondroitin, but not glucosamine or the combination, was associated with a statistically significant reduction in the number of patients found to have a joint effusion or swelling on clinical examination. In subjects with moderate to severe pain, the combination of glucosamine and chondroitin, but neither alone nor the cyclooxygenase inhibitor, was better than placebo at relieving symptoms in this group. The high placebo response in this trial, as well as the relatively mild degree of pain among many of the participants, makes meaningful interpretation of these findings limited.

The most recent meta-analysis to review the glucosamine literature was published through the Cochrane Collaboration.[27] This update reviewed 20 randomized, controlled trials that included 2570 subjects. Collectively, the studies showed that glucosamine favored placebo with a 28% improvement in pain and a 21% improvement in function using the Lequesne Index, but that WOMAC pain, function, and stiffness outcomes did not reach statistical significance. When the analysis was restricted to eight studies with adequate allocation concealment, none showed improvement in pain or function. Ten trials used the crystalline glucosamine preparation available from Rotta Pharmaceuticals. When these trials were analyzed separately, glucosamine was found to be superior to placebo in improving pain and function using the Lequesne Index. Two of the latter trials were also those that have suggested a slowing of radiographic progression. The authors noted that compared to the 1999 Cochrane review, this updated analysis suggested that there was high-quality evidence that glucosamine was not as useful for symptom improvement as had previously been thought. The potential impact of the involvement of glucosamine manufacturers in the sponsorship, design, or reporting of clinical trials of glucosamine has been discussed elsewhere.[28]

CHONDROITIN SULFATE

Like glucosamine, CS is an important constituent of normal joint tissue. CS levels are altered in OA cartilage, plasma, and synovial fluid.[29] In vitro work has similarly suggested a variety of mechanisms, in addition to a contribution to structural integrity, through which this glycosaminoglycan might be useful in the treatment of OA. However, the link between potential therapeutic effects and a definitive demonstration of efficacy in OA is no clearer for CS than for glucosamine. In part, this is because there have been fewer clinical trials examining the utility of CS than that of glucosamine, and the CS trials have generally been of short duration.

CS appears to be less readily absorbed after oral administration than glucosamine.[30] After oral administration of CS from shark cartilage, healthy volunteers showed considerable variability in absorption measured by disaccharide pattern evaluation on agarose gel electrophoresis and high performance liquid chromatography. All subjects had detectable levels of CS by 48 hours, but some had peak levels as early as 4 hours postingestion. The t_{max} of shark-derived cartilage was estimated to be 8.7 hours, compared with 2.4 hours for bovine CS.

Addition of CS to cultured chondrocytes derived from osteoarthritic joints results in significant increases in total proteoglycan production.[9,31] This effect occurs at concentrations as low as 100 µg/mL. When mixed in chondrocyte culture with interleukin-1β, CS will counteract the effects of IL-1β.[31] This includes reversing the decrease in proteoglycan production seen with IL-1β. Interestingly, although CS itself does not affect collagen II production, it inhibits the reduction in collagen II production caused by IL-1β. Furthermore, CS itself decreases prostaglandin E2 production and counters IL-1β–induced increases as well. Higher concentrations of CS, up to 500 to 1000 µg/mL, are needed to inhibit some of these IL-1β–induced effects. CS may also inhibit collagenolytic activity[9] and matrix metalloproteinase production in chondrocyte culture derived from patients with hip OA.[32] Data can be found to support and to refute the contention that CS has an effect on pretranslational regulation of genes for matrix metalloproteinases, aggrecanase, nitric oxide synthase, or cyclooxygenase.[18,33]

Animal studies have suggested that supplementation with CS can reduce the progression of articular cartilage lesions in the rabbit instability model, but not in the rabbit continuous immobilization model of OA. In the rabbit instability model, investigators found that CS supplementation fails to prevent osteophyte formation but did reduce cartilage lesions.[34] The combination of CS with glucosamine appeared synergistic and reduced the extent of both moderate and severe cartilage lesions more dramatically than either agent alone. Using a different model of OA, a subsequent study found different results. In this recent study using the rabbit continuous immobilization model, animals underwent limb immobilization for 12 weeks with half treated with CS. Osteophytes and subchondral cysts were not seen in these animals, but clefts, fibrillations, irregularity of the surface and chondrocyte disorganization and clusters, invasion of blood vessels, and erosions were seen. CS supplementation was not protective against these histological changes, and the results were similar in the chondroitin-treated and chondroitin-untreated groups.[35]

A meta-analysis of clinical trials evaluating the efficacy of CS prior to 2000 suggested that CS has modest efficacy for symptomatic management of OA.[20] Nine trials were analyzed and all found that CS was significantly more efficacious than placebo in the treatment of OA pain. However, when the studies were evaluated for quality, the authors found that the higher quality trials showed lower efficacy for CS. Methodological shortcomings included lack of intention to treat analysis, reporting of allocation concealment, and industry sponsorship. Nonetheless, the overall effect size for CS was considered large.

An abstract publication in 1998 suggested that administration of 1200 mg daily of CS was associated with a slowing of the progression of finger joint OA.[36] In this randomized, double-blind, placebo-controlled study, 119 subjects had anteroposterior radiographs of the hands at entry and at yearly intervals. At the conclusion of the study at 3 years, those treated with CS were found to have a significant reduction in the number of new erosive radiographic findings. In contrast, a more recent study of 24 subjects with erosive OA of the hands randomized participants to receive CS 800 mg daily plus naproxen or naproxen alone for 2 years.[37] Both groups significantly worsened over time in terms of radiographic changes and in terms of symptoms measured by the Dreiser index. The small size of this study makes it difficult to assess its generalizability.

One clinical trial used an intermittent dosing treatment schedule to test whether or not CS was efficacious in knee OA.[38] The authors felt this dosing schedule was reasonable given the hypothetically prolonged effect of CS. In this study, 120 subjects received either 800 mg daily of granulated bovine CS 4 and 6 sulfate mixed in water or an identical placebo with CS given from entry to month 3 and between months 6 and 9. In the intention to treat analysis, 110 participants were assessed and were found to have significantly greater improvements in the Lequesne index, visual analog scale measurements for pain and walking time than those in the placebo group. Radiographic evaluation showed that those in the placebo group had significant decreases in the joint space surface area, the mean joint space width, and the minimum joint space width. Those in the chondroitin-treated group showed no radiographic changes. CS had an excellent safety profile in this trial. The authors suggested that larger scale trials were warranted.

The largest trial of CS for the treatment of OA to date evaluated radiographic changes in knees.[39] In this randomized, double-blind, placebo-controlled trial, 300 participants received either CS 800 mg daily or placebo for 2 years. Using intention to treat analysis, the authors concluded that those who received CS had no significant change in joint space narrowing measured on anteroposterior radiographs of the knee in flexion. In contrast, the placebo-treated group had a mean progression of joint space narrowing of 0.14 ± 0.61 mm after 2 years, a statistically significant difference. Results were similar for minimum joint space width. However, there was no significant symptomatic effect measured by the WOMAC, and similar amounts of rescue drug were needed by chondroitin-treated and placebo-treated subjects alike. The authors suggested that this reflected the relatively low level of pain of those entered in the study. Adverse events did not differ significantly between the groups.

Whether the combination of glucosamine and CS is more efficacious than either alone for the treatment of symptoms or progression of radiographic change in OA remains unclear. Almost none of the in vitro or animal model data looks at the effects of the combination in comparison to either substance alone,[34] although the possibility of synergistic effects seems worthy of further investigation.[26]

VITAMINS

There has long been recognition that nutritional factors influence the maintenance of bone and joint health, but evidence to support the use of specific vitamin therapies for OA has not yet been compelling. Nonetheless, vitamin supplements remain among the most frequently used options chosen by patients from the CAM menu.[2]

Vitamin C is important for the growth, development, and enzymatic reactions of bone and cartilage. Vitamin C acts as an antioxidant in facilitating the hydroxylation of proline and lysine to hydroxyproline and hydroxylysine in procollagen. These products are essential to the maturation of collagen molecules and, thus, to the construction of the extracellular matrix of cartilage. This mechanism has been explored in the guinea pig model of surgically induced OA and in the spontaneous OA model. These animals, like humans, cannot synthesize ascorbic acid. Therefore they must obtain vitamin C through the diet. In guinea pigs fed a diet poor in vitamin C, proteoglycan synthesis declines. This may be related to alterations in enzymatic activity or reductions in proline hydroxylation or both.[40] Early work on a surgically induced model of OA in the guinea pig showed that animals who received low-dose supplementation with vitamin C (a dose adequate to prevent scurvy) had more severe OA that those on high-dose supplementation (60 times as much) over a several week period. Because animals receiving higher doses had higher cartilage weights, it was hypothesized that vitamin C protected against cartilage loss by stimulating collagen synthesis.[41] However, more recent work has suggested that long-term exposure to vitamin C supplementation might have deleterious effects.[42] In these experiments, no surgical procedures were performed and the animals developed spontaneous OA. Guinea pigs were supplemented with low, medium, and high doses of vitamin C for 8 months. On subsequent histological evaluation, the animals that had received the medium and high doses had more severe histological changes, including the formation of osteophytes. The investigators hypothesized that the process of chondrophyte formation, with evolution into osteophytes, may have been facilitated by the enhanced collagen synthesis afforded by higher doses of ascorbic acid.

On the basis of the most recent guinea pig data, it has been suggested that vitamin C supplementation above the currently recommended daily doses of 75 to 90 mg not be advised.[42] No prospective data are yet available to offer guidance in this area. The only human data comes from an epidemiological investigation using the Framingham population.[43] In this study, vitamin C intake was measured by food frequency questionnaire. The study compared 453 subjects without evidence of OA to 187 subjects with radiographic knee OA. The investigators found no correlation between vitamin C intake assessed at a single time point and the incidence of OA. However, they did identify a threefold reduction in the risk of OA (measured as radiographic evidence of cartilage loss) in the middle and highest tertiles of vitamin C intake. This observation suggests that further investigation is needed to clarify the role of vitamin C in human OA.

Whether or not additional mechanisms exist by which antioxidant supplements might be of benefit in OA is speculative,[44] but interest in the use of antioxidants as therapeutic agents remains high among patients. The potential link between antioxidants in the diet, other than vitamin C, and osteoarthritis was also investigated in the Framingham population.[43] Like vitamin C, β-carotene intake (OR = 0.3) and vitamin E intake (OR = 0.7) were associated, though more weakly, with a reduction in risk of OA progression. The role of β-carotene intake in the development or progression of OA has not been further investigated. Further work is available on vitamin E. Data from the Johnston County Osteoarthritis Project in North Carolina suggests that those with the highest ratios of serum α-tocopherol to γ-tocopherol had half the odds of radiographic knee OA.[45] This relationship was statistically significant in men and African Americans, but not for women or other ethnic groups among 400 participants studied. One prospective supplementation trial of vitamin E use for OA has been carried out. In this trial, 136 subjects were randomized to receive either vitamin E 500 IU or placebo for 2 years. Patients were followed with magnetic resonance imaging to measure tibial cartilage volume. There was no difference in medial or lateral tibial cartilage volume loss between the vitamin E supplemented group and those who got placebo at the end of the trial. Furthermore, there was no relationship between dietary levels of antioxidants and cartilage volume loss. Taken together, these findings suggest that simple supplementation with vitamins is unlikely to be a straightforward treatment for OA.

The role of vitamin D in bone health is clear and some epidemiological evidence suggests that vitamin D intake might be linked to the incidence or progression of OA as well. Framingham data[46] suggest that incident OA is not related to vitamin D intake. However, in a study of 556 subjects in which 75 had a new onset of OA and 62 had progression of OA, progression was related to vitamin D levels. Investigators found that the risk of progression increased threefold in those in the middle and lowest tertiles of vitamin D intake measured by serum levels of vitamin D and food frequency questionnaires. Low levels of serum vitamin D also predicted loss of cartilage assessed by joint space narrowing and the presence of osteophytes on knee radiographs. A second epidemiologic study suggested that incident OA in the hip was associated with vitamin D intake.[47] In the Study of Osteoporotic Fractures, investigators obtained baseline and followup hip radiographs an average of 8 years apart, and baseline serum vitamin D levels were obtained. The risk of incident hip OA, defined as the development of definite joint space narrowing, was increased in subjects in the middle and lowest tertiles for 25(OH) vitamin D, more than threefold compared to those with the highest vitamin D levels. The precise manner in which vitamin D should be supplemented in those at risk for OA or who have OA is unknown. No prospective treatment trials have been carried out.

HERBAL SUPPLEMENTS

A variety of herbal supplements have been investigated in well-designed, randomized, controlled trials for the treatment of osteoarthritis symptoms. However, they have generally been small in size and limited in duration. Some have suggested that the 1994 Dietary Supplement and Health Education Act (DSHEA) has had the unintended consequence of limiting research on herbal medicines. Under DSHEA, herbal medicines can be designated as "dietary supplements" and, as such, they are regulated like food, not drugs. Products having this designation are exempt from the safety and efficacy studies required of prescription drugs, and their manufacturers are not required to collect and report their postmarketing experience. The Act provides that dietary supplements are considered safe until proven otherwise. Because this legislation permits the sale of products for health promotion without rigorous studies to prove efficacy, there is no economic benefit to carrying out clinical trials. Nonetheless, several interesting plant-based supplements have been the subject of investigation.

Avocado Soybean Unsaponifiables

Laboratory evidence suggests that the unsaponifiable fractions of a mixture of 1 part avocado oil to 2 parts soybean oil has properties that might make it useful in the treatment of OA symptoms. In articular chondrocyte cultures, avocado soybean unsaponifiables (ASU) inhibits IL-1β and the stimulatory effects of IL-1β on matrix metalloproteinase, IL-6, IL-8, prostaglandin E$_2$, and collagenase. Further, it may stimulate collagen synthesis.[48] In one rabbit OA model, ASU significantly reduced the occurrence of postcontusion lesions. A few small studies have been carried out in patients with OA of the hip and knee. In one trial, subjects with radiographic evidence of disease who required NSAIDs for symptom management were enrolled, 114 with knee OA and 50 with hip OA.[49] They were randomized to receive either 300 mg ASU or placebo capsules daily for 6 months. The authors found that those who received ASU had significant improvements in pain and function as measured by the Lequesne index. However, they did not show a statistically significant reduction in NSAID requirements. Positive treatment effects were detected only after a delay of 2 months. A second trial evaluated whether or not structural effects could be attributed to the use of ASU.[50] In this study, 108 participants with hip OA were examined radiographically before and after 2 years of treatment with 300 mg ASU daily. No difference between the treated and placebo groups was detected overall, though a posthoc analysis showed that ASU was associated with less joint space narrowing in the group with more severe disease at baseline (i.e. baseline joint space width is $\le$ the median).

Ginger

Ginger is an ingredient in herbal medicinals used in the Chinese and Ayurvedic traditions for millennia. Often derived from several plants, ginger is frequently used in combination with a variety of herbs and the potentially pharmacologically active components and mechanisms of action are unclear. Anti-inflammatory effects have been suggested from in vitro and animal model experiments. Several trials have been carried out, all with manufacturer support. A study of 247 subjects with knee OA evaluated outcomes after 6 weeks of treatment with Eurovita ginger extract or placebo.[51] The percentage of responders with regard to reduction in knee pain on standing was larger in the treated group (63%) than in the placebo group (50%). Mean values for reduction in knee pain after walking 50 feet and WOMAC scores were also statistically significantly better in the treatment group. Another trial compared 3 weeks of treatment with Eurovita ginger extract to treatment with ibuprofen 1200 mg daily.[52] Ibuprofen was found to be superior using the Lequesne Index and pain visual analog scale (VAS) in the 56 subjects who completed the study. In a third trial, 29 subjects were randomly assigned to receive Zintona EC, a commercially available ginger extract or placebo.[53] This trial had a double-blind design with crossover after 3 months. At the 12 week time of crossover, no statistically significant differences were noted between the groups. Only 19 participants completed the trial. At 24 weeks, those who started placebo first had a statistically significant improvement in the level of their pain and functional disability measured by VAS compared to those who started Zintona EC first. The investigators suggested that this result supported the hypothesis that ginger might have a delayed onset of action.

Single small trials of a variety of herbal agents have appeared in the literature, but the very limited nature of the available data makes the efficacy of these agents and combination products difficult to assess. Many of these trials have been reviewed elsewhere.[54,55,56]

METHYLSULFONYL METHANE

Methylsulfonyl methane (MSM) is a common ingredient in many over-the-counter topical preparations and oral dietary supplements sold for a variety of health concerns including arthritis.[57] Marketed as a treatment for both RA and osteoarthritis, MSM gained initial popularity as an odorless, tasteless alternative to dimethylsulfoxide (DMSO) that had been in use for decades as a liniment for veterinary and human aches and pains. Despite multimillion dollar sales and tremendous popularity, fueled by lay publications and celebrity endorsements, very little evidence is available in the medical literature to evaluate the role of MSM in OA treatment. No data are available regarding potential mechanism(s) of action, but one study was unable to detect toxicity in rats given doses of MSM by gavage of either a single bolus of 2 g/kg or a 90-day course of 1.5 g/kg/day.[58] A recent report of use in humans suggested that MSM at a dose of 6 g/d for 12 weeks improved WOMAC pain and function.[59] The authors of this randomized, double-blind, placebo-controlled trial of 50 participants noted, however, that the effect they documented was so slight that it called into question whether or not it was clinically meaningful.

NONPHARMACOLOGIC INTERVENTIONS

Nonpharmacologic therapies are a mainstay of treatment in OA and a variety of interventions in this category are recommended by the American College of Rheumatology[60] and the European League Against Rheumatism.[61,62] Particularly prominent among the recommendations of both groups are a variety of exercises and physical interventions. CAM includes several possible modalities that might be candidates for addition to these lists of nonpharmacologic intervention.

Acupuncture

Acupuncture is a practice that began over 2000 years ago in China. It is based on the assumption that the placement of needles in certain locations on the body will permit the flow of energy or chi. The traditional concept is that disease blocks chi and that needle insertion along predefined channels, or meridia, unblocks chi. A considerable body of work has suggested that the mechanism of analgesia reported to result from acupuncture involves stimulation of endorphin production since the effect can be reduced by naloxone.[63] The evaluation of acupuncture as a viable therapy for OA has been hampered by the development of appropriate controls, given the impossibility of blinding the investigator and the difficulty of blinding the subject.

A meta-analysis of 7 acupuncture trials that included 393 OA patients[64] was performed. It showed that for pain and function there was limited evidence that acupuncture was more effective than being on a waiting list for treatment or receiving treatment as usual. For pain, there was strong evidence that acupuncture was superior to sham needling. However, for function, there was only inconclusive evidence of the efficacy of acupuncture. Data were insufficient to indicate whether or not acupuncture was similar in efficacy to other treatments for knee OA.

A large and well-designed trial of acupuncture for osteoarthritis has recently been published.[65] The acupuncture intervention used included needle placement at five local points (Yanglinquan, Yinlinquan, Zhusanli, Dubi, and Xiyan) and four distal points (Kunlun, Xuanzhong, Sanyinjiao, and Taixi) for a total of nine needles in each affected leg. Needles were 32 gauge and inserted to a depth of 0.6 to 1.0 inch. All participants who received true acupuncture were said to experience de chi, the local sensation of heaviness, soreness, numbness, or paresthesia that accompanies needle insertion. In addition to needle placement, electrical stimulation was applied at the knee points for 20 minutes. Two needles were also taped with adhesive tape to sham points on the abdomen. The design included both a form of sham acupuncture and an education control group. In the sham acupuncture group, needles were inserted into the sham abdominal points but only taped to the surface in the true acupuncture points. Electrical stimulation did not occur but the participants in this group attended sessions on the same schedule as the true acupuncture group. The education control group consisted of six 2-hour sessions based on the Arthritis Self-Management Program of the Arthritis Foundation. The

trial enrolled 570 participants with radiographic knee OA with at least one osteophyte and moderate to severe pain. Participants in the true and sham acupuncture groups received 25 sessions. Pain levels were statistically significantly reduced in the true acupuncture group compared to the sham acupuncture group at weeks 14 and 26. The true acupuncture group's improvement in function measured by WOMAC from baseline was statistically significantly greater than that in the sham group at 8, 14, and 26 weeks. There were no significant differences between the true and sham acupuncture groups with regard to patient global assessment, Short Form-36, or 6-minute walk time.

Yoga

Yoga is an ancient Indian practice that includes the assumption of physical postures, attention to breathing, and meditation in an attempt to harmonize mind, body, and spirit. A few small studies have assessed the efficacy of yoga for the treatment of symptoms of OA. The first of these involved the use of a variety of yoga postures for OA of the hand.[66] Compared to those who received no treatment, those who participated in an 8-week yoga program showed improvements in reported pain during activities, joint tenderness, and finger range of motion.

A pilot study exploring the feasibility of using yoga as a therapeutic intervention in symptomatic knee OA patients was recently published.[67] In this small trial, seven subjects were assessed by WOMAC before and after an 8-week course of Iyengar yoga modified to the needs of a group of obese, middle-aged women. When compared to their pre-intervention status, the participants had significant improvements in WOMAC pain and disability scores. Improvements in WOMAC stiffness and physician and patient VAS for pain following completion of the yoga intervention were not significant. Subsequent evaluation of a second small pilot group[68] by the same investigators suggested that a variety of temporal and distance footfall parameters and lower extremity three-dimensional kinematics and kinetics were altered by an 8-week course of yoga permitting an increase in walking speed. A second trial, which included formal gait analysis[69] before and after subjects with knee OA participated in a therapeutic yoga program, also found measurable differences in gait parameters.

Tai Chi

The practice of tai chi is an ancient Chinese form of exercise for health promotion and self-defense. It evokes cognitive, cardiovascular, and musculoskeletal responses that produce physiological and psychological alterations. Tai chi exercises include gentle flowing movements that are thought to enhance mobility and flexibility and that have been demonstrated to improve fitness and reduce falls in the elderly.[70,71] A study of 33 elderly subjects with lower extremity OA was performed. It showed that participation in two 1-hour tai chi classes for 12 weeks improved self-efficacy.[72] Self-efficacy for arthritis symptoms, total arthritis self-efficacy, level of tension, and satisfaction with general health significantly improved as measured by the Arthritis Self-Efficacy Scale.

A second small study randomized 43 subjects to a 12-week tai chi class or no intervention.[73] A high dropout rate was noted (41%). No significant differences were found in flexibility, upper body strength, or knee strength between the groups. However, the tai chi group did have significantly less pain and stiffness and perceived fewer difficulties with physical functioning. Significant improvements were measurable on physical fitness testing in balance and abdominal muscle strength. The authors suggested that a larger, longitudinal study would be appropriate.

CONCLUSION

As long as the majority of patients with osteoarthritis are choosing to use CAM therapies, most of them along with conventional medical treatments, it will remain important that physicians are well informed about which therapies are available and how well supported they are using rigorous scientific standards. Many dietary supplements, including a host of herbal products, as well as physical interventions are worthy of further study. In vitro and animal model data suggest some have potential effects on important pathways in the pathogenesis of OA. However, the current state of the literature makes the definition of clear guidelines for use in humans problematic.

REFERENCES

1. Eisenberg DM, Kessler RC, Foster C, et al. Unconventional medicine in the United States—Prevalence, costs, and patterns of use. NEJM 328:246–252, 1993.
2. Barnes PM, Powell-Griner E, McFann K, et al. Complementary and alternative medicine use among adults: United States, 2002. Advance Data from Vital and Health Statistics No. 343, May 27, 2004, Centers for Disease Control and Prevention National Center for Health Statistics.
3. Quandt SA, Chen H, Grzywacz JG, et al. Use of complementary and alternative medicine by persons with arthritis: results of the National Health Interview Survey. Arthritis Rheum:53:748–755, 2005.
4. Rao JK, Mihaliak K, Kroenke K, et al. Use of complementary therapies for arthritis among patients of rheumatologists. Ann Intern Med 131:409–416, 1999.
5. Kaboli PJ, Doebbeling BN, Saag KG, et al. Use of complementary and alternative medicine by older patients with arthritis: a population-based study. Arthritis Care Res:45:398–403, 2001.
6. Committee on the Framework for Evaluating the Safety of Dietary Supplements. Dietary supplements. a framework for evaluating safety. Washington: The National Academies Press, 2005.
7. Eisenberg DM, Davis RB, Ettner SL, et al. Trends in alternative medicine use in the United States, 1990–1997. JAMA 280:1569–1575, 1998.
8. Kolata G. 2 Top-selling arthritis drugs are found to be ineffective. NY Times Thursday, February 23, 2006.
9. Bassleer C, Henrotin Y, Franchimont P. In vitro evaluation of drugs proposed as chondroprotective agents. Int J Tissue React 14:231–240, 1992.
10. Mroz PJ, Silbert JE. Use of [³H]glucosamine and [³⁵S]sulfate with cultured human chondrocytes to determine effects of glucosamine concentration on formation of [³H]chondroitin. Arthritis Rheum 50:3574–3579, 2004.
11. Felson DT, McAlindon TE. Glucosamine and chondroitin for osteoarthritis: to recommend or not to recommend? Arthritis Care Res 13:179–182, 2000.
12. Aghazadeh-Habashi A, Sattari S, Pasutto F, et al. Single dose pharmacokinetics and bioavailability of glucosamine in the rat. J Pharm Pharm Sci 5:181–184, 2002.
13. Adebowale A, Du J, Liang Z, et al. The bioavailability and pharmacokinetics of glucosamine hydrochloride and low molecular weight chondroitin sulfate after single and multiple doses to beagle dogs. Biopharm Drug Dispos 23:217–225, 2002.
14. Biggee BA, Blinn CM, McAlindon TE, et al. Low levels of human serum glucosamine after ingestion of glucosamine sulfate relative to capability for peripheral effectiveness. Ann Rheum Dis 65:222–226, 2006.
15. Dodge GR, Jimenez SA. Glucosamine sulfate modulates the level of aggrecan and matrix metalloproteinase-3 synthesized by cultured human osteoarthritis articular chondrocytes. Osteoarthritis Cartilage 11:424–432, 2003.
16. Ilic MZ, Martinac B, Handley CJ. Effects of long term exposure to glucosamine and mannosamine on aggrecan degradation in articular cartilage. Osteoarthritis Cartilage 11:613–622, 2003.
17. Gouze JN, Bordji K, Gulberti S, et al. Interleukin-1beta down-regulates the expression of glucuronosyltransferase I, a key enzyme priming glycosaminoglycan biosynthesis: influence of glucosamine on interleukin-1beta-mediated effects in rat chondrocytes. Arthritis Rheum 44:351–360, 2001.
18. Neil KM, Orth MW, Coussens PM, et al. Effects of glucosamine and chondroitin sulfate on mediators of osteoarthritis in cultured equine chondrocytes stimulated by use of recombinant equine interleukin-1ß. Am J Vet Res 66:1861–1869, 2005.
19. Persiani S, Rotini R, Trisolino G, et al. Glucosamine plasma and synovial fluid concentrations before and after oral administration of crystalline glucosamine sulfate in knee osteoarthritis patients. Osteoarthritis Cartilage 13:S94, 2005.
20. McAlindon TE, LaValley MP, Gulin JP, et al. Glucosamine and chondroitin for treatment of osteoarthritis: a systematic quality assessment and meta-analysis. JAMA 283:1469–1475, 2000.
21. Reginster JY, Deroisy, R, Rovati LC, et al. Long-term effects of glucosamine sulfate on osteoarthritis progression: a randomized, placebo-controlled clinical trial. Lancet 357:251–256, 2001.
22. Pavelka K, Gatterova J, Olejarova M, et al. Glucosamine sulfate use and delay of progression of knee osteoarthritis. Arch Int Med 162:2113–2123, 2002.
23. Mazzuca SA, Brandt KD, Dieppe PA, et al. Effect of alignment of the medial tibial plateau and x-ray beam on apparent progression of osteoarthritis in the standing anteroposterior knee radiograph. Arthritis Rheum 44:1786–1794, 2001.
24. Mazzuca SA, Brandt KD, Lane KA, et al. Knee pain reduces joint space width in conventional standing anteroposterior radiographs of osteoarthritic knees. Arthritis Rheum 46:1223–1227, 2002.
25. Cibere J, Kopec JA, Thorne A, et al. Randomized, double-blind, placebo-controlled glucosamine discontinuation trial in knee osteoarthritis. Arthritis Rheum 51:738–745, 2004.
26. Clegg DO, Reda DJ, Harris CL, et al. Glucosamine, chondroitin sulfate and the two in combination for painful knee osteoarthritis. NEJM 354:795–808, 2006.
27. Towheed TE, Maxwell L, Anastassiades TP, et al. Glucosamine therapy for treating osteoarthritis. The Cochrane Database of Systematic Reviews 2005, Issue 2. Art. No.:CD002946.pub2.
28. McAlindon, T. Why are clinical trials of glucosamine no longer uniformly positive? Rheum Dis Clin North Am 29:789–801, 2003.
29. Lewis S, Crossman M, Flannelly J, et al. Chondroitin sulphation patterns in synovial fluid in osteoarthritis subsets. Ann Rheum Dis 58:441–445, 1999.
30. Volpi N. Oral absorption and bioavailability of ichthyic origin chondroitin sulfate in healthy male volunteers. Osteoarthritis Cartilage 11:433–441, 2003.
31. Bassleer CT, Combal JPA, Bougaret S, et al. Effects of chondroitin sulfate and interleukin-1ß on human articular chondrocytes cultivated in clusters. Osteoarthritis Cartilage 6:196–204, 1998.
32. Monfort J, Nacher M, Montel E, et al. Chondroitin sulfate and hyaluronic acid (500-730 kda) inhibit stromelysin-1 synthesis in human osteoarthritic chondrocytes. Drugs Exp Clin Res 31:71–76, 2005.

33. Chan PS, Caron JP, Rosa GJ, et al. Glucosamine and chondroitin regulate gene expression and synthesis of nitric oxide and prostaglandin E(2) in articular cartilage explants. Osteoarthritis Cartilage 13:387–394, 2005.
34. Lippiello L, Woodward J, Karpman R, et al. In vivo chondroprotection and metabolic synergy of glucosamine and chondroitin sulfate. Clin Ortho Related Res 381:229–240, 2000.
35. Torrelli SR, Rahal SC, Volpi RS, et al. Histopathological evaluation of treatment with chondroitin sulfate for osteoarthritis induced by continuous immobilization in rabbits. J Vet Med 52:45–51, 2005.
36. Verbruggen G, Goemaere S, Veys EM. Chondroitin sulfate: S/DMOAD (structure/disease modifying anti-osteoarthritis drug) in the treatment of finger joint OA. Osteoarthritis Cartilage 6 Suppl:A37–38, 1998.
37. Rovetta G, Monteforte P, Molfetta G, et al. A two-year study of chondroitin sulfate in erosive osteoarthritis of the hands: behavior of erosions, osteophytes, pain and hand dysfunction. Drugs Exptl Clin Res 30:11–16, 2004.
38. Uebelhart D, Malaise M, Marcolongo R, et al. Intermittent treatment of knee osteoarthritis with oral chondroitin sulfate: a one-year, randomized, double-blind multicenter study versus placebo. Osteoarthritis Cartilage 12:269–276, 2004.
39. Michel BA, Stucki G, Frey D, et al. Chondroitins 4 and 6 sulfate in osteoarthritis of the knee: a randomized, controlled trial. Arthritis Rheum 52:779–786, 2005.
40. Peterkofsky B. Ascorbate requirement for hydroxylation and secretion of procollagen: relationship to inhibition of collagen synthesis in scurvy. Am J Clin Nutr 54:1135S–1140S, 1991.
41. Schwartz ER, Oh WH, Leveille CR. Experimentally induced osteoarthritis in guinea pigs: metabolic responses in articular cartilage to developing pathology. Arthritis Rheum 24:1345–1355, 1981.
42. Kraus VB, Huebner JL, Stabler T, et al. Ascorbic acid increases the severity of spontaneous knee osteoarthritis in a guinea pig model. Arthritis Rheum 50:1822–1831, 2004.
43. McAlindon TE, Jacques P, Zhang Y, et al. Do antioxidant micronutrients protect against the development and progression of knee osteoarthritis? Arthritis Rheum 39:648–656, 1996.
44. Henrotin Y, Kurz G, Aigner T. Review: oxygen and reactive oxygen species in cartilage degradation: friends or foes? Osteoarthritis Cartilage 13:643–654, 2005.
45. Jordan JM, De Roos AJ, Renner JB, et al. A case-control study of serum tocopherol levels and the alpha- to gamma-tocopherol ratio in radiographic knee osteoarthritis: the Johnston County Osteoarthritis Project. Am J Epidemiol 159:968–977, 2004.
46. McAlindon TE, Felson DT, Zhanf Y, et al. Relation of dietary intake and serum levels of vitamin D to progression of osteoarthritis of the knee among participants in the Framingham study. Ann Intern Med 125:353–359, 1996.
47. Lane NE, Gore LR, Cummings SR, et al. Serum vitamin D levels and incident changes of radiographic hip osteoarthritis. A longitudinal study. Arthritis Rheum 42:854–860, 1999.
48. Henrotin YE, Sanchez C, Deberg MA, et al. Avocado/soybean unsaponifiables increase aggrecan synthesis and reduce catabolic and proinflammatory mediator production by human osteoarthritic chondrocytes. J Rheumatol 30:1825–1834, 2003.
49. Maheu E, Mazieres B, Valat J-P, et al. Symptomatic efficacy of avocado/soybean unsaponifiables in the treatment of osteoarthritis of the knee and hip. Arthritis Rheum 41:81–91, 1998.
50. Lequesne M, Maheu E, Cadet C, et al. Structural effects of avocado/soybean unsaponifiables on joint space loss in osteoarthritis of the hip. Arthritis Rheum 47:50–58, 2002.
51. Altman RD, Marcussen KC. Effects of ginger extract on knee pain in patients with osteoarthritis. Arthritis Rheum 44:2531–2538, 2001.
52. Bliddal H, Rosetzky A, Schlichting P, et al. A randomized, placebo-controlled cross-over study of ginger extracts and ibuprofen in osteoarthritis. Osteoarthritis Cartilage 8:9–12, 2000.
53. Wigler I, Grotto I, Caspi D, et al. The effects of Zintona EC (a ginger extract) on symptomatic gonarthritis. Osteoarthritis Cartilage 11:783–789, 2003.
54. Ernst E, Chrubasik S. Phyto-anti-inflammatories. A systematic review of randomized, placebo-controlled, double-blind trials. Rheum Dis Clin N Am 26:13–27, 2000.
55. Long L, Soeken K, Ernst E. Herbal medicines for the treatment of osteoarthritis: a systematic review. Rheum 40:779–793, 2001.
56. Setty AR, Sigal LH. Herbal medications commonly used in the practice of rheumatology: mechanisms of action, efficacy, and side effects. Semin Arthritis Rheum 34:773–784, 2005.
57. Kolasinski SL. Dimethylsulfoxide (DMSO) and methylmsulfonylmethane (MSM) for the treatment of arthritis. Altern Med Alert 3:115–119, 2000.
58. Horvath K, Noker PE, Somfai-Relle S, et al. Toxicity of methylsulfonylmethane in rats. Food Chem Toxicol 40:1459–1462, 2002.
59. Kim LS, Axelrod LJ, Howard P, et al. Efficacy of methylsulfonylmethane (MSM) in osteoarthritis pain of the knee: a pilot clinical trial. Osteoarthritis Cartilage 14:286–294, 2006.
60. American College of Rheumatology Subcommittee on Osteoarthritis Guidelines. Recommendations for the medical management of osteoarthritis of the hip and knee. Arthritis Rheum 43:1905–1915, 2000.
61. Jordan KM, Arden N, Doherty M, et al. EULAR recommendations 2003: an evidence based approach to the management of knee osteoarthritis: report of a task force of the standing committee for international clinical studies including therapeutic trials (ESCISIT). Ann Rheum Dis 62:1145–1155, 2003.
62. Zhang W, Doherty M, Arden N, et al. EULAR evidence based recommendations for the management of hip osteoarthritis: report of a task force of the EULAR standing committee for international clinical studies including therapeutics (ESCISIT). Ann Rheum Dis 64:669–681, 2005.
63. Chao DM, Shen LL, Tjen-A-Looi S, et al. Naloxone reverses inhibitory effect of electroacupuncture on sympathetic cardiovascular reflex responses. Am J Physiol 276:H2127–H2134, 1999.
64. Ezzo J, Hadhazy V, Circh S, et al. Acupuncture for osteoarthritis of the knee. Arthritis Rheum 44:819–825, 2001.
65. Berman BM, Lao L, Langenberg P, et al. Effectiveness of acupuncture as adjunctive therapy in osteoarthritis of the knee. A randomized, controlled trial. Ann Intern Med 141:901–910, 2004.
66. Garfinkel MS, Schumacher HR, Husain A, et al. Evaluation of a yoga based regimen for treatment of osteoarthritis of the hands. J Rheumatol 21:2341–2343, 1994.
67. Kolasinski SL, Garfinkel M, Gilden Tsai A, et al. Iyengar Yoga for Treating Symptoms of osteoarthritis of the knees: a pilot study. J Alt Complementary Med 11:689–693, 2005.
68. Evangelisto A, Kolasinski SL, Garfinkel M, et al. Changes in gait parameters after participation in a yoga program for treatment of symptoms of osteoarthritis (OA) of the knee: a pilot study. Osteoarthritis Cartilage 11:S44, 2003.
69. DiBenedetto M, Innes KE, Taylor AG, et al. Effect of the gentle Iyengar yoga program on gait in the elderly: an exploratory study. Arch Phys Med Rehabil 86:1830–1837. 2005.
70. Wolf SL, Barnhart HX, Kutner NG. Reducing frailty and falls in older persons: an investigation of tai chi and computerized balance training. J Am Geriatr Soc 44:489–497, 1996.
71. Lan C, Lai J, Wong M, et al. Cardiorespiratory function, flexibility, and body composition among geriatric tai chi chuan practitioners. Arch Phys Med Rehabil 77:612–616, 1996.
72. Hartman CA, Manos TM, Winter C, et al. Effects of tai chi training on function and quality of life indicators in older adults with osteoarthritis. J Am Geriatric Soc 48:1553–1559, 2000.
73. Song R, Lee EO, Lam P, et al. Effects of tai chi exercise on pain, balance, muscle strength, and perceived difficulties in physical functioning in older women with osteoarthritis: a randomized clinical trial. J Rheumatol 30:2039–2044, 2003.

Study Design and Outcome Measures in Osteoarthritis Clinical Trials

18

Vibeke Strand   *Marc C. Hochberg*

The typical patient with osteoarthritis (OA) is middle-aged or elderly and presents with the gradual onset of pain and stiffness accompanied by loss of function. Pain, gradual or insidious in onset, is usually moderate in intensity, worsened by use of involved joints, and improved or relieved with rest. Whereas pain at rest and nocturnal pain are thought to be features of severe disease, they may be indicative of both local inflammation and raised intraosseous pressure in the juxta-articular bone. The mechanism of pain in patients with OA is multifactorial. Pain may result from periosteal proliferation at sites of bone remodeling; subchondral microfractures; capsular irritation from osteophytes; periarticular muscle spasm; bone angina due to decreased blood flow and elevated intraosseous pressure; and synovial inflammation accompanied by the release of prostaglandins, leukotrienes, and various cytokines, including interleukin-1.[1] Morning stiffness and gel phenomenon, or stiffness after periods of rest and inactivity, are also common and usually resolve within 30 minutes and several minutes, respectively. Loss of function resulting from pain and other symptoms of OA may involve both activities of daily living, such as bathing, dressing, feeding, grooming, and toileting, and instrumental activities of daily living, and lead to a reduction in the patient's quality of life.[2,3] Indeed, recent work using the model of disablement developed by the Institute of Medicine shows that pain is the major determinant of physical disability, whereas physical disability is the major determinant of reduced quality of life in patients with OA.[4,5] Furthermore, pain is a predictor of both radiographic progression and need for total joint replacement in patients with OA.[6] Hence, contemporary management of OA is primarily focused on amelioration of pain and physical limitations; future treatment opportunities are likely to include slowing or arresting of the progression of the underlying disease.[7]

To determine whether new treatments for symptom and structure modification are effective, properly designed and conducted randomized controlled trials (RCTs) are necessary. This chapter reviews the design and conduct of clinical trials in patients with OA and the types of outcome measures used in these trials. Regulatory issues regarding registration of new therapies for OA in Europe and the United States are highlighted.

DESIGN OF CLINICAL TRIALS IN OSTEOARTHRITIS

Issues in the design of RCTs in patients with OA and limitations of published trials were discussed more than 20 years ago by Altman and Hochberg.[8] In 1996, the Osteoarthritis Research Society International (OARSI) produced recommendations for the design and conduct of clinical trials in patients with OA.[9,10] Outcome Measures in Rheumatology

Clinical Trials (OMERACT), an international consensus effort initiated in 1992, strives to improve outcome measures through a data driven, iterative consensus process of expert polls, committee discussion, literature review, validation studies, and data mining. In 2003, a joint effort sponsored by OARSI, OMERACT, representatives of regulatory agencies such as the U.S. Food and Drug Administration (FDA), and the pharmaceutical industry established the OARSI Standing Committee for Clinical Trials Response Criteria Initiative to produce a set of responder criteria to treatment in the three symptomatic domains: pain, function, and patient global assessment.[11,12] The concept of classification by symptom and structure modification is derived from a committee of the World Health Organization and International League of Associations of Rheumatology.[13]

Study Population

Selection of subjects relies not only on diagnostic criteria but also on identification of prognostic factors, which may predict responsiveness of the patient population to the therapeutic intervention being tested. Ideally, participants should fulfill validated criteria for the classification of symptomatic OA, such as those published by the American College of Rheumatology.[14–16] In addition, trials of symptom-modifying agents should include patients whose disease is likely to respond to treatment, for example, those with pain of at least moderate intensity. Trials of structure-modifying agents should include patients without end-stage disease; furthermore, these types of studies should strive to include patients at high risk of structural progression, for example, middle-aged overweight women with unilateral knee OA[17] or patients with an increased uptake on bone scintigraphy in the juxta-articular bone.[18] The role of serum levels of biochemical markers of bone and cartilage turnover as a predictor of structural progression in patients with symptomatic OA remains under investigation and is the subject of an ongoing multidisciplinary initiative coordinated by the National Institute of Arthritis and Musculoskeletal and Skin Diseases (http://www.niams.nih.gov/ne/oi/oabiomarwhipap.htm).

Study Joints

Which joints in patients with OA should be studied? In general, for studies of symptom-modifying agents, trials should focus on disease in the symptomatic or index joint; data on symptoms in other joints that may also be affected as part of a generalized osteoarthritic process should also be collected. For studies of structure-modifying agents, trials should also focus on the index joint; herein, data on both symptoms and structural change should also be collected for other affected joints. These additional data should be considered secondary outcomes when data on the index joint are the primary outcome measures.

Duration of Trials

Trial duration for demonstration of symptom improvement should be at least three months; product- or device-specific considerations (e.g., new classes of agents, agents with delayed onset) may lengthen the duration. Current recommendations stress that RCTs of symptom-modifying drugs should be at least 6 months in duration "to assess the maintenance of the therapeutic effect" and continued up to 1 year for collection of data on adverse events and to establish that the drug does not have a deleterious effect on cartilage.[9] Trials of structure-modifying agents should be of 1 to 2 years duration.[13]

Outcome Measures

Outcome measures in OA assess three primary domains: clinical, structural, and biochemical.[9] OMERACT 3 focused on the development of consensus recommendations for outcome measures to be used in clinical trials in OA; participants concluded that a core set should include those measures, with greater than 90% of individuals voting for inclusion, those items for which greater than 25% of individuals voted should be strongly recommended, and the remaining outcomes could be optional.[19] The final core set items, listed in Table 18–1, were pain, physical function, patient global assessment, and, for studies of at least 1 year in duration, joint imaging.[11,20] At OMERACT 6, meeting participants voted to ratify the OMERACT-OARSI set of criteria. It was subsequently found that successful trial designs must include both absolute and relative change, as well as measures of pain and function as primary domains.[12]

Studies of Symptom Modification

Disease-Specific Measures

As pain is the most important symptom of OA, measurement of pain and its improvement with therapy is often the primary outcome variable in RCTs of symptom-modifying therapy. In 1981, Bellamy undertook the development of an evaluative index, the Western Ontario and McMaster

---

TABLE 18–1

PROPORTION OF PARTICIPANTS VOTING FOR INCLUSION OF SPECIFIC OUTCOME DOMAINS IN THE CORE SET FOR PHASE III TRIALS IN PATIENTS WITH OSTEOARTHRITIS OF THE HAND, HIP, AND KNEE, OMERACT III (APRIL 1996)

Domain	Percentage
Pain	100
Physical function	97
Imaging (in studies of 12 months' duration or longer)	92
Patient global assessment	91
Physician global assessment	52
Generic quality of life	36
Morning stiffness	14
Measure of inflammation	8

Modified from Bellamy N, Kirwan J, Boers M, et al. Recommendations for a core set of outcome measures for future phase III clinical trials in knee, hip, and hand osteoarthritis. Consensus development at OMERACT III. J Rheumatol 24:799–802, 1997.

Universities (WOMAC) OA Index, using self-report to assess specifically OA of the knee and hip.[20-22] The conceptual basis of the index, derivation of the item inventory, and results of validation studies have been described extensively elsewhere and are only briefly reviewed here.[23] Questionnaire items were selected according to responses from 100 patients with OA on the basis of their prevalence, frequency, and importance to the patient. The final WOMAC includes a total of 24 questions divided into three sections: pain (five questions), stiffness (two questions), and function (seventeen questions) (Table 18–2). The questions probe symptoms of, and clinically important events affected by, lower limb OA and are answered by use of either a 5-point Likert scale or a 10-cm VAS. An eight-item short form of the WOMAC has been validated to enhance efficiency of use in RCTs and clinical practice.[24] The WOMAC has been translated into most European languages and has been shown to be valid, reliable, and responsive in studies of patients undergoing total joint arthroplasty and in clinical trials of nonsteroidal anti-inflammatory drugs (NSAIDs) and traditional Chinese acupuncture.[25-28] Although results have been reported on the basis of a single question in the pain section, such as pain with walking on a flat surface, and as a total WOMAC score summing the three subscales, the use of domain-specific scores, especially for pain and function, is preferable.

Creamer and colleagues[29] examined the relationship between the pain subscale of the WOMAC OA index, the McGill Pain Questionnaire, and a single 10-cm VAS pain-rating scale in 68 outpatients with OA of the knee. Although all three scales correlated with one another, the strongest correlation was between the WOMAC pain scale and the single 10-cm VAS pain scale. Severity of anxiety, depression, and fatigue all showed significant modest correlation with the McGill pain score, whereas none significantly correlated with the WOMAC pain score. On the other hand, total osteophyte score combining the tibiofemoral and patellofemoral joints correlated significantly with the WOMAC pain score but not with the McGill pain score. Largely on the basis of these findings, the authors concluded that the WOMAC pain scale should be the preferred measure of pain in clinical studies of patients with knee OA.

In the early 1980s, Lequesne and colleagues[30] developed two indices for measurement of severity of OA of the hip and knee that combine three domains: pain or discomfort (five questions), maximal distance walked, and activities of daily living (four items). These instruments were recommended as outcome measures for OA trials in the 1985 guidelines for antirheumatic drug research promulgated by the European League of Associations of Rheumatology.[31] The indices for knee and hip differ with regard to only one of the five pain items and in the four activities of daily living (Table 18–3). This instrument has been shown to be valid, reliable, and responsive in clinical trials of NSAIDs, slow-acting symptom-modifying drugs such as diacerein, and intra-articular agents and with traditional Chinese

TABLE 18–2
ITEMS IN THE WOMAC OSTEOARTHRITIS INDEX

Pain Subscale	Walking on a flat surface
	Going up or down stairs
	At night while in bed
	Sitting or lying
	Standing upright
Stiffness Subscale	Severity after first awakening in the morning
	Severity after sitting, lying, or resting later in the day
Physical Function Subscale	Going down stairs
	Going up stairs
	Standing up from sitting
	Standing
	Bending to the floor
	Walking on a flat surface
	Getting in or out of the car, or getting on or off a bus
	Going shopping
	Putting on your socks or stockings
	Rising from bed
	Taking off your socks or stockings
	Lying in bed
	Getting in or out of the bath
	Sitting
	Getting on or off the toilet
	Performing heavy domestic duties
	Performing light domestic duties

From Bellamy N. WOMAC Osteoarthritis Index: User's Guide III. London, Ontario, 1998.

TABLE 18–3
ITEMS IN THE LEQUESNE ALGOFUNCTIONAL INDICES FOR OSTEOARTHRITIS

Pain or discomfort
- During nocturnal bed rest
- Morning stiffness or regressive pain after rising
- After standing for 30 minutes
- While ambulating
- With prolonged sitting (hip index only)
- While getting up from sitting without the help of arms (knee index only)

Maximum distance walked (may walk with pain)

Activities of daily living (hip index only)
- Put on socks by bending forward
- Pick up an object from the floor
- Climb up and down a standard flight of stairs
- Get into and out of a car

Activities of daily living (knee index only)
- Able to climb up a standard flight of stairs
- Able to climb down a standard flight of stairs
- Able to squat or bend on the knees
- Able to walk on uneven ground

From Lequesne MG. The algofunctional indices for hip and knee osteoarthritis. J Rheumatol 24:779–781, 1997.

acupuncture.[32-34] The relative statistical efficiency of the WOMAC is similar to that of the Lequesne indices, although the WOMAC subscales and global score may be slightly more responsive than the comparable Lequesne sections and index.[35]

Several instruments have been developed and validated to evaluate hand OA: the Dreiser Functional Index for Hand Osteoarthritis,[36] the Australian/Canadian (AUSCAN) OA Hand Index modeled after the WOMAC OA index,[37,38] the Disabilities of the Arm, Shoulder, and Hand (DASH) questionnaire,[39] and the Cochin Index.[40] There is limited experience with their use. While all have been shown to be reliable, valid, and responsive to change in RCTs, there are no published data comparing their performance in the same study. Recommendations for the conduct of clinical trials in the hand, recently been published by the Osteoarthritis Research society International (OARSI), represent a significant addition to methodologic study approaches for this region of OA.[40a]

The Stanford Health Assessment Questionnaire (HAQ), a self-report questionnaire, has been used in clinical trials in rheumatoid arthritis, systemic lupus erythematosus, and progressive systemic sclerosis in addition to OA. The disability index contains 20 questions to assess eight categories of physical function (dressing and grooming, arising, eating, walking, hygiene, reach, grip, and activities); each question is scored by patients from 0 (without difficulty) to 3 (unable to do).[41] The worst scores in each category are then summed and divided by the number of categories to give the disability index. It has been extensively translated and shown to be valid, reliable, and responsive in clinical trials. In a comparative study of patients undergoing total knee arthroplasty, the WOMAC was slightly more responsive than the HAQ disability index.[42] The HAQ disability index should be especially useful in assessing treatment of patients with generalized OA because the range of activities captures both upper and lower extremity function. A shorter version of the HAQ disability index, the modified Health Assessment Questionnaire (MHAQ), is available as a single page of eight questions about functional activities performed on a daily basis; these are derived from the HAQ and are scored by patients from 0 (without difficulty) to 3 (unable to do).[43] The MHAQ has been shown to have responsiveness similar to that of the WOMAC OA Index.[44]

The Arthritis Impact Measurement Scale (AIMS), and the newer AIMS2, are comprehensive self-report questionnaires designed to evaluate mobility, physical activity, dexterity, social role, social activity, activities of daily living, pain, depression, and anxiety.[45,46] They are valid and reliable; however, their use has been limited in part because of the time required for completion and scoring. Like the HAQ disability index, the AIMS is slightly less responsive than the WOMAC in OA patients undergoing total knee arthroplasty.[42] It would also be a useful instrument in assessing treatment of patients with generalized OA.

Patient Global Assessment

The third element in the recommended core set of outcomes is patient global assessment of disease activity. The standard question, "Considering all of the ways your arthritis affects you, how are you doing today?" utilizes either a 5-point Likert scale (very good, good, fair, poor, very poor) or a 10-cm VAS.[47] Physician global assessment of disease activity is a subjective judgment queried as: "How would you describe the patient's disease activity today?" scored by a 5-point Likert scale (none, mild, moderate, severe, very severe) or 10-cm VAS. The clinimetric properties of both measures have been described by Bellamy.[21]

Health-Related Quality of Life Measures

Health-related quality of life (HRQoL) focuses on aspects of life that are directly affected by a health condition: physical, social/psychological functioning, work functioning, and vitality, but not personal values, socioeconomic status, environment, opportunity, or social network.[48] The Medical Outcomes Study 36-Item Short-Form Health Survey (SF-36) is a generic instrument designed to measure HRQoL with scores based on responses to individual questions, summarized into eight domains: physical functioning, role–physical, body pain, general health, vitality, social functioning, role–emotional, and mental health.[49,50] These eight domains are also combined into summary physical and mental component scores, again scored from 0 to 100; higher scores reflect better HRQoL. The SF-36 has been extensively translated, and normative data are available for a broad variety of cultural and disease-specific populations. It has been used in clinical trials in rheumatoid arthritis, OA, psoriatic arthritis, and systemic lupus erythematosus and shown responsive to change after 4 to 6 weeks of treatment.[51,52]

The European Quality of Life Questionnaire (EuroQOL), now named the EQ5D, is another generic measure of HRQoL. This instrument assesses five domains of health status: mobility, self-care, usual activities, pain and discomfort, and anxiety/depression; these are ranked from no problem to moderate to extreme difficulty, generating a potential 243 distinct health states.[53] It includes a feeling thermometer asking patients to rate their own health status from 0 to 100.

The Work Limitations Questionnaire was designed by Lerner et al. in 2001 to measure the impact of health problems on the daily work of people with chronic disease. The questionnaire uses 25 items to identify four domains (time, physical, mental-interpersonal, and output demands), and uses a demand-level methodology to address job content. It has been validated, although not yet published in RCTs.[54,55]

Utilizing both generic and disease or rheumatology-specific measures allow a more complete assessment of a therapeutic intervention. Specifically, generic HRQoL instruments facilitate economic analyses of new therapies, across differing disease states and afford a societal perspective.

Studies of Structure Modification

Agents that may retard, arrest, or reverse the degenerative process of OA in human cartilage have been defined as disease-modifying OA drugs (DMOADs).[13] To date, no therapeutic agent has met this definition, and it remains unclear how best to identify this benefit, whether by radiographs, magnetic resonance imaging (MRI), or direct visualization using arthroscopy.

Radiography

Although radiographs cannot directly visualize articular cartilage, several techniques have been developed to assess loss of joint space width (JSW). (*Note:* The term JSW is utilized here to distinguish it from "increased" joint space narrowing in RA, due to causes in addition to loss of articular cartilage.) To date, assessment of interbone distance using a plain radiograph of hip or knee remains the only validated measure of loss of JSW recommended for use in RCTs in OA, although the methodologic limitations are well recognized (Fig. 18–1).[56–58]

Specific weight-bearing methods to identify changes in JSW over time are valid only when the relevant articular surfaces remain in direct contact and are consistently assessed over time. It is challenging to reproducibly and precisely measure loss of JSW: 1) changes over time are small, on the order of 0.03 to 0.6 millimeters per year, and typically occur in only a subset of patients; 2) loss of JSW is often difficult to predict, as is the subset of "rapid progressors"; 3) identification of such a subset is dependent on the population accrued into the clinical trial; 4) conventional weight-bearing radiographs of hip and knee in full extension are poorly reproducible, especially in the knee (only one structural progression RCT has been conducted in hip OA); 5) varying degrees of flexion which inadvertently and all too frequently occur with repeated examinations of either joint may alter JSW width—in the absence of structural changes; and 6) intra-articular sites where deterioration most likely may occur expectedly differ across individuals.

Variability in assessment of JSW has been attributed to measurement techniques as well as heterogeneity across studied protocol populations. Simpler solutions, such as increasing sample sizes in RCTs of 2 to 3 years duration, or selecting treatment populations enriched for "risk factors" predicting progression, to overcome this high variability have so far proved impractical and prohibitively costly.[59–62]

A variety of methodologic approaches have been developed to improve the reproducibility of assessment of changes in JSW in RCTs of both hip and knee OA.[60] As no product has been proven disease modifying using a "regulatory definition," it remains unclear which approaches are preferable, or whether other imaging techniques may be more promising. Buckland-Wright and colleagues place the knee in a standing, semiflexed (7°–10° flexion) position, using fluoroscopy to achieve superimposition of the anterior and posterior lips of the medial tibial plateau, centering the tibial spines below the femoral notch (Fig. 18–1).[63]

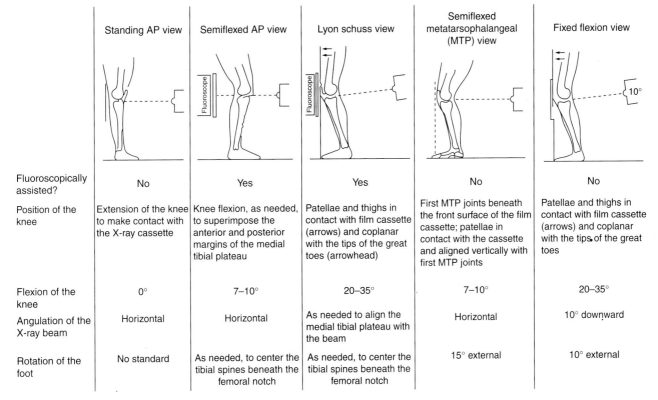

	Standing AP view	Semiflexed AP view	Lyon schuss view	Semiflexed metatarsophalangeal (MTP) view	Fixed flexion view
Fluoroscopically assisted?	No	Yes	Yes	No	No
Position of the knee	Extension of the knee to make contact with the X-ray cassette	Knee flexion, as needed, to superimpose the anterior and posterior margins of the medial tibial plateau	Patellae and thighs in contact with film cassette (arrows) and coplanar with the tips of the great toes (arrowhead)	First MTP joints beneath the front surface of the film cassette; patellae in contact with the cassette and aligned vertically with first MTP joints	Patellae and thighs in contact with film cassette (arrows) and coplanar with the tips of the great toes
Flexion of the knee	0°	7–10°	20–35°	7–10°	20–35°
Angulation of the X-ray beam	Horizontal	Horizontal	As needed to align the medial tibial plateau with the beam	Horizontal	10° downward
Rotation of the foot	No standard	As needed, to center the tibial spines beneath the femoral notch	As needed, to center the tibial spines beneath the femoral notch	15° external	10° external

Figure 18–1 Comparison of positioning of the subject for the conventional standing AP knee view and for fluoroscopically and nonfluoroscopically assisted protocols designated to standardize the positioning of the knee. (From Brandt KD, Mazzuca SA, Conrozier T, et al. Which is the best radiographic protocol for a clinical trial of a structure modifying drug in patients with knee osteoarthritis? J Rheumatol 29:1308–1320, 2002.)

After the radiograph is obtained, the foot is traced on the film jacket to facilitate repositioning during future examinations.[64] This method requires the technician to be specifically trained, adding another level of sophistication to the conduct of multicenter RCTs. Nonetheless, in a 1-year RCT examining 402 patients with knee OA, this method was shown feasible with good test/retest reliability.[65] Peterfy and colleagues developed a lightweight Plexiglas frame that reproducibly places the knee in a semiflexed weight-bearing "schuss" position with 10° angulation without requiring fluoroscopy.[66,67] Fluoroscopically determined standardizations of knee position, either in full extension or semiflexion, have been utilized in most RCTs seeking to demonstrate disease modification.[59–61,68–76] Nonetheless, it remains unclear the degree to which standing anteroposterior (AP) views may be altered by symptomatic improvements occurring during protocol treatment, as radiographic features of OA are only weakly associated, if at all, with pain in patients with knee OA.[59,77–80]

In hip OA, there is no definitive "gold-standard" for the most sensitive radiographic view or agreement on the number of readers to perform the measurements. Generally, either supine or standing radiographs are taken in one of three views: plain view of the pelvis with the feet in 10° to 15° of internal rotation, an AP view of the index hip, or an oblique or faux view of the index hip. In a recent RCT of 50 patients with hip OA, all three views provided similar results, although the plain view of the pelvis was the most sensitive in accurately measuring changes in JSW. The precision of the measurements depends more on the precision of the reader than on the view of the radiograph. In any trial, consistency of measurements from the reader over the course of the trial is essential, one of the reasons a single expert reader is preferable to multiple readers.[81]

Magnetic Resonance Imaging

MRI can delineate cartilage structure directly; several techniques modifying signal intensity allow assessment of its biochemical and biomechanical integrity.[56,82,83] MRI shows not only JSN reflective of cartilage loss but also cartilage volume, changes in cartilage contour and associated joint structures including bone, synovium, ligaments, menisci, and muscle. The fat-suppressed, T_1-weighted 3D gradient-echo technique is most useful for detailed evaluation of the articular cartilage surface—abnormal signal intensity, particularly with T_2-weighted images, in superficial and deep zones reflect biochemical changes in OA cartilage.[84] Delayed gadolinium-enhanced MRI offers a means to measure cartilage proteoglycan loss pre- and post-treatment.[85] Whole-organ evaluation (WORMS), assessing 14 articular features, provides a semiquantitative, multifeature system scoring structural damage over time.[82]

Whereas extensive data support the validity and reliability of MRI detecting cartilage defects in cross-sectional studies, few data exist to support its accuracy and reproducibility identifying longitudinal changes in structure.[86] Raynauld et al. showed that correlations between loss of cartilage volume by MRI and loss of JSW measured by radiographs over time are not strong.[87] MRI is not yet recommended as a

primary endpoint in structural modification RCTs in OA until additional supportive data become available.[88]

Direct Visualization of Articular Cartilage

Direct arthroscopic visualization of articular cartilage may arguably offer the best assessment of structural modification in OA. Chondroscopy has been shown valid, reliable, and sensitive to change in patients with OA of the knee.[89,90] However, there is increased risk with any invasive procedure, and it is difficult to assess volume and tensile strength of cartilage reproducibly.[85,91] Similarly, current methodology to evaluate healing of cartilage defects still requires validation.[92] Nonetheless, recent arthroscopic assessments show high sensitivity, specificity, and accuracy diagnosing articular chondropathy with high intra-observer reliability which compare well with nonarthroscopic assessments.[93–95]

Biochemical and Molecular Markers of Cartilage Turnover

Although the consensus reached at OMERACT 3 advocated continued study of biologic markers of bone and cartilage degradation and repair, none was recommended for inclusion in clinical trials.[96] Nonetheless, recognizing this active field of research and the value of biologic markers in identifying promising new therapies early in clinical development, it was recommended that serum and synovial fluid samples be collected in all pivotal trials and archived for future analyses of various markers. Particularly in view of the several-year duration required for phase 3 structure-modifying trials, identification of a surrogate marker for use in earlier phase 2 trials would considerably improve the safety, cost, and efficiency of clinical development programs. Osteoporosis trials provide a good example, in which molecular markers are increasingly used as adjunct measures of effect before initiation of several-year phase 3 trials. The role of biochemical markers as outcome measures reflecting structural change in OA trials remains, at this time, a topic of intense investigation and ongoing discussion without resolution.[97]

The choice of biologic markers must obviously depend on the specific mechanism of action of the potential therapeutic agent. Candidate molecular markers include measures of cartilage matrix repair, inflammation, regeneration, and degradation, as well as measures of subchondral bone synthesis and resorption.[98,99] Elevated serum levels of cartilage oligomeric matrix protein, hyaluronan, and C-reactive protein appear to predict future disease progression; they could be used to identify and select high-risk individuals for inclusion in early trials of structure-modifying agents.[100–102]

Time to Total Joint Replacement

Delaying or eradicating the need for total joint replacement has been used as a structural outcome measure, but it is a flawed measure due to so many personal, economic, and cultural variables which affect the decision to undergo surgery.[103] Pain and physical dysfunction are precursors to joint replacement and offer more standardized methods of measurement.

Interpreting Statistical Differences Clinically

Statistically significant differences between active treatment and control and across treatment groups over time may or may not represent clinically meaningful changes. The minimal clinically important difference (MCID) represents the minimum amount of improvement perceptible to patients, and may be used to determine whether changes inpatient-reported measures noted in RCTs are clinically meaningful.[59] MCID definitions have been derived and confirmed by statistical correlations with changes in patient-reported pain, global assessment of disease activity, and HRQoL in RCTs—and differ by intervention. Values are determined either by anchor-based methods based on direct observation or statistically determined distribution-based methods. When mean and median changes from baseline in a treatment group meet or exceed MCID, then it may be inferred that a majority of patients have reported clinically meaningful improvement or worsening. The minimal clinically important improvement (MCII) expresses results as the percentage of patients reporting improvement that meet or exceed MCID, thereby providing additional information on the effect size. These threshold values help clinical interpretation of results from RCTs, and may be utilized to monitor individual responses to treatment over time. The use of MCID or MCII in RCTs facilitates systematic reviews and meta-analyses of different interventions.[104]

Table 18–4 summarizes MCID ranges across RCTs assessing different therapeutic interventions in OA. MCID values for SF-36 and WOMAC (total score and subscales) in OA have been highly correlated.[59,104]

The Patient Acceptable Symptom State (PASS) is a complementary measure to MCID, although not yet widely used. While MCID denotes a clinically perceptible change in symptoms, that level of improvement may not be sufficient to be considered acceptable to the patient. Using both MCID and PASS, treatment results can be better interpreted clinically.[105]

Standardized response means (SRMs) and standardized effect sizes (SES) are used to define treatment effects based on changes in individual outcome measures. The SRM is the mean change in score from baseline divided by the standard deviation of the difference; the SES is the mean change in score divided by the standard deviation of the baseline scores. Large effect sizes indicate more responsive measures, and, therefore, require fewer subjects for detection. Smallest statistically detectable differences (SDD) allow interpretation of proposed MCID values. If MCID values exceed SDD, then the assumed effect is clinically meaningful and may be statistically significant. If MCID values are less than SDD, then the sample size of the trial was too small or the statistical or measurement method insufficiently sensitive to detect smaller effects.[59] MCID or MCII should complement, but not replace, SES because the effect size remains a more powerful approach.[104]

TABLE 18–4

COMPARISON OF MINIMAL CLINICALLY IMPORTANT DIFFERENCES (MCID): DEFINITIONS PUBLISHED FROM RANDOMIZED CONTROLLED TRIALS OF PHYSICAL THERAPY, COX-2, AND NS-NSAIDS IN OSTEOARTHRITIS

MCID	Actual (0–4)		Transformed (0–100)			VAS (0–100)			Comparison vs Ehrich**		
Author	Angst*	Zhao*	Angst[109]	Zhao[114]	Ehrich[115]	Tubach[104]	Tubach[104]	Publ.	Angst	Zhao	Tubach
Intervention	PT	COX-2	PT	COX-2	COX-2	NSAID hip	NSAID Knee	Var.			
		12 wk		12 wk	12 wk	4 wk	4 wk				
WOMAC total	0.67	0.42	16.75	10.50	9.30				1.80	1.13	
Pain	0.75	0.42	18.75	10.50	9.70				1.93	1.08	
Stiffness	0.72	0.60	18.00	15.00	10.00				1.80	1.50	
Phys function	0.67	0.38	16.75	9.50	9.30	12.00	12.00		1.80	1.02	1.29
% Change			[12–26]	[33–37]		[28]	[40]	[15]			
									Publ		
SF-36											
Phys function			3.3						5–10		
Pain			7.8			17.50	17.50		5–10		
PCS			2.0	4.3					2.5–5		
MCS				1.83					2.5–5		
Pt global					11.70	15.00	15.00		10.00		
MD global					10.75				10.00		
Pt pain						17.00	28.00		15.00		
% Change						[47]	[48]				

*Reported values divided by number of questions to yield 0–4 Likert scale.
**Comparability assessed by ratio of reported values to those defined by Ehrich et al.
Data from Strand V, Kelman A. Outcome measures in osteoarthritis: randomized controlled trials.
Curr Rheumatol Rep 6:20–30, 2004; refs 104, 109, 114, 115.

REGISTRATION OF THERAPEUTIC AGENTS FOR OSTEOARTHRITIS: THE REGULATORY PATHWAY

In developing new therapeutic products for OA, we are seeking to relieve symptoms, delay progression of disease, or prevent onset of disease in previously unaffected joints. At present, therapies have only been demonstrated to be symptom modifying.

Clinical trials accepted for FDA review include multiple procedures to ensure scientific integrity of the data and analyses: careful monitoring of investigational sites, adherence to "good clinical practices" (GCP) procedures, quality control and quality assurance standards, and cross-checking of case report form data against primary medical charts. The FDA performs detailed statistical and medical reviews of the data, typically independent, complete reanalyses—none of which are usually available when reports are submitted for peer review.

Guidance documents have been issued by the U.S. FDA and the European Agency for the Evaluation of Medicinal Products (EMEA).[106,107] The first draft guidance for industry, *Clinical Development Programs for Drugs, Devices and Biological Products Intended for the Treatment of Osteoarthritis*, was issued by the FDA in September 1998, and revised in July 1999. The first draft for Committee for Proprietary Medicinal Products (CPMP), *Points to Consider on Clinical Investigation of Medicinal Products Used in the Treatment of OA*, was issued in July 1997; the final version in July 1998. Recommendations outlined in these documents are summarized in the following sections.

Treatment of Symptoms

Pain and Function

For symptom relief, the FDA guidance document requires the completion of placebo RCTs of at least 3 months' duration, with use of endpoints for pain, function, and the patient's global assessment of disease severity. The EMEA guidance document similarly requests assessment of both pain and function with use of either the WOMAC or Lequesne indices, which evaluate pain, stiffness, and physical function. If benefit in pain relief alone is demonstrated, no deterioration in function must be observed. The EMEA document further recommends the conduct of three-arm placebo- and active-comparator–controlled trials including the most favorable comparator available. Both documents emphasize the importance of a sufficiently large database to support chronic use of the therapy. An important issue remains the generalizability of symptom relief beyond the signal joint. It is unclear at present how best to evaluate whether previously unaffected joints remain asymptomatic or become symptomatic; we think this can be achieved with the use of the patient's and physician's global assessment of the nonsignal joints. Patient questionnaires have been shown to be highly valid and reliable measures of disease status and change. Perhaps the best assessment of signal joint and nonsignal joint symptoms is to regularly ask the patient.[108]

The FDA document discusses trials using active comparators in more detail than the EMEA document, suggesting that parallel dose and placebo crossover designs should be employed. Although previous RCTs have utilized a flare design, whereby signs and symptoms are exacerbated after withdrawal of previous nonsteroidal anti-inflammatory drug therapy, this document suggests that this practice is suitable only for phase 2 dose-finding trials.

Structure Modification

The regulatory pathway to obtain labeling for both symptomatic relief and delay of structural progression of disease is less clear. No products, devices, or procedures have yet been proved to maintain cartilage structure and integrity. Furthermore, the goal of structure modification is not clear. Are we trying to reduce progression or induce healing in the affected joint? Are we trying to prevent development of OA in other joints? Are we concentrating on structural changes in cartilage, bone, or both? These are important issues that remain to be resolved.

Both regulatory documents are based on the postulate, supported by epidemiologic data, that stabilization or even improvement in structural damage during long-term observation should ultimately result in clinical benefit as measured by pain, function, or both. Thus, endpoints to assess symptomatic improvement as well as structural damage are to be included, although precedents from RCTs documenting stabilization or improvement in measures of structural damage are currently lacking. The FDA prefers Joint Space Narrowing (JSN) as the currently best-accepted marker for structural change.[106] After a short-term, randomized, placebo-controlled trial evaluating symptom relief, it is envisioned that data supporting maintenance of cartilage structure and function could be collected in the context of a long-term active controlled trial, in which placebo-treated patients would be switched to active therapy while the masking is maintained. Both documents emphasize that symptomatic outcome measures must be followed as well. The FDA document requires a minimum duration of 1 year for these trials; the EMEA guidance document requests 2-year data for both safety and efficacy.

The EMEA document also recommends inclusion of "hard clinical endpoints," such as necessity for joint replacement or delay of surgery. Although this may be an appealing outcome measure, there is no evidence-based consensus on when joint replacement surgery should be undertaken. Variations in practice, accessibility of patients, and economic forces further complicate decisions regarding joint replacement, making this approach unfeasible at present. OARSI has convened a task force to study the use of joint replacement surgery as an outcome measure in clinical trials.

Although these approaches hypothetically appear rational when viewed in the context of current clinical practice, several dilemmas present themselves and several questions arise. What is a clinically significant structural effect indicating lack of deterioration or even improvement? What is the best method to establish a link between delay of structural changes and compromise of function or

TABLE 18–5

COMPARISON OF OUTCOME MEASURES UTILIZED IN RCTS OF PHYSICAL THERAPY, ACUPUNCTURE, INTRA-ARTICULAR HYALURONANS, NSAIDs, COX-2 SELECTIVE AGENTS, GLUCOSAMINE, DOXYCYCLINE, RISEDRONATE, AND AUTOLOGOUS CHONDROCYTE IMPLANTATION

	Angst (2001)[109]	Berman (2004)[110]	Witt (2005)[111]	Day (2004)[112]	Tubach (2005)[104]	Zhao (1999)[114]	Pincus (2004)[116]	Cibere (2004)[117]	Brandt (2005)[60]	Spector (2005)[120]	Knutsen (2004)[119]
Intervention	PT	Acupuncture	Acupuncture	IA-HA	NSAID	COX-2	COX-2	Glucosamine	Doxycycline	Risedronate	Chondrocyte implantation
Primary outcome measure	Total WOMAC, SF-36	WOMAC pain and function	WOMAC	Total WOMAC	Pain VAS	Total WOMAC (Likert)	Total WOMAC	Disease flares	JSN in medial tibiofemoral compartment	WOMAC (VAS)	Lysholm, pain VAS, SF-36, histological analysis
Control	None	WOMAC pain and function	WOMAC	Total WOMAC	None	None	Total WOMAC				Microfracture
Pain	WOMAC (Likert)	WOMAC	WOMAC (VAS), Likert	WOMAC, Lequesne Index	VAS	WOMAC (Likert), Arthritis Pain–VAS, American Pain Soc. Patient Outcome Quest.	WOMAC (VAS)	WOMAC (VAS)	WOMAC (Likert), VAS	WOMAC (VAS)	VAS
Phys function	WOMAC (Likert)	WOMAC, SF-36, 6-minute walk	WOMAC (PDI)	WOMAC, knee examination	WOMAC (Likert)	WOMAC (Likert)	WOMAC (VAS)	WOMAC (VAS)	WOMAC (Likert)	WOMAC (VAS)	ICRS macroscopic evaluation
Pt global	None	AIMS2	None	Yes	VAS	Yes, OA Severity Index	MDHAQ	None	Likert	PGA (VAS)	None
MD global	None	None	None	Yes	None	Yes	None	Yes (Likert)	Yes (Likert)	None	None
Health-related quality of life	SF-36	None	SF-36	None	None	SF-36	SF-36	EQ-5D	None	None	SF-36
Joint imaging	None	None	None	Baseline X-rays	None	None	None	None	Standing AP, Semiflexed AP, Supine lateral, Skyline of patellofemoral joints	Semi-flexed	Weight-bearing, standing, Arthroscopy

Data from refs 60, 104, 109–112, 114, 116–120.

increased pain? What is the magnitude of structure preservation that would be clinically convincing and important? Would the results of a single study be applicable across differing products with unique mechanisms of action?

Perhaps the most challenging dilemma remains how to develop an agent with potential structural benefit that does not, in and of itself, offer symptom relief. In the context of the preceding trial designs, the FDA is considering offering an accelerated but preliminary approval based on demonstrated stabilization or even improvement in structure, contingent on demonstration of improvement during the long term in pain or function in a postmarketing continuation protocol. The authorities in the United Kingdom have suggested a variation of this theme, whereby data supporting structural benefit are collected as a surrogate measure.

Claims for the Prevention of Osteoarthritis

Considering a claim for prevention of disease is without precedent in rheumatology, with the exception of prevention of fracture in osteoporosis. Study of such a therapeutic agent in OA could imply treatment of healthy people to keep them healthy, endeavoring to include those at high risk for development of OA or to prevent the onset of disease in a second, previously uninvolved joint. Given the current state of the art, with the poor correlation between the degree of symptoms and the magnitude of structural damage, these trials are difficult to envision.

INSTRUCTIVE EXAMPLES FROM RECENT RANDOMIZED CONTROLLED TRIALS

Table 18–5 highlights the outcome measures used in recent RCTs of different interventions in OA. It is interesting to note how consistently the WOMAC and its subscales are used; it has clearly become the gold standard for measuring pain and physical function. Visual analog scale (VAS) measurements are also more commonly utilized than categorical Likert scales.

SUMMARY

At present, the regulatory path for developing therapeutic agents for symptom relief in OA is clear, and precedent has been established in the United States and the European Union with the approval of the COX-2 selective inhibitors and several intra-articular hyaluronan preparations. A regulatory pathway for approval of agents designed for structural modification is emerging, although no product has been demonstrated to delay structural loss by either radiography or magnetic resonance imaging. Currently, it is difficult to contemplate trials to demonstrate prevention of disease. Although disparities exist between the guidance documents issued by the American and European authorities, there is every reason to believe that these will be minimized as progressively more agents with novel mechanisms of action are studied.

REFERENCES

1. Creamer P, Hochberg MC. Why does osteoarthritis of the knee hurt—sometimes? Br J Rheumatol 37:726–728, 1997.
2. Jordan JM, Luta G, Renner J, et al. Knee pain and knee osteoarthritis severity in self-reported task specific disability: the Johnston County Osteoarthritis Project. J Rheumatol 24:1344–1349, 1997.
3. Jordan JM, Luta G, Renner J, et al. Self reported functional status and osteoarthritis of the knee in a rural Southern community: the role of sociodemographic factors, obesity and knee pain. Arthritis Care Res 9:273–278, 1996.
4. Creamer P, Lethbridge-Cejku M, Hochberg MC, et al. A model of the health effects of osteoarthritis of the knee. Arthritis Rheum 41:S229, 1998.
5. Lethbridge-Cejku M, Creamer P, Hochberg M. Quality of life in knee osteoarthritis. Arthritis Rheum 40:S174, 1997.
6. Hochberg MC. Progression of osteoarthritis. Ann Rheum Dis 55:685–688, 1996.
7. Creamer P, Hochberg MC. Management of osteoarthritis. In: Hazzard W, Blass JP, Ettinger WH Jr, et al, eds. Principles of Geriatric Medicine and Gerontology. 4th ed. New York, McGraw-Hill, 1999, 1155–1161.
8. Altman RD, Hochberg MC. Degenerative joint disease. Clin Rheum Dis 9:681–693, 1983.
9. Group for the Respect of Ethics and Excellence in Science: Osteoarthritis Section. Recommendations for the registration of drugs used in the treatment of osteoarthritis. Ann Rheum Dis 55:552–557, 1996.
10. Altman R, Brandt K, Hochberg M, et al. Design and conduct of clinical trials in patients with osteoarthritis: recommendations from a task force of the Osteoarthritis Research Society. Results from a workshop. Osteoarthritis Cartilage 4:217–243, 1996.
11. Pham T, Van Der Heijde D, Lassere M, et al. Outcome variables for osteoarthritis clinical trials: The OMERACT–OARSI set of responder criteria. J Rheumatol 30:1648–1654, 2003.
12. Pham T, van der Heijde D, Altman RD, et al. OMERACT-OARSI initiative: Osteoarthritis Research Society International set of responder criteria for osteoarthritis clinical trials revisited. Osteoarthritis Cartilage 12:389–399, 2004.
13. Lequesne M, Brandt K, Bellamy N, et al. Guidelines for testing slow acting drugs in osteoarthritis. J Rheumatol 21:65–71, 1994.
14. Altman RD, Asch E, Bloch D, et al. Development of criteria for the classification and reporting of osteoarthritis: classification of osteoarthritis of the knee. Arthritis Rheum 29:1039–1049, 1986.
15. Altman R, Alarcon G, Appelrouth D, et al. The American College of Rheumatology criteria for the classification and reporting of osteoarthritis of the hand. Arthritis Rheum 33:1601–1610, 1990.
16. Altman R, Alarcon G, Appelrouth D, et al. The American College of Rheumatology criteria for the classification and reporting of osteoarthritis of the hip. Arthritis Rheum 34:505–514, 1991.
17. Spector TD, Hart DJ, Doyle DV. Incidence and progression of osteoarthritis in women with unilateral knee disease in the general population: the effect of obesity. Ann Rheum Dis 53:565–568, 1994.
18. Dieppe P, Cushnaghan J, Young P, et al. Prediction of the progression of joint space narrowing in osteoarthritis of the knee by bone scintigraphy. Ann Rheum Dis 52:557–563, 1993.
19. Brooks P, Boers M, Tugwell P. OMERACT III: the ACT revisited. J Rheumatol 24:764–765, 1997.
20. Bellamy N. Osteoarthritis clinical trials: candidate variables and clinimetric properties. J Rheumatol 24:768–778, 1997.
21. Bellamy N. Musculoskeletal Clinical Metrology. Dordrecht, Kluwer Academic Publishers, 1993.
22. Bellamy N. Pain assessment in osteoarthritis: experience with the WOMAC osteoarthritis index. Semin Arthritis Rheum 18:14–17, 1989.
23. Bellamy N. WOMAC Osteoarthritis Index: User's Guide III. London, Ontario, 1998.
24. Tubach F, Baron G, Falissard B, et al. Using patients' and rheumatologists' opinions to specify a short form of the WOMAC function subscale. Ann Rheum Dis 64:75–79, 2005.

25. Bellamy N, Buchanan WW, Goldsmith CH, et al. Validation study of WOMAC: a health status instrument for measuring clinically important patient relevant outcomes to antirheumatic drug therapy in patients with osteoarthritis of the hip or knee. J Rheumatol 15:1833–1840, 1988.

26. Bellamy N, Buchanan WW, Goldsmith CH, et al. Validation study of the WOMAC: a health status instrument for measuring clinically-important patient relevant outcomes following total hip or knee arthroplasty in osteoarthritis. J Orthop Rheumatol 1:95–108, 1988.

27. Bellamy N, Kean WF, Buchanan WW, et al. Double blind randomized controlled trial of sodium meclofenamate (Meclomen) and diclofenac sodium (Voltaren): post validation reapplication of the WOMAC Osteoarthritis Index. J Rheumatol 19:153–159, 1992.

28. Berman BM, Singh BB, Lao L, et al. A randomized trial of acupuncture as an adjunctive therapy for osteoarthritis of the knee. Rheumatology (Oxford) 38:346–354, 1999.

29. Creamer P, Lethbridge-Cejku M, Hochberg MC. Determinants of pain severity in knee osteoarthritis: the effect of demographic and psychosocial variables using three different pain measures. J Rheumatol 26:1785–1792, 1999.

30. Lequesne MG, Mery C, Samsson M, et al. Indices of severity for osteoarthritis of the hip and knee. Validation — value in comparison with other assessment tests. Scand J Rheumatol 65:85–89, 1987.

31. Guidelines for the Clinical Investigation of Drugs Used in Rheumatic Diseases. European Drug Guideline Series 5. Copenhagen, World Health Organization, Regional Office for Europe, 1985.

32. Lequesne M. Indices of severity and disease activity for osteoarthritis. Semin Arthritis Rheum 20:48–54, 1991.

33. Lequesne MG. The algofunctional indices for hip and knee osteoarthritis. J Rheumatol 24:779–781, 1997.

34. Berman BM, Lao L, Greene M, et al. Efficacy of traditional Chinese acupuncture in the treatment of symptomatic knee osteoarthritis: a pilot study. Osteoarthritis Cartilage 3:139–142, 1995.

35. Theiler R, Sangha O, Schaeren S, et al. Superior responsiveness of the pain and function sections of the Western Ontario and McMaster Universities Osteoarthritis Index (WOMAC) as compared to the Lequesne–Algofunctional Index in patients with osteoarthritis of the lower extremities. Osteoarthritis Cartilage 7:515–519, 1999.

36. Dreiser RL, Maheu E, Guillou JB, et al. Validation of an algofunctional index for osteoarthritis of the hand. Rev Rheum Engl 6:43S–53S, 1995.

37. Bellamy N. AUSCAN Osteoarthritis Hand Index. London, Ontario, 1996.

38. Bellamy N, Campbell J, Haraoui B, et al. Clinimetric properties of the AUSCAN osteoarthritis hand index: an evaluation of reliability, validity and responsiveness. Osteoarthritis Cartilage 10: 863–869, 2002.

39. Gummesson C, Atroshi I, Ekdahl C. The disabilities of the arm, shoulder and hand (DASH) outcome questionnaire: longitudinal construct validity and measuring self-rated health change after surgery. BMC Musculoskelet Disord 16:4–11, 2003.

40. Poiraudeau S, Chevalier X, Conrozier T, et al. Reliability, validity, and sensitivity to change of the Cochin hand functional disability scale in hand osteoarthritis. Osteoarthritis Cartilage 9: 570–577, 2001.

40a. Maheu E, Altman R D and Bloch D. Design and conduct of clinical trials in patients with osteoarthritis of the hand: recommendations from a task force of the Osteoarthritis Research Society International. Osteoarthritis Cart 14:303–322, 2006.

41. Fries JF, Spitz P, Kraines RG, et al. Measurement of patient outcome in arthritis. Arthritis Rheum 23:137–145, 1980.

42. Griffiths G, Bellamy N, Bailey WH, et al. A comparative study of the relative efficiency of the WOMAC, AIMS, and HAQ instruments in evaluating the outcome of total knee arthroplasty. Inflammopharmacology 3:1–6, 1995.

43. Pincus T, Summey JA, Soraci SA Jr, et al. Assessment of patient satisfaction in activities of daily living using a modified Stanford Health Assessment Questionnaire. Arthritis Rheum 26:1346–1353, 1983.

44. Pincus T, Callahan LF, Wolfe F, et al. Arthrotec compared to acetaminophen (ACTA): a clinical trial in patients with osteoarthritis of the hip or knee. Arthritis Rheum 42:S404, 1999.

45. Meenan RF, Gertman PM, Mason JH. Measuring health status in arthritis: the Arthritis Impact Measurement Scales. Arthritis Rheum 23:146–152, 1980.

46. Meenan RF, Mason JH, Anderson JJ, et al. The content and properties of a revised and expanded Arthritis Impact Measurement Scales Health Status Questionnaire. Arthritis Rheum 35:1–10, 1992.

47. Bellamy N, Kirwan J, Boers M, et al. Recommendations for a core set of outcome measures for future phase III clinical trials in knee, hip, and hand osteoarthritis: consensus development at OMERACT III. J Rheumatol 24:799–802, 1997.

48. Beaton DE, Schemitsch E. Measures of health-related quality of life and physical function. Clin Orthop Relat Res 413:90–105, 2003.

49. Ware JE Jr, Sherbourne CD. The MOS 36-Item Short-Form Health Survey (SF-36). I. Conceptual framework and item selection. Med Care 30:473–481, 1992.

50. McHorney CA, Ware JE Jr, Raczek AE. The MOS 36-Item Short-Form Health Survey (SF-36). II. Psychometric and clinical tests of validity in measuring physical and mental health constructs. Med Care 31:247–263, 1993.

51. Ware JE, Kosinski M, Hatoum HT, et al. Is the SF-36 health survey a valid measure of osteoarthritis and rheumatoid arthritis? Arthritis Rheum S258, 1996.

52. Hatoum HT, Ware JE, Keller SD, et al. Effect of oxaprozin and nabumetone on health related quality of life of patients with osteoarthritis of the knee. Arthritis Rheum S258, 1996.

53. Hurst NP, Jobanputra P, Hunter M, and the Economic and Health Outcomes Research Group. Validity of EuroQOL—a generic health status instrument—in patients with rheumatoid arthritis. Br J Rheumatol 33:655–662, 1994.

54. Lerner D, Amick BC, Rogers WH, et al. The Work Limitations Questionnaire. Medical Care 39:72–85, 2001.

55. Lerner D, Reed J, Massarotti E, et al. The Work Limitations Questionnaire's validity and reliability among patients with osteoarthritis. J Clin Epidemiol 55:197–208, 2002.

56. Abadie E, Ethgen D, Avouac B, et al. Recommendations for the use of new methods to assess the efficacy of disease-modifying drugs in the treatment of osteoarthritis. Osteoarthritis Cartilage 12:263–268, 2004.

57. Brandt KD, Mazucca SA, Conrozier T, et al. Which is the best radiographic protocol for clinical trial of a structure modifying drug in patients with osteoarthritis? J Rheumatol 29:1308–1320, 2002.

58. Reginster JY, Bruyere O, Henrotin Y. New perspectives in the management of osteoarthritis. Structure modification: facts or fantasy? J Rheumatol 30:14–20, 2003.

59. Strand V, Kelman A. Outcome measures in osteoarthritis: randomized controlled trials. Curr Rheumatol Rep 6:20–30, 2004.

60. Brandt KD, Mazzuca SA, Katz BP, et al. Effects of doxycycline on progression of osteoarthritis: results of a randomized, placebo-controlled, double-blind trial. Arthritis Rheum 52:2015–2025, 2005.

61. Brandt KD, Mazzuca SA, Conrozier T, et al. Which is the best radiographic protocol for a clinical trial of a structure modifying drug in patients with knee osteoarthritis? J Rheumatol 29: 1308–1320, 2002.

62. Mazzuca SA, Brandt KD, Schauwecker DS, et al. Severity of joint pain and Kellgren-Lawrence grade at baseline are better predictors of joint space narrowing than bone scintigraphy in obese women with knee osteoarthritis. J Rheumatol 32:1540–1546, 2005.

63. Buckland-Wright JC, Macfarlane DG, Williams SA, et al. Accuracy and precision of joint space width measurements in standard and macroradiographs of osteoarthritic knees. Ann Rheum Dis 54:872–880, 1995.

64. Buckland-Wright J, Wolfe F, Ward R, et al. Substantial superiority of semiflexed (MTP) views in knee osteoarthritis; a comparative radiographic study, without fluoroscopy, of standing extended, semiflexed (MTP), and schuss views. J Rheumatol 26:2664–2674, 1999.

65. Buckland-Wright JC, Ward RJ, Peterfy C, et al. Reproducibility of the semiflexed (metatarsophalangeal) radiographic knee position and automated measurements of medial tibiofemoral joint space width in a multicenter clinical trial of knee osteoarthritis. J Rheumatol. 31:1588–1597, 2004.

66. Peterfy C, Li J, Duryea J, et al. Nonfluoroscopic method for flexed radiography of the knee that allows reproducible joint space width measurement. Arthritis Rheum 41:S, 1998.

67. Peterfy CG, Li J, Zaim S, et al. Comparison of fixed-flexion positioning with fluoroscopic semi-flexed positioning for quantifying radiographic joint space width in the knee: test-retest reproducibility. Skeletal Radiol 32:128–132, 2003.

68. Greenwald RA. Treatment of destructive arthritis disorders with MMP inhibitors. Ann NY Acad Sci 731:181–198, 1994.

69. Golub LM, Ramamurthy NS, McNamara TF, et al. inventors. Method to reduce connective tissue destruction. U.S. patent 5,258,371. Nov 3, 1993.

70. Spector TD, Hart DJ, Doyle DV. Incidence and progression of osteoarthritis in women with unilateral knee disease in the general population: the effect of obesity. Ann Rheum Dis 53: 565–568, 1994.

71. Altman R, Asch E, Bloch D, et al. Development of criteria for the classification and reporting of osteoarthritis: classification of osteoarthritis of the knee. Arthritis Rheum 29:1039–1049, 1986.

72. Kellgren JH, Lawrence JS. Radiographic assessment of osteoarthritis. Ann Rheum Dis 16:494–502, 1956.

73. National Health and Nutrition Examination Survey II: vital and health statistics anthropometric reference data and prevalence of overweight. U.S. Dept. of Health and Human Services, Oct 1987, p 21–22. Publication #PHS 87–1688.

74. Haynes RB, Dantes R. Patient compliance and the conduct and interpretation of therapeutic trials. Control Clin Trials 8:12–39, 1987.

75. Lang JM. The use of a run-in to enhance compliance. Stat Med 9:87–95, 1990.

76. Rudd P, Ahmed S, Szchary V, et al. Improved compliance measures: applications in an ambulatory hypertensive drug trial. Clin Pharmacol Ther 48:676–685, 1990.

77. Hochberg MC, Lawrence RC, Everett DF, et al. Epidemiological associations of pain in osteoarthritis of the knee. Semin Arthritis Rheum 18:4–9, 1989.

78. Lethbridge-Cejku M, Scott WW Jr, Reickle R, et al. Association of radiographic features of osteoarthritis of the knee with knee pain: data from the Baltimore Longitudinal Study of Ageing. Arthritis Care Res 8:182–188, 1995.

79. Bruyere O, Honore A, Rovati LC, et al. Radiologic features poorly predict clinical outcomes in knee osteoarthritis. Scand J Rheumatol 31:13–16, 2002.

80. Creamer P, Lethbridge-Cejku M, Hochberg MC, et al. Individual radiographic features are not associated with severity of pain and physical disability in patients with knee osteoarthritis. Arthritis Rheum 41:S87, 1998.

81. Maheu E, Cadet C, Marty M, et al. Reproducibility and sensitivity to change of various methods to measure joint space width in osteoarthritis of the hip: a double reading of three different radiographic views taken with a three-year interval. Arthritis Res Ther 7:R1375–R1385, 2005.

82. Peterfy CG, Guermazi A, Zaim S, et al. Whole-organ magnetic resonance imaging score (WORMS) of the knee in osteoarthritis. Osteoarthritis Cartilage 12:177–190, 2004.

83. Raynaud JP, Kauffman C, Beaudoins G, et al. Reliability of quantification imaging system using magnetic resonance images to measure cartilage thickness and volume in human normal and osteoarthritic knees. Osteoarthritis Cartilage 11:351–360, 2003.

84. Disler DG, McCauley TR, Wirth CR, et al. Detection of knee hyaline articular cartilage defects using fat-suppressed three-dimensional spoiled gradient-echo MR imaging: comparison with standard MR imaging and correlation with arthroscopy. Am J Radiol 165:377–382, 1995.

85. Moskowitz RW, Hooper M. State-of-the-art disease-modifying osteoarthritis drugs. Curr Rheumatol Rep 7:15–21, 2005.

86. Peterfy C, White D, Zhao J, et al. Longitudinal measurement of knee articular cartilage volume in osteoarthritis. Arthritis Rheum 41:S, 1998.

87. Raynauld JP, Martel-Pelletier J, Berthiaume MJ, et al. Quantitative magnetic resonance imaging evaluation of knee osteoarthritis progression over two years and correlation with clinical symptoms and radiologic changes. Arthritis Rheum 50:476–487, 2004.

88. Abadie E, Ethgen D, Avouac B, et al. Recommendations for the use of new methods to assess the efficacy of disease-modifying drugs in the treatment of osteoarthritis. Osteoarthritis Cartilage 12:263–268, 2004.

89. Ayral X, Dougados M, Listrat V, et al. Chondroscopy: a new method for scoring chondropathy. Semin Arthritis Rheum 22:289–297, 1993.

90. Ayral X, Dougados M, Listrat V, et al. Arthroscopic evaluation of chondropathy in osteoarthritis of the knee. J Rheumatol 23: 698–706, 1996.

91. Raynauld JP. Magnetic resonance imaging of articular cartilage: toward a redefinition of "primary" knee osteoarthritis and its progression. J Rheumatol 29:1809–1810, 2002.

92. Youn I, Fu F, Suh J-K. Determination of the mechanical properties of articular cartilage using a high frequency ultrasonic indentation technique. Trans Orthop Res Soc Abstract 162, 1999.

93. Oakley SP, Portek I, Szomor Z, et al. Arthroscopy—a potential "gold standard" for the diagnosis of the chondropathy of early osteoarthritis. Osteoarthritis Cartilage 13:368–378, 2005.

94. Ayral X, Pickering EH, Woodworth TG, et al. Synovitis: a potential predictive factor of structural progression of medial tibiofemoral knee osteoarthritis—results of a 1 year longitudinal arthroscopic study in 422 patients. Osteoarthritis Cartilage 13:361–367, 2005.

95. Ayral X, Mackillop N, Genant HK, et al. Arthroscopic evaluation of potential structure-modifying drug in osteoarthritis of the knee. A multicenter, randomized, double-blind comparison of tenidap sodium vs piroxicam. Osteoarthritis Cartilage 11: 198–207, 2003.

96. Lohmander LS, Felson DT. Defining the role of molecular markers to monitor disease, intervention, and cartilage breakdown in osteoarthritis. J Rheumatol 24:782–785, 1997.

97. Lohmander LS. What is the current status of biochemical markers in the diagnosis, prognosis and monitoring of osteoarthritis? Baillieres Clin Rheumatol 11:711–726, 1997.

98. Wollheim FA. Serum markers of articular cartilage damage and repair. Rheum Dis Clin North Am 25:417–432, 1999.

99. Myers SL. Synovial fluid markers in osteoarthritis. Rheum Dis Clin North Am 25:433–449, 1999.

100. Sharif M, Saxne T, Shepstone L, et al. Relationship between serum cartilage oligomeric matrix protein levels and disease progression in osteoarthritis of the knee joint. Br J Rheumatol 34:306–310, 1995.

101. Sharif M, George E, Shepstone L, et al. Serum hyaluronic acid level as a predictor of disease progression in osteoarthritis of the knee. Arthritis Rheum 38:760–767, 1995.

102. Spector TD, Hart DJ, Nandra D, et al. Low level increases in serum CRP are present in early osteoarthritis of the knee and predict progressive disease. Arthritis Rheum 40:723–727, 1997.

103. Maillefert JF, Dougados M. Is time to joint replacement a valid outcome measure in clinical trials of drugs for osteoarthritis? Rheum Dis Clin North Am 29:831–845, 2003.

104. Tubach F, Ravaud P, Baron G, et al. Evaluation of clinically relevant changes in patient reported outcomes in knee and hip osteoarthritis: the minimal clinically important improvement. Ann Rheum Dis 64:29–33, 2005.

105. Tubach F, Ravaud P, Baron G, et al. Evaluation of clinically relevant states in patient reported outcomes in knee and hip osteoarthritis: the patient acceptable symptom state. Ann Rheum Dis 64:34–37, 2005.

106. U.S. Department of Health and Human Services, Food and Drug Administration, Center for Drug Evaluation and Research, Center for Biologics Evaluation and Research, Center for Devices and Radiologic Health. Guidance for Industry: Clinical Development Programs for Drugs, Devices and Biological Products Intended for the Treatment of Osteoarthritis. Draft, July 1999.

107. European Agency for the Evaluation of Medicinal Products, Human Medicines Evaluation Unit, Committee for Proprietary

Medicinal Products. Points to Consider on Clinical Investigation of Medicinal Products Used in the Treatment of Osteoarthritis. Draft 8, July 16, 1998.

108. Pincus T, Wang X, Chung C, et al. Patient preference in a crossover clinical trial of patients with osteoarthritis of the knee or hip: face validity of self-report questionnaire ratings. J Rheumatol 32:533–539, 2005.

109. Angst F, Aeschlimann A, Stucki G. Smallest detectable and minimal clinically important differences of rehabilitation intervention with their implications for required sample sizes using WOMAC and SF-36 quality of life measurement instruments in patients with osteoarthritis of the lower extremities. Arthritis Care Res 45:384–391, 2001.

110. Berman BM, Lao L, Langenberg P, et al. Effectiveness of acupuncture as adjunctive therapy in osteoarthritis of the knee: a randomized, controlled trial. Ann Intern Med 141:901–910, 2004.

111. Witt C, Brinkhaus B, Jena S, et al. Acupuncture in patients with osteoarthritis of the knee: a randomised trial. Lancet 366: 136–143, 2005.

112. Day R, Brooks P, Conaghan PG, et al. Multicenter Trial Group. A double blind, randomized, multicenter, parallel group study of the effectiveness and tolerance of intraarticular hyaluronan in osteoarthritis of the knee. J Rheumatol 31:775–782, 2004.

113. Strand V, Conaghan PG, Lohmander LS, et al. An integrated analysis of five double-blind, randomized controlled trials evaluating the safety and efficacy of a hyaluronan product for intra-articular injections in osteoarthritis of the knee. Osteoarthritis Cartilage 14:859–866, 2006.

114. Zhao SZ, McMillen JI, Markenson JA, et al. Evaluation of the functional status aspects of health-related quality of life of patients with osteoarthritis treated with celecoxib. Pharmacotherapy 19:1269–1278, 1999.

115. Ehrich EW, Davies GM, Watson DJ, et al. Minimal perceptible clinical improvement with the Western Ontario and McMaster University Osteoarthritis Index questionnaire and global assessments in patients with osteoarthritis. J Rheumatol 27: 2635–2641, 2000.

116. Pincus T, Koch G, Lei H, et al. Patient Preference for Placebo, Acetaminophen (paracetamol) or Celecoxib Efficacy Studies (PACES): two randomised, double blind, placebo controlled, crossover clinical trials in patients with knee or hip osteoarthritis. Ann Rheum Dis 63:931–939, 2004.

117. Cibere J, Kopec JA, Thorne A, et al. Randomized, double-blind, placebo-controlled glucosamine discontinuation trial in knee osteoarthritis. Arthritis Rheum 51:738–745, 2004.

118. Spector TD, Conaghan PG, Buckland-Wright JC, et al. Effect of risedronate on joint structure and symptoms of knee osteoarthritis: results of the BRISK randomized, controlled trial [ISRCTN01928173]. Arthritis Res Ther 7:R625–R633, 2005.

119. Knutsen G, Engebretsen L, Ludvigsen TC, et al. Autologous chondrocyte implantation compared with microfracture in the knee. A randomized trial. J Bone Joint Surg Am 86:455–464, 2004.

Surgical Considerations in Osteoarthritis

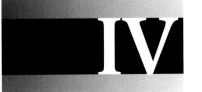

General Considerations, Indications, and Outcomes

19

Victor M. Goldberg

Osteoarthritis (OA) is the most common form of joint disease and is the second leading cause of disability in persons older than 50 years. It affects to some degree almost 90% of persons older than 65 years. Health care expenses for treatment of arthritis and other related chronic joint disorders in the United States are estimated at over $116 billion annually. In 2003, approximately 418,000 total knee replacements and over 220,000 hip replacements were performed in the U.S., and this number appears to be increasing at the rate of 11% for knee replacement and 2.5% for hip replacement per year. Although it can cause significant pain and loss of function over time, the treatment is usually nonoperative for the most part and consists of rest, physical therapy, analgesics, anti-inflammatory medication, and modifications of daily activities. For those patients who have significant pain and functional disability despite conservative treatment, carefully selected surgical procedures may provide substantial benefits.[1] Long-term studies evaluating the functional outcome of total joint replacement have demonstrated predictable and consistently satisfactory outcomes even in younger and more active patients.[2-9] These results provide the basis for an appealing therapeutic alternative for the patient suffering from the problems of OA. However, the beneficial results that can be seen after total joint replacement must be tempered by the possibility of failure secondary to mechanical and biologic problems. The end results of these complications may be less than optimal function, sometimes in a relatively young and active individual. Because of these possibilities, other surgical procedures should be considered that may improve the patient's symptoms and retard the progression of the disease. It is important to understand the indications and outcomes of other procedures that preserve the diarthrodial joint, such as osteotomy and joint débridement, to establish a complete treatment program for the patient with OA. This chapter provides the reader with an overview of the indications and expectations for the general types of surgical procedures that are presently available. Each anatomic area is discussed in detail in the sections that follow.

GENERAL CONSIDERATIONS

Before considering surgical treatment, the physician must weigh the risks and benefits of each procedure. This is especially important today, with the larger number of younger, active patients who are developing secondary arthritis after trauma or sports-related injuries. Although there are no absolute indications or contraindications for any surgical procedure, certain general concepts are important. For each individual patient, the physician should endeavor to develop a quantitative assessment of parameters of function to determine the appropriate therapeutic program. Not only is this an aid in the selection of the best therapeutic strategy, but it can also be of help in prospective studies evaluating the outcome of different surgical procedures. Figure 19-1 summarizes the scoring system for the evaluation of the knee as adapted by the Knee Society.

TKA EVALUATION DATA
02/25/98

UH NUMBER | PATIENT NAME: _____ | FORM COMPLETED BY:

SIDE: R L   Pre-Op Post-Op   SURGERY DATE ___/___/___   EXAM DATE ___/___/___

NOTE: All unshaded regions (KNEE SCORE and FUNCTION SCORE) MUST be completed if an evaluation score is to be calculated. The information in the shaded regions (MISCELLANEOUS) is merely requested, if available.

KNEE SCORE

PAIN

None/Ignores	50
Mild or occasional	45
Stairs only	40
Walking and Stairs	30
Moderate	
Occasional	20
Continuous	10
Severe	0

RANGE OF MOTION

From: _____ ° To: _____ °

STABILITY

Maximum movement in any position

Anteroposterior
< 5 mm	10
5 - 10 mm	5
> 10 mm	0

Mediolateral
< 5°	15
6 - 9°	10
10 - 15°	5
> 15°	0

DEDUCTIONS

Flexion Contracture
< 5°	0
5 - 10°	2
11 - 15°	5
16 - 20°	10
> 20°	15

Extension Lag
None	0
< 10°	5
10 - 20°	10
> 20°	15

Alignment
(circle type and write #°)

varus   0°   valgus

_____ °

Note: 0° is a 15 point deduction

FUNCTION SCORE

WALKING
Unlimited	50
> 10 blocks	40
5 - 10 blocks	30
< 5 blocks	20
Household, indoors	10
Unable, bed to chair	0

STAIRS
Normal, up and down	50
Up w/o rail, down w/rail	40
Up and down with rail	30
Up with rail, Unable down	15
Unable	0

(consider unable to reciprocate equivalent to using the rail in that direction)

DEDUCTIONS
None	0
Cane	5
Two Canes	10
Crutches or Walker	20

KNEE SOCIETY PATIENT CATEGORY

Unilateral (opposite knee normal) or Bilateral (opposite knee successfully replaced)	A
Unilateral (other knee symptomatic)	B
Multiple arthritis or medical infirmity	C

MISCELLANEOUS

LEVEL OF ACTIVITY
- ☐ Bedridden or confined to wheelchair
- ☐ Sedentary - minimum capacity for walking
- ☐ Semi-sedentary - white collar job, bench work, light housekeeping
- ☐ Light labor - heavy housekeeping, yard work, assembly line, or light sports (walking < 5 km)
- ☐ Moderate labor - lifts < 23 kg, moderate sports (walking, bicycling > 5 km)
- ☐ Heavy labor - frequently lifts 23-45 kg, vigorous sports

WALKING CAPACITY RESTRICTION
- ☐ NONE
- ☐ Right Knee
- ☐ Left Knee
- ☐ Other _____

NOTES:

MISCELLANEOUS (cont.)

WORK/ACTIVITY LAST 3 MONTHS

100%   75%   50%   25%   0%

MEDICATIONS
- ☐ NONE
- ☐ NSAIDS
- ☐ Narcotics
- ☐ Steroids/intra-articular
- ☐ Steroids/oral-current
- ☐ Steroids/oral-previous
- ☐ Antibiotics/current
- ☐ Antibiotics/previous

STATUS OF KNEES

	R	L
Normal	☐	☐
Abnormal	☐	☐
Primary TKA	☐	☐
Revision TKA	☐	☐
Unicompartmental	☐	☐
Internal Fixation	☐	☐
Fusion	☐	☐
Cement Spacer	☐	☐
Other (1)	☐	☐
Other (2)	☐	☐

(1) _____
(2) _____

STATUS OF HIPS

	R	L
Normal	☐	☐
Abnormal	☐	☐
THA	☐	☐
Hemiarthroplasty	☐	☐

OTHER ABNORMAL JOINTS

	R	L
NONE		☐
Shoulder	☐	☐
Elbow	☐	☐
Hand/Wrist	☐	☐
Ankle/Foot	☐	☐
Spine		☐

OTHER SIGNIFICANT DISEASE

_____

COMPLICATIONS
- ☐ Loosening
- ☐ Deep Infection
- ☐ Deep Venous Thrombosis (DVT)
- ☐ Urinary Tract Infection (UTI)
- ☐ Required Manipulation
- ☐ Other _____

Figure 19–1 Scoring system for evaluation of the knee for total knee arthroplasty. (From Insall JN, Dorr LD, Scott RD, et al. Rationale of the Knee Society Clinical Rating System. CORR 240:13–14, 1989.)

Similar scoring systems have been developed for the hip and other joints.

Pain is a key factor in the decision process. Rest pain, if it is present, poses a major problem for the patient and usually requires narcotics for control. Greater consideration for surgical intervention should be given in this circumstance. Activity-related discomfort is also important and may affect the patient's quality of life. However, many times these symptoms may be treated by nonoperative modalities, although lesser surgical procedures than total joint reconstruction may be of greater use during this stage of the disease.

Functional considerations are also central in the therapeutic decision process. Walking distance usually correlates with the anatomic severity of the joint disease. The need for external supports (e.g., canes) is an objective indication of the functional impairment experienced by the patient. The activities of daily living are also important. The ability to climb stairs and get into and out of an automobile or chair should be quantified. The physician should inquire about loss of time from work and the capability to perform household chores as well as recreational activities. This information gives the physician an estimate of the patient's quality of life and the socioeconomic problems the person may be experiencing. Many patients seek medical care because of the loss of their ability to participate in recreational sports such as golf or tennis. This also must be considered when developing a treatment plan.

Anatomic considerations include the range of joint motion, the presence or absence of extremity deformity, and an estimation of joint stability. This last function is easier to evaluate in the knee joint than in other joints. For example, in considering the hip, ligaments cannot be examined, and indirect techniques (e.g., evaluation of pain and deformity) may indicate joint integrity. The degree of motion or the extent of deformity is important not only in defining the stage of the disease but also in influencing the choice of the surgical procedure as described in subsequent chapters. The recent description of hip problems associated with femoral neck impingement on the anterior acetabular rim as a potential cause of secondary OA may, if recognized early in the natural history of hip disease, provide the indications for early intervention using arthroscopic techniques. Contouring the femoral neck as well as debriding any associated tears of the labrum may prevent further significant hip disease with the need for later joint arthroplasty.[10-11]

There have been a number of recent studies addressing the validity of several quantitative outcome assessments in hip and knee arthroplasty. Scoring systems that report categorical outcomes rather than numeric systems are less reliable in defining the hip or knee score. Additionally, studies have demonstrated that patients with a poorer preoperative status may not have as good an outcome as those with a higher level of preoperative function.[12] The Western Ontario and McMaster Universities Osteoarthritis Index (WOMAC), SF-36, and Oxford Twelve Item Knee Questionnaires have all been demonstrated to be valid systems to assess outcome measures. Studies have pointed to the WOMAC and SF-36 as better measures of pain and function and therefore are more reflective of patient-oriented outcomes than physician assessments.[12-14]

These data must be integrated into an overall evaluation of the present state of the patient's joint disease. Additional important considerations are the age and weight of the individual. For example, total joint arthroplasty has a higher chance of mechanical failure in a young, overweight, active individual, and other surgical procedures (e.g., arthrodesis) should be considered. By contrast, an elderly patient who may not have severe anatomic abnormalities but whose activities have had to be significantly modified because of pain may be a much better candidate for total joint replacement.

The ability of the patient to cooperate in any treatment plan is also important in surgical selection. Certain procedures (e.g., joint débridement or arthroplasty) require greater cooperation of the patient during the postoperative rehabilitation period compared with arthrodesis. In addition, the patient's knowledge of the disease and the possible outcomes of the surgical procedure must be understood. The patient's perception of what he or she hopes to obtain as a result of the surgery is central in the decision process. All too frequently, the physician does not ask the patient about his or her expectations. Although each person must be considered individually, information relative to the reported outcome of each surgical procedure is important in educating that individual. In some circumstances, an individual may desire a curative procedure, which may be unrealistic. At other times, cosmetic correction is foremost in the patient's mind. However, the patient may have become well adjusted to the malposition of the extremity, and if function is not compromised and the deformity does not constitute an anatomic threat to other joints, the mere presence of malposition may not be a reason for surgery. Specific quantitative assessment of the outcome of operative or nonoperative treatment will become more important in the future as the availability of health resources may become compromised.[15]

Long-term bed-bound or wheelchair-confined patients may desire a return to a community ambulatory status, but extra-articular anatomic factors may reduce the chance of a successful outcome. However, the improvement of function to an effective, household ambulatory status may be an attainable goal. These outcomes must be understood clearly by the patient and the physician.

The general health of the patient must be considered in evaluating surgical risk factors. Cardiovascular or respiratory disease may be severe enough to be a contraindication to general anesthesia and a major surgical procedure. However, regional or spinal anesthesia can often be substituted, thereby reducing the risk. One study assessing the results of randomized trials comparing epidural or spinal anesthesia to general anesthesia suggested that patient receiving regional anesthesia had a reduced rate of mortality and complications.[16-17] Many of the patients who are candidates for reconstructive surgery in the treatment of OA are elderly and are poor surgical and anesthetic risks. However, chronologic age alone should not be considered a contraindication; rather, the physiologic age of each patient must be considered in determining the risk/benefit ratio. It is important, however, to recognize, stabilize, and correct medical conditions that may exist before surgery. Some of the more common conditions include chronic obstructive lung disease, hypertension, angina pectoris, congestive heart failure, peripheral vascular disease, and diabetes mellitus. Any factors that predispose to infection (e.g., immunosuppressive drugs) should be considered and modified before surgery.

In addition to the risk/benefit ratio of any treatment, the cost/benefit relationships of a procedure must also be considered. Will the surgery enable the patient to become more self-sufficient or allow the individual to remain independent? If the surgical procedure is successful, can the person continue working or return to employment? The answers to these questions must be considered in the overall decision-making process. Care must be taken not to allow the decision to operate to depend heavily on socioeconomic considerations because many times surgery will reduce the dependence of the patient on a caregiver, which may be difficult to quantify.

There are no absolute indications for surgical intervention in OA. Many factors must be considered, and no one treatment algorithm is appropriate for any surgical treatment. The American Academy of Orthopaedic Surgeons (AAOS) has published care paths for the treatment of OA of the knee; however, within the pathway, flexibility is appropriate to treat individual patients.[18] Similarly, there are no absolute contraindications to surgery in patients with OA, although relative contraindications do exist. Active infection, overwhelmingly poor medical health, and inadequate anatomic structures (e.g., motor control) or available bone stock are reasons to reject surgical treatment. Other factors may increase the chances for a poorer outcome when a specific operative procedure is considered. For example, patients who are morbidly obese or whose joint in question is neuropathic usually do poorly when arthroplasties are performed, and suitable alternatives should be substituted, if possible.

More knowledge is being accumulated about the outcome of many operative procedures and which risk factors are most important in determining their long-term results; but clearly, the decision of which surgical procedure to use, when to use it, and on whom to use it must still be left to sound clinical judgment. Most important, each patient is an individual, and the positive and negative aspects of the treatment must be carefully considered for that patient. Finally, the availability of a large body of information on the internet has made patients more knowledgeable about their treatment alternatives. This does present a new challenge for physicians caring for these patients, as much of the data on this media has not been validated.

TYPES OF SURGICAL PROCEDURES

The surgical treatment modalities presently used for patients with OA may be classified into four broad categories: osteotomy, débridement, arthrodesis (fusion), and arthroplasty. General principles have evolved for each procedure that are applicable to its use in any OA joint problem. Table 19–1 provides the reader a comparison of surgical alternatives in OA detailing the indications and expected outcomes for each surgical category. The recent introduction of minimally invasive procedures for hip and knee arthroplasty has accelerated the postoperative rehabilitation and return of function. However, longer term studies to date have not demonstrated any ultimate advantage for this new approach.[19-20]

Osteotomy

One of the advantages of an osteotomy is that it addresses both biologic and mechanical problems without sacrificing the integrity of the joint. The two main goals of this procedure are to relieve pain and to prevent the progression of OA. If joint malalignment is present (e.g., genu varum of the knee), with resultant abnormal force distribution, an osteotomy to realign the joint in a more normal configuration will correct the abnormal mechanical loads causing progression of the disease. The aim of the procedure is to redistribute the forces in such a way that healthy cartilages on the relatively uninvolved side of the joint will be brought into apposition with each other. In addition, there is evidence that osteotomizing the bone changes the pattern of vascular supply to the joint, which may have a biologic effect on the OA process.[21]

Osteotomy was one of the earliest procedures to be used in the surgical management of OA. Although osteotomy is not curative, when patients are carefully selected, excellent pain relief, improved function, and maintenance of physiologic joint motion and stability may be expected.[22-35] It is especially applicable for the young, active individual when relatively normal articular cartilage is present. A functional range of motion must be present before surgery, because some motion may be lost after surgery. The knee joint, for example, should have close to 90° of flexion without a fixed flexion contracture of greater than 20° for osteotomy to be considered. If a deformity (e.g., genu valgum) is present, it should not be so excessive that correction to anatomic alignment cannot be obtained. Additional important considerations include satisfactory periarticular muscle control of the joint and intrinsic joint stability. Considerable cooperation of the patient and understanding are necessary for a successful outcome. The development of sophisticated instrumentation has provided the basis for improved surgical technique with the expectation of improved outcomes.[30,36] Further, the use of internal fixation devices lessens the postoperative need for casts and enables maintenance of joint motion. There have been reports of the combined use of osteotomy and débridement of the knee joint, with encouraging early results in difficult, more advanced problems of OA of the knee.[37-38] The application of specific additional biological procedures to encourage formation of new cartilage, such as microfracture, may improve the longer term outcome for knee osteotomy. This may delay the need for total knee replacement in younger patients. Osteotomy of the hip has enjoyed a resurgence lately with the recognition of subtle anatomical abnormalities in younger patients with very early OA. The periacetabular osteotomy described by Ganz has been reported to result in significant improvement in pain and function with a satisfactory rating of 90%.[11]

Débridement

The concept of smoothing irregular joint surfaces and removing the loose bodies and inflamed synovium that add to the destructive processes in OA of the knee was popularized by Magnuson[39] in 1946. In appropriate

TABLE 19–1
COMPARISON OF SURGICAL ALTERNATIVES IN OSTEOARTHRITIS

Procedure	Osteotomy	Débridement	Arthrodesis	Total Joint Replacement
Indications	Younger patient, activity pain, mild to moderate joint deformity with some preservation of articular cartilage, functional range of motion	Younger patient, little joint deformity, defined OA lesion	Young, active, heavy patient with single joint involved with OA; spinal arthrodesis is an adjunct to decompressive procedures	Significant pain, deformity, functional loss, with restricted range of motion or joint instability
Recovery period	Usually 3 months for knee; may be longer (6–12 months) for hip	Variable, depends on extent of procedure		
(3 weeks–3 months)	Depends on the rapidity of the arthrodesis to occur, usually 3–6 months	Usually rapid, 3–6 months		
Improvement in pain	Moderate improvement of activity pain	Variable, depends on extent of OA	Significant with successful arthrodesis	Significant, consistent, reproducible
Functional improvement	Pain relief usually improves function	Moderate, but may be for a short time	Excellent, but depends on joint (e.g., ankle arthrodesis, almost no functional loss)	Significant
Expected duration of improvement	Variable, depends on preoperative extent of OA	Highly variable, depends on extent of OA	Lifetime, but adjacent joints may degenerate	Durability improving; expectations now of clinical success for 10–15 years
Cost	Modest	Modest (least)	Modest	Most expensive
Options if procedure fails	Arthrodesis, total joint replacement	Osteotomy, arthrodesis, total joint replacement	Total joint replacement	Arthrodesis, excisional arthroplasty

circumstances, the hip, ankle, wrist, and elbow may also benefit from this surgical modality.[40–42] For this procedure to be considered, joint malalignment either should not be present or should be correctable with an osteotomy. A functional range of motion is necessary. It is also helpful to have preservation of at least 50% of the articular cartilage surface. The results are variable and depend a great deal on the careful selection of a motivated patient.[40] Pain relief can be impressive, but many times some joint mobility is lost after surgery. Insall[43] reported about 75% good results after knee joint débridement, with an average of 6.5 years of follow-up. A joint effusion is frequently present for a prolonged period after surgery, but this gradually subsides. Maximal improvement is usually not seen before 12 months after surgery. The addition of continuous passive motion in the postoperative rehabilitation phase may improve the results of débridement.[44] Advances in arthroscopic techniques, with their decrease in morbidity and postoperative recovery time, make débridement a more attractive approach in patients who present with early OA, and reports indicate an optimistic outcome in carefully

selected patients.[38,41–50] However, one recent Veteran's Administration study reporting the results of a randomized trial comparing arthroscopic lavage, débridement, or sham procedures in 180 patients demonstrated at a 2-year follow-up no statistical differences. There were a number of issues in this study that detracted from the conclusions including a 44% dropout rate, only male patients, and nonspecific indications for surgical intervention.[51] By contrast, Aaron reported a study of 122 consecutive patients who had failed conservative treatment and underwent arthroscopic débridement of the knee. At 34 months follow-up, 90% of the patients with objective mild arthritis demonstrated marked improvement by 6 months after surgery. However, there was little improvement in those patients with high grade OA according to clinical and radiographic signs.[52] Specific débridement techniques such as microfracture when used for local cartilage defects may be very effective in preserving joint function.[50] The use of débridement and newer biological treatments may prolong the patient's clinical course without the need for total joint replacement (see Chapter 23).

Arthrodesis (Fusion)

Although total joint replacement has become the treatment of choice for severe grade IV OA, there is still a place in the surgical management of OA for arthrodesis of joints. It must be understood by any patient about to undergo total joint replacement of the knee, for example, that fusion may be the only other alternative and may be the end result if failure occurs. However, there are specific instances in which arthrodesis may be the primary procedure of choice. OA of the cervical or lumbar spine that is unresponsive to medical management may require fusion of the involved segments, combined with decompression of the neutral elements.[53-55] Local intercarpal fusions may be extremely helpful in controlling the pain and instability of carpal OA without completely sacrificing wrist motion and function.[56]

If a single lower extremity joint is involved with OA in a young, overweight, active patient, arthrodesis may be the procedure of choice when the severity of joint destruction precludes use of a lesser procedure.[1] As long as the contiguous joints are mobile, function is usually maintained, and long-term pain relief is achieved. However, if OA is present in other joints (e.g., lumbar spine, hip, or knee), fusion may be contraindicated, and careful consideration should be given to the performance of an arthroplasty. Anatomic considerations are also important in the decision. For example, deficient bone stock or inadequate motor power may be a contraindication to other procedures and may make arthrodesis an attractive choice. If the shoulder joint lacks adequate rotator cuff and deltoid muscle power but has good scapular muscle stabilizers, fusion may be an effective surgical modality in relieving pain and improving upper extremity function. The use of internal fixation devices has made arthrodesis a more successful procedure and less dependent on prolonged cast immobilization. Care must be taken not to disturb the soft tissues around the joint so that satisfactory anatomy will be present if an arthroplasty is performed later.[57] A recent study of the conversion of a fused hip to a total hip arthroplasty (THA) reported a 96% survival rate at 10 years.[58]

Arthroplasty

The modern concepts of joint replacement have their origin in the Smith-Petersen cup arthroplasty,[59] but with the applications of sophisticated engineering principles to orthopedics, great strides in arthroplasty have been made since the 1970s. Charnley's adaptation of polymethylmethacrylate as a fixation interface between the metallic or plastic implant and the bone created a major impact on the surgical treatment of severe OA.[60]

Arthroplasty is indicated when severe pain and disability are present. Appropriate bone stock and muscle power must be present to technically accomplish the procedure and to expect satisfactory results. Because the failure of arthroplasty usually results in less than optimal function, lesser surgical procedures should be considered first, if feasible, and the patient should understand and be willing to accept, if necessary, the possible end-stage procedure.[61-64] Arthroplasty may be of the excisional, partial, or total replacement type. Biologic substitutes have been used to resurface confined destroyed articular surfaces in the knee joint, with encouraging early results.[65-67] Girdlestone[68] described a hip arthroplasty in which the head and neck of the femur were excised and a fibrous pseudarthrosis developed. The results of this procedure as a therapeutic modality are less than optimal, but patients who are candidates for total hip reconstruction must be willing to accept it as a possible consequence of the complications of the total joint arthroplasty. Excellent results are rarely seen after excisional arthroplasty, because most patients continue to complain of some pain, instability, and shortening of the extremity. External supports, such as a cane or crutches, are usually required for most activities.[69]

Excisional arthroplasty with the interposition of local tissue may be of greater use in small joints (e.g., the first carpometacarpal joint[70] or the first metatarsophalangeal joint[71]). Under these circumstances, the malalignment and pain resulting from OA of these joints are corrected, and function is improved. However, these joints are not usually subjected to the marked stresses seen in other large upper and lower extremity synovial joints.

The cup or mold arthroplasty was the first modern attempt to resurface destroyed articular surfaces.[59,72] The initial results were encouraging, but unfortunately, the long-term outcome has been inconsistent and too dependent on the technical expertise of the surgeon and on the postoperative rehabilitation program. Although satisfactory results may be expected in approximately 60% of patients, there are certain clinical situations in which the procedure should still be considered. Young patients with secondary OA after remote infection in a joint may benefit from this procedure with reduced pain but without a significant improvement in function.[73] The use of newer materials such as ceramics may improve the outcome of this procedure.

Another type of partial arthroplasty that has been used in the past with some success is the Austin-Moore or Thompson femoral head replacement. This procedure has been used extensively for treatment of the displaced femoral neck fracture in the elderly, with satisfactory results.[74] Its application to the surgical treatment of OA has been supplanted by the more dependable total replacement. However, in situations in which OA involves only the femoral articular surfaces (e.g., as a secondary manifestation of osteonecrosis), some consideration should be given to its use.[74,75] A bipolar femoral head replacement in which polymethylmethacrylate is used to fix the implant to bone has been employed in an attempt to prevent the problem of prosthesis loosening. Satisfactory results have been reported in selected problems, such as osteonecrosis.[76]

Biologic materials have also been used to resurface articular surfaces destroyed by OA. Osteochondral allografts have been used primarily in the knee joint.[65,66] The results have been variable, although satisfactory results have been reported when technical problems have been minimized and only a single compartment is replaced. Recently, other biological cartilage repair techniques have been introduced to clinical problems.[50] These include marrow stimulating procedures to promote the development of fibrocartilagenous surfaces by activating osteochondral stem cells in the bone marrow. Autologous osteochondral plugs have been used to repair focal small defects with reasonable early clinical outcomes.[49] Larger lesions greater than 2 cm^2 have been repaired using autologous chondrocyte transplants with satisfactory functional results.[49] The widespread applicability of this and other newer biologic treatment strategies using tissue engineering principles for articular problems in OA awaits improved techniques of cartilage preservation and fixation as well as a broader understanding of the molecular mechanisms leading to articular cartilage destruction[77] (see Chapter 23).

The surgical treatment of advanced OA currently centers primarily on total joint replacement. There is no doubt that this procedure is one of the most consistent and dependable operative techniques used in orthopedic surgery. The relief of pain and improved function that it affords are almost universal in technically satisfactory procedures. However, great care must be taken to consider other surgical treatment modalities in view of the possible complications, which fortunately occur relatively infrequently, and the poor outcome if failure does ensue. Although almost every diarthrodial joint has been replaced in the treatment of OA, the hip and knee have been the major foci.[61] More than 400,000 total hip and knee replacements are performed each year in the United States.[61,78-80] Several reports have related long-term follow-up of those procedures.[2,3,5,64,81,82] Many of the problems originally described have now been circumvented. Infection, a significant complication in the early days of replacement, can be controlled with antibiotic prophylaxis and the use of special operating facilities.[64] The expected incidence of periprosthetic infection should be less than 1%. Improvements in implant design and fixation methods have led to longer-lasting components with less loosening of hip and knee implants. Cementless methods to fix both hip and knee components to the bone were introduced during the 1980s. Advanced technologies such as hydroxyapatite coating on the implant have enhanced the fixation of these components.[83] Long-term studies have reported highly successful outcomes with use of this technology.[4,84,85] Techniques using minimally invasive surgical approaches and the use of computer-assisted navigation are newer technologies that appear to improve the early functional recovery of patients after total hip or knee replacement and assure excellent component alignment.[86,87] The long-term outcome of these technical modalities remains to be defined. Further, the cost-benefit ratio of new approaches to total joint arthroplasty must be justified to enable widespread use of these technologies.

Initially, total knee arthroplasty was considered a less satisfactory procedure than total hip replacement. However, long-term studies now suggest excellent sustained outcomes for total knee replacement.[82,88] Major advances in knee prosthetic design allow preservation of the major knee ligaments and provide physiologic range of motion and knee kinematics. Unicompartmental knee arthroplasty has recently become a viable alternative for single compartment OA because of improved designs, instruments, and surgical techniques. The 10-year survival rate has been reported as high as 98%.[89]

The advances in manufacturing techniques and improved metallurgical processes have encouraged renewed interest in metal-on-metal hip resurfacing.[90] The procedure does have a number of advantages including bone preservation, a reduced incidence of postoperative hip dislocation, and perhaps improved patient function. There is an added risk of femoral neck fracture and component loosening for these devices. The revision to a standard THA does not appear to be technically challenging. Although short-term results are generally good, longer follow-up is necessary.

The widespread use of arthroplasty in younger, active patients has resulted in excessive wear of the articulating surfaces and has become the most common complication after total hip and knee arthroplasty.[91-96] The particles that result from either the articulating surface or the surface of the implant itself are the primary cause of the subsequent bone resorption (osteolysis) that is seen.[93,97-99] Excessive quantities of these particles stimulate a biologic reaction that results in osteoclast differentiation, activation, and bone resorption. The osteolysis can ultimately result in implant loosening with significant loss of bone. This complication has led to the use of alternative materials as articulating surfaces.[94,100,101] Reports of ceramic-on-ceramic and metal-on-metal surfaces indicate a reduction in wear particles and osteolysis[102-103] (see Chapter 21A and 21B).

Reports of long-term follow-up of cemented total hip replacements indicate clinical results approaching a 90% survival.[2,104] However, during the second decade of follow-up, there appears to be an increased incidence of acetabular loosening. Because of the increased acetabular component loosening, a hybrid total hip replacement has emerged as the "gold standard."[81,105] This procedure uses a cementless acetabular component and a cemented femoral stem. The early clinical reports describing this procedure indicate a highly successful outcome.[106] Long-term assessments of fully cementless implants have also reported excellent component survivals.[107-108]

The increased costs of health care delivery have directed studies addressing hospital costs for total joint replacements during the last decade.[78-80] These studies have emphasized approaches to help reduce costs by institutional utilization reviews and the surgeon's involvement in the cost-containment process. The effect of total joint replacement on the quality of the life of patients has also been studied for total hip replacements in a randomized controlled trial.[78] The data from this study suggested that there is a significant improvement in the patient's function, social interaction, and overall health after hip replacement. This emphasizes the issue that the surgical treatment of OA is not primarily a quantity of life issue, but with the aging of the population, the quality of life that requires the patient's independence and the reduced dependence on caregivers for OA patients are important elements for a successful health care system. This becomes even more important with the availability of expensive advanced technologies for total joint replacement, such as alternative bearing surfaces and newer surfaces to improve component fixation. Their application must be evaluated in the context of their cost-effectiveness relative to outcomes for patients.

CONCLUSION

The present state of the art of surgical management of OA offers patients effective methods of alleviating the distressing symptoms of the disease. However, most individuals may obtain adequate relief with judicious nonoperative therapeutic modalities. Before surgical intervention, careful consideration should be given to the available surgical alternatives, and great effort should be made to educate the patient with regard to the risks and benefits of any procedure.

REFERENCES

1. Sponseller PD, McBeath AA, Perpich M, et al. Hip arthrodesis in young patients. A long-term follow-up study. J Bone Joint Surg Am 66:853–859, 1984.
2. Madey SM, Callaghan JJ, Olejniczak JP, et al. Charnley total hip arthroplasty with the use of improved techniques of cementing: the results after a minimum of fifteen years of follow-up. J Bone Joint Surg Am 79:53–64, 1997.
3. Engh CA Jr, Culpepper WJ III, Engh CA. Long-term results of use of the anatomic medullary locking prosthesis in total hip arthroplasty. J Bone Joint Surg Am 79:177–184, 1997.
4. Geesink RG, Hoefnagels NH. Six-year results of hydroxyapatite-coated total hip replacement. J Bone Joint Surg Br 77:534–547, 1995.
5. Mont MA, Hungerford DS. Proximally coated ingrowth prosthesis: a review. Clin Orthop 334:139–149, 1997.
6. Buechel FF: Long-term follow-up after mobile bearing total knee replacement. Clin Orthop 404:40–50, 2002.
7. Capello WN, D'Antonio JA, Freinberg, Manley MT. Ten-year results with hydroxyapatite-coated total hip femoral components in patients less than fifty years old: A concise follow-up of a previous report. J Bone Joint Surg Am 85:885–889, 2003.
8. Parvizi J, Sharkey PF, Hozack WJ, et al. Prospective matched-pair analysis of hydroxyapatite-coated and uncoated femoral stems in total hip arthroplasty: A concise follow-up of a previous report. J Bone Joint Am 86:783–786, 2004.
9. Whiteside LA: Long-term follow-up of the bone ingrowth Ortholoc knee system without a metal-backed patella. Clin Orthop 388:77–84, 2001.
10. Siebenrock KA, Schoeniger R, Ganz R, et al. Anterior femoro-acetabular impingement due to adetabular retroversion: Treatment with periacetabular osteotomy. J Bone Joint Surg Am 85:278–286, 2003.
11. van Bergayk AB, Garbuz DS. Quality of life and sports-specific outcomes after Bernese periacetabular osteotomy. J Bone Joing Surg Br 84:339–343, 2002.
12. Davies AP: Rating system for total knee replacement. Knee 9(4):261–266, 2002.
13. Kiebzak GM, Campbell M, Mauerhan DR. The SF-36 general health status survey documents the burden of osteoarthritis and the benefits of total joint arthroplasty: But why should we use it? Am J Manag Care 8(5):463–474, 2002.
14. Boardman DL, Dorey F, Thomas BJ, et al. The accuracy of assesing total hip arthroplasty outcomes: A prospective correlation study of walking ability and 2 validated measurement devices. J Arthroplasty 15(2):200–204, 2000.
15. Hunsaker FG, Cioffi DA, Amadio PC, et al. The American Academy of Orthopaedic Surgeons outcomes instruments: Normative values from the general population. J Bone Joint Surg Am 84:208–215, 2002.
16. Holte K, Sharrock NE, Kehlet H. Pathophysiology and clinical implications of perioperative fluid excess. Br J. Anaesth 89(4): 622–632, 2002.
17. Rodgers A, Walker N, Schug S, et al. Reduction of post-operative mortality and morbidity with epidural or spinal anaesthesia: Results from overview of randomised trials. BMJ 321 (7275): 1493, 2000.
18. Saleh KJ, Mulhall KJ, Hofmann AA, et al. Primary total knee arthroplasty outcomes. AAOS OKU 3:93–110, 2002.
19. Berry DJ, Berger RA, Callaghan JJ, et al. Minimally invasive total hip arthroplasty: Development, early results, and a critical analysis. J Bone Joint Surg Am 85:2235–2246, 2003.
20. Bonutti PM, McMahon M, Mont MA, et al. Minimally invasive total knee arthroplasty. J Bone Joint Surg Am 86:26–32, 2004.
21. Arnoldi CC, Lempreg R, Linderholm H, et al. Immediate effect of osteotomy on the intramedullary pressure in the femoral head and neck in patients with degenerative arthritis. Acta Orthop Scand 42:454–455, 1971.
22. Coventry MB. Osteotomy about the knee for degenerative and rheumatoid arthritis. Indications, operative technique, and results. J Bone Joint Surg Am 55:23–48, 1973.
23. Coventry MB. Upper tibial osteotomy for gonarthrosis. The evolution of the operation in the last 18 years and long term results. Orthop Clin North Am 10:191–210, 1979.
24. Insall J, Shoji J, Mayer V, et al. High tibial osteotomy. A five-year evaluation. J Bone Joint Surg Am 56:1397–1405, 1974.
25. Hansen FW, Hansen-Leth C, Jensen EG, et al. Intertrochanteric osteotomy with A.O. technique in arthrosis of the hip. Acta Orthop Scand 44:219–229, 1973.
26. Morrey BF. Upper tibial osteotomy for secondary osteoarthritis of the knee. J Bone Joint Surg Br 71:554–559, 1989.
27. Keene JS, Monson DK, Roberts MJ, et al. Evaluation of patients for high tibial osteotomy. Clin Orthop 243:157–165, 1989.
28. Hackenbroch MH. Intertrochanteric osteotomy for the treatment of coxarthrosis. Arch Orthop Trauma Surg 108:125–131, 1989.
29. Iwase T, Hasegawa Y, Kawamoto K, et al. Twenty years' followup of intertrochanteric osteotomy for treatment of the dysplastic hip. Clin Orthop 331:245–255, 1996.
30. Millis MB, Murphy SB, Poss R, et al. Osteotomies about the hip for the prevention and treatment of osteoarthritis. J Bone Joint Surg Am 77:626–647, 1995.
31. Nagel A, Insall J, Scuderi G. Proximal tibial osteotomy. J Bone Joint Surg Am 78:1353–1357, 1996.
32. Hernigou P, Medevielle D, Debeyre J, et al. Proximal tibial osteotomy for osteoarthritis with varus deformity. A ten-to thirteen-year follow-up study. J Bone Joint Surg Am 69:332–353, 1978.
33. Healy W, Anglen J, Wasielewski S, et al. Varus osteotomy of the distal part of the femur: a survivorship analysis. J Bone Joint Surg Am 78:1348–1352, 1996.
34. Amendola A: Uncompartmental osteoarthritis in the active patient: The role of high tibial osteotomy. Arthroplasty 19: 109–116, 2003.
35. Schramm M, Hohmann D, Radespiel-Troger M, et al. Treatment of the dysplastic acetabulum with Wagner sperical osteotomy: A study of patients followed for a minimum of twenty years. J Bone Joint Surg Am 85:808–814, 2003.
36. Siebenrock KA, Scholl E, Lottenbach M, et al. Bernese periacetabular osteotomy. Clin Orthop 363:9–20, 1999.
37. MacIntosh DL, Welsh RP. Joint débridement—a complement to high tibial osteotomy in the treatment of degenerative arthritis of the knee. J Bone Joint Surg Am 59:1094–1097, 1977.
38. Schonholtz GJ. Arthroscopic débridement of the knee joint. Orthop Clin North Am 20:257–263, 1989.
39. Magnuson PB. Technique of débridement of the knee joint for arthritis. Surg Clin North Am 26:149–166, 1946.
40. Edelson R, Burks R, Bloebaum RD, et al. Short-term effects of knee washout for osteoarthritis. Am J Sports Med 23:345–349, 1995.
41. Jackson R, Rouse D. The results of partial arthroscopic menisectomy in patients over 40 years of age. J Bone Joint Surg Br 64: 481–485, 1982.
42. Gibson J, White M, Chapman V, et al. Arthroscopy lavage and débridement for osteoarthritis of the knee. J Bone Joint Surg Br 74:534–537, 1992.
43. Insall JN. Intra-articular surgery for degenerative arthritis of the knee. A report of the work of the late K.H. Pridie. J Bone Joint Surg Br 49:211–228, 1967.
44. Coutts RD, Kaita J, Barr R, et al. The role of continuous passive motion in the postoperative rehabilitation of the total knee patient. Trans Orthop Res Soc 7:195, 1982.

45. Bert JM, Maschka K. The arthroscopic treatment of unicompartmental gonarthrosis: a five-year follow-up study of abrasion arthroplasty plus arthroscopic débridement and arthroscopic débridement alone. Arthroscopy 5:25–32, 1989.
46. Chang R, Falconer J, Stulberg S, et al. A randomized, controlled trial of arthroscopic surgery versus closed-needle joint lavage for patients with osteoarthritis of the knee. Arthritis Rheum 36:289–296, 1993.
47. Poss R. Current concepts review: the role of osteotomy in the treatment of osteoarthritis of the hip. J Bone Joint Surg Am 66:144–151, 1984.
48. Hangody L, Feczko P, Bartha L, et al. Masaicplasty for the treatment of articular defects of the knee and ankle. Clin Orthop 391S:328–336, 2201.
49. Aubin PP, Cheah HK, Davis AM, et al. Long-term followup of fresh femoral osteochondral allografts for posttraumatic knee defects. Clin Orthop 391S:318–327, 2001.
50. Steadman JR, Briggs KK, Rodrigo JJ, et al. Outcomes of microfracture for traumatic chondral defects of the knee: Average 11-year follow-up. Arthroscopy 19:447–484, 2003.
51. Moseley JB, O'Malley K, Petersen NJ, et al. A controlled trial of arthroscopic surgery for osteoarthritis of the knee. N Engl J Med 2002;347:81–88.
52. Aaron RK, Skolnick AH, Reinert SE, et al. Arthroscopic debridement for osteoarthritis of the knee. J Bone Joint Surg Am 88:936–943, 2006.
53. Dodge L, Bohlman HH, Rhodes R, et al. Concurrent lumbar spinal stenosis and peripheral vascular disease. Clin Orthop 230:141–148, 1988.
54. Paine KWE. Results of decompression for lumbar spinal stenosis. Clin Orthop 115:96–100, 1976.
55. Jacobs G, Krueger EG, Leivy DM. Cervical spondylosis with radiculopathy. Results of anterior diskectomy and interbody fusion. JAMA 211:2135–2139, 1970.
56. Watson HK, Hempton RF. Limited wrist arthrodesis I. The triscaphoid joint. J Hand Surg 5:320–327, 1980.
57. Stover MD, Beaule PE, Matta JM, et al. Hip arthrodesis: A procedure for the new millennium? Clin Orthop 418:126–133, 2004.
58. Joshi AB, Markovic L, Hardinge K, et al. Conversion of a fused hip to total hip arthroplasty. J Bone Joint Surg Am 84:1335–1341, 2002.
59. Smith-Petersen MN. Evolution of mould arthroplasty of the hip joint. J Bone Joint Surg Br 30:59–75, 1948.
60. Charnley J. The bonding of prosthesis to bone by cement. J Bone Joint Surg Br 46:518–529, 1964.
61. Kelsey JL. Epidemiology and impact. Presented at NIH Consensus Development Conference on Total Hip Joint Replacement, Bethesda, MD, March 1–3, 1981. In: Total Hip Joint Replacement. Program Abstracts. Washington, DC, U.S. Government Printing Office, 1981, pp 23–24.0-361-132/3806.
62. Charnley J. The long-term results of low-friction arthroplasty of the hip performed as a primary intervention. J Bone Joint Surg Br 54:638–647, 1969.
63. Stauffer RN. Ten year follow-up study of total hip replacement. With particular reference to roentgenographic loosening of the component. J Bone Joint Surg Am 64:983–990, 1982.
64. Salvati EA, Wilson PD, Jolley MN, et al. A ten-year follow-up of our first one hundred consecutive, Charnley total hip replacements. J Bone Joint Surg Am 63:753–767, 1981.
65. Gross AE, Silverstein EA, Falk J, et al. The allotransplantation of partial joints in the treatment of osteoarthritis of the knee. Clin Orthop 108:7–14, 1975.
66. Goldberg VM, Caplan AI. Biologic restoration of articular surfaces. Instructional Course Lectures. Vol 48. Rosemont, IL, American Academy of Orthopaedic Surgeons, 1999, pp 623–628.
67. Caplan AI, Golberg VM (guest editors). Orthopaedic Tissue Engineering. Overview. Association of Bone and Joint Surgeons Workshop. Special suppl., Clin Orthop 367S, 1999.
68. Girdlestone GR. Acute pyogenic arthritis of the hip: an operation giving free access and effective drainage. Lancet 1:419–424, 1943.
69. Bosquet MMJ, Duncan CP, Mulier JC, et al. Girdlestone excision arthroplasty of the hip. A review of 49 patients. Orthop Trans 6:336, 1982.
70. Jense JS. Operative treatment of chronic subluxation of the first carpometacarpal joint. Hand 7:269–271, 1975.
71. Wrighton JD. A ten-year review of Keller's operation. Review of Keller's operation at the Princess Elizabeth Orthopaedic Hospital, Exeter. Clin Orthop 89:207–214, 1972.
72. Harris WH. Traumatic arthritis of the hip after dislocation and acetabular fractures: treatment by mold arthroplasty. An end result study using a new method of result evaluation. J Bone Joint Surg Am 51:737–755, 1969.
73. Hunt DD, Larson CB. Treatment of the residual of hip infections by mold arthroplasty. An end result study of thirty-three hips. J Bone Joint Surg Am 48:111–125, 1966.
74. Anderson LD, Hamsa WR, Waring TL. Femoral-head prosthesis. A review of three hundred and fifty-six operations and their results. J Bone Joint Surg Am 46:1049–1065, 1964.
75. Apley AG, Millner WF, Porter DS. A follow-up study of Moore's arthroplasty in the treatment of osteoarthritis of the hip. J Bone Joint Surg Br 51:638–647, 1969.
76. Van Demark RE Jr, Cabanela ME, Henderson ED. The Bateman endoprosthesis: 104 arthroplasties. Orthop Trans 5:507, 1981.
77. Minas T. The role of cartilage repair techniques, including chondrocyte transplantation, in focal chondral knee damage. Instructional Course Lectures. Vol 48. Rosemont, IL, American Academy of Orthopaedic Surgeons, 1999, pp 629–643.
78. Laupacis A, Bourne R, Rorabeck C, et al. The effect of elective total hip replacement on health-related quality of life. J Bone Joint Surg Am 75:1619–1626, 1993.
79. Barber TC, Healy WL. The hospital cost of total hip arthroplasty. J Bone Joint Surg Am 75:321–325, 1993.
80. Kreder HJ, Deyo RA, Koepsell T, et al. Relationship between the volume of total hip replacements performed by providers and the rates of postoperative complications in the State of Washington. J Bone Joint Surg Am 79:485–494, 1997.
81. Maloney JB, Harris WH. Comparison of a hybrid with an uncemented total hip replacement: a retrospective matched-pair study. J Bone Joint Surg Am 72:1349–1351, 1990.
82. Goldberg VM, Figgie HE, Figgie MP, et al. Use of a total condylar knee prosthesis for treatment of osteoarthritis and rheumatoid arthritis. J Bone Joint Surg Am 70:802–811, 1988.
83. Maloney WJ, Galante JO, Anderson M, et al. Fixation, polyethylene wear and pelvic osteolysis in primary total hip replacement. Clin Orthop 369:157–164, 1999.
84. Bierbaum BE, Sweet R. Complications of resurfacing arthroplasty. Orthop Clin North Am 13:761–775, 1982.
85. Stern SH, Insall JN. Posterior stabilized prosthesis. Results after followup of nine to twelve years. J Bone Joint Surg Am 74:980–986, 1992.
86. Muir PF, DiGioia A III, Jaramaz B, et al. Computer-assisted orthopaedic surgery: Tools and technologies in clinical practice. MD Comput 17(5):34–43, 2000.
87. Saragaglia D, Picard F, Chaussard C, et al. Computer-assisted knee arthroplasty: Comparison with a conventional procedure: Results of 50 cases in a prospective randomized study. Rev Chir Orthop Reparatrice Appar Mot 87:18–28, 2001.
88. Rosenberg AG, Barden R, Galante JO. A comparison of cemented and cementless fixation with the Miller-Galante total knee arthroplasty. Orthop Clin North Am 20:97–111, 1989.
89. Berger RA, Meneghini RM, Jacobs JJ, et al. Results of unicompartmental knee arthroplasty at a minimum of ten years of follow-up. J Bone Joint 87(5):999–1006, 2005.
90. Goldberg, V.M.: Surface replacement solutions for the arthritic hip. Orthopedics, 28: 943–944, 2005.
91. Maloney WJ, Smith RL. Periprosthetic osteolysis in total hip arthroplasty: the role of particulate wear debris. J Bone Joint Surg Am 77:1448–1461, 1995.
92. Jasty M, Goetz DD, Bragdon CR, et al. Wear of polyethylene acetabular components in total hip arthroplasty: an analysis of 128 retrieved at autopsy or revision operation. J Bone Joint Surg Am 79:349–358, 1997.
93. Capello WN, D'Antonio JA, Manley MT, et al. Hydroxyapatite in total hip arthroplasty. Clin Orthop 336:286–296, 1997.
94. McKellop H, Shen F, Lu A, et al. Development of an extremely wear-resistant ultra high molecular weight polyethylene for total hip replacements. J Orthop Res 17:157–167, 1999.

95. Wright TM, Goodman SB (eds). Wear in Total Joint Replacement. Rosemont IL, American Academy of Orthopaedic Surgeons, 2000.

96. Dumbleton JH, Manley MT, Edidin AA, et al. A literature review of the association between wear rate and osteolysis in total hip arthroplasty. J Arthroplasty 17(5):649–661, 2002.

97. Howie DW, Vernon-Roberts B, Oakeshott R, et al. A rat model of resorption of bone at the cement-bone interface in the presence of polyethylene wear particles. J Bone Joint Surg Am 70:257–263, 1988.

98. Schmalzried TP, Kwong LM, Jasty M, et al. The mechanism of loosening of cemented acetabular components in total hip arthroplasty. Clin Orthop 274:60–78, 1992.

99. Maloney WJ, Smith RL, Schmalzried TP, et al. Isolation and characterization of wear particles generated in failed uncemented hip arthroplasty. J Bone Joint Surg Am 77:1301–1310, 1995.

100. Lerouge S, Yahia LH, Sedel L. Alumina ceramic in total joint replacement. In: Sedel L, Cabanela ME, eds. Hip Surgery: Materials and Developments. London, Martin Dunitz, 1998, pp 31–40.

101. Amstutz HC, Grigoris P. Metal on metal bearings in hip arthroplasty. Clin Orthop 329(suppl):11–34, 1996.

102. Dorr LD, Wan Z, Longjohn DB, et al. Total hip arthroplasty with use of the Metasusal metal-on-metal articulation. J Bone Joint Surg 82(6):789–798, 2000.

103. Hamadouche M, Boutin P, Daussange J, et al. Alumina-on-alumina total hip arthroplasty. A minimum 18.5 year follow-up study. J Bone Joint Surg Am 84:69–77, 2002.

104. Callaghan JJ, Templeton JE, Liu SS, et al. Results of Charnley total hip arthroplasty at a minimum of thirty years. J Bone Joint Surg 86:690–695, 2004.

105. Latimer HA, Lachiewicz PF. Porous-coated acetabular components with screw fixation: five to ten-year results. J Bone Joint Surg Am 78:975–981, 1996.

106. Goldberg VM, Ninomiya J, Kelly G, et al. Hybrid total hip arthroplasty. Clin Orthop 333:147–154, 1996.

107. Mallory TH, Lombardi AV, Leith JR, et al. Minimal 10-year results of a tapered cementless femoral component in total hip arthroplasty. J Arthroplasty 16(1):49–54, 2001.

108. Sinha RK, Dungy DS, Yeon HB. Primary total hip arthroplasty with a proximally porous-coated femoral stem. J Bone Joint Surg Am 86:1254–1261, 2004.

Upper Extremity Considerations: Osteoarthritis of the Shoulder

20A

Sara L. Edwards   John-Erik Bell   William N. Levine   Louis U. Bigliani

GLENOHUMERAL JOINT

The glenohumeral joint is a synovial joint comprised of the articulation between the round humeral head and the shallow cup-shaped glenoid process of the scapula. It has the greatest range of motion of any joint in the body.[1] Many arthritic conditions can disrupt the normally smooth, congruent, and lubricated articular surfaces of the glenohumeral joint, including osteoarthritis (OA), rheumatoid arthritis (RA), avascular necrosis, post-traumatic arthritis, rotator cuff tear arthropathy, and postcapsulorrhaphy arthropathy. The most common of these is OA, a slowly progressive disease that leads to cartilage thinning and ultimately complete cartilage loss. Advanced OA affecting the glenohumeral joint typically results in unremitting, achy pain and limitation of motion. The result is a significantly decreased level of function and impairment of general health status.[2–3] Multiple surgical procedures have been described for the treatment of painful glenohumeral arthritis. Prosthetic arthroplasty has proven to be an effective and reliable procedure with a well-established record of success.

ANATOMY AND PATHOPHYSIOLOGY

The glenoid process of the scapula is shaped like an inverted comma with 5° to 15° of retroversion relative to the scapular plane.[4–6] The articular surface is concave and covered with hyaline cartilage that is thinner centrally.[7] The articular surface area of the glenoid is only one third to one fourth that of the humeral head, and relatively little of the articulating ball is captured by the shallow glenoid cup.

Articular cartilage failure is the final common pathway of OA. It is unclear whether the cartilage failure is from the initial injury or from pathological processes due to changes in the mechanical and physical properties of the subchondral bone. As the subchondral plate stiffens, there is increased shear force in the cartilage layer. This alters the ultrastructure of the cartilage, increasing the water content and precipitating a cascade of events in the cartilage substance that results in an inability to tolerate applied forces. As the cartilage degrades, increasing friction within the affected joint induces mechanical destruction of the remaining cartilage. The adjacent bone is subjected to increased stress, which leads to subchondral sclerosis and microfissures in the bone surface. Synovial fluid is compressed through the small fissures and forms cysts. Incongruency of the joint leads to painful loss of motion.[8]

Loose bodies may be present. A large volume of clear yellow synovial fluid may be present that is high in catabolic markers of cartilage degradation.[9] While OA is primarily an osseous disease, the soft tissues of the shoulder are also affected, although less severely. Contracted anterior capsule and subscapularis tendon limit external rotation and force the humeral head posteriorly. Posterior glenoid wear and erosion result from posterior subluxation of the humeral head, with a reported incidence as high as 45%.[6,10]

Chronic posterior subluxation can lead to a redundant and attenuated posterior capsule. The synovium may be thickened, inflamed, and friable. Although the rotator cuff may be contracted, it is usually intact, as the incidence of full thickness rotator cuff tears in shoulders undergoing arthroplasty is exceedingly low.[10] In a recent series, only 4 of 110 shoulders (3.6%) undergoing replacement for OA had full thickness rotator cuff tears.[11]

CLINICAL EVALUATION

History

The chief complaint is often of a constant, dull ache in the shoulder that has an insidious onset and is unremitting in quality. Stiffness and loss of function are typical. Patients with severe OA will have difficulty performing activities of daily living. Patients with less severe involvement will present with muscle fatigue and difficulty with functions at the extreme of motion, such as fastening a bra strap or reaching for shelves. Patients may complain of positional night pain that is different from that of rotator cuff disease, which typically is unremitting. While uncommon, infection and tumor must be considered in the differential diagnosis. Cervical spondylosis is frequently coexistent in patients with OA and must be ruled out, as symptomatology from cervical disease can mimic primary glenohumeral disorders.

Physical Examination

The patient should be examined with both shoulders fully exposed. Inspection is made of shoulder contour, bony prominences, muscle atrophy, and deformity. A thorough examination of the cervical spine is done by assessing range of motion and performing Spurling's test. Neurologic sensory and motor function should be assessed. Active and passive range of motion in elevation, external rotation, and internal rotation is measured and recorded. When arthritis is advanced, capsular tightness and joint incongruity become severe. Shoulder motion may become restricted to scapulothoracic motion. Since scapular movement does not contribute significantly to glenohumeral rotation, limitation of external rotation is a very sensitive physical finding of shoulder arthritis.[12]

Imaging Studies

Radiographic views recommended include anteroposterior views in neutral, internal, and external rotations taken in the plane of the scapula, an axillary view, and a supraspinatus outlet view. Classic radiographic findings include joint space narrowing, irregular articular contours, subchondral sclerosis and cyst formation, flattening of the humeral and glenoid surfaces, and a ring of osteophytes around the humeral anatomic neck. The axillary view is most useful for evaluating posterior subluxation and glenoid wear and is the most sensitive view for detecting joint space narrowing.

Early shoulder arthritis is often clinically underappreciated because of the inability to radiographically demonstrate cartilage pathology. This is compounded by the fact that the shoulder is a nonweight-bearing joint. Weighted abduction views may be used to demonstrate cartilage loss and resultant joint space narrowing that may not be apparent on routine radiographs.[13]

Specialized studies such as computed tomography and magnetic resonance imaging are rarely necessary in routine cases. Computed tomography is useful for accurate assessment of the glenoid bone stock and version in cases of severe posterior glenohumeral subluxation and glenoid wear.[6,14,15]

This information is useful during preoperative planning for glenoid resurfacing. Magnetic resonance imaging may be used to evaluate for the presence of a rotator cuff tear.

TREATMENT OPTIONS

Conservative Treatment

The initial treatment of the patient presenting with glenohumeral OA should be symptomatic, consisting of activity modification, anti-inflammatory medications and acetaminophen, moist heat, and gentle physical therapy. Glenohumeral joint injections of corticosteroid can also be helpful in patients who wish to prolong surgical intervention. Injections of steroid may be most beneficial in patients with inflammatory disease and less effective in those with long-term pain, such as OA. Other variables affecting the outcome may be needle placement, anatomical site of inflammation, frequency and dose of injection, and type of corticosteroid delivered.[8]

Surgical Indications

The primary indication for surgical treatment of glenohumeral OA is pain and loss of function that has persisted despite nonoperative management. Shoulder arthroplasty is rarely performed solely to improve motion or function without concomitant pain. The health, activity, and motivation of the patient are important factors to consider. While patients are generally advised to delay reconstructive surgery as long as possible, the timing of shoulder arthroplasty is not always so straightforward. Absolute contraindications to arthroplasty are active infection and complete functional loss of both the rotator cuff and deltoid muscles.

While prosthetic arthroplasty has become the gold standard treatment for severe shoulder OA, other surgical options do exist and should be included in the surgeon's armamentarium.

Open Débridement and Soft Tissue Balancing

Neer reported uniformly poor results after open release, débridement, removal of osteophytes, and soft tissue balancing for OA.[16] However, MacDonald et al. successfully treated ten patients who had osteoarthritic changes following previous anterior instability surgery with an open release of the subscapularis and anterior capsule.[17] Each patient had decreased pain and increased external rotation an average 3.5 years after surgery. Goals of this procedure are to normalize the biomechanics of the shoulder joint through soft tissue balancing, so that joint forces are more evenly distributed and the articulation is altered to involve less affected cartilage surfaces.

Arthroscopic Débridement

Patients with early glenohumeral OA who are not candidates for prosthetic replacement may benefit from arthroscopic irrigation and débridement. Coexistent conditions that contribute to symptoms, such as subacromial impingement, may be addressed at the same time.[18] Intermediate-term results demonstrate significant pain relief, and the procedure may delay the need for arthroplasty.[19] Our experience in 49 cases of early glenohumeral OA treated arthroscopically has been 93% good to excellent results at an average 4.3 years follow-up.[19] Other authors have not demonstrated such positive results, with 75% of patients worsening following arthroscopic débridement. Arthroscopy is contraindicated in cases of severe arthritis, with complete loss of the joint space, large osteophytes, or posterior glenohumeral subluxation.[8]

Resection Arthroplasty

The success of prosthetic arthroplasty has significantly limited the indications for humeral head resection. This procedure is used today only in the presence of resistant infection or failed arthroplasty with extensive bone loss in which reimplantation is contraindicated. Although pain may be relieved in some cases, range of motion and function are uniformly poor as the fulcrum of the shoulder is lost.[20,21] According to Cofield, active forward elevation is typically limited to 40° to 90°, with minimal to no active internal or external rotation.[20] Resection arthroplasty has no role today in the treatment of primary OA.

Glenohumeral Arthrodesis

As with humeral head resection, the indications for glenohumeral arthrodesis have markedly diminished since the introduction of shoulder arthroplasty. Shoulder fusion is indicated in cases of combined deltoid and rotator cuff paralysis (as occurs in upper brachial plexus injuries), active chronic low-grade infection, failed reconstructive procedures, and in some cases of severe bone loss following radical shoulder girdle tumor resection. It is rarely indicated for the treatment of primary OA.

Humeral Hemiarthroplasty

Shoulder arthroplasty, either humeral hemiarthroplasty or total shoulder replacement, has become the standard treatment in most patients with painful OA.[22] Pain is relieved in a high percentage of patients. Restoration of function is somewhat less predictable and depends heavily on the surgical technique, the status of the soft tissues (especially the rotator cuff and deltoid muscles), and the postoperative rehabilitation. The decision whether to replace the humeral articular surface alone, or both the glenoid and humeral articular surfaces, is determined by the extent of arthritic change of the glenoid, the available glenoid bone stock, and the integrity of the rotator cuff muscles. Shoulder arthroplasty is contraindicated in the presence of combined rotator cuff and deltoid dysfunction and when active infection is present.

Prosthetic replacement of the humeral head is a satisfactory treatment option when arthritic change is confined to the humerus.[23] Better results with hemiarthroplasty are seen when the glenoid is concentric.[24] Shoulders with nonconcentric glenoids from posterior wear have limited forward elevation and external rotation compared to shoulders with concentric glenoids. Patients under 50 years of age with OA are candidates for humeral hemiarthroplasty, as they are often healthy and active and may outlive the longevity of a glenoid prosthesis. Burkhead and Hutton have described biologic resurfacing of the glenoid with autogenous fascia or capsule in young patients treated with hemiarthroplasty in an effort to relieve pain and avoid the complication of glenoid component loosening.[25]

Glenohumeral OA with a deficient rotator cuff is another fairly common indication for humeral hemiarthroplasty, as long-term studies have noted an association between glenoid component loosening and irreparable rotator cuff tears.[26–28] Franklin et al. postulated that eccentric loading of the glenoid, owing to superior migration of the humeral component as occurs when the head-depressing effect of the rotator cuff is lost, causes loosening of the glenoid component.[29]

Total Shoulder Arthroplasty

Total shoulder arthroplasty, in which both the humeral head and glenoid are replaced, is generally indicated when arthritic change involving the glenoid is advanced, glenoid bone stock is adequate, and the rotator cuff is intact and functional.[30] This is frequently the case in shoulders with primary OA (Fig. 20A–1). The potential advantages of glenoid resurfacing over humeral head replacement alone include a better fulcrum for improved strength and motion, increased stability, decreased friction, and elimination of arthritic glenoid pain. The disadvantages of glenoid resurfacing include increased operative time and blood loss, increased implant cost, and a slightly higher rate of revision.[31] A review of the literature by Rodosky and Bigliani has shown that total shoulder replacement provides more reliable pain relief and function than humeral hemiarthroplasty in patients with OA and rheumatoid arthritis.[31] Some studies have shown 30% to 50% better results with total shoulder arthroplasty compared to humeral hemiarthroplasty.[32,33]

RESULTS

Results of prosthetic replacement are superior to other forms of treatment for glenohumeral OA. Shoulder arthroplasty has been shown to result in a significant improvement in health status, by consistently relieving pain, increasing motion, and improving function.[34] Unfortunately, most published series reporting results of shoulder arthroplasty include mixed patient populations with multiple diagnoses in addition to OA, including post-traumatic arthritis, rheumatoid arthritis, avascular necrosis, and cuff tear arthropathy.[11,35–39]

Nevertheless, some important trends are apparent. Results of shoulder arthroplasty for treatment of OA with an intact rotator cuff are clearly superior to results of arthroplasty for other arthritic conditions like rheumatoid arthritis, cuff tear arthropathy, and post-traumatic arthritis (Table 20A–1).[11,35–43] This is likely due to the relatively preserved soft tissues in the osteoarthritic shoulder. Overall satisfactory results following shoulder arthroplasty for OA are greater than 90% in most

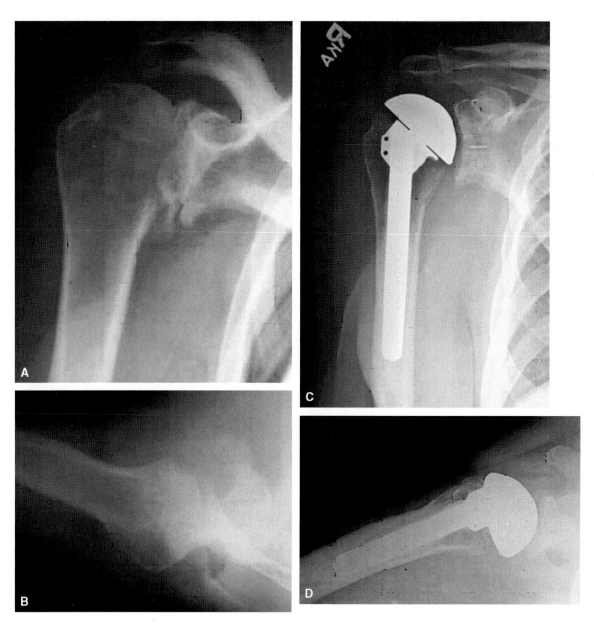

Figure 20A–1 *A, B,* Anteroposterior and axillary preoperative radiographs from a 60-year-old male with debilitating right shoulder pain and stiffness secondary to primary glenohumeral osteoarthritis demonstrate the hallmark radiographic features of the disease. Joint space narrowing, subchondral sclerosis and cyst formation, flattening of the articular surfaces, and inferior humeral osteophyte formation are evident on the anteroposterior view. The axillary view demonstrates loss of articular congruity and posterior subluxation of the humeral head resulting from wear of the posterior glenoid surface. The patient underwent a cemented total shoulder arthroplasty. At the time of surgery, the humeral head was severely arthritic, with exuberant osteophyte formation, loss of most of the articular cartilage, and eburnation of the exposed subchondral bone. Flattening of the humeral head was greater than suggested by the preoperative radiographs. *C, D,* Postoperative anteroposterior and axillary radiographs demonstrate replacement of the arthritic joint with a modular cemented total shoulder arthroplasty.

series.[11,24,35–39,42,43] Pain relief is predictable, with approximately 90% of patients reporting no or slight pain. Relief of pain is generally better with total shoulder arthroplasty than hemiarthroplasty.[44,45] Nearly full range of motion is restored in the osteoarthritic shoulder. The results of humeral head replacement alone, although not quite as good in most series, tend to deteriorate at a faster rate than total shoulder

replacement, even with the presence of glenoid lucent lines. It was found that more than 50% of a well-reviewed group of patients had pain and 26% required conversion to a total shoulder within 10 years of the initial procedure. Those requiring revision to a total shoulder did not have results as good as those patients treated with a primary total shoulder arthroplasty.[8]

TABLE 20–1

RESULTS OF SHOULDER ARTHROPLASTY FOR OSTEOARTHRITIS WITH INTACT ROTATOR CUFF

Author	Number of Shoulders	F/U Years	Satisfactory Results	Mild or No Pain	Forward Elevation Gain	External Rotation Gain
Neer,[39] 1982	40	3.25	100%	100%	57°	60°
Cofield,[36] 1984	31	3.3	74%	74%	55°	35°
Barrett,[35] 1987	33	3.5	78%	90%	44°	33°
Amstutz,[42] 1988	20	3.5	100%	100%	60°	40°
Hawkins,[38] 1989	29	2.4	90%	90%	77°	32°
Fenlin,[37] 1994	22	4.5	N/A	82%	39°	8°
Pollock,[11] 1995	67	4.7	97%	92%	48°	51°
Levine,[24] 1997	10	2.4	80%	N/A	35°	36°
Torchia,[43] 1997	34	12.2	71%	76%	47°	34°
Total	286	4.4	92% (weighted mean)	89% (weighted mean)	51°	37°

N/A, data not available.

Our experience with 68 osteoarthritic shoulders that underwent total shoulder arthroplasty documented 91% excellent results overall, excellent restoration of function, near total pain relief, 163° average active forward elevation, and 63° average active external rotation.[11] Other series have shown that an improvement in forward elevation of 50°, and external rotation of 35° to 40°, can be expected.[24,35–39,42,43]

COMPLICATIONS

The incidence of complications after shoulder arthroplasty has been less than for other major joint reconstructions.[46,47] A recent review by Cofield of 1183 shoulders in 22 series published since 1980 found the overall rate of complications to be 10.4%.[48] The most frequent complications, in decreasing order, were rotator cuff tear, instability, glenoid component loosening, intraoperative fracture, nerve injury, and infection.

Glenoid components have been in use for almost three decades, but the incidence and ramifications of lucent lines are often debated. The reported prevalence of lucent lines varies from 30% to 90% at 10 years postoperatively. The long-term implications are unknown, but clinical experience suggests that a patient becomes symptomatic only with gross failure.

Boileau et al.,[49] in a prospective, double-blind, randomized study, compared cemented all-polyethylene glenoids with uncemented metal-backed components. They found that, while the incidence of radiolucent lines was greater around cemented all-poly glenoid components (85%) than cementless metal-backed glenoid components (25%), the incidence of loosening of cementless metal-backed components was much greater (20% versus 0%). This increased loosening of metal-backed cementless components was associated with worsening functional results and increased pain. Boileau attributes this accelerated wear to insufficient polyethylene thickness, excessive thickness of the entire glenoid component leading to increased soft-tissue tension and increased load on the glenoid, and increased rigidity of the metal backing causing increased bone-implant peak

stresses. These authors stated that on the basis of their experience, they have abandoned the use of metal-backed cementless glenoid components.

A recent study by Martin et al.[50] reviewed a consecutive series of 140 uncemented metal-backed glenoid components fixed with screws at average follow-up of 7.5 years. Fifteen percent of the shoulders had radiographic evidence of glenoid failure, and clinical failure occurred in 11%. Common modes of failure included screw breakage, accelerated polyethylene wear, and loosening. The authors described their results as "troubling," since these failure rates were higher than those previously reported for uncemented glenoid components at shorter follow-up.

There is certainly a great deal of trepidation regarding cement fixation of all-poly glenoids because of the pervasiveness of radiolucent lines surrounding these components at follow-up. In fact, the rate is reported as high as 100%! However, the clinical relevance of the mere presence of these lines is not well defined, since progression is infrequently observed. By utilizing more modern cementing techniques, it may be possible to decrease the rate of radiolucent line formation. A recent article by Klepp[51] looked retrospectively at 68 patients who had undergone total shoulder arthroplasty by the same surgeon. Participants in the first group were cemented with a free-hand manual packing technique, and those in the second were cemented with a new instrument preparation and pressurization technique. The second pressurized group had a lower incidence of radiolucent lines based on blinded radiographic interpretation. Perhaps with more advanced cementation techniques, this aspect of cemented all-polyethylene glenoid components will become less worrisome.

SUMMARY

Efficient use of the upper extremity to position the hand in space requires a functional shoulder. OA of the glenohumeral joint is debilitating and painful. While many surgical procedures have been described over the years, unconstrained shoulder arthroplasty has become the treatment of choice for advanced glenohumeral OA. It has a well-established record of success for relieving pain, improving motion, and restoring function. Shoulder arthroplasty is technically demanding and highly dependent on the status of the soft tissues and surgical technique. With proper patient selection, good surgical technique, and supervised rehabilitation, excellent results can be achieved in greater than 90% of cases, with a low rate of complications.

ACROMIOCLAVICULAR JOINT

The acromioclavicular (AC) joint is a diarthrodial joint of varying inclination. The articular surface of the acromion is concave, directed medially and forward to face the convex lateral end of the clavicle. A fibrocartilaginous disc (meniscus) is often present as well, but is rarely a complete structure in adults.[52-54]

The AC joint is stabilized by a series of ligaments, made up predominantly of the AC capsule and ligaments, as well as the coracoclavicular ligaments (conoid and trapezoid). The superior AC ligament is thickest while the inferior AC ligament is relatively thin and provides less stability. The AC capsule and ligaments are important in preventing anteroposterior instability of the distal clavicle. The coracoclavicular ligament principally prevents superior instability of the lateral end of the clavicle.[55-58]

OA of the AC joint is common in the aging population. This degenerative problem most often occurs from overuse, but is sometimes associated with a history of trauma. A recent cadaveric study showed a distinctive pattern of degenerative changes in 560 AC joints over 40 years of age. On the acromial side, there is elongation of the joint in the sagittal plane, principally in the posterior aspect of the acromial facet. On the clavicular side there is a broadening and flattening-off of the distal clavicle in an anteroposterior direction conforming to the expanded surface of the acromial facet.[59]

Patients with AC joint pathology will often complain of anterosuperior pain—for women, directly under the bra strap. They will note difficulty reaching behind the back and across to the opposite axilla. Examination will show tenderness to direct palpation of the AC joint and pain with cross-body adduction. In addition, the patient may experience pain with humeral extension and internal rotation.

Radiographs may confirm the clinical suspicion but are often difficult to interpret. A silicone bag placed behind the affected shoulder helps to accentuate the AC joint and is routinely used at our institution. In addition, a 30° cephalic tilt view is helpful in better delineating the AC joint.[60] An axillary view is essential in traumatic cases to rule out posterior AC dislocation (type IV). Typical findings in acromioclavicular OA include joint space narrowing, subchondral sclerosis, and inferior osteophyte formation. In one study of 50 asymptomatic patients, MRI revealed 82% with changes consistent with acromioclavicular arthritis, a figure that rose to 93% in the over-30 age group. Osteolysis of the distal clavicle may also be encountered and is characterized by joint space widening, an irregular joint, and cyst formation.[61]

Nonoperative treatment includes rest, activity modification, nonsteroidal anti-inflammatory medications, and AC joint injections. There is little role for physical therapy in the treatment of AC OA. Although injections may provide temporary relief, long-term alleviation of symptoms is unlikely.

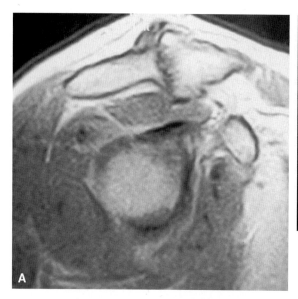
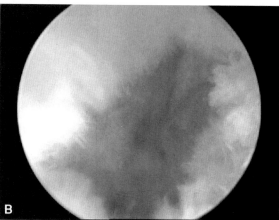

Figure 20A–2 A, Degeneration of the right acromioclavicular joint is seen in this anteroposterior radiograph of a 45-year-old male with anterosuperior shoulder pain. The joint space is narrowed and large inferior distal clavicle and medial acromion osteophytes are present. These osteophytes can impinge on the underlying rotator cuff tendons and lead to painful tendonitis, and in long standing cases, even frank rotator cuff tearing. B, The patient underwent arthroscopic subacromial decompression, anterior acromioplasty, and distal clavicle excision. The anterior acromial spur has been removed and 7 mm of distal clavicle has been resected.

If patients fail nonoperative treatment, surgery is indicated. Open distal clavicle excision as described independently by Mumford and Gurd in 1941 has been highly successful in treating patients with either OA or distal clavicle osteolysis.[57,62] A number of series have shown excellent results following open excision.[57,62-66] However, due to concern of increased morbidity, slower return to work, and cosmesis, attention has turned to arthroscopic resection of the distal clavicle.

Arthroscopic resection of the distal clavicle has been studied extensively in the last decade (Fig. 20A–2). Gartsman found the amount of bone resected arthroscopically to be equivalent to their standard open technique.[67] Flatow and others have shown that an even resection of minimal bone (5 to 7 mm) is preferable to an uneven resection that predisposes to posterior AC abutment.[68] Finally, care must be taken to preserve the coracoclavicular ligaments during resection of the lateral clavicle to maintain stability. Several series have shown that isolated distal clavicle resection is not indicated for the treatment of chronic grade III AC injuries. In addition, chronic grade II AC injuries should also be cautiously treated as inferior results have been observed due to residual distal clavicular instability.[68-70]

The results following arthroscopic resection of the distal clavicle have been equivalent or superior to those achieved with open resection.[71-76] There have been very few complications, especially when the indications are strictly adhered to as described above.

Sternoclavicular Joint

The sternoclavicular (SC) joint is incongruous with one half of the medial end of the clavicle articulating against the sternum and the other half forming one of the borders of the sternal notch. There is a variable disk and an extensive fibrous envelope. The costoclavicular ligament is crucial to medial clavicular stability and should be preserved whenever possible.[55,77]

Degenerative changes in the SC joint are common with advancing age. Several radiographic and cadaveric studies have shown a high incidence of arthritic changes in this joint. Fortunately, clinically significant symptoms are much rarer.[78-80]

Women may be more susceptible to noninflammatory sclerosis of the sternal end of the clavicle. In a small series, 14 females with this condition eventually developed osteoarthrosis of the SC joint. This condition may be due to avascular necrosis caused by strain or microtrauma, with sclerosis occurring during healing of the necrosis. Younger patients who suffer SC joint dislocations may be more susceptible to future degenerative changes due to increased activity.[81]

Physical exam findings include tenderness and edema at the SC joint, pain with shoulder abduction or forward elevation, prominence of proximal clavicular osteophytes, and crepitus with motion. Plain radiographs are typically obtained, but a computerized tomography scan is often necessary to accurately identify pathologic changes in the joint.

Treatment for symptomatic SC joint pain is usually nonoperative. Rest, NSAIDs, activity modification, and, rarely, corticosteroid injections are highly successful in treating the symptomatic SC joint. If nonoperative treatment fails, surgery may be necessary. The procedure performed depends entirely on the inherent stability of the medial clavicle. If the patient has had a severe SC joint dislocation, then the critically important costoclavicular ligament may be disrupted.[82] In this situation, the medial clavicle must be stabilized, either to the first rib or with a soft tissue interposition arthroplasty.[82-84] On the other hand, for symptomatic SC OA without trauma, medial clavicle resection has been highly successful.[85]

REFERENCES

1. Neer CS II. Anatomy of shoulder reconstruction. In: Shoulder Reconstruction. Philadelphia, WB Saunders, 1990, pp 1–40.
2. Gartsman GM, Brinker MR, Khan M, et al. Self-assessment of general health status in patients with five common shoulder conditions. J Shoulder Elbow Surg 7:228–237, 1998.
3. Matsen FA III, Ziegler DW, DeBartolo SE. Patient self-assessment of health status and function in glenohumeral degenerative joint disease. J Shoulder Elbow Surg 4:345–351, 1995.
4. Randelli M, Gambrioli PL. Glenohumeral osteometry by computed tomography in normal and unstable shoulders. Clin Orthop 208:151–156, 1986.
5. Rothman RH, Marvel JP Jr, Heppenstall RB. Anatomic considerations in the glenohumeral joint. Orthop Clin North Am 6: 341–352, 1975.
6. Badet R, Boileau P, Noel E, et al. Arthrography and computed arthrotomography study of seventy patients with primary glenohumeral osteoarthritis. Rev Rhum Engl Ed 62:555–562, 1995.
7. Soslowsky LJ, Flatow EL, Bigliani LU, et al. Articular geometry of the glenohumeral joint. Clin Orthop 285:181–190, 1992.
8. Brems, JJ. Management of osteoarthritis of the shoulder. In Orthopaedic Knowledge Update: Shoulder and Elbow, 2nd ed. Tom Norris, ed. Rosemont, Illinois, AAOS, 2002.
9. Ratcliffe A, Flatow EL, Roth N, et al. Biochemical markers in synovial fluid identify early osteoarthritis of the glenohumeral joint. Clin Orthop 330:45–53, 1996.
10. Walch G, Boulahia A, Boileau P, et al. Primary glenohumeral osteoarthritis: Clinical and radiographic classification. The Aequalis group. Acta Orthop Belg 64S:46–52, 1998.
11. Pollock RG, Higgs GB, Codd TP, et al. Total shoulder replacement for the treatment of primary glenohumeral osteoarthritis. J Shoulder Elbow Surg 4:S12, 1995.
12. Neer CS II. Glenohumeral arthroplasty. In: Shoulder Reconstruction. Philadelphia, WB Saunders, 1990, pp 143–272.
13. Apple AS, Pedowitz RA, Speer KP. The weighted abduction Grashey shoulder method. Radiol Technol 69:151–156, 1997.
14. Friedman RJ, Hawthorne KB, Genez BM. The use of computerized tomography in the measurement of glenoid version. J Bone Joint Surg 74:1032–1037, 1992.
15. Mullaji AB, Beddow FH, Lamb GH. CT measurement of glenoid version in arthritis. J Bone Joint Surg 76:384–388, 1994.
16. Neer CS II. Replacement arthroplasty for glenohumeral arthritis. J Bone Joint Surg 56A:1–13, 1974.
17. MacDonald PB, Hawkins RJ, Fowler PJ, et al. Release of the subscapularis for internal rotation contracture and pain after anterior repair for recurrent anterior dislocation of the shoulder. J Bone Joint Surg 74A:734–737, 1992.
18. Ellman H, Harris E, Kay SP. Early degenerative joint disease simulating impingement syndrome: arthroscopic findings. Arthroscopy 8:482–487, 1992.
19. Maxy RJ, Wiater JM, Marra G, et al. Arthroscopic debridement of glenohumeral osteoarthritis: intermediate term results. 18th Annual Meeting of the Arthroscopy Association of North America, Vancouver, BC, 1999.
20. Cofield RH. Shoulder arthrodesis and resection arthroplasty. Instr Course Lect 34:268–277, 1985.
21. Neer CS II, Brown TH Jr, McLaughlin HL. Fracture of the neck of the humerus with dislocation of the head fragment. Am J Surg 85:252–258, 1953.

22. Fenlin JM Jr, Frieman BG. Indications, technique, and results of total shoulder arthroplasty in osteoarthritis. Orthop Clin North Am 29:423–434, 1998.

23. Brostrom LA, Kronberg M, Wallensten R. Should the glenoid be replaced in shoulder arthroplasty with an unconstrained Dana or St. Georg prosthesis? Ann Chir Gynaecol 81:54–57, 1992.

24. Levine WN, Djurasovic M, Glasson J-M, et al. Hemiarthroplasty for glenohumeral osteoarthritis: Results correlated to degree of glenoid wear. J Shoulder Elbow Surg 6:449–454, 1997.

25. Burkhead WZ Jr, Hutton KS. Biologic resurfacing of the glenoid with hemiarthroplasty of the shoulder. J Shoulder Elbow Surg 4: 263–270, 1995.

26. DiGiovanni J, Marra G, Park J-Y, et al. Hemiarthroplasty for glenohumeral arthritis with massive rotator cuff tears. Orthop Clin North Am 29:477–489, 1998.

27. Pollock RG, Deliz ED, McIlveen SJ, et al. Prosthetic replacement in rotator-cuff deficient shoulders. J Shoulder Elbow Surg 1: 173–186, 1992.

28. Williams GR, Rockwood CA Jr. Hemiarthoplasty in rotator cuff-deficient shoulders. J Shoulder Elbow Surg 5:362–367, 1996.

29. Franklin JL, Barrett WP, Jackins SE, et al. Glenoid loosening in total shoulder arthroplasty: association with rotator cuff deficiency. J Arthroplasty 3:39–46, 1988.

30. Smith KL, Matsen FA III. Total shoulder arthroplasty versus hemiarthroplasty: Current trends. Orthop Clin North Am 29:491–506, 1998.

31. Rodosky MW, Bigliani LU. Indications for glenoid resurfacing in shoulder arthroplasty. J Shoulder Elbow Surg 5:231–248, 1996.

32. Bell SN, Gschwend N. Clinical experience with total arthroplasty and hemiarthroplasty of the shoulder using the Neer prosthesis. Int Orthop 10:217–222, 1986.

33. Clayton ML, Ferlic DC, Jeffers PD. Prosthetic arthroplasties of the shoulder. Clin Orthop 164:184–191, 1982.

34. Matsen FA III. Early effectiveness of shoulder arthoplasty for patients who have primary glenohumeral degenerative joint disease. J Bone Joint Surg 78A: 260–264, 1996.

35. Barrett WP, Franklin JL, Jackins SE, et al. Total shoulder arthroplasty. J Bone Joint Surg 69A:865–872, 1987.

36. Cofield RH. Total shoulder arthroplasty with the Neer prosthesis. J Bone Joint Surg 66A:899–906, 1984.

37. Fenlin JM, Ramsey ML, Allardyce TJ, et al. Modular total shoulder replacement. Clin Orthop 307:37–46, 1994.

38. Hawkins RJ, Bell RH, Jallay B. Total shoulder arthroplasty. Clin Orthop 242:188–194, 1989.

39. Neer CS II, Watson KC, Stanton FJ. Recent experience in total shoulder replacement. J Bone Joint Surg 64A:319–337, 1982.

40. Dines DM, Warren RF, Altchek DW, et al. Posttraumatic changes of the proximal humerus: malunion, nonunion, and osteonecrosis. Treatment with modular hemiarthroplasty or total shoulder arthroplasty. J Shoulder Elbow Surg 2:11–21, 1993.

41. Norris TR, Green A, McGuigan FX. Late prosthetic shoulder arthroplasty for displaced proximal humerus fractures. J Shoulder Elbow Surg 4:271–280, 1995.

42. Amstutz HC, Thomas BJ, Kabo JM, et al. The Dana total shoulder arthroplasty. J Bone Joint Surg 70A:1174–1182, 1988.

43. Torchia ME, Cofield RH, Settergren CR. Total shoulder arthroplasty with the Neer prosthesis: long term results. J Shoulder Elbow Surg 6:495–505, 1997.

44. Norris TR, Iannotti JP. A prospective outcome study comparing humeral head replacement and total shoulder replacement for primary osteoarthritis of the shoulder. 12th Open Meeting of the American Shoulder and Elbow Surgeons, Atlanta, GA, 1996.

45. Zuckerman JD, Cofield RH. Proximal humeral prosthetic replacement in glenohumeral osteoarthritis. Orthop Trans 10: 231, 1986.

46. Miller SR, Bigliani LU. Complications of total shoulder replacement. In: Bigliani LU (ed): Complications in Shoulder Surgery. Baltimore, Williams & Wilkins, 1993, pp 59–72.

47. Wirth MA, Rockwood CA Jr. Current concepts review. Complications of total shoulder replacement arthroplasty. J Bone Joint Surg 78A:603–616, 1996.

48. Cofield RH. Complications of total shoulder arthroplasty. Instructional Course Lecture 148. 65th Annual Meeting of the American Academy of Orthopaedic Surgeons, New Orleans, 1998.

49. Boileau P, Avidor C, Krishnan SG, et al. Cemented polyethylene versus cemented metal-backed glenoid components in total shoulder arthroplasty: a prospective, double-blind, randomized study. J Shoulder Elbow Surg 11:351–359, 2002.

50. Martin SD, Zurakowski D, Thornhill TS. Uncemented glenoid component in total shoulder arthroplasty: survivorship and outcomes. J Bone Joint Surg 87:1284–1292.

51. Klepp S, Chiang AS, Miller S, et al. Incidence of early radiolucent glenoid lines in patients having total shoulder replacements. Clin Orthop Related Res 435:118–125, 2005.

52. DePalma AJ. Degenerative Changes in the Sternoclavicular and Acromioclavicular Joints in Various Decades. Springfield, Charles C Thomas, 1957.

53. Oppenheimer A. Arthritis of the acromioclavicular joint. J Bone Joint Surg 25A:867–870, 1942.

54. Worcester JN, Green DP. Osteoarthritis of the acromioclavicular joint. Clin Orthop 58:69–73, 1968.

55. Flatow EL. The biomechanics of the acromioclavicular, sternoclavicular, and scapulothoracic joints. Inst Course Lect 42:237–245, 1993.

56. Fukuda K, Craig EV, An K, et al. Biomechanical study of the ligamentous system of the acromioclavicular joint. J Bone Joint Surg 68A:434–440, 1986.

57. Mumford EB. Acromioclavicular dislocation: a new operative treatment. J Bone Joint Surg 23:799–801, 1941.

58. Salter EG, Nasca RJ, Shelley BS. Anatomical observations on the acromioclavicular joint and supporting ligaments. Am J Sports Med 15:199–206, 1987.

59. Edelson JG. Patters of degenerative change in the acromioclavicular joint. J Bone Joint Surg 78B:242–243, 1996.

60. Rockwood CA Jr, Young DC. Disorders of the acromioclavicular joint. In: Rockwood CA Jr, Matsen FA III (eds). The Shoulder. Philadelphia, WB Saunders, 1990, 413–476.

61. Auge WK II, Fischer RA. Arthroscopic distal clavicle resection for isolated atraumatic osteolysis in weight lifters. Am J Sports Med 26:189–192, 1998.

62. Gurd FB. The treatment of complete dislocation of the outer end of the clavicle: a hitherto undescribed operation. Ann Surg 63: 1094, 1941.

63. Cook FF, Tibone JE. The Mumford procedure in athletes: an objective analysis of function. Am J Sports Med 16:97–100, 1988.

64. Eskola A, Santavirta S, Viljakka T, et al. The results of operative resection of the lateral end of the clavicle. J Bone Joint Surg 78A:584–587, 1996.

65. Petersson C. Resection of the lateral end of the clavicle: A 3 to 30-year follow-up. Acta Orthop Scand 54:904–907, 1983.

66. Taylor GM, Tooke M. Degeneration of the acromioclavicular joint as a cause of joint pain. J Bone Joint Surg 59B:507, 1977.

67. Gartsman GM, Combs AH, Davis PF, et al. Arthroscopic acromioclavicular joint resection. Am J Sports Med 19:2–5, 1991.

68. Flatow EL, Duralde XA, Nicholson GP, et al. Arthroscopic resection of the distal clavicle with a superior approach. J Shoulder Elbow Surg 4:41–50, 1995.

69. Gartsman GM. Arthroscopic resection of the acromioclavicular joint. Am J Sports Med 21:71–77, 1993.

70. Levine WN, Barron OA, Yamaguchi K, et al. Arthroscopic distal clavicle resection from a bursal approach. Arthroscopy 14:52–56, 1998.

71. Bigliani LU, Nicholson GP, Flatow EL. Arthrscopic resection of the distal clavicle. Orthop Clin N Am 24:133–141, 1993.

72. Flatow EL, Cordasco FA, Bigliani LU. Arthroscopic resection of the outer end of the clavicle from a superior approach: a critical, quantitative radiographic assessment of bone removal. Arthroscopy 8:55–64, 1992.

73. Henry MH, Liu SH, Loffredo AJ. Arthroscopic management of the acromioclavicular joint disorder. A review. Clin Orthop 316: 276–283, 1995.

74. Jerosch J, Castro WHM. Arthroscopic Mumford operation: surgical technique and results. J Bone Joint Surg 75B(suppl):189–190, 1993.

75. Jerosch J, Steinbeck J, Schroeder M, et al. Arthroscopic resection of the acromioclavicular joint. Knee Surg Sports Traum Arthroplasty 1:209–215, 1993.

76. Kay SP, Ellman H, Harris E. Arthroscopic distal clavicle excision: technique and early results. Clin Orthop 301:181–184, 1994.

77. Bearn JG. direct observations on the function of the capsule of the sternoclavicular joint in clavicular support. J Anat 101:159–170, 1967.

78. Jurik AG, Albrechtsen J. Spiral CT with three-dimensional and multiplanar reconstruction in the diagnosis of anterior chest wall joint and bone disorders. Acta Radiol 35:468–472, 1994.

79. Kier R, Wain SL, Apple J, et al. Osteoarthritis of the sternoclavicular joint. Radiographic features and pathologic correlation. Invest Radio 21:227–233, 1986.

80. Louvel JP, Duvey A, DaSilva F, et al. Computed tomography of sternoclavicular joint lesions in spondyloarthropathies. Skel Radiol 26:419–423, 1997.

81. Jurik AG. Noninflammatory sclerosis of the sternal end of the clavicle: a follow-up study and review of the literature. Skel Radiol 23:373–378, 1994.

82. Lunseth PA, Chapman KW, Frankel VH. Surgical treatment of chronic dislocation of the sterno-clavicular joint. J Bone Joint Surg 57B:193–196, 1975.

83. Barth E, Hagen R. Surgical treatment of dislocations of the sternoclavicular joint. Acta Orthop Scand 54:746–747, 1983.

84. Lowman CL. Operative correction of old sternoclavicular dislocation. J Bone Joint Surg 10:740, 1928.

85. Acus RW III, Bell RH, Fisher DL. Proximal clavicle excision: an analysis of results. J Shoulder Elbow Surg 4:182–187, 1995.

Upper Extremity Considerations: Hand, Wrist, and Elbow

Roderick J. Bruno   *Jason M. McKean*   *Steven H. Goldberg*
Robert J. Strauch   *and*   *Melvin P. Rosenwasser*

It has been estimated that by the year 2020, 18.2% or 59.4 million Americans will be affected by osteoarthritis (OA).[1] The causes of OA are multifactorial,[2] and in the upper extremity, the majority of cases result from a post-traumatic or idiopathic etiology. The prevalence of OA in the hand has been shown to increase with advancing age and at a higher rate in women, especially in patients older than 50 years.[3] Radiographic evaluation of the hand confirms a higher incidence of OA in women, but the joints most frequently affected are the same in both sexes.[4] The distal interphalangeal, thumb carpometacarpal (CMC), proximal interphalangeal, and metacarpophalangeal joints are most frequently affected in that order.[4] A study has reported an association of obesity with the development of OA in the hand.[5] Appearance of OA at an earlier age (younger than 50 years) may be indicative of a familial or genetic predisposition.[6] Autosomal dominant transmission[7] has been described for hereditary arthritic changes of OA. Recent studies have revealed a genetic component that can also be transmitted in a nonmendelian manner. Some investigators have shown joint-specific genetic susceptibility in hand OA.[8,9] The products of genes that play a role in the regulation of chondrocyte differentiation and survival have been implicated in OA susceptibility, including interleukin 1 (IL1), IL-4 receptor alpha-chain, frizzle-related protein 3 gene (FRZB), and the asporin gene (ASPN).[10–12]

The goals of treatment of OA in any joint must include the relief of pain, suppression of inflammation, maintenance of function, and prevention of deformities.[13] Activity modification, nonsteroidal anti-inflammatory medications, analgesics,[14] and occupational therapy are the most commonly used nonsurgical modalities for the management of upper extremity OA.[15] Because acetaminophen has been shown to be effective in many patients with mild to moderate pain and has minimal side effects when appropriately prescribed in patients without hepatic dysfunction, it is often the first-line drug of choice.[16] In patients with more severe pain or in the presence of inflammation, nonsteroidal anti-inflammatory agents may be more effective and merit consideration for initial therapy or use in combination with acetaminophen.[17] The role of antibiotics in OA is also being examined. A study demonstrated that oral administration of doxycycline inhibited collagenase and gelatinase activity in human cartilage with preexisting OA.[18] In addition to oral administration of drugs, topical or intra-articular corticosteroids can provide pain relief. Intra-articular corticosteroid injections into the thumb basal joint have shown to be well tolerated and reduce pain,[19] but significant long-term benefits have only been shown in early arthritis.[20,21] Hand therapy encompasses activity modification, splinting, and modalities including hot soaks, paraffin baths, and strengthening exercises. By providing local pain relief and alternately resting and using the joints, joint function can be preserved.

There has been recent interest in alternative treatments of OA, such as use of nutraceuticals.[22–25] Short-term trials have demonstrated benefits in the treatment of OA with glucosamine and chondroitin sulfate.[26,27] However, studies using meta-analysis of the available data have stated that definitive evaluation is not possible.[24,25,28,29] The source of the glucosamine may have an effect on its efficacy.[30] Because these compounds are not considered drugs, they are not subjected to the same rigorous safety and efficacy testing by the Federal Drug Administration as other medications. Therefore, the specific components of a preparation may vary considerably, leading to variable degrees of efficacy and safety. Glucosamine and chondroitin sulfate may play some role in the moderation of symptoms in OA, but their effects are modest in most populations of patients.

DISTAL INTERPHALANGEAL JOINT

Degenerative OA of the distal interphalangeal joint is most commonly seen in men and women older than 40.[31] Arthritis of this joint presenting at an earlier age has been recognized to have an autosomal dominant inheritance pattern.[32] Isolated trauma, such as chronic untreated mallet finger, may mimic degenerative OA in the distal interphalangeal joint.

Early radiographic evidence of OA is joint space narrowing secondary to thinning of articular cartilage. Bone spur formation with erosion and joint obliquity may cause malalignment and instability of the distal phalanx. As the disease progresses, the base of the phalanx may broaden, and cysts may form. Hypertrophy of capsular and ligamentous structures contribute to the bulbous appearance of the joint.

The Heberden node, a prominent and often painful exostosis, is characterized by osteophyte formation on the dorsal and lateral aspects of the distal finger joint (Fig. 20B–1). Heberden nodes, which are typically large and painless after their initial emergence, cause a cosmetic deformity with the joint fixed in a slightly flexed position. This results in attenuation of the terminal extensor tendon by osteophytes, creating an apparent pseudo-mallet finger deformity with an extensor lag.

Surgical treatment options include arthrodesis, cheilectomy, and arthroplasty. Arthrodesis achieves a stable joint, free of pain and deformity, but sacrifices function (Fig. 20B–2). Provided that the proximal interphalangeal and metacarpophalangeal joints in the finger are supple and relatively asymptomatic, arthrodesis of the distal

interphalangeal joint has only small effects on grip and pinch activities. At the distal interphalangeal joint, full extension is the most common position of fusion, although slight flexion for the border digits is acceptable. A multitude of fusion techniques have been advocated.[33-35] Complications from distal interphalangeal joint arthrodesis have been reported to be as high as 30% and are mainly nonunion and malunion.[36-37]

Cheilectomy with removal of excessive bone is an alternative to fusion. Cheilectomy can improve joint motion in certain cases but more reliably serves to improve cosmesis. It is routinely performed as part of the treatment of mucous cysts which are ganglion-like masses that arise most commonly from the distal interphalangeal joint (Fig. 20B–3). They are associated with underlying osteophytes. The cyst may rupture through the overlying skin as it enlarges and may lead to septic arthritis. Excision of the cysts is recommended when the patient has pain or when skin compromise has occurred. Recurrence rates of up to 50% have been reported, especially if the underlying osteophytes are not removed.[38] In fact, mucous cyst and underlying osteophyte removal is one of the most commonly performed surgical treatments for distal interphalangeal joint arthritis. Specific technical portions of the procedure include elevating the proper collateral ligaments from their attachments as a sleeve from the distal phalanx joint to prevent iatrogenic instability. The osteophytes are débrided on either side of the extensor tendon. The extensor tendon should not be disturbed or split longitudinally to facilitate bone removal or the tendon will attenuate, resulting in an irreparable mallet finger.

Because arthrodesis of the distal interphalangeal joint is well tolerated, implant arthroplasty is rarely performed. Success has been reported in long-term follow-up studies of silicone arthroplasty; an average of 33° of range of motion is preserved at 6- and 10-year follow-up, with a 10% implant removal rate in one study.[39,40]

PROXIMAL INTERPHALANGEAL JOINT

Proximal interphalangeal joint primary OA, so-called Bouchard nodes, is pathoanatomically similar to distal interphalangeal joint OA but occurs with much less frequency. OA of this joint displays familial tendency and is more common in women and with aging beyond 50 years. Mucous cysts are less commonly associated with OA in the proximal interphalangeal joint than in the distal interphalangeal joint. Patients present clinically with swelling, loss of motion, and characteristically little pain. Swan-neck or boutonniere deformities with tendon imbalance such as that seen in rheumatoid arthritis are unusual.[41]

Radiographic evidence supports the tenet of mirror OA lesions across similar joints in the hand[4,42] (Fig. 20B–4). Isolated arthritis of one proximal interphalangeal joint suggests an etiology other than idiopathic arthritis. However, early in the course of the disease process, one-joint involvement may be a sentinel of developing OA. Post-traumatic arthritis in this joint is often secondary to intra-articular fracture or fracture-dislocations resulting in chronic joint

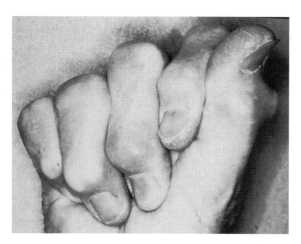

Figure 20B–1 Heberden nodes in a patient with distal interphalangeal joint arthritis.

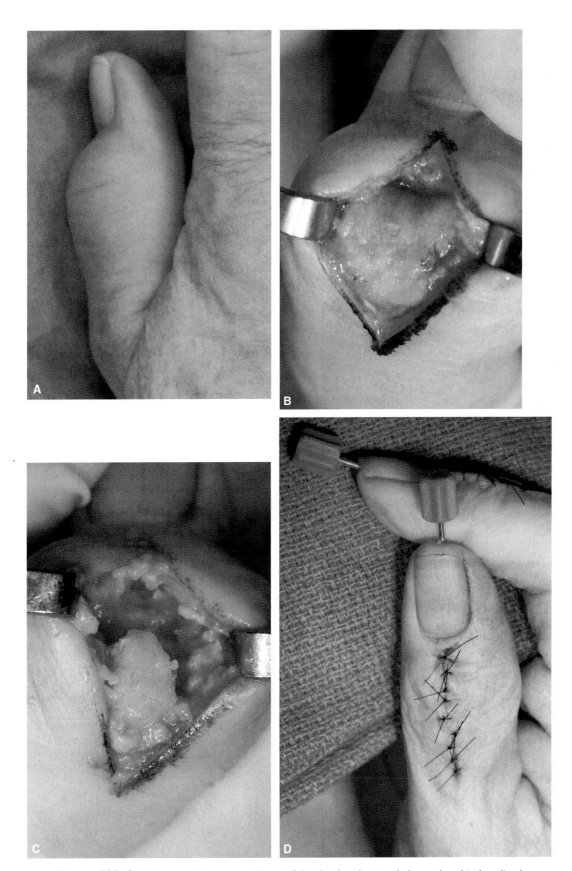

Figure 20B–2 A 70-year-old woman with painful right thumb interphalangeal and index distal interphalangeal joint arthritis. *A,* Note periarticular swelling at thumb joint from osteophyte formation, synovial hypertrophy, and synovitis. *B,* Intraoperative photograph shows eburnated bone and osteophytes on the proximal phalanx head. *C,* Any remaining cartilage and subchondral bone were removed and contoured to create a cup-in-cone articulation to increase surface area and stability for joint fusion. *D,* Temporary Kirschner wires with blue caps maintain alignment during bone healing. Note the improved cosmesis of the thumb after osteophyte removal.

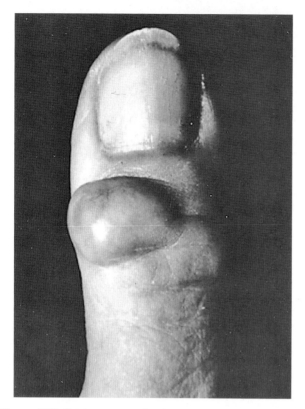

Figure 20B–3 Mucous cyst, distal interphalangeal joint.

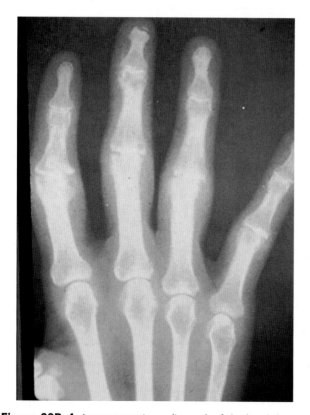

Figure 20B–4 Anteroposterior radiograph of the hand demonstrating proximal interphalangeal joint OA.

subluxation or dislocation that causes cartilage degeneration. Conservative treatments including heat modalities, mild analgesics, and activity modification may palliate the early stages of the disease. Advanced disease, especially with pain and stiffness, may need surgery, including cheilectomy, arthroplasty, and arthrodesis. Large lateral osteophytes may displace the lateral bands, precluding tight fist closure of the hand. Volar osteophytes may also contribute to the loss of flexion motion. Cheilectomy offers a temporizing procedure to improve joint mechanics. Osteophyte excision is usually through a palmar incision, with release of the volar plate and resection of the accessory collateral ligaments. Palmar plate resection arthroplasty, when combined with flexor tenodesis, can provide a stable joint with preserved motion[43] and a range of motion from 5° to 95° in 87% of patients with a 94% satisfaction rating by patients.[44]

As with the distal interphalangeal joint, arthrodesis of the proximal interphalangeal joint provides a pain-free, stable joint. Arthrodesis is the preferred method of treatment of any digit that presents with instability, but it is used primarily in the radial digits, particularly the index finger, because it provides additional stability for pinch.[45] In a review of a variety of fusion techniques, including Herbert screws, Kirschner wires, tension band wiring, and plating, Leibovic and Strickland[46] reported that Herbert screw fixation had the most predictable outcome. Tension band wiring is preferred by others,[47] with fusion rates from 86% to 97%.[46,47] Fusion angle is variably based on the natural cascade of flexion from radial to ulnar: 25° to 30° for the index finger, 30° to 35° for the long finger, 35° to 40° for the ring finger, and 40° to 45° for the small finger.

Arthroplasty of the proximal interphalangeal joint is best reserved for the central digits (long and ring), which are protected from shear and angular stress by the adjacent digits. Implant material and durability limit indications in manual laborers with high physical demands. Implants are constructed out of various materials including silicone, titanium, pyrolytic carbon, or combinations of materials. The most commonly implanted material is silicone. The implants may be secured by press-fit, cement, or they may be allowed to piston within the bone. In most studies, regardless of the type of implant, pain is relieved, but range of motion is unchanged.[48] However, each implant has different complications and modes of failure. Silicone implants are associated with implant fracture, bone resorption, and instability.[45,49] Cemented, hinged biomeric devices had well-fixed stems, but had an early failure rate at an average of 2.25 years due to symptomatic device failure at the elastomer hinge leading to prosthesis dissociation, particulate debris, joint instability, and angular deviation of the finger.[45] Early studies using osseointegrated prostheses[50] and surface-replacing arthroplasties[51] are promising, but long-term results are not available. In a retrospective study involving 18 proximal interphalangeal joint arthroplasties in 8 women using pyrolytic carbon implants, range of motion decreased in half the patients and satisfaction was only 50%.[52] Another study that included 25 joints in 19 patients investigated the use of titanium implants with silicone spacers.[53] While there was adequate osteointegration into 94% of the titanium implants, there was a 68% fracture rate of the silicone spacers. Despite the fracture rate, 80% of the patients were satisfied with pain relief. There is no single current arthroplasty design or material that is superior. Whereas objective parameters of success of arthroplasty may not be evident, patient-based subjective satisfaction, particularly with pain relief, remains high and may be the primary benefit of this procedure.[54]

METACARPOPHALANGEAL JOINT

Primary OA of the metacarpophalangeal joint is rare, and an underlying cause should be investigated, particularly a history of trauma or an underlying systemic disease.[55] There is likely a genetic predisposition to metacarpophalangeal joint OA, and mutations in the HFE gene have been shown to be associated with OA of the index and middle metacarpophalangeal joints.[56] The loosely constrained cam configuration of the metacarpophalangeal joint allows abduction-adduction in addition to flexion-extension. Restoration of mobility is the treatment goal for OA of this joint. Grasp is greatly affected by loss of active flexion, particularly when only one of the metacarpophalangeal joints is affected. Post-traumatic ligamentous injuries may lead to joint instability and subsequent cartilaginous injury. Impaction injuries to the cartilage can occur with activities such as boxing and the martial arts. Intra-articular fractures, fracture-dislocations, and osteonecrosis after fracture have been implicated in the cause of secondary OA in the joint.[57] The risk of post-traumatic OA of the metacarpophalangeal joint can be minimized if displaced intra-articular fractures are stabilized and early motion is allowed.[58]

Unlike the distal interphalangeal joint, metacarpophalangeal joint arthrodesis results in significant loss of function. Therefore, treatment of this joint focuses on maintenance of range of motion with some type of arthroplasty. When the joint articular surface is severely damaged, one surgical option is interposition palmar plate arthroplasty. For post-traumatic or postseptic OA, palmar plate arthroplasty has been shown to provide a stable, pain-free joint up to 4 years postoperatively, with a joint flexion arc of 55°.[59] If the volar plate arthroplasty fails, implant arthroplasty can still be performed.

Most of the literature on arthroplasty for the metacarpophalangeal joint has been written in regard to rheumatoid arthritis. However, silicone arthroplasty for degenerative arthritis has also proved successful. Modifications to enhance the durability of these flexible implants, including the use of grommets, are controversial.[60,61] The surgical technique described by Swanson[62] emphasizes soft tissue rebalancing as integral to the success of the hinged implant. Active motion within a few days of surgery, as dictated by skin healing, combined with dynamic splinting, has achieved good results.[63]

The Swanson silicone implant with or without grommets is the most widely used implant for metacarpophalangeal joint replacement and is the preferred implant of the authors.[64-65] However, newer designs with more anatomic features have been introduced and show promise. In a study of joint mechanics of three silicone implants, the NeuFlex (DePuy Orthopaedics, Warsaw, IN) implant appears to more closely reproduce joint motions than the other two implants.[66] There was no statistically significant difference between the kinematics of the metacarpophalangeal joints

with the preflexed implant and the joints that were not operated on.[67] Unconstrained pyrolytic carbon metacarpophalangeal joint implants have shown excellent long-term results without the need for revision or significant particulate debris.[68] Implant stem stabilization by osseointegration is being evaluated,[69] but the long-term efficacy of these devices is unproven.

Fusion of the metacarpophalangeal joint at any angle of flexion causes a loss of hand function but may still be indicated, particularly for an unstable index or middle metacarpophalangeal joints. Fusion is a last resort, but when it is required (under such conditions as massive bone loss after infection, mutilating injury, or failed implant arthroplasty), the position of fusion should follow the resting posture of the flexed hand, with the index finger in 20°, the long finger in 25°, the ring finger in 30°, and the small finger in 35° of flexion.

Degenerative changes in the thumb metacarpophalangeal joint are more common and may be seen after high-grade injuries with disruption of the ulnar or radial collateral ligaments. Collateral ligament injury can lead to subluxation of the joint and to changes in normal contact forces, which lead to cartilaginous wear. Late repair of the ulnar or radial collateral ligaments of the thumb metacarpophalangeal joint has been successful in restoring normal joint mechanics and should be considered unless the articular cartilage wear is severe. Secondary arthritis of the thumb metacarpophalangeal joint may also result from chronic hyperextension in a patient with motion-limiting thumb basilar joint arthritis. Thumb metacarpophalangeal joint fusion will predictably result in excellent function with power grasp and pinch as long as there is preservation of CMC motion. However, concomitant OA at the CMC joint would need to be addressed simultaneously with any metacarpophalangeal arthrodesis in order to fully address the arthritis of the entire ray and achieve long-term pain relief and function. Fusion of the thumb metacarpophalangeal joint in 10° of flexion is recommended for painful instability.

CARPOMETACARPAL JOINTS

Sometimes less-invasive measures, such as injections, can be effective in pain control with CMC joint OA. Local corticosteroid injection can be done safely in an office setting based on anatomical landmarks[70] and may alleviate symptoms.

Carpal bossing of the second or third CMC joint may occur in conjunction with or may be misdiagnosed as an isolated dorsal ganglion (Fig. 20B–5). This often results from subacute trauma such as extreme radial or ulnar deviation forces, as in taking a divot with a golf swing. The bone prominence of the carpal boss with associated soft tissue hypertrophy may be painful. Osteophytes may irritate the overlying extensor tendons; however, simple cheilectomy may not provide lasting relief. Early studies reported that simple excision of osteophyte and degenerative tissue provided symptomatic relief.[71,72] A later study demonstrated a 77% failure of boss excision or arthrodesis to relieve symptoms, contrasting with previously reported findings.[73]

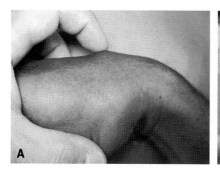
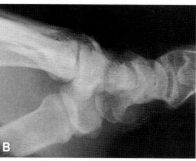

Figure 20B–5 Carpal bossing. *A*, Clinical photograph localizing area of bossing. *B*, Lateral radiograph; carpal bossing is visible at the carpometacarpal joint.

Cadaveric analysis has shown that dorsal wedge excision approximately doubles the passive range of motion of the CMC joint, disturbing the normal anatomy and creating instability.[74] For the rare symptomatic carpal boss, excision with CMC fusion is recommended.

THUMB CARPOMETACARPAL JOINT

OA of the thumb CMC joint is a common and debilitating condition second in incidence only to distal interphalangeal joint arthritis.[31] Epidemiologic studies have shown an overall gender differential in prevalence, with women affected six times more frequently than men.[75] However, a recent study demonstrated an elevated first CMC joint OA rate in men (9%) compared to women (5%) within the age group of 40 to 49 years of age.[31] This difference may be due to anatomic variation, hormones, or other factors.[76-78] Although an idiopathic etiology is most common, there are known genetic predispositions to thumb CMC joint OA. A relatively strong association between OA of the first CMC joint and chromosome 15 has been implicated, with candidate genes around including cartilage intermediate-layer protein (CLIP), aggrecan core protein precursor, fibrillin 1, fibroblast growth factor 7, and insulin-like growth factor 1 receptor.[79]

The thumb CMC joint consists of the articular surfaces of the distal trapezium and the proximal thumb metacarpal with two reciprocally opposed saddles. This unique shape in the human body allows the prehensile capability of the thumb. Passive stability is provided by the bony anatomy and six defined ligaments: the anterior oblique, palmar beak, posterior oblique, dorsoradial, ulnar collateral, and intermetacarpal ligaments. The extrinsic and intrinsic muscles of the thumb also contribute to the active stability of the CMC joint.

Unlike a ball and socket joint, the CMC joint has a certain degree of incongruity that allows its physiologic motion. The saddle shape allows flexion-extension, abduction-adduction, and axial rotation. The saddle-shaped anatomy and the kinematics of the joint are believed to be related to the pathogenesis and development of OA.[80] Imaeda and colleagues[81] have demonstrated that the center of rotation of the joint is not fixed; rather, it moves from the trapezium to the metacarpal as the thumb assumes flexion-extension and abduction-adduction attitudes.

The pathogenesis of OA in the thumb CMC joint is multifactorial. High focal stresses on joint cartilage may

be a primary cause.[82] Ligamentous laxity may play a role as well. A common deformity in advanced basal joint arthritis is dorsal subluxation and adduction of the metacarpal on the trapezium with compensatory metacarpophalangeal joint hyperextension. The primary restraint to dorsal subluxation is the dorsoradial ligament, although detachment or attenuation of the anterior oblique ligament also alters joint mechanics, may lead to arthritis.[68,69,83] Because ligaments provide optimal stability at different joint positions, they all play a role in joint stabilization, and the deterioration of thumb CMC cartilage is dependent on pathologic changes in multiple ligaments.[83]

Changes in biochemical composition of cartilage in the CMC joint relative to baseline normal values occurs with OA and directly affects the biomechanical properties of cartilage.[84] Additionally in OA, articular cartilage injury has been shown to occur in common patterns. It begins radially on the metacarpal base and dorsoradially on the trapezium then progresses palmarly in both in later stages.[85] This has been demonstrated in cadavers showing regional variation in contact areas during different joint positions which are associated with regional variation in cartilage thickness.[82] Thus, there are high and low load-bearing areas in positions of pinch and grasp. Pinching and gripping generate large loads across the CMC joint and contribute to the development of OA.[86] Thumb adduction with tip pinch may accentuate the incongruity of the joint and promote wear. The joint reactive force may be ten times the tip pinch force of the thumb and can exceed 1500 Newtons during strong grasp.

Radiographs are the most common and useful initial diagnostic study to evaluate the thumb CMC joint for OA. Pronated anteroposterior, lateral, and oblique views centered over the trapezium are routinely obtained. It is often useful to image both hands on the same film to assess for symmetry. The Eaton classification is based on the degree of degenerative changes noted on the radiograph and the presence or absence of scaphotrapezial arthritis.[87] In stage 1 disease, the joint space is preserved or mildly widened, indicative of synovitis or effusion. Stage 2 involves joint space narrowing with subchondral changes and osteophytes smaller than 2 mm (Fig. 20B–6A). In stage 3, there are more advanced degenerative changes with osteophytes larger than 2 mm. Stage 4 represents advanced joint destruction with involvement of the scaphotrapezial joint (Fig. 20B–6B).

However, radiographs tend to underestimate the severity of the disease both at the trapeziometacarpal joint and especially at the scaphotrapezial joint.[88] A full thickness cartilage erosion in one area of the joint may not be appreciated

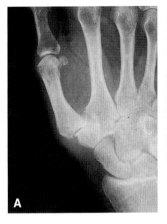
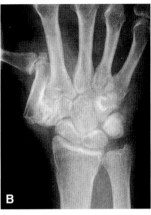

Figure 20B–6 Radiographic staging of thumb basilar joint arthritis. *A*, Eaton stage 2 changes in the thumb carpometacarpal joint. Note loss of joint space with subchondral cysts and osteophyte formation (<2 mm). *B*, Eaton stage 4 thumb carpometacarpal arthritis. There is advanced joint destruction with pantrapezial arthritis.

since the intact articular cartilage can preserve the joint space width. Additionally, since the thumb CMC joint is out of plane with the hand, it is difficult to obtain reproducible positions over sequential studies. A study quantified that radiographic staging can lag behind pathologic staging by more than one stage.[89] Radiographic severity has been associated with decreased grip and pinch strength.[90]

Symptomatic thumb CMC arthritis usually presents with dorsal and palmar basal joint pain at the thenar eminence, exacerbated by tip pinch and grasp. Deformity may also be present (Fig. 20B–7). Clinically advanced OA demonstrates the "shoulder sign" with dorsoradial subluxation of the first metacarpal on the trapezium. Pain can be elicited by palpation of the dorsal radial aspect of the trapeziometacarpal joint, adduction of the thumb, or with rotation of the axially loaded joint (grind test).

Compensatory deformities, such as collapse of the thumb-index web space with hyperextension of the metacarpophalangeal joint, should be noted because they will affect the treatment plan. Confounding diagnoses such

as de Quervain tenosynovitis, carpal tunnel syndrome, and radioscaphoid arthritis must be ruled out.

Initial treatment is focused on rest, limited immobilization, behavior modification, and nonsteroidal anti-inflammatory medicines. Several randomized, prospective studies demonstrate the efficacy of nonoperative treatment for early, mild basal joint arthritis. Seventy percent of patients in a group that was waiting for basal joint arthroplasty never underwent surgery during a 7-year study period when they were treated with occupational therapy, splinting, technical accessories, and advice on how to improve function through activity modification.[91] Other studies have shown that soft splints made of prefabricated neoprene, for example, are better tolerated with equal efficacy with respect to pain relief than more rigid splints, even when custom made.[67,92]

Intra-articular steroid efficacy has been shown to be inversely related to stage of disease. Splinting and steroid injection are superior to either alone; they are more effective and last longer in milder stages of OA. This was confirmed in a randomized, double-blind study comparing corticosteroid and saline in patients with moderate to severe CMC joint OA in which no difference in pain relief was observed.[21] Pain relief with intra-articular steroids may be delayed several weeks.[19-22] The major disadvantages of frequent steroid injections are possible injection site depigmentation and degradation of articular cartilage or the joint capsule.[93] Intra-articular hyaluronic acid also provides equivalent pain relief as steroids within 1 month of injection and improved strength and function from 3 to 6 months.[94] Another randomized, blinded controlled trial that the senior authors recently submitted for publication showed injections of hylan provided greater pain relief based on visual analog scores than both saline and steroid injections after 27 months.

The above nonoperative measures are usually used for at least a 3-month trial in an attempt to minimize pain and avoid contractures; however, response is variable and may be related to the patient's workload, activity level, and extent of arthritis.[95] Failure to control pain or inability or unwillingness to accept activity limitations are major indications for surgical treatment. Constitutional or acquired ligamentous laxity also affects the success of nonoperative and operative treatments. Most patients who elect surgery are in the advanced stages of OA. A host of surgical alternatives have been described, including arthrodesis, osteotomy, resection arthroplasty, ligament reconstruction with or without tendon interposition, and prosthetic replacement. Most techniques report good to excellent pain relief with a wide range of recovery of strength and functional capacity.

For early basilar thumb joint disease with instability but preservation of cartilage, Eaton has reported good results with an extra-articular ligament reconstruction using the flexor carpi radialis tendon.[69] Ligament reconstruction has been shown to preserve function and retard progression of OA.[96] Metacarpal extension osteotomy can also be performed in early disease.[97] Cadaver studies have shown metacarpal osteotomy shifts contact forces in the joint, which may unload and alleviate symptoms of arthritis; compared to ligament reconstruction, osteotomy may more comprehensively reduce thumb laxity.[98,99] Finally, arthroscopic procedures have also been described for early

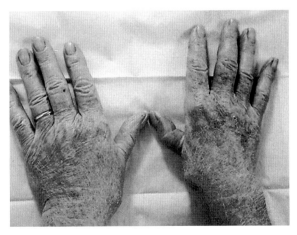

Figure 20B–7 Clinical photograph in a patient with advanced thumb basilar joint arthritis.

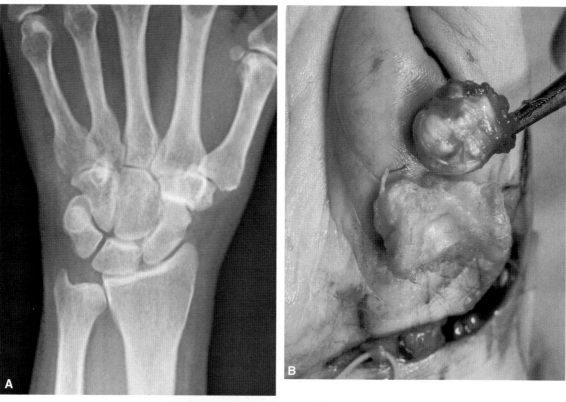

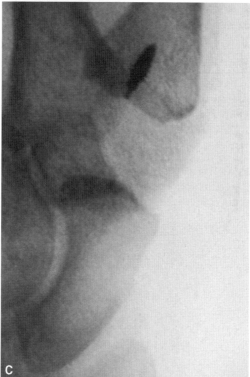

Figure 20B–8 *A,* Intraoperative photo showing excised trapezium on right and a harvested tendon to be interposed in the trapezial space between the distal scaphoid and metacarpal base. *B,* Intraoperative image of the wrist showing the absence of the trapezium. Tendon has been interposed in this space and secured to the metacarpal using a 2.5 mm suture anchor, which can be visualized in *C* Tendon has been interposed in this space and secured to the metacarpal using a 2.5 mm suture anchor, which can be visualized in *C.*

arthritis. These include debridement, thermal capsular shrinkage, interpositional arthroplasty, and hemitrapeziectomy or complete trapeziectomy.[100-104] No prospective randomized trials have evaluated the efficacy of arthroscopic treatment, but a small series of 24 thumbs in 22 patients treated arthroscopically had successful results and 8 patients who had an open arthroplasty on the contralateral side preferred their arthroscopic procedure.[105]

In more advanced basal joint arthritis, there are multiple treatment options that center around a complete trapeziectomy to remove the painful bone contact with variations in reconstruction of the ligaments and interposition of tissue into the trapezial space (Fig. 20B–8). Several randomized, prospective studies analyze various surgical treatments for basal joint arthritis. Although many of the studies are small and do not include a power analysis, the following conclusions can be reasonably drawn. Trapeziectomy is the primary critical element of surgical treatment of advanced basal joint arthritis because it removes the painful trapezial-metacarpal articulation. Trapeziectomy alone may be all that is necessary to treat basal joint arthritis since there is no difference in patient outcomes between patient groups who underwent trapeziectomy, trapeziectomy with tendon interposition, or trapeziectomy with ligament reconstruction.[106-110] However, all five of these studies recommending trapeziectomy alone were performed by two groups and only short-term results up to 1 year have been evaluated. Thus, the outcome of trapeziectomy alone in the long-term is unknown, and isolated trapeziectomy seems to have the highest risk for progressive collapse and pain over time from metacarpal-scaphoid contact, which occurred in several patients who did not have stabilization of the thumb metacarpal with either ligament reconstruction or tendon interposition.[110] Revision procedures have been described more commonly after isolated trapeziectomy for metacarpal-scaphoid arthritis,[111] whereas only one metacarpal-scaphoid painful articulation has been described in the randomized, prospective studies in which ligament reconstruction was performed.[112-114] The primary reasons to perform ligament reconstruction and/or tendon interposition is to maintain trapezial space height, thumb ray length, and to stabilize the thumb metacarpal for use during pinch. Ligament reconstruction with tendon interposition can maintain trapezial height better than ligament reconstruction alone.[113] However, the maintenance of trapezial height may not correlate with pain relief, strength, or function on validated tests at one year after surgery.[113] If trapeziectomy and tendon reconstruction is performed, ligament interposition could be superfluous as some studies have found that it does not improve patient outcome, requires more surgical dissection, more operative time, and may decrease range of motion.[112] One study randomized patients to trapeziectomy with ligament interposition or silicone arthroplasty and concluded both procedures were equivalent in partially relieving pain at 48 months postsurgery, but prosthesis subluxation or dislocation was common.[115] Length of postoperative immobilization has not been systematically studied, but one study suggests immobilization for only 1 week after surgery is all that is necessary for trapeziectomy alone.[116]

Both senior authors (RJS and MPR) routinely perform a complete trapezial excision for symptomatic advanced CMC arthritis. Additionally, one senior author (RJS) performs a ligament reconstruction using flexor carpi radialis secured to the metacarpal through bone suture anchors and interposition of the remaining tendon in the trapezial space,[117] while the other (MPR) favors interposition of the palmaris longus with imbrication of the dorsal capsule and dynamic stabilization with advancement of the flexor carpi radialis to the abductor pollicis brevis origin. An assessment of metacarpophalangeal motion is performed intraoperatively. If significant metacarpophalangeal hyperextension is present (>10°), the metacarpophalangeal joint is temporarily stabilized with a transarticular Kirschner wire to prevent subluxation of the base of the metacarpal during postoperative rehabilitation. For metacarpophalangeal hyperextension of 10° to 30°, we perform a volar plate advancement or plication. The thumb is splinted in an abducted position for 2 to 3 weeks to protect the soft tissue repair. An active motion rehabilitation protocol with supervised occupational therapy is then initiated.

True thumb CMC joint arthroplasties with metal or polyethylene prosthetic devices or silicone spacer implants have been developed. Excellent short-term results with more rapid return to function have been reported; however, long-term complications, which include wear, bone resorption with loss of height, instability, loosening, and silicone synovitis, continue to be a problem.[118-120] Long-term results of the de la Caffinière arthroplasty have been excellent in women older than 60 years, but higher failure rates were observed in more active individuals, including men and young women[121-124] (Fig. 20B–9).

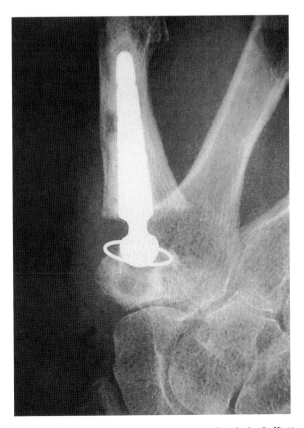

Figure 20B–9 Radiograph demonstrating the de la Caffinière thumb basilar joint arthroplasty.

Arthrodesis of the CMC joint has been shown to relieve pain and provide a strong and stable thumb for pinch and grip.[125] Arthrodesis is most commonly indicated for young, high-demand manual laborers, often with a post-traumatic etiology. The major limitation of arthrodesis is the fixed position of the thumb ray in relation to the palmar digits. The recommended position of fusion is 35° to 40° of palmar abduction with 10° to 15° of extension.[126]

SCAPHOTRAPEZIOTRAPEZOIDAL JOINT

OA of the thumb basilar joint is a common and frequently disabling condition, and extensive research has focused on the CMC joint. However, the more proximal joints, particularly the scaphotrapezial, scaphotrapezoidal, and trapeziotrapezoidal joints, have been less well examined. Isolated scaphotrapeziotrapezoidal pain may be differentiated from CMC disease by selective anesthetic injections into the joints. However, thumb basilar joint pain often results from pantrapezial arthritis, and treatment must address both the scaphotrapeziotrapezoidal and the CMC joints.

North and Eaton[127] performed an anatomic study of the thumb basal joint comparing it with radiographic evaluation. They reported that when trapeziometacarpal arthritis was seen on x-ray examination, concomitant scaphotrapeziotrapezoidal arthritis was seen 73% of the time. Anatomic dissection of the same specimens demonstrated pantrapezial arthritis in only 46%. These discordant results led to their conclusion that degenerative joint disease in the scaphotrapeziotrapezoidal joint is rare and that routine radiographs can be misleading. Other studies have agreed, reporting 39% to 76% concurrence of radiographs with direct visualization of scaphotrapezial arthritis.[88,128] A study evaluating the scaphotrapezoidal joint in patients undergoing trapezium excision arthroplasty similarly found that the sensitivity and specificity of radiographic diagnosis for the scaphotrapezoidal joint were only 44% and 86%, respectively.[129]

The known coexistence of scaphotrapeziotrapezoidal and trapeziometacarpal OA[88] has led authors to recommend direct visualization of both joints when a procedure is contemplated that only addresses one joint. In contrast, Glickel[128] stated that even if moderate scaphotrapezial arthritis was present at the time of surgery, at an average of 8 years of follow-up, there was no evidence of progression of degenerative changes at the scaphotrapezial joint and consideration of a procedure for only the trapeziometacarpal arthritis can be considered. The role of arthroscopy in directly visualizing the articular cartilage at both joints may increase as instrumentation, surgeon skill, and experience with small joint arthroscopy continues to evolve.

Techniques used to address the scaphotrapezial arthritis are dependent on the extent of arthritis at each trapezial articulation. The scaphotrapezial component of pantrapezial disease is most commonly treated by resection of the entire trapezium and some type of interpositional or ligament reconstruction arthroplasty. Scaphotrapezial and trapeziometacarpal arthrodesis can also be performed, but is uncommon due to the need for fusion to occur at two surfaces.[130–134]

Isolated scaphotrapeziotrapezoidal OA can be successfully treated with partial distal scaphoid removal and is the preferred procedure for one of the senior authors (RJS) (Fig. 20B–10).[135] This eliminates the painful contact between the distal scaphoid and proximal trapezium and trapezoid. The newly created space can be interposed with capsule, tendon, gelfoam, or be left empty to fill in with hematoma and scar tissue. In one clinical series of 21 patients at an average follow-up of 29 months, grip and pinch strength improved by an average of 26% and 40% respectively, 13 patients were pain free, and 8 patients had mild discomfort.

The scaphotrapeziotrapezoidal joint can also be fused to treat isolated disease. However, fusion must be performed with the bones in proper alignment, with particular attention to establishing a normal scapholunate angle (approximately 57°) and maintaining the joint space widths within the fusion mass. A long-term follow-up study[136] of triscaphe fusion reported that complication rates were high, and even anatomic scaphoid position did not preclude adjacent joint arthrosis. A loss of wrist motion is common, particularly in radial deviation.

RADIOCARPAL JOINT

The seminal paper by Linscheid and Dobyns[137] described the patterns of carpal instability that arise from degenerative arthritis or trauma. Similarly, Viegas[138,139] has described the normal and altered kinematics of the wrist after ligament disruption. Scaphoid flexion posture and triquetrum extension are dynamically balanced through the lunate. The proximal carpal row, controlled by the scaphoid, undergoes obligatory flexion with radial deviation and extension with ulnar deviation. When the scapholunate joint is dissociated, the lunate assumes an extended position because of intact ligament attachment to the triquetrum. This is commonly known as the dorsal intercalated segmental instability pattern. This collapse deformity may also develop after scaphoid fracture or nonunion with displacement as well as with markedly displaced distal radius fractures. Lunotriquetral dissociation obligates the lunate to assume a flexed posture through its attachment to the scaphoid and is recognizable as volar intercalated segmental instability. Although the scaphoid and lunate normally move congruently, there is some motion between them. A cadaver study of wrist kinematics demonstrated approximately 25° of rotation between the scaphoid and lunate in flexion-extension and 10° of rotation in radial-ulnar deviation.

Standard posteroanterior radiographs of the wrist may reveal static scapholunate dissociation. The lateral radiograph is used to assess the scapholunate angle, which averages 46°, with a normal range from 30° to 60°.[140] The lateral radiograph also allows measurement of the radiolunatocapitate angle, which is normally colinear or zero degrees.[141] The clenched fist or "gripping" view anteroposterior radiograph may reveal dynamic scapholunate diastasis with capitate descent and intrusion into the scapholunate gap.[142]

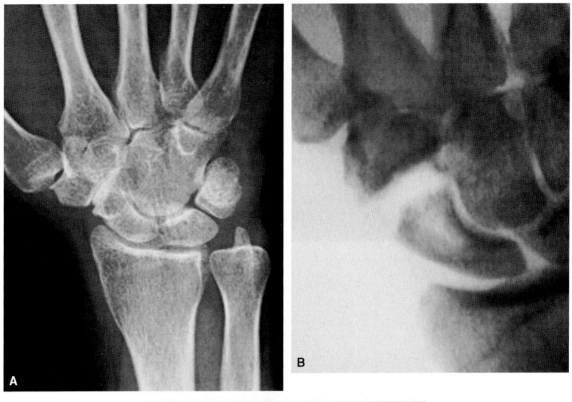

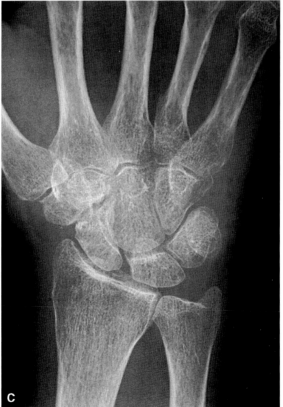

Figure 20B–10 A 41-year-old woman with scaphotrapeziotrapezoidal arthritis. *A*, Posteroanterior radiograph of the wrist shows joint space narrowing of the scaphotrapezial joint with sparing of the trapeziometacarpal joint. *B*, A postoperative posteroanterior radiograph shows resection of the distal pole of the scaphoid, which removes the painful scaphotrapezial articulation. *C*, Posterioanterior radiograph 4 months after surgery.

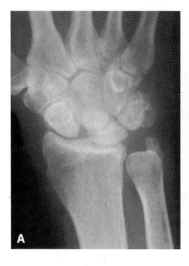

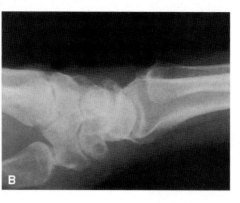

Figure 20B–11 Radiographs demonstrating scapholunate dissociation and the early scapholunate advanced collapse (SLAC) pattern of wrist degenerative arthritis. *A,* Anteroposterior radiograph of the wrist with static scapholunate dissociation and early degenerative changes at the radial styloid–scaphoid articulation. *B,* Lateral radiograph with increased scaphoid flexion and lunate extension illustrating the dorsal intercalated segmental wrist instability pattern.

The anteroposterior radiograph with the wrist in ulnar deviation places the scaphoid in its most extended position, allowing the most complete view of scaphoid bony architecture. Cinefluoroscopy may also be used to demonstrate dynamic instability[143] (Fig. 20B–11).

Degenerative arthritis of the wrist occurs in predictable patterns. The most frequent form of arthritis in the wrist is the spectrum of scapholunate advanced collapse (SLAC) wrist.[144] SLAC describes a disease evolution and does not specify the basic cellular events that contribute to its typical pattern. Chronic scapholunate dissociation can lead to the formation of a SLAC wrist and the dorsal intercalated segmental instability pattern of carpal instability.[145] The patient often has a limited range of motion and a positive scaphoid shift test result.[146] There are many additional associations or causes of radiocarpal arthritis, such as intra-articular distal radius fractures, scaphoid nonunion, Kienböck disease (osteonecrosis of the lunate), and perilunate dislocations.

The pattern of SLAC wrist degeneration is initiated with arthritic changes between the radial styloid and distal pole of the scaphoid, followed by wear at the radioscaphoid articulation. This may be due to primary scapholunate ligament injury or secondary attenuation after articular cartilage wear with altered joint contact forces and stresses. The final common pathway is capitate carpal descent and ultimate panradiocarpal disease.[144] The radiolunate articulation is spared secondary to the highly concentric congruent articulation between these two bones and the unloading of the radiolunate joint by the disease process on the radioscaphoid articulation.

Watson[144] initially described scaphoid excision, capitolunate fusion with or without inclusion of the hamate and triquetrum, and scaphoid replacement with a silicone implant as treatment of advanced SLAC wrist. Silicone scaphoid replacement has been abandoned because of particulate wear, synovitis, and cyst formation[147] (Fig. 20B–12).

Numerous techniques for treatment of SLAC wrist have evolved and been advocated, including proximal row carpectomy (PRC), scaphoidectomy with capitate-lunate-hamate-triquetrum arthrodesis (four-corner fusion), variations of intercarpal arthrodeses, total wrist fusion, and

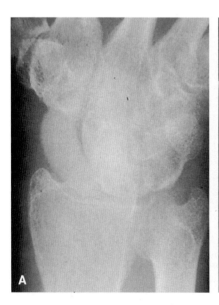

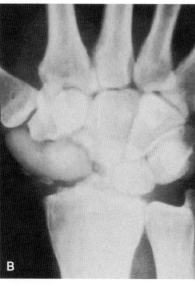

Figure 20B–12 Anteroposterior radiographs of a patient after scaphoid excision and replacement with a silicone arthroplasty. *A,* Early postoperative radiograph demonstrating silicone arthroplasty replacing the excised scaphoid. *B,* Late radiograph illustrating silicone collapse, cyst formation in the adjacent carpal bones, and progression of arthritic changes.

wrist arthroplasty.[147-153] PRC, in which the arthritic scaphoid, lunate, and triquetrum are removed allowing the distal carpal row to collapse proximally so the capitate articulates with the lunate facet of distal radius. It is a highly effective treatment for diffuse radiocarpal arthritis with preservation of a moderate amount of wrist motion and does not require the successful fusion of multiple joint surfaces as in the four-corner fusion. A comparative study of treatment methods for SLAC wrist found that PRC best preserved wrist motion;[148] a satisfaction rate of 82% was reported in one multicenter study,[153] and another study reported no revisions with 94% preserved motion compared with the contralateral uninvolved normal wrist.[149] However, a different study comparing PRC and four-corner fusion found similar success and outcomes.[154] A long-term, average 14-year follow-up study of PRC was recently performed and found all patients over 35 had satisfactory range of motion, grip strength, and pain relief.[155-156] However, a failure rate of 18% in patients under 35 years of age led the authors to caution against use in patients under 35 years of age.[156] To our knowledge, there is no similar long-term study on four-corner fusion. The presence of capitolunate arthritis is a relative contraindication to PRC, as the arthritic capitate will articulate with the distal radius. In this setting, either a four-corner fusion or a PRC with soft-tissue interposition would be indicated.[150]

Although different intercarpal or radiocarpal fusions for the treatment of degenerative changes in the wrist have had good success,[147,148,151,157] each fusion method alters the stress on the remaining articulations and will demonstrate wear and arthritic progression at adjacent joints. Furthermore, they entail a loss of wrist motion. In a long-term follow-up study of scaphotrapeziotrapezoidal fusion, Fortin and Louis[136] reported that at 62 months, 11 of 14 patients had complications including radiocarpal arthrosis, trapeziometacarpal arthrosis, and nonunion. The authors reported that scaphotrapeziotrapezoidal fusion with the scaphoid malpositioned predicted a poor outcome, and even excellent reduction of the scaphoid did not ensure joint preservation. Wyrick[149] reported that in 5 of 17 patients, four-corner fusions failed, necessitating total wrist fusion; these patients had on average decreased grip strength and range of motion compared with patients who had a proximal row carpectomy.

The reduction and association of the scaphoid and lunate (RASL) procedure using a cannulated headless bone screw between the scaphoid and lunate reduces the scapholunate dissociation, but preserves nearly normal carpal kinematics by allowing some obligatory rotation motion between the scaphoid and lunate (Fig. 20B–13).[158] Part of the procedure involves a radial styloidectomy, making the RASL procedure a viable treatment for early SLAC in which focal radial styloid-scaphoid arthritis is present. Progression of arthritis or failure of the RASL procedure does not preclude later salvage procedures, including proximal row carpectomy, intercarpal fusions, and total wrist fusion.

Scaphoid nonunion with displacement may lead to degenerative changes across the wrist.[159] Scaphoid nonunion with preservation of articular cartilage is usually treated with repair or screw stabilization and bone grafting (Fig. 20B–14). If the scaphoid has already undergone ebur-

nation with collapse, salvage options such as resection with or without intercarpal fusions are employed. Prosthetic replacement of the scaphoid with materials like Silastic cannot withstand the normal forces without fragmentation and have fallen into disfavor. When identified, scaphoid nonunion should be repaired before the development of OA, which necessitates subsequent salvage procedures.[159-162]

Another condition of the proximal carpal row that can lead to OA is Kienböck disease or osteonecrosis of the lunate. Numerous factors have been implicated in the etiology of Kienböck disease. Negative ulnar variance, acute trauma or repetitive microtrauma, and presence of aberrant vascular channels to the lunate may contribute to the osteonecrosis seen in Kienböck disease.[163-165] Szabo[166] reported that the clinical presentation of Kienböck disease in its early stages may be localized pain; normal radiographs do not allow confirmation. The study of choice to facilitate definitive diagnosis is magnetic resonance imaging, and it is also useful in assessing the course of treatment. Plain radiography is best used for staging (Fig. 20B–15).

Stage I Kienböck disease is characterized by mild pain, no loss of motion, and normal radiographs with possible disruption of trabecular lines within the lunate.[167] Stage II presents with increased pain, soft tissue swelling, some loss of motion, and radiographs revealing increased lunate density and possibly some early collapse. In stage III, patients have more chronic pain and may complain of clicking or a "clunk" with wrist motion. Radiographs demonstrate complete lunate collapse without scapholunate dissociation (stage IIIA) or with scapholunate dissociation (stage IIIB) and proximal migration of the capitate.[168] Stage IV is characterized by generalized wrist pain and pancarpal arthrosis.[167] Clinical progression may not correlate with radiographic findings, but the most accurate way to follow progression of disease is through measurement of radioscaphoid angle.[169] Many patients with stage III disease have few or no symptoms.

Early treatment of Kienböck disease is based on symptoms. Synovitis may lead to median nerve symptoms. Stage I or stage II disease is treated with rest, nonsteroidal anti-inflammatory drugs, or electrical stimulation by ultrasound. Later stages (IIIA, IIIB) may necessitate more extensive joint leveling surgical procedures which decrease force on the lunate and may indirectly promote revascularization or the performance of a direct vascularization procedure. In patients with negative ulnar variance (the distal ulna articular surface is shorter than the radius), a radial shortening[135,136] or ulnar lengthening[170] osteotomy is often performed. In patients with neutral or ulnar positive variance, a radial osteotomy that changes radial inclination,[171] a distal radial decompression,[172] or a capitate shortening osteotomy[173,174] can be performed. Revascularization of the lunate has been performed by transferring a vascularized pedicle with bone from the pisiform or distal radius, for example.[175] At the 12-year follow-up of 23 patients who underwent a vascularized pisiform transfer to lunate, pain improved in 87% of patients, grip power was 84% of unaffected side, and range of motion increased.[176] When lunate healing is not likely or the lunate is significantly collapsed, salvage options include silicone arthroplasty,[177,178] lunate excision with fascial or tendon interposition arthroplasty,[179]

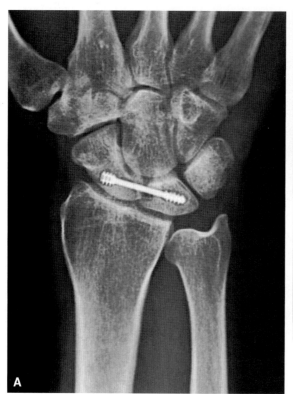

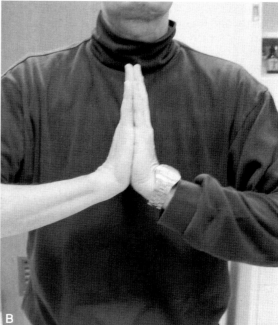

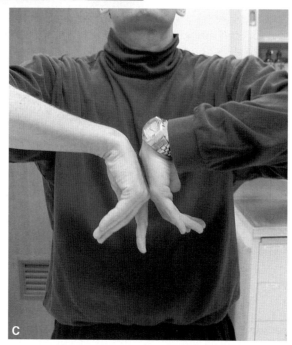

Figure 20B–13 A 31-year-old patient had chronic wrist pain due to a scapholunate ligament tear that was unrelieved by oral medication, therapy, and arthroscopic débridement. *A,* Posterioranterior radiograph 8 years after a reduction and association of the scapholunate (RASL) procedure. Note the headless bone screw maintains the scaphoid and lunate relationship and no radiographic arthritis is evident. Clinical photographs show near symmetric wrist extension *B* and flexion *C* in the patient who has no pain or activity limitations.

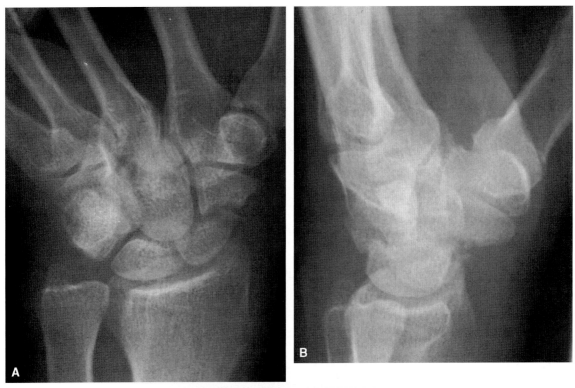

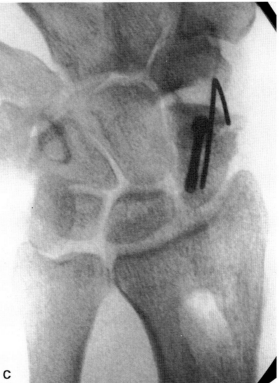

Figure 20B–14 *A,* A posteroanterior radiograph in ulnar deviation illustrates a scaphoid nonunion following four months of casting. Note the resorption of bone at the fracture site with displacement and preservation of the radiocarpal and midcarpal joint spaces. *B,* An intraoperative fluoroscopic image shows a distal radius lucency that corresponds to the bone graft donor site, which was harvested through a dorsal approach. *C,* The corticocancellous bone graft was placed through a separate, palmar approach and then a cannulated headless bone screw and supplemental temporary Kirschner wire were inserted through a palmar approach.

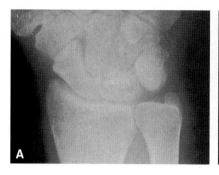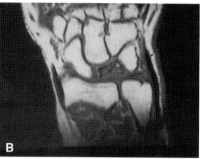

Figure 20B–15 Imaging studies in a patient with osteonecrosis of the lunate (Kienböck disease). *A,* Anteroposterior radiograph of the wrist showing fragmentation and collapse of the lunate. *B,* Magnetic resonance imaging in the same patient. This coronal section of the wrist shows the collapse and fragmentation of the lunate, with loss of signal.

arthroscopic débridement of the necrotic lunate,[180] proximal row carpectomy,[181-183] scaphotrapeziotrapezoidal fusion,[181,184] scaphocapitate fusion,[185] and total wrist arthrodesis.[183]

Prosthetic wrist arthroplasty for primary or post-traumatic arthritis is uncommon (Fig. 20B–16). This is related to the limited number of prosthetic designs. Unconstrained total joint designs are not indicated for heavy, unrestricted use. Therefore, the most common indication for a total wrist arthroplasty is in a patient with bilateral arthritis, such as rheumatoid, in which bilateral wrist fusions may excessively limit activities of daily living. Thus, a wrist fusion and contralateral wrist arthroplasty provides the patient with a good compromise.

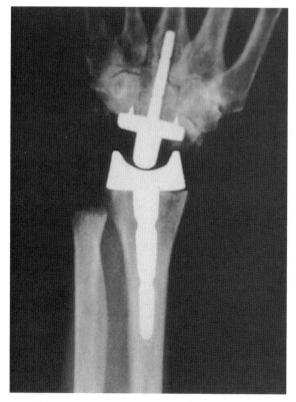

Figure 20B–16 Anteroposterior radiograph in a patient after total wrist arthroplasty (Volz II total wrist implant, Howmedica, Rutherford, NJ) for advanced degenerative arthritis.

Progress has been made with new implant designs restoring a functional range of motion, providing pain relief, and having lower rates of complications or revisions than older designs.[185-187] However, most implants have been reported in patients with severe rheumatoid arthritis, rather than OA. Meuli[188,189] introduced a metal and plastic wrist joint with cement fixation in 1972 and reported that good results can be obtained if adequate bone stock is present. Figgie and Ranawat[190] developed a trispherical arthroplasty, and Beckenbaugh[191] developed a biaxial arthroplasty with a semi-constrained design. In patients with rheumatoid arthritis, 8-year survival of the biaxial total wrist replacement was 83% with revision as the endpoint and 78% if radiographic loosening was considered the endpoint.[192] In another study, there were no revisions at an average 6-year follow-up in 17 patients.[191] In the patients with a contralateral wrist fusion, over half would have preferred another wrist arthroplasty. A multicenter study including 53 patients showed good results at early 1- to 5-year follow-up. Complications with total wrist joint implants are still present including loosening, instability, and fracture.[185,192,193] Silicone implant use in the wrist has been associated silicone particle-induced implant failure and progressive erosive synovitis at adjacent articulations, leading to diminished enthusiasm for the use of silicone implants.[194,195] At present, there are rare indications for the use of total wrist arthroplasty in the treatment of advanced radiocarpal OA.[196]

Wrist fusion remains the standard salvage procedure for painful end-stage arthritis of the radiocarpal joint, regardless of the inciting cause.[197] Wrist arthrodesis may be used for failed intercarpal fusions, proximal row carpectomy with persistent symptoms, and failed wrist arthroplasty.[196,198-204] Wrist fusion has a high success rate, providing a painless, strong wrist at the expense of mobility in the arc of flexion and extension and radial and ulnar deviation. However forearm pronation and supination are preserved after a total wrist arthrodesis.

DISTAL RADIOULNAR JOINT

Patients with established distal radioulnar joint OA can have significant pain and functional impairment. Physical findings include restricted painful forearm rotation, instability, and decreased grip strength. The distal radius and ulna must maintain a proper orientation to allow full forearm rotation. Intra-articular fractures involving the distal radioulnar joint or malunion of forearm fractures can lead to significant alterations in the biomechanics of both the radiocarpal and the distal radioulnar joints. In 565 patients with distal radius fractures, distal radioulnar joint arthritis (4.8%) may be a more frequent cause of long-term morbidity than radiocarpal joint arthritis (1.8%).[205] In fact, 70% of the patients with distal radioulnar joint arthritis eventually required surgical treatment.

The radiographic assessment includes the posteroanterior view with the shoulder abducted 90°, the elbow flexed 90°, and the wrist in neutral. A true lateral view of the wrist with the arm abducted to the side and the forearm in neutral supination-pronation can be compared with the uninjured side to assess distal radioulnar joint subluxation. Plain radiographs are usually sufficient to show degenerative changes and subluxation of the distal radioulnar joint; but in equivocal cases, an axial computed tomographic scan can be helpful in assessing the congruity of the distal radioulnar joint articulation.[206]

Before the development of joint incongruity or arthritis, attempts at realignment of the distal radioulnar joint through soft tissue procedures, osteotomy at the site of malunion, or ulnar shortening osteotomy[207] should be considered. After arthritis has developed, salvage procedures including resection arthroplasty, Darrach resection of the distal ulna,[208] hemiresection of the distal ulna, arthroplasties of Bowers[209] and Watson,[210] Sauvé-Kapandji arthrodesis,[211] and a distal ulnar head replacement[207–209] can be performed. The choice of procedure depends on the patient's functional status and the degree of impingement and instability.

Adams[212] performed a cadaver experiment to study the kinematics of the distal radioulnar joint and found that radial shortening caused the greatest alteration in kinematics. Werner[213] showed in a cadaver model that radial shortening and ulnar lengthening caused increased pressure in the distal radioulnar joint and a shift in joint contact. Jupiter[214] reported that more than 6 mm of shortening caused decreased forearm rotation with pain in the region of the distal radioulnar joint. Restoration of radial length with an external fixator may also decrease the incidence of subsequent distal radioulnar joint arthrosis.[205]

Treatment of the distal radius malunion is dependent on the status of the articular cartilage of the sigmoid notch and the ulnar seat.[215–217] With no or mild distal radioulnar joint arthrosis, soft tissue reconstruction and ulnar shortening osteotomy can reliably restore distal radioulnar joint stability and relieve ulnocarpal abutment.[215] With more advanced distal radioulnar joint arthrosis, a distal ulna ablation procedure may be warranted[217] (Fig. 20B–17).

The amount of ulnar resection should be determined intraoperatively and is tailored to the patient's anatomy. The results of the Darrach procedure reported in the literature have been variable, with good results ranging from 50% to 91%.[218–220] Dingman[221] has shown improved results when the length of ulna resected is limited to the area of the sigmoid notch. From cadaver biomechanical studies, the Darrach procedure has shown greater instability compared to hemiresection interposition arthroplasty,[222] and clinical symptomatic instability appears to

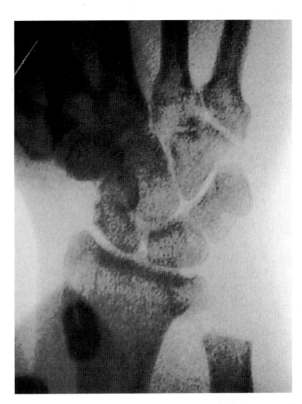

Figure 20B–17 Posteroanterior radiograph of the wrist after distal ulnar resection, the Darrach procedure, for distal radioulnar joint arthrosis and ulnocarpal impaction. Note resection of distal ulna to just proximal to the level of the distal radioulnar joint of the radius.

be more of a problem in the younger, high-demand patient or in one with ligamentous laxity. The Darrach procedure should be avoided in these patients. In the senior authors' experience (RJS and MPR), symptomatic radioulnar convergence and instability have not been encountered when the soft tissue envelope (distal radioulnar joint capsule, the dorsal and palmar radioulnar ligaments, triangular fibrocartilage complex, and extensor carpi ulnaris subsheath) is meticulously preserved or repaired. A retrospective study comparing 20 Darrach, 25 Sauvé-Kapandji, and 16 hemiresection-interposition arthroplasty procedures with an average follow-up of 10 years[223] showed the Darrach had less improvement in grip strength and motion. Supination and pronation showed improvement in all procedures studied.

Replacement of the ulnar head is becoming more popular, and the indications for its use are expanding. This procedure has been used for failed resection arthroplasty[208,224] with good results. The rationale for the development of such a procedure is based on the biomechanics of the distal radioulnar joint. Resection of the distal ulna may reduce pain, but patients who are relatively more active may have a significant reduction in stability, torque strength, and upper limb function. In a study with 22 patients over 2 years, distal radioulnar joint stability was achieved in all patients, with good to excellent results in 82%.[209] There were two cases of prosthesis failure due to stem loosening. In another study of patients with complications after a partial or total distal ulna resection, replacement with an ulnar head implant resulted in symptomatic improvement and joint stability in all 23 patients.[208]

ELBOW

The primary role of the elbow is to position the hand in space. Elbow dysfunction may be compensated for by motion at other joints in the extremity, and disability may become apparent only with strenuous activity.[225] Clinically significant primary OA of the elbow joint is exceedingly rare (only 1% to 2% of all patients with elbow arthritis).[226] Primary OA of this joint is seen predominantly in middle-aged male laborers.[227–229] More common causes of elbow arthritis are post-traumatic changes, crystalline deposition (gout and pseudogout), inflammation, osteonecrosis, osteochondritis dissecans, and infection.[230–234] Two long-term follow-up studies of osteochondritis dissecans demonstrated that late findings of OA in the elbow joint, with residual symptoms associated with activities of daily living and loss of motion, were present in approximately 50% of joints.[235,236] For reasons not known, primary OA of the elbow has a higher reported prevalence in the Japanese literature.[228,236]

The elbow joint consists of three separate articulations that together form a complex ginglymus joint: ulnohumeral, radiocapitellar, and radioulnar. Flexion of the elbow locks the tip of the coronoid process into the coronoid fossa and the radial head in its radial fossa; extension locks the olecranon tip posteriorly in its fossa. The capsule and ligaments of the elbow also provide stability to the articulations in elbow motion and in the statically loaded joint. Injuries to these structures from trauma or a surgical procedure may also subject the articular cartilage to abnormal loads, leading to early degeneration and OA. Patients with OA of the elbow can present with painful motion in both terminal flexion and extension. However, if there is soft tissue or bone encroachment into the olecranon or coronoid fossae, there may be loss of motion, particularly early in the course of the disease. These patients may have a mild flexion contracture at presentation.

The elbow should be inspected for effusion and alignment. Range of motion including flexion-extension and pronation-supination is recorded. Localized tenderness associated with ligament or tendinous injuries should be assessed. Varus and valgus stability is tested. Neurologic examination and strength assessment findings are recorded. Osteophytes along the posteromedial ulnohumeral joint are commonly seen and may impinge on the ulnar nerve.

Radiographs are essential to assess bone alignment, joint congruity, loose bodies, and osteophytes. Osteochondral loose bodies may not be visible on radiographs,[237] but mechanical symptoms including crepitance, locking, and intermittent synovitis may suggest their presence. Computed tomography can give a more accurate picture of the joint surfaces, especially when there is post-traumatic deformity or heterotopic bone (Fig. 20B–18). Magnetic resonance imaging is useful to assess osteonecrosis of the articular surfaces as well as to visualize the capsuloligamentous structures important to elbow function, such as the medial and lateral

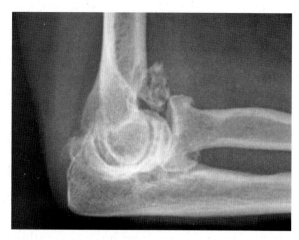

Figure 20B–18 Lateral radiograph of the elbow shows a large anterior loose body and osteophyte formation of the radial head, olecranon, and coronoid.

humeroulnar ligaments. We have used magnetic resonance arthrography with gadolinium contrast enhancement to evaluate injuries to the medial collateral ligament complex.

Like arthritis in other joints of the upper extremity, elbow arthritis is initially treated with conservative management. In addition to physical therapy and non-narcotic pain medication, specific measures such as static splinting may be helpful. Intra-articular injections of corticosteroids may provide temporary pain relief and allow therapy to advance through plateaus. However, we do not recommend multiple injections because they may allow overuse and exacerbate joint degeneration.

Indications for surgical intervention are marked loss of motion, osteochondral loose bodies, ulnar neuropathy, and joint articular cartilage loss with joint space obliteration. Elbow arthroscopy is a common treatment option in the surgical treatment of elbow OA.[238] The most common indication for elbow arthroscopy is removal of loose bodies.[238a,239] Other indications are débridement of posterior impinging lesions, capsular release, radial head excision, and fenestration of the olecranon fossa.[185,187–192] Elbow arthroscopy should be performed by experienced surgeons to minimize the risk of injury to neurovascular structures.[238,240]

Advanced global humeroulnar arthritis may require extensive open procedures. Débridement arthroplasty facilitates anterior and posterior soft tissue releases, capsular excision, bone spur removal, and restoration of the coronoid and olecranon fossae.

Post-traumatic changes in the radial head articulations with the humerus and ulna are a common cause of degenerative arthritis. These may occur after displaced radial head fractures that require excision. Radial head replacement with a metallic prosthesis has been advocated to prevent these secondary changes (Fig. 20B–19).[241–243] Most commonly the implants are placed in a press-fit manner and may be a monoblock or modular, bipolar[244] (separate head and neck) design. Proper sizing of the implant is important, with care taken to not place an implant that is too large, as it could impinge and limit flexion or cause

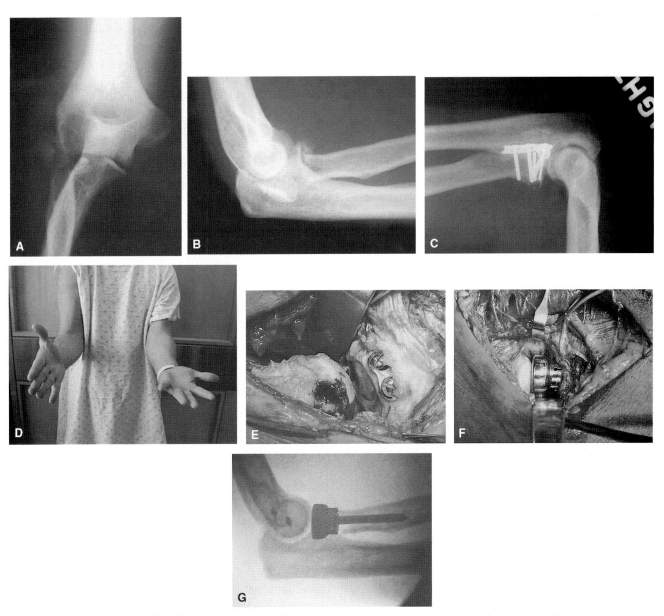

Figure 20B–19 Radiographs and clinical and intraoperative photographs of a patient with post-traumatic radiocapitellar arthritis. *A, B,* Anteroposterior and lateral radiographs of the elbow after the initial injury. A comminuted, displaced radial head fracture is visible. *C,* Postoperative lateral radiograph of the elbow after open reduction and internal fixation (ORIF) of the radial head fracture. *D,* Clinical photograph 6 months after ORIF. The patient has markedly limited supination of the operative side. *E,* Intraoperative photograph. The radial head with the plate and screws from the ORIF is visible. Note the loss of articular congruity of the radial head and degenerative changes in the radiocapitellar joint. *F,* Intraoperative photograph with a metallic radial head implant in place. *G,* Postoperative lateral radiograph of the elbow. The radial head replacement demonstrates excellent congruity with the capitellum. Two suture anchors are visible in the distal humerus. The suture anchors were placed as part of the repair of the lateral ulnar collateral ligament of the elbow.

premature wear of the capitellar cartilage.[245,246] In a study with an average of 12-year follow-up and 20 patients with metallic radial head prostheses, the results were excellent in 60%, good in 20%, fair in 10%, and poor in 10%.[306] Silicone prostheses do not withstand the loading forces at the radiocapitellar joint, may promote particulate silicone synovitis, and are primarily historical.[247]

For elbow OA that is beyond débridement procedures, options include distraction arthroplasty, fascial interposition arthroplasty, resection arthroplasty, and total elbow replacement. Morrey[234,248-249] has advocated the use of distraction arthroplasty with or without interposition arthroplasty, with 85% to 96% good results, but noted that release of elbow contractures is necessary. Resection arthroplasty is largely

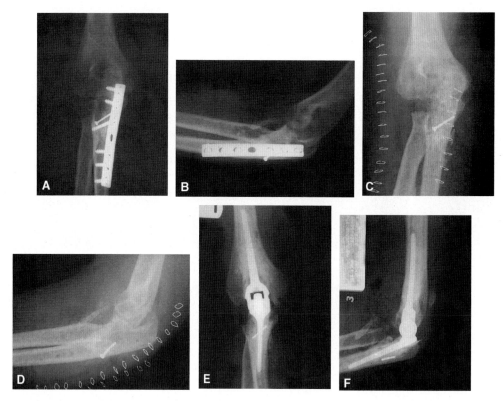

Figure 20B–20 Radiographic series in a patient with post-traumatic elbow arthritis. *A, B,* Anteroposterior and lateral radiographs of the patient after open reduction and internal fixation of a proximal ulna fracture. Note on the lateral radiograph that the radial head does not appear to be congruent with the capitellum. There is also evidence of early heterotopic bone formation. This injury probably represents an unrecognized or untreated Monteggia injury. *C, D,* Anteroposterior and lateral radiographs after removal of the internal fixation. The radial head has been excised. The radiocapitellar articulation remains unreduced, and gross instability with subluxation of the ulnohumeral joint is evident on the lateral radiograph. *E, F,* Anteroposterior and lateral radiographs of the same patient after total elbow arthroplasty (Solar total elbow implant, Howmedica, Rutherford, NJ). A stable, functional elbow joint has been restored. The patient has an active elbow arc of motion of 20° to 130°.

avoided because of the resultant dysfunction from a flail elbow. As a result of the success of total elbow arthroplasty for post-traumatic arthritis in less active or older patients,[232,233,250] indications for elbow replacement have been expanded[251] (Fig. 20B–20).

Elbow arthroplasty is a successful treatment for end-stage ulnohumeral arthritis. Pain relief and improved range of motion is predictable.[252-254] Because patients with rheumatoid arthritis are typically lower demand, results and long-term prosthesis survival may be better in these patients compared to post-traumatic or OA. Elbow implants are cemented in place and most prostheses in current use are classified with two different degrees of constraint between the humeral and ulnar components.[255] Unlinked designs rely on component geometry and soft-tissue balance for stability and thus they have a relatively higher subluxation or dislocation rate.[256] Semi-constrained designs have a formal linkage between the humeral and ulnar components with a "sloppy" hinge allowing varus-valgus motion, but providing improved stability. This motion at the articulation has been found to be important in preventing force transfer to the bone-cement interface which caused early loosening and failure in the constrained

designs with a more rigid articulation. Each company has multiple generations of prostheses that continue to improve the long-term outcomes with lower rates of loosening and mechanical failure leading to failure of the linkage systems.[255,257,258] However, patient selection and a thorough discussion with the patient about life-long lifting and activity limits is critical in order to maximize the chances of a successful outcome since the complication rate is higher, prosthesis survival length is lower, and the ease of performing revision procedures may be more difficult than the more commonly performed hip and knee arthroplasties.[254,258-260]

Arthrodesis of the elbow is rarely used because fusion in any position places significant restrictions on the functional activity of the limb.[261,262] Elbow arthrodesis may be the only alternative to a flail elbow. However, if possible, fusion should be avoided if there is contralateral upper extremity involvement that would place severe functional limitations on the patient. Elbow arthrodesis is reserved for salvage for severe infections, particularly tuberculosis, or for extensive bone loss after trauma or failed total elbow arthroplasty.[263,264] There is no ideal position of fusion of the elbow. Nagy and colleagues[261] tested healthy volunteers with elbow immobilizers and found that the preferred position was 90° of flexion. Shoulder motion, particularly abduction and internal rotation, is essential to maintenance of limb function after elbow fusion.

SUMMARY

OA can be a painful and debilitating disease. It may leave the patient with feelings of helplessness and can make daily functions, such as getting dressed, more difficult. As the average age of the population increases, the incidence of this condition will increase as well.

Treatment methods to mitigate the effects of OA range from nonsurgical modalities (such as therapy, nonsteroidals, analgesics, and activity modification) to surgical options (soft tissue reconstruction, cheilectomy, arthroplasty, and fusion). The preferred method of treatment depends on a variety of factors including the patient's health, primary outcome goal, and joints affected.

Although efforts have been made to diminish the impact of OA, no completely successful treatment has emerged. As we move through the twenty-first century, research is focused on the development of novel treatment methods, including gene therapy and cartilage regeneration, and the identification of factors that precipitate OA. Not only does this research address the effects of the disease, but more important, it may allow further identification of the underlying cause of OA. This may ultimately enable the clinician to prevent the development and progression of debilitating OA.

REFERENCES

1. Lawrence RC, Helmick CG, Arnett FC, et al. Estimates of the prevalence of arthritis and selected musculoskeletal disorders in the United States [see comments]. Arthritis Rheum 41:778–799, 1998.
2. Moskowitz RW. Clinical and laboratory findings in osteoarthritis. In: McCarty DJ, Koopman WJ, eds. Arthritis and Allied Conditions. Philadelphia, Lea & Febiger, 1993, pp 1735–1760.
3. Oliveria SA, Felson DT, Reed JI, et al. Incidence of symptomatic hand, hip, and knee osteoarthritis among patients in a health maintenance organization. Arthritis Rheum 38:1134–1141, 1995.
4. Chaisson CE, Zhang Y, McAlindon TE, et al. Radiographic hand osteoarthritis: incidence, patterns, and influence of pre-existing disease in a population based sample. J Rheumatol 24:1337–1343, 1997.
5. Oliveria SA, Felson DT, Cirillo PA, et al. Body weight, body mass index, and incident symptomatic osteoarthritis of the hand, hip, and knee. Epidemiology 10:161–166, 1999.
6. Jimenez SA, Dharmavaram RM. Genetic aspects of familial osteoarthritis. Ann Rheum Dis 53:789–797, 1994.
7. Kellgren JH, Lawrence JS, Bier F. Genetic factors in generalized osteoarthritis. Ann Rheum Dis 22:237–255, 1963.
8. Stefansson SE, et al. Genomewide scan for hand osteoarthritis: a novel mutation in matrilin-3. Am J Hum Genet 72(6):1448–1459, 2003.
9. Hunter DJ, Demissie, Cupples S et al. A genome scan for joint-specific hand osteoarthritis susceptibility: The Framingham Study. Arthritis Rheum 50(8):2489–2496, 2004.
10. Loughlin J, Genetics of osteoarthritis and potential for drug development. Curr Opin Pharmacol 3(3):295–299, 2003.
11. Kizawa H, et al. An aspartic acid repeat polymorphism in asporin inhibits chondrogenesis and increases susceptibility to osteoarthritis. Nat Genet 37(2):138–144, 2005.
12. Pelletier JP, Martel-Pelletier J, Abramson SB. Osteoarthritis, an inflammatory disease: potential implication for the selection of new therapeutic targets. Arthritis Rheum 44(6):1237–1247, 2001.
13. Swanson AB, Swanson GD. Osteoarthritis in the hand. J Hand Surg Am 8(2):669–675, 1983.
14. Blackburn WD. Management of osteoarthritis and rheumatoid arthritis: prospects and possibilities. Am J Med 100:24S–30S, 1996.
15. Goldberg SH, Von Feldt JM, Lonner JH. Pharmacologic therapy for osteoarthritis. Am J Orthop 31(12):673–680, 2002.
16. Bradley JD, Brandt KD, Katz BP, et al. Comparison of an antiinflammatory dose of ibuprofen, an analgesic dose of ibuprofen, and acetaminophen in the treatment of patients with osteoarthritis of the knee [see comments]. N Engl J Med 325:87–91, 1991.
17. Altman RD, Hochberg MC, Moskowitz RW, et al. Recommendation for the medical management of osteoarthritis of the knee: 2000 update. Arthritis Rheum 43:1905–1915, 2000.
18. Smith GN Jr, Yu LP Jr, Brandt KD, et al. Oral administration of doxycycline reduces collagenase and gelatinase activities in extracts of human osteoarthritic cartilage. J Rheumatol 25:532–535, 1998.
19. Joshi R. Intraarticular corticosteroid injection for first carpometacarpal osteoarthritis. J Rheumatol 32(7):1305-1306, 2005.
20. Day CS, et al. Basal joint osteoarthritis of the thumb: a prospective trial of steroid injection and splinting. J Hand Surg Am 29(2):247–251, 2004.
21. Meenagh GK, et al. A randomised controlled trial of intra-articular corticosteroid injection of the carpometacarpal joint of the thumb in osteoarthritis. Ann Rheum Dis 63(10):1260–1263, 2004.
22. Gaby AR. Natural treatments for osteoarthritis. Altern Med Rev 4:330–341, 1999.
23. Fillmore CM, Bartoli L, Bach R, et al. Nutrition and dietary supplements. Phys Med Rehabil Clin North Am 10:673–703, 1999.
24. McAlindon TE, LaValley MP, Gulin JP, et al. Glucosamine and chondroitin for treatment of osteoarthritis: a systematic quality assessment and meta-analysis [see comments]. JAMA 283:1469–1475, 2000.
25. Deal CL, Moskowitz RW. Nutraceuticals as therapeutic agents in osteoarthritis. The role of glucosamine, chondroitin sulfate, and collagen hydrolysate. Rheum Dis Clin North Am 25:379–395, 1999.
26. Leffler CT, Philippi AF, Leffler SG, et al. Glucosamine, chondroitin, and manganese ascorbate for degenerative joint disease of the knee or low back: a randomized, double-blind, placebo-controlled pilot study. Mil Med 164:85–91, 1999.
27. Rovetta G, et al. A two-year study of chondroitin sulfate in erosive osteoarthritis of the hands: behavior of erosions, osteophytes, pain and hand dysfunction. Drugs Exp Clin Res 30(1):11–16, 2004.
28. Towheed TE, Anastassiades TP. Glucosamine therapy for osteoarthritis [editorial; comment]. J Rheumatol 26:2294–2297, 1999.
29. Towheed TE, Anastassiades TP. Glucosamine and chondroitin for treating symptoms of osteoarthritis: evidence is widely touted but incomplete [editorial; comment]. JAMA 283:1483–1484, 2000.
30. Towheed TE, et al. Glucosamine therapy for treating osteoarthritis. Cochrane Database Syst Rev 2:CD002946, 2005.
31. Wilder FV, JP Barrett JP, Farina EJ. Joint-specific prevalence of osteoarthritis of the hand. Osteoarthritis Cartilage 14(9):953–957, 2006.
32. Stecher RM, Hersh AH, Hauser H. Heberden's nodes. The family history and radiographic appearance in large family. Am J Hum Genet 5:46–69, 1953.
33. Watson HK, Shaffer SR. Concave-convex arthrodeses in joints of the hand. Plast Reconstr Surg 46:368–371, 1970.
34. Burton RI, Margles SW, Lunseth PA. Small-joint arthrodesis in the hand. J Hand Surg Am 11:678–682, 1986.
35. Carroll RE, Hill NA. Small joint arthrodesis in hand reconstruction. J Bone Joint Surg Am 51:1219–1221, 1969.

36. Stern PJ, Fulton DB. Distal interphalangeal joint arthrodesis: an analysis of complications. J Hand Surg Am 17:1139–1145, 1992.

37. Brutus JP, et al. Use of a headless compressive screw for distal interphalangeal joint arthrodesis in digits: clinical outcome and review of complications. J Hand Surg Am 31(1):85–89, 2006.

38. Dodge LD, Brown RL, Niebauer JJ, et al. The treatment of mucous cysts: long-term follow-up in sixty-two cases. J Hand Surg Am 9:901–904, 1984.

39. Wilgis EF. Distal interphalangeal joint silicone interpositional arthroplasty of the hand. Clin Orthop 342:38–41, 1997.

40. Zimmerman NB, Suhey PV, Clark GL, et al. Silicone interpositional arthroplasty of the distal interphalangeal joint. J Hand Surg Am 14:882–887, 1989.

41. Stern PJ, Ho S. Osteoarthritis of the proximal interphalangeal joint. Hand Clin 3:405–413, 1987.

42. Plato CC, Norris AH. Osteoarthritis of the hand: age-specific joint-digit prevalence rates. Am J Epidemiol 109:169–180, 1979.

43. Ostgaard SE, Weilby A. Resection arthroplasty of the proximal interphalangeal joint. J Hand Surg Br 18:613–615, 1993.

44. Durham-Smith G, McCarten GM. Volar plate arthroplasty for closed proximal interphalangeal joint injuries. J Hand Surg Br 17:422–428, 1992.

45. Pellegrini VD Jr, Burton RI. Osteoarthritis of the proximal interphalangeal joint of the hand: arthroplasty or fusion? [see comments]. J Hand Surg Am 15:194–209, 1990.

46. Leibovic SJ, Strickland JW. Arthrodesis of the proximal interphalangeal joint of the finger: comparison of the use of the Herbert screw with other fixation methods. J Hand Surg Am 19:181–188, 1994.

47. Stern PJ, Gates NT, Jones TB. Tension band arthrodesis of small joints in the hand. J Hand Surg Am 18:194–197, 1993.

48. Takigawa S, et al. Long-term assessment of Swanson implant arthroplasty in the proximal interphalangeal joint of the hand. J Hand Surg Am 29(5):785–795, 2004.

49. Lin HH, Wyrick JD, Stern PJ. Proximal interphalangeal joint silicone replacement arthroplasty: clinical results using an anterior approach. J Hand Surg Am 20:123–132, 1995.

50. Moller K, Sollerman C, Geijer M, et al. Early results with osseointegrated proximal interphalangeal joint prostheses. J Hand Surg Am 24:267–274, 1999.

51. Linscheid RL, Murray PM, Vidal MA, et al. Development of a surface replacement arthroplasty for proximal interphalangeal joints. J Hand Surg Am 22:286–298, 1997.

52. Tuttle HG, Stern PJ. Pyrolytic carbon proximal interphalangeal joint resurfacing arthroplasty. J Hand Surg Am 31(6):930–939, 2006.

53. Johnstone BR. Proximal interphalangeal joint surface replacement arthroplasty. Hand Surg 6(1):1–11, 2001.

54. Hage JJ, Yoe EP, Zevering JP, et al. Proximal interphalangeal joint silicone arthroplasty for posttraumatic arthritis. J Hand Surg Am 24:73–77, 1999.

55. Feldon P, Belsky MR. Degenerative diseases of the metacarpophalangeal joints. Hand Clin 3:429–447, 1987.

56. Lundborg G, Branemark PI. Osseointegrated proximal interphalangeal joint prostheses with a replaceable flexible joint spacer—long-term results. Scand J Plast Reconstr Surg Hand Surg 34(4):345–353, 2000.

57. McElfresh EC, Dobyns JH. Intra-articular metacarpal head fractures. J Hand Surg Am 8:383–393, 1983.

58. Light TR, Bednar MS. Management of intra-articular fractures of the metacarpophalangeal joint. Hand Clin 10:303–314, 1994.

59. Bolis GU, Oni JA, Davis TR. Palmar plate interposition (Tupper) arthroplasty for post-traumatic metacarpophalangeal osteoarthritis. J Hand Surg Br 22:94–95, 1997.

60. Schmidt K, Willburger R, Ossowski A, et al. The effect of the additional use of grommets in silicone implant arthroplasty of the metacarpophalangeal joints. J Hand Surg Br 24:561–564, 1999.

61. Swanson AB, de Groot Swanson G, Ishikawa H. Use of grommets for flexible implant resection arthroplasty of the metacarpophalangeal joint. Clin Orthop 342:22–33, 1997.

62. Swanson AB. Distal interphalangeal joint implant arthroplasty. In: Swanson AB, ed. Surgical Techniques for Flexible Implant Arthroplasty in the MP, PIP, DIP Joints of the Hand. Grand Rapids, MI, Orthopaedic and Reconstructive Surgeons, PC, 1980, pp 25–26.

63. Kirkpatrick WH, Kozin SH, Uhl RL. Early motion after arthroplasty. Hand Clin 12:73–86, 1996.

64. Beevers DJ, Seedhom BB. Metacarpophalangeal joint prostheses. A review of the clinical results of past and current designs. J Hand Surg Br 20:125–136, 1995.

65. DeHeer DH, Owens SR, Swanson AB. The host response to silicone elastomer implants for small joint arthroplasty. J Hand Surg Am 20(pt 2):S101–S109, 1995.

66. Weiss, A.P., et al. Metacarpophalangeal joint mechanics after 3 different silicone arthroplasties. J Hand Surg Am 29(5):796–803, 2004.

67. Elhassan B, et al. Experimental investigation of finger dynamics before and after metacarpophalangeal joint arthroplasty. J Hand Surg Am 31(2):228–235, 2006.

68. Eaton RG, Littler JW. Ligament reconstruction for the painful thumb carpometacarpal joint. J Bone Joint Surg Am 55:1655–1666, 1973.

69. Pellegrini VD Jr, Olcott CW, Hollenberg G. Contact patterns in the trapeziometacarpal joint: the role of the palmar beak ligament. J Hand Surg Am 18:238–244, 1993.

70. Mandl LA, et al. Can the carpometacarpal joint be injected accurately in the office setting? Implications for therapy. J Rheumatol 33(6):1137–1139, 2006.

71. Cuono CB, Watson HK. The carpal boss: surgical treatment and etiological considerations. Plast Reconstr Surg 63:88–93, 1979.

72. Fusi S, Watson HK, Cuono CB. The carpal boss. A 20-year review of operative management. J Hand Surg Br 20:405–408, 1995.

73. Clarke AM, Wheen DJ, Visvanathan S, et al. The symptomatic carpal boss. Is simple excision enough? J Hand Surg Br 24:591–595, 1999.

74. Citteur JM, Ritt MJ, Bos KE. Carpal boss: destabilization of the third carpometacarpal joint after a wedge excision. J Hand Surg Br 23:76–78, 1998.

75. Peyron JG, Altman RD. The epidemiology of osteoarthritis. In: Moskowitz RW, Howell DS, Goldberg VM, Mankin HJ, eds. Osteoarthritis: Diagnosis and Medical/Surgical Management. Philadelphia, WB Saunders, 1992, pp 233–252.

76. Xu L, Strauch RJ, Ateshian GA, et al. Topography of the osteoarthritic thumb carpometacarpal joint and its variations with regard to gender, age, site, and osteoarthritic stage. J Hand Surg Am 23:454–464, 1998.

77. Ateshian GA, Rosenwasser MP, Mow VC. Curvature characteristics and congruence of the thumb carpometacarpal joint: differences between female and male joints. J Biomech 25:591–607, 1992.

78. Cooley HM, Stankovich J, Jones G. The association between hormonal and reproductive factors and hand osteoarthritis. Maturitas 45(4):257–265, 2003.

79. Hunter DJ, Demissie S, Cupples LA. A genome scan for joint-specific hand osteoarthritis susceptibility: The Framingham Study. Arthritis Rheum 50(8):2489–2496, 2004.

80. Imaeda T, Niebur G, Cooney WP III, et al. Kinematics of the normal trapeziometacarpal joint. J Orthop Res 12:197–204, 1994.

81. Imaeda T, An KN, Cooney WP III. Functional anatomy and biomechanics of the thumb. Hand Clin 8:9–15, 1992.

82. Ateshian GA, Ark JW, Rosenwasser MP, et al. Contact areas in the thumb carpometacarpal joint. J Orthop Res 13:450–458, 1995.

83. Xu L, Cohen NP, Roglic H, et al. A computer simulation of laxity of the thumb carpometacarpal joint. Transactions of the 44th Annual Meeting of the Orthopaedic Research Society, New Orleans, LA, 1998, p 288.

84. Rivers PA, et al. Osteoarthritic changes in the biochemical composition of thumb carpometacarpal joint cartilage and correlation with biomechanical properties. J Hand Surg Am 25(5):889–898, 2000.

85. Koff MF, et al. Sequential wear patterns of the articular cartilage of the thumb carpometacarpal joint in osteoarthritis. J Hand Surg Am 28(4):597–604, 2003.

86. Cooney WP III, Chao EY. Biomechanical analysis of static forces in the thumb during hand function. J Bone Joint Surg Am 59:27–36, 1977.

87. Eaton RG, Glickel SZ. Trapeziometacarpal osteoarthritis. Staging as a rationale for treatment. Hand Clin 3:455–471, 1987.
88. Brown GD III, et al. Radiography and visual pathology of the osteoarthritic scaphotrapezio-trapezoidal joint, and its relationship to trapeziometacarpal osteoarthritis. J Hand Surg Am 28(5):739–743, 2003.
89. Brown G, Rosenwasser MP. Topography, radiography, and pathology of the scaphotrapezio-trapezoidal joint and its relationship to thumb carpometacarpal arthritis. Transactions of the 45th Annual Meeting of the Orthopaedic Research Society, Anaheim, CA, February 1999.
90. Dominick KL, et al. Relationship of radiographic and clinical variables to pinch and grip strength among individuals with osteoarthritis. Arthritis Rheum 52(5):1424–1430, 2005.
91. Berggren M, et al. Reduction in the need for operation after conservative treatment of osteoarthritis of the first carpometacarpal joint: a seven year prospective study. Scand J Plast Reconstr Surg Hand Surg 35(4):415–417, 2001.
92. Buurke JH, et al. Usability of thenar eminence orthoses: report of a comparative study. Clin Rehabil 13(4):288–294, 1999.
93. Burton RI, Pellegrini VD Jr. Surgical management of basal joint arthritis of the thumb. Part II. Ligament reconstruction with tendon interposition arthroplasty. J Hand Surg Am 11:324–332, 1986.
94. Stahl S, et al. Comparison of Intraarticular Injection of Depot Corticosteroid and Hyaluronic Acid for Treatment of Degenerative Trapeziometacarpal Joints. J Clin Rheumatol 11(6): 299–302, 2005.
95. Poole JU, Pellegrini VD Jr. Arthritis of the thumb basal joint complex. J Hand Ther 13(2):91–107, 2000.
96. Deitch MA, Stern PJ. Ulnocarpal abutment. Treatment options. Hand Clin 14:251–263, 1998.
97. Tomaino MM. Treatment of Eaton stage I trapeziometacarpal disease. Ligament reconstruction or thumb metacarpal extension osteotomy? Hand Clin 17(2):197–205, 2001.
98. Koff MF, et al. An in vitro analysis of ligament reconstruction or extension osteotomy on trapeziometacarpal joint stability and contact area. J Hand Surg Am 31(3):429–439, 2006.
99. Shrivastava N, et al. Simulated extension osteotomy of the thumb metacarpal reduces carpometacarpal joint laxity in lateral pinch. J Hand Surg Am 28(5):733–738, 2003.
100. Menon J. Arthroscopic evaluation of the first carpometacarpal joint. J Hand Surg Am 23(4):757, 1998.
101. Menon J. Arthroscopic management of trapeziometacarpal joint arthritis of the thumb. Arthroscopy 12(5):581–587, 1996.
102. Orellana MA, Chow JC. Arthroscopic visualization of the thumb carpometacarpal joint: introduction and evaluation of a new radial portal. Arthroscopy 19(6):583–591, 2003.
103. Walsh EF, et al. Thumb carpometacarpal arthroscopy: a topographic, anatomic study of the thenar portal. J Hand Surg Am 30(2):373–379, 2005.
104. Berger RA. A technique for arthroscopic evaluation of the first carpometacarpal joint. J Hand Surg Am 22(6):1077–1080, 1997.
105. Culp RW, Rekant MS. The role of arthroscopy in evaluating and treating trapeziometacarpal disease. Hand Clin 17(2):315–319, x-xi, 2001.
106. Davis TR, Brady O, Barton NJ, et al. Trapeziectomy alone, with tendon interposition or with ligament reconstruction? J Hand Surg Br 22:689–694, 1997.
107. Davis TR, O. Brady O, Dias JJ. Excision of the trapezium for osteoarthritis of the trapeziometacarpal joint: a study of the benefit of ligament reconstruction or tendon interposition. J Hand Surg Am 29(6):1069–1077, 2004.
108. Belcher HJ, Nicholl JE. A comparison of trapeziectomy with and without ligament reconstruction and tendon interposition. J Hand Surg Br 25(4):350–356, 2000.
109. Horlock N, Belcher HJ. Early versus late mobilisation after simple excision of the trapezium. J Bone Joint Surg Br 84(8):1111–1115, 2002.
110. Downing ND, Davis TR. Trapezial space height after trapeziectomy: mechanism of formation and benefits. J Hand Surg Am 26(5):862–868, 2001.
111. Conolly WB, Rath S. Revision procedures for complications of surgery for osteoarthritis of the carpometacarpal joint of the thumb. J Hand Surg Br 18(4):533–539, 1993.
112. Gerwin M, Griffith A, Weiland AJ, et al. Ligament reconstruction basal joint arthroplasty without tendon interposition. Clin Orthop 342:42–45, 1997.
113. Kriegs-Au G, et al. Ligament reconstruction with or without tendon interposition to treat primary thumb carpometacarpal osteoarthritis. A prospective randomized study. J Bone Joint Surg Am 86-A(2):209–218, 2004.
114. Belcher HJ, Nicholl JE. A comparison of trapeziectomy with and without ligament reconstruction and tendon interposition. J Hand Surg Br 25(4):350–356, 2000.
115. Tagil M, Kopylov P. Swanson versus APL arthroplasty in the treatment of osteoarthritis of the trapeziometacarpal joint: a prospective and randomized study in 26 patients. J Hand Surg Br 27(5):452–456, 2002.
116. Horlock N, Belcher HJ. Early versus late mobilisation after simple excision of the trapezium. J Bone Joint Surg Br 84(8):1111–1115, 2002.
117. Taylor NA, Strauch RJ. Suture anchor arthroplasty for thumb carpometacarpal osteoarthritis. J Am Soc Surg Hand 5(3):153–158, 2005.
118. Pellegrini VD Jr, Burton RI. Surgical management of basal joint arthritis of the thumb. Part I. Long-term results of silicone implant arthroplasty. J Hand Surg Am 11:309–324, 1986.
119. Hofammann DY, Ferlic DC, Clayton ML. Arthroplasty of the basal joint of the thumb using a silicone prosthesis. Long-term follow-up. J Bone Joint Surg Am 69:993–997, 1987.
120. Ashworth CR, Blatt G, Chuinard RG, et al. Silicone-rubber interposition arthroplasty of the carpometacarpal joint of the thumb. J Hand Surg Am 2:345–357, 1977.
121. van Cappelle HG, Elzenga P, van Horn JR. Long-term results and loosening analysis of de la Caffiniere replacements of the trapeziometacarpal joint. J Hand Surg Am 24:476–482, 1999.
122. Nicholas RM, Calderwood JW. De la Caffiniere arthroplasty for basal thumb joint osteoarthritis. J Bone Joint Surg Br 74: 309–312, 1992.
123. Chakrabarti AJ, Robinson AH, Gallagher P. De la Caffiniere thumb carpometacarpal replacements. 93 cases at 6 to 16 years follow-up [see comments]. J Hand Surg Br 22:695–698, 1997.
124. Kuschner SH, Lane CS. Surgical treatment for osteoarthritis at the base of the thumb. Am J Orthop 25:91–100, 1996.
125. Carroll RE, Hill NA. Arthrodesis of the carpo-metacarpal joint of the thumb. J Bone Joint Surg Br 55:292–294, 1973.
126. Leach RE, Bolton PE. Arthritis of the carpometacarpal joint of the thumb. Results of arthrodesis. J Bone Joint Surg Am 50: 1171–1177, 1968.
127. North ER, Eaton RG. Degenerative joint disease of the trapezium: a comparative radiographic and anatomic study. J Hand Surg Am 8:160–166, 1983.
128. Glickel SZ, Kornstein AN, Eaton RG. Long-term follow-up of trapeziometacarpal arthroplasty with coexisting scaphotrapezial disease. J Hand Surg Am 17:612–620, 1992.
129. Tomaino MM, Vogt M, Weiser R. Scaphotrapezoid arthritis: prevalence in thumbs undergoing trapezium excision arthroplasty and efficacy of proximal trapezoid excision. J Hand Surg Am 24:1220–1224, 1999.
130. Barron OA, Eaton RG. Save the trapezium: double interposition arthroplasty for the treatment of stage IV disease of the basal joint. J Hand Surg Am 23:196–204, 1998.
131. Freeman GR, Honner R. Silastic replacement of the trapezium. J Hand Surg Br 17:458–462, 1992.
132. Sennwald GR, Segmuller G. The value of scapho-trapezio-trapezoid arthrodesis combined with "de la Caffiniere" arthroplasty for the treatment of pantrapezial osteoarthritis. J Hand Surg Br 18:527–532, 1993.
133. Trumble TE, Rafijah G, Gilbert M, et al. Thumb trapeziometacarpal joint arthritis: partial trapeziectomy with ligament reconstruction and interposition costochondral allograft. J Hand Surg Am 25: 61–76, 2000.
134. Watson HK, Hempton RF. Limited wrist arthrodeses. I. The triscaphoid joint. J Hand Surg Am 5:320–327, 1980.
135. Garcia-Elias M, et al. Resection of the distal scaphoid for scaphotrapeziotrapezoid osteoarthritis. J Hand Surg Br 24(4):448–452, 1999.

136. Fortin PT, Louis DS. Long-term follow-up of scaphoid-trapezium-trapezoid arthrodesis. J Hand Surg Am 18:675–681, 1993.
137. Linscheid RL, Dobyns JH, Beabout JW, et al. Traumatic instability of the wrist. Diagnosis, classification, and pathomechanics. J Bone Joint Surg Am 54:1612–1632, 1972.
138. Viegas SF, Tencer AF, Cantrell J, et al. Load transfer characteristics of the wrist. Part I. The normal joint. J Hand Surg Am 12:971–978, 1987.
139. Viegas SF, Tencer AF, Cantrell J, et al. Load transfer characteristics of the wrist. Part II. Perilunate instability. J Hand Surg Am 12:978–985, 1987.
140. Moskal MJ, Savoie FH III, Field LD. Arthroscopic treatment of posterior elbow impingement. Instr Course Lect 48:399–404, 1999.
141. Palmer AK, Dobyns JH, Linscheid RL. Management of post-traumatic instability of the wrist secondary to ligament rupture. J Hand Surg Am 3:507–532, 1978.
142. Dobyns JH, Linscheid RL, Chao EYS, et al. Traumatic instability of the wrist. Instructional Course Lectures. St. Louis, CV Mosby, 1975, pp 182–199.
143. Rosenwasser MP, Paul SB, Froimson AI. Arthroplasty of the hand and wrist. Hand Clin 5:487–505, 1989.
144. Watson HK, Ballet FL. The SLAC wrist: scapholunate advanced collapse pattern of degenerative arthritis. J Hand Surg Am 9:358–365, 1984.
145. Linscheid RL, Dobyns JH, Beckenbaugh RD, et al. Instability patterns of the wrist. J Hand Surg Am 8(Pt 2):682–686, 1983.
146. Watson HK, Ashmead D 4th, Makhlouf MV. Examination of the scaphoid. J Hand Surg Am 13:657–660, 1988.
147. Ashmead D 4th, Watson HK, Damon C, et al. Scapholunate advanced collapse wrist salvage. J Hand Surg Am 19:741–750, 1994.
148. Krakauer JD, Bishop AT, Cooney WP. Surgical treatment of scapholunate advanced collapse. J Hand Surg Am 19:751–759, 1994.
149. Wyrick JD, Stern PJ, Kiefhaber TR. Motion-preserving procedures in the treatment of scapholunate advanced collapse wrist: proximal row carpectomy versus four-corner arthrodesis. J Hand Surg Am 20:965–970, 1995.
150. Salomon GD, Eaton RG. Proximal row carpectomy with partial capitate resection. J Hand Surg Am 21:2–8, 1996.
151. Rotman MB, Manske PR, Pruitt DL, et al. Scaphocapitolunate arthrodesis. J Hand Surg Am 18:26–33, 1993.
152. Tomaino MM, Delsignore J, Burton RI. Long-term results following proximal row carpectomy. J Hand Surg Am 19:694–703, 1994.
153. Culp RW, McGuigan FX, Turner MA, et al. Proximal row carpectomy: a multicenter study. J Hand Surg Am 18:19–25, 1993.
154. Cohen MS, Kozin SH. Degenerative arthritis of the wrist: proximal row carpectomy versus scaphoid excision and four-corner arthrodesis. J Hand Surg Am 26(1):94–104, 2001.
155. DiDonna ML, Kiefhaber TR, Stern PJ. Proximal row carpectomy: study with a minimum of ten years of follow-up. J Bone Joint Surg Am 86-A(11):2359–2365, 2004.
156. Stern PJ, et al. Proximal row carpectomy. J Bone Joint Surg Am 87(Suppl 1, Pt 2):166–174, 2005.
157. Minami A, Kato H, Iwasaki N, et al. Limited wrist fusions: comparison of results 22 and 89 months after surgery. J Hand Surg Am 24:133–137, 1999.
158. Lipton CB, et al. Reduction and association of the scaphoid and lunate for scapholunate ligament injuries (RASL). Atlas of the Hand Clinics 8:249–260, 2003.
159. Malerich MM, Clifford J, Eaton B, et al. Distal scaphoid resection arthroplasty for the treatment of degenerative arthritis secondary to scaphoid nonunion. J Hand Surg Am 24:1196–1205, 1999.
160. Herbert TJ, Fisher WE. Management of the fractured scaphoid using a new bone screw. J Bone Joint Surg Br 66:114–123, 1984.
161. Inoue G, Shionoya K, Kuwahata Y. Herbert screw fixation for scaphoid nonunions. An analysis of factors influencing outcome. Clin Orthop 343:99–106, 1997.
162. Gabl M, Reinhart C, Lutz M, et al. Vascularized bone graft from the iliac crest for the treatment of nonunion of the proximal part of the scaphoid with an avascular fragment. J Bone Joint Surg Am 81:1414–1428, 1999.
163. Bonzar M, Firrell JC, Hainer M, et al. Kienböck disease and negative ulnar variance [see comments]. J Bone Joint Surg Am 80:1154–1157, 1998.
164. Panagis JS, Gelberman RH, Taleisnik J, et al. The arterial anatomy of the human carpus. Part II. The intraosseous vascularity. J Hand Surg Am 8:375–382, 1983.
165. Williams CS, Gelberman RH. Vascularity of the lunate. Anatomic studies and implications for the development of osteonecrosis. Hand Clin 9:391–398, 1993.
166. Szabo RM, Greenspan A. Diagnosis and clinical findings of Kienböck's disease. Hand Clin 9:399–408, 1993.
167. Lichtman DM, Alexander AH, Mack GR, et al. Kienböck's disease—update on silicone replacement arthroplasty. J Hand Surg Am 7:343–347, 1982.
168. Bourne MH, Linscheid RL, Dobyns JH. Concomitant scapholunate dissociation and Kienböck's disease. J Hand Surg Am 16:460–464, 1991.
169. Keith PP, Nuttall D, Trail I. Long-term outcome of nonsurgically managed Kienbock's disease. J Hand Surg Am 29(1):63–67, 2004.
170. Armistead RB, et al. Ulnar lengthening in the treatment of Kienböck's disease. J Bone Joint Surg Am 64(2):170–178, 1982.
171. Iwasaki N, et al. Radial osteotomy for late-stage Kienbock's disease. Wedge osteotomy versus radial shortening. J Bone Joint Surg Br 84(5):673–677, 2002.
172. Illarramendi AA, De Carli P. Radius decompression for treatment of kienbock disease. Tech Hand Up Extrem Surg 7(3):110–113, 2003.
173. Horii E, et al. Effect on force transmission across the carpus in procedures used to treat Kienbock's disease. J Hand Surg Am 15(3):393–400, 1990.
174. Moritomo H, Murase T, Yoshikawa H. Operative technique of a new decompression procedure for Kienbock disease: partial capitate shortening. Tech Hand Up Extrem Surg 8(2):110–115, 2004.
175. Shin AY, Bishop AT. Pedicled vascularized bone grafts for disorders of the carpus: scaphoid nonunion and Kienböck's disease. J Am Acad Orthop Surg 10(3):210–216, 2002.
176. Daecke W, et al. Occurrence of carpal osteoarthritis after treatment of scaphoid nonunion with bone graft and herbert screw: a long-term follow-up study. J Hand Surg Am 30(5):923–931, 2005.
177. Swanson AB, de Groot Swanson G. Implant resection arthroplasty in the treatment of Kienböck's disease. Hand Clin 9:483–491, 1993.
178. Kaarela OI, Raatikainen TK, Torniainen PJ. Silicone replacement arthroplasty for Kienböck's disease. J Hand Surg Br 23:735–740, 1998.
179. Carroll RE. Long-term review of fascial replacement after excision of the carpal lunate bone. Clin Orthop 342:59–63, 1997.
180. Menth-Chiari WA, Poehling GG, Wiesler ER, et al. Arthroscopic débridement for the treatment of Kienböck's disease. Arthroscopy 15:12–19, 1999.
181. Nakamura R, Horii E, Watanabe K, et al Proximal row carpectomy versus limited wrist arthrodesis for advanced Kienböck's disease. J Hand Surg Br 23:741–745, 1998.
182. Begley BW, Engber WD. Proximal row carpectomy in advanced Kienböck's disease. J Hand Surg Am 19:1016–1018, 1994.
183. Lin HH, Stern PJ. "Salvage" procedures in the treatment of Kienböck's disease. Proximal row carpectomy and total wrist arthrodesis. Hand Clin 9:521–562, 1993.
184. Watson HK, Fink JA, Monacelli DM. Use of triscaphe fusion in the treatment of Kienböck's disease. Hand Clin 9:493–499, 1993.
185. Divelbiss BJ, Sollerman C, Adams BD. Early results of the Universal total wrist arthroplasty in rheumatoid arthritis. J Hand Surg Am 27(2):195–204, 2002.
186. Rahimtoola ZO, Hubach P. Total modular wrist prosthesis: a new design. Scand J Plast Reconstr Surg Hand Surg 38(3):160–165, 2004.
187. Rizzo M, Beckenbaugh RD. Results of biaxial total wrist arthroplasty with a modified (long) metacarpal stem. J Hand Surg Am 28(4):577–584, 2003.
188. Meuli HC. Meuli total wrist arthroplasty. Clin Orthop 187:107–111, 1984.
189. Meuli HC. Total wrist arthroplasty. Experience with a noncemented wrist prosthesis. Clin Orthop 342:77–83, 1997.

190. Figgie HE III, Ranawat CS, Inglis AE, et al. Preliminary results of total wrist arthroplasty in rheumatoid arthritis using the trispherical total wrist arthroplasty. J Arthroplasty 3:9–15, 1988.

191. Beckenbaugh RD, Linscheid RL. Arthroplasty in the hand and wrist. In: Green DP, ed. Operative Hand Surgery. Vol 1. New York, Churchill Livingstone, 1993, pp 167–184.

192. Takwale VJ, et al. Biaxial total wrist replacement in patients with rheumatoid arthritis. Clinical review, survivorship and radiological analysis. J Bone Joint Surg Br 84(5):692–699, 2002.

193. Vogelin E, Nagy L. Fate of failed Meuli total wrist arthroplasty. J Hand Surg Br 28(1):61–68, 2003.

194. Peimer CA, Medige J, Eckert BS, et al. Reactive synovitis after silicone arthroplasty. J Hand Surg Am 11:624–638, 1986.

195. Smith RJ, Atkinson RE, Jupiter JB. Silicone synovitis of the wrist. J Hand Surg Am 10:47–60, 1985.

196. Beer TA, Turner RH. Wrist arthrodesis for failed wrist implant arthroplasty. J Hand Surg Am 22:685–693, 1997.

197. Carlson JR, Simmons BP. Total wrist arthroplasty. J Am Acad Orthop Surg 6:308–315, 1998.

198. Carlson JR, Simmons BP. Wrist arthrodesis after failed wrist implant arthroplasty. J Hand Surg Am 23:893–898, 1998.

199. Weiss AP, Hastings H II. Wrist arthrodesis for traumatic conditions: a study of plate and local bone graft application. J Hand Surg Am 20:50–56, 1995.

200. Lee DH, Carroll RE. Wrist arthrodesis: a combined intramedullary pin and autogenous iliac crest bone graft technique. J Hand Surg Am 19:733–740, 1994.

201. Moneim MS, Pribyl CR, Garst JR. Wrist arthrodesis. Technique and functional evaluation. Clin Orthop 341:23–29, 1997.

202. Richterman I, Weiss AP. Wrist fusion. Hand Clin 13:681–687, 1997.

203. Clayton ML, Ferlic DC. Arthrodesis of the arthritic wrist. Clin Orthop 187:89–93, 1984.

204. Divelbiss BJ, Baratz ME. The role of arthroplasty and arthrodesis following trauma to the upper extremity. Hand Clin 15:335–345, ix, 1999.

205. Cooney WP III, Dobyns JH, Linscheid RL. Complications of Colles' fractures. J Bone Joint Surg Am 62:613–619, 1980.

206. Staron RB, Feldman F, Haramati N, et al. Abnormal geometry of the distal radioulnar joint: MR findings. Skeletal Radiol 23: 369–372, 1994.

207. Scheker LR, Severo A. Ulnar shortening for the treatment of early post-traumatic osteoarthritis at the distal radioulnar joint. J Hand Surg Br 26(1):41–44, 2001.

208. van Schoonhoven J, et al. Salvage of failed resection arthroplasties of the distal radioulnar joint using a new ulnar head prosthesis. J Hand Surg Am 25(3):438–446, 2000.

209. Berger RA, Cooney WP III. Use of an ulnar head endoprosthesis for treatment of an unstable distal ulnar resection: review of mechanics, indications, and surgical technique. Hand Clin 21(4):603–620, 2005.

210. Watson HK, Gabuzda GM. Matched distal ulna resection for posttraumatic disorders of the distal radioulnar joint. J Hand Surg Am 17:724–730, 1992.

211. Taleisnik J. The Sauvé-Kapandji procedure. Clin Orthop 275: 110–123, 1992.

212. Adams BD. Effects of radial deformity on distal radioulnar joint mechanics. J Hand Surg Am 18:492–498, 1993.

213. Werner FW, Murphy DJ, Palmer AK. Pressures in the distal radioulnar joint: effect of surgical procedures used for Kienböck's disease. J Orthop Res 7:445–450, 1989.

214. Jupiter JB, Masem M. Reconstruction of post-traumatic deformity of the distal radius and ulna. Hand Clin 4:377–390, 1988.

215. Hunt TR, Hastings H 2nd, Graham TJ. A systematic approach to handling the distal radio-ulnar joint in cases of malunited distal radius fractures. Hand Clin 14:239–249, 1998.

216. Deitch MA, Stern PJ. Ulnocarpal abutment. Treatment options. Hand Clin 14:251–263, 1998.

217. Lichtman DM, Ganocy TK, Kim DC. The indications for and techniques and outcomes of ablative procedures of the distal ulna. The Darrach resection, hemiresection, matched resection, and Sauvé-Kapandji procedure. Hand Clin 14:265–277, 1998.

218. Hartz CR, Beckenbaugh RD. Long-term results of resection of the distal ulna for post-traumatic conditions. J Trauma 19:219–226, 1979.

219. Tulipan DJ, Eaton RG, Eberhart RE. The Darrach procedure defended: technique redefined and long-term follow-up. J Hand Surg Am 16:438–444, 1991.

220. Field J, Majkowski RJ, Leslie IJ. Poor results of Darrach's procedure after wrist injuries. J Bone Joint Surg Br 75:53–57, 1993.

221. Dingman PC. Resection of the distal end of the ulna: an end-result of twenty-four cases. J Bone Joint Surg Am 34:893–899, 1952.

222. Sauerbier M, et al. The dynamic radioulnar convergence of the Darrach procedure and the ulnar head hemiresection interposition arthroplasty: a biomechanical study. J Hand Surg Br 27(4): 307–316, 2002.

223. Minami A, et al. Treatments of osteoarthritis of the distal radioulnar joint: long-term results of three procedures. Hand Surg 10(2-3): 243–248, 2005.

224. Fernandez DL, Joneschild ES, Abella DM. Treatment of failed Sauve-Kapandji procedures with a spherical ulnar head prosthesis. Clin Orthop Relat Res 445:100–107, 2006.

225. Colman WW, Strauch RJ. Physical examination of the elbow. Orthop Clin North Am 30:15–20, 1999.

226. Calandruccio JH, Collins ED, Hanel DP, et al. Wrist and Hand Trauma. Rosemont, IL, American Academy of Orthopaedic Surgeons, 1999, 392.

227. Morrey BF. Primary degenerative arthritis of the elbow. Treatment by ulnohumeral arthroplasty. J Bone Joint Surg Br 74:409–413, 1992.

228. Tsujino A, Itoh Y, Hayashi K, et al. Cubital tunnel reconstruction for ulnar neuropathy in osteoarthritic elbows. J Bone Joint Surg Br 79:390–393, 1997.

229. Doherty M, Preston B. Primary osteoarthritis of the elbow. Ann Rheum Dis 48:743–747, 1989.

230. Josefsson PO, Gentz CF, Johnell O, et al. Dislocations of the elbow and intraarticular fractures. Clin Orthop 246:126–130, 1989.

231. Ippolito E, Tudisco C, Farsetti P, et al. Fracture of the humeral condyles in children: 49 cases evaluated after 18–45 years. Acta Orthop Scand 67:173–178, 1996.

232. Schneeberger AG, Adams R, Morrey BF. Semiconstrained total elbow replacement for the treatment of post-traumatic osteoarthrosis. J Bone Joint Surg Am 79:1211–1222, 1997.

233. Lee DH. Posttraumatic elbow arthritis and arthroplasty. Orthop Clin North Am 30:141–162, 1999.

234. Morrey BF. Post-traumatic contracture of the elbow. Operative treatment, including distraction arthroplasty. J Bone Joint Surg Am 72:601–618, 1990.

235. Bauer M, Jonsson K, Josefsson PO, et al. Osteochondritis dissecans of the elbow. A long-term follow-up study. Clin Orthop 284: 156–160, 1992.

236. Takahara M, Ogino T, Sasaki I, et al. Long term outcome of osteochondritis dissecans of the humeral capitellum. Clin Orthop 363:108–115, 1999.

237. Garcia-Elias M, Lluch A. Partial excision of scaphoid: is it ever indicated? Hand Clin 17(4):687–695, 2001.

238. Baker CL, Brooks AA. Arthroscopy of the elbow. Clin Sports Med 15:261–281, 1996.

238a. Oka Y. Débridement for osteoarthritis of the elbow in athletes. Int Orthop 23:91–94, 1999.

239. O'Driscoll SW. Arthroscopic treatment for osteoarthritis of the elbow. Orthop Clin North Am 26:691–706, 1995.

240. Ruch DS, Poehling GG. Anterior interosseous nerve injury following elbow arthroscopy. Arthroscopy 13:756–758, 1997.

241. Carn RM, Medige J, Curtain D, et al. Silicone rubber replacement of the severely fractured radial head. Clin Orthop 209:259–269, 1986.

242. Knight DJ, Rymaszewski LA, Amis AA, et al. Primary replacement of the fractured radial head with a metal prosthesis. J Bone Joint Surg 75:572–576, 1993.

243. King GJ. Management of comminuted radial head fractures with replacement arthroplasty. Hand Clin 20(4):429–441, 2004.

244. Brinkman JM, et al. Treatment of sequelae of radial head fractures with a bipolar radial head prosthesis: good outcome after 1-4 years follow-up in 11 patients. Acta Orthop 76(6):867–872, 2005.

245. Doornberg JN, et al. Reference points for radial head prosthesis size. J Hand Surg Am 31(1):53–57, 2006.

246. Birkedal JP, Deal DN, Ruch DS. Loss of flexion after radial head replacement. J Shoulder Elbow Surg 13(2):208–213, 2004.

247. Vanderwilde RS, Morrey BF, Melberg MW, et al. Inflammatory arthritis after failure of silicone rubber replacement of the radial head. J Bone Joint Surg Br 76:78–81, 1994.

248. Cobb TK, Morrey BF. Use of distraction arthroplasty in unstable fracture dislocations of the elbow. Clin Orthop 312:201–210, 1995.

249. Morrey BF. Posttraumatic stiffness: distraction arthroplasty. Orthopedics 15:863–869, 1992.

250. Morrey BF, Adams RA, Bryan RS. Total replacement for post-traumatic arthritis of the elbow. J Bone Joint Surg Br 73:607–612, 1991.

251. Cobb TK, Morrey BF. Total elbow arthroplasty as primary treatment for distal humeral fractures in elderly patients. J Bone Joint Surg Am 79:826–832, 1997.

252. Chafik D, Lee TQ, Gupta R. Total elbow arthroplasty: current indications, factors affecting outcomes, and follow-up results. Am J Orthop 33(10):496–503, 2004.

253. Morrey BF, et al. Total elbow arthroplasty. A five-year experience at the Mayo Clinic. J Bone Joint Surg Am 63(7):1050–1063, 1981.

254. van der Lugt JC, Geskus RB, Rozing PM. Limited influence of prosthetic position on aseptic loosening of elbow replacements: 125 elbows followed for an average period of 5.6 years. Acta Orthop 76(5):654–661, 2005.

255. Wright TW, Wong AM, Jaffe R. Functional outcome comparison of semiconstrained and unconstrained total elbow arthroplasties. J Shoulder Elbow Surg 9(6):524–531, 2000.

256. Thillemann TM, et al. Long-term results with the Kudo type 3 total elbow arthroplasty. J Shoulder Elbow Surg 15(4):495–499, 2006.

257. Figgie MP, et al. Locking mechanism failure in semiconstrained total elbow arthroplasty. J Shoulder Elbow Surg 15(1):88–93, 2006.

258. Aldridge JM III, et al. Total elbow arthroplasty with the Coonrad/Coonrad-Morrey prosthesis. A 10- to 31-year survival analysis. J Bone Joint Surg Br 88(4):509–514, 2006.

259. Goldberg SH, et al. Thermal tissue damage caused by ultrasonic cement removal from the humerus. J Bone Joint Surg Am 87(3):583–591, 2005.

260. Hastings H II, Theng CS. Total elbow replacement for distal humerus fractures and traumatic deformity: results and complications of semiconstrained implants and design rationale for the Discovery Elbow System. Am J Orthop,. 32(9 Suppl):20–28, 2003.

261. Nagy SM III, Szabo RM, Sharkey NA. Unilateral elbow arthrodesis: the preferred position. J South Orthop Assoc 8:80–85, 1999.

262. O'Neill OR, Morrey BF, Tanaka S, et al. Compensatory motion in the upper extremity after elbow arthrodesis. Clin Orthop 281:89–96, 1992.

263. Rashkoff E, Burkhalter WE. Arthrodesis of the salvage elbow. Orthopedics 9:733–738, 1986.

264. Arafiles RP. A new technique of fusion for tuberculous arthritis of the elbow. J Bone Joint Surg Am 63:1396–1400, 1981.

Lower Extremity Considerations: Hip

21A

Michael N. Kang   Daniel J. Berry   William J. Maloney III

INTRODUCTION

There has been much debate whether OA of the hip is a primary or secondary process. A pre-existing condition such as hip dysplasia, slipped capital femoral epiphysis, Perthes disease, and previous trauma are well-recognized processes that lead to osteoarthritis (OA).[1] Ganz and colleagues have proposed a different primary process referred to as *femoroacetabular impingement*. Regardless of the underlying etiology, the end result of OA is loss of articular cartilage and subsequent joint deformity. Clinically, the patient experiences progressively increasing frequency and severity of pain with loss of range of motion. First-line therapy includes medications such as acetaminophen and non-steroidal anti-inflammatory medications, nutritional supplements such as glucosamine and chondroitin sulfate, activity modification, weight loss, physical therapy, and a walking aid such as a cane.

This chapter focuses on the surgical considerations for treatment of OA of the hip—primary and secondary. Surgical options depend on the diagnosis, severity of arthritis, patient age and activity level, patient occupation, patient medical health, and patient expectations. Surgical options are grouped into five main categories. Hip arthroscopy is utilized for the pre-arthritic hip with labral lesions. Surgical débridement and reshaping of the femoral head and neck through open and arthroscopic approaches is used to treat femoroacetabular impingement in the early stages of arthritis. Hip arthrodesis or fusion is indicated in the very young patient with end stage arthritis. Osteotomy is an option mainly in patients who have hip dysplasia. An osteotomy realigns the acetabulum, normalizing the forces that are transmitted through the hip joint and subsequently relieve pain. Finally, hip joint arthroplasty involves replacing all or parts of the diseased joint with artificial components. Each category will be discussed individually.

ARTHROSCOPY

The development of arthroscopic surgery of the hip has been slower to evolve in comparison to other joints such as the knee or shoulder due to more complex anatomic constraints as well as the fact that conditions of the hip like labral pathology can go unrecognized and untreated. As a less invasive tool to diagnose and treat hip pathology, the indications for hip arthroscopy most commonly include labral tears, capsular laxity, chondral injury, ligamentum teres avulsions, and removal of loose bodies. Less commonly, they can include management of osteonecrosis, inflammatory synovial processes, infection, and possibly early to mild OA.[2,3]

Advanced imaging studies such as computed tomography (CT), magnetic resonance imaging (MRI), and magnetic resonance arthrography (MRA) have improved the ability to diagnose bony and soft tissue pathology about the hip. However, Edwards and colleagues[4] reported that MRI was relatively poor in the diagnosis of chondral fibrillation or defects under 1 cm. Furthermore, MRI did not reliably diagnose loose bodies and labral tears. Gadolinium-enhanced MRA has improved diagnostic sensitivity and accuracy.[5] The gold standard of diagnosis remains visualization via arthroscopy.

Keeney and colleagues[6] evaluated the effectiveness of MRA as a diagnostic tool. In 102 hips, MRA was obtained in order to confirm the diagnosis of labral pathology as well as exclude other conditions that could contribute to hip pain. MRA was able to diagnose 71 out of 102 hips with labral pathology. The sensitivity is 71%, while the positive predictive value is 93%. Articular pathology was also assessed, and MRA demonstrated a sensitivity of 47%, specificity of 89%, and a positive predictive value of 84%. The authors conclude that MRA is an effective tool to diagnose labral pathology; however, a negative study does not exclude intra-articular pathology that can be treated arthroscopically.

375

For the patient 1) who complains of mechanical symptoms in the hip, 2) has physical exam consistent with an intra-articular process, and 3) has supporting imaging studies, arthroscopic débridement of labral tears has shown to be effective in nearly 90% by Philippon et al.[7] It is important to differentiate an intra-articular process versus external pathology, such as psoas tendon irritation over the iliopectineal eminence or femoral head.[8] McCarthy and colleagues[9] performed 436 hip arthroscopies and determined that 55% had labral tears. In the labral tear group, 73% were found to have associated chondral injury, and chondral injury was more prevalent in older patients. The authors hypothesize that the altered biomechanics of the hip joint lead to labral tears and subsequent degenerative changes in the cartilage.

Femoro-Acetabular Impingement

Femoro-acetabular impingement is a concept that has been championed by Ganz as a cause of secondary OA.[10] Abnormal or excessive contact between the proximal femur and acetabular rim leads to lesions in the labrum and chondral surfaces that can result in degenerative changes of the entire hip joint. Initial radiographic work-up may appear relatively normal. Physical examination involves provocative tests to cause the bony impingement. Anterior impingement can be assessed with hip flexion and internal rotation, while posterior impingement can be re-created by extension and external rotation.

Radiographic examination often demonstrates a bony prominence on the anterolateral aspect of the femoral neck as well as possible herniation pits in this region. Other bony abnormalities, such as acetabular retroversion, acetabular protrusion, hip dysplasia, and coxa vara or valga, can also be present. MRA should be routinely obtained in this patient population as there is a high incidence of labral and chondral pathology.[11]

Two types of impingement have been described: cam impingement and pincer impingement. Cam impingement is caused by an abnormal femoral head with a larger radius being forced into a smaller acetabulum, especially in flexion.[12] This produces shear forces that produce abrasion of the cartilage or avulsion of the labrum at the anterosuperior rim. Pincer impingement involves over-coverage anteriorly by the acetabulum leading to impingement and subsequent labral degeneration. Chronic abutment can lead to further ossification of the anterior rim which deepens the acetabulum, worsening this condition. Chronic impingement leads to a "lever" effect and chondral injury in the posteroinferior aspect of the acetabulum.

When conservative therapy is inadequate, surgical dislocation of the femoral head via a trochanteric flip osteotomy, as described by the Swiss group, is suggested.[13] Surgical treatment includes débridement of the femoral neck to improve offset in order to alleviate the cam impingement. Care must be taken to avoid the retinacular vessels as they enter the superior portion of the femoral neck region. Anterior acetabular bony impingement can also be reduced (pincer impingement). Intra-articular pathology can be treated as well (Fig. 21A–1A, B).

Ganz et al.[14] reviewed the surgical treatment in 19 hips with an average follow-up of a minimum of 4 years. The average age of the patients was 36 years. At the latest follow-up, there was significant improvement in the Merle d'Aubigne hip score and pain score. There was an increase in range of motion, though not significant. Thirteen patients had considerable improvement in pain, while two patients had no change. Four patients developed increasing pain in the hip. These four patients and one other went on to total hip arthroplasty. The grade of OA was important in the long-term prognosis of these patients. Of the five hips that underwent conversion to total hip arthroplasty, two hips had grade 2 arthritis, and the other three hips had extensive acetabular cartilage degeneration as well as focal defects in the femoral head.

Other groups have demonstrated similar results. Murphy and colleagues[15] describe their experience with débridement of the neck with surgical dislocation in 23 patients. Fifteen patients were satisfied with the procedure.

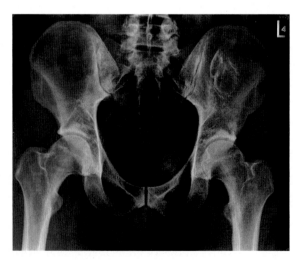

Figure 21A–1A Preoperative radiograph of femoro-acetabular impingement.

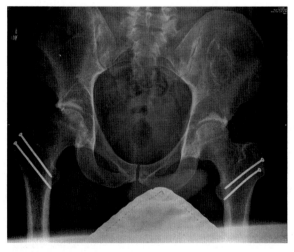

Figure 21A–1B Postoperative radiograph after surgical dislocation and recontouring of femoral neck.

Seven patients went on to total hip replacement between 6.4 and 9.5 years, while one patient had an arthroscopic procedure for recurrent labral pathology. The Merle d'Aubigne hip score was significantly improved postoperatively in the 15 patients with well-functioning hips. Clohisy and McClure[16] describe a different surgical technique to treat anterior impingement. The patients undergo arthroscopic evaluation of the hip joint with debridement of any chondral and labral pathology, followed by a decompression of any bony impingement via an anterior approach. The authors report good results with this technique (Clohisy, unpublished data).

Acetabular retroversion has become more commonly diagnosed as a cause of femoroacetabular impingement. Radiographic diagnosis can be performed by the "cross-over and posterior wall" signs.[17] Siebenrock et al.[18] reported on 29 patients with acetabular retroversion who underwent periacetabular osteotomy to relieve the anterior femoroacetabular impingement. Any intra-articular pathology was also addressed. Twenty-six patients had good to excellent results with significant increase of range of motion. One patient had recurrent anterior impingement, while one had posterior impingement due to overcorrection. In summary, it is important to diagnose the underlying etiology of femoro-acetabular impingement as well as any intra-articular pathology in order to determine the appropriate surgical procedure.

ARTHRODESIS

Arthrodesis of the hip is a reliable procedure to eliminate pain in young patients (ages 16 to 30) who have prematurely developed end stage arthritis. Due to the successful functional outcomes of total hip arthroplasty (THA) in the older patient, the indications for THA have been stretched to this younger population with the advent of newer, more durable materials. Furthermore, THA is better accepted as it preserves joint mobility and improved gait mechanics, sitting comfort, and sexual function. However, numerous authors have reported on THA failure rates of 33% to 45% in this young patient population.[19-22] The higher failure rate has been attributed to increased activity, leading to increased wear.

A successful hip arthrodesis can provide an active lifestyle that can be later converted to THA.[23,24] The indications for hip fusion are young age (<30 years) with noninflammatory, monoarticular, end stage arthritis, especially if any neurologic or muscle (abductor) imbalances exist. Absolute contraindications include active infection, inflammatory arthritis, and radiographic evidence of arthrosis with symptomatic stiffness of the ipsilateral knee, spine, or contralateral hip.[25]

The position of hip fusion affects outcome. The optimal position for hip fusion is 20° to 30° of hip flexion, 5° to 7° of adduction, and 5° to 10° of external rotation.[26] As noted, hip position is important, as too much extension can prevent a comfortable sitting position, while too much flexion can cause increased lumbar lordosis with standing. Discrepancies in abduction or adduction can lead to pelvic obliquity as well as apparent limb length discrepancies.

It is recommended that an intraoperative radiograph be performed prior to finalizing position.

The surgical techniques have evolved, however, the principles remain: maximize bone contact, rigid internal fixation, and slightly medialize the hip center. Intra-articular contact with rigid fixation of the ilium to the proximal femur allows initial stability of the fusion, while permitting mobilization of adjacent joints.[27-30] Early accepted techniques included stripping the abductors and placing a lateral cobra plate contoured to the anatomy of the pelvic brim. Matta et al.[28] describe a different technique of anterior plating which spares scarring of the abductors during subsequent conversion to THA. External fixation has been described in the pediatric literature.[31,32] In the modern literature, nonunion rates have ranged from 10% to 20%. Nonunions typically require reoperation.

Several groups have reported good results for hip fusion in terms of pain relief and functional ability; however, nearly 70% felt that their activity level was below their respective age group.[23,33] Functionally speaking, patients have an asymmetric, arrhythmic gait that is pain free.[34,35] The majority of patients lead productive lives without limitations except for activities requiring the extremes of hip flexion. The major long-term complication of hip arthrodesis is ipsilateral knee and lower back arthrosis. Hauge[36] reported that 65% of 200 patients developed radiographic evidence of OA of the ipsilateral knee. Callaghan et al.[33] had similar results with 60% of the patients experiencing either lower back or ipsilateral knee pain. Furthermore, they noted that there was a trend toward increased arthrosis with malposition of the hip fusion.

A hip fusion, whether it be spontaneous or iatrogenic, can be converted to a THA.[24] The primary indications are to relieve symptoms of increasing pain in the lumbar spine, ipsilateral knee, or contralateral hip. It is important to maintain hip abductor function in the index hip fusion and during the subsequent takedown of the hip fusion to permit normal gait. Patients with damage to the abductor muscles will experience a chronic Trendelenburg gait following THA. In addition, adequate tension of the abductors is important during the conversion to THA to diminish the risk of postoperative dislocation. Abductor function can be assessed preoperatively by palpating the contraction of the abductors. Finally, choice of implants (constrained implant) may be affected by a poorly functioning abductor mechanism that may compromise the long-term efficacy and survival of the implants.

Hardinge et al.[37] reported on 112 patients converted to THA from either a spontaneous or surgical hip fusion, excluding ankylosing spondylitis. Limb length discrepancies remained in 11.5% of patients, however, only 5% of all patients were dissatisfied with the results. The authors noticed that patients who had fusions prior to skeletal maturity had underdeveloped greater trochanters, and subsequently, abductor function was poor after conversion to THA. Kilgus et al.[38] reported that relief of back pain was higher than the relief in ipsilateral knee pain, or contralateral hip or knee pain. The UCLA hip function scores did not improve after THA, reflecting the high level of activity of the patients with a hip fusion. Only 33% of the patients were able to use a less restrictive ambulatory aid.

Caution should be undertaken when performing an arthroplasty of the ipsilateral knee of a fused hip. Garvin et al.[39] reported on nine patients who received total knee replacements under a fused hip. Seven patients were available for follow-up; all required at least one postoperative manipulation, and two were unable to flex to at least 90 degrees. The overall complication rate was 65%. Consideration for the takedown of the hip fusion and conversion to a THA prior to knee replacement must be undertaken.

In summary, hip fusion is a reliable operation to eliminate hip pain in the very young patient. Patients can be converted to THA to obtain pain relief in adjacent joints, correct leg length discrepancies, and improve hip mobility. It is important to maintain abductor function during conversion to THA. Although patients are satisfied after conversion to THA, hip function scores do not improve significantly.

OSTEOTOMY

Osteotomies around the hip joint are joint-preserving procedures that are an acceptable alternative to joint replacement surgery in younger patients for the appropriate diagnoses.[40] The underlying diagnoses in whom one would consider an osteotomy include young patients with secondary OA from hip dysplasia and residual deformities from childhood conditions such as Perthes disease and Slipped Capital Femoral Epiphysis (SCFE). Other indications for osteotomies include partial osteonecrosis of the femoral head and femoral neck fracture nonunions; however, these fall outside of the scope of this chapter.

In the 1960s, the introduction of THA markedly diminished the utilization of osteotomy for OA. However, as long-term studies demonstrated that THA lacked durability past 15 to 20 years, especially in younger patients, hip osteotomies have become more attractive as they have the potential to provide excellent results with good long-term durability in the appropriately selected patient. The goal of an osteotomy is to relieve pain by redirecting the distribution of load and changing the stress gradients, but there is little change in the actual joint loads.[41] Hip osteotomies can provide durable pain relief by one or a combination of the following mechanisms: 1) improvement in joint congruity leading to increased joint contact area and decreased joint contact stress; 2) improvement in hip biomechanics decreasing joint contact forces; 3) rotation of intact articular cartilage into the weight-bearing dome, thus loading more normal cartilage; and 4) reduction in joint subluxation decreasing shear stresses on the articular cartilage.

Osteotomies around the hip joint can be performed on the pelvic or the femoral side. Pelvic osteotomies can be categorized as reconstructive or salvage procedures. Proximal femoral osteotomies are generally performed in the intertrochanteric region, and the descriptive terms describe the mechanical effect of the osteotomy. These terms include varus, valgus, flexion, and extension osteotomies. Osteotomies of the greater trochanter can be performed as well, but these are not used to address osteoarthritic conditions.

PELVIC OSTEOTOMY

Pelvic osteotomies are traditionally performed in children as treatment of residual hip dysplasia and have produced successful results. The Salter and Pemberton pelvic osteotomies restore the normal anatomy and biomechanical forces around the hip joint. These single and double osteotomies are possible in children as the flexibility of the symphysis pubis and the triradiate cartilage allow for rotation around these points.

The role of reconstructive pelvic osteotomies is an extension of pediatric hip experience. In recent years, they have become more popular as more surgeons are trained and become familiar with this procedure. They have been popularized in Europe and Asia, mainly Japan. The main indications for pelvic osteotomies are young patients with a symptomatic hip secondary to developmental dysplasia of the hip. The dysplastic hip typically has an acetabulum that is shallow, lateralized, and anteverted with deficient coverage anteriorly and superiorly. The proximal femur is usually anteverted with an increased neck-shaft angle and a small femoral head and canal. The patients usually complain of locking or catching symptoms as the femoral head subluxates with extension and external rotation. Radiographic examinations including a faux profile view are important to determine the anatomic abnormalities. The center edge angle of Wieberg,[42] adult acetabular angle of Sharp, and the acetabular depth are employed to describe the amount of uncoverage existing superolaterally. A patient is a candidate for an osteotomy if they have a reasonable range of motion with mild degenerative changes graded radiographically. Usually, the deformity is located on the acetabular side, thus the correction is usually performed on this side. However, femoral osteotomies may be necessary where there are concomitant abnormalities. Complications can be significant and include neurovascular injury, intra-articular damage, delayed union, and heterotopic ossification. Thus, osteotomies for developmental dysplasia should be performed only in patients who are symptomatic.

Reconstructive Pelvic Osteotomies

The reconstructive pelvic osteotomies in the young adult patient include the spherical osteotomy, triple osteotomy, and the Bernese peri-acetabular osteotomy. Spherical osteotomies have been described by numerous authors.[43,44] They provide good lateral coverage, but may lack the ability to gain anterior coverage as well as medialize the hip. Due to close proximity to the articular surface, these osteotomies are difficult to reproduce, and oftentimes, the osteotomy may encroach into the articular surface. Furthermore, the vascular supply to the acetabular fragment is dependent on the vascular supply of the hip capsule due to the nature of the osteotomy. In experienced hands, Ninomiya and Tagawa[45] initially reported on 41 patients of an average age of 24 years who had an average 4-year follow-up after a spherical acetabular osteotomy. Their reported results were 35 patients with no pain and 6 patients with occasional mild pain. Prior to surgery, all patients had some form of limp requiring a cane or crutches. Postoperatively, 23 patients had no limp, 15 had mild limp, and 3 had moderate limp. The authors noted that poor results were obtained with inadvertent penetration through the articular cartilage. Contraindications include an open tri-radiate cartilage and poor abductor function that may compromise postoperative recovery.

Schramm and associates[45] evaluated the Wagner spherical osteotomy in 22 patients with a minimum of 20 years of follow-up. At 20 years, only three patients went on to progress to THA. At final follow-up of an average of 23.9 years, seven patients required THA, and two patients had developed severe OA. The 13 patients who did not have arthrosis demonstrated a mean Harris Hip Score of 91. Clinical success was related to the amount of joint congruency that was obtained on the postoperative radiograph. The authors also reported that the severity of the dysplasia was a prognostic indicator of worse outcomes as the osteotomy did not perform a sufficient correction. Again, because of the technical challenges involved in performing a spherical osteotomy, this procedure is performed in a limited number of centers.

The triple or Steele osteotomy is performed through three separate incisions, and the osteotomies of the pubis, ischium, and ilium are performed some distance from the acetabulum. The downside is that to achieve any degree of correction, it is necessary to create some pelvic deformity. Tonnis et al.[46] described a juxta-articular triple osteotomy that allowed more correction with less pelvic obliquity; however, the defect that is created between the ischium and the acetabulum may be great, and stabilization techniques between the two fragments may be difficult. As a result of these problems, triple osteotomies are currently rarely performed.

The Bernese periacetabular osteotomy developed by Ganz in the early 1980s has become the preferred technique of most surgeons today. The procedure is performed through one incision with extra-articular cuts that are reproducible and allow for lateralization and anterior rotation of the acetabular fragment as well as medialization of the hip joint without creating pelvic obliquity. Furthermore, the posterior column is left intact, which preserves the inferior gluteal artery and subsequently the vascularity of the articular fragment. The surgical technique includes performing a hip joint arthrotomy to visualize the labrum. Fixation is usually adequate with screws alone, and due to the stability of the entire construct, immobilization with a brace or cast is usually not necessary (Fig. 21A–2A, B).

Siebenrock and associates[47] reported on Ganz's experience on 71 hips with an average 11.3 year follow-up. At last follow-up, 82% had preservation of the hip joint, with 52 demonstrating good or excellent results and 6 with fair results using the Merle d'Aubigne clinical rating system. Prognostic indicators of poorer outcome included older age at time of operation, radiographic grade of arthritis, and presence of labral lesion. In review of their technique, the authors emphasize the importance of avoiding overcorrection of the pelvis as this may cause anterior femoroacetabular impingement.

Trousdale et al.[48] described 42 patients followed for an average of 4 years after osteotomy. Thirty-two out of thirty-three patients with stage I or II arthritis had good to excellent results, while only eight out of nine patients with moderate to severe arthritic findings had Harris Hip Scores less than 70 or poor results. Six of these patients went on to THA. Clohisy and colleagues[49] reported on 16 patients that underwent a Bernese periacetabular osteotomy for treatment of hip dysplasia. In the group, the average Harris Hip Score increased from 73.4 to 91.3 at an average of 4.2 years follow-up. Fourteen of the sixteen patients were satisfied with the results. There were two complications: loss of fixation requiring reoperation and overcorrection leading to ischial nonunion.

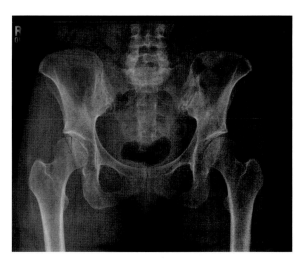

Figure 21A–2A Preoperative radiograph demonstrating hip dysplasia.

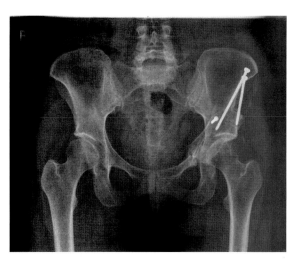

Figure 21A–2B Postoperative radiograph of Bernese periacetabular osteotomy.

Salvage Pelvic Osteotomies

"Salvage" osteotomies such as the Chiari and the shelf osteotomy are performed in patients with severe dysplasia in whom joint congruency cannot be obtained with a reconstructive osteotomy. The Chiari osteotomy medializes the hip center producing a biomechanical advantage and provides better coverage of the femoral head. Windhager and associates[50] reported on their series of 236 patients undergoing a Chiari osteotomy. Their results demonstrate that 215 patients did not need further surgery at a mean of 24.8 years. In this group, 51% had good results, 30% had fair results, and 18% had poor results. Other groups have documented somewhere between 60% and 75% clinical success at the latest follow-up.[51-53] In summary, the authors concluded that 1) increased arthritis led to poorer results, 2) older patients did worse than younger ones, and 3) the results deteriorate with time.[54]

The Shelf procedure is described as corticocancellous augmentation to the anterolateral dome of the acetabulum in order to increase femoral head coverage. It is postulated that the bone augmentation undergoes metaplasia becoming a fibrocartilaginous structure. Migaud et al.[55] reported on 56 shelf arthroplasties with an average 17 years follow-up. Survival at 20 years was 37%. When there was no preop evidence of arthrosis, the survivorship increased to 83% at 20 years. Furthermore, the patients that required conversion to THA had sufficient bone stock for conventional placement of the acetabular socket.

In summary, the most predictable indicator of outcome after osteotomy is the amount of arthritis present at the time of osteotomy. Therefore, it is important to identify the appropriate patients with dysplasia of the hip early. Patients who do not demonstrate significant radiographic evidence of arthrosis are ideal candidates. Results also correlate with achieving adequate correction of the deformity. Careful preoperative evaluation and surgical planning as well as skilled technical execution contribute to the likelihood of a successful osteotomy.

Femoral Osteotomy

Proximal femoral osteotomies can be performed in conjunction with an acetabular osteotomy or in isolation when the primary site of deformity is in the femur. Conditions that must be met to perform a femoral osteotomy includes 1) ability to perform a satisfactory correction of the deformity; 2) ability to maintain a satisfactory range of motion after the correction; and 3) joint congruency after correction. Furthermore, the surgeon must keep in mind that these patients may progress to THA and should try to avoid fragment translation, as this may require a second osteotomy at the time of arthroplasty.

The most common deformities of proximal femur/femoral neck are valgus deformity, spherical femoral head, and slight acetabular dysplasia. Historically, the osteotomy is usually performed through the intertrochanteric region in order to minimize the nonunion rate. The most frequently used hardware is a blade plate which allows for rigid fixation and facilitates rotation and angulation. In addition to varus, the usual osteotomy is placed in slight extension in order to gain increased anterior femoral head coverage. Flexion osteotomies are generally performed to rotate out small anterior lesions secondary to osteonecrosis. Valgus intertrochanteric osteotomies are indicated with flattened femoral heads with a large medial femoral head osteophyte. A valgus osteotomy can decrease the joint reactive forces through medialization of the center of hip rotation, increased leg length, and improved abductor function.[56] Patients should be warned about the leg length discrepancy that may occur.

The results of proximal femoral osteotomies have been varied. Varus osteotomies have produced better results than valgus osteotomies as these patients usually have mild dysplasia with minimal accompanied arthritis as described earlier. Iwase et al.[57] reported on long-term results of both valgus and varus intertrochanteric osteotomies. In the varus group, survivorship from clinical failure was 89%, 87%, and 82% at 10, 15, and 20 years, respectively, while in the valgus group, the numbers were strikingly worse at 66%, 38%, and 19% at the same time points. In a meta-analysis of all current data regarding valgus and varus proximal femoral osteotomies, at 10 to 15 years, about 25% of varus osteotomies require hip arthroplasty, while nearly 50% of valgus osteotomies require arthroplasty.[58,59] Today, proximal femoral osteotomies are performed less commonly, as these cases with acetabular dysplasia are usually addressed with an acetabular osteotomy.

HIP JOINT ARTHROPLASTY

History

THA remains the standard of care in the treatment of end stage arthrosis. Hip joint arthroplasty has been in a constant state of evolution in terms of implant design, biomaterials, and surgical technique for the past 40 years or more. Initial attempts to treat arthritic conditions interposed tissues (interpositional arthroplasty) between the worn articular surfaces.[60] In the 1920s, Smith-Peterson introduced the concept of "mould arthroplasty."[61] This concept was spurred by an observation that he made when a piece of glass was embedded in the subcutaneous tissue of a patient. He noticed that "it was lined by a glistening synovial sac, containing a few drops of clear yellow fluid" and compared this to the normal synovial lining of the hip joint. The cup arthroplasty era began in 1923 when he implanted his first glass mold. His goal was to induce formation of a cartilaginous material, then to remove the glass mold. The initial attempts had problems with breakage of the glass mold which led to the experimentation and the development of Vitallium, a metal alloy.

The first total hip replacement is attributed to Phillip Wales.[49] He implanted a stainless steel cup to the femoral neck that was fixed with a bolt and a similar sized stainless steel socket into the acetabulum fixed to the pelvis with screws. These large metal-to-metal articulations became dominant in use for many years. Sir John Charnley pioneered the modern era of THA with his work in bone cement for fixation, introduction of polyethylene as a bearing material, use of aseptic techniques, and his diligence in recording patient follow-up.[62–65]

Hemiresurfacing and Total Hip Resurfacing

Hip resurfacing is a renewal of an old concept that began with the cup arthroplasty as described by Smith-Peterson and subsequent bone preserving arthroplasties. Hip resurfacing is theoretically an attractive option as a time buying procedure for young patients with disabling OA but no other factor that would limit physical activity.

Hemiresurfacing is a cemented hemispherical femoral head implant that is an option in patients without evidence of acetabular arthrosis. Clinical results from hemiresurfacing have not been reliable clinically as only approximately two thirds of patients experience pain relief.[66,67] This is most likely related to implant articulating on intact acetabular cartilage.

Older generation total resurfacing was a failure due to volumetric polyethylene wear, but modern metal-on-metal articulations have demonstrated reduced wear and renewed interest in this implant. Mesko et al.[68] described their experience with the older generation total articular replacement that included a femoral head resurfacing and a cemented all polyethylene acetabular component. From a total of 174 hips, 23 underwent revision surgery for component failure at an average of 5.1 years. Survivorship was 84.5% at 9 years. The reason for failure was high volumetric wear due to the large size of the femoral head. In addition, the large size of the femoral head led to a thin polyethylene as well as increased reaming of the acetabular bone stock in order to gain adequate fixation.

More recently, Amstutz et al.[69] reported on 400 metal-on-metal total hip resurfacings performed on patients of an average age of 48 (Fig. 21A–3). The implant consisted of a porous-coated hemispherical acetabular component and a cemented femoral component that resurfaced the head. This system had the benefits of a low wear articulation, large diameter femoral head to reduce the chance for

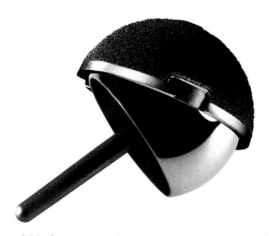

Figure 21A–3 Conserve Plus metal-on-metal total resurfacing prosthesis.

dislocation, and preservation of bone stock. Four-year survivorship has been 94%. No revisions have been performed due to the acetabular component; however, ten hips were revised to THA secondary to femoral component loosening or femoral neck fracture. The clinical results have been promising with an average Harris Hip Score of 93.5. Strict contraindications of this procedure include metaphyseal cysts (seen in osteonecrosis) and osteoporosis. The early results seem promising with reliable clinical results; however, longer follow-up is necessary to determine the durability of the prosthesis. In addition, patient selection has to be carefully defined to limit these early failures as total resurfacing is not as versatile as total hip replacement.

Total Hip Arthroplasty

Epidemiology

The prevalence of THA has steadily increased between 1990 and 2002 according to the National Hospital Discharge Survey (NHDS).[70] Over this time period, the rate of total hip replacement has increased nearly 50% per 100,000 patients. In contrast, total knee replacement has tripled. When comparing total hip revision to total knee revision surgery, the revision rate for hips (17.5%) was twice that of knees (8.2%).

In the health care environment today, health care costs and the ratio of cost and benefit are critically analyzed for every given procedure. Total hip replacement is one of the most beneficial surgical procedures that we currently perform.[71,72] Barber and Healy[73] reported that the actual cost of THA rose approximately 46.5% between 1981 and 1990. However, once adjusted for inflation, the actual increase was only 2%. When the components of the cost were examined, the cost of implants during this same time period had increased 212%, and the increase was 117% when adjusted for inflation. In 1981, the cost of the implant was 11% of the cost, while in 1990, the cost had become 24%. In order to maintain cost, surgical time has become more efficient, hospital stays have been shortened, and ancillary services have been employed more judiciously. Bozic et al.[74] examined the actual costs of primary THA at their institution. The mean total costs were $24,170, with a mean hospital stay of 5.6 days. Worse preoperative medical health was a predictive factor of higher resource utilization.

Surgeon as well as hospital efficiency has also been examined, as the majority of total hip replacements are done by surgeons who perform fewer than 15 per year. A statewide registry for the state of Washington was examined to define a relationship between surgical volume and postoperative complications.[75] The study identified that surgeons and hospitals below the fortieth percentile for surgical volume had a patient profile with the worst health profile. However, when comorbid conditions were stratified, there was a statistically significant increase in complications in surgeons who performed less than two total hip arthroplasties per year. Low volume surgeons tended to have higher mortality rates, more infections, higher infection rates, and more serious complications. The authors suggested that perhaps regional high volume centers should be considered. Lavernia and Guzman[76] identified similar findings with low volume providers having a higher mortality rate as well as higher average charges and increased hospital stay.

Katz and colleagues[77] examined patients 3 years after THA from both high and low volume surgical centers. Functionally speaking, there was no statistical difference of functional level when preoperative medical health was stratified. However, there was a significantly higher rate of patient satisfaction when their surgery was performed at a high volume center. The authors (rheumatologists) suggested that they may refer their patients to high volume centers for the procedure.

These studies suggest that surgeon experience and institution volume tend to lead to beneficial outcomes. However, it is easy to misinterpret the data. Databases that are used by these authors are based on codes for THA, and coding may differ from one institution to another. Furthermore, complications once a patient is discharged are difficult to track. In the high volume surgical center with shorter hospital stay, the rate of deep venous thrombosis and pulmonary embolus may be diminished during the hospital stay, however, the overall rate regardless of whether the patient is an outpatient or inpatient may not differ.

Outcome measures have increased in importance as evidence-based medicine has come to the forefront.[78] The Harris Hip Score has become the widely used disease-specific tool to assess arthritic conditions of the hip as well as outcomes in THA.[79] The Harris Hip Score has components that quantify pain, function, and physical examination findings. Functional data include walking tolerance, need for supports, ability to climb stairs as well as sitting tolerance, ability to use public transportation, and ability to put on shoes and socks. Physical exam parameters include the existence of limp and range of motion. A perfect score is 100. Traditionally, these scores were tabulated by the surgeon, leading to a bias in the score. Most clinical studies now have a combination of physician assessments and patient self-administered questionnaires to provide a balanced assessment of outcome.

Surgical Management

The main indication for hip arthroplasty is pain that cannot be controlled by conservative means (Fig. 21A–4A, B). Conservative therapy usually entails activity modification, weight loss, nonsteroidal anti-inflammatory medication as tolerated, and in certain circumstances corticosteroid injections into the hip joint. Surgical intervention is indicated when there is a significant level of pain that usually limits normal functional activities of daily living such as the ability to walk, stand, maneuver stairs, climb in and out of a car, and put on shoes and socks. The pain in combination with restricted lifestyle limits the quality of life and health status of this subset of patients.

The Socket

Cemented Fixation

In North America, the standard has become cementless socket fixation for primary THA. However, cemented fixation is still prevalent in parts of the world. The two designs of cemented fixation include an all-polyethylene socket and a metal-backed design. The initial Charnley design was a cemented THA with a stainless steel flat-backed stem with a polished surface and a nonmodular 22.25 mm head mated to an ultra-high molecular weight all-polyethylene cup that was cemented.

Hozack and colleagues[80] examined 1041 Charnley THA and predicted a 96% survival at 10 years with acetabular revision as the endpoint. When the follow-up was extended to 30 years in younger, more active patients, Wroblewski et al.[81] discovered that the revision rate of the cemented socket for aseptic loosening was 11.7%. Callaghan et al.[82] reported a Kaplan-Meier survivorship of 85% at 30 years.

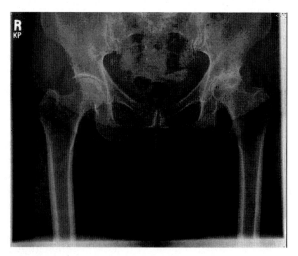

Figure 21A–4A Preoperative radiograph of hip arthritis.

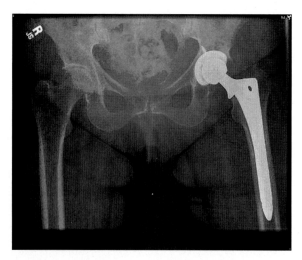

Figure 21A–4B Postoperative radiograph of extensively porous-coated total hip arthroplasty.

Cemented all-polyethylene sockets have demonstrated a linear increase in clinical failure over time with failure rates reaching 45% at 20 years. The process of loosening cemented PE sockets has been described as a progressive radiolucency around the bone-cement interface that becomes circumferential and leads to aseptic loosening. Schmalzried et al.[83] performed retrieval studies of cemented sockets that failed at the cement-bone interface. The foreign body response leads to erosion of the bone at the cement-bone interface. This erosion progresses from the periphery circumferentially until the socket is completely destabilized from the pelvis and becomes loose. Modern cement techniques may not improve the incidence of radiographic failure.[84]

With the poor long-term results of cemented polyethylene sockets, the etiology of failure was proposed to be mechanical—related to alterations in stress distribution in the acetabulum. Metal-backed components were proposed to provide a more uniform stress distribution which would reduce the peak magnitude of stresses and theoretically reduce the fatigue failure and subsequent aseptic loosening. This was proven in the laboratory setting.[85] Chen et al.[86] described their results of cemented metal-backed acetabular components in 86 hips at an average of 10-year follow-up. In their study, 40% of the patients had radiographic evidence of loosening or revision surgery. Other groups have had similar poor results with cemented metal-backed components with failure rates as high as 86% at 15-year follow-up.[87] The proposed mechanism of failure was the trend toward larger femoral heads that created volumetric wear. In addition, the metal backing reduced the thickness of the polyethylene which increased contact stresses and wear. Furthermore, the rigid metal backing actually may increase the stresses placed on the polyethylene.

Ritter et al.[88] compared cemented metal-backed components with cemented all-polyethylene sockets in two groups of patients. When these two cohorts were examined for wear rate, radiographic loosening, and revision rate, all three were higher in the metal-backed components. With these poor results, many surgeons who wish to cement sockets have returned to the all-polyethylene sockets. The theoretical advantages of the metal-backed cemented components were never realized.

Cementless Fixation

Cementless fixation was initially proposed in order to eliminate cement from the equation. The loosening that was encountered with cemented implants was attributed to a biologic reaction to the bone cement and commonly referred to as "cement disease." Further work demonstrated that the bone resorption or osteolysis was associated with wear debris, whether it be titanium, cobalt-chrome, or polyethylene. Polyethylene debris has been considered the main particle associated with this inflammatory response to propagate bone resorption.[89-93]

The goals of cementless fixation on both the acetabular and femoral sides are to provide stable, reliable fixation of the implant into the bony surfaces (osseointegration)[94]

and achieve biologic fixation. Different fixation surfaces have been employed, namely titanium fiber mesh, cobalt-chrome beads, titanium beads, and titanium plasma-sprayed surfaces. Furthermore, osteoconductive materials have been employed such as hydroxyapatite and calcium phosphate to induce bone ingrowth and ongrowth. Each porous coating surface must be independently evaluated as survivorship has varied in intermediate to long-term follow-up.[95-98]

Osseointegration, coined by Branemark, is a term employed of an implant that is able to provide functional support under physiologic loads of activities of daily living. The implant must be able to transmit physiologic loads of daily living without causing pain. In order to accomplish this goal, biomechanically there must be a functional connection between the implant and the bone that is able to transmit these loads as a unit. Joint reactive forces about the hip are commonly three to four times the body weight of the person and can rise to six to seven times the body weight with activities such as running and jumping. Large amounts of stress are placed at this interface. On histologic analysis, osseous integration implies direct contact between the bone and the implant. There is no intervening gap, nor intervening fibrous tissue bridging this gap.

Osseointegration of both the socket and the femur with cementless fixation is accomplished by numerous steps. First, the bone must be machined so that an adequate area of host bone is in direct contact with the implant surface. Secondly, the bone surface must be viable. Necrotic bone will not produce bone ingrowth, and osseointegration will not occur. Finally, there must be stable fixation between the implant and bone surfaces. Jasty et al.[99] demonstrated that micromotion between the implant and bone surfaces of more than 40 µm tends to induce fibrous ingrowth as opposed to bony ingrowth. Therefore, it is important to obtain stable fixation in the operating room to achieve osseointegration.

Cementless socket fixation is achieved by a variety of surgical techniques. Most commonly, the acetabulum is reamed into a hemisphere of viable cancellous bone to fit a hemispherical metal shell. The acetabular bed is prepared by slightly underreaming the diameter of the acetabulum to the actual size of the acetabular component. This can provide the required initial stability, or supplemental fixation can be provided with screws, spikes, or fins.

As a result of the relatively poor results of cemented sockets that were attributed to "cement disease," there has been a push toward cementless socket fixation. Maloney and colleagues[95] reported on a multicenter study of 1081 primary total hip replacements that employed the Harris-Galante I cementless acetabular component with screw fixation. Patients had a minimum of 5-year follow-up with a mean of 81 months. Pelvic osteolysis was seen in 2.3% of the patients. Cup migration occurred in four patients. Revision surgery was performed in 18 patients for polyethylene wear and pelvic osteolysis. All 18 had well ingrown sockets during the time of surgery. The overall mechanical failure rate that includes socket revisions, liner exchanges, and radiographically loose sockets was 2.4%. The mean linear wear rate of the polyethylene was 0.11 mm per year with a trend toward increased wear rates related to younger age.

Pelvic osteolysis was also associated with younger age, as 22% of the patients who were younger than 50 at the time of the index procedure developed pelvic osteolysis. For the most part, these lesions were located at the periphery and were relatively small lesions that did not compromise fixation. In contrast, the prevalence of osteolysis in patients who were older than 50 was 7.8% at 10 years. The association of wear and osteolysis can be attributed to the increased activity level of younger patients.

Della Valle and colleagues[100] reviewed a single surgeon experience of 335 primary total hip replacements performed with second-generation cementless modular sockets. Improvements included better locking mechanisms of the modular liner, a smooth undersurface on the shell, increased conformity between the metal socket and polyethylene, and clustered screw holes. At 4- to 7-year follow-up, 2.4% required reoperation for aseptic loosening (6) or infection (2). Of the 262 hips with radiographic follow-up, 259 (99%) had well-fixed, bone-ingrowth sockets in place. Osteolysis was present in 5% of the hips at latest follow-up.

The follow-up data with cementless sockets have become sufficient to objectively compare it with cemented fixation. With over 20 years of experience, near hemispherical sockets with nearly continuous materials for porous ingrowth supplemented with screws have provided a successful design. Clohisy and Harris[101] performed a matched pair analysis of 45 patients with either cemented or cementless socket fixation in primary total hip replacements. They demonstrated that at 9- to 12-year follow-up, 31% of the cemented sockets were found to be radiographically loose, while none were loose in the cementless sockets. Pelvic osteolysis was also more prevalent in the cemented group at 20% versus 7% in the cementless group. Clinically speaking, both groups had good results.

Rorabeck et al.[102] performed a prospective randomized trial comparing cemented to cementless socket fixation in 147 patients. None of the acetabular sockets had been revised in either group. In the cemented group, 3% were definitely loose, and 24% were probably loose. Only one cementless socket was radiographically loose. However, pelvic osteolysis was more prevalent in the cementless group at 14% versus 8% in the cemented group.

Cementless socket designs must be evaluated individually, as the fixation surfaces differ. Engh and colleagues[103] described their experience with the anatomic medullary locking (AML) socket with a minimum 10-year follow-up. This is a cobalt-chrome socket with a beaded surface. There is supplemental fixation with three spikes instead of screws. Survivorship at 10 years after the index operation was 92%. Seven of 174 sockets (4%) were loose. Revision surgery was most commonly associated with polyethylene wear and pelvic osteolysis.

Moskal and colleagues[104] reported on the porous-coated anatomic (PCA) socket with a minimum of 12-year follow-up. Thirteen percent of the acetabular components were deemed failures, while osteolysis behind the socket was visualized 7.5% of the time. Failure was attributed to a considerable amount of deformation of the polyethylene insert that accounted for backside wear. In addition, thin polyethylene liners that were gamma-sterilized in air in

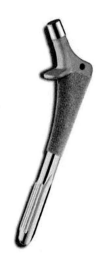

Figure 21A–5A Proximally coated femoral component.

conjunction with large femoral heads (32 mm) accounted for increased wear and osteolysis.

The Femur

Fixation on the femoral side is broadly categorized into cement and cementless fixation. Similar to the acetabulum, with cementless fixation there are multiple different types of fixation surfaces. Implant designs also vary considerably in cementless stems (Fig. 21A–5A, B, C). One of the more important variables remains the extent of porous coating. Implants are generally classified as proximally coated or extensively porous coated stems. Stem shape and geometry can also differ. There are curved stems that are designed to approximate the anatomic bow of the femur. Also, there are straight stems that have a cylindrical distal

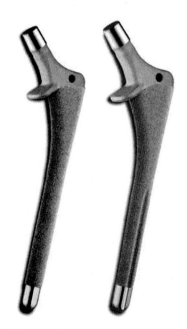

Figure 21A–5B Extensively porous coated femoral component.

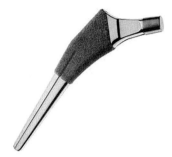

Figure 21A–5C Tapered femoral component.

component. Implant choices are surgeon and patient specific with each stem requiring a different surgical technique of bone preparation and implant insertion.

Cemented Femoral Fixation

The initial technique of femoral fixation as described by Charnley employed cemented fixation. Subsequent published results with cemented fixation have had varying results. In order to interpret these results, one must evaluate the evolution of cementing techniques. First-generation cement technique refers to finger packing doughy cement into an unplugged femoral canal. This was prevalent in the 1970s and early 1980s. In addition, poor machining skills led to sharp corners of the implant which resulted in stress risers at the cement-implant interface. Furthermore, implant materials were prone to breakage because they were not made of superalloys.

Second-generation cementing introduced the idea of pressurized insertion of cement down the femoral canal. The medullary canal was plugged, followed by pressurized lavage of the canal. The cement was inserted in retrograde fashion with a cement gun. By using the cement gun, the cement was introduced evenly through the canal which would reduce the incidence of deficient cement mantles. The cement plug allows for better pressurization of the cement as the implant is inserted so that there is better cement interdigitation into the bone. This increases the interfascial shear strength. Finally, pressurized lavage removes marrow and fat elements from the canal and allows for deeper intrusion of the bone cement into the remaining medullary bone of the proximal femur which increases the shear strengths. This also limits systemic embolization of marrow contents during cement pressurization and implant insertion. Furthermore, implant designs and materials were improved. Implants were made of superalloys, and sharp corners were eliminated from the prosthesis.

Third-generation cement technique improved the porosity of the cement, improved pressurization of the cement, and made changes in implant surfacing. The cement was vacuum mixed in order to diminish large voids in the cement. The surface of the implants was modified to provide a macrotexturing to improve bond strength between the implant and the cement. Precoating the component also improves the bond strength.

A bonded interface between the cement and the implant has been shown to decrease the stresses within the cement mantle.[105-108] A good cement-implant interface should improve implant survivorship.[109,110] However, clinical data have not been consistent with these laboratory findings. Polymethylmethacrylate has been applied to stems to enhance the bond between the cement and implant. This factory process is referred to as precoating. To precoat a femoral stem, the finish of the stem must be relatively rough. Surface roughness of implants is measured in microinches. In general, three types of finishes are currently used in cemented femoral components: polished surface, matte finish, and grit blasted surface. Typically, polished surfaces have a surface roughness of less than 10 microinches; a matte finish surface, approximately 20 to 30 microinches; and a grit blasted surface, approximately 70 to 100 microinches. Also, there are rougher macrotextured implants that have a surface roughness greater than 300 microinches. When reviewing the results of cemented femoral components, the surface finish may play a role in the long-term survivorship. The results must be evaluated individually based on the shape and surface texture of the implant.

When reviewing the literature, rough stems have not fared well clinically. Once a rough stem debonds from the cement mantle evidenced by radiolucencies at the cement-implant interface, clinical failure follows rapidly, through the production of particles.[111-113] The high particle load tends to destabilize the implant via femoral osteolysis. This cycle of increased particle production continues until the implant is completely debonded. Although smooth femoral components are more likely to have a higher prevalence of debonding from the cement mantle noted radiographically, a debonded smooth femoral stem is more likely to be better tolerated clinically.[114] Though there is no consensus on the optimal surface finish, recent trends are toward smoother surfaces.

Though it is difficult to compare studies with different implant designs, it is possible to compare defined endpoints such as failure. Failure can be subdivided into clinical failure, radiographic failure, and revision surgery. Clinical failure represents the pain and disability that the patient undergoes, while radiographic failure is demonstrated by implant loosening. Harris and McGann[115] reviewed 104 patients with a minimum 5-year follow-up who underwent cemented THA with second-generation cement techniques. The average age of the patients was 58. The overall failure rate was 2% on the femoral side. This represents a sevenfold increase in overall survivorship as compared to historical data with first-generation techniques.[116] When this patient population was observed at a minimum 14 year follow-up, 102 of the patients were still alive for examination.[87] Two percent of the patients had been revised, and an additional seven components were loose radiographically for a combined mechanical failure rate of 9%. When a subset of younger patients (<50 years) was examined, only 1 out of the 51 patients required revision surgery. Roberts and colleagues[117] found a more significant difference in first- versus second-generation cementing techniques. When two matched-pair groups were compared, patients with second-generation techniques had a mechanical failure rate of 0% versus 21% with first-generation techniques. The authors concluded the obvious effect of cement technique on implant survivorship.

With the importance of cement techniques, attempts have been made to qualitatively grade cement mantles with the use of radiographs. Barrack et al.[118] formulated an outline on grading cement mantles. A grade A cement mantle is one in which there is a complete filling of the proximal portion of the medullary canal with no distinction between the cortical bone and bone cement in the diaphysis. A grade B cement mantle has a complete distribution of cement, but the cortical bone and cement can be distinguished in some areas. A grade C cement mantle is subdivided into C1 and C2. A C1 grade is one in which there is an extensive radiolucent line of more than 50% of the cement-bone interface or large voids in the cement. A C2 mantle has a mantle thickness of less than 1 mm radiographically, or an obvious cement mantle defect in which the implant is in direct contact with the cortical bone. Finally, a grade D mantle indicates a gross mantle defect, with no cement distal to the tip of the stem. The goal of this classification system is to predict how cement technique will affect survivorship. Several studies have demonstrated that C2 and D mantles have a statistically higher rate of failure.[119,120] This has been confirmed in autopsy studies where there is a correlation between thin cement mantles and cement mantle fracture.[121] These studies emphasize the importance of stem centralization both proximally and distally. The goal with stem centralization is to ensure a continuous cement mantle that is at least 1 mm thick. The ability to reproduce this type of cement mantle would improve survivorship.

Proximally Porous-Coated Femoral Fixation

The first-generation cementless porous-coated femoral implants were either extensively coated or proximally coated. In general, the older generation, proximally coated stems did not provide reliable fixation. In the proximally coated stems, the porous coating was not circumferential, which allowed wear particles to access the endosteal canal of the femoral diaphysis. This resulted in a rather high prevalence of osteolysis.[122,123] A patch porous-coated stem was followed at two time intervals of 44 and 71 months. At 44 months, the prevalence of femoral osteolysis was 22%. This increased to 52% at a mean of 71 months in this same patient population. Two thirds of the lesions diagnosed at the first time point had increased in size at the second time point. Femoral osteolysis tends to slowly increase in size. Similar problems occurred with other patch porous-coated implants. As a result, most proximally coated stems now have circumferential porous coating.

Sinha and associates[124] reviewed 88 hips at an average age of 53.8 years that received a second-generation circumferentially proximally coated stem. At a minimum of 5-year follow-up, all but one stem were found to be biologically stable. Three stems were found to have a stable fibrous fixation. One third had minimal proximal osteolysis, while none demonstrated diaphyseal osteolysis, given the high activity level of these relatively young patients. Other second-generation proximally coated stems have similar successful results at 5- to 10-year follow-up.[125,126]

Extensively Porous-Coated Femoral Fixation

The longest follow-up and largest series of extensively porous-coated stems in North America has been the AML prosthesis. This is a cobalt-chrome beaded stem with extensive porous coating down to the diaphysis. Engh and colleagues[127] have reported their series at a mean follow-up of 13.9 years on 223 consecutive AML femoral prostheses. Three stems were revised secondary to loosening. Radiographically, three additional stems were found to be loose with four stems found to have a stable fibrous ingrowth. Younger patients had statistically significant increased rate of wear and osteolysis. They also had a higher revision rate, most secondary to severe polyethylene wear. When these stems were analyzed in autopsy retrieval studies, approximately 35% of the fixation surface had bone ingrowth.[128,129] In areas of bone ingrowth, about 67% of the pore space was occupied by bone. This degree of osseointegration leads to long-term implant fixation. Although implant fixation has shown good long-term results, proximal stress shielding as well as the higher rates of thigh pain have subjected these stems to some criticism.

Tapered Stems

Widely employed in Europe, tapered stems such as the Zweymuller stem design have become increasingly popular in North America. Over 700,000 Zweymuller stems have been implanted worldwide.[130] First implanted in 1979, the Zweymuller stem achieves stability axially via a dual longitudinal taper and rotationally by contact between the corners of the implant and cortical bone. Secondary stability is maintained by osseointegration. Surgical technique for optimal stability relies on fit but not fill of the femoral canal. Mid-term results of 10 to 13 years of two studies with a combined 345 hips demonstrated that none of the stems were loose.[131,132] Though its design prinicples are different from traditional canal-filling American concepts, these promising results have funneled increased American interest into this stem design.

Pervizi et al.[133] reported on 129 hips that underwent primary THA with the Taperloc stem. The Taperloc has a circumferential proximal plasma spray that is collarless. At a mean follow-up of 11 years, only one stem was revised for extensive femoral osteolysis. The Kaplan-Meier survival estimate was 99.1%. Five patients (3.6%) experienced thigh pain that was worse with activity. The acetabular component did not fare as well with a revision rate for aseptic loosening or wear at 20%. Bourne et al.[134] have reproduced similar results with the Mallory-Head tapered stem. No femoral stem was revised for aseptic loosening, with one each being revised for sepsis and periprosthetic fracture. Poor acetabular design including polyethylene irradiated in an oxygen-rich environment and titanium femoral heads led to poor survivorship of the acetabular component. In conclusion, tapered stems have a long track record of success, with aseptic loosening and wear of the acetabular component and/or liner being the primary cause for revision.

COMPLICATIONS

A complete discussion of all perioperative complications of THA is beyond the scope of this chapter; however, a discussion of several new trends that affect surgical technique will be discussed.

Dislocation

Recurrent dislocation is a common cause of revision surgery in total hip replacement. Scrutiny has been intense on surgical technique, increased femoral stem offset, larger femoral head articulations, and rehabilitation protocols. Surgical techniques have varied based on surgeon comfort and training as well as the success of their results. Traditionally, the majority of dislocations occur posteriorly as the leg is placed in a flexed, internally rotated, and adducted position. Modern studies with emphasis on correct implant position have shown dislocation to be minimal, especially with anterolateral-based approaches. Employing an anterolateral approach, Peak et al.[135] demonstrated in 265 patients that total hip precautions were not necessary in the acute postoperative period. The authors had one acute dislocation in this group, and this occurred during transfer from the operating room bed to the hospital bed. Posterior approaches have traditionally reported higher dislocation rates as violation of the posterior capsule and external rotators have attenuated these structures. Pellicci and colleagues[136] performed a capsular repair that decreased their dislocation rate from 4% to 0% in two groups of 395 patients.

With the popularity of modular acetabular liners, liners with elevated rims have increased in popularity. Cobb and associates[137] described the experience at the Mayo Clinic in 5167 total hip replacements with 2469 hips receiving an elevated rim liner. The dislocation rate was significantly decreased from 3.85% to 2.19%. With the advent of alternative bearings, the amount of wear debris particles has diminished in comparison to the traditional metal on polyethylene bearings from days past. In the past, larger femoral heads permitted increased range of motion before implant impingement; however, due to the higher volumetric contact at the interface, there was more wear debris that subsequently led to aseptic loosening. Alternative bearings and highly cross-linked polyethylene have diminished the wear rates significantly. The traditional Charnley total hip replacement employed a 22.25 mm femoral head. In contrast, with these new bearings, femoral heads up to 44 mm can be employed in the primary setting.

Periprosthetic Bone Resorption

Periprosthetic bone resorption is a mechanical phenomenon that is induced secondary to 1) bone remodeling as a result of stress alterations in the proximal femur after hip implantation, and 2) a biologic reaction to particulate wear debris.[131,138] Osteolysis was initially seen with Charnley cemented hip arthroplasty and was referred to as "cement disease." Analysis of these granulomas as well as the observation of this same phenomenon with cementless implants helped to elucidate this biologic reaction now known as osteolysis.

Osteolysis has emerged as the most common long-term complication after THA.[95,139] Three important pathophysiologic components must be considered: 1) generation of wear debris, 2) access of wear debris to the implant-bone interface, and 3) biologic reaction to wear debris. These wear particles in sufficient quantity can stimulate a biologic cascade that results in osteoclastic activation with bone resorption being the end result (Fig. 21A–6).

There are many potential sources of particulate wear debris. The largest wear generator is the head-liner articulation. With standard polyethylene and cobalt-chrome articulations, the average wear rate has typically ranged from 0.1 to 0.2 mm per year. Modularity has introduced another potential interface that can create wear debris. Cook and associates[140] demonstrated corrosion between the Morse taper connection of the femoral head and neck region. Burnishing has also been demonstrated at junctions of modular implants. Other potential sources of wear particles are the implant–cement interface in debonded components and the implant–bone interface in cementless implants. Laboratory studies have shown that the majority of these wear particles (>90%) are less than 1 μm in size.[89,91]

Schmalzried and associates[83] have suggested that the "effective joint space" is the area in which these wear particles have access to cause osteolysis. This is not only the articulation, but encases the entire periprosthetic region accessible to joint fluid and wear debris. This includes access behind the socket into the pelvis as well as the endosteal canal of the femur in noncircumferential-coated femoral implants. Bobyn and colleagues[141] demonstrated that areas of bone ingrowth act as a barrier to wear debris migration.

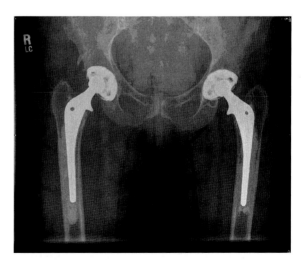

Figure 21A–6 Osteolysis from wear debris.

Histologic evaluation of these osteolytic membranes have demonstrated abundant macrophages and giant cells consistent with foreign body granuloma.[142,143] Cell cultures of these retrieved membranes have demonstrated inflammatory markers such as prostaglandin E_2, collagenase, interleukin-1, and tumor necrosis factor. These laboratory findings are applied to the clinical setting, researchers are evaluating drug therapies such as osteoclast inhibitors that may decrease osteolysis.[144] However, no drug is currently approved for such therapy.

Alternative Bearing Surfaces

Highly Cross-Linked Polyethylene

To decrease the prevalence of osteolysis, wear debris must be reduced. Basic science and clinical research are ongoing to investigate different materials. Hard bearing surfaces including ceramic-on-ceramic (alumina) and metal-on-metal (cobalt-chrome) have recently been approved for use in the United States. In addition, research focused on the oxidation of polyethylene when gamma-irradiated in an oxygen-rich environment has shown that gamma irradiation also forms cross-links in polyethylene that decrease wear rates[145] (Fig. 21A–7A, B, C). D'Lima and associates[146] performed an in vitro wear simulator study evaluating highly cross-linked polyethylene against traditional polyethylene. They determined that highly cross-linked polyethylene was significantly more resistant to wear versus traditional polyethylene. In vitro studies have also demonstrated that cross-linking has decreased wear versus conventional polyethylene even when there are third-body particles such as bone cement.[147] Furthermore, volumetric wear is also decreased even with femoral heads up to 46 mm in diameter.[148]

When employed in the clinical setting, early results have been consistent with the findings in the laboratory. Manning and colleagues[149] examined 138 patients who had highly cross-linked polyethylene (HXLPE) implanted versus 111 age-matched controls who had traditional polyethylene inserts. The steady-state wear as determined by Martell wear analysis was 0.007 mm/year in the HXLPE versus 0.174 mm/year in the traditional group. This was significant. Digas et al.[150] performed bilateral total hip arthroplasties in 32 patients with HXLPE on one side and conventional polyethylene on the contralateral side. Twenty-seven patients had completed a 2-year follow-up.

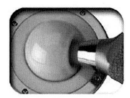

Figure 21A–7B Ceramic-on-ceramic articulation.

Radiostereometric analysis was performed at interval time periods. At 1-year follow-up, head penetration was 0.08 mm in the highly cross-linked group and 0.12 mm in the conventional group. At the second year, the highly cross-linked group remained at 0.08 mm, while the conventional group was 0.21 mm in penetration. This was statistically significant. In a second arm of the study, 49 patients were randomized to receive either cemented highly cross-linked or conventional polyethylene unilaterally. The femoral heads used in all these patients were 28 mm. For the first 6 months, there was no difference in the proximal penetration in either group; however, by 3 years, the proximal penetration of the conventional polyethylene (0.25 mm) had doubled that of the HXLPE (0.13 mm). Early clinical results indicate that the wear rates are significantly diminished with HXLPE.[151,152] Short-term results are promising; however, one must be cautious as early retrieval studies have also demonstrated evidence of scratching, pitting, abrasion, surface cracks, deformation, and delamination.[153]

Cross-linking has also been associated with decreased resistance to fatigue crack propagation. Birman et al.[154] analyzed 120 liners of traditional polyethylene that were retrieved. They found neck-liner impingement to be evident in 32% of the liners. Crack initiation was present in 70% at the region of impingement. By using highly cross-linked liners that are less resistant to crack propagation, impingement may lead to fracture.

Ceramic-on-Ceramic

Alumina ceramic-on-ceramic couplings were first introduced by Boutin in 1970. Ceramic-on-ceramic bearings have the structural properties of 1) hardness, 2) wetability, 3) brittleness, and 4) biocompatibility. The proposed advantages are less wear debris as well as smaller wear particles that may be less biologically active. However, Yoon

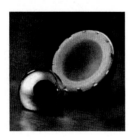

Figure 21A–7A Metal polyethylene articulation.

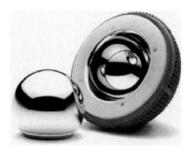

Figure 21A–7C Metal-on-metal articulation.

and colleagues[155] reported that ceramic particles can induce an inflammatory reaction and osteolysis. The brittleness of ceramic has been a concern of catastrophic fracture. Hannouche and colleagues[156] have had 13 ceramic head fractures in 4500 documented total hip replacements. They propose that the load necessary for crack propagation may be far less than the fatigue limit of ceramics. These loads may be encountered with implant impingement or recurrent dislocation. The current ceramics are third generation, and its documented fracture rate is approximately 0.01%. And finally, the clinical wear rates have ranged from 0.02 to 0.03 mm/year as compared to traditional bearings at about 0.1 mm/year.[157,158] Though the wear rates are low, the phenomenon of microseparation during daily activity can produce stripe wear.[159]

There are other concerns with ceramic articulations as well. First, revision surgery of ceramic bearings can be difficult due to the overload of abrasive debris particles that are retained. Secondly, the metal trunnion of the femoral stem is usually damaged by the ceramic head due to modular wear. Replacement of a new head may not be possible due to an incompetent morse taper. And finally, component placement must be optimized as ceramic is unforgiving with neck-liner impingement. The brittleness of ceramic also does not permit the ability to employ modularity to its fullest due to the risk of catastrophic fracture.

D'Antonio et al.[160] have reported an update on ceramic-on-ceramic articulations. Six surgeons have randomized 316 patients to receive a ceramic articulation or a traditional metal-on-polyethylene articulation. At 5 year follow-up, the revision rate for any reason was 2.7% for the ceramic coupling and 7.5% for the control group. The incidence of osteolysis was 1.4% in the ceramic group and 14% in the control group. They have not encountered a ceramic head fracture. Yoo et al.[161] evaluated 100 primary total hips with ceramic bearings at a minimum of 5 year follow-up. The mean Harris Hip Score was 97. There were no revisions performed, and no periprosthetic osteolysis was identified. Only one femoral head and insert fracture occurred in a patient who was involved in a motor vehicle accident.

Metal-on-Metal

Metal-on-metal articulations such as the McKee-Farrar were developed in the 1960s but fell out of favor in the 1970s due to high failure rates. This was attributed to the success of the Charnley metal-polyethylene articulation as well as poor implant design, including head-socket frictional torque, concern of metal carcinogenesis, and increased strain rates in trabecular periprosthetic bone.[162] However, many McKee-Farrar total hip arthroplasties have survived over 25 years. August et al.[163] reported their experience on 808 McKee-Farrars. At an average of 13.9 years follow-up, they had a survivorship of 83.4%. However, due to intolerances, high implant-bone stresses led to cup migration greater than 5 mm in 40% of hips.

In 1988, Bernard Weber developed a new metal-on-metal design with Sulzer (Switzerland) from a forged cobalt chrome alloy with a high carbon content. Preliminary work in hip simulators demonstrated low wear rates in the range of 10 to 20 μm per million cycles.[164] Tighter manufacturing tolerances have provided more consistent metal hardness and optimal head clearance that allows for increased fluid lubrication and clearance of wear debris. Dorr and associates[165] have described their experience in 96 hips with the Metasul hip. At 5- to 11-year follow-up, no areas of focal osteolysis have been noted. Calcar resorption has been noted in 6.3% of the hips. One acetabular component was revised for loosening. Only three patients did not have good or excellent results by self-assessment. Similar results have been reported by Lombardi and associates.[166]

Concerns with the McKee-Farrar THA focused on early loosening, metal carcinogenesis, and metal sensitivity. Improved designs appear to have addressed the issue of premature loosening. Jacobs et al.[167] addressed metal carcinogenesis and reported that high doses of cobalt-chrome particles were toxic to macrophages; however, at sublethal doses metallic debris stimulate an inflammatory response.

Histologic analysis of failed metal-on-metal couplings have determined that there is a preponderance of perivascular infiltration of lymphocytes.[168] The authors noted that there was more extensive surface ulceration in the tissues around metal-on-metal implants. In contrast, metal-on-polyethylene implants demonstrated more commonly giant cells and macrophages. From these findings, metal-on-metal couplings may invoke a different biologic response; however, the end result is unchanged—namely, osteolysis. When applied clinically, Willert et al.[169] identified the predominance of lymphocytes in periprosthetic tissues in 19 failed metal-on-metal total hip replacements. The acetabular or femoral components were revised if loose. In 14 patients, the bearing surfaces were switched to conventional metal and polyethylene or ceramic-on-ceramic. In five patients, a new metal-on-metal bearing was placed. These five patients continued to have groin pain postoperatively. Two patients underwent a second revision to conventional bearings, and their clinical symptoms resolved. The authors theorize that the immunologic lymphocytic response may lead to a different pathway toward aseptic loosening as well as possibly a clinically relevant metal hypersensitivity reaction.

Remote dissemination of metal particles is a concern with metal-on-metal articulations. MacDonald and colleagues[170] have performed a randomized study comparing metal levels in urine and erythrocytes between traditional couplings and metal-on-metal couplings at 2 years follow-up. Patients with metal-on-metal articulations were found to demonstrate increased urine levels of cobalt as well as chrome as compared with patients with traditional metal on polyethylene. Ladon et al.[171] performed a prospective study on patients with metal couplings. Cytogenetic data reflected significantly greater aneuploidy and translocations in peripheral blood lymphocytes. Clinically relevant changes have not been noted at this time.

Gillespie and associates[172] reported that there was an increased risk for lymphatic and hematopoietic tumors in patients with total hip replacements. However, one fourth of these tumors were identified in the first year after surgery—much too short a latency period for the replacement to be a causative factor. Mathieson and colleagues[173] were not able to establish an association between cancer and total hip replacement in the first 10 years after surgery. At this point, there is no clear-cut consensus regarding the carcinogenesis of metal products either locally or remote.

SUMMARY

Total hip replacement has been dissected in every possible manner, from surgical technique and implant choices to cost efficiency. The risks of perioperative and short-term complications have been minimized; however, long-term fixation continues to be a problem. Implant choices have evolved to improve long-term fixation, and alternative bearings seem to provide promising short-term data to battle the most common long-term reason for revision—aseptic loosening from wear debris. Further work to decrease wear should improve an already statistically successful operation.

REFERENCES

1. Reijman M, Hazes JM, Pols HA, et al. Acetabular dysplasia predicts incident osteoarthritis of the hip: the Rotterdam study. Arthritis Rheum 52:787–793, 2005.
2. Kelly BT, Williams RJ, Philippon MJ. Hip arthroscopy: Current indications, treatment options, and management issues. AJSM, 31:1020–1037, 2003.
3. McCarthy JC, Busconi B. The role of hip arthroscopy in the diagnosis and treatment of hip disease. Orthopedics 18:753–756, 1995.
4. Edwards DJ, Lomas D, Villar RN. Diagnosis of the painful hip by magnetic resonance imaging and arthroscopy. JBJS 77B:374–376, 1995.
5. Czerny C, Kramer J, Neuhold A, et al. Magnetic resonance imaging and magetic resonance arthrography of the acetabular labrum: Comparison with surgical findings [in German]. Rofo Fortschr Rontgenstr Neuen Bildgeb Verfahr 173:702–707, 2001.
6. Keeney JA, Peelle, Jackson, J, et al. Magnetic resonance arthrography versus arthroscopy in the evaluation of articular hip pathology. Clin Orthop 429:163–169, 2004.
7. Philippon MJ. Debridement of acetabular labral tears with associated thermal capsulorrhaphy. Oper Tech Sports Med 10:215–218, 2002.
8. Dobbs MB, Gordon JE, Luhmann SJ, et al. Surgical correction of the snapping iliopsoas tendon in adolescents. JBJS 84A:420–424, 2002.
9. McCarthy JC, Noble PC, Schuck MR, et al. The role of labral lesions to development of early degenerative hip disease. Clinical Orthop Relat Res 393:25–37, 2001.
10. Ganz R, Parvizi J, Beck M, et al. Femoroacetabular impingement. A cause for osteoarthritis of the hip. Clin Orthop 417:112–120, 2003.
11. Ito KI, Leunig M, Ganz R. Histopathologic features of the acetabular labrum in femoroacetabular impingement. Clin Orthop 429:262–271, 2004.
12. Ito K, Minka MA II, Leunig M, et al. Femoroacetabular impingement and the cam-effect: A MRI-based quantitative study of the femoral head-neck offset. JBJS 83B:171–176, 2001.
13. Lavigne M, Parvizi J, Beck M, et al. Anterior femoroacetabular impingement. Part I. Techniques of joint preserving surgery. Clin Orthop 418:61–66, 2004.
14. Beck M, Leunig M, Parvizi J, et al. Anterior femoroacetabular impingement. Part II. Midterm results of surgical treatment. Clin Orthop 418:67–73, 2004.
15. Murphy S, Tannast M, Kim Y, et al. Debridement of the adult hip for femoroacetabular impingement. Clin Orthop 429:178–181, 2004.
16. Clohisy JC, McClure JT. Treatment of anterior femoroacetabular impingement with combined hip arthroscopy and limited anterior decompression. Iowa Orthop J 25:164–171, 2005.
17. Reynolds D, Lucas J, Klaue K. Retroversion of the acetabulum. A cause of hip pain. JBJS 81B:281–288, 1999.
18. Siebenrock KA, Schoeniger R, Ganz R. Anterior femoro-acetabular impingement due to acetabular retroversion. JBJS 85A:278–286, 2003.
19. Dorr LD, Luckett M, Conaty JP. Total hip arthroplasties in patients younger than 45 years: A nine to ten year follow-up study. Clin Orthop 260:215–219, 1990.
20. Ortiguera CJ, Pulliam IT, Cabanela ME. Total hip arthroplasty for osteonecrosis: Matched-pair analysis of 188 hips with long-term follow-up. J Arthroplasty 14:21–28, 1999.
21. Sochart DH, Porter ML. Long term results of cemented Charnley low friction arthroplasty in patients aged less than 30 years. J Arthroplasty 13:123–131, 1998.
22. Torchia ME, Klassen RA, Bianco AJ. Total hip arthroplasty with cement in patients less than twenty years old: Long-term results. JBJS 78A:995–1003, 1996.
23. Sponseller PD, McBeath AA, Perpich M. Hip arthrodesis in young patients. A long term follow-up study. JBJS 66A:853–859, 1984.
24. Strathy GM, Fitzgerald RH Jr. Total hip arthroplasty in the ankylosed hip. A ten year follow-up. JBJS 70A:963–966, 1988.
25. Gudmundsson G. Function following arthrodesis for coxarthrosis with special reference to the mobile hip. Acta Orthop Scand Suppl 141:1–79, 1972.
26. Stover MD, Beaule PE, Matta JM, et al. Hip arthrodesis: A procedure for the new millennium? Clin Orthop 418:126–133, 2004.
27. Iobst CA, Stanitski CL. Hip arthrodesis: Revisited. J Ped Orthop 21:130–134, 2001.
28. Matta JM, Siebenrock KA, Gautier E, et al. Hip fusion through an anterior approach with the use of a ventral plate. Clin Orthop 337:129–178, 1997.
29. Morris JB. Charnley compression arthrodesis of the hip. JBJS 48A:260–279, 1966.
30. Schoenecker PL, Johnson LO, Martin RA, et al. Intra-articular hip arthrodesis without subtrochanteric osteotomy in adolescents: Technique and short-term follow-up. Am J Orthop 26:257–264, 1997.
31. Scher DM, Jeong GK, Grant AD, et al. Hip arthrodesis in adolescents using external fixation. J Ped Orthop 21:194–197, 2001.
32. Tavares JO, Frankovitch KF. Hip arthrodesis using the AO modular external fixator. J Ped Orthop 18:651–656, 1998.
33. Callaghan JJ, Brand RA, Pedersen DR. Hip arthrodesis: A long term follow-up. JBJS 67A:1328–1335, 1985.
34. Gore DR, Murray MP, Sepic SB, et al. Walking patterns of men with unilateral surgical hip fusion. JBJS 57A:759–765, 1975.
35. Karol LA, Halliday SE, Gourineni P. Gait and function after intra-articular arthrodesis of the hip in adolescents. JBJS 82A:561–569, 2000.
36. Hauge MF. The knee in patients with hip joint ankylosis: Clinical survey and bio-mechanical aspects. Acta Orthop Scand 44:485–495, 1973.
37. Hardinge K, Murphy JC, Frenyo S. Conversion of hip fusion to Charnley low-friction arthroplasty. Clin Orthop 211:173–179, 1986.
38. Kilgus DJ, Amstutz HC, Wolgin MA, et al. Joint replacement for ankylosed hips. JBJS 72A:45–54, 1990.
39. Garvin KL, Pellicci PM, Windsor RE, et al. Contralateral total hip arthroplasty or ipsilateral total knee arthroplasty in patients who have a long-standing fusion of the hip. JBJS 71:1355–1362, 1989.
40. Millis MB, Murphy SB, Poss R. Osteotomies about the hip for the prevention and treatment of osteoarthritis. JBJS 77A:626–647, 1995.
41. Brand RA. Hip osteotomies: A biomechanical consideration. JAAOS 5:282–291, 1997.
42. Wieberg G. Studies on dysplastic acetabula and congenital subluxation of the hip joint: With special reference to the complication of osteoarthritis. Acta Chir Scand Suppl 58:7–135, 1939.
43. Wagner H. Experiences with spherical acetabular osteotomy for the correction of the dysplastic acetabulum. In: Weil UH, ed. Acetabular Dysplasia: Skeletal Dysplasias in Childhood. Berlin, Springer-Verlag, 1978, pp 131–145.

44. Ninomiya S, Tagawa H. Rotational acetabular osteotomy for the dysplastic hip. JBJS 66A:430–436, 1984.
45. Schramm M, Hohmann D, Radespiel-Troger M, et al. Treatment of the dysplastic acetabulum with Wagner Spherical Osteotomy. JBJS 85A:808–814, 2003.
46. Tonnis D, Behrens K, Tscharani F. A modified technique of the triple pelvic osteotomy. J Ped Orthop 1:241–249, 1981.
47. Siebenrock KA, Leunig M, Ganz R. Periacetabular osteotomy: The Bernese experience. JBJS 83A:449–455, 2001.
48. Trousdale RT, Ekkernkamp A, Ganz R, et al. Periacetabular and intertrochanteric osteotomy for the treatment of osteoarthrosis in dysplastic hips. JBJS 77A:73–85, 1995.
49. Clohisy JC, Barrett SE, Gordon E, et al. Periacetabular osteotomy for the treatment of severe acetabular dysplasia. JBJS 87A:254–259.
50. Windhager R, Pongracz N, Schoenecker W, et al. Chiari osteotomy for congenital dislocation and subluxation of the hip. Results after 20 to 34 years of follow up. JBJS 73B:890–895, 1991.
51. Lack W, Windhager R, Kutschera HP, et al. Chiari pelvic osteotomy for osteoarthritis secondary to hip dysplasia: Indications and long-term results. JBJS 73B:229–234, 1991.
52. Calvert PT, August AC, Albert JS, et al. The Chiari pelvic osteotomy: a review of the long term results. JBJS 69B:551–555, 1987.
53. Hogh J, MacNicol MF. The Chiari Osteotomy. A long term review of clinical and radiographic results. JBJS 69B:365–373, 1987.
54. Cabanela ME, Chiari osteotomy. In: Sedel L, Cabanela ME, eds. Hip Surgery: Materials and Developments. London, Martin Dunitz, 1998, pp. 149–157.
55. Migaud H, Chantelot C, Giraud F, et al. Long-term survivorship of hip shelf arthroplasty and Chiari osteotomy in adults. Clin Orthop 418:81–86, 2004.
56. Sanchez-Sotelo J, Trousdale RT, Berry DJ, et al. Surgical treatment of developmental dysplasia of hip in adults: I. Non-arthroplasty options. JAAOS 10:321–333, 2002.
57. Iwase T, Hasegawa Y, Kawamoto K, et al. Twenty years' follow-up of intertrochanteric osteotomy for treatment of the dysplastic hip. Clin Orthop 331:245–255, 1996.
58. Pellicci PM, Hu S, Garvin KL, et al. Varus rotational femoral osteotomies in adults with hip dysplasia. Clin Orthop 272:162–166, 1991.
59. Perlau R, Wilson MG, Poss R. Isolated proximal femoral osteotomy for treatment of residua of congenital dysplasia or idiopathic osteoarthrosis of the hip: Five to ten-year results. JBJS 78A: 1462–1467, 1996.
60. Fielding JW, Stillwell WT. The evolution of total hip arthroplasty. In: Stillwell WT, ed. The Art of Total Hip Arthroplasty. New York, Grune & Stratton, 1987, pp 1–24.
61. Smith-Peterson MN. Arthroplasty of the hip. A new method. JBJS 21:269, 1939.
62. Charnley J. The lubrication of animal joints. New Scientist 6:60, 1969.
63. Charnley J. Anchorage of the femoral head prosthesis to the shaft of the femur. JBJS 42B:28, 1960.
64. Charnley, J. The bonding of prosthesis to bone by cement. JBJS 46B:518, 1964.
65. Charnley J. Low friction arthroplasty of the hip joint. JBJS 53B:149, 1971.
66. Hungerford MW, Mont MA, Scott R, et al. Surface Replacement Hemiarthroplasty for the Treatment of Osteonecrosis of the Femoral Head. JBJS 80-A: 1656–1664, 1998.
67. Amstutz HC, Grigoris P, Safran MR, et al. Precision-fit surface hemiarthroplasty for femoral head osteonecrosis. In Osteonecrosis: Etiology, Diagnosis, and Treatment. Rosemont, IL, AAOS, 1997, pp 373–383.
68. Mesko JW, Goodman FG, Stanescu S. Total articular replacement arthroplasty. Clin Orthop 300:168–177, 1994.
69. Amstutz HC, Beaule PE, Dorey FJ, et al. Metal-on-metal hybrid surface arthroplasty: two to six-year follow-up study. JBJS 86A: 28–39, 2004.
70. Kurtz S, Mowat F, Ong K, et al. Prevalence of primary and revision total hip and knee arthroplasty in the United States from 1990 through 2002. JBJS 87A:1487–1497, 2005.
71. Laupacis A, Bourne R, Rorabeck C, et al. The effect of elective total hip replacement on health-related quality of life. JBJS 75:1619–1626, 1993.
72. Wiklund I, Romanus B. A comparison of quality of life before and after arthroplasty in patients who had arthrosis of the hip joint. JBJS 73A:765–769, 1991.
73. Barber TC, Healy WL. The hospital cost of total hip arthroplasty. JBJS 75A:321–321, 1993.
74. Bozic KJ, Katz P, Cisternas M, et al. Hospital resource utilization for primary and revision total hip arthroplasty. JBJS 87A: 570–576, 2005.
75. Kreder HJ, Deyo RA, Koepsell T, et al. Relationship between the volume of total hip replacements performed by providers and the rates of postoperative complications in the state of Washington. JBJS 79A:485–494, 1997.
76. Lavernia CJ, Guzman JF. Relationship of surgical volume to short-term mortality, morbidity, and hospital charges in arthroplasty. J Arthroplasty 10:133–140, 1995.
77. Katz JN, Phillips CB, Baron JA, et al. Association of hospital and surgeon volume of total hip replacement with functional status and satisfaction three years following surgery. Arthritis Rheum 48:560–568, 2003.
78. Callaghan JJ, Dysart SH, Savory CF, et al. Assessing the results of hip replacement: a comparison of five different rating systems. JBJS 72B:1008–1009, 1990.
79. Harris WH. Traumatic arthritis of the hip after dislocation and acetabular fractures: treatment by mold arthroplasty. An end result study using a new method of result evaluation. JBJS 51A:737–755, 1969.
80. Hozack WJ, Rothman RH, Booth RE, et al. Survivorship analysis of 1041 Charnley total hip arthroplasties. J Arthroplasty 5:41–47, 1990.
81. Wroblewski BM, Siney PD, Flemin PA. Charnley low-frictional torque arthroplasty in patients under the age of 51 years. JBJS 84B:540–543, 2002.
82. Callaghan JJ, Templeton JE, Liu SS, et al. Results of Charnley total hip arthroplasty at a minimum of thirty years. JBJS 86A:690–695, 2004.
83. Schmalzried TP, Kwong LM, Jasty M, et al. The mechanism of loosening of cemented acetabular components in total hip arthroplasty. Clin Orthop 274:60–78, 1992.
84. Mulroy RD, Harris WH. The effect of improved cementing techniques on component loosening in total hip replacement: an 11-year radiographic review. JBJS 72B:757, 1990.
85. O'Connor D, Maloney WJ, Burke D, et al. Cement strain profile in cemented acetabular components: the effects of metal-backing. Orthop Trans 18:613, 1994.
86. Chen FS, Di Cesare PE, Kale AA, et al. Results of cemented metal-backed acetabular components: A 10-year average follow-up study. J Arthroplasty 13:867–873, 1998.
87. Mulroy WF, Estok DM, Harris WM: Total hip arthroplasty with use of so-called second-generation cementing techniques. JBJS 77:1845, 1995.
88. Ritter MA, Keating EM, Faris PM, et al. Metal-backed acetabular cups in total hip arthroplasty. JBJS 72A:672–677, 1990.
89. Maloney WJ, Smith RL, Schmalzried TP, et al. Isolation and characterization of wear particles generated in failed uncemented hip arthroplasty. JBJS 77A:1301–1310, 1995.
90. Maloney WJ, Smith RL. Periprosthetic osteolysis in total hip arthroplasty: the role of particulate wear debris. JBJS 77A: 1448–1461, 1995.
91. McKellop HA, Campbell P, Park SH, et al. The origin of submicron polyethylene wear debris in total hip arthroplasty. Clin Orthop 31:3–20, 1995.
92. Jasty M, Bragdon CR, Burke D, et al. In vivo skeletal responses to porous-surfaced implants subjected to small induced motions. JBJS 79A:707–714, 1997.
93. Jasty M, Goetz DD, Bragdon CR, et al. Wear of polyethylene acetabular components in total hip arthroplasty: an analysis of 128 retrieved at autopsy or revision operation. JBJS 79A:349–358, 1997.
94. Branemark P-I. Introduction to osseointegration. In: Branemark P-I, Zarb G, Albrekttson T, eds. Tissue-Integrated Prostheses: Osseointegration in Clinical Dentistry. Chicago, Qunitessence, 1985, pp 11–76.

95. Maloney WJ, Galante JO, Anderson M, et al. Fixation, polyethylene wear, and pelvic osteolysis in primary total hip replacement. Clin Orthop 369:157–164, 1999.
96. Engh CA Jr, Culpepper WJ III, Engh CA. Long-term results of use of the anatomic medullary locking prosthesis in total hip arthroplasty. JBJS 79A:177–184, 1997.
97. Astion DJ, Saluan P, Stulberg BN, et al. The porous-coated anatomic total hip prosthesis: failure of the metal-backed acetabular component. JBJS 78A:755–766, 1996.
98. Manley MT, Capello WN, D'Antonio JA, et al. Fixation of acetabular cups without cement in total hip arthroplasty: a comparison of three different implant surfaces at a minimum duration follow-up of 8 years. JBJS 80A:1175–1185, 1998.
99. Jasty M, Bragdon CR, Burke D, et al. In vivo skeletal responses to porous surfaced implants subjected to small induced motions. JBJS 79A:707–714, 1997.
100. Della Valle AG, Zoppi A, Peterson M, et al. Clinical and radiographic results associated with a modern, cementless modular cup design in total hip arthroplasty. JBJS 86A:1998–2003, 2004.
101. Clohisy JC, Harris WH. Matched-pair analysis of cemented and cementless acetabular reconstruction in primary total hip arthroplasty. J Arthroplasty 16:697–705, 2001.
102. Rorabeck CH, Bourne RB, Mulliken BD, et al. The Nicolas Andry Award: Comparative results of cemented and cementless total hip arthroplasty. Clin Orthop 325:330–344, 1996.
103. Engh CA, Jr, Culpepper WJ III, Engh CA. Long term results of use of the anatomic medullary locking prosthesis in total hip arthroplasty. JBJS 79A:177–184, 1997.
104. Moskal JT, Jordan L, Brown TE. The porous-coated anatomic total hip prosthesis: 11- to 13-year results. J Arthroplasty 19:837–844, 2004.
105. Ahmed AM, Raab S, Miller JE. Metal/cement interface strength in cemented stem fixation. J Orthop Res 2:105–118, 1984.
106. Crowninshield RD, Tolbert JR. Cemented strain measurement surrounding loose and well-fixed femoral component stems. J Biomed Mater Res. 17:819–828, 1983.
107. Crowninshield RD, Brand RA, Johnston RC, et al. An analysis of femoral component stem design in total hip arthroplasty. JBJS 62A:68–78, 1980.
108. Stone MH, Wilkinson R, Stother IG. Some factors affecting the strength of the cement-metal interface. JBJS 71B:217–221, 1989.
109. Mohler CG, Kull LR, Martell JM, et al. Total hip replacement with insertion of an acetabular component without cement and a femoral component with cement: four to seven year results. JBJS 77A:86–96, 1995.
110. Oishi CS, Walker RH, Colwell CW Jr. The femoral component in total hip arthroplasty. Six to eight year follow-up of one hundred consecutive patients after use of a third-generation cementing technique. JBJS 76A:1130–1136, 1994.
111. Mohler CG, Callaghan JJ, Collis DK, et al. Early loosening of the femoral component at the cement-prosthesis interface after total hip replacement. JBJS 77A:1315–1322, 1995.
112. Woolson ST, Haber DF. Primary total hip replacement with insertion of an acetabular component without cement and a femoral component with cement: follow-up study at an average of six years. JBJS 78A:698–705, 1996.
113. Crowninshield RD, Jennings JD, Larent ML, et al. Cemented femoral component surface finish mechanics. Clin Orthop 355:90–102, 1998.
114. Berry DJ, Harmsen WS, Ilstrup DM. The natural history of debonding of the femoral component from the cement and its effect on long-term survival of Charnley total hip replacement. JBJS 80A:715–721, 1998.
115. Harris WH, McGann WA. Loosening of the femoral component after use of the medullary-plug cementing technique. JBJS 68A:1064–1066, 1986.
116. Sutherland CJ, Wilde AH, Borden LS, et al. A ten-year follow-up of 100 consecutive Muller curved-stem total hip replacement arthroplasties. JBJS 64A:970–982, 1982.
117. Roberts DW, Poss R, Kelley K. Radiographic comparison of cementing techniques in total hip arthroplasty. J Arthroplasty 1:241–247, 1986.
118. Barrack RL, Mulroy RD, Harris WH. Improved cementing techniques and femoral component loosening in young patients with hip arthroplasty. JBJS 74B:385–389, 1992.
119. Dowd JE, Cha CW, Traku S, et al. Failure of total hip arthroplasty with a precoated prosthesis. Clin Orthop 355:123–136, 1998.
120. Callaghan JJ, Forest EE, Olejniczak JP, et al. Charnley total hip arthroplasty in patients less than fifty years old. JBJS 80A:704–714, 1998.
121. Kawate K, Maloney WJ, Bragdon CA, et al. Importance of a thin cement mantle: autopsy studies of eight hips. Clin Orthop 355:70–76, 1998.
122. Woolson ST, Maloney WJ. Cementless total hip arthroplasty using a porous-coated prosthesis for bone ingrowth: a $3\frac{1}{2}$ year follow-up. J Arthroplasty 7:381–387, 1992.
123. Maloney WJ, Woolson ST. The increasing incidence of femoral osteolysis in association with uncemented Harris-Galante total hip arthroplasty: A follow-up report. J Arthroplasty 11:130–134, 1996.
124. Sinha RK, Dungy DS, Yeon HB. Primary total hip arthroplasty with a proximally porous-coated femoral stem. JBJS 86A:1254–1261, 2004.
125. Archibeck MJ, Berger RA, Jacobs JJ, et al. Second generation total hip arthroplasty. Eight to eleven year results. JBJS 83A: 1666–1673, 2001.
126. Kang JS, Dorr LD, Wan Z. The effect of diaphyseal biologic fixation on clinical results and fixation of the APR II stem. J Arthroplasty 15:730–735, 2000.
127. Engh CA Jr, Claus AM, Hopper RH, et al. Long-term results using the anatomic medullary locking hip prosthesis. Clin Orthop 393:137–146, 2001.
128. Engh CA, Hooten JP Jr, Zettl-Schaffer KF, et al. Evaluation of bone ingrowth in proximally and extensively porous-coated anatomic medullary locking prostheses retrieved at autopsy. JBJS 77A: 903–910, 1995.
129. Maloney WJ, Sychterz C, Bragdon C, et al. Skeletal response to well-fixed femoral components inserted with and without cement. Clin Orthop 333:15–26, 1996.
130. Swanson TV. The tapered pressfit total hip arthroplasty. A European alternative. J Arthroplasty 20:63–67, 2005.
131. Garcia-Cimbrelo E, Cruz-Pardos A, Madero R, et al. Total hip arthroplasty with use of the cementless Zweymuller alloclassic system. JBJS 85A: 296–303, 2003.
132. Vervest T, Anderson PG, van Hout F, et al. Ten to twelve-year results with the Zweymuller cementless total hip prosthesis. J Arthroplasty 20:362–368, 2005.
133. Parvizi J, Keisu KS, Hozack WJ, et al. Primary total hip arthroplasty with an uncemented femoral component. A long term study of the Taperloc stem. J Arthroplasty 19:151–156, 2004.
134. Bourne RB, Rorabeck CH, Patterson JJ, et al. Tapered titanium cementless total hip replacements. A 10 to 13-year follow-up study. Clin Orthop 393:112–120, 2001.
135. Peak EL, Parvizi J, Ciminiello M, et al. The role of patient restrictions in reducing the prevalence of early dislocation following total hip arthroplasty. A randomized, prospective study. JBJS 87A:247–253, 2005.
136. Pellicci PM, Bostrom M, Poss R. Posterior approach to total hip replacement using enhanced posterior soft tissue repair. Clin Orthop 355:224–228, 1998.
137. Cobb TK, Morrey BF, Ilstrup DM. The elevated-rim acetabular liner in total hip arthroplasty: relationship to postoperative dislocation. JBJS 78A:80–86, 1996.
138. Maloney WJ, Smith RL. Periprosthetic osteolysis in total hip arthroplasty: the role of particulate wear debris. JBJS 77A:1448–1461, 1995.
139. Joshi R, Eftekhar N, McMahon D, et al. Osteolysis after Charnley primary low friction arthroplasty. JBJS 80B:585–590, 1998.
140. Cook SD, Barrack RL, Baffes GC, et al. Wear and corrosion of modular interfaces in total hip replacements. Clin Orthop 298:80–88, 1994.
141. Bobyn JD, Jacobs JJ, Tanzer M, et al. The susceptibility of smooth implant surfaces to periimplant fibrosis and migration of polyethylene wear debris. Clin Orthop 311:21–39, 1995.
142. Goldring SR, Jasty M, Roelke MS, et al. Formation of a synovial-like membrane at the bone-cement interface. Its role in bone resorption and implant loosening after total hip replacement. Arthritis Rheum 29:836–842, 1986.
143. Goodman SB, Chin RC, Chiou SS, et al. A clinical-pathologic-biochemical study of the membrane surrounding loosened and nonloosened total hip arthroplasties. Clin Orthop 244:182–187, 1989.

144. Schwarz EM, Benz EB, Lu AP, et al. Quantitative small animal surrogate to evaluate drug efficacy in preventing wear debris-induced osteolysis. J Orthop Res 18:849–855, 2000.

145. Muratoglu OK, Bragdon CR, O'Connor DO, et al. A novel method of cross-linking ultra-high molecular weight polyethylene to improve wear, reduce oxidation, and retain mechanical properties. Recipient of the 1999 HAP Paul Award. J Arthroplasty 16:149–160, 2001.

146. D'Lima DD, Hermida JC, Chen PC, et al. Polyethylene cross-linking by two different methods reduces acetabular liner wear in a hip joint wear simulator. J Orthop Res 21:761–766, 2003.

147. Bragdon CR, Jasty M, Muratoglu OK, et al. Third-body wear of highly cross-linked polyethylene in a hip simulator. J Arthroplasty 18:553–561, 2003.

148. Muratoglu OK, Bragdon CR, O'Connor D, et al. Larger diameter femoral heads used in conjunction with a highly cross-linked ultra-high molecular weight polyethylene: a new concept. J Arthroplasty 16:24–30, 2001.

149. Manning DW, Chiang PP, Martell JM, et al. In vivo comparative wear study of traditional and highly cross-linked polyethylene in total hip arthroplasty. J Arthroplasty 20:880–886, 2005.

150. Digas G, Karrholm J, Thanner J, et al. Highly cross-linked polyethylene in total hip arthroplasty. Clin Orthop 429:6–16, 2004.

151. Krushell RJ, Fingeroth RJ, Cushing MC. Early femoral head penetration of a highly cross-linked polyethylene liner vs a conventional polyethylene liner: A case-controlled study. J Arthroplasty 20(S3):73–76, 2005.

152. Dorr LD, Wan Z, Shahrdar C, et al. Clinical performance of a Durasul highly cross-linked polyethylene acetabular liner for total hip arthroplasty at five years. JBJS 87A:1816–1821, 2005.

153. Bradford L, Baker DA, Graham J, et al. Wear and surface cracking in early retrieved highly cross-linked polyethylene acetabular liners. JBJS 86A:1271–1282, 2004.

154. Birman MV, Noble PC, Conditt MA, et al. Cracking and impingement in ultra-high-molecular-weight polyethylene acetabular liners. J Arthroplasty 20(S3):87–92, 2005.

155. Yoon TR, Rowe SM, Jung ST, et al. Osteolysis in association with ceramic total hip arthroplasty. JBJS 80A:1459–1468, 1998.

156. Hannouche D, Nich C, Bizot P, et al. Fractures of ceramic bearings. CORR 417:19–26, 2003.

157. Hamadouche M, Boutin P, Daussange J, et al. Alumina-on-alumina THA. A minimum 18.5 year follow-up study. JBJS 84: 69–77, 2002.

158. Wroblewski BM, Siney PD, Dowson D, et al. Prospective clinical and joint simulator studies of a new total hip arthroplasty using alumina ceramic heads and crosslinked polyethylene cups. JBJS 78B:280–285, 1996.

159. Barrack RL, Burak C, Skinner HB. Concerns about ceramics in THA. Clin Orthop 429:73–79, 2004.

160. D'Antonio J, Capello W, Manley M, et al. Alumina ceramic bearings for total hip arthroplasty: five-year results of a prospective randomized study. Clin Orthop 436:164–171, 2005.

161. Yoo JJ, Kim YM, Yoon KS, et al. Alumina-on-alumina total hip arthroplasty. JBJS 87A:530–534, 2005.

162. Amstutz HC, Grigoris P. Metal on metal bearings in hip arthroplasty. CORR 329S:11–34, 1996.

163. August AC, Aldam CH, Pynsent PB. The McKee-Farrar hip arthroplasty. A long-term study. J Bone Joint Surg 68B:520–527, 1986.

164. Semlitsch M, Streicher RM, Weber H. The wear behavior of capsules and heads of CoCrMo casts in long term implanted all-metal hip prostheses. Orthopade 18:377–381, 1989.

165. Dorr LD, Wan Z, Sirianni LE, et al. Fixation and osteolysis with Metasul metal-on-metal articulation. J Arthroplasty 19:951–955, 2004.

166. Lombardi AV Jr, Mallory TH, Cuckler JM, et al. Mid-term results of a polyethylene-free metal-on-metal articulation. J Arthroplasty S2:42–47, 2004.

167. Jacobs JJ, Hallab NJ, Skipor AK, et al. Metal degradation products: A cause for concern in metal-metal bearings? CORR 417:139–147, 2003.

168. Davies AP, Willert HG, Campbell, PA, et al. An unusual lymphocytic perivascular infiltration in tissues around contemporary metal-on-metal joint replacements. JBJS 87A:18–27, 2005.

169. Willert H, Buchhorn GH, Fayyazi DA, et al. Metal-on-metal bearings and hypersensitivity in patients with artificial hip joints. JBJS 87A:28–36, 2005.

170. MacDonald SJ, McCalden RW, Chess DG, et al. Metal-on-metal versus polyethylene in hip arthroplasty: A randomized clinical trial. CORR 406:282–296, 2003.

171. Ladon D, Doherty A, Newson R, et al. Changes in metal levels and chromosome aberrations in the peripheral blood of patients after metal on metal arthroplasty. J Arthroplasty 19(S3):78–83, 2004.

172. Gillespie WJ, Frampton CMA, Henderson RJ. The incidence of cancer following total hip replacement. JBJS 70B:539–542, 1988.

173. Mathieson EB, Ahlborn A, Bermann G, et al. Total hip replacement and cancer. JBJS 77B:345–350, 1995.

Lower Extremity Considerations: Knee

21B

Brian J. Cole   *Richard Berger*   *Victor M. Goldberg*   *Aaron Rosenberg*

OSTEOARTHRITIS OF THE KNEE

Osteoarthritis (OA) of the knee is a disease with profound physical and economic impact. As the most common form of arthritis, it (along with hip OA) accounts for more dependency and disability of the lower extremity than any other disease. OA is considered a spectrum of cartilage failure ranging from the symptomatic focal chondral defect to established arthrosis. Clinically, OA consists of joint symptoms due to articular cartilage structural changes that are generally demonstrated on plain radiographs.[1] OA is characterized pathologically as cartilage erosion, and it is defined epidemiologically through radiographic evaluation because this is the most readily available means to assess joints on a large scale. Not uncommonly, however, radiographic evidence of OA does not correlate with the patient's symptoms.

The inability of cartilage to repair itself after traumatic injury and the progression of the untreated osteoarthritic process, once it is initiated, are discussed elsewhere in this book. The etiology of OA is controversial and seems to represent a combination of qualitative biologic change with loss of biochemical homeostasis and biomechanical failure of the joint cartilage due to physical forces. Independent of the etiology, OA is heralded by damage to the articular cartilage with diffuse fraying and fibrillation and hypertrophic changes in adjacent bone.

Epidemiology

The incidence and prevalence of OA in any joint are correlated with age. Before the age of 50 years, men have a higher incidence and prevalence, but after the age of 50 years, women have a higher incidence and prevalence. Gender differences increase progressively with advancing age until approximately 80 years.[2]

OA of the knee can be either primary or secondary. Primary OA is a progressive "wear and tear" degenerative condition that increases in prevalence nonlinearly with age after 50 years. It is estimated that 25% to 30% of people 45 to 64 years of age and more than 85% of individuals older than 65 years have radiographically detectable OA.[3]

Secondary OA of the knee may occur much earlier, however, after significant injury resulting in varus or valgus malalignment, intra-articular fracture, or ligamentous and meniscal deficiency.[4,5] Rangger and colleagues[6] reported radiographic increases in OA after partial arthroscopic medial (38% increase) and lateral (24% increase) meniscectomy at an average follow-up of 53.5 months in 284 consecutive patients. The effect of focal articular damage on joint function and the development of secondary OA is difficult to predict.[7] The progression to arthrosis from focal articular damage is believed to be exacerbated when it is associated with meniscectomy.[8]

Cross-racial studies can often produce insights, but with respect to knee OA, there is conflicting evidence. The greater relative body weight of African-American women may predispose them to higher rates of knee OA. Generalized OA appears to have a strong genetic susceptibility, and knee OA may develop more as a function of inheritance than as a result of repeated mechanical insults or other lifestyle factors.[9]

The Framingham study demonstrated that men with jobs that require both carrying and kneeling or squatting have twice the risk of developing knee OA than that of men whose jobs do not require those activities. Elite athletes in several sports have increased risk of knee OA, even those without a history of injury.[10] However, there is no evidence that recreational running predisposes to OA. Despite a lifetime of activity, no data to date support the development of or association with premature arthrosis of the knee in active patients.[11]

By any definition of OA, overweight individuals develop knee OA more often than do those who are not overweight.

395

Furthermore, studies confirm that increased weight precedes the occurrence of OA. Obese women with unilateral disease are at increased risk for development of bilateral disease, and overweight persons are at higher risk of experiencing progressive disease. These strong relationships between obesity and knee OA persist even when other factors associated with obesity are adjusted for. Weight loss has been associated with reduction in risk for development of symptomatic knee OA and improvement in symptoms in those with this condition.[12]

The Meniscus and Osteoarthritis

It is estimated that the lateral meniscus normally carries 70% of the lateral compartment load and the medial meniscus 50% of the medial compartment load with the knee fully extended.[13] The interrelationship between the loss of the load-bearing role of the meniscus after meniscectomy and the development of arthritis is well documented, with loads increasing up to threefold in the involved compartment.[8,14,15] Patients who have had total meniscectomies have high risk of subsequent knee OA; those who receive partial meniscectomy also appear to be at increased risk.[16] Not uncommonly, the young and previously active patient presents with disabling unicompartmental arthritis with progressive deformity as a result of previous subtotal or total meniscectomy. As discussed in the section on surgical options, these patients pose a treatment challenge with additional surgical options available, such as allograft meniscal transplantation, osteotomy, and unicompartmental knee replacement.

Biomechanics of Osteoarthritis of the Knee

Standing weight-bearing anteroposterior radiographs that include both extremities from the hips to the ankles determine mechanical and anatomic axes of the limb. The mechanical axis is based on a line connecting the center of the femoral head and the center of the tibiotalar joint; it averages 1.2° of varus and generally passes through the center of the knee. The anatomic axis represents the longitudinal orientation of the femur with respect to the longitudinal orientation of the tibia; it is the angle formed by the intersection of the anatomic axes of the femoral and tibial shafts (Fig. 21B–1). The difference between the anatomic and mechanical axes is usually between 3° and 7°.[17,18]

A relatively neutral mechanical axis alignment allows the stress on the knee to be evenly distributed during weight bearing. With varus or valgus deformity, a line drawn between the center of the femoral head and the center of the ankle falls medial or lateral to the center of the knee, respectively. Therefore, in the varus knee, more forces are transmitted to the medial compartment; in the valgus knee, more forces are transmitted to the lateral compartment. This situation leads to a vicious circle once the arthritic process is initiated.

During activities of daily living, the knee is subjected to forces ranging between three and seven times body weight. Under these normal circumstances, the medial side of the knee is loaded about 50% more than the lateral side of the knee. This relative difference is due to the adduction moment

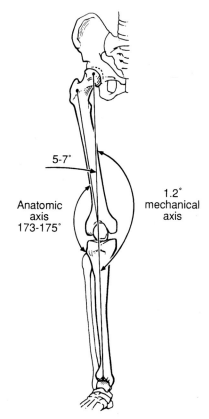

Figure 21B–1 Mechanical and anatomic axes of the lower extremity. The mechanical axis represents a line drawn between the center of the femoral head and the center of the tibiotalar joint; it averages 1.2° of varus relative to the center of gravity. The anatomic axis is the angle formed by the intersection of lines drawn along the longitudinal axes of the femur and tibia; it averages 5° of valgus in normal individuals. (From Hanssen A, Chao EYS. High tibial osteotomy. In: Fu FH, Harner CD, Vince KG, eds. Knee Surgery. Baltimore, Williams & Wilkins, 1994, p 1123.)

normally produced at the knee during weight bearing and ambulation. These factors help to explain why 90% of knee arthritis begins in the medial compartment whereas only 10% of knee arthritis begins in the lateral compartment.

Conditions that increase the stress (or pressure) on the articular surface of the knee can lead to mechanical and biologic breakdown of the articular cartilage. Although the initiation of this process may be subject to conjecture or be purely idiopathic, once the process begins, progression of disease is affected by biomechanical abnormalities leading to relative increases in joint stress or pressure.

The interplay between biomechanical abnormalities and OA is complex and self-perpetuating. Factors such as primary articular cartilage degeneration, the effects of meniscectomy, and developmental deformities such as post-traumatic arthritis and fracture malunion often lead to a vicious circle of progressive degeneration with associated deformity.

Conditions such as a flexion deformity, which develops as a result of the arthritic condition, may similarly adversely affect the knee. For example, a flexion contracture of the knee reduces the contact area between the tibia and femur; this is because the largest area of contact between the tibia and femur occurs with the knee in nearly full extension and decreases with flexion. Therefore, fixed flexion deformity, which is common in the arthritic process, can further accelerate the degeneration process by increasing the stresses across the knee as the forces are distributed over a smaller surface area.

Because individuals often compensate with the use of assistive devices, reduced activity levels, and adaptive changes in activities of daily living, progressive arthritis does not occur in all cases of abnormal knee biomechanics. Similarly, predicting who will develop progressive arthritis in the setting of abnormal biomechanics is difficult and dependent on many factors including genetics, habitus, activity levels, ligamentous stability, alignment, status of the meniscus, and overall condition of the articular cartilage.

Evaluation

There are several causes of knee arthrosis that are most often determined by the findings of the history, physical examination, and plain radiographs. If the findings are inconsistent, alternative diagnoses such as primary disease of the hip or back with referred pain to the knee, osteonecrosis, and stress fractures around the knee should be entertained. A complete history and physical examination of the spine, neurovascular system, and contiguous joints are imperative to avoid missing additional sources of knee symptoms.

History

A comprehensive history focusing on the patient's symptoms includes factors commonly elicited during any evaluation of the musculoskeletal system (Table 21B–1). A patient's employment, activity level, and symptoms are important factors in determining the appropriate treatment option. The patient's occupation and current and desired activity levels are determined. Questioning the patient about activities that require adequate knee function, such as getting out of a chair or car, climbing stairs, and walking on level ground, provides insight into the patient's ability to function on a daily basis.

Response to medical management (i.e., nonsteroidal anti-inflammatory drugs, analgesics, and injections) is sought. The response to modalities such as physical therapy, recent body weight or activity level changes, and assistive devices is reviewed.

Clinical Manifestations

The main symptoms of OA of the knee are joint pain and stiffness. The pain is generally related to activity and tends to worsen throughout the day. Rest pain implies severe OA, and sharp pains occasionally occur with particular activities. Pain localized to one compartment (i.e., unicompartmental) of the knee is common early in the disease process, especially in secondary OA. Alternatively, in long-standing OA, pain may be more diffuse. Atypical, severe pain should alert the clinician to other possibilities, such as osteonecrosis, inflammatory arthritis, or mechanical symptoms due to an intra-articular pathologic process (e.g., loose bodies, unstable meniscal or articular cartilage flap tears). In some patients with disorders of the spine and hip, pain can be

TABLE 21B-1
COMPONENTS OF A COMPREHENSIVE HISTORY

Symptom location
  Isolated
    Medial
    Lateral
    Patellofemoral
  Diffuse
Symptom type
Pain
Swelling
Decreased range of motion
Mechanical
  Crepitus
  Locking
  Pseudolocking
  Catching
  Giving way
Symptom timing
  Onset
    Sudden
    Insidious
    Duration
    Exacerbating and ameliorating factors
Symptom intervention and response
  Lifestyle modification
  Rehabilitation
  Shoe wear
  Assistive devices
  Prior treatment
    Nonsteroidal anti-inflammatory drugs
    Injections
    Bracing
    Rehabilitation
    Surgery
Past medical history
Past surgical history
Family history

referred to the knee. Patients with periarticular disorders such as anserine, infrapatellar, or prepatellar bursitis may be incorrectly diagnosed as having knee OA.

Stiffness in the morning is usual but brief, in contradistinction to inflammatory arthritis such as rheumatoid arthritis. The signs of OA include joint swelling, crepitus, reduced range of motion, pain on active movement and at the extremes of movement, and joint tenderness. A mild inflammatory reaction is sometimes present. Periarticular syndromes such as bursitis and tendinitis are common, as are muscle wasting and weakness. Weakness may be an important cause of both symptoms and disability.

Swelling related to a joint effusion or synovitis may be intermittent or constant. Small or moderate joint effusions are common; large effusions are rare. The synovial fluid has less than 2000 white blood cells/mm^3, but cartilage fragments or calcium pyrophosphate crystals are common. Active OA results in the release of abnormal quantities of cartilage matrix molecules into the synovial fluid and in turn into blood.[19] The value and meaning of these biochemical markers of OA are under investigation (see Chapter 12).

Mechanical symptoms of intermittent catching or locking may suggest gross articular surface irregularity, a loose osteochondral fragment, or meniscal disease commonly seen in secondary OA. It is important to consider the patient's complaints of instability, pain, or a combination of both when ligamentous deficiency and arthrosis coexist. In addition, instability due to pain, effusion, and subsequent quadriceps inhibition is to be differentiated from instability due to ligamentous insufficiency, which may or may not be associated with pain.

Physical Examination

The components of a comprehensive physical examination are outlined in Table 21B–2. Body habitus and gait are observed. Antalgia, medial or lateral thrusts, and other dynamic compensatory gait patterns (quadriceps avoidance, out-toeing) are determined. Clinically, static limb alignment and deformity serve as a rough index of the duration and severity of the disease process. In long-standing primary OA or secondary OA after trauma or meniscectomy, genuvarum suggests medial compartment involvement and genu valgum suggests lateral compartment involvement. With long-standing deformity, patients may exhibit pseudolaxity due to stretching of the collateral ligaments on the contralateral side of the affected compartment.

Range of motion with side-to-side comparison is assessed in the supine and prone positions. Patients may commonly present with a mild flexion contracture (i.e., <10°) and lack full flexion (i.e., by >20°). Larger losses of motion are unusual in active individuals. Patients may complain of swelling or perceive stiffness due to swelling. Patellofemoral or joint line crepitus is a common finding.

Patellofemoral evaluation includes patellar tilt, lateral and medial patellar glide, and patellar facet tenderness as described in the section on anterior knee pain and patellofemoral disorders. Stability in the coronal plane (i.e., varus or valgus at 0° and 30° of flexion) and sagittal (anteroposterior) plane is determined. Positive results of the Lachman and pivot shift tests may indicate chronic anterior cruciate ligament insufficiency. Similarly, loss of the normal 5 to 10 mm of anteromedial tibial step-off relative to the medial femoral condyle or the presence of a tibial "sag sign" with the hip and knee held in 90° of flexion in the supine position may be indicative of chronic posterior cruciate ligament insufficiency.

Evaluation for joint line tenderness and swelling, and provocative meniscal tests such as the McMurray test are performed.[20] The McMurray test is performed with the patient in the supine position with the hip and knee flexed to 90° while the axially loaded foot is maneuvered from a position of abduction and external rotation to one of adduction and internal rotation to elicit a painful "pop" or "click" in the affected compartment. The hip, back, and neurovascular status are evaluated for additional pathologic changes including losses in motion, with the need for radiographic imaging of these regions if a concomitant pathologic process is suspected.

Diagnostic Imaging

Plain Radiographs

Reproducible radiographs are examined in a systematic manner (Table 21B–3). Careful comparison of affected and unaffected knees helps to document subtle radiographic changes. A standard anteroposterior view with the patient

---

TABLE 21B–2
COMPONENTS OF A PHYSICAL EXAMINATION

Habitus
  Height
  Weight
Alignment
  Varus
  Valgus
Gait
  Antalgic
  Flexed-knee
  Recurvatum
  Compensatory
    Adduction or abduction moment
    Out-toeing or in-toeing
  Thrust
    Varus (lateral) or valgus (medial)
Laxity
  Anteroposterior
  Medial-lateral
    Pseudolaxity
    True laxity
    Rotary
Range of motion
Specific compartments
  Tibiofemoral
  Patellofemoral
Meniscal
  Joint line
    Tenderness
    Swelling
  Provocative
Related joints
  Spine
  Hips
  Ankles, hindfoot, forefoot
Neurovascular

TABLE 21B–3
PLAIN RADIOGRAPHIC SERIES

Anteroposterior	45° weight-bearing posteroanterior view of both knees[21]
Lateral	45° non–weight-bearing flexion lateral view of affected knee
Patellar	45° axial view of both knees[22]
Alignment	Long cassette view of both knees from hip to ankle

standing with the body weight evenly distributed on both legs is commonly obtained, but a 45° flexion weight-bearing posteroanterior radiograph as described by Rosenberg and colleagues[21] is particularly valuable. In addition, a non–weight-bearing true 45° flexion lateral view and a 45° axial view of both patellae according to Merchant[22] are obtained.

The 45° flexion weight-bearing posteroanterior radiograph may demonstrate subtle loss of joint space indicative of early arthrosis that traditional extension views fail to show (Fig. 21B–2), especially in the lateral compartment. The earliest loss of cartilage is typically in the 30° to 60° flexion zone and thus is easily overlooked with radiographs obtained in full extension. Symptoms of joint line

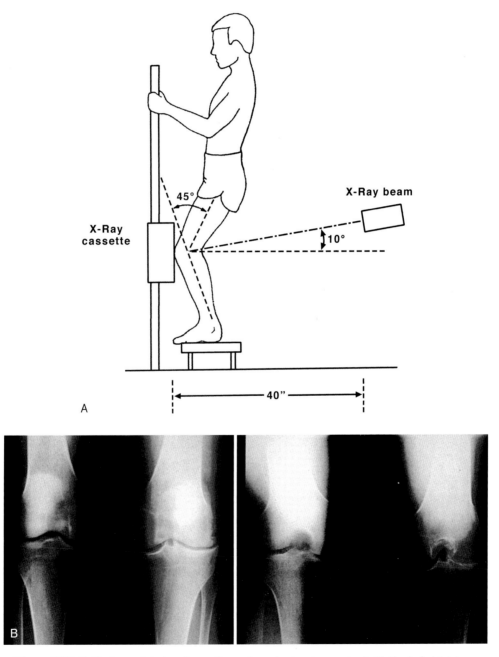

Figure 21B–2 Flexion weight-bearing radiograph method and example. *A*, Method of obtaining a flexion weight-bearing radiograph to bring the weight-bearing portion of the femoral condyles into view, demonstrating subtle changes of joint space narrowing. (From Rosenberg TR, Paulos L, Parker R, et al. The 45 degree PA flexion weight-bearing radiograph of the knee. J Bone Joint Surg Am 70:1479–1483, 1988.) *B*, Joint space narrowing not seen on a traditional anteroposterior extension weight-bearing radiograph (*left*) is best appreciated on a posteroanterior 45° flexion weight-bearing radiograph (*right*) in the same patient.

pain and a loss of cartilage clear space by 2 mm or more are likely to be due to chondrosis rather than meniscal disease.[21] Because the 45° posteroanterior view provides a view of the notch, changes consistent with chronic anterior cruciate ligament deficiency are also evaluated, such as peaking of the tibial spines and narrowing of the intercondylar notch. Several important findings are determined from these views (Table 21B–4). For example, Fairbank[23] changes seen after meniscectomy include osteophyte formation along the periphery of the tibia, flattening of the femoral condyles, and joint space narrowing.

A history of prior meniscectomy, tibial plateau fracture, or clinically significant angular deformity is evaluated by standing, weight-bearing anteroposterior radiographs that include both extremities from the hips to the ankles to determine mechanical and anatomic axes of the limb (Fig. 21B–1).

Magnetic Resonance Imaging

Magnetic resonance imaging (MRI) scans of patients with knee arthritis are not routinely ordered. However, if there is a question of mechanical derangement such as a meniscal or cruciate ligament tear, or osteochondral fracture, osteonecrosis, or an isolated chondral defect, MRI may be informative. MRI is most useful in the setting of minimal arthritic change on radiographs in patients with localized pain and clinical findings consistent with meniscal disease. Not uncommonly, degenerative meniscal tears are present with OA, and one should avoid the temptation to operate solely on this finding without clinical correlation. Special MRI techniques to evaluate articular cartilage, including proton-density images, fat suppression or saturation techniques, and gradient-echo techniques with or without intra-articular gadolinium contrast enhancement, are gaining greater acceptance.[24] In most cases, however, if joint space narrowing is present on the 45° flexion weight-bearing view, MRI is not indicated.

Bone Scintigraphy

Technetium scintigraphy may be useful in difficult cases in which plain radiographs are normal despite a clinical scenario consistent with "arthritis-like" symptoms.[25] For example, abnormal osseous activity detected by a bone scan (i.e., increased uptake in the patellofemoral compartment) may support findings of a periarticular pathologic process in the setting of a normal radiograph or normal findings on MRI. Abnormal findings on bone scans are likely in the presence of symptomatic OA, meniscal tears, osteonecrosis, and osteochondral lesions. Alternatively, diffuse soft tissue uptake may be associated with reflex sympathetic dystrophy.

Treatment Options

No treatment has yet been shown to definitively stop the osteoarthritic process; thus, the therapeutic goals must focus on reducing pain and improving function. Before considering therapeutic options in an individual with OA of the knee, the physician should be certain that the patient's knee pain is attributable to OA. If the physician is in doubt about the diagnosis, consultation with a specialist is recommended.

Chronologic age is clearly only a relative consideration, and physiologic age often drives decision-making. Nonsurgical management (Table 21B–5) includes

---

TABLE 21B–4
RADIOGRAPHIC FINDINGS

Bone
  Fairbank[23] changes
  Osteophytes
  Subchondral sclerosis
  Osteonecrosis
  Osteochondritis dissecans
  Notch narrowing
  Peaked tibial spines
  Loose bodies
  Avulsion fracture
    Segond fracture of lateral tibia
    Pellegrini-Stieda lesion of medial collateral ligament femoral insertion
Cartilage
  Joint space narrowing
  Chondrocalcinosis
  Focal articular contour irregularities
Soft tissue
  Swelling
  Atrophy
  Effusion
  Gas
  Myositis ossificans
  Ectopic calcification
Alignment
  Coronal plane deformity (varus or valgus)
  Sagittal plane deformity
  Patellar height
  Patellar tilt/subluxation

TABLE 21B–5
NONSURGICAL MANAGEMENT OF OSTEOARTHRITIS

Nonpharmacologic modalities
  Lifestyle modification
    Education of the patient
    Activity modification
    Weight loss
    Ambulatory assist devices
  Rehabilitation
  Shoe wear, orthoses
  Brace wear
Pharmacologic modalities
Analgesics
Nonsteroidal anti-inflammatory agents
Topical analgesics
Intra-articular therapy
  Corticosteroids
  Hyaluronans

TABLE 21B–6
SURGICAL MANAGEMENT OF OSTEOARTHRITIS

Arthroscopy, débridement, lavage
Osteotomy
    Tibial
    Femoral
Arthroplasty
    Unicondylar knee replacement
    Total knee replacement
Arthrodesis
Resection arthroplasty
Symptomatic focal chondral defect
    Arthroscopy, débridement, lavage
    Marrow-stimulating techniques
    Autologous chondrocyte implantation
    Osteochondral autograft or allograft
Meniscal allograft transplantation

nonpharmacologic (rehabilitation, lifestyle modification, shoe wear modifications, orthotics, bracing) and pharmacologic modalities. Intolerable lifestyle changes or a poor response to nonsurgical management may ultimately dictate surgical treatment.

Surgical modalities (Table 21B–6) include joint arthroscopy and reconstructive procedures (osteotomy, arthroplasty, arthrodesis, resection arthroplasty) and may include preventive measures, such as meniscal transplantation and articular cartilage restoration (marrow-stimulating techniques, osteoarticular allografts or autografts, and autologous chondrocyte implantation). Knowledge of the indications and outcomes for each of these procedures is important for appropriate management of the patient's potentially unrealistic goals and expectations.

Nonsurgical Management

Nonsurgical therapy is divided into nonpharmacologic and pharmacologic modalities. The treatment plan is determined by numerous factors, including the presence of comorbid conditions, which may influence decisions about drug therapy. Details regarding nonsurgical approaches are provided in Chapters 14 to 17.

Surgical Management

When nonoperative treatment of OA of the knee fails to alleviate pain and knee function is compromised, operative intervention is warranted. The timing of and recommendation for the most appropriate surgical procedure require great skill and cooperation between the patient and physician. Patients with severe symptomatic OA of the knee who have pain that has failed to respond to medical therapy and have progressive limitations in activities of daily living should be referred for surgical consideration (Table 21B–6).

Surgical options include arthroscopy and joint reconstruction. Joint reconstruction options include osteotomy, replacement, and arthrodesis. Joint replacement can be in the form of either unicompartmental or total knee arthroplasty. The symptomatic focal chondral defect limited to one of the femoral condyles or trochlea can be managed by a variety of techniques, and allograft meniscal transplantation may be a viable option when arthritis is unicompartmental and less severe.

The principles of management of the adult arthritic knee follow a relatively intuitive algorithm. Arthroscopy is primarily indicated as a first-time procedure in patients who often present with a relatively acute or subacute onset in pain. Mechanical symptoms caused by unstable articular cartilage flap tears, meniscal tears, or loose bodies are common indications to proceed with arthroscopy and débridement. To improve the prognosis after arthroscopy and débridement, patients should not have significant malalignment, ligament instability, or end-stage arthritis.

Osteotomy is principally indicated for unicompartmental arthritis and corresponding malalignment or for symptomatic post-traumatic malunions about the knee associated with painful knee arthritis. Unicompartmental knee arthroplasty is primarily indicated for the patient with lower physical demands and arthritis of a single compartment. Arthroplasty (total knee replacement) is indicated in the patient who is not a candidate for arthroscopy or osteotomy, in patients with more diffuse arthritic involvement, and for salvage of the failed osteotomy or unicompartmental knee replacement. Last, arthrodesis is most commonly indicated for the salvage of failed arthroplasty.

Arthroscopy

In OA, degenerating articular cartilage and synovium release proinflammatory cytokines (e.g., interleukin-1, tumor necrosis factor-α, transforming growth factor-β). These cytokines induce chondrocytes to release lytic enzymes leading to type II collagen and proteoglycan degradation. Arthroscopic lavage and débridement may "wash out" or dilute these inflammatory mediators.[26] The effectiveness of joint lavage alone has been suggested by Livesley and colleagues.[27] These authors compared the results of 37 painful arthritic knees treated with lavage by one surgeon with the results of 24 knees treated with physiotherapy alone by a second surgeon and suggested that there was better pain relief in the lavage group at 1 year. Edelson and coworkers[28] demonstrated that lavage alone had good or excellent results in 86% at 1 year and in 81% at 2 years with use of the Hospital for Special Surgery score.

Jackson and Rouse[29] reported the results of arthroscopic lavage alone versus lavage combined with débridement with 3-year follow-up. In the 65 cases treated with lavage alone, 80% showed initial improvement, whereas only 45% maintained improvement at follow-up. Of the 137 cases treated with lavage plus débridement, 88% showed initial improvement and 68% maintained improvement at follow-up. Gibson and associates[30] demonstrated no significant improvement with either method, even in the short term. Patients who present with flexion deformities associated with pain or discomfort with osteophyte formation around the tibial spines may benefit from osteophyte removal and notchplasty as demonstrated by Puddu and colleagues.[31]

The efficacy of lavage with or without débridement is controversial; some studies suggest that arthroscopic lavage and débridement, when appropriately indicated, will provide pain relief in 50% to 70% of patients lasting several months to several years (i.e., 2 to 4 years).[32–35] In a recent Veterans Administration randomized trial comparing arthroscopic lavage, débridement, or sham procedures involving 180 patients, no statistically significant differences between study arms was demonstrated at a 2-year follow-up. Caveats related to the study included a 44% dropout rate; recruitment of only male patients; and nonspecific indications for surgical intervention.[36] By contrast, Aaron reported a study of 122 consecutive patients who had failed conservative treatment and underwent arthroscopic débridement of the knee.[37] At 34 months follow-up, 90% of the patients with objective mild arthritis demonstrated marked improvement by 6 months after surgery. However, there was little improvement in those patients with high grade OA according to clinical and radiographic signs. Specific débridement techniques such as microfracture when used for local cartilage defects may be very effective in preserving joint function.

Drilling and abrasion arthroplasty do not appear to offer additional benefit to arthroscopic débridement, although intermediate-term results in noncontrolled trials suggest that microfracture may offer some benefit.[38,39] Arthroscopy is also a sensitive way to evaluate the extent and location of articular disease when osteotomy or unicompartmental knee arthroplasty is contemplated because plain radiographs and MRI often underestimate the extent of OA.[40]

Several factors may be relevant to prognosis after lavage and débridement (Table 21B–7). Those who appear to benefit most present with a history of mechanical symptoms, symptoms of short duration (i.e., <6 months), normal alignment, and only mild to moderate radiographic evidence of OA.[32–34] It is not uncommon for patients to have unrealistic expectations after arthroscopic débridement. Thus, it is important to counsel patients about the limited indications and often palliative results. Patients who have undergone a minimum of 3 months of supervised nonsurgical treatment with normal alignment and only mild to moderate OA on 45° flexion weight-bearing posteroanterior radiographs may be considered candidates for arthroscopic débridement.

Osteotomy

Varus Malalignment. In the younger active patient with varus malalignment and medial arthrosis, our recommendation is to perform a valgus-producing high tibial osteotomy to decrease medial compartment loads, diminish symptoms, and improve function. In general, it is better to perform the osteotomy sooner rather than later (i.e., when <5° of varus is present) and to overcorrect by 2° to 3°. Mild to moderate patellofemoral OA is still compatible with a successful result after high tibial osteotomy.

Indications for osteotomy and unicompartmental knee replacement are similar in some respects. The two are similar in that mild preoperative deformity is acceptable, ligamentous stability is required, and no significant joint subluxation can be present. Compared with unicompartmental knee replacement, osteotomy is better suited for the younger patient with higher demands and when extended longevity is required. Although thin patients have better results after osteotomy, any body weight is acceptable. In addition, because motion is less likely to be improved after osteotomy (unlike with unicompartmental knee replacement, in which

TABLE 21B–7
PROGNOSTIC FACTORS FOR ARTHROSCOPIC DÉBRIDEMENT

Prognosis	History	Physical Examination	Radiographic Findings	Arthroscopic Findings
Good	Short duration	Medial tenderness	Unicompartmental	Outerbridge grade I or II
	Associated trauma	Effusion	Normal alignment	Meniscal flap tear
	First arthroscopy	Normal alignment	Minimal Fairbank changes	Chondral fracture/flap
	Mechanical symptoms	Ligaments stable	Loose bodies	Loose bodies
			Relevant osteophytes	Osteophyte at symptom site
Poor	Long duration	Lateral tenderness	Bi-/tricompartmental	Outerbridge grade III or IV
	Insidious onset	No effusion	Malalignment	Degenerative meniscus
	Multiple procedures	Malalignment	Significant Fairbank changes	Diffuse chondrosis
	Rest pain	Varus >10°	Irrelevant osteophytes	Osteophyte away from symptom site
	Litigation	Valgus >15°		
	Work related	Ligaments unstable		

preoperative motion is improved postoperatively), the osteotomy candidate requires at least 90° of motion without flexion contracture. Today, most osteotomy patients are younger individuals with relatively high physical demands. They generally have early arthritis involving a single tibiofemoral compartment, minimal patellofemoral involvement, more than 100° of flexion, no fixed flexion deformity, and no instability or subluxation.

Contraindications to osteotomy include panarthrosis, severe patellofemoral disease, severely restricted range of motion (i.e., extension loss of more than 15° to 20° or flexion <90°), instability, and inflammatory arthritis.

Most proximal tibial osteotomies are performed with a lateral closing wedge with rigid fixation, allowing early mobilization, although recently it has been suggested that opening wedge osteotomy has benefits including the ability to correct biplaner deformities. An advantage of osteotomy is minimal activity restriction because no prosthetic material is used. However, the results of proximal tibial osteotomy are successful only when mechanical alignment is adequately corrected. Compared with unicompartmental arthroplasty, pain relief and motion restoration are not as predictable. Finally, if the osteotomy fails, conversion to a total knee arthroplasty can be more difficult than primary replacement because of secondary deformity and soft tissue scarring.[41]

Valgus Malalignment. Distal femoral osteotomy is indicated for valgus deformity of the knee with lateral compartment arthritis. If significant valgus deformity correction (i.e., >10°) is attempted in the tibia rather than in the distal femur, joint line obliquity will result. Indications, complications, and features of the distal femoral osteotomy are similar to those for varus deformity with unicompartmental arthritis. The procedure is most commonly performed with a medial wedge closing osteotomy in the femur with blade plate fixation. However, a lateral opening wedge approach is commonly used in Europe. Rigid fixation allows early motion. Results are somewhat better than for varus arthrosis treated with tibial osteotomy.

The most common problem with both proximal tibial osteotomy and distal femoral osteotomy is undercorrection leading to inadequate stress transfer to the opposite compartment, resulting in insufficient pain relief. Other common problems are nonunion, malunion, intraarticular fracture, thromboembolic events, and infection. In addition, patella infra or contracture with associated motion loss can occur.

Results of Osteotomy. Coventry[42] determined that 61% of his patients had less pain and 65% had better function 10 years after high tibial osteotomy. Noyes and coworkers[43] noted in a prospective study of 41 patients who underwent high tibial osteotomy that 88% were satisfied at a mean of 58 months postoperatively and would undergo the operation again, and 78% thought that their knee condition was improved by the operation. Nagel and associates[44] concluded that activities that may be inappropriate after total knee arthroplasty (climbing, jumping, impact sports, and jogging) were possible in their patients who were symptomatic but able to perform these activities before osteotomy surgery. In a comparative study by Broughton and

colleagues,[45] only 46% of knees that had proximal tibial osteotomy and 76% of knees that had a unicompartmental replacement maintained a good result at a follow-up of 5 to 10 years.

In a compilation of 1364 cases of proximal tibial osteotomy at up to 10 years of follow-up, 76% had good to excellent results, 19% had fair results, and 14% had poor results. Overall, 60% of the patients were satisfied with their proximal tibial osteotomy after 10 years.[46] However, these results compare poorly with total knee arthroplasty, which may explain why proximal tibial osteotomy has dropped by 10% to 15% per year each year since introduction of total knee replacement and its application to relatively younger patients with unicompartmental OA.

Outcomes of greater than 80% good or excellent results have been reported after the treatment of valgus deformities.[47] Finkelstein and colleagues[48] determined that the probability of symptom relief after a distal femoral varus-producing osteotomy at 19 years was 64%. After this procedure, activity levels are maintained but not improved.

Arthroplasty Versus Osteotomy

Any joint replacement is at risk for mechanical failure and loosening because of heavy or prolonged cyclic loads. Patients who are obese but relatively young and active or heavy laborers should be considered for osteotomy and not for joint arthroplasty. Arthroplasty and osteotomy most reliably relieve pain that is produced by weight-bearing activities. Best results for both procedures are achieved when preoperative rest pain is minimal. Appreciable pain at rest usually indicates that there is an inflammatory process. Patients with unicompartmental disease secondary to inflammatory arthritis, such as rheumatoid arthritis and possibly chondrocalcinosis, are best treated with a total knee arthroplasty because the other compartments may subsequently become involved.

Although proximal tibial osteotomy is still preferred for young, active patients with unicompartmental disease, unicompartmental arthroplasty and total knee arthroplasty have advantages. Compared with proximal tibial osteotomy, arthroplasty has fewer postoperative complications and a higher rate of early and long-term successful results. After knee replacement surgery, a patient is able to walk with a more normal range of motion sooner than after an osteotomy.[45] Arthroplasty has an additional advantage of removing osteophytes, releasing intra-articular adhesions, and improving postoperative range of motion. Lastly, in patients with bilateral disease, arthroplasties can be performed simultaneously or staged during a short period. Conversely, bilateral osteotomies must be done 3 to 6 months apart, leading to a prolonged total recovery period.

Unicompartmental Knee Arthroplasty

Unicompartmental knee replacement for the treatment of OA of the knee has gained increased acceptance. Early reports of the procedure with primitive designs were conflicting, and the efficacy of unicompartmental knee replacements was in doubt; its use has become a more viable alternative for single compartment disease based on improved designs, instruments, and surgical techniques. The 10-year survival rate has been reported as high as 98%.[49-51] Additional reports of unicompartmental knee replacement demonstrate excellent clinical results even after 10 years, stimulating increased interest in this treatment option.[52-54] Reduced implant costs, shorter lengths of hospital stay, and less use of blood products offer additional advantages of unicompartmental knee replacement over total knee replacement.

Compared with both proximal tibial osteotomy and total knee replacement, unicompartmental knee replacement has potential advantages. Unicompartmental knee replacement is a bone stock– and cartilage-preserving procedure. If necessary, a technically well-performed unicompartmental knee replacement can be easily revised to a total knee replacement.

Selection of patients for unicompartmental knee replacement, as with most procedures, is arguably the most important factor to achieve a successful result. Unicompartmental knee replacement is indicated for patients with OA limited primarily to either the medial or the lateral compartment. Selection criteria for unicompartmental knee replacement include the patient's age, weight, and physical demands. Additional criteria are preoperative range of motion and minimal angular deformity. The final determinant is the operative inspection for additional disease in other compartments of the knee that may contraindicate a unicompartmental knee replacement.

The angular deformity of the knee should be between 10° of varus and 15° of valgus. Patients should have a preoperative range of motion of at least 90° of flexion with a minimal flexion contracture (i.e., <5°). The best candidates for a unicompartmental knee arthroplasty are older than 55 years with noninflammatory arthritis who are not obese and who have a relatively low activity level demand. Ultimately, the final decision to perform a unicompartmental knee replacement is made at the time of the surgical inspection of the articular surfaces.

At the time of surgery, both cruciate ligaments should be examined and intact to ensure the best results for a unicompartmental knee replacement. Patellofemoral joint pain is a relative contraindication to unicompartmental knee replacement, but asymptomatic chondromalacia of the patella is not. The opposite tibiofemoral compartment and the patellofemoral joint should have no more than Outerbridge grade II changes. If more extensive disease exists, a unicompartmental replacement should be abandoned and a total knee replacement should be performed.

Another limited arthroplasty approach for medial OA is the UniSpacer implant. However, one recent report after 26 months of follow-up indicates an unacceptable percentage of unsatisfactory results. The procedure does not offer a viable alternative to a standard unicompartmental replacement.[52]

Results of Unicompartmental Knee Replacement. The clinical results of unicompartmental arthroplasty are generally comparable with those of total knee replacement and better than those of osteotomy.[42,52-55] In a prospective study, Mackinnon and colleagues[53] reported that 86% of 115 knees had an excellent or good result after a mean follow-up of 4.8 years. Marmor[52] reported that 70% of 60 consecutive unicompartmental knee replacements had a satisfactory result, and 87% had continued relief of pain 10 to 13 years postoperatively. Sullivan and coworkers[56] described 107 patients in whom only four revisions occurred and 96% had no limitation of activities 5 to 11 years postoperatively. Recent longer term follow-up indicates satisfactory outcomes even in community-based practices. Gioe reported an 89% 10-year survival for 516 knees using nine different designs.[57] Another report describing a newer design, a meniscal bearing unicompartmental arthroplasty, to treat OA of the medial compartment indicated a 10-year survival rate of 95% for 95 knees.[58] All of the studies suggest that patient selection is the key to a successful outcome. In comparing unicompartmental with total knee arthroplasty, many patients who had bilateral procedures report that the knee with the unicompartmental replacement feels better and more normal than the knee with a total replacement. It appears that postoperative range of motion is also greater after unicompartmental replacement compared with total knee replacement.[59]

Total Knee Arthroplasty

Total knee arthroplasty is one of the most successful procedures in orthopedic surgery today. Introduced as a simple concept in the late 1960s by Gunston,[60] it has evolved into a fairly sophisticated procedure. The indications for total knee arthroplasty are well defined and are universally accepted; subsequently, the results have been uniformly excellent. The procedure has met wide acceptance by the orthopedic community as reflected by the steadily increasing number of total knee replacements performed annually in the United States and now exceeds the number of hip replacements by 50%.

Long-term reports of excellent pain relief and function of total knee replacement have now made it the treatment of choice for the most end-stage arthritic conditions of the knee, depending on the patient's age, the extent of disease, and a paucity of indications for alternative procedures. The indications are expanding to include younger patients, otherwise candidates for osteotomy, and older patients, otherwise candidates for unicompartmental knee replacement. In addition, as the results have improved, many surgeons have lowered the age criteria for total knee replacement and have eliminated obesity as a relative contraindication. However, as the population ages (toward an average life expectancy of 84 years for women and 78 years for men), an increasing number of patients may live long enough to see the failure of these knee prostheses. Total knee replacement is readily performed after a failed unicompartmental arthroplasty if standard bone-sparing cuts are made during the original implantation and if the holes for fixation with cement do not deeply invade the condylar bone stock.

The recent introduction of minimally invasive total knee replacement techniques has sparked considerable debate concerning the value of this procedure. The early reports[61,62] suggest that the early recovery of the patient is accelerated; however, by 1 year after surgery, there are no significant differences compared to standard surgical techniques. Computer-assisted surgery also has been introduced as an adjunctive technique to enhance the implantation of total knee components in optimal alignment.[63] The early experience is optimistic, but additional developmental work is required to establish the role of computer assistance in total knee arthroplasty.

Results of Total Knee Arthroplasty. Total knee arthroplasty provides reliable pain relief and improved function for patients with degenerative and inflammatory arthritis of the knee. Implant survival is reported to be greater than 94% at 10 years.[64–67] Longer various series report that, at least in the short term, the results of cemented total knee arthroplasty in young patients are comparable to those for the general population.[68–72]

Studies of total knee arthroplasty comparing cemented and cementless fixation in patients of all ages reveal no significant difference in the clinical results at short-term follow-up.[73–75] Similarly excellent results have been reported in several series of cementless tibial and femoral components with minimal follow-up ranging from 24 to 108 months.[76–80] Longer follow-ups indicated a 97% survival at 11 years in very active patients.[81] Even at 18 years, the survival rates for cementless components have been 98% in one report.[82]

With the use of aseptic loosening of the femoral or tibial component as the endpoint, Whiteside[76] reported that a 10-year survivorship was 99.5%. Rosenberg and associates[83] prospectively compared 139 cemented and 132 cementless Miller-Galante total knee arthroplasties with a minimum of 3 years of follow-up and found no differences in the results. However, longer term follow up demonstrated a significantly higher incidence of revision for peri-prosthetic osteolysis. This reflects a common finding, long term fixation of the implant has in general less of a problem than the development of osteolysis generated by the response to particulate debris, which may be the result of primary and secondary polyethylene bearing wear. These studies demonstrate that both cemented fixation and cementless fixation for total knee arthroplasty provide excellent functional and durable results. Continued follow-up will answer the question of which fixation is preferred for the younger patient.

Knee Arthrodesis

Because of the reproducibly excellent results with total knee arthroplasty compared with the dysfunction of a knee arthrodesis (knee fusion), arthrodesis is no longer routinely considered a primary treatment of the arthritic knee. The disabilities that follow knee arthrodesis include increased energy and oxygen consumption during ambulation, hip circumduction during stair climbing, difficulties in sitting, and difficulty using foot controls for driving. However, in rare cases, knee arthrodesis is still a viable option, particularly in the youngest, most active patient. In the patient in whom arthroplasty is not possible owing to the unreconstructable bone, soft tissue, or extensor mechanism loss, knee fusion may provide better results than arthroplasty. In addition, loss of tissue compliance, a significant risk factor for postoperative ankylosis after arthroplasty, may be an indication for arthrodesis. Last, arthrodesis may be the only viable treatment of persistent sepsis. Today, the most common indication for knee arthrodesis is for salvage of the failed, usually infected, total knee replacement.

Management of the Focal Chondral Defect

An estimated 900,000 Americans suffer cartilage injuries each year.[84] In an attempt to delineate the prevalence of chondral lesions, Curl and associates[85] reviewed 31,516 arthroscopies during a 4-year period. They noted 53,569 articular cartilage lesions in 19,827 patients. Lesions amenable to some form of cartilage restoration technique are ideally full thickness and located on the weight-bearing surface of the femoral condyle. In patients younger than 40 years, full-thickness lesions of the femur were present in only 5% of all arthroscopies.[85] Clinical studies relative to cartilage restoration are described elsewhere in this text, as are concepts related to cartilage injury and repair (see Chapters 19 and 23). A brief review of the issues will be discussed here.

Isolated superficial cartilage injuries that do not penetrate the vascular subchondral bone do not heal and may enlarge for several years after the initial injury, potentially leading to overt degenerative arthritis. Full-thickness cartilage injuries that penetrate the more vascular subchondral bone permit local access to an undifferentiated cell pool ("primitive mesenchymal stem cells") capable of forming fibrocartilage or "scar cartilage." Fibrocartilage is composed predominantly of type I collagen and is biochemically and mechanically inferior to normal hyaline articular cartilage composed predominantly of type II collagen. Fibrocartilage formation is the biologic basis of marrow-stimulating techniques commonly used to treat symptomatic full-thickness cartilage defects.

Full thickness defects of the femoral cartilage typically result from shear stress due to a twisting injury, and patellofemoral joint lesions result from direct trauma to the front of the knee. The natural history of an asymptomatic full-thickness cartilage defect and the relationship to the development of secondary degenerative changes typically seen in OA are poorly understood. However, lesions that become symptomatic will inexorably progress, leading to degenerative changes typical of OA with the development of reciprocal changes at the opposing articular surface.[86–89] The ultimate goal of any surgical option used to treat articular cartilage defects is to restore the joint surface, leading to a knee with a full range of painless motion with the hope of halting cartilage degeneration. Conceptually, surgical options differ on the basis of their ability to be palliative (arthroscopic débridement and lavage), reparative (marrow-stimulating techniques), or restorative (autologous chondrocyte implantation and osteochondral grafts obtained from the patient [autografts] or from cadaveric donors [allografts]). Arthroscopic débridement and lavage is discussed earlier because most literature to date reflects outcomes that follow the treatment of established OA and not the isolated focal chondral defect.

Determining the appropriate surgical option is a complex process and is the topic of a comprehensive review by Cole and associates.[90] Decision making is related to the size of the defect (smaller or larger than 2 cm²), the number and type of previous surgeries (primary or secondary), the location of the defect (femoral condyle, trochlea, or patella), the patient's demands and expectations, and any coexisting pathologic change (e.g., ligament tears, malalignment) (Table 21B–8).

Reparative Treatment Options

Marrow-Stimulating Techniques. Unlike partial-thickness cartilage injuries that do not extend to the underlying bone, full-thickness cartilage injuries can undergo some

TABLE 21B–8
SURGICAL TREATMENT OPTIONS FOR THE SYMPTOMATIC FOCAL CARTILAGE DEFECT

Lesion	Treatment	Rehabilitation*	Comments
PRIMARY TREATMENT			
<2 cm^2	Débridement and lavage	Straightforward	Provides short-term symptomatic relief
	Marrow stimulation technique (MST)	Significant	Ideal for smaller lesions located on the femoral condyle; provides intermediate-term relief; low cost
	Osteochondral autograft	Moderate	Relatively new procedure; probably as good as if not better than MST; provides potentially long-term relief
>2 cm^2	Débridement and lavage	Straightforward	Provides short-term symptomatic relief
	Marrow stimulation technique	Significant	Has lower success rate for larger lesions; good choice for symptomatic relief in low-demand individuals; intermediate-term relief is possible; low cost
	Cartilage biopsy for future autologous chondrocyte implantation	Straightforward	Staged procedure
	Osteochondral autograft	Significant	With larger lesions, potential for donor site morbidity exists; results are variable
	Osteochondral allograft	Significant	Useful for larger lesions with significant bone stock loss; small concern for disease transmission and allograft availability; provides potentially long-term relief
SECONDARY TREATMENT †			
<2 cm^2	Osteochondral autograft	Moderate	Relatively new procedure; probably as good as if not better than MST; provides potentially long-term relief
	Autologous chondrocyte implantation	Significant	High success rate for return to activities; potentially long-term relief; relatively high cost
>2 cm^2	Osteochondral autograft	Significant	With larger lesions, potential for donor site morbidity exists; results are variable
	Osteochondral allograft	Significant	Useful for larger lesions with significant bone stock loss; small concern for disease transmission and allograft availability; provides potentially long-term relief
	Autologous chondrocyte implantation	Significant	High success rate for return to activities; potentially long-term relief; relatively high cost

*Straightforward: early weight bearing and return to activities within 4 weeks; moderate: short-term protected weight bearing and return to activities within 12 weeks; significant: prolonged protected weight bearing and significant delay until return to activities (6 to 8 months).
†Follows failed primary treatment.
From Cole BJ, Fredericks RW, Levy AS, et al. Management of a 35-year-old male with recurrent knee pain. J Clin Outcomes Management 5:46–57, 1999.

degree of repair from marrow-derived primitive mesenchymal stem cell migration and vascular ingrowth.[91] This limited capacity to form repair cartilage provides the rationale for marrow-stimulating techniques. Despite a variety of techniques (abrasion arthroplasty, subchondral drilling, and microfracture), the common goal is to penetrate the subchondral zone of vascularization within the cartilage defect, allowing a conduit and site for clot formation containing mesenchymal stem cells capable of forming fibrocartilage repair tissue.[39,89,92] Postoperatively, partial weight bearing may be required for a time with the use of continuous passive motion to enhance the extent and quality of the repair tissue within the defect.[93,94] Authors have cited symptom relief in about two thirds of patients at 2 to 3 years of follow-up.[39,89,92] One report of longer follow-up indicated that even at 7 years, 80% of the patients were satisfied with the procedure.[95] Results may deteriorate with time, however, because fibrocartilage is biochemically (i.e., predominantly type I collagen) and biomechanically inferior to normal articular cartilage.

Restorative (Transplantation) Treatment Options

Autologous Chondrocyte Implantation. Autologous chondrocyte implantation is a technique that biologically resurfaces the knee in the presence of focal cartilage damage. With autologous chondrocyte implantation, the cartilage defect in the knee joint is repaired with the patient's own healthy cartilage cells originally harvested through an arthroscopic procedure from a separate, minor load-bearing area in the knee. These cells are expanded and transformed into biologically active cells through cell culturing techniques and subsequently implanted during a second procedure. At the time of implantation, a small arthrotomy (incision) is made in the knee, and the cells are injected beneath a periosteal (the soft tissue covering bone) patch obtained from the upper tibia that is sewn over the defect.

Research indicates that this repair tissue looks and acts more like the normal hyaline articular cartilage than does the fibrocartilage formed with the marrow-stimulating techniques. Outcomes of this procedure are discussed in Chapter 23.

Osteochondral Autografts and Allografts. In the technique of osteochondral plugs or mosaicplasty, small dowels of bone and cartilage are taken from a non–weight-bearing portion of the femoral trochlea and press-fit into a recipient hole made by removal of the cartilage defect. This is analogous to a hair-plug transplant, and is a relatively successful means to manage small areas of cartilage damage on the weight-bearing portion of the medial or lateral femoral condyle. Similarly, larger areas of bone and cartilage loss can be managed with fresh or fresh-frozen bulk allografts, but the risk of disease transmission and immune response remains a concern. Authors report good and excellent results in at least 75% between 2 and 10 years of follow-up.[96–101]

Allograft Meniscal Transplantation

In patients who are meniscal deficient, implanting a meniscus is potentially an ideal solution before progressive arthritis ensues. Meniscus transplantation is indicated in patients with prior meniscectomy, persistent pain, intact cartilage or low-grade arthrosis (< Outerbridge grade III), normal alignment, and a stable joint. Ligament reconstruction or realignment procedures are performed simultaneously or in a staged fashion as indicated.

A cryopreserved or fresh-frozen meniscus is size matched to the patient's plain radiographs, taking magnification into account. The procedure is typically performed by an arthroscopically assisted approach with a small arthrotomy to place the meniscus into the joint. The meniscus is anchored by either a bone block (laterally) or bone plugs (medially), and repair is performed by standard meniscal repair techniques (Fig. 21B–3). To date, several reports of good and excellent results exist in the literature. A series by Cameron and Saha[102] described 63 patients with greater than 85% good and excellent results at a mean follow-up of 31 months. Other authors have reported similar results during similar time periods and indicate that allograft meniscus transplantation has a role

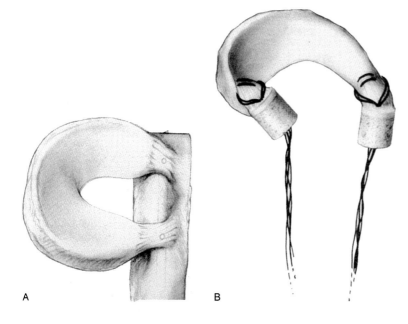

A   B

Figure 21B–3 Examples of prepared meniscus allograft before placement. *A,* Lateral meniscus based on a bone block, maintaining the closeness of the anterior and posterior horns. *B,* Medial meniscus based on separate bone plugs.

in this population of difficult patients improving function and reducing pain.[103-107]

PATELLOFEMORAL JOINT DISORDERS

Patellofemoral disorders encompass a large differential diagnosis including but not limited to nonarthritic (nonpatellofemoral) causes of anterior knee pain, patellofemoral malalignment, and patellofemoral arthritis. Diagnosis and treatment of nonpatellofemoral causes of anterior knee pain are challenging and directed toward the specific pathologic process in question. Patellofemoral malalignment and arthritis require accurate diagnosis to predicate a treatment plan. Rehabilitation focusing on the extensor mechanism, if unsuccessful, may lead to one of several realignment-type procedures. The term *chondromalacia patellae* as defined by Outerbridge[108] describes the pathologic changes often occurring concomitantly with patellofemoral pain. It should not be used as a synonym for anterior knee pain or patellofemoral symptoms.

Biomechanics of the Patellofemoral Joint

Soft tissue stabilizers of the patellofemoral joint circumferentially converge on the patella and include 1) cephalad, the quadriceps tendon; 2) distal, the patellar tendon; 3) medial, the vastus medialis obliquus (VMO), retinaculum, and patellofemoral ligament; and 4) lateral, the vastus lateralis tendon, retinaculum, and iliotibial band. The medial patellofemoral ligament is the major restraint to lateral displacement (53%). Capsular thickenings, patellomeniscal ligaments (Kaplan ligaments), are thought to be the cause of referred joint line pain in patellofemoral disorders. Nociceptive pain fibers within the lateral retinaculum are believed to be a cause of anterior and patellofemoral knee pain.[109]

Normal function of the patellofemoral joint depends on the intrinsic balance between lower extremity alignment and static (retinaculum, bone anatomy, Q angle) and dynamic (VMO) stabilizers. The patella increases the moment arm (the distance between the extensor mechanism and the center of the knee), increasing quadriceps strength by one third to one half. Large forces as much as seven times body weight are generated across the patellofemoral joint. Coronal (lateral) plane contact forces are greatest at low flexion angles (<30°). In general, sagittal (posterior) plane patellofemoral contact forces increase with knee flexion between 0° and 90°.

The quadriceps angle (Q angle) is defined in extension as the angle between the line of pull of the quadriceps (anterior superior iliac spine to center of patella) and patellar (center of patella to center of tibial tubercle) tendons (Fig. 21B–4). Angles greater than 20° are considered abnormal, reflecting a net lateral moment during quadriceps contraction. The lateral moment is normally counteracted by the VMO and static restraints. Measurement of the tubercle-sulcus Q angle (the relative position of the tibial tubercle to the inferior pole of the patella at 90°) is preferred by many because it accounts for the effects of

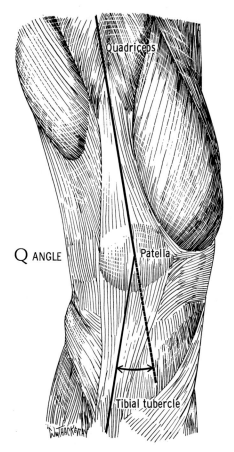

Figure 21B–4 Quadriceps angle (Q angle). The Q angle is formed by the intersection of the quadriceps tendon vector and the patellar tendon vector. More than 20° is considered abnormal. (From Insall JN. Surgery of the Knee. New York, Churchill Livingstone, 1984, p 195.)

malalignment. Angles greater than 8° to 10° are consistent with a lateralized distal patella vector primarily due to malalignment.

Clinical Evaluation

Patients with anterior knee pain and patellofemoral dysfunction often present with a history of direct trauma, patellar subluxation, or dislocation. Pain is often poorly localized and described as a dull ache exacerbated by prolonged sitting ("movie sign") or stair climbing, and it is often bilateral and of insidious onset. Pain locations most commonly include anteromedial, retropatellar, and posterior. Pain in long-standing patellofemoral disease may be from soft tissue contractures, lateral retinacular pain fibers, and arthrosis.

Giving way of the knee may occur with patellar instability or be secondary to painful quadriceps inhibition, unlike that occurring secondary to ligamentous instability in which the knee "comes apart." Patellofemoral crepitus, although often bothersome to the patient, is not commonly associated with pain and should not be overtreated. Sources of patellofemoral crepitus include malalignment, synovium, quadriceps tendon irritation, and chondrosis.

Patients may complain of a catching sensation during active extension. Swelling implies intra-articular disease and is less common with anterior knee pain than with patellofemoral arthrosis.

Physical Examination

In addition to tests specific for patellofemoral disorders (discussed later, later), the patellofemoral physical examination should include tests necessary to establish other pathologic conditions that may coexist as described previously.

Patients should be observed and evaluated for hindfoot pronation, external tibial torsion, genu valgum, femoral anteversion (hip internal rotation), gynecoid pelvis, flexion contractures, and patellar subluxation. The Q angle is measured in extension and flexion.

The knee is palpated for effusions and tenderness in all anterior knee structures including the extensor mechanism, medial and lateral patellar facets (arthrosis), retinaculum, epicondyles, iliotibial band, pes anserinus, joint line, and fat pad. Flexibility, strength, and crepitus should be assessed for side-to-side differences. Crepitus may be indicative of chondromalacia. Patellofemoral joint compression with the palm of the hand may re-create symptoms. Crepitus alone, however, does not confirm patellofemoral dysfunction.

Several special tests are used in evaluating the patellofemoral joint. The *lateral pull sign* occurs when VMO insufficiency leads to disproportionate superolateral pull of the patella with quadriceps contraction with the knee in extension. The *J sign*, which occurs with patellofemoral malalignment, is demonstrated by persistent lateral patellar movement with active flexion rather than the normal inferomedial movement. The *passive patellar tilt test* is performed with the knee in full extension to assess for side-to-side differences in the ability to elevate the lateral edge of the patella. The inability to elevate the lateral edge of the patella beyond neutral (i.e., parallel to the floor) is consistent with a tight lateral retinaculum (negative tilt). The *patellar glide test* is performed with the knee in 30° of flexion to engage the patella into the trochlear groove. The patella can normally be displaced medially or laterally by 50% without pain or apprehension (subjective feeling that the patella will dislocate). *Patellofemoral apprehension* is determined with the knee in 30° to 45° of flexion, with firm pressure applied to the medial edge of the patella, attempting to displace it laterally.[110] Abnormal findings are consistent either with patellofemoral instability (i.e., apprehension) or with excessive lateral compression syndrome or a tight lateral retinaculum.

Diagnostic Aids

Radiographic Evaluation

Radiographic evaluation of the knee is described previously. Specific views exist to evaluate the patellofemoral joint. Lateral displacement of the patella may be normal from 0° to 20° of flexion. Excessive patellar tilt is best demonstrated at 20° to 30° of flexion using Laurin's view.[111]

Subluxation decreases from 0° to 30° of flexion and is best measured using Merchant's view taken at 45° of knee flexion.[22] Lateral facet arthrosis is seen as subchondral sclerosis, cyst formation, perpendicular trabeculae, facet collapse, lateral margin patellar osteophytes or fractures, and calcification within the lateral retinaculum. Medial facet osteoporosis may also be present from relative patellofemoral joint stress shielding. A sunrise view is taken with the knee flexed to 60° to 90° such that the x-ray beam is tangential to the patellofemoral joint to image most of the femoral condyles. This view is helpful for the demonstration of patellar fractures, dislocations, loose bodies, and articular irregularities, but it is not particularly helpful in the evaluation of patellofemoral malalignment.

Computed Tomography

Detection of patellofemoral malalignment is more sensitive earlier in flexion before the patella engages in the trochlea. Midpatellar transverse computed tomographic (CT) scans performed in 15°, 30°, and 45° of flexion prevent the image overlap or distortion seen in plain radiographs. A CT scan demonstrates subluxation (a congruence angle with the central ridge of the patella well medial to the bisected trochlea) and tilt (lateral patellofemoral tilt angle of more than 12°) more accurately when these measures are referenced from the posterior condyles of the femur.

Diagnosis and Treatment Options

Nonpatellofemoral Causes of Anterior Knee Pain

Common to the many causes of anterior and patellofemoral pain are quadriceps atrophy, weakness, and chronic effusions. Radiographic evaluation is used to rule out malalignment and unsuspected bone disease. Evaluation and treatment are problem specific and include a specific differential diagnosis (Table 21B–9).

TABLE 21B–9
NONPATELLOFEMORAL CAUSES OF ANTERIOR KNEE PAIN

Plica
Tendinitis
Bursitis
Fat pad syndrome
Chronic effusion/synovitis
Iliotibial band friction syndrome
Tumorous conditions
Referred pain
Patellar osteochondritis dissecans
Saphenous neuralgia and varices
Cruciate ligament insufficiency
Adolescent anterior knee pain
Reflex sympathetic dystrophy

Patellofemoral Disorders

The term *patellar instability* is specific to patients with a history of lateral subluxation or dislocation, but it may also include patients with excessive lateral compression syndrome. Articular damage is a common sequela of long-standing patellar tilt and recurrent instability. A history of trauma, effusion, and crepitus with reproduction of symptoms with patellofemoral compression is common.

Operative treatment assumes that at least 3 months of nonoperative treatment has failed. Treatment of patellofemoral instability includes lateral release, proximal realignment, and medial tubercle transfer. Treatment of articular degeneration includes chondroplasty, tubercle elevation, patellectomy, and arthroplasty. In general, tubercle elevation reduces sagittal plane forces, and lateral release, proximal realignment, and medialization of the tubercle reduce coronally directed forces. Combinations of these procedures should be used when appropriate.

There are a number of problems that may predispose the patellofemoral articulation to arthrosis. These include excessive lateral compression syndrome with patellar tilt and overt patellofemoral instability. Patients usually complain of activity-related anterior knee pain, with or without a shifting of the patella during rotational activities. Physical and radiological signs reflect abnormal patellofemoral orientation. Treatment options include arthroscopy, débridement, lateral release, medial tubercle transfer, and anteromedialization of the tubercle. Often these procedures are combined with tightening of the medial soft tissue structure.

Patellofemoral Instability. This is a spectrum of patellofemoral disease ranging from patellar subluxation to frank dislocation. Patients typically present with complaints that the patella shifts laterally during cutting maneuvers and often relate a history of direct patellofemoral trauma. On physical examination, patients present with apprehension to lateral translation of the patella in full extension, increased lateral patellar glide, and negative patellar tilt with lateral retinacular tightness.

Patellofemoral Arthrosis. Patients with patellofemoral arthrosis may have a history of both direct patellofemoral trauma and chronic instability with malalignment. Patients complain primarily of pain while stair climbing and with active extension. On physical examination, patients may demonstrate malalignment, retropatellar crepitus exacerbated by posteriorly directed palmar pressure, facet tenderness, and effusion. Patellar arthrosis is best seen on axial and lateral radiographs, and bone scans show increased uptake within the patellofemoral joint. Treatment options include arthroscopic débridement, tibial tubercle anteromedialization, patellectomy, and arthroplasty.

Rehabilitation for Patellofemoral Disorders

Symptomatic patellofemoral pain is successfully managed in most patients with nonoperative means. Individualized and pain-free rehabilitation is performed for at least 3 months before surgical intervention is considered. Variations of this protocol are used for postoperative rehabilitation with relative protection of surgical reconstructions.

Phase I. Goals for phase I rehabilitation are to reduce inflammation and effusion (nonsteroidal anti-inflammatory drugs, multimodality physical therapy); to improve VMO control of patellar tracking, flexibility, and soft tissue stretching; and to correct soft tissue imbalances by McConnell taping techniques. Patellar sleeves or dynamic braces are controversial but sometimes helpful.

Phase II. Supervised isotonic eccentric and concentric strengthening is prescribed with emphasis on muscle endurance and adduction facilitating VMO contraction. Closed chain exercises in extension and open chain exercises in flexion are emphasized while avoiding isokinetics.

Phase III. Proprioceptive and sport-specific functional training is encouraged with the use of plyometrics, aquatics, running, and agility drills.

Operative Approaches for Patellofemoral Disorders

Figure 21B–5 represents a three-arm algorithm for surgical decision making should conservative measures fail to resolve the patient's symptoms. Procedure selection is based on the degree of articular arthrosis and the presence of patellofemoral malalignment.

Diagnostic Arthroscopy. The goal of diagnostic arthroscopy is to define the specific pathologic process, facilitating definitive treatment; it is generally considered an adjunct to additional procedures. At the time of arthroscopy, chondral débridement of patellofemoral arthrosis is performed to judiciously remove unstable chondral flaps with occasional use of marrow-stimulating techniques (e.g., microfracture) when it is considered appropriate. The best results are with isolated patellar chondromalacia or traumatic focal chondral defects.

Lateral Release. The goals of the lateral release are to relieve posterolateral patellar tether and tilt, to decrease lateral facet stress, to improve congruence in combination with other realignment procedures, and to improve dynamic VMO function. The primary indication for lateral release is for isolated patellar tilt (i.e., excessive lateral compression syndrome), minimal patellar subluxation, low-grade arthrosis, minimal patellar hypermobility, and nearly normal Q angle. Success rates of 85% to 90% are seen in properly chosen patients.[112] Long-term results deteriorate with higher grades of chondrosis, patellar instability, and hypermobility. Complications include hemarthrosis, infection, reflex sympathetic dystrophy, arthrofibrosis, neuroma, medial subluxation of the patella, and worsened pain without evidence of tilt.[113] Increased contact pressures on the distal medial patellar facet in the presence of articular lesions may cause crepitus after lateral release.

Proximal Realignment. The goals of a proximal realignment are to increase the static posteromedial restraint to limit patellar subluxation. Proximal realignment has only a minor and unproven benefit in altering dynamic restraints to patellofemoral stability. The Q angle is not altered, but patellofemoral incongruence is corrected. The indications

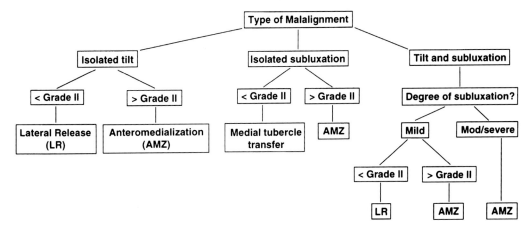

Figure 21B–5 Algorithm for surgical treatment of patellofemoral malalignment and arthritis. (From Post WR. Surgical decision making in patellofemoral pain and instability. Oper Tech Sports Med 2:280, 1994.)

are a need for greater static restraint (i.e., preoperative subluxation) in the presence of lateral tilt when a lateral release alone is thought to be insufficient. Combined with lateral release, proximal realignment offers no clear benefit to lateral release alone.[114] Complications include quadriceps dysfunction, phlebitis, hematoma, arthrofibrosis, recurrent instability, and potentially increased medial patellofemoral contact stress when it is performed in isolation.

Distal Realignment Procedures. In general, as the tibial tubercle is osteotomized and translated medially, more effective prevention of patellofemoral instability results. When the tubercle is translated anteriorly, more effective unloading of the patellofemoral joint results. Thus, a spectrum of distal realignment procedures exists.[115] These include straight medial tubercle transfer and tubercle anteromedialization with or without elevation. The indications for each procedure depend on the extent of patellofemoral instability and the degree of arthrosis.

Each of these procedures demonstrates between 70% and 90% excellent or good results in patients who are appropriately selected.[115] Complications of distal realignment procedures include inadvertent posterior tubercle displacement, increasing patellofemoral contact force, and arthrosis. Anteromedialization may cause proximal medial patellar pain if lesions exist there. Inadequate correction, nonunion, infection, arthrofibrosis, recurrent instability, skin necrosis, and growth arrest in the skeletally immature have all been reported.

Patellectomy. The principal goal of a patellectomy is to relieve pain with relative improvement in overall function. It is indicated for severe pain from extensive articular lesions limiting quadriceps function and not otherwise amenable to distal realignment. The results are between 33% and 60% good and excellent at follow-up beyond 5 years.[116,117] Complications include strength deficits of 30% to 50% with symptoms of giving way.

Patellofemoral Arthroplasty. The goal of patellofemoral arthroplasty is to relieve pain with relative improvement in overall function. It is indicated for isolated patellofemoral

arthritis in elderly individuals or patients with low physical demands. There are no strict age criteria. It should be avoided in patients with significant uncorrectable patellar maltracking. Further, if tibiofemoral arthrosis is present, the arthroplasty should not be performed. Most commonly, total joint replacement is performed because only limited success is documented for isolated patellofemoral arthroplasty. Reports demonstrate up to 85% good or excellent results at 2 to 17 years of follow-up.[118-120] Complications include loosening, wear, and infection.

SUMMARY

Knee arthritis in the active individual is common. It can be disabling, compromising activities of daily living and participation in sports. Carefully prescribed treatment with nonoperative modalities such as medications, activity modification, and physical therapy is often successful but palliative in nature. Once it is symptomatic, OA usually progresses. Arthroscopy is performed only with a clear understanding of the prognostic factors determining success and failure. Osteotomy of the tibia or femur is an excellent alternative when deformity and symptoms coexist, especially when it is performed early in the disease process. Unicompartmental arthroplasty has an important place in the contemporary treatment algorithm. Total knee arthroplasty is the last alternative and is considered when all other options have been exhausted; however, it is not performed with the expectation that patients will return to high-impact activities. Today, arthrodesis is rarely performed. In selected cases, meniscus transplantation may prevent or delay the need for more definitive procedures such as arthroplasty. Combining procedures that address a combination of meniscal and articular cartilage disease to prevent progressive arthrosis is likely to become more commonplace as indications and results become better defined.

Anterior knee pain may have a variety of causes, only some of which are due to patellofemoral disorders (e.g., malalignment, arthrosis). Diagnosis and treatment are difficult and are predicated on a systematic history and physical examination. Radiographic evaluation may offer additional information for diagnosis and treatment of patellofemoral disorders. Chondromalacia should not be used as a substitute term to describe anterior knee or patellofemoral pain. Performing a lateral release as a panacea for all conditions presenting with anterior knee pain is to be condemned. Rigorous attempts at rehabilitation are usually successful. In the event that surgical intervention is required, malalignment (tilt, instability) and arthrosis must be completely evaluated and addressed by the chosen procedure.

REFERENCES

1. Hannan M, Anderson J, Zhang Y, et al. Bone mineral density and knee osteoarthritis in elderly men and women. The Framingham Study. Arthritis Rheum 36:1671–1680, 1993.
2. van Saase J, van Romunde L, Cats A, et al. Epidemiology of osteoarthritis: Zoetermeer survey. Comparison of radiological osteoarthritis in a Dutch population with that in 10 other populations. Ann Rheum Dis 48:271–280, 1989.
3. Chang R, Falconer J, Stulberg S, et al. A randomized, controlled trial of arthroscopic surgery versus closed-needle joint lavage for patients with osteoarthritis of the knee. Arthritis Rheum 36:289–296, 1993.
4. King D. The function of semilunar cartilages. J Bone Joint Surg Am 18:1069–1076, 1936.
5. Daniel D, Stone M, Dobson B, et al. Fate of the ACL-injured patient. A prospective outcome study. Am J Sports Med 22:632–644, 1994.
6. Rangger C, Klestil T, Gloetzer W, et al. Osteoarthritis after arthroscopic partial meniscectomy. Am J Sports Med 23:240–244, 1995.
7. Messner K, Maletius W. The long-term prognosis for severe damage to weight-bearing cartilage in the knee. Acta Orthop Scand 67:165–168, 1996.
8. Maletius W, Karola M. The effect of partial meniscectomy on the long-term prognosis of knees with localized, severe chondral damage. A twelve- to fifteen-year followup. Am J Sports Med 24:258–262, 1996.
9. Felson D. The epidemiology of knee and hip osteoarthritis. Epidemiol Rev 10:1–28, 1988.
10. Spector T, Harris P, Hart D, et al. Risk of osteoarthritis associated with long-term weight bearing sports: a radiologic survey of the hips and knees in female ex-athletes and population controls. Arthritis Rheum 39:988–995, 1996.
11. Konradsen L, Hansen E-MB, Sondergaard L. Long distance running and osteoarthrosis. Am J Sports Med 18:379–381, 1990.
12. Felson D, Zhang Y, Naimark A, et al. Weight loss reduces the risk for symptomatic osteoarthritis in women: the Framingham study. Ann Intern Med 116:535–539, 1992.
13. Seedhom B, Wright V. Functions of the menisci—a preliminary study. J Bone Joint Surg Br 56:381–382, 1974.
14. Dandy D, Jackson R. The diagnosis of problems after meniscectomy. J Bone Joint Surg Br 57:349–352, 1975.
15. Johnson R, Kettelkamp D, Clark W, et al. Factors affecting late results after meniscectomy. J Bone Joint Surg Am 56:719–729, 1974.
16. Sommerlath K, Gillquist J. The long-term course of various meniscal treatments in anterior cruciate ligament deficient knees. Clin Orthop 283:207–214, 1992.
17. Port J, DiGioia A, Kwoh C, et al. A technique for valgus high tibial osteotomy. J Am Knee Surg 6:135–144, 1993.
18. Moreland J, Bassett L, Hanker G. Radiographic analysis of the axial alignment of the lower extremity. J Bone Joint Surg Am 69:745–749, 1987.
19. Lohmander L. Markers of cartilage metabolism in arthrosis. A review. Acta Orthop Scand 62:623–632, 1991.
20. McMurray T. The semilunar cartilages. J Bone Joint Surg Br 29:407, 1941.
21. Rosenberg T, Paulos L, Oarker R, et al. The 45-degree PA flexion weightbearing radiograph of the knee. J Bone Joint Surg Am 70:1479–1483, 1988.
22. Merchant A, Mercer R, Jacobsen R, et al. Roentgenographic analysis of patellofemoral congruence. J Bone Joint Surg Am 56:1391–1396, 1972.
23. Fairbank T. Knee joint changes after meniscectomy. J Bone Joint Surg Br 30:664–670, 1948.
24. Heron C, Calvert P. Three-dimensional gradient-echo MR imaging of the knee: comparison with arthroscopy in 100 patients. Radiology 183:839–844, 1992.
25. Dye S, Chew M. The use of scintigraphy to detect increased osseous metabolic activity about the knee. J Bone Joint Surg Am 75:1388–1406, 1993.
26. Doherty M, Richards N, Hornby J, et al. Relationship between synovial fluid C3 degradation products and local joint inflammation in rheumatoid arthritis, osteoarthritis and crystal associated arthropathy. Ann Rheum Dis 47:190–197, 1988.
27. Livesley P, Doherty M, Needoff M, et al. Arthroscopic lavage of osteoarthritic knees. J Bone Joint Surg Br 73:922–926, 1991.
28. Edelson R, Burks R, Bloebaum RD. Short-term effects of knee washout for osteoarthritis. Am J Sports Med 23:345–349, 1995.
29. Jackson R, Rouse D. The results of partial arthroscopic meniscectomy in patients over 40 years of age. J Bone Joint Surg Br 64:481–485, 1982.
30. Gibson J, White M, Chapman V, et al. Arthroscopic lavage and débridement for osteoarthritis of the knee. J Bone Joint Surg Br 74:534–537, 1992.
31. Puddu G, Cipolla M, Cerullo G, et al. Arthroscopic treatment of the flexed arthritic knee in active middle-aged patients. Knee Surg Sports Traumatol Arthrosc 2:73–75, 1994.
32. Merchant E, Galindo E. Arthroscopic-guided surgery versus nonoperative treatment for limited degenerative osteoarthritis of the femorotibial joint in patients over 50 years of age: a prospective study. Arthroscopy 9:663–667, 1993.
33. Wouters E, Bassett FI, Hardaker W, et al. An algorithm for arthroscopy in the over-50 age group. Am J Sports Med 20:141–145, 1992.
34. Yang S, Nisonson B. Arthroscopic surgery of the knee in the geriatric patient. Clin Orthop 316:50–58, 1995.
35. Bonamo J, Kessler K, Noah J. Arthroscopic meniscectomy in patients over the age of 40. Am J Sports Med 20:422–428, 1992.
36. Moseley JB, O'Malley K, Petersen NJ, et al. A controlled trial of arthroscopic surgery for osteoarthritis of the knee. N Engl J Med 34;7:81–88, 2002.
37. Aaron RD, Skolnick AH, Reinert SE, et al. Arthroscopic debridement for osteoarthritis of the knee. J Bone Joint Surg Am 88:936–943, 2006.
38. Bert J, Maschka K. The arthroscopic treatment of unicompartmental gonarthrosis: a five-year follow-up study of abrasion arthroplasty plus arthroscopic débridement and arthroscopic débridement alone. Arthroscopy 5:25–32, 1989.
39. Steadman J, Rodkey W, Singleton S, et al. Microfracture technique for full-thickness chondral defects: technique and clinical results. Op Tech Orthop 7:300–304, 1997.
40. Blackburn W, Bernreuter W, Rominger M, et al. Arthroscopic evaluation of knee articular cartilage. A comparison with plain radiographs and magnetic resonance imaging. J Rheumatol 21:675–679, 1994.
41. Katz M, Hungerford D, Krackow K, et al. Results of total knee arthroplasty after failed proximal tibial osteotomy for osteoarthritis. J Bone Joint Surg Am 69:225–233, 1987.
42. Coventry M. Upper tibial osteotomy for gonarthrosis. The evolution of the operation in the last 18 years and long term results. Orthop Clin North Am 10:191–210, 1979.
43. Noyes F, Barber S, Simon R. High tibial osteotomy and ligament reconstruction in varus angulated, anterior cruciate ligament–deficient knees. Am J Sports Med 21:2–12, 1993.
44. Nagel A, Insall J, Scuderi G. Proximal tibial osteotomy. J Bone Joint Surg Am 78:1353–1357, 1996.
45. Broughton N, Newman J, Baily R. Unicompartmental replacement and high tibial osteotomy for osteoarthritis of the knee. A

comparative study after 5–10 years follow-up. J Bone Joint Surg Br 63:447–452, 1985.

46. Hernigou P, Medevielle D, Debeyre J, et al. Proximal tibial osteotomy for osteoarthritis with varus deformity. A ten- to thirteen-year follow-up study. J Bone Joint Surg Am 69:332–353, 1987.

47. Healy W, Anglen J, Wasilewski S, et al. Distal femoral varus osteotomy. J Bone Joint Surg Am 70:1348–1352, 1996.

48. Finkelstein A, Gross A, Davis A. Varus osteotomy of the distal part of the femur: a survivorship analysis. J Bone Joint Surg Am 78:1348–1352, 1996.

49. Berger RA, Meneghini RM, Jacobs JJ, et al. Results of unicompartmental knee arthroplasty at a minimum of ten years of follow-up. J Bone Joint Surg Am 87(5):999–1006, 2005.

50. Insall J, Aglietti P. A five to seven-year follow-up of unicompartmental arthroplasty. J Bone Joint Surg Am 62:1329–1337, 1980.

51. Laskin R. Unicompartmental knee arthroplasty using an uncemented, polyethylene tibial implant. A seven-year follow-up study. Clin Orthop 288:270–276, 1978.

52. Marmor L. Unicompartmental knee arthroplasty. Ten to 13-year follow-up study. Clin Orthop 226:14–20, 1987.

53. Mackinnon J, Young S, Bailey R. The St. George Sledge unicompartmental replacement of the knee. A prospective study of 115 cases. J Bone Joint Surg Br 70:217–223, 1988.

54. Knutson J, Lindstrand A, Lidgren L. Survival of knee arthroplasties. A nationwide multicenter investigation of 8000 cases. J Bone Joint Surg Br 68:795–803, 1986.

55. Sisto DJ, Mitchell IL. UniSpacer arthroplasty of the knee. J Bone Joint Surg Am. 2005;87:1706–1711.

56. Sullivan P, Hugus J, Johnston R. Long-term Follow-up of Unicompartmental Knee Arthroplasty. Atlanta, Georgia, American Academy of Orthopaedic Surgeons, 1988.

57. Gioe TJ, Killeen KK, Hoeffel DP, et al. Analysis of unicompartmental knee arthroplasty in a community-based implant registry. Clin Orthop Relat Res 416:111–119, 2003.

58. Svard UC, Price AJ. Oxford medial unicompartmental knee arthroplasty. A survival analysis of an independent series. J Bone Joint Surg Br 83:191–194, 2001.

59. Kozinn S, Scott R. Current concepts review. Unicompartmental knee arthroplasty. J Bone Joint Surg Am 71:145–150, 1989.

60. Gunston P. Polycentric knee arthroplasty: prosthetic simulation of normal knee movement. J Bone Joint Surg Am 53:272–275, 1979.

61. Bonutti PM, Mont MA, McMahon M, et al. Minimally invasive total knee arthroplasty. J Bone Joint Surg Am 86-A(Suppl 2):26–32, 2004.

62. Laskin RS, Beksac B, Phongjunakorn A, et al. Minimally invasive total knee replacement through a mini-midvastus incision: an outcome study. Clin Orthop Relat Res 428:74–81, 2004.

63. Chauhan SK, Scott RG, Breidahl W, et al. Computer-assisted knee arthroplasty versus a conventional jig-based technique. A randomised, prospective trial. J Bone Joint Surg Br 86:372–377, 2004.

64. Ranawat C, Boachie-Adjei O. Survivorship analysis and results of total condylar knee arthroplasty. Eight- to 11-year follow-up period. Clin Orthop 226:6–13, 1988.

65. Vince K, Insall J, Kelly M. The total condylar prosthesis: 10 to 12 year results of a cemented knee replacement. J Bone Joint Surg Br 71:793–797, 1989.

66. Scuderi G, Insall J, Windsor R, et al. Survivorship of cemented knee replacements. J Bone Joint Surg Br 71:798–803, 1989.

67. Scott R, Volatile T. Twelve years' experience with posterior cruciate–retaining total knee arthroplasty. Clin Orthop 205:100–107, 1986.

68. Ewald F, Christie M. Results of cemented total knee replacement in young patients. Orthop Trans 11:442, 1987.

69. Carmichael E, Chaplin D. Total knee arthroplasty in juvenile rheumatoid arthritis. A seven-year follow-up study. Clin Orthop 210:192–200, 1986.

70. Sarokhan A, Scott R, Thomas W, et al. Total knee arthroplasty in juvenile rheumatoid arthritis. J Bone Joint Surg Am 65:1071–1080, 1983.

71. Stern S, Bowen M, Insall J, et al. Cemented total knee arthroplasty for gonarthrosis in patients 55 years old or younger. Clin Orthop 260:124–129, 1990.

72. Lonner JH, Hershman S, Mont M, et al. Total knee arthroplasty in patients 40 years of age and younger with osteoarthritis. Clin Orthop Relat Res 380:85–90, 2000.

73. Rand J. Cement or cementless fixation in total knee arthroplasty? Clin Orthop 273:52–62, 1991.

74. Dodd C, Hungerford D, Krackow K. Total knee arthroplasty fixation. Comparison of the early results of paired cemented versus uncemented porous coated anatomic knee prostheses. Clin Orthop 260:66–70, 1990.

75. Khaw FM, Kirk LM, Morris RW, et al. A randomised, controlled trial of cemented versus cementless press-fit condylar total knee replacement. Ten-year survival analysis. J Bone Joint Surg Br 84(5):658–666, 2002.

76. Whiteside L. Four screws for fixation of the tibial component in cementless total knee arthroplasty. Clin Orthop 299:72–76, 1994.

77. Wright R, Lima J, Scott R, et al. Two- to four-year results of posterior cruciate–sparing condylar total knee arthroplasty with an uncemented femoral component. Clin Orthop 260:80–86, 1990.

78. Rorabeck C, Bourne R, Nott L. The cemented kinematic-II and the non-cemented porous-coated anatomic prosthesis for total knee replacement. A prospective evaluation. J Bone Joint Surg Am 70:483–490, 1988.

79. Laskin R. Total knee arthroplasty using an uncemented, polyethylene tibial implant. A seven-year follow-up study. Clin Orthop 288:270–276, 1993.

80. Hoffman A, Wyatt R, Beck S, et al. Cementless total knee arthroplasty in patients over 65 years old. Clin Orthop 271:28–34, 1991.

81. Schroder HM, Berthelsen A, Hassani G, et al. Cementless porous-coated total knee arthroplasty: 10-year results in a consecutive series. J Arthroplasty 16(5):559–567.

82. Whiteside LA. Long-term followup of the bone-ingrowth Ortholoc knee system without a metal-backed patella. Clin Orthop Relat Res 388:77–84, 2001.

83. Rosenberg A, Barden R, Galante J. Cemented and ingrowth fixation of the Miller-Galante prosthesis. Clinical and roentgenographic comparison after three- to six-year follow-up studies. Clin Orthop 260:71–79, 1990.

84. Minus T, Nehrer S. Current concepts in the treatment of articular cartilage defects. Orthopedics 20:525–538, 1997.

85. Curl W, Krome J, Gordon E, et al. Cartilage injuries: a review of 31,516 knee arthroscopies. Arthroscopy 13:456–460, 1997.

86. Dandy D. Arthroscopic débridement of the knee for osteoarthritis [editorial]. J Bone Joint Surg Br 73:877–888, 1991.

87. Gillogly S, Voight M, Blackburn T. Treatment of articular cartilage defects of the knee with autologous chondrocyte implantation. J Orthop Sports Phys Ther 28:241–251, 1998.

88. Johnson L. Arthroscopic abrasion arthroplasty historical and pathologic perspective: present status. Arthroscopy 2:341–360, 1986.

89. Johnson L. Arthroscopic abrasion arthroplasty. In: McGinty J, ed. Operative Arthroscopy. New York, Raven Press, 1991, pp 341–360.

90. Cole BJ, Fredericks RW, Levy AS, et al. Management of a 35 year-old male with recurrent knee pain. J Clin Outcomes Management 5:46–57, 1999.

91. Furakawa T, Eyre D, Koide S, et al. Biochemical studies on repair cartilage resurfacing experimental defects in the rabbit knee. J Bone Joint Surg Am 62:79–89, 1980.

92. Tippet J. Articular cartilage drilling and osteotomy in osteoarthritis of the knee. In: McGinty J, ed. Operative Arthroscopy. New York, Raven Press, 1991, pp 325–339.

93. Rodrigo J, Steadman J, Silliman J, et al. Improvement of full-thickness chondral defect healing in the human knee after débridement and microfracture using continuous passive motion. Am J Knee Surg 70:595–606, 1994.

94. O'Driscoll S, Keeley F, Salter R, et al. Durability of regenerated articular cartilage produced by free autogenous periosteal grafts in major full-thickness defects in joint surfaces under the influence of continuous passive motion. J Bone Joint Surg Am 70:595–606, 1988.

95. Steadman JR, Briggs KK, Rodrigo JJ, et al. Outcomes of microfracture for traumatic chondral defects of the knee: average 11-year follow-up. Arthroscopy. 19(5):477–484, 2003. Review.

96. Convery F, Meyers M, Akeson W. Fresh osteochondral allografting of the femoral condyle. Clin Orthop 273:139–145, 1991.

97. Bobic V. Arthroscopic osteochondral autograft in anterior cruciate ligament reconstruction: a preliminary clinical study. Arthroscopy 3:262–264, 1996.

98. Garrett J. Osteochondral allografts for reconstruction of articular defects. In: McGinty J, Caspari R, Jackson R, Poehling G, eds. Operative Arthroscopy. Philadelphia, Lippincott-Raven, 1996, pp 395–403.

99. Zukor D, Gross A. Osteochondral allograft reconstruction of the knee. Am J Knee Surg 2:139–149, 1989.

100. Hangody L, Feczko P, Bartha L, et al. Mosaicplasty for the treatment of articular defects of the knee and ankle. Clin Orthop Relat Res 391(Suppl):S328–S336, 2001. Review.

101. Aubin PP, Cheah HK, Davis AM, et al. Long-term followup of fresh femoral osteochondral allografts for posttraumatic knee defects. Clin Orthop Relat Res 391(Suppl):S318–S327, 2001.

102. Cameron J, Saha S. Meniscal allograft transplantation for unicompartmental arthritis of the knee. Clin Orthop 337:164–171, 1997.

103. Veltri D, Warren R, Wickiewicz T, et al. Current status of allograft meniscal transplantation. Clin Orthop 303:44–55, 1994.

104. van Arkel E, deBoer H. Human meniscal tansplantation. Preliminary results at 2- to 5-year follow-up. J Bone Joint Surg Br 77:589–595, 1995.

105. Garrett J, Stevenson R. Meniscal transplantation in the human knee: a preliminary report. Arthroscopy 7:57–62, 1991.

106. Cole BJ, Carter TR, Rodeo SA. Allograft meniscal transplantation: background, techniques, and results. Instr Course Lect. 2003;52:383–396. Review.

107. Yoldas EA, Sekiya JK, Irrgang JJ, et al. Arthroscopically assisted meniscal allograft transplantation with and without combined anterior cruciate ligament reconstruction. Knee Surg Sports Traumatol Arthrosc 11(3):173–182, 2003. Epub 2003 May 9.

108. Outerbridge R. The etiology of chondromalacia patellae. Bone Joint Surg Br 43:752–757, 1961.

109. Fulkerson J. Evaluation of the peripatellar soft tissues and retinaculum in patients with patellofemoral pain. Clin Sports Med 8:197–202, 1989.

110. Jacobson KE, Flandry FC. Diagnosis of anterior knee pain. Clin Sports Med 8(2):179–195, 1989.

111. Laurin C, Dussault R, Levesque H. The tangential x-ray investigation of the patellofemoral joint: x-ray technique, diagnostic criteria, and their interpretation. Clin Orthop 144:16–26, 1979.

112. Bigos S, McBride G. The isolated lateral retinacular release in the treatment of patellofemoral disorders. Clin Orthop 186:75–80, 1984.

113. Busch M, Dehaven K. Pitfalls of the lateral retinacular release. Clin Sports Med 8:279–290, 1989.

114. Insall J, Bullough P, Burstein A. Proximal tube realignment of the patella for chondromalacia patellae. Clin Orthop 144:63–69, 1979.

115. Fulkerson J, Hungerford D. Disorders of the Patellofemoral Joint. Baltimore, Williams & Wilkins, 1990.

116. Kelly M, Insall J. Patellectomy. Orthop Clin North Am 17:289–295, 1986.

117. Geckler E, Quaranta A. Patellectomy for degenerative arthritis of the knee. J Bone Joint Surg Am 44:1109–1114, 1962.

118. Harrington K. Long-term results for the McKeever patellar resurfacing prosthesis used as a salvage procedure for severe chondromalacia patellae. Clin Orthop 279:201–213, 1992.

119. Kooijman HJ, Driessen AP, van Horn JR. Long-term results of patellofemoral arthroplasty. A report of 56 arthroplasties with 17 years of follow-up. J Bone Joint Surg Br 85(6):836–840, 2003.

120. Lonner JH. Patellofemoral arthroplasty: pros, cons, and design considerations. Clin Orthop Relat Res 428:158–165, 2004. Review.

Lower Extremity Considerations: Foot and Ankle

James Michelson

OVERVIEW OF OSTEOARTHRITIS IN THE FOOT AND ANKLE

Normal Biomechanics

The entire complex of the foot and ankle encompasses 30 bones having 38 distinct articulations, all of which must work in smooth coordination to withstand peak loads in excess of one body weight for each normal stride. Relatively small alterations in the functioning of any of these articulations, such as in osteoarthritis (OA), can lead to significant disability (Fig. 21C–1). The joints in the foot and ankle have two functional roles: to bear load and to provide for motion. These two activities are interactive in the sense that an alteration in the range of motion of a given joint will alter its ability to bear load. Table 21C–1 summarizes the phases of gait during which there is load bearing for the various articulations in the foot and ankle and details the primary directions of motion. The gait cycle for walking is divided into a swing phase, when the limb is elevated off the ground, and a stance phase, during which the limb is in contact with the ground. The stance phase is further subdivided into heel strike, foot flat (or mid-stance), heel rise, and toe-off. The process of advancing from heel strike through toe-off requires motion of the foot and ankle complex in the sagittal plane to decrease the impact loading to the rest of the lower extremity. The inversion-eversion motion of the hindfoot and supination-pronation of the forefoot allow the foot to accommodate to uneven ground. It is considerably more difficult to walk on uneven ground, such as pebbles or grass, if the joints providing these functions (subtalar joint, transverse tarsal joint) are impaired by OA.

Effect of Osteoarthritis on Biomechanics

OA can have a primary effect on both the motion and the load-bearing functions of the joints of the foot and ankle. With the development of secondary osteophytes about any given articulation, the range of motion of the joint can be significantly compromised. This can cause significant pain from impingement of the osteophytes on surrounding bone and soft tissues (Fig. 21C–2). Pain can also result from a transfer of load from the affected joint to the surrounding joints, leading to pain in the overloaded secondary joints, which can result in a confusing clinical presentation.

The load-bearing function of a joint can obviously be primarily affected by OA. This will result in pain with weight bearing, frequently accompanied by a functional decrease in range of motion despite an absence of osteophytes. The load-bearing pain can also result in an apparent loss of motor control and instability due to the reflex inhibition of the controlling muscles when loading of the joint causes significant pain. In addition, as OA progresses, significant deformity and malalignment of the joints of the foot and ankle complex may develop (Fig. 21C–3).

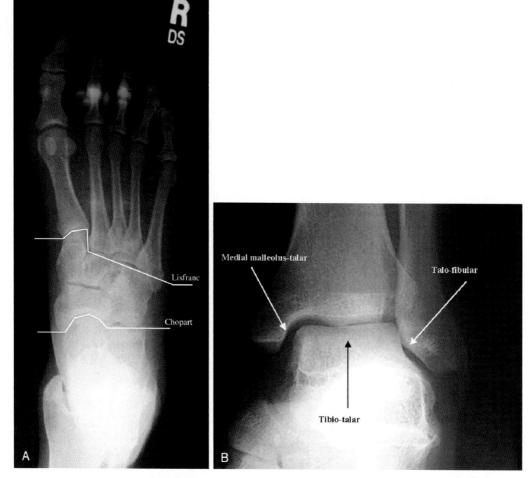

Figure 21C–1 Radiographs of a normal foot and ankle. *A,* Anteroposterior view of the foot. The foot can be divided into three zones: the forefoot (all the metatarsals and toes), the midfoot (all the tarsal bones except the calcaneus and talus), and the hindfoot (the calcaneus and talus). The midfoot-forefoot articulation is named the Lisfranc joint. The hindfoot-midfoot articulation is called the Chopart (or transverse tarsal) joint. The majority of sagittal motion (plantar flexion and dorsiflexion) occurs at the ankle joint and Chopart joint. *B,* Anteroposterior view of the ankle. There are three distinct articulations: the tibiotalar (black arrows), the medial malleolar–talar (white arrow), and the talofibular (white arrowheads).

TABLE 21C–1
THE RELATIONSHIP OF FOOT AND ANKLE LOADING AND MOTION TO THE PHASES OF GAIT

	Gait Phase									
	Heel Strike		Foot Flat		Heel Rise		Toe Off		Swing Phase	
Articulation	**Loaded***	**Motion†**	**Loaded**	**Motion**	**Loaded**	**Motion**	**Loaded**	**Motion**	**Loaded**	**Motion**
Ankle	Yes	PF	Yes	DF	Yes	DF	No	PF	No	DF
Hindfoot-Midfoot	Yes	Ever	Yes	Ever	Yes	Inver	Yes	Inver	No	Inver
Forefoot	No	Pron	Yes	Pron	Yes	Supin	Yes	Supin	No	Supin

*Denotes if there is force being applied (loading) to the indicated articulations.
†Denotes direction of motion of the articulation at each instance of the gait cycle. It is not the absolute position of the joint (e.g., if the ankle is in a dorsiflexed position but is moving in a plantarflexion direction, then the motion is noted as plantarflexion). The directions of motion are as defined in Figure 21C–2.
PF, plantarflexion; DF, dorsiflexion; Ever, eversion; Inver, inversion; Pron, pronation; Supin, supination.

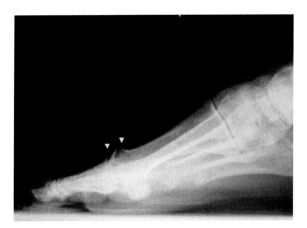

Figure 21C–2 Clinical and radiographic appearance of hallux rigidus. Lateral weight-bearing radiograph in which the dorsal exostosis is observed (arrowhead) but also in which the reluctance to bear weight on the hallux is noted by the elevation of the first ray off the standing board (black line) relative to the fifth metatarsal (white line).

Differential Diagnosis of Osteoarthritis of the Foot and Ankle

The differential diagnosis of OA of the foot and ankle essentially includes everything else that can possibly occur to these structures. In many instances, the key to determining a diagnosis is based on localizing the source of pain and its temporal pattern. Pain that is not related to weight bearing is unlikely to be OA but is more probably due to neuritis, infection, or inflammatory diseases. Weight-bearing pain that is worse initially and then gets better with further activity is also unlikely to be OA but may be related to tendinitis or inflammatory arthritis. In contrast, typical osteoarthritic pain gradually increases with progressive weight bearing. A complete absence of pain by history and on physical examination of the suspected joints makes OA unlikely, although it can be seen in individuals exhibiting pure complaints of

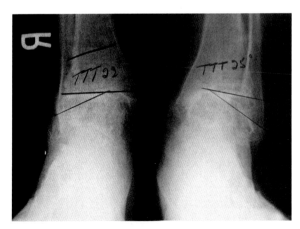

Figure 21C–3 Anteroposterior radiographs of ankles with severe degeneration and resultant varus deformities of the tibial plafond from erosion of the medial articulations.

instability. The distinction between a low-grade infection and OA can be difficult clinically. Hematogenous spread of infection to bones of the foot and ankle in the nonpediatric age group is extremely unusual. Consequently, infection in the absence of a local source would not be likely. Pain related to weight bearing in the context of acute trauma should, of course, raise the suspicion of a fracture. One final possible etiology of weight-bearing–associated pain is that of avascular necrosis. This is most common in the talus and presents in three forms: osteochondritis dissecans (involving a small part of the talar dome,), post-traumatic (especially after a talar neck fracture), and idiopathic (most commonly associated with steroid use, diabetes, or alcoholism).

Diagnostic Assessment

In most cases, the diagnosis of OA can be made on the basis of the history of symptoms. As noted earlier, pain that is weight bearing in nature and has a monotonically increasing severity with continued weight bearing is classic for OA and serves to differentiate it from tendinitis, neuritis, and inflammatory conditions. The pain should be localized to a joint and should not have radiation of significance either proximally or distally. This can be a bit complicated in long-standing cases of OA in which there may be fairly generalized pain. A change in visible foot shape should also be directly queried because it may be the first clue to conditions such as Lisfranc OA causing midfoot collapse (Fig. 21C–4). Finally, a specific question should be asked about the existence of similar symptoms in the contralateral foot. Although bilateral symptoms can occur in primary OA, they raise the possibility of an underlying inflammatory diathesis.

The physical examination should include observations of the patient standing barefoot, walking barefoot, and sitting. The standing examination allows assessment of symmetry as well as of any weight-bearing deformity or malalignment that would not otherwise be appreciated. The patient should also be asked to do both a heel rise (single- and double-limbed) and forefoot rise to test the strength of the posterior and anterior musculature, respectively. Pain elicited with either of these maneuvers can pinpoint the joint or joints affected by OA. Observing the gait provides insight into limping from either pain (antalgic gait) or weakness. It may also reveal a tendency for the patient to protect one part of the foot by shifting weight elsewhere on the foot. When this occurs, the patient can be specifically asked to bear weight more normally to elicit symptoms.

For the last part of the examination, the patient is sitting with the legs dangling. The passive range of motion of the ankles, subtalar joints, midfoot articulations, and toes should be assessed and recorded. A motor examination of the posterior, tibialis anterior, peroneal, and Achilles tendons is also performed. This is to elicit tenderness in the tendons more than to assess strength. A gross sensory examination should include testing to light touch in the distributions of the deep peroneal (first web space dorsally), superficial peroneal (medial hallux and dorsal lateral midfoot), sural (lateral foot), medial plantar (plantar

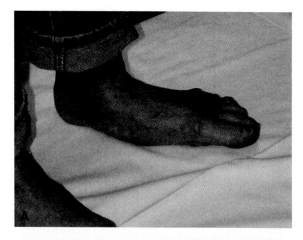

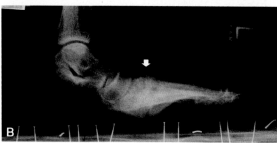

Figure 21C–4 Clinical and radiographic appearance of severe midfoot collapse. *A*, Clinical view of new onset pes planus with characteristic medial prominence of bone at the midfoot. *B*, Lateral radiograph of the same patient demonstrating collapse at the Lisfranc articulation (*arrowhead*).

medial midfoot and forefoot), and lateral plantar (plantar lateral midfoot and forefoot) nerves. The L5 nerve root is tested by sensation on the medial forefoot and strength of the extensor hallucis longus; the S1 nerve root is tested by sensation on the lateral border of the foot and the Achilles reflex. A systematic palpation examination of each joint of the ankle and foot should then be undertaken to determine the presence of tenderness. The entire physical examination takes between 3 and 4 minutes. The establishment of a personal routine of the complete examination of the foot and ankle will effectively guard against missing significant pathologic processes in this region.

Imaging of the Foot and Ankle

The most useful imaging modality for foot and ankle problems is the plain radiograph. Because most of the symptoms are related to weight bearing, such films should be obtained with the patient standing. Significant shifts in the articulations can occur with weight bearing, making non–weight-bearing films particularly unhelpful in OA.[1] For the foot, the films are obtained in anteroposterior, oblique, and lateral views. For the ankle, anteroposterior, mortise, and lateral views are standard.

Computed tomography (CT) is not a sensitive, specific, or cost-effective way to screen for foot and ankle problems. On the other hand, it is the best method to define bone and joint anatomy in the presence of subtle intra-articular

malalignments that can cause OA. The two joints most commonly assessed by CT are the Lisfranc and subtalar joints, both of which are nonlinear, multiplanar, complex articulations. As with CT, screening with MRI is exceedingly unhelpful given the wide variation of normal findings. MRI can be helpful in delineating soft tissue disease, such as posterior tibial tendon ruptures, but it does not add to the clinical assessment of OA. Bone scans typically show abnormalities in osteoarthritic joints, but this does not add any information that cannot be easily obtained by less expensive means, such as by a physical examination.

PRINCIPLES OF NONOPERATIVE TREATMENT OF OSTEOARTHRITIS OF THE ANKLE AND FOOT

Recognition of the Sources of Pain

There are three primary sources of pain on patient presentation. The most common in OA is pain directly related to axial loading of a joint compromised by degenerative changes within the articular surfaces (Fig. 21C–5). In this instance, mere weight bearing frequently elicits the symptoms. The second major source, which may coexist with the first, is pain related to mechanical limitation of motion. This is a consequence of osteophytic change in the periarticular region, which mechanically interferes with a normal range of motion (Fig. 21C–6). These patients primarily have complaints related to ambulation, which requires a functional range of motion that exceeds the limits of the involved articulations. It is important to distinguish these two sources of pain because the surgical treatment of osteophytic change is frequently much less destructive than that of degenerative change. Last, pain may be a consequence of the architectural loss of integrity accompanying OA. This results in clinical instability, such as the midfoot collapse seen in the Lisfranc arthritis, which can be a source of great pain (Fig. 21C–3, Fig. 21C–4).

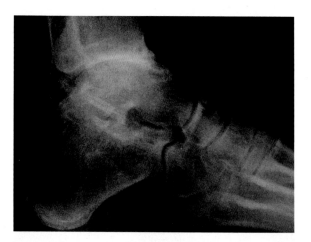

Figure 21C–5 Lateral radiograph of patient with complete loss of articular cartilage at the ankle and subtalar joints. There is no significant deformity or osteophyte formation, but any motion of either joint is painful due to the compromised articular surfaces.

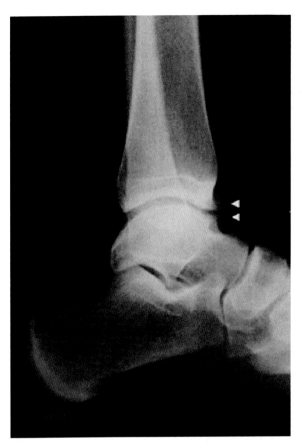

Figure 21C–6 Lateral radiograph of patient with moderate ankle degeneration and primarily anterior ankle pain. The pain results from the anterior ankle osteophytes that have formed (arrowheads) and impinge during the dorsiflexion that occurs during normal walking.

Biomechanical Rationale of Nonoperative Treatment (With Specific Examples)

The nonoperative treatment of OA of the foot and ankle can be divided into mechanical and biologic regimens. In those patients for whom loading of a compromised arthritic joint is causing pain, the treatment goal is to shunt the forces away from the defective joint to decrease painful loading. For the ankle, this is exemplified by the use of a patella tendon–bearing brace in which the axial loads are supported by the brace and the surrounding soft tissues. Loading across the midfoot joints can be diminished by the use of a stiff-soled rocker-bottom shoe that decreases the bending of the midfoot. External support, such as a cane in the opposite hand or crutches, is also effective in decreasing loading by transferring the load to an upper extremity.

Joints with motion limited by osteoarthritic changes can be made less symptomatic by similar means. A rigid ankle-foot orthosis serves to limit motion in the ankle joint, thereby decreasing painful anterior impingement from osteophytes. Such braces can frequently be obtained off the shelf and used with normal shoes. Hallux rigidus is a prototypical example of how a mechanically limited joint can cause a great deal of pain during normal gait (Fig. 21C–2). The use of a steel shank shoe protects the first

metatarsophalangeal joint from dorsiflexion forces, thereby alleviating many of the symptoms of this condition. An interesting example of how shoe wear can provide accommodation to a limited range of motion is the use of a rocker-bottom shoe in patients with anterior ankle osteophytes. The rocker bottom allows the foot to roll off the floor as one progresses from midstance to toe-off without forcing the ankle into a dorsiflexed position. The overall pattern of gait is therefore preserved while the range of motion necessary at the ankle is minimized.

The use of external supports in cases of instability is fairly obvious. It may be possible to provide support for the midfoot by a combination of a stiff-soled shoe with soft arch support. Such modalities are designed to prevent further collapse and are incapable of restoring normal architecture to the foot. Similarly, a lace-up ankle splint may provide enough support for the ankle and subtalar joint to allow greater functional activities.

On the biologic side of the equation, various anti-inflammatory medications can be helpful in alleviating symptoms. The results of such treatments are unpredictable because the underlying source of pain is mechanical and the medications are employed solely to alleviate symptoms.

With increasing experience in treating OA of the foot and ankle, one appreciates a remarkable discontinuity between the radiographic findings and symptoms. It is not unusual for joints exhibiting marked degenerative changes to have minimal clinical symptoms (Fig. 21C–7). This highlights the importance of ensuring that the presenting symptoms are, in fact, related to the radiographic findings. In other words, remember to treat the patient, not the radiographs.

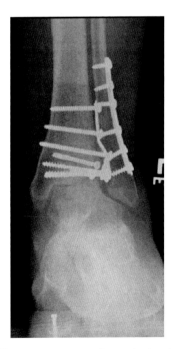

Figure 21C–7 Anteroposterior radiograph of patient's ankle with significant degeneration following an intra-articular ankle fracture. Note the loss of the lateral plafond height and resultant valgus alignment of the talus. The patient has very few clinical symptoms.

PRINCIPLES OF OPERATIVE TREATMENT OF OSTEOARTHRITIS OF THE FOOT AND ANKLE

Relationship of Surgical Methods to Underlying Biomechanical Dysfunction

The guiding principle of surgery is to directly address the biomechanical consequences of the affected osteoarthritic joint. In the case of the joint that is unable to sustain loads because of intra-articular destruction, this is usually achieved by an arthrodesis. A fusion resects and stabilizes the compromised articulation, thereby allowing load transmission directly through the fused bone. The other method by which the loading of an arthritic joint can be surgically alleviated is joint replacement. Although this has been successful in the knee and hip, joint replacement about the foot and ankle has limited indications (primarily for the ankle and first metatarsophalangeal joint), with uncertain long-term results.[2] There are some new developments on this front, but the studies to date are too short term to justify the routine recommendation of these implants. The situation for replacement of the first metatarsophalangeal joint is similar. Multiple attempts at designing such joints, ranging from Silastic implants to titanium and polyethylene implants that look like miniature total knees, have not been successful except in patients with low functional demands (Fig. 21C–8).[3] Consequently, the current standard of operative treatment of severe degeneration of joints in the foot and ankle is a fusion.

When an arthrodesis is chosen to treat a degenerated joint with associated collapse, attention must also be paid to the overall malalignment that exists. Increased stresses will be placed on adjacent, otherwise normal joints as a consequence of the alteration in mechanical alignment and loading. The surgery to stabilize the collapsed arthritic joint must therefore also restore the normal alignment of the foot and ankle to decrease the destructive mechanical forces on other joints. One of the more common applications of this principle is the use of a calcaneal osteotomy in conjunction with a subtalar fusion in the presence of hindfoot varus.

The surgical outlook for osteoarthritic pain due to limitation of motion is much brighter. In the most common scenario of impinging osteophytes, the goal of surgery is simply to excise the impinging periarticular osteophytes. This is an effective treatment of virtually all of the joints of the foot and the ankle.

Rehabilitation after Surgery

After limited surgical interventions such as osteophyte removal, the primary perioperative goal is to obtain healing of the soft tissues. Once this has occurred, usually in 1 to 2 weeks, an aggressive range-of-motion program can be instituted. Most patients can begin weight bearing immediately postoperatively.

More extensive surgeries that involve arthrodesis and osteotomy require a greater degree of external protection. This usually consists of 6 weeks of non–weight-bearing immobilization in a short-leg cast followed by another 6 weeks of immobilization in a weight-bearing short-leg cast. Other than the initial physical therapy for crutch walking instruction, postoperative physical therapy is not typically needed.

The potential complications from these surgeries are similar to that of any surgery: infection (the risk is generally between 0.5% and 1%), bleeding (but almost never requiring a transfusion), and nerve damage (generally causing altered sensation in the toes or dorsal foot without any weakness). The anesthetics used range from an ankle block with sedation, to regional block (spinal), to general, with the choice made by the patient in consultation with the anesthesiologist.

Treatment of Osteoarthritis by Anatomic Site

What follows is a brief overview of modalities that have been found useful in the management of OA of various joints. Each section is grouped by those treatments that are appropriate for mild to moderate OA versus those reserved for more severe cases. These descriptions are intended to provide an overview of the indications and specific surgical techniques involved. The reader is referred to several excellent surgical textbooks for more specific technical discussions.[4–6]

Ankle

Mild to moderate ankle arthritis that impairs some activities of daily living, usually without widespread loss of the joint space, is initially treated by mild immobilization (lace-up ankle splints, high-top shoes) with appropriate additions of anti-inflammatory medications. Adding a

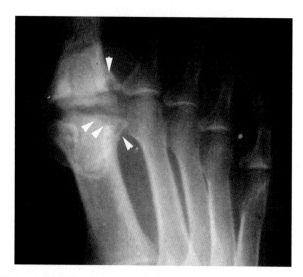

Figure 21C–8 Anteroposterior radiograph of a Silastic first metatarsophalangeal joint arthroplasty implant. There is fragmentation of the implant, and the resultant silicon synovitis has caused bone resorption around the implant. The clinical consequences are pain, while the surgical treatment typically requires a substantial iliac crest bone graft to substitute for the resorbed bone.

rocker-bottom sole to the shoe can also effectively relieve pain because it decreases the required ankle motion during normal gait. Patients who have impinging osteophytes anteriorly may benefit from surgical resection of the osteophytes if this is the primary source of their pain (Fig. 21C–6). Most people will regain motion and have decreased pain, with arthroscopic and open techniques yielding equivalent functional results.[7] Abrasion chondroplasty of localized areas of degeneration within the ankle has not proved to be beneficial. There has been some interest in the use of osteochondral transplants from the femoral condyles (called the mosaicplasty or osteoarticular transplantation [OATS] procedure) as a method of restoring normal articular cartilage to the talar dome.[8] The transplanted cartilage does not biologically heal to the surrounding cartilage, and the long-term results of this procedure are not yet known.

Patients with severe ankle arthritis unresponsive to conservative therapy can be offered an ankle arthrodesis. This surgery has a predictable, functionally successful result in 90% of patients. There have been many surgical techniques for this procedure over the years, but the direct lateral transfibular approach has become the most widely practiced during the last decade.[9]

The direct lateral transfibular approach can be accomplished with a single incision that runs along the lateral border of the fibula, then curves anteriorly distally. Once the fibula is exposed, it is osteotomized in the proximal part of the wound and either excised or reflected inferiorly to expose the lateral tibia and ankle joint. This provides wide exposure of the ankle joint, which can be thoroughly débrided, including the talar–medial malleolar articulation. Care is taken to minimize the loss of bone during the débridement of articular cartilage and subchondral bone. If present, the normal contours of the articulation are preserved to minimize the loss of height at the level of the ankle. The fusion is then placed in a position of 0° plantar flexion, 5° valgus, and 10° external rotation to achieve the optimal functional result.[10] Many methods of fixation can be employed. I have found the placement of two parallel screws running from the anterior lateral ridge of the talus in a superior-medial direction to engage the medial cortex of the tibia to be simple and highly effective (Fig. 21C–9). The osteotomized fibula can be morselized for autologous bone graft or used as a biologic plate that is fixed to the lateral surfaces of the tibia and talus.

The fusion rate for this procedure is above 90%. Earlier techniques that used suboptimal methods such as external fixation suffered nonunion rates as high as 30%. The functional results are excellent in most patients, provided that the arthrodesis is placed in the optimal position, as detailed before. The resulting gait is limp-free, with a slightly shortened stride length. I also offer patients the use of a rocker-bottom shoe, which allows the limb to accommodate to the lack of motion at the ankle. Many patients will develop compensatory increased sagittal motion at the transverse tarsal joint. Although this can be functional, it places added stresses at these articulations that may lead to premature arthritis after 15 to 20 years.

The development of a successful total ankle arthroplasty holds the promise of alleviating pain in the arthritic ankle

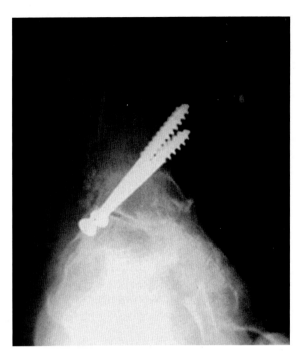

Figure 21C–9 Anteroposterior radiograph of an ankle fusion. This demonstrates the typical position of the fixation screws and the resected distal fibula, which is used for bone graft.

while preserving functional motion. Current intermediate-term clinical studies with up to 9 years of average follow-up have been encouraging, with revision rates in the largest study being 11%.[11] However, with a reoperation rate of 58% at 5 years,[12] this still remains a procedure for which the clinical expectations are guarded, particularly in younger patients.[13-15] Consequently, the indications for their use is primarily in low-demand patients, which includes severely debilitated patients with rheumatoid disease and the relatively inactive elderly patient.[15,16] Even in these populations of patients, the long-term results are not uniformly excellent.

Hindfoot (Subtalar Joint, Calcaneocuboid Joint, Talonavicular Joint)

Treatment of mild to moderate hindfoot arthritis revolves around supportive measures to decrease the impact loading to the hindfoot as well as to limit the imposed range of motions in this region during normal activities. Placing cushioned heels in the shoe serves to diminish the loading of the hindfoot during heel strike and can be helpful. Braces that limit inversion and eversion of the hindfoot may also be beneficial. These can take the form of lace-up ankle splints, U splints, or double upright braces attached to the shoe. Bracing is particularly useful for patients who need to walk on uneven surfaces, such as grass or unpaved regions.

Localized injections of corticosteroids may alleviate symptoms, particularly in acute exacerbations. The calcaneocuboid and talonavicular joints can be injected by use of a direct approach. The subtalar joint is injected through the sinus tarsi with the needle angled in a posterior-medial direction so that the medicine is deposited adjacent to the posterior and medial facets of the subtalar joint. Long-term alleviation of symptoms should not be anticipated with such injections.

The decision-making process in treating severe OA of the hindfoot is centered on deciding which joints should be fused. Fusions should be limited to those joints that are affected, as determined by the presence of radiographic findings correlated to clinical symptoms and physical examination findings. The three joints of the hindfoot are mechanically interdependent, so that fusing one or more joints can have a profound effect on the remaining motion in the unfused joints. Fusing the calcaneocuboid joint will diminish subtalar motion by less than 10°, whereas a similar procedure on the talonavicular joint will decrease subtalar motion by roughly 50%. There has been some enthusiasm for fusing both articulations of the Chopart joint to spare the subtalar joint from surgical intervention. However, such a procedure virtually eliminates all motion from the subtalar joint, so the mechanical consequences are indistinguishable from a triple arthrodesis, in which all three joints are fused.

There are several approaches for performing a triple arthrodesis. An oblique sinus tarsi incision that runs along the lines of Langer from the peroneal tendons posteriorly to the lower border of the extensor tendons dorsally centered over the soft spot of the sinus tarsi provides excellent exposure of all three joints to be fused. The intermediate branch of the superficial peroneal nerve, which is encountered at the medial aspect of the incision, is retracted medially or can be sharply incised if necessary. The investing fascia of the extensor brevis muscle is preserved for the deep layer of the closure; the deeper muscle belly and sinus tarsi contents can be excised as needed for exposure. Through this approach, the subtalar and calcaneocuboid joints can be exposed in their entirety. The talonavicular joint can also be satisfactorily exposed in the most medial aspect of the incision by incising its lateral joint capsule and placing a retractor dorsally to reveal the articulation. One should also observe the articulation between the navicular and cuboid bones, which is also easily seen and should be débrided to achieve fusion. In most cases, an additional dorsomedial incision is made over the talonavicular joint just medial to the tibialis anterior to complete the exposure of the talonavicular joint. Débridement of the articulation is done by a combination of curettage and burr, with an emphasis placed on minimizing the loss of bone and maintaining the normal joint contours. Screw fixation is generally satisfactory for stabilization of the fusions; a 6.5-mm screw is used for the subtalar joint, and 4.5-mm screws are used elsewhere (Fig. 21C–10). Although there is some disagreement among surgeons on the placement of the subtalar screw, I find the placement from the talar neck in an inferior-posterior direction to engage the calcaneus to be easily done with no risk posed to the ankle joint. The desired positioning of the fusion is to achieve hindfoot valgus of 5°, with a neutral forefoot with respect to supination-pronation. Fusion of any of the three individual joints of the hindfoot is accomplished by a limited approach using one of the other incisions described for the triple arthrodesis.

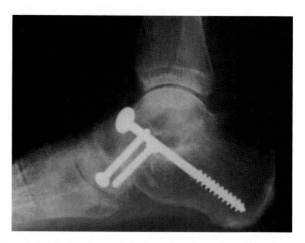

Figure 21C–10 Lateral radiograph of the foot after a triple arthrodesis. The subtalar (6.5-mm screw), talonavicular (retrograde 4.5-mm screw), and calcaneocuboid (antegrade 4.5-mm screw) joints have been fused in this procedure.

In addition to the usual potential complications with surgery, there has been some concern about the predisposition to development of arthritis in the joints adjoining a triple arthrodesis. In particular, it is noted that up to 30% of patients can have radiographic signs of OA in the ankle after triple arthrodesis.[17] Although this is certainly a potential issue that is consistent with the altered biomechanics consequent to a triple arthrodesis, closer examination of the data seems to indicate that the risk of ankle arthritis after triple arthrodesis is probably closer to 10% in those patients without other comorbidities, such as neuromuscular diseases or inflammatory arthritis. Studies with long-term follow-up (up to 44 years) have found that although radiographic evidence of arthritis in adjacent joints is observed, this does not correlate with the patients' clinical symptoms, nor their satisfaction with the clinical outcome.[18,19]

Midfoot (Chopart Joint to Lisfranc Joint)

Midfoot arthritis of mild to moderate degree is extremely common in a general orthopedic or medical practice. The majority of patients complain of occasional achiness in their feet that increases with strenuous activity. Reassurance, activity modification, and anti-inflammatory medications are frequently all that is needed for treatment. For recalcitrant cases without a great deal of radiographic degeneration, the symptoms may be amenable to the use of a rocker-bottom sole with the steel shank added to immobilize the midfoot during normal gait.

There is a subset of patients in whom the joint spaces are well preserved but significant dorsal osteophytes have developed at the affected joints (Fig. 21C–11). These osteophytes can cause impingement pain during normal gait. Pain can also be caused by tightly tying shoes, which places pressure over the dorsal prominence. Finally, the osteophytes can cause pressure against the more superficial nerves, particularly the deep peroneal as it runs across the tarsometatarsal joint into the first web space. If nonoperative treatment is unsuccessful in these patients, resection of the offending

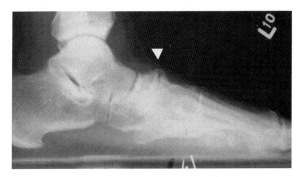

Figure 21C–11 Lateral foot radiograph demonstrating dorsal osteophytes at the naviculocuneiform joint (*arrowhead*). Pain can be caused by mechanical impingement between the osteophytes, by tight-fitting shoes that press on the bone prominence, or by increased pressure placed on the deep peroneal nerve that runs dorsal to the osteophytes.

osteophytes can be undertaken. This is accomplished through direct dorsal incisions over the symptomatic exostoses.

More severe OA of the midfoot that is unresponsive to conservative care can be treated by arthrodesis of the affected joints. The surgery should be limited to those joints that are symptomatic, because extending the fusion to the entire lateral set of articulations can frequently result in a stiff foot that is uncomfortable to walk on. The surgical principles for fusion of these joints include two longitudinal dorsal incisions over the second and fourth rays as necessary to achieve exposure. Care is taken to protect the dorsalis pedis artery and deep peroneal nerve through the medial incision. The articulations, which are much deeper than is commonly appreciated, are then débrided, with care taken to minimize the loss of bone. Fixation is by 4.5-mm lag screws and is generally augmented by bone grafting. If there is collapse at the Lisfranc joint, the arch can be restored by placement of a plantar plate under the first tarsometatarsal joint through a separate direct medial incision. Although high rates of fusion have been reported with these surgeries, they are technically demanding and require precise apposition of the fusion surfaces for a successful result to be achieved. Following a successful fusion, the patient will perceive his or her foot to be stiff but should be able to pursue normal activities of daily living. Non–impact-loading athletics, such as bicycling, elliptical trainer, hiking, and swimming, should also be possible.

Forefoot

The most common site of OA in the forefoot is the first metatarsophalangeal joint. This typically manifests as a painful limitation of motion of the joint (called hallux rigidus) that is due to a dorsal metatarsal head osteophyte (see Fig. 21C–2). The presenting complaints consist of hallux pain with push-off and an inability to wear high-heeled shoes (which force the hallux into a dorsiflexed position). On physical examination, patients have pain with extremes

of dorsiflexion and plantar flexion. Pain with plantar flexion is due to the pressure exerted on the extensor tendon by the dorsal osteophytes when the toe is plantar flexed.

In early stages, the symptoms can be adequately controlled by activity modification, refraining from the use of high-heeled shoes, and the use of a stiff-soled shoe. The indication for any surgical intervention is an unacceptable level of activity restriction or pain as determined by the patient. The first surgical option in such patients is a dorsal cheilectomy of the osteophytes. The results of this are satisfactory in 80% of patients, with the recognition that other surgical options are not compromised should a cheilectomy fail. Interestingly, the results of cheilectomy can be satisfactory even in the presence of significant joint loss radiographically. However, it is important to educate the patients that long-term pain in the joint may recur as a consequence of the underlying OA.

The surgical approach to a cheilectomy is a straight dorsal incision centered on the metatarsophalangeal joint. Care is taken to stay out of the extensor hallucis longus tendon sheath to minimize postoperative adhesions. The goal of surgery is to obtain a minimum of 70° of dorsiflexion of the joint at the time of surgery. This typically requires a resection of the dorsal 25% to 30% of the metatarsal head. The main technical cause of failure is an inadequate resection. Attention should also be paid to the osteophytes medially and laterally on the metatarsal head, which will also limit motion by restricting the excursion of the collateral ligaments. The dorsal osteophytes on the base of the proximal phalanx should also be resected because these can cause pain during plantar flexion. The key to the surgical result is the postoperative treatment. Once the incision has healed, at 1 to 2 weeks, the patient is instructed in aggressive-passive range-of-motion exercises to maximize the ultimate dorsiflexion range of motion. Failure to pursue this is likely to result in arthrofibrosis, which will restrict the range of motion.

In more severe cases of OA of the hallux metatarsophalangeal joint, after failure of cheilectomy, or in the presence of significant valgus deformity, other surgical options can be pursued. The choices at this stage are arthrodesis, resection arthroplasty (Keller procedure), and joint replacement. In younger patients and in those who are more active, fusion is the procedure of choice. Because of the consequent derangement of foot mechanics (in the case of a resection arthroplasty) or the limited longevity (for the arthroplasty), the other procedures are primarily intended for elderly patients with low functional demands.

The surgical approach for any of these three operations is identical to that for the cheilectomy. The structure at risk during these procedures is the dorsal medial sensory nerve, which should be medial to the location of the incision. The optimal position of arthrodesis is approximately 15° relative to the plantar surface of the foot, 15° of valgus, and neutral pronation. Fixation can be accomplished by either crossed screws or a dorsal third tubular plate. These patients can be managed postoperatively in a weight-bearing walking boot until fusion, which is typically 6 weeks. Once healed, the only significant functional restriction is difficulty wearing shoes with a heel height greater than about three fourths of an inch.

A Keller arthroplasty differs from arthrodesis in that the resection is limited to the base of the proximal phalanx. The position is held postoperatively by a longitudinal Steinmann pin, which is removed several weeks later.

OA of the lesser toe metatarsophalangeal joints is generally associated with the formation of hammertoes. This opens up the semantic argument as to whether this arthritis is primary OA or secondary to the hammertoe deformity. The definition is not important for the diagnosis or treatment, so I will not make the distinction. Another cause of OA, particularly in the second metatarsophalangeal joint, is avascular necrosis of the metatarsal head, known as Freiberg infraction.

The first stage of symptoms is a synovitis of one or more metatarsophalangeal joints without associated deformity. This is frequently misdiagnosed as a Morton neuroma but is distinguished from it by tenderness localized to the affected joint rather than to the intermetatarsal space. Initial treatment of this is by immobilization by such methods as a Budin splint or a stiff-soled shoe. The joint can also be injected with cortisone in an effort to quiet the synovitis.[20]

Once deformity has occurred with dorsiflexion at the metatarsophalangeal joint, conservative treatment revolves around having the patient wear shoes that accommodate the deformity. This is accomplished by using extra-depth shoes with a high, wide toe box and good cushioning of the metatarsal heads plantarly. Because these deformities are flexible, one can also use the Budin splint to correct the position of the toe so that it does not rub dorsally on the shoe. Fairly impressive hammertoe deformities can be satisfactorily treated by these simple means.

If a deformity is flexible but unresponsive to such conservative methods, soft tissue realignment is undertaken to surgically correct the position of the joint. A simple extensor tenotomy with or without capsulotomy and medial and lateral collateral ligament resection can be done, but this has a fairly high incidence of recurrence. A better option is a Girdlestone-Taylor procedure, which involves distal transection of the flexor digitorum longus (FDL) plantarly, rerouting the two slips around the medial and lateral base of the proximal phalanx and reattaching the slips dorsally just distal to the metatarsophalangeal joint. In this manner, the FDL actively corrects the dorsiflexion deformity at the metatarsophalangeal joint, serving to decrease the chance of long-term recurrence of the deformity. The tendon transfer is performed by use of two incisions. The FDL is harvested by a longitudinal plantar incision starting at the proximal flexor crease. The medial and lateral bands of the FDL are then passed about either side of the base of the proximal phalanx and anastomosed through a small dorsal incision just distal to the metatarsophalangeal joint. The position of the toe is stabilized postoperatively by a percutaneous K wire, which is taken out 3 to 4 weeks later.

In a small percentage of patients, the pain at the metatarsophalangeal joint is due to a dorsal exostosis on the metatarsal, which causes impingement similar to that seen in hallux rigidus. This can be treated by a dorsal cheilectomy.

More severe arthritis of the lesser metatarsophalangeal joint is marked by an irreducible dorsal dislocation of the joint. The main bastion of conservative care for this remains the use of an accommodative shoe with a soft insole. If this is not successful, the toes can be reduced by a complete capsulotomy of the joint in association with resection of a small portion of the metatarsal head (the DuVries procedure). This is carried out through a standard dorsal incision, and the toe is stabilized postoperatively with a K wire for several weeks. Alternatively, one may elect to resect the base of the proximal phalanx and then hold the affected toe in a reduced position by performing a syndactylization to the adjacent toe.[21] This has the advantage of not requiring postoperative pin stabilization, but it does have the theoretical disadvantage that the original deformed toe may pull the initially uninvolved toe into a deformed position.

Almost universally, the presence of deformity at the metatarsophalangeal joint is accompanied by a flexion deformity at the proximal interphalangeal joint. The conservative treatment of these deformities is similar to that of the metatarsophalangeal joint deformities. Accommodative shoes with a variety of dorsal pads to protect the toe can be helpful. If the symptoms are persistent or if surgery is undertaken to correct the metatarsophalangeal joint deformity, surgical intervention can be entertained. If the interphalangeal joint deformity is flexible, the surgical correction of the metatarsophalangeal joint position should correct the interphalangeal joint deformity. If the interphalangeal joint deformity is fixed, it is corrected by a resection arthroplasty in which the distal condyles of the proximal phalanx are removed. This is done through a dorsal transverse elliptic incision, which allows excellent exposure of the joint and provides a dermadesis effect to maintain the position of the toe postoperatively. The toe is further stabilized by a temporary percutaneous pin.

For all of the lesser toe surgeries, the affected toe is frequently permanently swollen and it will be stiffer than normal. This does not alter shoe wear and is not a functional problem, but patients may be concerned about the resulting appearance.

SUMMARY

Although assessment of the painful osteoarthritic foot and ankle can be somewhat daunting, the diagnostic and anatomic possibilities can be considerably narrowed by resorting to the primary principles of the examination of the foot and ankle. The development of a systematic process for the history taking and physical examination ensures that attention is paid to the relevant structures and that the appropriate assessment and treatment are undertaken. Foot and ankle complaints are exceedingly common in a general medical practice, and most treatment is nonoperative in nature. Consequently, an understanding of the underlying principles of diagnosis and treatment of arthritis in the foot and ankle should be an integral part of the primary care physician's and general orthopedist's knowledge base.

REFERENCES

1. Innis PC, Krackow KA. Weightbearing roentgenograms in arthritis of the ankle: a case report. Foot Ankle 9(1):54–58, 1988.
2. Lewis G. The ankle joint prosthetic replacement: clinical performance and research challenges. Foot Ankle Int 15(9): 471–476, 1994.
3. Granberry WM, Noble PC, Bishop JO, et al. Use of a hinged silicone prosthesis for replacement arthroplasty of the first metatarsophalangeal joint [see comments]. J Bone Joint Surg [Am] 73(10):1453–1459, 1991.
4. Jahss M. Disorders of the Foot and Ankle. Medical and Surgical Treatment. 2nd ed. Philadelphia, W.B. Saunders Co., 1991.
5. Johnson KA. Surgery of the Foot and Ankle. New York: Raven Press, 1989.
6. Mann RA, Coughlin MJ. Surgery of the Foot and Ankle. 7th ed. St. Louis, Mosby, 1999.
7. Cheng JC, Ferkel RD. The role of arthroscopy in ankle and subtalar degenerative joint disease. Clin Orthop 349:65–72, 1998.
8. Kish G, Modis L, Hangody L. Osteochondral mosaicplasty for the treatment of focal chondral and osteochondral lesions of the knee and talus in the athlete. Rationale, indications, techniques, and results. Clin Sports Med 18(1):45–66, vi, 1998.
9. Dennis DA, Clayton ML, Wong DA, et al. Internal fixation compression arthrodesis of the ankle. Clin Ortho Rel Res 253: 212–220, 1990.
10. Buck P, Morrey BF, Chao EY. The optimum position of arthrodesis of the ankle. A gait study of the knee and ankle. J Bone Joint Surg Am 69:1052–1062, 1987.
11. Knecht SI, Estin M, Callaghan JJ, et al. The Agility total ankle arthroplasty. Seven to sixteen-year follow-up. J Bone Joint Surg Am 86-A(6):1161–1171, 2004.
12. Spirt AA, Assal M, Hansen ST, Jr. Complications and failure after total ankle arthroplasty. J Bone Joint Surg Am 86-A(6): 1172–1178, 2004.
13. Haskell A, Mann RA. Ankle arthroplasty with preoperative coronal plane deformity: short-term results. Clin Orthop 424: 98–103, 2004.
14. SooHoo NF, Kominski G. Cost-effectiveness analysis of total ankle arthroplasty. J Bone Joint Surg Am 86-A(11):2446–2455, 2004.
15. Clare MP, Sanders RW. Preoperative considerations in ankle replacement surgery. Foot Ankle Clin 7(4):709–720, 2002.
16. Su EP, Kahn B, Figgie MP. Total ankle replacement in patients with rheumatoid arthritis. Clin Orthop 424:32–38, 2004.
17. Graves SC, Mann RA, Graves KO. Triple arthrodesis in older adults. Results after long-term follow-up. J Bone Joint Surg Am 75(3):355–362, 1993.
18. Saltzman CL, Fehrle MJ, Cooper RR, et al. Triple arthrodesis: twenty-five and forty-four-year average follow-up of the same patients. J Bone Joint Surg Am 81(10):1391–1402, 1999.
19. Smith RW, Shen W, Dewitt S, et al. Triple arthrodesis in adults with non-paralytic disease. A minimum ten-year follow-up study. J Bone Joint Surg Am 86-A(12):2707–2713, 2004.
20. Mizel MS, Michelson JD. Nonsurgical treatment of monarticular nontraumatic synovitis of the second metatarsophalangeal joint. Foot Ankle Int 18(7):424–426, 1997.
21. Daly PJ, Johnson KA. Treatment of painful subluxation or dislocation at the second and third metatarsophalangeal joints by partial proximal phalanx excision and subtotal webbing. Clin Ortho Rel Res 278:164–170, 1992.

Osteoarthritis of the Spine

22

Sanford E. Emery   Vytautas M. Ringus

CERVICAL SPINE

Pathoanatomy

Osteoarthritis (OA) of the cervical spine is primarily a result of aging changes related to disk degeneration.[1,2] Progressive loss of proteoglycans, particularly chondroitin sulfate, leads to slow desiccation of the disk. Small microfissures or frank herniation of the nucleus pulposus occurs with resultant settling and alteration of the biomechanical environment of that motion segment. The osseous structures respond with spur formation where the annular fibers insert near the end plate, in the facet joints, and importantly, at the uncovertebral joints. Chondroosseous spurs at these uncovertebral regions narrow the foramen and commonly cause nerve root impingement. These degenerative changes of the cervical spine are termed cervical *spondylosis*. Other pathoanatomic changes that can be associated with cervical spondylosis are herniated disks, dynamic instability, and kyphosis, all of which can be important clinically (Fig 22–1A, B).

Clinical Syndromes

Cervical Radiculopathy

The most common clinical manifestation of OA in the cervical spine that may require surgical consideration is termed cervical *radiculopathy*. This denotes nerve root compression, typically from hard disk and osteophytic changes, although soft disk herniations certainly occur in the arthritic neck (Fig. 22–2). The hallmark of cervical radiculopathy is arm pain. This is often associated with neurologic symptoms, such as weakness or paresthesias. In most patients, cervical root impingement produces axial neck pain as well. Neck tenderness and limited range of motion are typically found on physical examination. A full neurologic examination should be performed, looking for motor weakness and sensory findings as well as evidence of hyporeflexia.[3] Symptoms and signs may suggest a specific root involvement, but neuroradiologic corroboration is necessary. The C5-6 disk and C6-7 disk are most commonly involved with cervical spondylosis, probably because these two segments have the greatest range of motion and sustain the highest loads in the cervical spine.

Cervical Myelopathy

If disk herniations, osteophytes, kyphosis, or instability causes spinal cord compression, *myelopathy* can result (Fig. 22–3).[4,5] Chronic cord compression can lead to demyelinization and ultimately cell death. This occurs first in the central gray matter where the small transverse endarterioles provide less blood supply and only later in the white matter tracts. The earliest symptoms of cervical myelopathy are often subtle changes in gait or balance. Subjective arm or leg weakness as well as global numbness of the arms or hands is common in more moderate to severe cases. Although most patients do have neck and often arm pain, one series documented an approximately 15% incidence of no pain in patients with cervical myelopathy, so this should not confuse the clinician in the diagnostic work-up.[6]

Physical examination should include full neurologic testing to look for motor weakness, sensory changes, and long tract signs (Hoffmann, Babinski, and clonus). Gait and balance should also be tested, such as toe-walking, heel-walking, and toe-to-heel tandem gait (walking a tightrope). An isolated reflex may be decreased because of anterior horn cell necrosis or concomitant root impingement, but patients with myelopathy are generally hyperreflexic with the pathologic reflexes noted before.

427

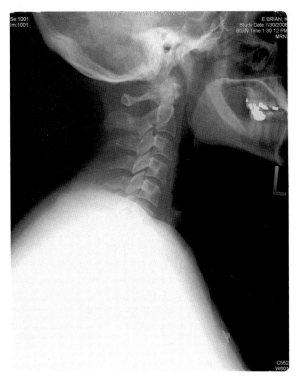

Figure 22–1A A lateral radiograph of a normal cervical spine. There is normal disc height at each level and no evidence of osteophytic changes.

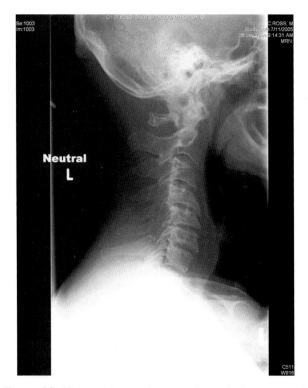

Figure 22–1B Lateral cervical spine radiograph showing significant cervical spondylosis. Note the loss of disc space height, loss of normal lordosis, and osteophytes present at the posterior aspect of the end plates as well as the anterior part of the vertebral bodies.

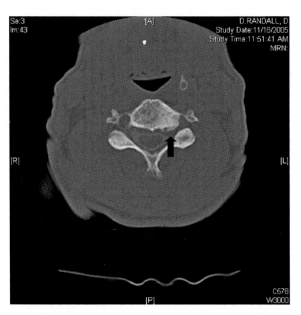

Figure 22–2 (Cervical radiculopathy) A CT myelogram cross-section demonstrating a left-sided disc herniation in the typical posterolateral position (arrow). This will compress the exiting nerve root typically producing radiculopathy.

Neck Pain Alone

Many patients with cervical spondylosis have neck pain without symptoms or signs of radiculopathy or myelopathy. In patients with cervical spondylosis, this axial neck pain is usually from degenerative disks or facet arthritis. At times, patients with moderate to severe cervical stenosis from spondylotic changes have significant neck pain but

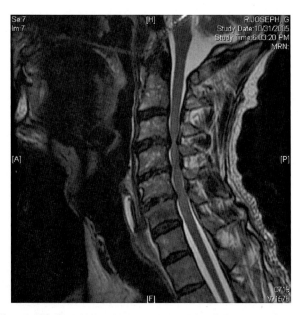

Figure 22–3 A sagittal T_2-weighted MRI of the cervical spine demonstrating multiple levels of cervical spondylosis producing canal narrowing and cord compression at three different levels. Clinically this patient had severe signs and symptoms of cervical myelopathy.

no evidence of myelopathy or radiculopathy on examination.[7] This is a reason to consider neuroradiologic investigation of patients with significant, debilitating neck pain alone because if stenosis is present, it can be surgically addressed with good results.

Diagnostic Evaluation

Plain radiographs remain the cornerstone of the diagnostic work-up for OA of the cervical spine.[8] Disk space narrowing, posterior osteophytes, and size of the spinal canal can be determined from a plain lateral radiograph. Oblique films can visualize foraminal spurring, although they are not routinely necessary. Flexion and extension lateral views are helpful and can pick up instability that may not be evident on a neutral lateral view.

The next diagnostic study in symptomatic patients is magnetic resonance imaging (MRI). This modality provides excellent visualization of the soft tissues, including disks and the neural elements.[9–11] Bone detail, such as osteophytic ridging, can be seen but not to the extent that computed tomographic (CT) imaging allows. Plain CT scans do not show the neural structures adequately, so if further evaluation is needed, myelography plus CT-myelography is recommended. A well-done myelogram can demonstrate root impingement that may not be appreciated on MRI. CT-myelography delineates cord compression as well; often these more invasive studies are obtained to decide which levels need to be included in multilevel fusion procedures.

Electrodiagnostic studies can be helpful in confirming cervical radiculopathy or clarifying peripheral nerve entrapment syndromes, such as carpal tunnel or thoracic outlet syndrome. Brachial plexopathy is another entity that can mimic acute cervical radiculopathy in which evaluation by electromyography and nerve conduction velocity studies is useful. In straightforward cases of cervical radiculopathy or stenosis, however, electrodiagnostic studies are not necessary. These tests are of little or no value in the diagnostic work-up of cervical myelopathy.

Nonoperative Treatment

For patients with cervical radiculopathy or neck pain alone, there are three main nonoperative treatment measures: 1) soft collar immobilization, 2) anti-inflammatory medication, and 3) physical therapy modalities including traction.

A soft collar limits extremes in range of motion and rests the overworked paraspinal musculature. Nonsteroidal medications are initially used, and a short steroid taper can be effective for pinched nerve symptoms. Physical therapy methods of heat, ultrasound, and massage may relieve some muscle symptoms as well; traction can sometimes promote resolution of radicular symptoms, particularly in younger patients. With home traction kits, care should be taken to instruct patients to "face the door" in traction with use of a rope and water bag; this ensures slight flexion of the neck rather than extension, the latter of which closes down the spinal canal and usually exacerbates the symptoms. Epidural steroid injections are performed at some centers, but the physician must be well trained in this technique given the proximity of the spinal cord; patients with a narrow spinal canal should probably avoid injection treatments in the cervical spine.

Patients with cervical myelopathy are more difficult to treat nonoperatively because frank spinal cord compression is present. A soft collar and nonsteroidal anti-inflammatory medications may be used for pain flare-ups, but traction or manipulation should be avoided. Symptoms and documented cord impingement consistent with moderate to severe myelopathy are generally treated operatively.

Indications for Surgery

Patients with neck pain alone from spondylotic changes are preferably managed with anti-inflammatory medications and physical therapy measures as needed. At times, however, patients without radiculopathy or myelopathy but with significant, intractable neck pain have cervical stenosis. This subset of patients with neck pain only responds well to anterior decompression and fusion, provided that months of nonoperative treatment efforts have failed.[12]

Symptoms of radiculopathy from a soft disk herniation or spondylosis usually resolve in 2 to 3 months with (or often without) treatment. If pain persists longer than this and if nonoperative measures have failed, and the symptoms are not tolerable for the patient, surgery is indicated.[13] Mild weakness can be observed closely and often resolves as well. Moderate to severe weakness with substantial pathologic changes on neuroradiologic studies may need decompression to optimize neural recovery. Patients with mild cervical myelopathy may remain stable for years and can be observed. They should have long-term follow-up, however, because the natural history of myelopathy in the majority of patients is slow, stepwise deterioration.[14,15] If moderate to severe myelopathy is present with cord compression evident on studies, surgical decompression is indicated to at least stabilize and usually improve the neurologic status of the patient.

Surgical Treatment

Anterior Approach

For many spine surgeons, the anterior surgical approach is the preferred method for operative treatment of degenerative conditions of the neck.[6,16–19] Because most spinal cord or nerve root compression is anterior as a result of ridging of the vertebral end plates, disk herniations, or uncovertebral hypertrophy, the anterior approach is a direct way of removing the pathologic process and relieving compression. It is useful for patients with radiculopathy, myelopathy, instability, and deformities such as kyphosis.[20]

The most commonly performed procedure is the anterior cervical discectomy and fusion (ACDF). This technique can well address pathologic changes limited to the disk space or adjacent end plates. The operative approach is through the fascial planes of the anterior neck and is straightforward.[21] After decompression of the neural elements, the end plates are abraded with a burr to provide a raw bleeding surface, which increases the fusion rate.[22] A horseshoe-shaped tricortical iliac crest bone graft is harvested from the patient's iliac crest and carefully fitted into place after some gentle distraction of the disk space. With successful arthrodesis, that segment is stabilized and foraminal height is maintained. Autograft has superior healing properties;[23] however, many surgeons use allograft in one-level ACDF procedures or in instrumented cases; good results have been reported with allograft material.[24-27]

Anterior Plate Fixation

Anterior instrumentation of the cervical spine for degenerative conditions has increased in popularity during the past 10 years. Initially developed for use in traumatic injuries, anterior plates can help stabilize the grafted segments in degenerative disease and promote a higher fusion rate for multilevel ACDF procedures (Fig. 22–4).[28-32] Their use may also decrease the need for rigid postoperative bracing. Anterior instrumentation is typically used for two- or three-level ACDF procedures. One-level anterior cervical ACDF operations have a high union rate, and though many surgeons use a plate in these cases, in the absence of other circumstances such as adjacent fused levels,[33] history of a pseudarthrosis, or smoking, a plate is probably unnecessary.[34] As with any instrumentation, there is some increased risk of loosening and malposition or the need to remove the plate on rare occasions.[35]

Anterior Cervical Corpectomy and Strut Graft Fusions

For many patients with severe degenerative conditions, particularly those with spinal cord compression and myelopathy, ACDF techniques alone may not address all the compressive disease. Many patients with cervical spondylotic myelopathy or ossified posterior longitudinal ligament may need one or more corpectomies followed by a longer strut graft placement.[6,36-39]

Corpectomy procedures are designed to remove compressive disease behind the vertebral bodies. The initial exposure and technique are similar to those for ACDF. For a corpectomy, the middle portion of the vertebral body is removed. This is often done over two or three levels, because many patients with severe spondylosis have multi-level disease. This long channel is then spanned with a strut graft. Anterior instrumentation is useful for one-level corpectomy and strut grafting procedures; however, longer constructs become biomechanically unfavorable for long anterior plates,[40,41] and patients with these long reconstruction procedures need rigid bracing to protect the graft and maximize healing. Concomitant posterior fusion may be performed to maximize stability with circumferential arthrodesis (Fig. 22–5).[42] These are often complex procedures in patients with severe myelopathy and should be performed by spine surgeons with experience in this area and with significant ancillary backup, such as spinal cord monitoring.

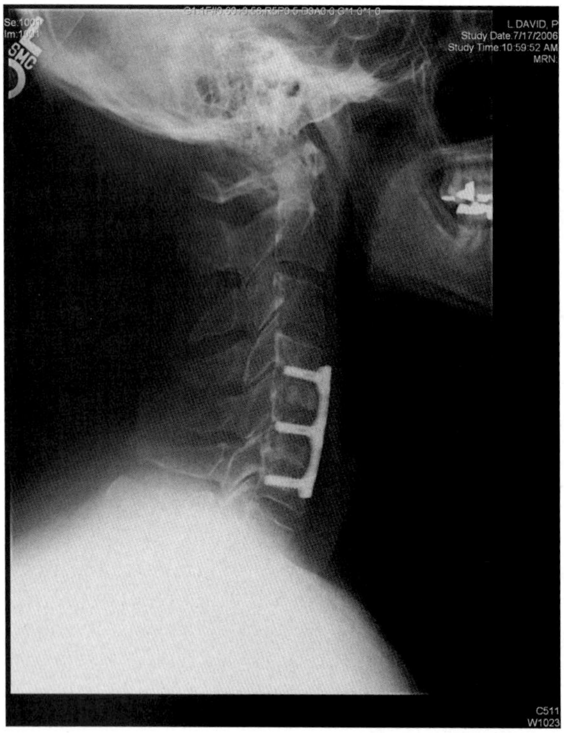

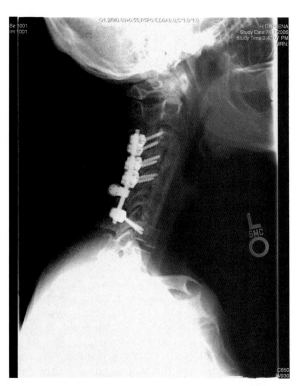

Figure 22–4 A lateral cervical spine radiograph approximately 1 year following a two-level anterior cervical discectomy and fusion with allograft plus anterior plating. The patient's cervical radiculopathy was completely relieved.

Figure 22–5 A lateral cervical radiograph approximately 1 year post-op following a three-level anterior cervical corpectomy, fibula strut grafting followed by posterior instrumentation for stabilization. This patient was treated for severe cervical myelopathy with resultant improvement of clinical symptoms.

Posterior Approach

The simplest posterior approach is that for a lateral soft disk herniation.[43-45] A keyhole laminotomy is performed by thinning a lamina with a burr. Then, using a Kerrison rongeur to perform a foraminotomy, the surgeon visualizes the takeoff of the nerve root. Epidural veins need to be controlled, and the disk can be incised by gently retracting the nerve root cephalad. If most of the facet joint has been preserved, no fusion is needed and the patient can use a soft collar postoperatively for comfort. If there is any cord deformation, the posterior laminotomy approach is typically avoided because the herniated disk is more safely accessible from an anterior approach.

For multilevel spondylotic disease with cervical stenosis, a laminectomy can be performed.[46,47] This procedure should be reserved for patients without deformity or pre-existing instability and for those with severe anterior cord impingement.[48] Because of the difficult problem of post-laminectomy kyphosis in some patients who have had multilevel laminectomies, a technique called laminoplasty has evolved in the last 20 years. This was developed in Japan to address severe cord compression in patients with continuous ossified posterior longitudinal ligament. Its indications have expanded to include patients with cervical spondylotic myelopathy. Laminoplasty is a canal-expanding procedure in which the posterior laminae are hinged open and held there by bone grafts or suture until healing occurs (Fig. 22-6).[49-53] The spinal canal is then enlarged and cervical stenosis thus relieved. Laminoplasty is a satisfactory technique for patients with normal lordosis (so the spinal cord can float posteriorly),[54,55] with no instability, and without significant neck pain. Because the soft tissues can heal to a residual bone roof, the incidence of postoperative kyphosis has decreased. A laminoplasty is not as technically demanding as long anterior corpectomy and strut graft procedures are, and does not require a fusion. Both laminoplasty and anterior decompression and strut graft methods have had satisfactory neural recovery rates.[36,56] Corpectomy and strut grafting procedures can correct deformity and stabilize the neck; they seem to have better pain results than those suggested by laminoplasty reports.[6,57]

Results

Both anterior and posterior decompression procedures have been demonstrated to provide satisfactory neurologic recovery.[55] Patients with cervical spondylosis and radiculopathy can achieve particularly good results with anterior cervical ACDF techniques.[16,58-60] Patients with cervical spondylotic myelopathy often require longer, more extensive decompression procedures, either anterior or posterior.[61] Improvement can be expected in most of these patients with myelopathy, resulting in increased strength, improved gait, and better overall function.[6,37,39,62] Neurologic recovery in patients with myelopathy largely depends on the degree of myelopathy existing preoperatively as well as other factors, including degree of cord compression on preoperative studies and duration of symptoms.

Pain relief for patients undergoing cervical spine procedures for degenerative disorders is most consistent for arm pain. For patients with significant arthritic changes in the neck, we prefer anterior decompression and fusion for best relief of pain, although posterior laminotomy and discectomy with or without a foraminotomy can provide good results for radiculopathy as well. Whereas radicular pain is relieved in approximately 90% of patients, axial neck pain can be expected to be relieved in approximately 80% of patients.[16,63,64] In the older population, certainly other degenerative levels can contribute to persistent axial symptoms. Patients with recurrent pain after fusion procedures should be evaluated to rule out a pseudarthrosis or problems at adjacent levels.

THORACIC SPINE

Due to the rib cage, the thoracic spine is more stable and has less range of motion than the other regions of the spine. This added stability results in less degenerative changes and less clinical problems than seen in the cervical or lumbar areas. Certainly degenerative disc disease does occur in thoracic levels and some facet changes can occur, however, these aging changes are usually well tolerated. There are two main clinical syndromes that result from degenerative changes of the thoracic spine: thoracic *disc herniations* and thoracic *spinal stenosis*.

Thoracic Disc Herniations

Presumably due to less motion and lower loads, thoracic disc herniations are less frequent than those in the lumbar or even cervical regions. Clinicians have become more

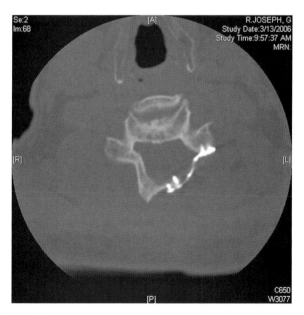

Figure 22–6 A post-operative axial CT image showing expansion of the spinal canal following laminoplasty. The small titanium plate helps maintain the posterior elements in the open trap door position. Typically this would be done over several levels to address all areas of cervical stenosis.

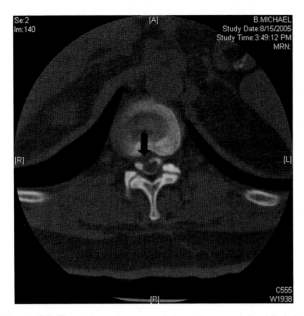

Figure 22–7 A CT myelogram axial cut shows a right-sided thoracic disc herniation (arrow). Note there is some deformation of the spinal cord. Because of physiologic thoracic kyphosis, the spinal cord normally rests against the posterior vertebral bodies, thus a small- to medium-sized thoracic disc herniation can produce cord deformation with symptoms.

aware of thoracic disc pathology, however, since the introduction of MRI technology and the ability to easily image this area (Fig. 22–7). As with disc herniations anywhere in the spine, thoracic disc herniations are usually asymptomatic. Whether or not they will cause symptoms depends primarily on size and location.[65] Because of the kyphotic nature of the thoracic spine, the spinal cord will usually rest against the posterior aspect of the vertebral body when patients are upright. A central disc herniation in the thoracic region can more easily produce cord deformation, even though the protrusion itself may not be terribly large. Cord compression can cause pain that is typically in the midline of the back. Patients may also describe a boring type pain that radiates through the chest to the sternal area. Other reasons for thoracic pain, such as thoracic or intra-abdominal visceral causes, must be kept in mind. Pain, however, may be minimal or nonexistent, yet enough cord compression can cause thoracic myelopathy. These patients present with gait imbalance, weakness of the lower extremities, and/or numbness of the lower extremities. Severe compression may cause sphincter dysfunction as well. The pattern would be that of an upper motor neuron lesion since the spinal cord is involved. Posterolateral disc protrusions in the thoracic spine may not cause cord compression at all, but if large enough can pinch the exiting nerve root and cause radicular pain radiating around the rib cage at the level of the herniation.

Diagnostic Evaluation

Radiographic imaging is the basis of evaluation for these patients. Plain films may show evidence of thoracic disc disease which will not be terribly helpful.[66,67] However, fractures or evidence of bone destruction such as with neoplastic disorders or infection will often be readily visible on plain x-rays. The next study of choice is MRI. This allows for excellent visualization of soft tissue such as disc herniations and a good view of bone pathology as well.[68–70] A good quality image can detect disc protrusions and cord deformation if present. At times, signal changes within the cord are visible, suggesting acute injury with edema or more commonly chronic compression causing histologic changes termed myelomylacia. The predictive value of signal changes while in the spinal cord itself and of degenerative conditions is debatable at this time.

Plain CT scans are typically not helpful for evaluation of thoracic disc pathology. CT myelography does give an excellent outline of the spinal cord and is still helpful for preoperative planning. Electromyography (EMG) nerve conduction studies are not helpful for the diagnosis of thoracic disc herniation in order to evaluate myelopathy or radiculopathy; however, it may be of use for differential diagnosis considerations such as Guillain-Barré syndrome, peripheral neuropathy, or amyotrophic lateral sclerosis. Evoked potential studies in these authors' opinion have been of little diagnostic or prognostic value for thoracic disc pathology.

Nonoperative Treatment

Nonoperative treatment of thoracic disc herniations will follow similar guidelines for low back pain. Mild to moderate symptoms can be treated with nonsteroidal anti-inflammatories, narcotic pain medicine for short periods, and muscle relaxers. Passive modalities such as heat, ice, ultrasound, and electrical stimulation have all been used and may promote short-term relief. Thoracic strengthening exercises plus aerobic conditioning may promote pain relief in the longer term. These authors would not recommend epidural steroid injections for a central disc herniation with cord compression; however, intercostal root blocks may give some relief for a more posterolateral disc herniation with radicular symptoms radiating around the rib cage.

Operative Treatment

Indications for surgery include intolerable pain unresponsive to conservative measures and evidence of thoracic myelopathy from cord compression.[71] Because the surgical treatment of thoracic disc herniations requires a fairly large operation, most surgeons will allow for many months or even years for pain symptoms to resolve on their own before recommending operative intervention.[72]

Because thoracic disc herniations usually produce anterior cord compression, the anterior surgical approach is typically favored.[73,74] This allows for a no-touch technique such that the disc herniation is pulled away from the dura thus relieving the anterior compression on the cord without manipulation of the neural structures. Many, but not all, spine surgeons perform an arthrodesis of that motion segment after the discectomy, though there are no hard data to suggest that fusion is necessary.[75,76] Usually this anterior approach to the spine requires an open thoracotomy, which is not without morbidity including late incisional pain. Some spine surgeons have more recently pioneered thorocoscopic surgical treatment of thoracic disc herniations.[77,78] This also requires an anterior approach but through much smaller incisional portals with thoracoscopic instruments. The steep learning curve and questions regarding ultimate improvement in outcomes compared to standard open techniques have kept this technique from becoming mainstream.

Thoracic Spinal Stenosis

Unlike thoracic disc herniations, the pathoanatomy for thoracic stenosis arises from the posterior elements. Posterior facet hypertrophy and occasionally ossification of the ligamentum flavum produce dorsal compression.[79-83] Circumferential canal compromise can occur if there are associated bulging discs or endplate osteophytes (Fig. 22–8). Typically this occurs over several levels and is more common in the lower thoracic spine. These degenerative changes occur slowly over time and significant compression may be present before clinical symptoms arise. Presentation usually develops as a gait disturbance, weakness in the lower extremities, or numbness. Sphincter dysfunction is a late sign usually associated with severe compression. Hyperreflexia and pathological reflexes consistent with upper motor neuron pathology will be present in moderate to severe myelopathy.

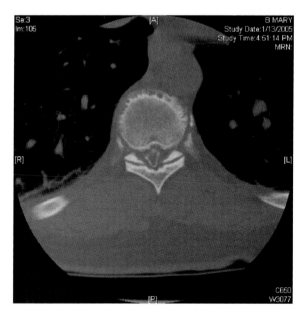

Figure 22–8 A CT myelogram axial cut showing a severely deformed spinal cord. Note the thin rim of dye around the cord itself. There is almost circumferential compression with some bulging of the disc as well as hypertrophic facet changes producing the thoracic stenosis.

Diagnostic Imaging

MRI is the study of choice for initial evaluation of suspected thoracic spinal stenosis. Because the pathology is often bony in nature with hypertrophic osteoarthritic facet changes, CT myelography may allow better visualization of the pathoanatomy, which can be useful for preoperative planning.

Because of the difference in pathoanatomy, thoracic spinal stenosis is typically treated by a posterior approach as opposed to anterior surgery for thoracic disc herniations as described earlier.[84] A laminectomy at the appropriate number of pathological levels will typically decompress the spinal cord and allow for neural recovery or at least stop the neurologic deterioration.[85] Many surgeons will add a posterior instrumented fusion over the decompressed levels if there are instability, kyphotic deformity, or obesity issues.[86-88]

LUMBAR SPINE

Introduction

For many patients and physicians alike, problems related to the lumbar spine may be considered the bane of human existence. Low back pain and degenerative conditions of the lumbar region are ubiquitous, with symptoms ranging from a minor annoyance to incapacitating pain. Though imaging techniques have certainly given us better anatomic views of the lumbar spine and associated pathological conditions, there is often a disconnect between patient symptoms and radiographic findings.[89-91] Add this variability to a plethora of nonoperative and operative treatment options with less than clear-cut outcomes, and one is left with a difficult area in health care. This section will attempt to provide clarity and acknowledge the limitations in both knowledge and clinical practice.

Incidence

It is estimated that 50% to 80% of the adult population will at some time suffer from low back pain.[92,93] One study documented a true incidence of 34% of men and 37% of women will develop new onset of low back pain over a 1-year period of the study.[94] Not only is low back pain common but it can also be functionally limiting, leading to significant time lost at work.[95-99] Twelve and a half percent of all illness-related absent days during a 10-year period were due to back pain in a Swedish study.[100] This has a huge socioeconomic impact on the economy. Using 1996 data, the total annual productivity losses from chronic back pain were estimated to be $28 billion in the United States alone.[101] More recently, the total annual direct and indirect costs for chronic low back pain were $2,900 and $16,600, respectively.[102] Spine disorders were the most frequent main cause of work limitation in adults in 1998, followed by heart disease, OA, and respiratory diseases.[96] In 1999, six large U.S. employers were evaluated for conditions generating the largest health and productivity cost burdens; it was found that for physical diseases, low back pain ranked fourth behind angina pectoris, essential hypertension, and diabetes mellitus.[103]

Risk Factors

Certain factors have been shown to contribute to the development of disorders of the lumbar spine.[104-108] One study demonstrated earlier radiographic degenerative changes in masonry workers doing heavy labor as compared to house painters.[109] There is also some evidence, however, that people who are sedentary may have a greater incidence of degenerative disc disease.[106,110] People who drive a bus or truck for a living have also been shown, in some studies, to have a higher incidence of low back disorders, perhaps because of vibrational stress—although other studies seem to show no correlation.[111-114]

Other factors such as obesity[115,116] and smoking[117] have been associated with a higher risk of degenerative disc disease. As in any clinical disorders, genetics is also believed to play a role.[118-120] A study comparing monozygotic and dizygotic twins[121] suggests that a strong genetic influence on intervertebral disc degeneration. A defect in collagen IX was recently reported in certain patients with lumbar disc herniations.[122,123] Additional studies found that the Trp 3 allele acted synergistically with obesity to increase disc bulging and height loss in the lumbar spine.[124] Elevated levels of collagen II degradation may also play a role in postmenopausal women.[125,126]

Pathoanatomy

The underlying cause of degenerative conditions in the lumbar spine is due to aging of the intervertebral disc (Fig. 22–9A, B, C).[127,128] Normal discs are excellent shock

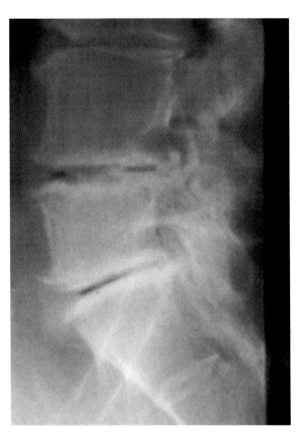

Figure 22–9B This lateral radiograph of the lumbar spine demonstrates typical degenerative changes. Note severe disc narrowing at L4-5 and L5-S1 with anterior and posterior osteophytes evident at the end plates. A dark streak in the disc at these two levels is felt to represent nitrogen gas related to disc degeneration.

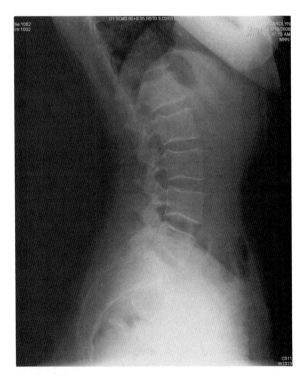

Figure 22–9A A lateral radiograph of the lumbar spine showing normal disc height, normal alignment, and lack of osteophyte changes.

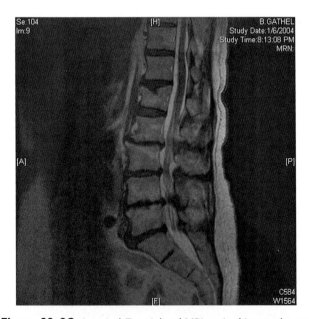

Figure 22–9C A typical T_2-weighted MRI sagittal image demonstrating lumbar disc degeneration. Note disc narrowing, irregularities of the end plates in the low lumbar spine, with small- to medium-sized disc bulges evident at the four lowest levels. Note some inward buckling of hypertrophic ligamentum flavum particularly at the L4-5 level.

absorbers and allow motion at multiple segments in the entire spine. The center of the disc is the nucleus pulposus, which consists of proteoglycans, type II collagen, and water, with small contributions from type IX and other collagens. The nucleus is concentrically surrounded by the multilayered annulus fibrosis. This is composed of strong type I collagen that is attached to the end plates of the vertebral body above and below. Biochemical changes occur within the nucleus pulposus primarily with loss of water content and a relative shift of chondrotin sulfate to keratin sulfate which makes up the proteoglycan matrix.[129-131] Loss of hydrostatic pressure and fluid-like properties of the nucleus compromises the ability of the disc to resist compression and shear forces.[132,133] Bulging of the disc occurs and the annulus develops tears or fissures.[134-136] When the nucleus pulposus protrudes posteriorly, either elevating the annulus or penetrating through it, a *disc herniation* has occurred. Though many disc herniations occur in young individuals with seemingly healthy discs, most disc herniations occur in slightly degenerative discs where the annulus cannot contain the herniation of nucleus pulposus material.

Simple bulging of the disc with loss of height will slightly alter the biomechanics of that motion segment.[137,138] This will directly affect the facet joints posteriorly over the long term. These joints are true synovial joints and here is where true OA can occur, with hypertrophic bony changes and loss of cartilage.[139-145] These degenerative changes can lead to thickening of the soft tissues with hypertrophic capsule and ligamentum flavum developing. These posterior element changes, in conjunction with bulging (or herniated) discs, can compromise the volume of the spinal canal and the neural elements leading to lumbar *spinal stenosis*. Facet arthritis and capsular changes can lead to incompetence of the facet joints as stabilizing structures.[139] If the disc is unable to control shear forces, then a degenerative *spondylolisthesis* can slowly develop. This is very common in the older population at the L4-5 level, more so in females than males. Asymmetric degenerative changes in the lumbar spine structures can lead to *degenerative scoliosis*.

Clinical Syndromes

Mechanical Low Back Pain

Low back pain is a general term that includes many pathologic conditions and spans many patient age groups. It is well known that low back pain can occur with totally normal radiographic studies including MRI. This is believed to be due to soft tissue strain on muscle, ligament, or capsular tissues.[146] Tears of the outer annulus fibrosis can at times be seen on MRI. This is felt to be a possible cause of low back pain in some individuals, but the correlation of symptoms with these radiographic findings are limited.[147] There is reasonably good evidence, however, that degeneration of the intervertebral discs is responsible for mechanical back pain in many patients. One study[148] documented that in a group of 20-year-old patients, one or more lumbar discs were abnormal in 57% of those with low back pain

symptoms versus only 35% of asymptomatic patients. However, the incidence of radiographic disc degeneration is certainly much higher than that of symptomatic lumbar disorders.[149,150] In a study of asymptomatic patients using MRI, approximately one third of subjects were found to have substantial abnormalities. In patients 60 years of age or more, abnormal findings were present on 57% of these MRI scans.[151] Even patients younger than 40 years of age showed a 19.5% incidence of disc degeneration or other radiographic abnormalities.[152]

Mechanical low back pain may develop acutely or in a more insidious pattern. Often there is a history of excessive activities or minor trauma though this certainly is not always the case. Body position and lifting maneuvers have been shown to significantly increase loads on lumbar discs.[153,154] Patients may have the perception that low back pain due to degenerative processes or soft tissue injury should be mild or always self-limiting.[155-159] On the contrary, episodic low back pain can be quite severe with debilitating pain or muscle spasm that can interfere with activities of daily living or even ambulation.[160] Severe pain should always be investigated and persistence of significant low back pain may herald a more sinister diagnosis such as neoplasm, infection, or pathologic fracture.

Low back pain due to degenerative disc disease is typically located in the midline, though it is often painful across the whole width of the lumbar area. Mechanical low back pain can radiate down into the buttocks and even the proximal thigh areas. This is often called *referred* pain.[161,162] It typically should not go below the knee, which would signify a more *radicular* pattern of pain and suggest nerve root compression rather than a mechanical etiology. Sensory symptoms, motor complaints, or sphincter disturbance are all symptoms of neurologic compression and should not be associated with pure mechanical back pain. Severe back pain will usually cause the patient to lie down for relief since standing or sitting may be difficult.[163,164] Pain waking the patient at night would be more suggestive of neoplastic disease.

In patients over 40, OA of the hips should always be entertained in a differential diagnosis in this patient population. Though most patients with hip arthritis will present with groin pain and, often, anterior thigh pain, a certain percentage of patients with hip disease will present with only low back pain. Careful examination and radiographic evaluation should clarify the diagnosis, though at times an intra-articular lidocaine plus steroid injection into the hip joints proper can help differentiate hip OA versus lumbar spine disease as a cause of low back and leg symptoms.

Physical Examination

Most patients with chronic low back pain can easily ambulate in a normal fashion, but those with severe acute episodes may have difficulty.[165,166] Most patients will be tender in the paraspinal muscles, and range of motion, particularly in flexion, will be limited.[167-169] Hypersensitivity to touch and exaggerated response to the examination may suggest psychosomatic overlay to complicate the picture.[170]

Motor, sensory, and reflex examination as part of the neurologic evaluation should be unremarkable in patients with isolated mechanical low back pain without neurologic compromise. As mentioned above, examination of the hips should always be performed looking for OA or hip bursitis as an etiology of the patient's symptoms.

Diagnostic Evaluation

Though an acute lumbar strain does not always need initial radiographs, if the low back pain persists for more than 1 to 2 weeks, radiographs are usually indicated. We would recommend AP, lateral, and oblique lumbar films for initial evaluation. Flexion/extension views can be obtained if any instability needs to be evaluated. Oblique films are important since spondylolysis (established stress fracture of the pars interarticularis) is present in about 5% of the U.S. population. This typically causes mechanical low back pain, particularly in younger patients, and most likely will require more treatment efforts than a simple strain; it is important to make this diagnosis (Fig. 22–10).[148] Plain radiographs of the hips are recommended for older patients since hip OA may present primarily as low back pain as previously mentioned.

CT scanning is sometimes used as the next step in diagnostic evaluation of mechanical low back pain. This can show evidence of disc degeneration and gives a cross-sectional view of the spinal canal. It also provides excellent visualization of facet joint arthritis and chronic pars interarticularis defects that may be difficult to see on plain x-rays. Because of its superior capability to image the disc, neural elements, and soft tissues, MRI is generally more valuable and utilized more frequently for evaluation of low back symptoms. MRI is the study of choice for diagnosing degenerative disc disease, spinal stenosis, synovial cysts, as well as infections and neoplasms.[171,172] It is also useful for diagnosing vertebral body compression fractures that in the older population frequently present as mechanical low back pain. Though MRI gives us an excellent view of the pathoanatomy, it does not always help localize the pain source, particularly in patients with mechanical back pain without radiculopathy.[173] It must be remembered that both young and old patients commonly have abnormal MRI findings of their lumbar spine without any symptoms whatsoever, so it remains the clinician's task to link pathoanatomy to clinical symptoms.[174] This is a crucial point to note.

A particularly vexing problem for clinicians and patients alike is that of low back symptoms caused by "discogenic pain." The outer fibers of the annulus are innervated, and as the discs degenerate it is believed that this can cause low back pain in some patients.[175-180] In an attempt to learn which disc might be the source of pain, *discography* evolved decades ago as a diagnostic tool. A needle is introduced into the disc space and dye is injected. Leakage out through the annulus indicates disc degeneration but has little if any value in localizing the pain source. Since discography is done with the patient awake, the *concordant pain* response to the increased fluid pressure created in the degenerative disc space is believed by some authors to have utility in localizing the painful disc. We avoid discography in patients with multiple levels of lumbar degenerative disc disease, though it has been found to be of some benefit as a confirmatory test for patients with one-level pathology in the absence of psychosomatic issues.

Nonoperative Treatment

Most low back pain is acute in nature and self-limiting. For these patients, treatment is symptomatic in order to try to keep the patients functional during their episode. One or two days of bed rest may help severe symptoms, but prolonged bed rest is counterproductive because of deconditioning and overemphasizing the illness.[155,160] There are many treatment options for low back pain, including medications, passive and active physical therapy modalities, chiropractic treatments, acupuncture, and bracing. Some of these options have been shown to be effective, though most have either not been rigorously tested or, in fact, have been shown equivalent to the natural history of recovery. For an acute bout of low back pain, we recommend nonsteroidal anti-inflammatories, muscle relaxers as needed, and even a short course of oral narcotics as needed.[158,159,180,181] Decreasing activities is appropriate though complete bed rest should be avoided. As the patient's symptoms begin to settle down, physical therapy efforts can be of benefit. Passive modalities such as heat, ice, electrical

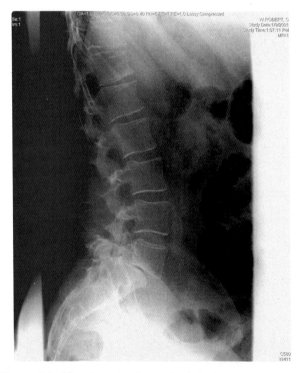

Figure 22–10 A lateral radiograph of the lumbar spine showing an isthmic spondylolisthesis at L5-S1. The chronic pars interarticularis defect allows for slippage of the L5 vertebrae. This can occur at other levels but L5-S1 is by far the most common. Note significant disc degeneration at this lowest level as well. This pathology can be a cause of significant low back pain with or without radiculopathy.

stimulation, and massage can certainly provide some relief in the short run for many patients though this is difficult to prove in scientific studies. As the patient can tolerate, active core strengthening combined with stretching and aerobic conditioning has the best chance of providing sustained relief or at least minimizing recurrent episodes.[182-191] Whether active exercise such as aerobic conditioning promotes relief based on increased endogenous endorphins, treatment of underlying depression, or physiologically helping at the source of the pain is unclear. Use of a lumbar corset or other type of brace may be of some benefit for patients with mechanical low back pain, particularly in the manual labor population. An effort should be made to maintain these patients on an exercise program, however, so their muscles do not get deconditioned from use of the brace.[192-195] In a Norwegian study, it was found that early rehabilitation led to less time off work and diminished productivity losses.[196] Individualized therapy that addressed the patients' realization of back pain seemed to offer some advantages.

Trigger point injections into areas of maximal tenderness in the lumbar region may provide some temporary relief, but are so nonspecific that we believe they are of little value. Facet blocks, with injection of an anesthetic plus steroid, can also provide some short-term relief in an older population with facet arthritis.[197-199] Though these are commonly done in some centers, these authors have found them to be of only transient benefit and are of lasting value for only an occasional patient.

Chronic low back pain is typically defined as symptoms greater than 3 months in duration. This entity is difficult to treat and results in huge socioeconomic losses from loss of work time. Many of these patients are part of a workers' compensation support system that actually promotes the prevalence of this disorder in industrialized nations. In some studies, return to work in chronic low back pain patients is correlated more with job satisfaction and managing the fear of recurrent injury as opposed to actual physical disability.[170,200,201] Rehabilitation efforts have focused not only on the physical component with programs such as active exercise and work hardening, but also psychological counseling and job modification for this patient population.[202] Pain management has evolved into a discipline of its own, which is well beyond the scope of this topic.

Operative Treatment

Successful surgical treatment of low back pain syndromes will depend on 1) the specific diagnosis and 2) patient selection. If a patient with mechanical low back pain unresponsive to nonoperative measures has an L5 bilateral spondylolysis, then that patient may respond very well to a one-level arthrodesis. Similarly, if a young patient has severe degenerative disc disease at one level with incapacitating mechanical symptoms and no secondary gain issues, then anterior interbody fusion can achieve excellent results. However, in that same patient with a degenerative disc who is on workers' compensation, and who smokes and dislikes his job, even a technically successful

arthrodesis is much less likely to result in a satisfactory outcome or return to work.

For the patient with discogenic pain and one or even two levels of severe pathology, if the patient has failed all nonoperative measures for 6 to 12 months and psychosomatic issues or secondary gain are absent or minimized, lumbar fusion is a reasonable option.[203-208] This patient population with only mechanical back pain typically does not have spinal stenosis or other evidence of neural compression. This means a posterior approach, which is the typical surgical approach for decompressive procedures, is not required.[209-211] Anterior interbody fusion is often the procedure of choice in these patients since it avoids stripping of the posterior paraspinal muscles and actually eliminates the suspected source of pain with arthrodesis of the disc space itself.[212] Various techniques of interbody fusion have been utilized for decades, including iliac crest bone graft, cylindrical or polygonal metal cages, or composite cages (Fig. 22–11).[213] Bone graft, typically autogenous but at times allogeneic, would be added anteriorly with these constructs. Bone morphogenic proteins (BMPs) have in recent years been utilized to promote bone formation and obviate the need for autograft harvest. This has been shown to be quite successful for anterior interbody fusion in the lumbar spine when used with either structural cages or allograft cortical rings.[214-220]

Newer alternatives to fusion include lumbar disc arthroplasty or nucleoplasty. Currently, disc arthroplasty

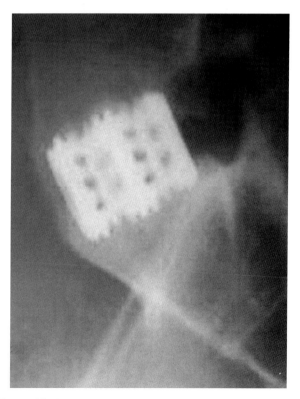

Figure 22–11 A postoperative lateral radiograph with a healed L5-S1 interbody fusion using a cage device plus bone graft. Appropriate patient selection is the key factor in obtaining good results with interbody fusion for discogenic back pain.

techniques include surgical removal of the disc from an anterior approach and replacing this with a metal and polyethylene prosthesis. This is typically press-fit into the disc space with contact on the end plate above and below. The engineered surfaces allow motion to be maintained at that level as an alternative to fusion. There is relatively long term European data on some of these implants and shorter term follow-up data from North America to suggest satisfactory results in properly selected patients.[221-223] In contrast to total disc arthroplasty, nucleoplasty is a research effort designed to replace or enhance the shock absorber function of the nucleus pulposus. Research in hydrogels and compressible synthetics that can be inserted into the disc is being done but has not yet been shown to be effective in the clinical situation.[224-226] The goal of these technologies is to avoid absolute stiffening of the motion segment, which in turn may avoid adjacent segment degenerative changes that can occur in a significant percentage of postfusion patients in the long term.

Lumbar Disc Herniation

Clinical Presentation

Herniation of a lumbar disc is one of the more common causes of symptoms in the lumbar spine. Disc herniations that are large enough can mechanically pinch a nerve root producing back and leg pain or leg pain alone.[227-229] The leg pain component of a low lumbar disc herniation is commonly termed sciatica. The more proper term for leg symptoms involved with nerve root compression manifesting as pain, numbness, or weakness is *radiculopathy*. By definition, this term means symptoms are originating from a nerve root source. The mechanical squeeze on the root is believed to be the main problem in symptomatic disc herniations; however, it has been well established there is a chemical component to radiculopathy.[230-232] Several cytokine mediators including phospholipase A, substance P, and tumor necrosis factor have been shown in animal studies to promote inflammation of the adjacent neural

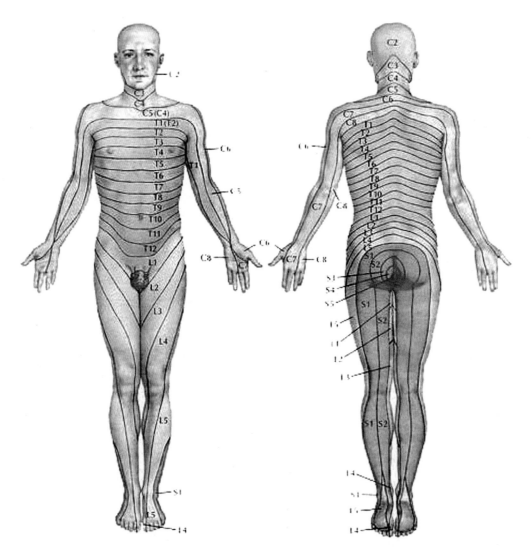

Figure 22–12 A listing of human sensory dermatomes and their distributions.

tissue even in the absence of mechanical compression, which could manifest as radicular signs or symptoms in humans.[233-236] This chemical component may help explain why some patients with an obvious pinched nerve on imaging may or may not be symptomatic.

Most but not all patients who sustain a lumbar disc herniation will have some traumatic episode be it lifting or twisting or bending over. They may or may not feel a pop or some sensation in their low back. Oftentimes, low back pain will be immediate, but the radicular symptoms radiating into the buttock and leg may be delayed for a few days. Either or both the back pain and leg pain may be mild, moderate, or severe. The vast majority of patients will have pain, but, occasionally, a patient may present with frank neurologic deficits such as a foot drop with sensory loss (Fig. 22–12) and have no pain whatsoever. Clinically, we often speak of radicular pain as opposed to referred pain. Referred pain associated with a disc herniation is a deep pain that is felt in the buttocks, sacroiliac joint area, or posterior thigh. It will not radiate below the knee, as this would imply a radicular or nerve root pattern. Referred pain is believed to arise from mechanical or cytokine induced irritation of soft tissue structures such as ligaments, joint capsule, and annulus. Injection of hypertonic saline into these structures has been shown to elicit referred pain into these regions.[161,162]

Typically, disc herniations are unilateral in nature and thus the clinical presentation is that of unilateral buttock and leg symptoms.[237] However, a broad-based large disc herniation can produce bilateral leg symptoms. Severe compression of both sides of the cauda equina with a large midline disc can produce the *cauda equina syndrome*.[238] This syndrome can be somewhat variable with respect to the severity of symptoms, but the hallmark signs and symptoms include some combination of bilateral leg pain, weakness, sensory loss, and sphincter dysfunction.[239,240] Any bilateral weakness or loss of bladder or bowel control warrants emergent neuroradiologic evaluation to rule out a possible cauda equina syndrome. If present from a disc herniation or other mechanical cause, this typically is a true surgical emergency requiring prompt decompression of the thecal sac in order to prevent further loss of neurologic function and promote recovery.

Pathoanatomy

Classically, lumbar disc herniations occur when the nucleus pulposus, which is under significant load in a standing or a sitting position, herniates into the annulus fibrosis or all the way through the annulus fibrosis. This usually occurs in the posterolateral position of the annulus, because the posterior longitudinal ligament is directly in the midline providing some increased strength centrally (Fig. 22–13A, B).[241] Annular fissures are felt to be more common in the posterolateral region as well. The vast majority of lumbar disc herniations occur at the two lowest levels, L4-L5 and L5-S1, probably because these levels sustain the greatest loads and provide the most motion in the low back. Patients in their 60s and 70s are slightly more prone to herniate an upper lumbar disc, such as L1-L2 or

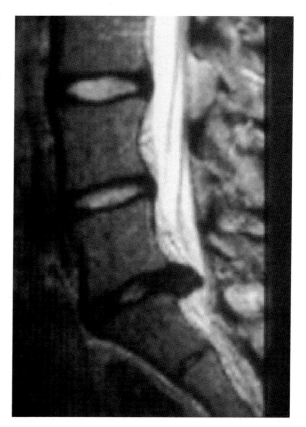

Figure 22–13A A sagittal T_2-weighted MRI image showing a large L5-S1 disc herniation. Note the decreased signal intensity at L5-S1 indicating a lesser water content of that disc.

L2-L3, because these are the only remaining levels with enough moisture in the nucleus pulposus to allow a herniation. Of course, upper lumbar discs will cause more proximal symptoms in patients, causing either groin pain or anterior thigh pain in an upper lumbar root dermatome.

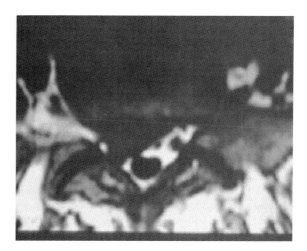

Figure 22–13B This axial T_2-weighted MRI image showing the large disc herniation in the typical posterolateral position. This will cause significant compression of the S1 nerve root with an L5-S1 disc herniation.

Disc herniations run the entire spectrum of size and shape, and this contributes to confusion in terminology as well as variability in clinical syndromes. Simple disc degeneration with loss of water content will result in settling of the disc and bulging of the annulus (much like letting air out of a tire). This simple bulging is not a true disc herniation, though large bulges certainly can take some room away from the spinal canal. Partial herniation of the nucleus pulposus into the annulus will result in a disc herniation called a *protrusion*. By definition, a disc protrusion is not broken through the outer covering of the annulus. If the fragmented nucleus pulposus does protrude through the outer annulus yet still has its tail within the disc, then it is called an *extruded* disc herniation. Fragments that have totally been propelled through the annulus and are no longer in continuity with the disc are called *sequestered* or free disc fragments. Extruded or free fragments tend to be larger and cause more severe symptoms though this is not always true. The exact position of the disc herniation will also dictate which nerve root may be compressed. The most common posterolateral position for herniation will affect the nerve root exiting at the next lowest foramen. For example, an L5-S1 disc herniation in the posterolateral position will produce an S1 radiculopathy. However, a more lateral disc herniation such as an intraforamenal or far lateral herniation will pinch the root in the foramen above the disc, i.e., the L5 nerve root for an L5-S1 lateral disc herniation.

Natural History

It is very important for clinicians to understand the natural history of a lumbar disc herniation with sciatica. Because this syndrome is so very common, knowledge of the natural history can help prevent both nonoperative and operative overtreatment. It has been shown that approximately 80% of patients presenting with sciatica and a disc herniation will resolve their symptoms over 6 to 12 weeks regardless of treatment. This can be quite reassuring to patients that even though their symptoms may be quite severe initially, most of the time the symptoms will get better in a self-limiting fashion.[155,242–245] Why the back and leg pain, or even neurologic symptoms, resolve is not totally understood. It is believed that if the chemical component of nerve root inflammation resolves even though there is no immediate change in any mechanical component, then the symptoms may abate. It has also been well documented that some disc herniations will shrink away over time.[246] This generally takes months to years if it occurs at all. It is believed that extruded or sequestered disc herniation fragments have a better chance of being partially or completely resorbed, probably since it is easier for macrophages to attack the fragment when it is outside the relatively avascular confines of the annulus fibrosis. Slow adaptation of the nerve root itself to compression as well as any degradation of the herniated fragment over time may help explain why the longer term naturally history of symptomatic disc herniations is also relatively favorable. Many patients' symptoms will slowly abate over years, and studies have shown that the results of nonoperative versus operative treatment

of radiculopathy from lumbar disc herniations at 5 years and 10 years seem to be quite similar.[247,248]

Physical Examination

Patients with a lumbar disc herniation and radiculopathy may have difficulty walking secondary to pain. Young patients may present with a list to one side or the other, which suggests they are trying to find a position that minimizes the root compression. Tenderness to palpation in the paraspinal muscles as well as the sciatic notch on the symptomatic side is common. Limitation in lumbar range of motion is also typical. A full neurologic examination should always be performed in evaluation of these patients. Because lumbar disc herniations are most common at the two lowest levels, weakness would usually be present in an L4, L5, or S1 motor group. Similarly, dermatomal sensory findings would most commonly be present for these three root levels. The knee jerk reflex is mediated mostly by L4 and the Achilles reflex is modulated by the S1 level. These reflexes would be decreased (hyporeflexia) in most significant disc herniations with radiculopathy. The hallmark diagnostic finding on examination is the straight leg raising test.[249–251] Typically this is done with a patient supine and both the asymptomatic and symptomatic leg individually elevated with the knee in full extension. This puts mechanical tension on the lumbar roots via the sciatic nerve, and on the ipsilateral side it creates increased buttock and leg pain, typically from 20° to 70° depending on the severity of the root compression. This is considered a positive straight leg raise test. A cross straight leg raise test is when the asymptomatic leg is elevated; if radicular symptoms are reproduced on the opposite (symptomatic) leg, it is a positive test and has been shown to be the most reliable physical examination sign for a lumbar disc herniation.[252–253] Typically these are large disc herniations with significant root compression, where even a slight amount of increased tension on the cauda equina will result in worsening of the symptoms on the opposite side. Examination of rectal tone and perianal sensation should be performed to evaluate for a cauda equina syndrome as described earlier in the appropriate clinical situation.

Diagnostic Studies

Plain radiographs are still important for initial evaluation of patients with a suspected lumbar disc herniation. Though they do not always need to be obtained initially given a favorable natural history of this problem, at some point the patient should have lumbar films to help rule out spondylolysis, spondylolisthesis, scoliosis, or destructive processes such as infection or tumor. Plain films also give a reasonable indication of the degree of disc degeneration present. Dynamic flexion/extension radiographs will help identify instability if that is a concern. Dynamic instability is usually less of a problem in the younger age group where disc herniations are common as opposed to the older population.

Plain CT scans are of limited utility in diagnosing lumbar disc herniations. It can be difficult to see the interface between the disc itself and the thecal sac. Because of the soft tissue limitations, plain CT scanning has largely been replaced by MRI.[171] When combined with myelography, however, CT myelography can indeed be very helpful. This provides the contrast to delineate the neural structures within the canal and identify areas of compression. This is most helpful for areas of central pathology and less helpful for intraforaminal or far lateral disc herniations.[174,197] Again, MRI is superior but may not always be possible for some patients such as those with pacemakers or metal fragments in the eye.

Because MRI has excellent soft tissue visualization and can provide both sagittal and axial images, it is by far the study of choice for evaluating the pathoanatomy in the lumbar spine. T_2-weighted MRIs have been shown to correlate with decreases in proteoglycan content and chondroitin sulfate/keratin sulfate ratios in the nucleus pulposus.[132] Sagittal cuts allow visualization of the nerve root in the foramen with excellent diagnostic capability for identifying intraforaminal and far lateral disc protrusions. Again we will note that because many asymptomatic patients have MRI findings including frank disc herniations, it is up to the clinician to correlate the patient's symptoms with the MRI findings for any given patient.

EMG can be a useful test for accurate diagnosis of symptomatic lumbar disc herniations. Though certainly not indicated for all patients, it is most useful for differential diagnosis considerations such as peripheral neuropathy or a lumbosacral plexopathy, which can mimic intraspinal disease. EMGs are not felt to be accurate enough to pinpoint a given level of symptomatic pathology so they have limited utility in preoperative planning.

A psychological evaluation can play a role in patients with lumbar spine problems including disc herniations. Patients who have had chronic, disabling low back pain may have symptom magnification, hysteria, or associated depression which can be measured on certain psychological tests such as the Minnesota Multiphasic Personality Inventory (MMPI).[255] It has been noted that increased scores in hysteria or hypochondriasis from the MMPI correlate with poor surgical outcomes.[254,255] Though these tests are not routinely used, pain-drawing diagrams are indeed common and simple for office use. A patient depicting entire body pain or large areas in a nondermatonal distribution usually have other psychosomatic issues and not just symptoms from a focal lumbar disc herniation.[256,257]

Nonoperative Treatment

Myriad treatment options exists for lumbar disc herniation patients with many of them lacking in evidence-based efficacy. Because of the favorable natural history of sciatica in most patients, several nonoperative treatment options may successfully make patients more comfortable though not necessarily alter the ultimate outcome. Medications used for low back pain symptoms can also be used for lumbar disc symptoms, including narcotic pain medicine, anti-inflammatories, and muscle relaxers as

needed. Another type of medication that has become relatively popular in treatment of radiculopathy is gabapentin or the next generation pregabalin. Originally designed as an anti-seizure medication, gabapentin can help control neuropathic or radicular pain. A short course of oral steroids can also be quite useful for patients with severe radiculopathy.

Physical therapy efforts can include passive modalities such as heat, ultrasound, electrical stimulation, or massage. None of these modalities are wrong to utilize as they may enhance short-term functioning, though it is unlikely they affect the long-term outcome. More active therapy options include stretching, strengthening, and aerobic conditioning. Typically these are utilized once the severe pain has lessened so that the patient can indeed tolerate and possibly gain benefit from active exercise. Sitting on a stationary bike may not be well tolerated by a patient with a lumbar disc herniation as sitting generally makes the symptoms worse. A treadmill, stair stepper, or aquatic program may be more appropriate for this patient group. Chiropractic manipulation has long been utilized for lumbar spine problems including disc herniations. Though some articles suggest benefit, more rigorous studies show less success for manipulation in patients with lumbar disc.[258-265]

Corticosteroid epidural injections or the similar technique of nerve root blocks have also long been used to treat lumbar radiculopathy. Some studies have shown no benefit compared to placebo, yet other investigators have suggested it can change the natural history and help a portion of the patients avoid surgical intervention.[266] Regardless of the strength of the science behind corticosteroid injections, complications from this method are unusual and it is a well-accepted nonsurgical option for the management of patients with lumbar disc herniations.[267-271]

Operative Treatment

Despite the favorable history of sciatica, lumbar disc herniations are so widespread that a surgical discectomy is a common procedure for this clinical problem. Knowing the time course of the natural history of sciatica suggests that surgical intervention should be delayed 6 to 12 weeks at the minimum if possible, as many patients will resolve their symptoms in this time period. The indications for earlier surgery include cauda equina syndrome,[272] significant or progressive neurologic deficit (typically motor paresis), or severe pain that cannot be controlled with narcotics. Certainly the most common indication for operative treatment is pain, with the second reason being neurologic deficit such as foot drop. As discussed above, cauda equina syndrome is felt to be a surgical emergency and warrants decompression as soon as possible; fortunately this clinical problem is uncommon.

A standard open discectomy involves removal of ligamentun flavum and usually some of the superior lamina, followed by excision of the protruded part of the herniated disc. Despite the term "discectomy," typically only the herniated fragment and any loosely attached fragments of nucleus pulposus in the posterolateral corner of the disc are removed. This leaves the remainder of the disc as a functioning shock absorber to varying degrees, but studies have also shown a 5% to 10% incidence of a recurrent disc herniation at that same level.[273,274] Microdiscectomy evolved as an improved technique using smaller incisions and more limited dissection to preserve the bony architecture and minimize scar tissue formation. Typically a microscope is utilized for this technique, though the actual removal of the disc herniation fragment is essentially the same as a standard open discectomy.

Percutaneous methods of partial discectomy have waxed and waned in popularity over the last 20 years. Suffice it to say for this venue, percutaneous methods have not attained wide popularity.[275–277] The safety, efficacy, and same day surgery results of microdiscectomy have kept that as the procedure of choice for most spine surgeons.

Surgical Results

Studies examining the outcome of patients with lumbar disc herniations having surgical treatment will vary primarily according to patient selection. In patients with a clear cut radiculopathy, a large disc with root compression evident on imaging studies, and no secondary gain issues such as worker's compensation, will have a 90% to 95% success rate for resolution of radiculopathy. Back pain is slightly more problematic in that mechanical symptoms resulting from degenerative disc disease will not be altered by discectomy and relief of root compression. However, most patients with sciatica also have low back pain due to their root compression and thus most of these symptoms will resolve. Certainly some of these surgical patients will have problems later on such as recurrent disc herniations or mechanical low back pain. With some deterioration of surgical results over years and some improvement of radicular symptoms treated nonoperatively over years, the results of some studies show outcomes converging at these late time points, i.e., with 5 or 10 years of follow-up.[247,248]

Lumbar Spinal Stenosis

Although not as highly publicized as OA of the hips or knees, lumbar stenosis is an extremely common degenerative condition in the older age groups. Degenerative changes in the disc, soft tissues, and posterior facets of each motion segment can hypertrophy and encroach on the spinal canal.[278,279] This is most common in the low lumbar spine where motion and loads are greatest.[167–169] Chronic compression of the cauda equina classically produces symptoms termed *neurogenic claudication*. This symptom complex is pain in the low back and buttocks, aggravated by standing or walking distances, with or without pain radiating distally into the legs that may be accompanied by numbness or tingling in the legs and feet. As degenerative changes slowly accrue in the low lumbar spine, patients with stenosis will typically cut back on their walking until they can only walk a block or two.[164] Typically they will sit down for relief or even lean over, as these maneuvers flex the lumbar spine and slightly expand the canal. Patients note they can walk much better in the grocery store leaning over their shopping cart than they can without the cart. Whereas standing in place will relieve vascular claudication, relief of neurogenic claudication will require the patient to sit or bend forward.[163,166] Most patients with lumbar stenosis will have tolerated their low grade back pain for years, but when their walking capabilities reach a point where their day-to-day function is limited, they often seek medical attention. Lumbar stenosis may present with numbness in the legs as mentioned, and the feet may be involved; however, chronic constant numbness of the feet or a painful sensation of the feet with weight bearing is more commonly due to peripheral neuropathy rather than spinal stenosis. Unilateral or bilateral weakness may be present and is typically in the L4 and L5 distribution with tibialis anterior or extensor hallacis longus weakness. Patients may note dragging of their feet consistent with a partial or complete foot drop in severe cases.

Although the classic presentation of lumbar stenosis is that of neurogenic claudication, it is not uncommon to have a radicular component in any given patient. One or more nerve roots can be pinched enough to produce radicular pain all the way down the leg with or without neurologic deficit.[167,280] This pinching typically occurs in the lateral recess area of the spinal canal underneath the facet joints or more laterally in the neural foramen.

Pathoanatomy

In some patients there is a congenital component to lumbar spinal stenosis. These patients have congenitally short pedicles and thus less space in the spinal canal. The shape of the canal may also contribute to stenosis with a trefoil or triangular shape being potentially problematic. Far and away the most common cause of canal stenosis, however, is degenerative change in the low lumbar spine. Bulging of the intervertebral discs, thickening of ligamentum flavum, and hypertrophy of the facet joints and facet capsule tissues all contribute to decreasing the diameter of the spinal canal (Fig. 22–14A, B). Because of this pathoanatomy, spinal stenosis is typically the worst at the level of the disc space as opposed to behind the mid portion of the vertebral bodies. Further compromise at any level can result from a degenerative spondylolisthesis, which is usually seen at the L4-L5 motion segment. Because compression of the cauda equina from these pathoanatomic changes occurs very slowly, the nerve roots are quite tolerant until there is significant compromise of the spinal canal.

Natural History

The degenerative changes in the bony and soft tissues of the lumbar spine that produce spinal stenosis represent a permanent structural change of the spinal canal. Thus spinal stenosis will not typically improve over time, as might a soft lumbar disc herniation. The symptoms of spinal stenosis, however, are known to wax and wane. Patients can smolder for long periods of time without definitive worsening of their symptoms.[281] Usually, however, a slow progression of symptoms will occur depending on

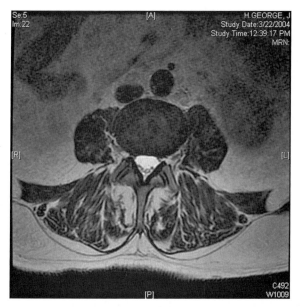

Figure 22–14A An axial T_2-weighted MRI image demonstrating the normal cross-sectional area of the spinal canal in the lumbar spine.

the patients' activity levels. Whether or not they seek treatment will depend on their requirements for function from a walking standpoint and sometimes whether or not they have weakness or radicular pain associated with their lumbar spinal stenosis.

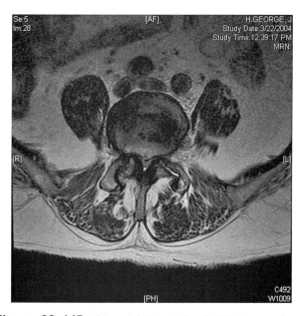

Figure 22–14B This axial T_2-weighted MRI image shows severe spinal stenosis. Note the hypertrophic, irregular facet changes. This, in combination with thickening of the ligamentum flavum and typical bulging of the disc at that level, produces severe narrowing of the lumbar spinal canal as demonstrated here. Note the decrease in size of the canal available for the cauda equina.

Physical Examination

These patients may exhibit a stooped forward posture since this relieves some of their stenosis. Lumbar tenderness is usually mild, and buttock tenderness may or may not be present. Forward flexion is usually painless, but hyperextension typically aggravates the symptoms.[282] If the patient has concomitant radiculopathy, he or she may have a positive straight leg raise test; however, the vast majority of patients with spinal stenosis will have a negative straight leg raise test. This makes sense given that this maneuver tends to flex the lumbar spine and thus increases the canal diameter. Neurologic testing may reveal weakness that is typically in the tibialis anterior or extensor hallacis longus, as the L4 and L5 roots are commonly involved. Dermatomal sensory loss may be present, and reflexes are typically absent or hyporeflexic in significant lumbar stenosis.

Diagnostic Studies

Patients in older age groups with symptoms consistent with spinal stenosis should have lumbar plain films including flexion/extension views. Disc degeneration and hypertrophic facet changes can be seen on these simple studies. Degenerative spondylolisthesis is an important diagnosis to make, as there will almost always be stenosis present at the level of the slipped vertebrae if it is more than a few millimeters. Flexion/extension views also help with identifying dynamic instability that may be contributing to the patient's symptoms.[283–286] Oblique films are helpful for identifying pars interarticularis defects, which will diagnose the isthmic type of spondylolisthesis. This type of spondylolisthesis is usually seen in younger patients and will not be covered in this chapter.

CT and CT myelography play a somewhat limited role in the diagnosis and treatment of lumbar spinal stenosis. Certainly CT scans can give a reasonable picture of bony stenosis and disc degeneration.[278] It is difficult to visually separate the thecal sac from the soft tissue such as ligamentum flavum and hypertrophic capsule. CT myelography gives an excellent picture of central spinal stenosis and is very helpful in patients who cannot get an MRI or in patients having had prior surgery.

MRI remains the study of choice for identifying and evaluating the degree of lumbar spinal stenosis. Bone is visualized fairly well and all the soft tissues can be identified. Sagittal views are excellent for diagnosing foraminal stenosis, much better than plain CT or even CT myelography. MRIs with gadolinium help delineate scar tissue versus recurrent disc herniation or recurrent stenosis in patients having had prior surgery. MRI is somewhat limited in patients with significant degenerative scoliosis as the sagittal cuts weave in and out of plane, thus CT myelography may be a better choice for this subset of patients.

Electrodiagnostic studies such as electromyography may be useful in differential diagnosis for these patients. Peripheral neuropathy and lumbar plexopathy can overlap in symptoms and may be best identified by careful history, physical examination, and an experienced electromyography professional.[287]

Nonoperative Treatment

The success of nonoperative treatment of lumbar spinal stenosis depends primarily on the degree of stenosis present and the clinical symptomatology. Though symptoms may wax and wane over time, the pathoanatomy of stenosis does not spontaneously improve as in some soft disc herniations.[318] Thus if symptoms are severe, "buying time" with nonoperative modalities does not usually pay off in the long run. Certainly anti-inflammatories or an exercise program[288,289] may help patients with mild neurogenic claudication symptoms. Typically a flexibility and strengthening program is recommended for the low back in patients with stenosis, relying on flexion exercises and avoiding extension maneuvers because of the tight lumbar canal. Whereas walking may not be well tolerated, either water exercises or an exercise bike (because of the sitting position) may allow for endurance training and help with back and leg pain. Epidural steroid injections are commonly used for patients with neurogenic claudication symptoms from spinal stenosis, but the longer term efficacy of injections for these patients is minimal. However, selected individuals with a radicular pain component may achieve some relief with epidural steroid injections or selective nerve root blocks by settling down the local inflammation around the pinched nerve root causing the radiculopathy.[290] Patients with severe stenosis causing intolerable functional limitations, neurologic deficits such as a foot drop, or significant radicular pain will often require surgical intervention to relieve the mechanical compression on the cauda equina.

Operative Treatment

The classic surgical procedure for treatment of lumbar spinal stenosis is termed a lumbar decompression.[291] Most commonly this requires one or more level laminectomies which decompress the central part of the canal. Usually the large hypertrophic facet joints and thickened ligamentum flavum need to be partially removed in the lateral gutters of the spinal canal in order to eliminate the lateral recess stenosis caused by these enlarged tissues. Enlarging of the individual foramen (called foraminotomies) may or may not be needed depending on that patient's specific pathoanatomy. Technically it is important to preserve the pars interarticularis which preserves the inferior facet joint. This minimizes the chance of iatrogenic postoperative instability if no fusion is planned for that given patient.

Most studies suggest good surgical outcome in 70% to 80% of patients treated operatively for lumbar stenosis.[291-300] Because the decompressive procedure relieves the pinching of the neural elements, the walking capability of most patients typically improves and radicular leg pain should resolve if the roots are adequately decompressed. Because the patient still has degenerative discs and arthritic facet joints, the relief of back pain is much less consistent for patients undergoing a lumbar decompression. For this reason, some surgeons opt to perform an arthrodesis with a lumbar decompression; however, the more standard treatment reserves fusion for those patients with specific indications such as spondylolisthesis, scoliosis, or revision procedures.

Degenerative Spondylolisthesis

Degenerative changes in the lumbar spine leading to lumbar spinal stenosis can also commonly produce a degenerative spondylolisthesis. This is a slipping forward of one vertebrae on another due to degenerative changes of the posterior facet joints (Fig. 22–15).[301,302] The joints become incompetent over time and allow forward subluxation, typically occurring at the L4-5 motion segment.[286] Because the spinal canal is made up essentially of bony rings stacked on each other, with a degenerative spondylolisthesis one ring slides forward on another and the diameter of the spinal canal will obligatorily be decreased. This will significantly contribute to narrowing of the canal at that level. Degenerative spondylolisthesis and the associated pathoanatomy typically occur very slowly and the degree of narrowing that many patients tolerate without significant symptoms can be surprising.[303] As with lumbar stenosis, indications for surgery are primarily intolerable functional limitations with walking, intolerable pain, or significant neurologic deficit. Many patients with lumbar stenosis and a degenerative spondylolisthesis who undergo only a lumbar decompression will tend to slip farther over time, as this is a relatively destabilizing procedure. Thus the classic surgical treatment for this combination is a lumbar decompression and fusion, typically performed with autogenous bone graft and pedicle screw instrumentation (Fig. 22–16).[304-307] Recombinant human bone morphogenetic protein is a commercially available alternative to autogenous bone

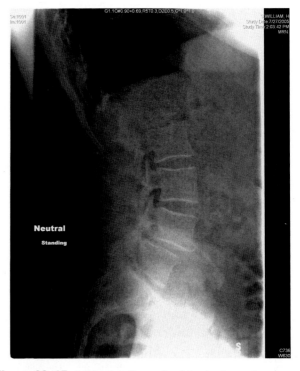

Figure 22–15 A lateral radiograph of the lumbar spine demonstrating a typical degenerative spondylolisthesis at L4-5. There is no pars interarticularis defect in this type of slippage, which most commonly occurs in older individuals at the L4-5 level. It usually produces spinal stenosis at the level of the slip.

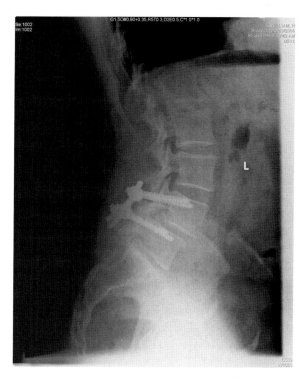

Figure 22–16 A postoperative lateral radiograph of the lumbar spine. This patient had undergone a lumbar decompression for stenosis. If a spondylolisthesis is present, then typically a bone graft plus instrumentation is utilized for stabilization purposes as shown here.

graft. Results for posterolateral lumbar fusions using BMP are promising, though at this time the cost of the product remains an issue.

Degenerative Scoliosis

Some patients with lumbar degenerative disease will develop a deformity of the lumbar spine in the coronal plane termed degenerative scoliosis. There is some rotational deformity (though not typically as much as with idiopathic scoliosis), and a lateral listhesis may occur. The development of this is based on asymmetric wear and tear of the disc and facet joints. Varying degrees of scoliosis can result. Mild cases usually do not require any special surgical treatment; however, patients with typically more than 20° of scoliosis may warrant a concomitant arthrodesis when any lumbar decompression procedures are performed. Decisions on the number of levels to include in a fusion for these patients can be very challenging, as both shorter and longer lumbar fusions have their potential drawbacks.[308,309]

REFERENCES

1. Bohlman HH, Emery SE. The pathophysiology of cervical spondylosis and myelopathy. Spine 13:843–846, 1988.
2. Payne EE, Spillane JD. The cervical spine: an anatomico-pathological study of 70 specimens (using a special technique) with particular reference to the problem of cervical spondylosis. Brain 80:571–596, 1957.
3. Bohlman HH. The neck. In: D'Ambrosia RD, ed. Musculoskeletal Disorders: Regional Examination and Differential Diagnosis. Philadelphia, JB Lippincott, 1977, pp 178–244.
4. Nurick S. The pathogenesis of the spinal cord disorder associated with cervical spondylosis. Brain 95:87–100, 1972.
5. Brain WR, Northfield D, Wilkinson M. The neurological manifestations of cervical spondylosis. Brain 75:187–225, 1952.
6. Emery SE, Bohlman HH, Bolesta MJ, et al. Anterior cervical decompression and arthrodesis for the treatment of cervical spondylotic myelopathy: two-to seventeen-year follow-up. J Bone Joint Surg Am 80:941–951, 1998.
7. Rao R. Neck pain, cervical radiculopathy, and cervical myelopathy: pathophysiology, natural history, and clinical evaluation. Instr Course Lect. 52:479–488, 2003.
8. Kellgren JH, Lawrence JS. Osteo-arthritis and disk degeneration in an urban population. Ann Rheum Dis 17:388–397, 1958.
9. Boden SD, McCowin PR, Davis DO, et al. Abnormal magnetic-resonance scans of the cervical spine in asymptomatic subjects. A prospective investigation. J Bone Joint Surg Am 72:1178–1184, 1990.
10. Bell GR, Ross JS. Diagnosis of nerve root compression. Myelography, computed tomography, and MRI. Orthop Clin North Am 23(3):405–419, 1992.
11. Wolansky LJ, Parikh DD, Shah KJ, et al. Magnetic resonance imaging protocols for cervical disc disease: what is your neighbor up to? J Neuroimaging 15(2):183–187, 2005.
12. Demir A, Ries M, Moonen CT, et al. Diffusion-weighted MR imaging with apparent diffusion coefficient and apparent diffusion tensor maps in cervical spondylotic myelopathy. Radiology 229(1):37–43, 2003.
13. Ahn NU, Ahn UM, Andersson GB, et al. Operative Treatment of the patient with neck pain. Phys Med Rehabil Clin N Am14(3): 675–692, 2003.
14. Clarke E, Robinson PK. Cervical myelopathy: a complication of cervical spondylosis. Brain 79:483–510, 1956.
15. Lees F, Turner JWA. Natural history and prognosis of cervical spondylosis. Br Med J 5373:1607–1610, 1963.
16. Bohlman HH, Emery SE, Goodfellow DB, et al. Robinson anterior cervical discectomy and arthrodesis for cervical radiculopathy. Long-term follow-up of one hundred and twenty-two patients. J Bone Joint Surg Am 75:1298–1307, 1993.
17. Riley LH Jr, Robinson RA, Johnson KA, et al. The results of anterior interbody fusion of the cervical spine. Review of ninety-three consecutive cases. J Neurosurg 30:127–133, 1969.
18. Gore DR, Sepic SB. Anterior discectomy and fusion for painful cervical disc disease. A report of 50 patients with an average follow-up of 21 years. Spine 23(19):2047–2051, 1998.
19. Yue WM, Brodner W. Long-term results after anterior cervical discectomy and fusion with allograft and plating: a 5- to 11-year radiologic and clinical follow-up study. Spine 30(19): 2138–2144, 2005.
20. Zdeblick TA, Bohlman HH. Cervical kyphosis and myelopathy: treatment by anterior corpectomy and strut-grafting. J Bone Joint Surg Am 71:170–182, 1989.
21. Robinson RA, Smith GW. Anterolateral cervical disc removal and interbody fusion for cervical disc syndrome [abstract]. Bull Johns Hopkins Hosp 96:223–224, 1955.
22. Emery SE, Bolesta MJ, Banks MA, et al. Robinson anterior cervical fusion: comparison of the standard and modified techniques. Spine 19:660–663, 1994.
23. Zdeblick TA, Ducker TB. The use of freeze-dried allograft bone for anterior cervical fusions. Spine 16:726–729, 1991.
24. Martin GJ Jr, Haid RW Jr, MacMillan M, et al. Anterior cervical discectomy with freeze-dried fibula allograft. Overview of 317 cases and literature review. Spine 24:852–858, 1999.
25. Shapiro S. Banked fibula and the locking anterior cervical plate in anterior cervical fusions following cervical discectomy. J Neurosurg 84:161–165, 1996.
26. Ryu SI, Lim JT, Kim SM, et al. Comparison of the biomechanical stability of dense cancellous allograft with tricortical iliac autograft and fibular allograft for cervical interbody fusion. Eur Spine J 15(9):1339–1345, 2006.
27. Malloy KM, Hilibrand AS. Autograft versus allograft in degenerative cervical disease. Clin Orthop Relat Res. 2002 Jan;(394):27–38.

28. Emery SE, Fisher JR, Bohlman HH. Three-level anterior cervical discectomy and fusion: radiographic and clinical results. Spine 22:2622–2624, 1997.

29. Wang JC, McDonough PW, Endow KK, et al. Increased fusion rates with cervical plating for two-level anterior cervical discectomy and fusion. Spine 25:41–45, 2000.

30. Connolly PJ, Esses SI, Kostuik JP. Anterior cervical fusion: outcome analysis of patients fused with and without anterior cervical plates. J Spinal Disord 9:202–206, 1996.

31. Kaiser MG, Haid RW JR, Subach BR, et al. Anterior cervical plating enhances arthrodesis after discectomy and fusion with cortical allograft. Neurosurgery 50(2):229–236, 2002; discussion 236–238.

32. Bolesta MJ, Rechtine GR II, Chrin Am. One- and two-level anterior cervical descectomy and fusion: the effect of plate fixation. Spine J 2(3):197–203, 2002.

33. Hilibrand AS, Yoo JU, Carlson GD, et al. The success of anterior cervical arthrodesis adjacent to a previous fusion. Spine 22:1574–1579, 1997.

34. Wang JC, McDonough PW, Endow K, et al. The effect of cervical plating on single-level anterior cervical discectomy and fusion. J Spinal Disord 12:467–471, 1999.

35. Emery SE, Bolesta MJ. Complications of cervical spine surgery. In: Bridwell KH, DeWald RL, eds. The Textbook of Spinal Surgery. 2nd ed. Philadelphia, Lippincott-Raven, 1997, pp 1427–1438.

36. Yonenobu K, Hosono N, Iwasaki M, et al. Laminoplasty versus subtotal corpectomy: a comparative study of results in multisegmental cervical spondylotic myelopathy. Spine 17:1281–1284, 1992.

37. Okada K, Shirasaki N, Hayashi H, et al. Treatment of cervical spondylotic myelopathy by enlargement of the spinal canal anteriorly, followed by arthrodesis. J Bone Joint Surg Am 73: 352–364, 1991.

38. Kalfas IH. Role of corpectomy in cervical spondylosis. Neurosurg Focus 12(1):E11, 2002.

39. Mayr MT, Subach BR, Comey CH, et al. Cervical spinal stenosis: outcome after anterior corpectomy, allograft reconstruction, and instrumentation. J Neurosurg 96(1 Suppl):10–16, 2002.

40. Vaccaro AR, Falatyn SP, Scuderi GJ, et al. Early failure of long segment anterior cervical plate fixation. J Spinal Disord 11:410–415, 1998.

41. Albert TJ, Anderson DG. Bone grafting, implants, and plating options for anterior cervical fusions. Orthop Clin North Am 33(2):317–328, 2002.

42. Sasso RC, Ruggiero RA Jr, Reilly TM, et al. Early reconstruction failures after multilevel cervical corpectomy. Spine 28(2): 140–142, 2003.

43. Scoville WB, Dohrmann GJ, Corkill G. Late results of cervical disc surgery. J Neurosurg 45:203–210, 1976.

44. Herkowitz HN, Kurz LT, Overhold DP. Surgical management of cervical soft disc herniation. A comparison between the anterior and posterior approach. Spine 15(10):1026–1030, 1990.

45. Aldrich F. Posterolateral microdisectomy for cervical monoradiculopathy caused by posterolateral soft cervical disc sequestration. J Neurosurg 72(3):370–377, 1990.

46. Epstein JA, Janin Y, Carras R, et al. A comparative study of the treatment of cervical spondylotic myeloradiculopathy. Experience with 50 cases treated by means of extensive laminectomy, foraminotomy, and excision of osteophytes during the past 10 years. Acta Neurochir 61:89–104, 1982.

47. Hansen-Schwartz J, Kruse-Larsen C, Nielsen CJ. Follow-up after cervical laminectomy, with special reference to instability and deformity. Br J Neurosurg 17(4):301–305, 2003.

48. Epstein NE. Laminectomy for cervical myelopathy. Spinal Cord 41(6):317–327, 2003.

49. Hirabayashi K, Satomi K. Operative procedure and results of expansive open-door laminoplasty. Spine 13:870–876, 1988.

50. Kurokawa T. Enlargement of the spinal canal by the sagittal splitting of spinous processes. Bessatsu Seikeigeka 2:249–252, 1982.

51. Nakano K, Harata S, Suetsuna F, et al. Spinous process–splitting laminoplasty using hydroxyapatite spinous process spacer. Spine 17(suppl):S41–S43, 1992.

52. O'Brien MF, Peterson D, Casey AT, et al. A novel technique for laminoplasty augmentation of spinal canal area using titanium miniplate stabilization: a computerized morphometric analysis. Spine 21:474–484, 1996.

53. Patel CK, Cunningham BJ, Herkowitz HN. Techniques in cervical laminoplasty. Spine J 2(6):450–455, 2002.

54. Kimura I, Shingu H, Nasu Y, et al. Long-term follow-up of cervical spondylotic myelopathy treated by canal-expansive laminoplasty. J Bone Joint Surg Br 77:956–961, 1995.

55. Iwasaki M, Kawaguchi Y, Kimura T, et al. Long-term results of expansive laminoplasty for ossification of the posterior longitudinal ligament of the cervical spine: more than 10 years follow up. J Neurosurg. 96(2 Suppl):180–189, 2002.

56. Edwards CC 2nd, Heller JG, Marukami H. Corpectomy versus laminoplasty for multilevel cervical myelopathy: an independent matched-cohort analysis. Spine 27(11):1168–1175, 2002.

57. Hosono N, Yonenobu K, Ono K. Neck and shoulder pain after laminoplasty: a noticeable complication. Spine 21:1969–1973, 1996.

58. Gore DR, Sepic SB. Anterior cervical fusion for degenerated or protruded discs: a review of one hundred forty-six patients. Spine 9:667–671, 1984.

59. Simmons EH, Bhalla SK. Anterior cervical discectomy and fusion: a clinical and biomechanical study with eight-year follow-up. J Bone Joint Surg Br 51:225–237, 1969.

60. Maurice-Williams RS, Elsmore A. Extended anterior cervical decompression without fusion: a long-term follow-up study. Br J Neurosurg 13(5):474–479, 1999.

61. Truumees E, Herkowitz HN. Cervical spondylotic myelopathy and radiculopathy. Instr Course Lect 49:339–360, 2000.

62. Saunders RL, Bernini PM, Shirreffs TG Jr, et al. Central corpectomy for cervical spondylotic myelopathy: a consecutive series with long-term follow-up evaluation. J Neurosurg 74:163–170, 1991.

63. Eck JC, Humphreys SC, Hodges SC, et al. A comparison of outcomes of anterior cervical discectomy and fusion in patients with and without radicular symptoms. J Surg Orthop Adv 15(1): 24–26, 2006.

64. Albert TJ, Murrell SC. Surgical management of cervical radiculopathy. J Am Acad Orthop Surg 7(6):368–376, 1999.

65. Vanichkachorn JS, Vaccaro AR. Thoracic disk disease: diagnosis and treatment. J Am Acad Orthop Surg 8:159–169, 2000.

66. Symmons DP, van Hemert AM, Vandenbroucke JP, et al. A longitudinal study of back pain and radiological changes in the lumbar spines of middle aged women. II. Radiographic findings. Ann Rheum Dis 50:162–166, 1991.

67. O'Neill TW, McCloskey EV, Kanis JA, et al. The distribution, determinants, and clinical correlates of vertebral osteophytosis: a population based survey. J Rheumatol 26:842–848, 1999.

68. Bruckner FE, Greco A, Leung AW. 'Benign thoracic pain' syndrome: role of magnetic resonance imaging in the detection and localization of thoracic disc disease. J R Soc Med 82:81–83, 1989.

69. Wood KB, Garvey TA, Gundry C, et al. Magnetic resonance imaging of the thoracic spine. Evaluation of asymptomatic individuals. J Bone Joint Surg Am 77:1631–1638, 1995.

70. Girard CJ, Schweitzer Me, Morrison WB, et al. Thoracic spine disc-related abnormalities: longitudinal MR imaging assessment. Skeletal Radiol 33:216–222, 2004.

71. Brown CW, Deffer PA Jr, Akmakjian J, et al. The natural history of thoracic disc herniation. Spine 17(suppl):S97–S102, 1992.

72. Stillerman CB, Chen TC, Couldwell WT, et al. Experience in the surgical management of 82 symptomatic herniated thoracic discs and review of the literature. J Neurosurg 88:623–633, 1998.

73. Ohnishi K, Miyamoto K, Kanamori Y, et al. Anterior decompression and fusion for multiple thoracic disc herniation. J Bone Joint Surg Br 87: 356–360, 2005.

74. Bohlman HH, Zdeblick TA. Anterior excision of herniated thoracic discs. J Bone Joint Surg Am 70:1038–1047, 1988.

75. Korovessis PG, Stamatakis MV, Baikousis A, et al. Transthoracic disc excision with interbody fusion. 12 patients with symptomatic disc herniation followed for 2–8 years. Acta Orthop Scand Suppl 275:12–16, 1997.

76. Debnath U.K., McConnell JR, Sengupta DK, et al. Results of hemivertebrectomy and fusion for symptomatic thoracic disc herniation. Eur Spine J 12: 292–299, 2003.

77. Regan JJ, Mack MJ, Picetti GD 3rd. A technical report on video-assisted thoracoscopy in thoracic spinal surgery. Preliminary description. Spine 20(7):831–837, 1995.

78. Osman SG, Marsolais EB. Posterolateral arthroscopic discectomies of the thoracic and lumbar spine. Clin Orthop 304:122–129, 1994.
79. Bazin A, Rousseaux P, Bernard MH, et al. Myelopathies caused by dorsal spinal canal spondylotic stenosis. 3 cases and a review of the literature. Neurochirurgie 35:229–235, 1989.
80. Smith DE, Godersky JC. Thoracic spondylosis: an unusual cause of myelopathy. Neurosurgery 20:589–593, 1987.
81. Rosenbloom SA. Thoracic disc disease and stenosis. Radiol Clin North Am 29:765–775, 1991.
82. Barnett GH, Hardy RW Jr, Little JR, et al. Thoracic spinal canal stenosis. J Neurosurg 66:338–344, 1987.
83. Irwin ZN, Hilibrand A, Gustavel M, et al. Variation in surgical decision making for degenerative spinal disorders. Part I: lumbar spine. Spine 30(19):2208–2213, 2005.
84. Palumbo MA, Hilibrand AS, Hart RA, et al. Surgical treatment of thoracic spinal stenosis: a 2- to 9-year follow-up. Spine 26(5):558–566, 2001.
85. Gupta MC. Degenerative scoliosis. Options for surgical management. Orthop Clin North Am 34(2):269–279, 2003.
86. Ben Hamouda K, Jemel H, Haouet S, et al. Thoracic myelopathy caused by ossification of the ligamentum flavum: a report of 18 cases. J Neurosurg 99(2 Suppl):157–161, 2003.
87. Chang U.K., Choe WJ, Chung CK, et al. Surgical treatment for thoracic spinal stenosis. Spinal Cord 39(7):362–369, 2001.
88. Yamazaki M, Mochizuki M, Ikeda Y, et al. Clinical results of surgery for thoracic myelopathy caused by ossification of the posterior longitudinal ligament: operative indication of posterior decompression with instrumented fusion. Spine 31(13):1452–1460, 2006.
89. Thomas E, Silman AJ, Croft PR, et al. Predicting who develops chronic low back pain in primary care: a prospective study. BMJ 318:1662–1667, 1999.
90. Symmons DP, van Hemert AM, Vandenbroucke JP, et al. A longitudinal study of back pain and radiological changes in the lumbar spines of middle aged women. II. Radiographic findings. Ann Rheum Dis 50:162–166, 1991.
91. O'Neill TW, McCloskey EV, Kanis JA, et al. The distribution, determinants, and clinical correlates of vertebral osteophytosis: a population based survey. J Rheumatol 26:842–848, 1999.
92. Frymoyer JW, Pope MH, Clements JH, et al. Risk factors in low-back pain: an epidemiological survey. J Bone Joint Surg Am 65:213–218, 1983.
93. Svensson HO, Andersson GBJ. Low-back pain in 40- to 47-year-old men: work history and work environment factors. Spine 8:272–276, 1983.
94. Croft PR, Papageorgiou AC, Thomas E, et al. Short-term physical risk factors for new episodes of low back pain. Prospective evidence from the South Manchester Back Pain Study. Spine 24:1556–1561, 1999.
95. Grazier KL, Holbrook TL, Kelsey JL, et al. The frequency of occurrence, impact, and cost of musculoskeletal conditions in the United States. Chicago, American Academy of Orthopaedic Surgeons, 1984.
96. Stoddard S, Jans L, Ripple JM, et al. Chartbook on work and disability in the United States. Section 3. Washington, DC, National Institute on Disability and Rehabilitation Research, 1998.
97. Gheldof EL, Vinck J, Vlayen JW, et al. The differential role of pain, work characteristics and pain-related fear in explaining back pain and sick leave in occupational settings. Pain 113:71–81, 2005.
98. Hoogendoorn WE, Bongers PM, de Vet HC, et al. High physical work load and low job satisfaction increase the risk of sickness absence due to low back pain: results of a prospective cohort study. Occup Environ Med. 60:306, 2003.
99. Hestbaek L, Larsen K, Weidick F, et al. Low back pain in military recruits in relation to social background and previous low back pain. A cross-sectional and prospective observational survey. BMC Musculoskelet Disord 6:25, 2005.
100. Svensson HO, Andersson GBJ. Low-back pain in 40- to 47-year-old men: work history and work environment factors. Spine 8:272–276, 1983.
101. Rizzo JA, Abbott TA III, Berger ML. The labor productivity effects of chronic backache in the United States. Med Care 36:1471–1488, 1998.
102. Goetzel RZ, Hawkins K, Ozminkowski RJ, et al. The health and productivity cost burden of the "top 10" physical and mental health conditions affecting six large U.S. employers in 1999. J Occup Environ Med 45:5–14, 2003.
103. Ekman M, Jonhagen S, Hunsche E, et al. Burden of chronic lower back pain in Sweden: a cross-sectional, retrospective study in primary care setting. Spine 30:1777–1785, 2005.
104. Frymoyer JW, Pope MH, Costanza MC, et al. Epidemiologic studies of low-back pain. Spine 5:419–423, 1980.
105. Luoma K, Riihimaki H, Raininko R, et al. Lumbar disc degeneration in relation to occupation. Scand J Work Environ Health 24:358–366, 1998.
106. Evans W, Jobe W, Seibert C. A cross-sectional prevalence study of lumbar disc degeneration in a working population. Spine 14:60–64, 1989.
107. Harreby M, Hesselsoe G, Kjer J, et al. Low back pain and physical exercise in leisure time in 38-year-old men and women: a 25-year prospective cohort study of 640 school children. Eur Spine J 6:181–186, 1997.
108. Thomas E, Silman AJ, Croft PR, et al. Predicting who develops chronic low back pain in primary care: a prospective study. BMJ 318:1662–1667, 1999.
109. Riihimaki H, Mattsson T, Zitting A, et al. Radiographically detectable degenerative changes of the lumbar spine among concrete reinforcement workers and house painters. Spine 15:114–119, 1990.
110. Hartvigsen J, Bakketeig LS, Leboeuf-Yde C, et al. The association between physical workload and low back pain clouded by the "healthy worker" effect: population-based cross-sectional and 5-year prospective questionnaire study. Spine 26:1788–1792, 2001.
111. Anderson R. The back pain of bus drivers. Prevalence in an urban area of California. Spine 17:1481–1488, 1992.
112. Battie MC, Videman T, Gibbons LE, et al. Occupational driving and lumbar disc degeneration: a case-control study. Lancet 360:1369–1374, 2002.
113. Drerup B, Granitzka M, Assheuer J, et al. Assessment of disc injury in subjects exposed to long-term whole-body vibration. Eur Spine J 8:458–467, 1999.
114. Holm S, Nachemson A. Nutrition of the intervertebral disc: effects induced by vibrations. Orthop Trans 9:451, 1985.
115. Croft PR, Papageorgiou AC, Thomas E, et al. Short-term physical risk factors for new episodes of low back pain. Prospective evidence from the South Manchester Back Pain Study. Spine 24:1556–1561, 1999.
116. Heliovaara M. Risk factors for low back pain and sciatica. Ann Med 21:257–264, 1989.
117. Battie MC, Videman T, Gill K, et al. 1991 Volvo Award in clinical sciences. Smoking and lumbar intervertebral disc degeneration: an MRI study of identical twins. Spine 16:1015–1021, 1991.
118. Videman T, Battie MC, Gibbons LE, et al. Lifetime exercise and disk degeneration: an MRI study of monozygotic twins. Med Sci Sports Exerc 29:1350–1356, 1997.
119. Simmons ED Jr, Guntupalli M, Kowalski JM, et al. Familial predisposition for degenerative disc disease. A case-control study. Spine 21:1527–1529, 1996.
120. Matsui H, Kanamori M, Ishihara H, et al. Familial predisposition for lumbar degenerative disc disease. A case-control study. Spine 23:1029–1034, 1998.
121. Sambrook PN, MacGregor AJ, Spector TD. Genetic influences on cervical and lumbar disc degeneration: a magnetic resonance imaging study in twins. Arthritis Rheum 42:366–372, 1999.
122. Annunen S, Paassilta P, Lohiniva J, et al. An allele of COL9A2 associated with intervertebral disc disease. Science 285:409–412, 1999.
123. Solovieva S, Lohiniva J, Leino-Arjas P, et al. COL9A3 gene polymorphism and obesity in intervertebral disc degeneration of the lumbar spine: evidence of gene-environment interaction. Spine 27:2691–2696, 2002.
124. Paassilta P, Lohiniva J, Goring HH, et al. Identification of a novel common genetic risk factor for lumbar disk disease. JAMA 285:1886–1888, 2001.
125. Garnero P, Sornay-Rendu E, Arlot M, et al. Association between spine disc degeneration and type II collagen degradation in postmenopausal women: the OFELY study. Arthritis Rheum 50:3137–3144, 2004.

126. Vogt MT, Rubin D, Valentin RS, et al. Lumbar olisthesis and lower back symptoms in elderly white women. The Study of Osteoporotic Fractures. Spine 23:2640–2647, 1998.

127. Fujiwara A, Tamai K, Yamato M, et al. The relationship between facet joint osteoarthritis and disc degeneration of the lumbar spine: an MRI study. Eur Spine J 8:396–401, 1999.

128. Rauschning W. Normal and pathologic anatomy of the lumbar root canals. Spine 12:1008–1019, 1988.

129. Antoniou J, Steffen T, Nelson F, et al. The human lumbar intervertebral disc: evidence for changes in the biosynthesis and denaturation of the extracellular matrix with growth, maturation, ageing, and degeneration. J Clin Invest 98:996–1003, 1996.

130. Johnstone B, Bayliss MT. The large proteoglycans of the human intervertebral disc. Changes in their biosynthesis and structure with age, topography, and pathology. Spine 20:674–678, 1995.

131. Lyons G, Eisenstein SM, Sweet MB. Biochemical changes in intervertebral disc degeneration. Biochim Biophys Acta 673:443–453, 1981.

132. Tertti M, Paajanen H, Laato M, et al. Disc degeneration in magnetic resonance imaging. A comparative biochemical, histologic, and radiologic study in cadaver spines. Spine 16:629–634, 1991.

133. Ritchie JH, Fahrni WH. Age changes in lumbar intervertebral discs. Can J Surg 13:65–71, 1970.

134. Fujita Y, Duncan NA, Lotz JC. Radial tensile properties of the lumbar annulus fibrosus are site and degeneration dependent. J Orthop Res 15:814–819, 1997.

135. Hirsh C, Schajowicz F. Studies of structural changes in the lumbar annulus fibrosus. Acta Orthop Scand 22:184, 1952.

136. Osti OL, Vernon-Roberts B, Moore R, et al. Annular tears and disc degeneration in the lumbar spine. A post-mortem study of 135 discs. J Bone Joint Surg Br 74:678–682, 1992.

137. Morgan FP, King T. Primary instability of the lumbar vertebrae as a common cause of low back pain. J Bone Joint Surg Br 39:6, 1957.

138. Haughton VM, Schmidt TA, Keele K, et al. Flexibility of lumbar spinal motion segments correlated to type of tears in the annulus fibrosus. J Neurosurg 92(suppl):81–86, 2000.

139. Macnab I. The traction spur: an indication of segmental instability. J Bone Joint Surg Am 53:663, 1971.

140. Holm S, Maroudas A, Urban JP, et al. Nutrition of the intervertebral disc: solute transport and metabolism. Connect Tissue Res 8:101–119, 1981.

141. Ogab K, Whiteside LA. Nutritional pathways of the intervertebral disc. Spine 6:211–216, 1981.

142. Roberts S, Urban JP, Evans H, et al. Transport properties of the human cartilage endplate in relation to its composition and calcification. Spine 21:415–420, 1996.

143. Roberts S, Menage J, Urban JP. Biochemical and structural properties of the cartilage end-plate and its relation to the intervertebral disc. Spine 14:166–174, 1989.

144. Yasuma T, Suzuki F, Koh S, et al. Pathological changes in the cartilaginous plates in relation to intervertebral disc lesions. Acta Pathol Jpn 38:735–750, 1988.

145. Modic MT, Steinberg PM, Ross JS, et al. Degenerative disk disease: assessment of changes in vertebral body marrow with MR imaging. Radiology 166(pt 1):193–199, 1988.

146. Parkkola R, Rytokoski U, Kormano M. Magnetic resonance imaging of the discs and trunk muscles in patients with chronic low back pain and healthy control subjects. Spine 18:830–836, 1993.

147. Brinckmann P. Injury of the annulus fibrosus and disc protrusions. An in vitro investigation on human lumbar discs. Spine 11:149–153, 1986.

148. Paajanen H, Erkintalo M, Kuusela T, et al. Magnetic resonance study of disc degeneration in young low-back pain patients. Spine 14:982–985, 1989.

149. Borenstein DG, O'Mara JW Jr, Boden SD, et al. The value of magnetic resonance imaging of the lumbar spine to predict low-back pain in asymptomatic subjects: a seven-year follow-up study. J Bone Joint Surg Am 83:1306–1311, 2001.

150. Elfering A, Semmer N, Birkhofer D, et al. Risk factors for lumbar disc degeneration: a 5-year MRI study in asymptomatic individuals. Spine 27:125–134, 2002.

151. Boden SD, Davis DO, Dina TS, et al. Abnormal magnetic-resonance scans of the lumbar spine in asymptomatic subjects. A prospective investigation. J Bone Joint Surg Am 72:403–408, 1990.

152. Wiesel SW, Tsourmas N, Feffer HL, et al. A study of computer-assisted tomography. I. The incidence of positive CAT scans in an asymptomatic group of patients. Spine 9:549–551, 1984.

153. Videman T, Nurminen M, Troup JD. 1990 Volvo Award in clinical sciences. Lumbar spinal pathology in cadaveric material in relation to history of back pain, occupation, and physical loading. Spine 15:728–740, 1990.

154. Anderson GBJ, Ortengren R, Nachemson A, et al. Lumbar disc pressure and myoelectric back activity during sitting. Scand J Rehabil Med 6:128, 1974.

155. Deyo RA. Conservative therapy for low back pain. JAMA 250: 1057–1062, 1983.

156. Van Tulder MW, Koes BW, Bouter LM. Conservative treatment of acute and chronic non-specific low back pain. Spine 22: 2128–2156, 1997.

157. Wheeler AH, Hanley EN. Spine update: non-operative treatment for low back pain. Spine 20:375–378, 1995.

158. Deyo RA. Drug therapy for back pain. Spine 21:2840–2849, 1996.

159. Berry H, Hutchinson DR. Tizanidine and ibuprofen in acute low-back pain. J Int Med Res 16:83–91, 1988.

160. Deyo RA, Diehl AK, Rosenthal M. How many days of bedrest for acute low back pain? N Engl J Med 315:1064–1070, 1966.

161. McCall IW, Park WM, O'Brien JP. Induced pain referral from posterior lumbar elements in normal subjects. Spine 4:441–446, 1979.

162. Hirsch C, Ingelmark B-E, Miller M. The anatomical basis for low back pain: studies on the presence of sensory nerve endings in ligamentous capsular and intervertebral disc structures in the human lumbar spine. Acta Orthop Scand 33:1–17, 1963.

163. Hawkes CH, Roberts GM. Neurogenic and vascular claudication. J Neurol Sci 38:337–345, 1978.

164. Deen HG Jr, Zimmerman RS, Lyons MK, et al. Measurement of exercise tolerance on the treadmill in patients with symptomatic lumbar spinal stenosis: a useful indicator of functional status and surgical outcome. J Neurosurg 83:27–30, 1995.

165. Deen HG, Zimmerman RS, Lyons MK, et al. Use of the exercise treadmill to measure baseline functional status and surgical outcome in patients with severe lumbar spinal stenosis. Spine 23: 244–248, 1998.

166. Fritz JM, Erhard RE, Delitto A, et al. Preliminary results of the use of a two-stage treadmill test as a clinical diagnostic tool in the differential diagnosis of lumbar spinal stenosis. J Spinal Disord 10:410–416, 1997.

167. Inufusa A, An HS, Lim TH, et al. Anatomic changes of the spinal canal and intervertebral foramen associated with flexion-extension movement. Spine 21:2412–2420, 1996.

168. Dai LY, Yu YK, Zhang WM, et al. The effect of flexion-extension motion of the lumbar spine on the capacity of a spinal canal. An experimental study. Spine 14:523–525, 1989.

169. Takahashi K, Kagechika K, Takino T, et al. Changes in epidural pressure during walking in patients with lumbar spinal stenosis. Spine 20:2746–2749, 1995.

170. Waddell G, Main CJ, Morris EW, et al. Chronic low back pain, psychologic distress, and illness behavior. Spine 9:209–213, 1984.

171. Ross JS, Modic MT. Current assessment of spinal degenerative disease with magnetic resonance imaging. Clin Orthop 279: 68–81, 1992.

172. Jackson RP, Cain JE Jr, Jacobs RR, et al. The neuroradiographic diagnosis of lumbar herniated nucleus pulposus: II. A comparison of computed tomography (CT), myelography, CT-myelography, and magnetic resonance imaging. Spine 14:1362–1367, 1989.

173. Savage RA, Whitehouse GH, Roberts N. The relationship between the magnetic resonance imaging appearance of the lumbar spine and low back pain, age and occupation in males. Eur Spine J 6:106–114, 1997.

174. Forristall RM, Marsh HO, Pay NT. Magnetic resonance imaging and contrast CT of the lumbar spine. Comparison of diagnostic methods and correlation with surgical findings. Spine 13: 1049–1054, 1988.

175. Saifuddin A, Mitchell R, Taylor BA. Extradural inflammation associated with annular tears: demonstration with gadolinium-enhanced lumbar spine MRI. Eur Spine J 8:34–39, 1999.

176. Haldeman S. Why one cause of back pain? In: Buerger AA, Tobis JS, eds. Approaches to the Validation of Manipulation Therapy. Springfield, IL, Charles C Thomas, 1977, p 187.
177. Wyke BD. The neurology of low back pain. In: Jayson MIV, ed. The Lumbar Spine and Back Pain. 3rd ed. Edinburgh, Churchill Livingstone, 1987, p 56.
178. Lewin P. Backache and Sciatic Neuritis. Philadelphia, Lea & Febiger, 1943, p 43.
179. Wheeler AH, Hanley EN. Spine update: non-operative treatment for low back pain. Spine 20:375–378, 1995.
180. Lee HM, Weinstein JN, Meller ST, et al. The role of steroids and their effects on phospholipase A2. Spine 23:1191–1196, 1998.
181. Tewari R, Boswell MV, Rosenberg SK. Therapeutic drugs for neuropathic pain. J Back Musculoskeletal Rehabil 9:247–254, 1997.
182. Risch SV, Norvell NK, Pollock ML, et al. Lumbar strengthening in chronic low back pain. Spine 18:232–238, 1993.
183. Manniche C, Lundberg E, Christensen I, et al. Intensive dynamic back exercises for chronic low back pain. Pain 47:53–63, 1991.
184. Khalil TM, Asfour SS, Martinez LM, et al. Stretching in the rehabilitation of low-back pain patients. Spine 17:311–317, 1992.
185. Handa N, Yamamoto H, Tani T, et al. The effect of trunk muscle exercises in patients over 40 years of age with chronic low back pain. J Orthop Sci. 5:210–216, 2000.
186. Donelson R. The McKenzie approach to evaluating and treating low back pain. Orthop Rev 19:681–686, 1990.
187. Stankovic R, Johnell O. Conservative treatment of acute low back pain. A 5-year follow-up study of two methods of treatment. Spine 20:469–472, 1995.
188. Saal JA. Dynamic muscular stabilization in the nonoperative treatment of lumbar pain syndromes. Orthop Rev 19:691–700, 1990.
189. Nutter P. Aerobic exercise in the treatment and prevention of low back pain. Occup Med 3:137–145, 1988.
190. Soukup MG, Glomsrod B, Lonn JH, et al. The effect of a Mensendieck exercise program as secondary prophylaxis for recurrent low back pain. Spine 24:1585–1591, 1999.
191. Mannion AF, Muntener M, Taimela S, et al. 1999 Volvo Award winner in clinical studies. A randomized clinical trial of three active therapies for chronic low back pain. Spine 24:2435–2438, 1999.
192. Galloway MT, Jokl P. Aging successfully: the importance of physical activity in maintaining health and function. J Am Acad Orthop Surg 8:37–44, 2000.
193. Mitchell RI, Carmen GM. The functional approach to the treatment of chronic pain in patients with soft tissue and back injuries. Spine 6:633–642, 1994.
194. Liemohn W. Exercise and arthritis. Exercise and the back. Rheum Dis Clin North Am 16:945–970, 1990.
195. Kong WZ, Goel VK, Gilbertson LG, et al. Effects of muscle dysfunction on lumbar spine mechanics. Spine 21:2197–2206, 1996.
196. Molde Hagen E, Grasdal A, Eriksen HR. Does early intervention with a light mobilization program reduce long-term sick leave for low back pain: a 3-year follow-up study. Spine 28:2309–2315, 2003.
197. Jackson RP. The facet syndrome, myth or reality? Clin Orthop 279:110–121, 1962.
198. Dreyer SJ, Dreyfuss P, Cole AJ. Zygapophyseal (facet) joint injections. Phys Med Rehabil Clin North Am 6:715–741, 1995.
199. Carette S, Marcoux S, Truchon R, et al. A controlled trial of corticosteroid injections into facet joints for chronic low back pain. N Engl J Med 325:1002–1007, 1991.
200. Gatchel RW, Polatin PB, Mayer TG, et al. Psychopathology and the rehabilitation of patients with chronic low back pain. Ach Phys Med Rehabil 75:666–670, 1994.
201. Cohen JE, Goel V, Frank JW, et al. Group education interventions for people with low back pain. Spine 11:1214–1222, 1994.
202. Indahl A, Haldorsen EH, Holm S, et al. Five-year follow-up study of a controlled clinical trial using light mobilization and an informative approach to low back pain. Spine 23: 2625–2630, 1998.
203. Lorenz M, Zindrick M, Schwaegler P, et al. A comparison of single-level fusions with and without hardware. Spine 16(suppl): 455–458, 1991.
204. Stauffer RN, Coventry MD. Posterolateral lumbar-spine fusion. Analysis of Mayo Clinic series. J Bone Joint Surg Am 54: 1195–1204, 1972.
205. McCulloch JA. Uninstrumented posterolateral lumbar fusion for single level isolated disc resorption and/or degenerative disc disease. J Spinal Disord 12:34–39, 1999.
206. Thomsen K, Christensen FB, Eiskjaer SP, et al. 1997 Volvo Award winner in clinical studies. The effect of pedicle screw instrumentation on functional outcome and fusion rates in posterolateral lumbar spinal fusion: a prospective, randomized clinical study. Spine 22:2813–2822, 1997.
207. France JC, Yaszemski MJ, Lauerman WC, et al. A randomized prospective study of posterolateral lumbar fusion. Outcomes with and without pedicle screw instrumentation. Spine 24: 553–560, 1999.
208. Greenough CG, Peterson MD, Hadlow S, et al. Instrumented posterolateral lumbar fusion. Results and comparison with anterior interbody fusion. Spine 23:479–486, 1998.
209. Parker LM, Murrell SE, Boden SD, et al. The outcome of posterolateral fusion in highly selected patients with discogenic low back pain. Spine 21:1909–1916, 1996.
210. Nachemson A, Zdeblick TA, O'Brien JP. Lumbar disc disease with discogenic pain. What surgical treatment is most effective? Spine 21:1835–1838, 1996.
211. Weber BR, Grob D, Dvorak J, et al. Posterior surgical approach to the lumbar spine and its effect on the multifidus muscle. Spine 22:1765–1772, 1997.
212. Penta M, Fraser RD. Anterior lumbar interbody fusion. A minimum 10-year follow-up. Spine 22:2429–2434, 1997.
213. Vamvanij V, Fredrickson BE, Thorpe JM, et al. Surgical treatment of internal disc disruption: an outcome study of four fusion techniques. J Spinal Disord 11:375–382, 1998.
214. Ray CD. Threaded titanium cages for lumbar interbody fusions. Spine 22:667–679, 1997.
215. Hacker RJ. Comparison of interbody fusion approaches for disabling low back pain. Spine 22:660–665, 1997.
216. Linson MA, Williams H. Anterior and combined anteroposterior fusion for lumbar disc pain. A preliminary study. Spine 16: 143–145, 1991.
217. Leufven C, Nordwall A. Management of chronic disabling low back pain with 360 degrees fusion. Results from pain provocation test and concurrent posterior lumbar interbody fusion, posterolateral fusion, and pedicle screw instrumentation in patients with chronic disabling low back pain. Spine 24:2042–2045, 1999.
218. Whitecloud TS 3rd, Castro FP Jr, Brinker MR, et al. Degenerative conditions of the lumbar spine treated with intervertebral titanium cages and posterior instrumentation for circumferential fusion. J Spinal Disord 11:479–486, 1998.
219. Gertzbein SD, Hollopeter M, Hall SD. Analysis of circumferential lumbar fusion outcome in the treatment of degenerative disc disease of the lumbar spine. J Spinal Disord 11:472–478, 1998.
220. Okuyama K, Abe E, Suzuki T, et al. Posterior lumbar interbody fusion: a retrospective study of complications after facet joint excision and pedicle screw fixation in 148 cases. Acta Orthop Scand 70:329–334, 1999.
221. Enker P, Steffee A, Mcmillin C, et al. Artificial disc replacement. Preliminary report with a 3-year minimum follow-up. Spine 18:1061–1070, 1993.
222. Griffith SL, Shelokov AP, Buttner-Janz K, et al. A multicenter retrospective study of the clinical results of the LINK SB Charité intervertebral prosthesis. The initial European experience. Spine 19:1842–1849, 1994.
223. Cinotti G, David T, Postacchini F. Results of disc prosthesis after a minimum follow-up period of 2 years. Spine 21:995–1000, 1996.
224. Bertagnoli R, Sabatino CT, Edwards JT, et al. Mechanical testing of a novel hydrogel nucleus replacement implant. Spine J. 5: 672–681, 2005.
225. Allen MJ, Schoonmaker JE, Bauer TW, et al. Preclinical evaluation of a poly (vinyl alcohol) hydrogel implant as a replacement for the nucleus pulposus. Spine 29:515–523, 2004.
226. Klara PM, Ray CD. Artificial nucleus replacement: clinical experience. Spine 27:1374–1377, 2002.
227. Takahashi K, Shima I, Porter RW. Nerve root pressure in lumbar disc herniation. Spine 24:2003–2006, 1999.

228. Kobayashi S, Baba H, Uchida K, et al. Effect of mechanical compression on the lumbar nerve root: localization and changes of intraradicular inflammatory cytokines, nitric oxide, and cyclooxygenase. Spine 30:1699–1705, 2005.

229. Takata K, Inoue S, Takahashi K, et al. Swelling of the cauda equina in patients who have herniation of a lumbar disc. A possible pathogenesis of sciatica. J Bone Joint Surg Am 70:361–368, 1988.

230. Habtemariam A, Virri J, Gronblad M, et al. The role of mast cells in disc herniation inflammation. Spine 24:1516–1520, 1999.

231. Nygaard OP, Mellgren SI, Osterud B. The inflammatory properties of contained and noncontained lumbar disc herniation. Spine 22:2484–2488, 1997.

232. Kang JD, Stefanovic-Racic M, McIntyre LA, et al. Toward a biochemical understanding of human intervertebral disc degeneration and herniation. Contributions of nitric oxide, interleukins, prostaglandin E2, and matrix metalloproteinases. Spine 22:1065–1073, 1997.

233. Weiler C, Nerlich AG, Zipperer J, et al. 2002 SSE Award Competition in Basic Science: expression of major matrix metalloproteinases is associated with intervertebral disc degradation and resorption. Eur Spine J. 11:308–320, 2002.

234. Kang JD, Georgescu Hi, McIntyre-Larkin L, et al. Herniated lumbar intervertebral discs spontaneously produce matrix metalloproteinases, nitric oxide, interleukin-6, and prostaglandin E2. Spine 21:271–277, 1996.

235. Takahashi H, Suguro T, Okazima Y, et al. Inflammatory cytokines in the herniated disc of the lumbar spine. Spine 21:218–224, 1996.

236. Piperno M, Hellio le Graverand MP, et al. Phospholipase A_2 activity in herniated lumbar discs. Clinical correlations and inhibition by piroxicam. Spine 22:2061–2065, 1997.

237. Matsui H, Kanamori M, Kawaguchi Y, et al. Clinical and electrophysiologic characteristics of compressed lumbar nerve roots. Spine 22:2100–2105, 1997.

238. Shapiro S. Cauda equina syndrome secondary to lumbar disc herniation. Neurosurgery 32:743–746, 1993.

239. Nielsen B, de Nully M, Schmidt K, et al. A urodynamic study of cauda equina syndrome due to lumbar disc herniation. Urol Int 35:167–170, 1980.

240. Perner A, Andersen JT, Juhler M. Lower urinary tract symptoms in lumbar root compression syndromes: a prospective survey. Spine 22:2693–2697, 1997.

241. Aprill C, Bogduk N. High-intensity zone: a diagnostic sign of painful lumbar disc on magnetic resonance imaging. Br J Radiol 65:361–369, 1992.

242. Hakelius A. Prognosis in sciatica: a clinical follow up of surgical and non-surgical treatment. Acta Orthop Scand Suppl 129:1–76, 1970.

243. Zentner J, Schneider B, Schramm J. Efficacy of conservative treatment of lumbar disc herniation. J Neurosurg Sci 41:263–268, 1997.

244. Saal JA, Saal JS. Nonoperative treatment of herniated lumbar intervertebral disc with radiculopathy. Spine 4:431–437, 1989.

245. The natural history of herniated nucleus pulposus with radiculopathy. Spine 21: 225–229, 1996.

246. Yukawa Y, Kato F, Matsubara Y, et al. Serial magnetic resonance imaging follow-up study of lumbar disc herniation conservatively treated for average 30 months: relation between reduction of herniation and degeneration of disc. J Spinal Disord 9:251–256, 1996.

247. Atlas SJ, Keller RB, Chang Y, et al. Surgical and nonsurgical management of sciatica secondary to a lumbar disc herniation: five-year outcomes from the Maine Lumbar Spine Study. Spine 26: 1179–1187, 2001.

248. Atlas SJ, Keller RB, Wu YA, et al. Long-term outcomes of surgical and nonsurgical management of sciatica secondary to a lumbar disc herniation: 10 year results from the Maine Lumbar Spine Study. Spine 30:847–849, 2005.

249. Jonsson B, Stromqvist B. The straight leg raising test and the severity of symptoms in lumbar disc herniation. A preoperative evaluation. Spine 20:27–30, 1995.

250. Thelander U, Fagerlund M, Friberg S, et al. Straight leg raising test versus radiologic size, shape, and position of lumbar disc hernias. Spine 17:395–399, 1992.

251. Supik LF, Broom MJ. Sciatic tension signs and lumbar disc herniation. Spine 19:1066–1069, 1994.

252. Vroomen PC, de Krom MC, Knottnerus JA. Diagnostic value of history and physical examination in patients suspected of sciatica due to disc herniation: a systematic review. J Neurol 246: 899–906, 1999.

253. Hudgins WR. The crossed straight leg raising test: a diagnostic sign of herniated disc. J Occup Med 21:407–408, 1979.

254. Spengler DM, Ouellette EA, Battie M, et al. Elective discectomy for herniation of a lumbar disc. Additional experience with an objective method. J Bone Joint Surg Am 72:230–237, 1990.

255. Herron LD, Turner JA, Weiner P. Lumbar disc herniations: the predictive value of the Health Attribution Test (HAT) and the Minnesota Multiphasic Personality Inventory (MMPI). J Spinal Disord 1:2–8, 1988.

256. Buttermann GR. The effect of spinal steroid injections for degenerative discdisease. Spine J 4(5):495–505, 2004.

257. Ohnmeiss DD. Repeatability of pain drawings in a low back pain population. Spine 25(8):980–988, 2000.

258. Geisser ME, Wiggert EA, Haig AJ, et al. A randomized, controlled trial of manual therapy and specific adjuvant exercises for chronic low back pain. Clin J Pain 21:463–470, 2005.

259. Hawk C, Long CR, Rowell RM, et al. A randomized trial investigating a chiropractic manual placebo: a novel design using standardized forces in the delivery of active and control treatments. J Altern Complement Med. 11:109–117, 2005.

260. McMorland G, Suter E. Chiropractic management of mechanical neck and low-back pain: a retrospective, outcome-based analysis. J Manipulative Physiol Ther 23:307–311, 2000.

261. Lisi AJ, Holmes EJ, Ammendolia C. High-velocity low-amplitude spinal manipulation for symptomatic lumbar disc disease: a systematic review of the literature. J Manipulative Physiol Ther 28:429–442, 2005.

262. Haas M, Sharma R, Stano M. Cost-effectiveness of medical and chiropractic care for acute and chronic low back pain. J Manipulative Physiol Ther 28:555–563, 2005.

263. Oliphant D. Safety of spinal manipulation in the treatment of lumbar disc herniations: a systematic review and risk assessment. J Manipulative Physiol Ther 27:197–210, 2004.

264. Kuo PP, Loh ZC. Treatment of lumbar intervertebral disc protusions by manipulation. Clin Orthop Relat Res 215:47–55, 1987.

265. Haldeman S. Spinal manipulative therapy. A status report. Clin Orthop Relat Res 179:62–70, 1983.

266. Wang JC, Lin E, Brodke DS, et al. Epidural injections for the treatment of symptomatic lumbar herniated discs. J Spinal Disord Tech 15(4):269–272, 2002.

267. Cannon DT, April CN. Lumbosacral epidural steroid injections. Arch Phys Med Rehabil 81(suppl):S87–S98, 2000.

268. Weinstein SM, Herring SA, Derby R. Contemporary concepts in spine care. Epidural steroid injections. Spine 20:1842–1846, 1995.

269. Brown FW. Management of diskogenic pain using epidural and intrathecal steroids. Clin Orthop Relat Res 129:72–28, 1977.

270. Woodward JL, Weinstein SM. Epidural injections for the diagnosis and management of axial and radicular pain syndromes. Phys Med Rehabil Clin North Am 6:691–713, 1995.

271. Botwin KP, Baskin M, Rao S. Adverse effects of fluoroscopically guided interlaminar thoracic epidural steroid injections. Am J Phys Med Rehabil 85:14–23, 2006.

272. Kostuik JP, Harrington I, Alexander D, et al. Cauda equina syndrome and lumbar disc herniation. J Bone Joint Surg Am 68:386–391, 1986.

273. Dahl B, Gerhchen PM, Kiaer T, et al. Nonorganic pain drawings are associated with low psychological scores on the preoperative SF-36 questionnaire in patients with chronic low back pain. Eur Spine J 10(3):211–214, 2001.

274. Carragee EJ, Han MY, Suen PW, et al. Clinical outcomes after lumbar discectomy for sciatica: the effects of fragment type and anular competence. J Bone Joint Surg Am 85-A(1):102–108, 2003.

275. Sahlstrand T, Lonntoft M. A prospective study of preoperative and postoperative sequential magnetic resonance imaging and early clinical outcome in automated percutaneous lumbar discectomy. J Spinal Disord 12:368–374, 1999.

276. Dullerud R, Nakstad PH. Side effects and complications of automated percutaneous lumbar nucleotomy. Neuroradiology 39:282–285, 1997.

277. Nerubay J, Caspi I, Levinkopf M. Percutaneous carbon dioxide laser nucleolysis with 2- to 5-year followup. Clin Orthop 337:45–48, 1997.

278. Schonstrom N, Bolender NF, Spengler DM. The pathomorphology of spinal stenosis as seen on CT scans of the lumbar spine. Spine 10:806–811, 1985.

279. Schonstrom N, Bolender NF, Spengler DM. Dynamic changes in the dimension of the lumbar spinal canal. An experimental study in vitro. J Orthop Res 7:115–121, 1988.

280. Rydevik BL, Pedowitz RA, Hargens AR, et al. Effects of acute, graded compression on spinal nerve root function and structure. An experimental study of the pig cauda equina. Spine 16:487–493, 1991.

281. Johnsson KE, Rosen I, Uden A. The natural course of lumbar spinal stenosis. Clin Orthop 279:82–86, 1992.

282. Hall S, Bartleson JD, Onofrio BM, et al. Lumbar spinal stenosis. Clinical features, diagnostic procedures, and results of surgical treatment in 68 patients. Ann Intern Med 103:271–275, 1985.

283. Boden SD, Riew KD, Yamaguchi K, et al. Orientation of the lumbar facet joints: association with degenerative disc disease. J Bone Joint Surg Am 78:403–411, 1996.

284. Nagaosa Y, Kikuchi S, Hasue M, et al. Pathoanatomic mechanisms of degenerative spondylolisthesis. A radiographic study. Spine 23:1447–1451, 1998.

285. Berlemann U, Jeszenszky DJ, Buhler DW, et al. The role of lumbar lordosis, vertebral end-plate inclination, disc height, and facet orientation in degenerative spondylolisthesis. J Spinal Disord 12:68–73, 1999.

286. Laus M, Tigani D, Alfonso C, et al. Degenerative spondylolisthesis: lumbar stenosis and instability. Chir Organi Mov 77:39–49, 1992.

287. Carragee EJ, Spinnickie AO, Alamin TF, et al. A prospective controlled study of limited versus subtotal posterior discectomy: short-term outcomes in patients with herniated lumbar intervertebral discs and large posterior anular defect. Spine 31(6): 653–657, 2006.

288. Simotas AC, Dorey FJ, Hansraj KK, et al. Non-operative treatment for lumbar spinal stenosis. Spine 25:197–203, 2000.

289. Jackson CP, Brown MD. Analysis of current approaches and a physical guide to prescription of exercise. Clin Orthop 179: 46–54, 1983.

290. Plastaras CT. Electrodiagnostic challenges in the evaluation of lumbar spinal stenosis. Phys Med Rehabil Clin North Am 14(1): 57–69, 2003.

291. Amundsen T, Weber H, Nordal HJ, et al. Lumbar Spinal Stenosis: Conservative or surgical management?: A prospective 10 year study. Spine 25(11):1424–1435, 2000.

292. Herron LD, Mangelsdorf C. Lumbar spinal stenosis: results of surgical treatment. J Spinal Disord 4:26–33, 1991.

293. Atlas SJ, Deyo RA, Keller RB, et al. The Maine Lumbar Spine Study, Part III. 1-year outcomes of surgical and nonsurgical management of lumbar spinal stenosis. Spine 21:1787–1794, discussion 1794–1795, 1996.

294. Tuite GF, Stern JD, Doran SE, et al. Outcome after laminectomy for lumbar spinal stenosis. Part I. Clinical correlations. J Neurosurg 81:699–706, 1994.

295. Javid MJ, Hadar EJ. Long-term follow-up review of patients who underwent laminectomy for lumbar stenosis: a prospective study. J Neurosurg 89:1–7, 1998.

296. Katz JN, Lipson SJ, Chang LC, et al. Seven- to 10-year outcome of decompressive surgery for degenerative lumbar spinal stenosis. Spine 21:92–98, 1996.

297. Airaksinen O, Herno A, Turunen V, et al. Surgical outcome of 438 patients treated surgically for lumbar spinal stenosis. Spine 22:2278–2282, 1997.

298. Mauersberger W, Nietgen T. Surgical treatment of lumbar stenosis: long-term results. Neurosurg Rev 12:291–295, 1989.

299. Caputy AJ, Luessenhop AJ. Long-term evaluation of decompressive surgery for degenerative lumbar stenosis. J Neurosurg 77:669–676, 1992.

300. Postacchini F, Cinotti G, Gumina S, et al. Long-term results of surgery in lumbar stenosis. 8-year review of 64 patients. Acta Orthop Scand Suppl 251:78–80, 1993.

301. Boden SD, Riew KD, Yamaguchi K, et al. Orientation of the lumbar facet joints: association with degenerative disc disease. J Bone Joint Surg Am 78:403–411, 1996.

302. Berlemann U, Jeszenszky DJ, Buhler DW, et al. The role of lumbar lordosis, vertebral end-plate inclination, disc height, and facet orientation in degenerative spondylolisthesis. J Spinal Disord 12:68–73, 1999.

303. Nagaosa Y, Kikuchi S, Hasue M, et al. Pathoanatomic mechanisms of degenerative spondylolisthesis. A radiographic study. Spine 23:1447–1451, 1998.

304. Lombardi JS, Wiltse LL, Reynolds J, et al. Treatment of degenerative spondylolisthesis. Spine 10:821–827, 1985.

305. Herkowitz HN, Kurz LT. Degenerative lumbar spondylolisthesis with spinal stenosis. A prospective study comparing decompression and intertransverse process arthrodesis. J Bone Joint Surg Am 73:802–808, 1991.

306. Bridwell KH, Sedgewick TA, O'Brien MF, et al. The role of fusion and instrumentation in the treatment of degenerative spondylolisthesis with spinal stenosis. J Spinal Disord 6:461–472, 1993.

307. Fischgrund JS, Mackay M, Herkowitz HN, et al. 1997 Volvo Award winner in clinical studies. Degenerative lumbar spondylolisthesis with spinal stenosis: a prospective, randomized study comparing decompressive laminectomy and arthrodesis with and without spinal instrumentation. Spine 22:2807–2812, 1997.

308. Cooper G, Lutz GE, Boachie-Adjei O, et al. Effectiveness of transforaminal epidural steroid injections in patients with degenerative lumbar scoliotic stenosis and radiculopathy. Pain Physician 7(3):311–317, 2004.

309. Irwin ZN, Hilibrand A, Gustavel M, et al. Variation in surgical decision making for degenerative spinal disorders. Part I: lumbar spine. Spine 30(19): 2208–2213, 2005.

New Frontiers in Surgery of Osteoarthritis

23

Tom Minas *Andreas H. Gomoll*

INTRODUCTION

Since Hunter's famous statement over 250 years ago describing cartilage as a "troublesome thing and once destroyed, it is not repaired,"[1] medicine has directed considerable effort toward improving the limited repair potential of chondral lesions. Partial thickness lesions that do not penetrate the subchondral bone are avascular, therefore do not heal, and may enlarge over time. Full-thickness defects, especially with injury to the underlying vascular bone, have the potential to fill with a fibrocartilaginous scar formed by mesenchymal stem cells invading from the marrow cavity. This fibrocartilage, however, is predominantly composed of type I collagen, resulting in inferior mechanical properties compared to the type II collagen-rich hyaline cartilage.

Long implicated in the subsequent development of osteoarthritis (OA), focal chondral defects result from various etiologies. The exact incidence of chondral defects is still poorly established. Traumatic events and developmental etiologies such as osteochondritis dissecans (OCD) predominate in the younger age groups. Traumatic hemarthroses in young athletes with knee injuries are associated with chondral defects in up to 10% of cases;[2] the incidence of OCD is estimated at 30 to 60 cases per 100,000 people.[3] Several large studies have found high-grade chondral lesions (Outerbridge grade III and IV) in 5% to 11% of younger patients (less than 40 years), and up to 60% in the older age groups.[4-6] The most common locations for these defects are the medial femoral condyle and the patella,[4,6] and most present as incidental findings during procedures such as meniscectomy or anterior cruciate ligament reconstruction.[5,7]

Since articular cartilage lesions have no spontaneous repair potential if left untreated, different techniques have evolved in an attempt to stimulate filling of these defects,

ideally with hyaline articular cartilage. Even today, the treatment of chondral defects remains a challenge, and none of the conventional techniques discussed in this chapter has provided predictable long-term clinical results. These conventional techniques, such as abrasion arthroplasty, drilling, or microfracture, attempt to fill the defect with a fibrocartilaginous scar produced by marrow-derived pluripotent stem cells. This scar cartilage, however, is of lesser biological and mechanical quality than the articular, or hyaline cartilage. More recently developed techniques used in current clinical practice, such as autologous chondrocyte implantation (ACI) or matrix autologous chondrocyte implantation (MACI), achieve a tissue that more closely resembles the original hyaline cartilage. Several challenges remain, such as the integration of regenerated cartilage with the surrounding host tissue, and the development of sufficient long-term stability and wear characteristics that will allow the repair tissue to withstand the stresses of physical activity over years.

This chapter will provide a concise overview of current techniques for cartilage repair, and subsequently present several of the more promising new developments in this evolving area.

SURGICAL TREATMENT OF CHONDRAL DEFECTS

Underlying Abnormalities and Predisposing Factors for Chondropenia

On careful evaluation, the majority of chondral defects is associated with coexisting abnormalities of the knee, including limb malalignment, patellar maltracking, and insufficiency of the ligamentous and meniscal structures.

Varus or valgus malalignment of the lower extremity shifts the load-bearing axis to one compartment, thus resulting in local overload and accelerated degeneration of the articular surface. Ligamentous insufficiency, most commonly of the anterior cruciate ligament, increases shear forces in the knee joint and thus contributes to chondral wear. Meniscal insufficiency, such as after subtotal meniscectomy, increases contact stresses by up to 300% in the respective compartment, and is predictably associated with the development of OA. More recently, the disappointing early results of cartilage repair have been explained by the failure to diagnose and correct these associated bony and ligamentous abnormalities; for example, in early studies of patellar defects treated with ACI alone, good and excellent results were found in only one third of patients.[8] Later studies, however, identified patellar maltracking as an important associated abnormality, and performance of a corrective osteotomy concurrently with cartilage repair led to 71% good or excellent results.[9] These reports emphasize the importance of a thorough patient evaluation to correctly identify and treat all associated abnormalities to ensure the long-term success of chondral repair.

When performed concurrently with cartilage repair, osteotomy around the knee should restore the mechanical axis to neutral alignment in cases where the radiographic joint space is maintained. Coventry's early work with osteotomies popularized this technique for the treatment of OA. However, the population treated for chondral defects is predominantly athletic and cannot tolerate large overcorrection, as has been successfully used in osteoarthrosis patients. Therefore, even in patients with early joint space narrowing, overcorrection of the mechanical axis should be limited to 2 degrees or less.

Subtotal meniscectomy significantly alters the biomechanical environment and frequently results in secondary OA. In carefully selected patients with meniscal insufficiency, meniscal allograft transplantation can provide pain relief and improved function. The ideal candidate for allograft transplantation has a history of prior total or subtotal meniscectomy with persistent pain localized to the involved compartment. Associated abnormalities such as malalignment, discrete chondral defects, or ligamentous instability can be addressed in either staged or concomitant procedures. Following meniscal allograft transplantation, good to excellent results are achieved in nearly 85% of cases, and patients demonstrate a measurable decrease in pain and increase in activity level.[10]

Conventional Cartilage Repair Techniques

Prior to the development of modern bioengineering techniques, orthopedists were restricted to procedures that either aimed to palliate the effects of chondral lesions or attempted to stimulate a healing response of the subchondral bone, resulting in the formation of scar tissue to fill the defect. Simple arthroscopic lavage and débridement of arthritic joints has been used since the 1940s[11] in an effort to reduce symptoms resulting from loose bodies and cartilage flaps. While lavage alone has not been found to be effective, in combination with débridement it can result in

adequate pain reduction in slightly more than half of patients.[12,13] The goal of débridement of chondral defects is to remove any loose flaps, and to create a defect shouldered by a stable rim of intact cartilage, thus reducing mechanical stresses in the defect bed. Currently, its use is limited to the treatment of small cartilage lesions that are incidental findings during arthroscopic treatment of meniscal or ligamentous pathology.

Marrow stimulation techniques, such as drilling, abrasion arthroplasty, and microfracture, attempt to induce a reparative response in the avascular cartilage. This is achieved by perforation of the subchondral bone after radical débridement of damaged cartilage and removal of the tide mark zone, thus enhancing the integration of repair and surrounding tissue. Perforation of the subchondral bone results in the extravasation of blood and marrow elements with formation of a blood clot in the defect. Over time, this blood clot, and the primitive mesenchymal cells contained within, differentiate into a fibrocartilaginous repair tissue that fills the defect, but may also form bone resulting in an intralesional osteophyte. Unlike hyaline cartilage, this fibrocartilage predominantly consists of type I collagen, and exhibits inferior wear characteristics. Postoperatively, all marrow-stimulating techniques require extended periods of strict non–weight-bearing for 6 weeks or more, as well as the use of continuous passive motion (CPM) therapy for up to 6 hours per day to enhance maturation of the repair tissue, as do other techniques intended to produce hyaline cartilage. Even though marrow stimulation techniques result in a repair tissue with inferior wear characteristics, treatment of smaller defects (<4 cm^2) results in good outcomes in 60% to 70% of patients.[14]

New Cartilage Repair Techniques

Cartilage Restoration

Restorative cartilage repair techniques introduce chondrogenic cells into the defect area, resulting in the formation of a repair tissue that more closely resembles articular (hyaline) cartilage. The original technique of ACI was developed over 15 years ago, and has been used in the United States to treat more than 10,000 patients since its approval by the FDA in 1997. Second-generation techniques that involve the use of resorbable carrier matrices are available in Europe with over 5-year follow-up results. These techniques offer the benefit of a less-invasive surgical approach, and have demonstrated excellent early results without periosteum-related problems seen in conventional ACI.

Autologous Chondrocyte Implantation

ACI is a technique aimed at treating medium to large size chondral defects by in vitro expansion of an autologous chondrocyte biopsy, followed by staged reimplantation. Originally reported in 1994[8] for the treatment of chondral defects in the knee, it has more recently been applied to other joints such as the shoulder[15] and ankle.[16]

ACI in its current form is a two-stage procedure in which a cartilage biopsy of approximately 200 mg is harvested during an initial arthroscopic procedure. The biopsy is usually obtained from a non–weight-bearing area of the knee, commonly from the superior medial edge of the trochlea or the area of the intercondylar notch. The approximately 200,000 to 300,000 chondrocytes contained within the tissue are released by enzymatic digestion of the surrounding matrix, and expanded in a monolayer culture for several weeks. Initial concerns over cell dedifferentiation and loss of type II collagen expression were addressed by early studies that demonstrated re-expression of the chondrocyte phenotype when the expanded cells were cultured in agarose gels.[17]

After successful culture expansion, the patient returns to the operating room for reimplantation, which necessitates open arthrotomy. The chondral defect is exposed and carefully debrided of cartilage remnants, including the layer of calcified cartilage, down to the subchondral plate, which should not be violated. The defect should be bordered by stable shoulders of surrounding cartilage, and have a healthy and nonbleeding bed of subchondral bone. A patch of periosteum, harvested from the proximal tibia, is then sewn to the adjacent cartilage to cover the defect, with the cambium layer facing inward. Fibrin glue is added to the suture line to achieve a watertight seal prior to injection of the chondrocyte suspension into the covered defect.[18] While the ideal cell density for reimplantation is controversial, in current practice reimplantation of approximately 12 million cells is attempted for an average size lesion of 4 to 6 cm^2.

Rehabilitation

The rehab protocol after ACI is divided into three phases. These are based on the slow maturation of the repair tissue, which at the same time has to be protected from overloading, and stimulated to encourage tissue maturation. The three phases of the healing process are the proliferative (fill) phase, the transitional (integration) phase, and the remodeling (hardening) phase, each of which can accommodate increasing amounts of load. During the initial proliferative phase, protection of the graft is paramount, and the patient is limited to touchdown weight bearing for 6 weeks. During this phase, patients also utilize a CPM machine for 6 to 8 hours per day to reduce the likelihood of adhesions and aid in maturation of the transplant. This initial period is followed by the transitional stage in which patients advance to full weight bearing over the course of several weeks. Additional exercises are prescribed based on the specific location and type of the defect. During the final remodeling phase that begins approximately 3 months after transplantation, the joint is increasingly loaded with strengthening and impact-loading activities. A full return to high-impact and pivoting activities should be delayed for at least 12 months until near-complete graft maturation has been achieved. Complete maturation is not expected until 12 to 24 months.

Results

Several long-term studies have reported good to excellent results in over 80% of patients after ACI for the treatment of chondral lesions in the knee (Table 23–1). Several studies have critically reviewed the results of ACI in comparison with other forms of treatment, such as débridement,[19] microfracture,[20] mosaicplasty,[21] and osteochondral autograft transfer[22] (Table 23–2).

Hypertrophy of the periosteal patch resulting in mechanical symptoms such as clicking and popping occurs in up to 15% to 20% of patients, and typically occurs 7 to 9 months after the procedure.[23] This hypertrophy is treated

TABLE 23-1
RESULTS OF SELECTED ACI STUDIES

Author	Patients [n]	Age [Years]	Follow-up [Years]	Defect Size [cm^2], Location/Type	Results
Brittberg[32] (2003)	57	32.9	4	4.2 FC	51 (89%) exc./good, 4 fair, 2 poor
Peterson[33] (2003)	58	26.4	5.6	5.7 OCD	53 (91%) exc./good, 4 fair, 1 poor
Bentley[21] (2003)	58	31.3	1.7	4.7 FC, PAT, TRO	51 (87%) exc./good, 7 fair, 0 poor
Mithoefer[34] (2005)	20	15.9	3.9	6.4 FC, PAT, TRO, TP	19 (95%) exc./good, 1 fair, 0 poor
Minas[9] (2005)	45	38	3.9	10.5 FC, PAT, TRO	32 (71%) exc./good, 10 fair, 3 poor
Browne[35] (2005)	100	37	5	4.9 FC, TRO	62 patients improved, 6 pts. no change, 19 pts. worsened

FC, femoral condyle; PAT, patella; TRO, trochlea; TP, tibial plateau; exc., excellent.

TABLE 23-2

COMPARISON OF ACI WITH OTHER TREATMENTS

Author	Age [Years]	Follow-up [Years]	Defect Size [cm²]	Patients [n]	Treatment	Results
Bentley[21] (2003)	30.9			58	ACI	51 (88%) exc./good, 7 fair, 0 poor
		1.7	4.7			
	31.6			42	Mosaicplasty	29 (69%) exc./good, 6 fair, 7 poor
Fu[19] (2005)	37.9		5	54	ACI	81% of patients improved
	35.9	3	4.5	42	Débridement	60% of patients improved (p <0.05)
Knutsen[20] (2004)	33.3		5.1	40	ACI	No significant differences between groups. Defects >4 cm² treated with micro fx did worse than smaller defects.
		2				
	31.1		4.5	40	Microfracture	
Horas[22] (2003)	31.4		3.9	20	ACI	No significant differences between groups. ACI patients with slower recovery
		2				
	35.4		3.6	20	OATS	

with simple arthroscopic débridement of the hypertrophic tissue. The most common complications following ACI are postoperative stiffness (2%) and graft detachment or delamination (1%).

CARTILAGE REPLACEMENT TECHNIQUES

Cartilage replacement techniques remove damaged cartilage along with subchondral bone and replace it with osteochondral grafts harvested from the patient or a tissue donor.

Osteochondral Autograft

Osteochondral autograft transplantation is used in procedures such as osteochondral autograft transplantation (OATS) or mosaicplasty to address medium size defects (1 to 4 cm²), often with associated bone loss. In this technique, multiple small cylinders of cartilage and subchondral bone are harvested from non–weight-bearing areas of the knee joint. The chondral defect is prepared with a punch to create a recipient hole that matches the graft cylinders, which are then press-fitted into the defect. Commonly, multiple cylinders have to be transplanted to fill larger defects. Osteochondral autografting is limited by the amount of cartilage that can be harvested without violating the weight-bearing articular surface.[24] The main advantage lies in its autogeneity, thus avoiding the risk of disease transmission, immediate graft availability through harvesting of the patient's own tissue, and decreased cost of this single-stage procedure.

Osteochondral Allograft

More than 750,000 musculoskeletal allografts were transplanted in 1999, mainly for the treatment of bone defects and for the reconstruction of the anterior cruciate ligament. More recently, the treatment of chondral defects with fresh osteochondral allografts has garnered significant attention because of its potential to restore and resurface even extensive areas of damaged or diseased cartilage. Unfortunately, the supply of osteochondral allograft tissue remains limited since it should be transplanted fresh to retain cartilage viability. However, improved preservation techniques have been developed that allow storage times of up to 3 weeks, which has begun to improve graft availability.

Allograft transplantation is mainly used to repair large osteochondral lesions resulting from OCD, osteonecrosis, or traumatic osteochondral fractures, but can also be used to treat peripherally uncontained cartilage and bone defects. Furthermore, osteochondral allografting presents a viable salvage option after failure of other cartilage resurfacing procedures. When it is used for the salvage of failed cartilage (surface) lesions, a thin subchondral bone graft (5 to 7 mm) results in the most rapid integration and best chance of success, since osteochondral allografts fail due to creeping substitution and collapse of the transplanted osseous bed, and not through failure of the cartilage itself.

The main advantages over autograft transplantation are the ability to very closely match the curvature of the articular surface by harvesting the graft from a corresponding location in the donor condyle, the ability to transplant large grafts, and the avoidance of donor site morbidity. The main concern with allograft transplantation is the risk, albeit small, of disease transmission, which is estimated at 1 in 1.6 million for the transmission of HIV.[25]

NEW DEVELOPMENTS

Autologous Chondrocyte Implantation—Matrix-Assisted

A relatively recent technique in cartilage repair, MACI™, was developed as the logical next step after ACI to improve upon a number of perceived shortcomings of that procedure. Similarly to ACI, MACI is also performed as a two-stage procedure, with an initial arthroscopic chondral biopsy, which is expanded in cell culture. Subsequently, however, instead of remaining in a two-dimensional culture, the chondrocytes are seeded onto a type I/type III porcine-derived collagen carrier matrix. During the second stage of the procedure, this carrier matrix is sized to match the defect, and then implanted either open or arthroscopically with fibrin glue fixation. The use of a pre-seeded matrix obviates the need to harvest and suture a periosteal patch to cover the defect, thus decreasing surgical time and morbidity associated with a wide exposure. MACI also addresses disadvantages of the ACI procedure that are associated with cell delivery in a liquid medium, such as the risk of cell leakage from the defect and the potentially uneven cell distribution within the defect. In addition, there is a significantly reduced risk of graft hypertrophy with the MACI procedure. Besides the above-mentioned porcine collagen matrix, hyaluronic acid[26] has also been used as a carrier substance (Hyalograft C™).

Early studies of MACI from Europe have shown clinical results that are comparable to current ACI techniques, with lower reoperation rates for graft hypertrophy.[27] However, similarly to ACI, MACI is limited by the slow cell growth and differentiation, which precludes early aggressive rehabilitation. MACI has been used in Europe for several years, but is not yet available in the United States due to pending FDA approval.

Other Matrix-Associated Techniques

The successful application of biologic matrices as carrier devices for autologous chondrocytes (MACI) has led several groups to investigate the use of such matrices in conjunction with marrow-stimulation techniques (MST). Here, a resorbable matrix is placed into a chondral defect after performance of a marrow-stimulation technique such as microfracture. The matrix acts to stabilize the resultant blood clot and allows cell adherence. In comparison to ACI and MACI, no initial harvest procedure is needed to obtain a cartilage biopsy, and the technique can be performed all-arthroscopic. Most importantly, the decision to perform this type of chondral repair can be made intraoperatively, since the acellular carrier matrix has an extended shelf-life, and is not patient specific. Early work with such a technique, however, has not been able to demonstrate any improvement in results over conventional MST alone.[28] Future research to modify these matrices with growth factors to enhance cell adherence and differentiation holds promise to improve the results of this technology.

Synthetic Plugs

Synthetic PLA-PGA CaSO4 (OBI TruFit™) plugs have been FDA approved to back-fill donor sites and thus decrease morbidity after osteochondral autograft procedures. Studies investigating the use of this plug technology for the primary treatment of chondral defects are currently being conducted in animal models. Currently, this plug technology has not received FDA approval to treat chondral defects.

Tissue-Engineered Cartilage

Autologous articular cartilage engineered by pressure perfusion is presently undergoing clinical trials in the United States (Histogenics) for small lesions (2 to 3 cm^2). The chondrocytes are harvested arthroscopically in an initial staging procedure. The cells are then grown to confluence in 2 to 3 days, seeded on a type I bovine collagen membrane, and then placed in a fluid chamber that pressure-cycles nutrients through the matrix until near-mature tissue is produced. During reimplantation, the tissue is cut to fit the templated defect and secured to the subchondral bone with a collagen-based glue. The patient follows an accelerated rehabilitation protocol that includes immediate full weight bearing. The early results are encouraging.

Allogenic tissue-engineered cartilage that is derived from immature donors younger than 12 years of age has apparent excellent promise for nonimmunogenic incorporation into mature recipients (ISTO Technologies, Zimmer Inc.). The harvested tissue is morselized and prepared in a serum-free environment to form near-mature tissue. It is then surgically implanted and secured with allogenic fibrin glue. The results to date are limited to animal models and are unpublished as of this time. Clinical trials are set to begin in the near future in the United States.

Gene Therapy and Growth Factors

The ideal cartilage repair technique would be performed as a single stage procedure, in which autologous pluripotent mesenchymal cells are obtained, either from peripheral blood or locally through MST, and combined with a carrier matrix that provides a mechanical and biological environment conducive to chondrocyte differentiation. To succeed, several areas have to be addressed, including improved differentiation of mesenchymal cells into chondroblasts, production and maintenance of a hyaline cartilage matrix, and successful integration with the surrounding cartilage. The use of growth factors offers a potential solution to these issues. Several growth factors have been identified, such as the transforming growth factor beta (TGF-β), fibroblast growth factor (FGF), and bone morphogenic protein (BMP) families, which can influence cell differentiation (e.g., TGF-β1 and 2), proliferation (FGF-2, IGF-I), and matrix production (IGF-I, BMP-2, and -7).[29] However, as polypeptides, growth factors have a short half-life, limiting their use as injectable agents or even when bound to a carrier matrix. Gene therapy offers a potential solution to this problem by creating cells that can locally produce and deliver growth factors in higher concentrations for prolonged time. Initial experiments have shown promise, but current techniques remain limited by the only transient production of growth factors. Prior to clinical application, additional studies are required to refine the optimal combination of growth factors, and optimize gene transfer and expression.

Stem Cells

The use of autologous chondrocytes for the treatment of chondral defects requires a two-stage procedure for the harvest and subsequent reimplantation of the expanded chondrocytes, and is associated with a donor site morbidity, potentially low numbers of cells harvested, and cell dedifferentiation during culture. Mesenchymal stem cells (MSC) have been suggested as a possible solution to the above-mentioned issues. MSCs are stromal cells that have the ability to differentiate into many diverse cell lineages such as myoblasts, osteoblasts, and chondrocytes. Initially thought to reside only in the bone marrow, MSCs have more recently been isolated from other tissues such as fat, umbilical cord blood, skin, and peripheral blood. MSCs offer several advantages since they are autogenous, can now be obtained through means other than bone marrow biopsy, and can be expanded more than 500-fold with a potential cell yield in the billions.[30] Ideally, stem cells will be extracted from donated autologous blood, expanded in culture, seeded onto a suitable carrier matrix, and then treated with a combination of environmental factors such as hypoxia and hydrostatic pressure, and biochemical agents such as growth factors to commit the cells to the chondrogenic pathway[31] prior to surgical implantation.

SUMMARY

Before the advent of ACI in 1982, and its first implementation in humans in 1987, the concepts and results of cartilage repair were humbling. It is an exciting time that we live in that these troublesome lesions can now be addressed successfully and with a hyaline repair response. Next-generation techniques are evolving that will expand these technologies to other joints, utilizing less invasive techniques and offering more predictable results. The future is here.

REFERENCES

1. Hunter W. On the structure and diseases of articulating cartilage. Philos Trans R Soc Lond 42b:514-4-21, 1743.
2. Noyes FR, Bassett RW, Grood ES, et al. Arthroscopy in acute traumatic hemarthrosis of the knee. Incidence of anterior cruciate tears and other injuries. J Bone Joint Surg Am 62(5):687–695, 757, 1980.
3. Federico DJ, Lynch JK, Jokl P. Osteochondritis dissecans of the knee: a historical review of etiology and treatment. Arthroscopy 6(3):190–197, 1990.
4. Curl WW, Krome J, Gordon ES, et al. Cartilage injuries: a review of 31,516 knee arthroscopies. Arthroscopy 13(4):456–460, 1997.
5. Aroen A, Loken S, Heir S, et al. Articular cartilage lesions in 993 consecutive knee arthroscopies. Am J Sports Med 32(1):211–215, 2004.
6. Hjelle K, Solheim E, Strand T, et al. Articular cartilage defects in 1,000 knee arthroscopies. Arthroscopy 18(7):730–734, 2002.
7. Piasecki DP, Spindler KP, Warren TA, et al. Intraarticular injuries associated with anterior cruciate ligament tear: findings at ligament reconstruction in high school and recreational athletes. An analysis of sex-based differences. Am J Sports Med 31(4):601–605, 2003.
8. Brittberg M, Lindahl A, Nilsson A, et al. Treatment of deep cartilage defects in the knee with autologous chondrocyte transplantation. N Engl J Med 331(14):889–895, 1994.
9. Minas T, Bryant T. The role of autologous chondrocyte implantation in the patellofemoral joint. Clin Orthop Relat Res 436:30–39, 2005.
10. Cole BJ, Carter TR, Rodeo SA. Allograft meniscal transplantation: background, techniques, and results. Instr Course Lect 52: 383–396, 2003.
11. Magnusson P. Technique for débridement of the knee joint for arthritis. Surg Clin North Am 26:226–249, 1946.
12. Baumgaertner MR, Cannon WD, Jr., Vittori JM, et al. Arthroscopic débridement of the arthritic knee. Clin Orthop Relat Res 253:197–202, 1990.
13. Hubbard MJ. Articular débridement versus washout for degeneration of the medial femoral condyle. A five-year study. J Bone Joint Surg Br 78(2):217–219, 1996.
14. Mithoefer K, Williams RJ, III, Warren RF, et al. The microfracture technique for the treatment of articular cartilage lesions in the knee. A prospective cohort study. J Bone Joint Surg Am 87(9):1911–1920, 2005.
15. Romeo AA, Cole BJ, Mazzocca AD, et al. Autologous chondrocyte repair of an articular defect in the humeral head. Arthroscopy 18(8):925–929, 2002.
16. Whittaker JP, Smith G, Makwana N, et al. Early results of autologous chondrocyte implantation in the talus. J Bone Joint Surg Br 87(2):179–183, 2005.
17. Benya PD, Shaffer JD. Dedifferentiated chondrocytes reexpress the differentiated collagen phenotype when cultured in agarose gels. Cell 30(1):215–224, 1982.
18. Minas T, Peterson L. Advanced techniques in autologous chondrocyte transplantation. Clin Sports Med 18(1):13–44, v–vi, 1999.
19. Fu FH, Zurakowski D, Browne JE, et al. Autologous chondrocyte implantation versus débridement for treatment of full-thickness chondral defects of the knee: an observational cohort study with 3-year follow-up. Am J Sports Med 33(11):1658–1666, 2005.
20. Knutsen G, Engebretsen L, Ludvigsen TC, et al. Autologous chondrocyte implantation compared with microfracture in the knee. A randomized trial. J Bone Joint Surg Am 86-A(3):455–464, 2004.
21. Bentley G, Biant LC, Carrington RW, et al. A prospective, randomised comparison of autologous chondrocyte implantation versus mosaicplasty for osteochondral defects in the knee. J Bone Joint Surg Br 85(2):223–230, 2003.
22. Horas U, Pelinkovic D, Herr G, et al. Autologous chondrocyte implantation and osteochondral cylinder transplantation in cartilage repair of the knee joint. A prospective, comparative trial. J Bone Joint Surg Am 85-A(2):185–192, 2003.
23. Micheli LJ, Browne JE, Erggelet C, et al. Autologous chondrocyte implantation of the knee: multicenter experience and minimum 3-year follow-up. Clin J Sport Med 11(4):223–228, 2001.
24. Garretson RB, III, Katolik LI, Verma N, et al. Contact pressure at osteochondral donor sites in the patellofemoral joint. Am J Sports Med 32(4):967–974, 2004.

25. Gitelis S, Cole BJ. The use of allografts in orthopaedic surgery. Instr Course Lect 51:507–520, 2002.
26. Nehrer S, Domayer S, Dorotka R, et al. Three-year clinical outcome after chondrocyte transplantation using a hyaluronan matrix for cartilage repair. Eur J Radiol Sep 23 2005.
27. Bartlett W, Skinner JA, Gooding CR, et al. Autologous chondrocyte implantation versus matrix-induced autologous chondrocyte implantation for osteochondral defects of the knee: a prospective, randomised study. J Bone Joint Surg Br 87(5): 640–645, 2005.
28. Dorotka R, Bindreiter U, Macfelda K, et al. Marrow stimulation and chondrocyte transplantation using a collagen matrix for cartilage repair. Osteoarthritis Cartilage 13(8):655–664, 2005.
29. Cucchiarini M, Madry H. Gene therapy for cartilage defects. J Gene Med Sep 5 2005.
30. Magne D, Vinatier C, Julien M, et al. Mesenchymal stem cell therapy to rebuild cartilage. Trends Mol Med 11(11):519–526, 2005.
31. Mackay AM, Beck SC, Murphy JM, et al. Chondrogenic differentiation of cultured human mesenchymal stem cells from marrow. Tissue Eng 4(4):415–428, 1998.
32. Brittberg M, Peterson L, Sjogren-Jansson E, et al. Articular cartilage engineering with autologous chondrocyte transplantation. A review of recent developments. J Bone Joint Surg Am 85-A Suppl 3:109–115, 2003.
33. Peterson L, Minas T, Brittberg M, et al. Treatment of osteochondritis dissecans of the knee with autologous chondrocyte transplantation: results at two to ten years. J Bone Joint Surg Am 85-A Suppl 2:17–24, 2003.
34. Mithofer K, Minas T, Peterson L, et al. Functional outcome of knee articular cartilage repair in adolescent athletes. Am J Sports Med 33(8):1147–1153, 2005.
35. Browne JE, Anderson AF, Arciero R, et al. Clinical outcome of autologous chondrocyte implantation at 5 years in U.S. subjects. Clin Orthop Relat Res 436:237–245, 2005.

Index

Page numbers followed by *f* or *t* indicate figures or tables, respectively.